Drugs and nursing implications

This book

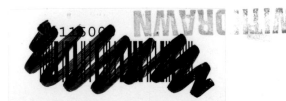

Drugs and nursing implications

LAURA E. GOVONI   Ph.D., R.N.

Lecturer and Consultant, Medical-Surgical Nursing and Pharmacology
Formerly Professor of Nursing, Graduate Division
School of Nursing, University of Connecticut

JANICE E. HAYES   Ph.D., R.N.

Distinguished Visiting Scholar in Nursing
Worcester State College
Lecturer and Consultant, Pathophysiology and Pharmacology
Formerly Associate Dean and Professor of Nursing, Graduate Division
School of Nursing, University of Connecticut

Adapted for the United Kingdom by

JILL A. DAVID   B.Sc., M.Sc., R.G.N., H.V.

Formerly Director of Nursing Research
Royal Marsden Hospital
London

Prentice Hall
New York   London   Toronto   Sydney   Tokyo   Singapore

Published 1990 by
Prentice Hall International (UK) Ltd,
66 Wood Lane End, Hemel Hempstead,
Hertfordshire, HP2 4RG
A division of
Simon & Schuster International Group
Original edition published by Appleton & Lange

Printed and bound in Great Britain.

British Library Cataloguing in Publication Data

David, Jill A.
  Drugs and nursing implications.
  1. Medicine. Drug therapy – For nursing
  I. Title   II. Govoni, Laura E. Drugs and nursing
  implications
  615.58024613

  ISBN 0-13-221003-7

1 2 3 4 5 94 93 92 91 90

CONTENTS

PREFACE

Drugs and Nursing Implications is a well established text from the USA which was written with the conviction that a total understanding of the pharmacotherapeutic regimen is an essential part of nursing care. The nursing implications detailed in the text provide a basis for care planning and patient education which is particularly relevant in long-term drug therapy.

Adaptation of this text for the British reader has involved the obvious changes in drug names, both generic and proprietary as well as changes in drug use and dose; language, culture and idiom. Some aspects that are generally not covered in British texts have been retained, for example the advice on the use of sun protection products. Increased concern about the effects of ultraviolet irradiation on the skin has made this information about sensitizing drugs more relevant. Similarly, the inclusion of advice on the use of 'over-the-counter' medicines (OTC) was felt to be important as it is a subject which is often considered irrelevant in spite of the fact that many patients continue to take their own self prescribed drugs in addition to prescribed drugs even while in hospital. In this adaptation, the *British National Formula* and *Data Sheet Compendium* have been used to check the route and dosage of drugs. However, the author must point out that the use and dosage given, is only a guideline which may be varied in practice. Whenever the nurse is unfamiliar with a drug or unsure about the route or dosage these should be checked with the doctor concerned or the hospital pharmacist.

Within a handbook such as this, space and the time available to the reader are always of importance, and for this reason abbreviations have been used in places to reduce the text. Should these be unfamiliar a list of abbreviations used is found on pages viii. In nursing records, written course work or in student education abbreviations should not be used as this can lead to misunderstanding.

The aim of this text is to provide a day to day reference for drugs commonly used in the UK together with practical guidelines for care. It is not intended to replace the classical pharmacology textbooks which detail the physiological effects of drugs in the body, details of which are found in the bibliography. Every effort has been made to ensure that the information in this book is up to date at the time of going to press and the author and publishers cannot accept responsibility for errors or omissions.

ABBREVIATIONS

ABG	arterial blood gases
a.c.	before meals (ante cibom)
ACh	acetylcholine
ACT	activated clotting time
ACTH	adrenocorticotropic hormone
ADH	antidiuretic hormone
ad lib	freely as desired (ad libitum)
ADR	adverse drug reaction
$AgNO_3$	silver nitrate
AL	activities of living
ALT	alanine aminotransferase (formerly SGPT)
ANA	antinuclear antibodies
APTT	activated partial thromboplastin time
ASHD	arteriosclerotic heart disease
AST	aspartate aminotransferase (formerly SGOT)
AV	atrioventricular
b.i.d.	two times a day (bis in die)
BBT	basal body temperature
BP	blood pressure
BMR	basal metabolic rate
BNF	British National Formulary
BP	British Pharmacopoeia
BPM/bpm	beats per minute
BSP	bromsulphalein
BT	bleeding time
BUN	blood urea nitrogen
C	centigrade, Celsius
Ca	calcium
CBC	complete blood count
CCr	creatinine clearance
CHF	congestive heart failure
Cl	chloride
cm	centimeter
CNS	central nervous system
COMT	catechol-o-methyltransferase
COPD/COAD	chronic obstructive pulmonary (airways) disease
CPK	creatinine phosphokinase
CPR	cardiopulmonary resuscitation
CSF	cerebrospinal fluid
CSM	Committee on Safety of Medicines
CT	clotting time
CTZ	chemoreceptor trigger zone
Cu	copper

CV	cardiovascular
CVA	cerebrovascular accident
CVP	central venous pressure
Derm	dermatological
D&C	dilatation and curettage
DIC	disseminated intravascular clotting
dl	decilitre (100 ml or 0.1 litre)
DM	diabetes mellitus
DNA	deoxyribonucleic acid
DSD	dry sterile dressing
DTRs	deep tendon reflexes
ECG	electrocardiogram
ECT	electroconvulsive therapy
End	endocrine
EEG	electroencephalogram
EENT	eye, ear, nose, throat
ENT	ear, nose, throat
EPS	extrapyramidal symptoms (or syndrome)
ESR	erythrocyte sedimentation rate
F	Fahrenheit
FBS	fasting blood sugar
Fe	iron
Fl	fluoride
FSH	follicle stimulating hormone
GABA	gamma-aminobutyric acid
GFR	glomerular filtration rate
GH	growth hormone
GI	gastrointestinal
Gm	gram
gr	grain
GU	genito-urinary
Gyn	gynaecological
G6PD	glucose-6-phosphate dehydrogenase (deficiency)
HCG	human chorionic gonadotropin
HCl	hydrochloride
HCO_3	bicarbonate
Hct	haematocrit
HDL	high density lipoprotein
Hem	haematological
Hg	mercury
Hgb	haemoglobin
5-HIAA	5-hydroxyindoleacetic acid
HMG	human menopausal gonadotropin
HPA	hypothalamic-pituitary-adrenocortical (axis)
h.s.	hour of sleep (hora somni)
HSV	herpes simplex virus
Hx	history
I	iodine
I&O	intake and output
IBW	ideal body weight
Ig	immunoglobulin
IM	intramuscular
IOP	intraocular pressure
IPPB	intermittent positive pressure breathing (respiration)
IU	international unit

IUD	intrauterine device
IV	intravenous
IVH	intravenous hyperalimentation
K	potassium
kg	kilogram
17-KGS	17-ketogenic steroids
17-KS	17-ketosteriods
KVO	keep vein open
L	litre
lb	pound
LDH	lactic dehydrogenase
LDL	low density lipoprotein
LE	lupus erythematosus
LH	leuteinizing hormone
Li	lithium
LVEDP	left ventricular end-diastolic pressure
m^2	square meter (of body surface area)
MAO	monamine oxidase
MAOI	monamine oxidase inhibitor
MBD	minimal brain dysfunction
MDR	minimum daily requirements
μCi or μC	microcurie
mCi or mC	millicurie
μg or mcg	microgram (1/1,000 of a milligram)
mEq	milliequivalent
mg	milligram
Mg	magnesium
MI	myocardial infarction
MIC	minimum inhibitory concentration
ml	millilitre (1/1,000 of a litre)
N	nitrogen
N&V	nausea and vomiting
Na	sodium
NaCl	sodium chloride
NAPA	N-acetyl procainamide
ng	nanogram (1/1,000 of a microgram)
NPN	nonprotein nitrogen
NPO/NBM	nothing by mouth (nil per orum)
NS	nervous system
NSAID	nonsteroidal antiinflammatory drug
NSR	normal sinus rhythm
17-OHCS	17-hydroxycorticosteriods
Oph	ophthalmic
OTC	over-the-counter
P	phosphorus
PABA	para-aminobenzoic acid
PAS	para-aminosalicylic acid
PAWP	pulmonary artery wedge pressure
Pb	lead
PBI	protein bound iodine
p.c.	after meals (post cibum)
PERLA	pupils equal, react to light and accommodation
PG	prostaglandin
Ph	hydrogen ion concentration
PKU	phenylketonuria

PND	paroxysmal nocturnal dyspnoea
PO	by mouth (per orum)
POR	problem oriented record
PPI	patient packet insert
PRN	when required (pro re nata)
PSP	phenolsulphonphthalein
PSVT	paroxysmal supraventricular tachycardia
PT	prothrombin time
PTT	partial thromboplastin time
PUO	Pyrexia of unknown origin
PVC	premature ventricular contraction
qv	which see (quode vide)
RAI	radioactive iodine
RDA	recommended (daily) dietary allowance
REM	rapid eye movement
Reprod	reproductive
RIA	radioimmunoassay
RNA	ribonucleic acid
ROM	range of motion
RTA	renal tubular acidosis
SA	sinoatrial
SBE	self-breast examination
SC	subcutaneous
SGOT	serum glutamic-oxaloacetic transaminase (*see* AST)
SGPT	serum glutamic-pyruvic transaminase (*see* ALT)
SIADH	syndrome of inappropriate antidiuretic hormone
SL	sublingual
SLE	systemic lupus erythematosus
SMA	sequential multiple analysis
SOAP	subjective, objective, assessment, planning (*see* POR)
SPF	sun protection factor
SR	sedimentation rate
SRS-A	slow-reacting substance of anaphylaxis
t1/2	half-life
TCA	tricyclic antidepressant
TIA	transient ischaemic attack
t.i.d.	three times a day (ter in die)
TPN	total parenteral nutrition
TPR	temperature, pulse, respirations
TSH	thyroid-stimulating hormone
URI/UTI	urinary tract infection
VDRL	veneral disease research laboratory
vital signs	temperature, pulse, respirations, blood pressure
VLDL	very low density lipoprotein
VMA	vanillylmandelic acid
VS	vital signs (qv)
WBC	white blood (cell) count
WBCT	whole blood clotting time
Zn	zinc

GLOSSARY

Acid rebound   Hypersecretion of gastric acid induced by excessive buffering of stomach acid (e.g., by calcium carbonate).

Adverse effect   An unintended, unpredictable, and potentially injurious response to drug action. Adverse effects generally result from direct toxic drug effects, idiosyncrasies, hypersensitivity reactions, and noncompliance.

Agonist   A drug with high affinity for the receptor and high intrinsic activity; causes a pharmacologic effect by its interaction with a specific receptor.

Antagonist   A drug with high affinity for the receptor, but minimal or no intrinsic activity. Capable of preventing or reducing activity at the receptor site.

Atopy   An inherited predisposition to allergies (e.g., asthma, acute urticaria, allergic dermatitis, hay fever).

Bioavailability   The fraction of unchanged drug that reaches the systemic circulation.

Biotransformation   Metabolic changes that occur following drug absorption and distribution convert the drug into products that are usually less active and that can be more readily excreted.

Drug abuse   Self-administered drug use that deviates from prescribed medical, social, or cultural patterns. Implicit in the definition is the notion of social disapproval.

Drug addition   *See* Drug dependence.

Drug dependence   A state of physical or psychological dependence or both on a drug that occurs following repeated use of that drug. *Physical dependence* is an altered physiological state that results following repeated drug use such that withdrawal symptoms appear when drug dose is reduced or drug discontinued. *Psychological dependence* is an emotional reliance on a drug. Drug dependence is characterized by compulsive drug seeking and drug taking behaviour and a high risk of recurrence following drug withdrawal.

Enterohepatic circulation   (A route of elimination) Drugs or drug metabolites released in the bile enter the small intestine where they may be totally or partially reabsorbed, returned to the liver, and again secreted to the bile. The metabolite may be enzymatically broken down by intestinal bacteria to release unchanged drug which is then reabsorbed.

First-pass effect   The extensive metabolism of a drug that occurs during its passage through the gut wall and/or through the liver before reaching the systemic circulation. As a result of first-pass metabolism, the amount of drug reaching the active sight is reduced and the effectiveness of the oral drug is decreased.

Fixed drug eruption   A drug-induced circumscribed skin lesion that persists or recurs in the same site. Residual pigmentation may remain following drug withdrawal.

Half-life   The time required for drug concentration in plasma or total body to decline by one-half. The concept of half-life is important in time determinations of steady state and clearance of drug from the body.

Lipoatrophy   Atrophy of subcutaneous fat caused by repeated injections of insulin in the same site, over prolonged periods.

Microsomal enzyme system A catalytic system that generally inactivates drugs and makes them more water soluble so they can be readily eliminated by the kidneys.

Minimum inhibitory concentration (MIC) Minimum drug concentration that inhibits microbial growth.

Nadir Pharmacological expression of the lowest point reached in the blood count; for example, thrombocytes and leucocytes in response to cytotoxic drug effects on haematopoietic tissues.

Pharmacodynamics Study of the time required for drug actions to occur in the body through processes of absorption, distribution, metabolism, and elimination.

Pharmacokinetics The study of how a drug reaches its site of action and is removed from the body through processes of absorption, distribution, metabolism, and elimination.

Photosensitivity Drug-induced skin changes resulting in unusual susceptibility to effects of sun or ultraviolet light.

Physical dependence An altered physiological state resulting from repeated drug use such that withdrawal symptoms appear with dose redirection or when the drug is discontinued.

Pressure effect Haemodynamic effect reflected in changes in blood pressure.

Protein binding A reversable drug-protein complex in equilibrium with free (active) drug in the plasma. Only the free drug can diffuse to the action sight, thus factors that decrease protein binding (for example, displacement of bound drug by another drug, or hypoalbumenism). May raise the potential for increased pharmacological effect.

Psychological dependence An emotional reliance on a drug.

Recall phenomenon Skin reaction due to prior radiotherapy.

Sequential multiple analysis (SMA) An automated electronic system that performs comprehensive blood studies rapidly and economically. For example, SMA 12/60 can make 12 determinations on 60 serum specimens in 1 hour.

Side effects An expected or predictable drug response caused by the pharmacological action of a drug.

Smogi effect A rebound phenomenon caused by accelerated release of hormone normally covered with plasma glucose regulation. Smogi effect develops when patient chronically receives unnecessarily large insulin doses. As a result, the body attempts to compensate by producing unrecognized hypoglycaemia.

Smoking–drug interaction Interaction which occurs when smoking interferes with the pharmacokinetics of the drug.

Steady-state (plateau) During continued drug administration amount of drug in the body rises until average rate of drug elimination (drug clearance) equals average rate of drug intake. Plateau remains as long as drug intake is maintained.

Tachyphylaxis A sudden resistance to pharmacological effectiveness of a drug. Initial drug response cannot be restored by increasing the dose.

Therapeutic window Effective serum drug level is close to toxic level.

Tolerance Reduced responsiveness during repeated administration of a drug requiring increasingly larger doses.

Acebutolol

(Sectral)

Beta-adrenoceptor blocking agent; Antihypertensive; antianginal; anti-arrhythmic

For further information *see* Propranolol

ROUTE AND DOSAGE Oral: *Hypertension*: 400 mg once a day or 200 mg twice a day initially increased to 400 mg twice a day after two weeks. *Angina*: 400 mg once a day or 200 mg twice a day (300 mg may be given 3 times a day in severe cases) maximum dose 1.2 g per day. *Arrhythmia*; 0.4–1.2 g daily in divided doses. **Intravenous**: Severe arrhythmia, 20 mg over 3–5 min with two further doses of 20 mg at 10 min intervals. Subsequent doses may be given orally.

Acetazolamide

(Diamox, Diamox sustets)

Anticonvulsant; carbonic anhydrase inhibitor; diuretic alkalizer (systemic, urinary); sulphonamide derivative

Acetazolamide sodium

(Diamox parenteral)

ACTIONS AND USES Nonbacteriostatic sulphonamide derivative. Diuretic effect is due to inhibition of carbonic anhydrase activity in proximal renal tubule resulting in alkaline diuresis with conservation of chloride and ammonia. After 3 or 4 days of continuous inhibition, mild metabolic acidosis develops with concomitant reduction in diuresis. Inhibition of carbonic anhydrase in the eye reduces rate of aqueous humour formation with consequent lowering of intraocular pressure. This effect is apparently independent of systemic acid–base balance and diuretic action. Mechanism of anticonvulsant action unknown, but thought to involve inhibition of CNS carbonic anhydrase, which retards abnormal paroxysmal discharge from CNS neurons.

Used adjunctively in treatment of several forms of epilepsy, especially absence seizures (petit mal), generalized tonic–clonic (grand mal), and focal seizures; to reduce intraocular pressure in open- and closed-angle glaucoma, and secondary glaucoma; for preoperative treatment of acute closed-angle glaucoma prior to laser iridotomy; and in treatment of oedema. Also used to correct metabolic alkalosis, to treat hypokalaemic and hyperkalaemic forms of familial periodic paralysis, and to relieve symptoms of acute mountain sickness.

ROUTE AND DOSAGE Adults: *Glaucoma*: Oral: 250 mg every 6 hours (extended-release preparations may be prescribed every 12 to 24 hours); **Intravenous, intra-**

ACETAZOLAMIDE SODIUM (continued)

muscular: *Initial*: 500 mg repeated in 2 to 4 hours; if necessary. *Anticonvulsant, diuretic*: 250 mg to 1 g daily in divided doses.

ABSORPTION AND FATE   Rapidly absorbed from GI tract. Effects begin in 30 minutes to 1 hour; plasma levels peak within 2 to 4 hours and persist for 8 to 12 hours. **Sustained-release form**: onset: 2 hours; peaks in 8 to 12 hours with duration: 18 to 24 hours. Acts within 2 minutes after IV administration. **Duration of action**: 4 to 5 hours. Wide distribution including CNS penetration; especially high concentrations in erythrocytes, pancreas, gastric mucosa, and renal cortex. Highly bound to plasma proteins. **Half-life**: 2.4 to 5.8 hours. Excreted unchanged in urine (90 to 100%) within 24 hours. Crosses placenta.

CONTRAINDICATIONS AND PRECAUTIONS   Hypersensitivity to sulphonamides; renal and hepatic dysfunction; Addison's disease or other types of adrenocortical insufficiency, hyponatraemia, hypokalaemia, hyperchloraemic acidosis, prolonged administration to patients with hyphaema, or chronic noncongestive angle closure glaucoma. Safe use in fertile women or during pregnancy not established.

ADVERSE/SIDE EFFECTS   Paraesthesias (especially of tongue, lips, anus, and extremities) and drowsiness are common; disorientation, depression, nervousness, excitement, fatigue, flaccid paralysis, headache, dizziness, convulsions. Transient myopia, tinnitus. Anorexia, nausea, vomiting, weight loss, constipation, diarrhoea, melaena. *Haematologic/electrolyte imbalance (as for other sulphonamides)*: bone marrow depression with agranulocytosis, thrombocytopenic purpura, haemolytic anaemia, leucopenia, pancytopenia; increased serum bilirubin. Increased excretion of Ca, K, Mg, Na, thiamine, pyridoxine; hyperchloraemic acidosis, hyperglycaemia, hyperuricaemia. *Hypersensitivity*: pruritus, rash, urticaria, fever. *Renal*: glycosuria, urinary frequency, polyuria, dysuria, alkaline urine, haematuria, crystalluria, ureteral colic, nephrolithiasis. *Other*: fatigue, weakness, hirsutism, loss of libido, impotence, exacerbation of gout, altered taste and smell; thirst, hepatic dysfunction, hyperpnoea, cyanosis, pain at IM injection site.

NURSING IMPLICATIONS
- Not to be confused with acetohexamide.
- Acetazolamide may be taken with food to minimize possibility of GI upset.
- The long-acting preparation (Diamox sustets) may be opened but contents should not be crushed, chewed, or swallowed dry. It may be spread on soft food.
- If necessary, one regular tablet (not sustained release form) may be softened in 2 tsp of hot water and added to 2 tsp of honey or syrup (e.g., chocolate, raspberry, cherry) to disguise bitter taste. The drug does not dissolve in fruit juices. Alternatively, tablet(s) may be crushed and suspended in syrup (250 to 500 mg per 5 ml syrup).
- High alkalinity (pH approximately 9.2) of the parenteral solution causes intense pain when injected IM; this route is not commonly used.
- Adequate fluid intake (1.5 to 2.5 L/24 hr) should be maintained during acetazolamide therapy to reduce risk of kidney stone formation. Check with physician.
- Transient nearsightedness (myopia) may occur following initiation of therapy. Re-

ACETAZOLAMIDE SODIUM (continued)

port to physician. Symptom usually responds readily to dosage reduction or drug withdrawal.

■ Advise patient to report numbness, tingling, burning, and other paraesthesias, and drowsiness (common side-effects). Note implications for the ambulatory patient. Caution patient to avoid driving a car and other potentially hazardous activities if these symptoms are prominent.

■ Caution patient to report sore throat or mouth, unusual bleeding, fever, skin or renal problems (indications to discontinue acetazolamide).

■ Acetazolamide may cause substantial increases in blood glucose in diabetics and in prediabetics. Observe these patients closely. Changes in antidiabetic drug dose or diet may be indicated.

■ Hypokalaemia and severe metabolic acidosis are direct extensions of the pharmacological actions of acetazolamide. Note that concomitant use of steroids or ACTH may contribute to hypokalaemia. Hypokalaemia can sensitize the heart to toxic effects of digitalis.

■ Observe for and advise patient to report signs of *hypokalaemia* (malaise, fatigue, depressed reflexes, muscle weakness and cramps, rapid, irregular pulse, vomiting, mental confusion, abdominal distention, polyuria), and signs of metabolic acidosis (lethargy, headache, weakness, abdominal pain, nausea, vomiting, dyspnoea, hyperpnoea progressing to Kussmaul breathing, dehydration).

■ When acetazolamide is given in high doses or for prolonged periods physician may prescribe potassium-rich diet and K supplement. *See Index: Food sources.*

■ Excessive salt intake should be avoided. *See Index: Food sources.*

■ The sustained release drug form is not recommended for treatment of epilepsy.

■ When used as an anticonvulsant, drug withdrawal, if contemplated, should be gradual to prevent precipitating seizure activity.

■ Because the parenteral solution contains no antibacterial preservative, its use within 24 hours of reconstitution is strongly recommended by manufacturer.

■ Oral preparations are preserved in tightly covered, light-resistant containers. Store preferably between 15° and 30°C (59° and 86°F) unless otherwise directed by manufacturer.

Diagnostic test interferences   False-positive urinary protein determinations; falsely high values for urine urobilinogen; depressed iodine uptake values (exception: hypothyroidism).

DRUG INTERACTIONS *Acetazolamide*

PLUS	INTERACTIONS
Amphetamines	Enhanced amphetamine effect. (Drug-induced alkaline urine decreases amphetamine excretion rate)
Amphotericin ⎫ Corticosteroids ⎬ Corticotropin ⎭	Concurrent use may cause severe hypokalaemia

ACETAZOLAMIDE SODIUM (continued)

PLUS (continued)	INTERACTIONS
Anticonvulsants	Predisposes patient to anticonvulsant-induced osteomalacia (adult rickets) by increasing calcium excretion rate
Digitalis glycosides	Acetazolamide-induced hypokalaemia may predispose patient to digitalis toxicity
Insulins and oral antidiabetic agents	Hypoglycaemic effect may be reduced (possibly because of hypokalaemia)
Lithium	Drug-induced alkaline urine increased lithium excretion and decreases plasma levels
Hexamine compounds	Drug-induced alkaline urine inhibits antibacterial effect of hexamine (requires acid urine to be effective)
Primidone	Decreased anticonvulsant (reduced GI absorption of primidone). *See Anticonvulsants*
Procainamide	Enhanced procainamide effect (drug-induced alkaline urine delays procainamide excretion)
Pseudoephedrine	Risk of pseudoephedrine toxicity (drug-induced alkaline urine delays pseudoephedrine excretion). Concurrent use generally avoided
Quinidine	Drug-induced alkaline urine decreases rate of quinidine excretion with possible toxicity
Salicylates	Increased risk of salicylate toxicity in patients receiving large salicylate doses. Concurrent use generally avoided

Acetohexamide

(Dimelor)

Antidiabetic agent (oral); hypoglycaemic; sulphonlyurea

ACTIONS AND USES   Intermediate-acting sulphonylurea that promotes-increased effectiveness of endogenous insulin. Chemically related to sulphonamides, but has no antibacterial action. More potent and has longer action than tolbutamide (qv), but uses, precautions, and adverse reactions are similar. Also has moderate uricosuric effect, probably due to its primary metabolite, hydroxyhexamide.

Used in mild to moderately severe stable non-insulin-dependent diabetes mellitus (NIDDM).

For further information *see* Tolbutamide.

ROUTE AND DOSAGE   Oral (highly individualized): 250 mg daily before breakfast. May be increased every 5 to 7 days by 250 to 500 mg as needed to maximum of 1.5 g daily. Patients on 500 mg/day or less usually can be controlled on once daily dosage. Those receiving 1.5 g/day usually benefit from twice daily dosage given before morning and evening meals.

Acetylcysteine ─────────────────────────

(Acetylcysteine fabrol, Parvolex)   *Mucolytic; antidote*

ACTIONS AND USES   Derivative of naturally occurring amino acid L-cysteine. Probably acts by disrupting disulphide linkages of mucoproteins in purulent and nonpurulent secretions, thereby lowering viscosity and facilitating their removal. Acetylcysteine is a precursor of hepatic glutathione, which normally inactivates an hepatotoxic metabolite of paracetamol.

Used as adjuvant therapy in patients with abnormal, viscid, or inspissated mucous secretions in acute and chronic bronchopulmonary diseases, and in pulmonary complications of cystic fibrosis and surgery, tracheostomy, atelectasis. Also used in diagnostic bronchial studies.

ROUTE AND DOSAGE   Oral: Adults and children over 6 yrs (granules) 200 mg 3 times a day in water for 5–10 days. May be continued for 6 months or longer. **Child:** 2–6 yrs 200 mg twice a day, less than 2 yrs 200 mg daily. Paracetamol overdose: IV infusion in 5% glucose 150 mg/kg in 200 ml given over 15 min, then 50 mg/kg in 500 ml over 4 hrs, then 100 mg/kg in 1,000 ml over 16 hrs.

ABSORPTION AND FATE   Liquefaction of mucus occurs within 1 minute after inhalation or instillation; maximum effects in 5 to 10 minutes. Most drug appears to participate in sulphhydryl-disulphide reaction; remainder is absorbed from epithelium, deacetylated by liver to cysteine and subsequently metabolized.

CONTRAINDICATIONS AND PRECAUTIONS   Hypersensitivity to acetylcysteine. Safe use during pregnancy and in nursing mothers not established. **Cautious Use:** patients with asthma, the elderly, debilitated patients with severe respiratory insufficiency.

ADVERSE/SIDE EFFECTS   Drowsiness. Nausea, vomiting, stomatitis. **Respiratory**: bronchospasm, rhinorrhoea, bronchorrhoea, burning sensation in upper respiratory passages, haemoptysis. **Other**: fever, chills, clamminess, sensitization (rarely), transient maculopapular rash (after frequent and extended use).

NURSING IMPLICATIONS
- Have suction apparatus immediately available. Following drug administration, increased volume of respiratory tract fluid may be liberated. If patient cannot cough adequately, suction or endotracheal aspiration will be necessary to establish and maintain an open airway. Elderly and debilitated patients require close monitoring to prevent aspiration of excessive secretions.
- Unpleasant odour of the drug (rotten egg odour of hydrogen sulphide) and excess volume of liquefied bronchial secretions may cause nausea and possibly vomiting, particularly when face mask is used. Assure patient that the odour becomes less noticeable with continued inhalation.
- Bronchospasm is most likely to occur in patients with asthma, and it may happen unpredictably. If it occurs, drug should be discontinued immediately. Consult physician beforehand about emergency use of bronchodilator (by nebulization) such as isoprenaline.

A

ACETYLCYSTEINE (continued)

- Solutions of acetylcysteine release hydrogen sulphide and become discoloured when autoclaved and upon contact with rubber and certain metals (particularly iron and copper). When administering by nebulization, it is recommended to use equipment made of plastic, glass, stainless steel, aluminium, chromed metal, sterling silver, or other nonreactive metals. Silver may tarnish, but this does not affect drug potency.
- When drug is administered by nebulization, compressed air should be used to provide pressure. Oxygen may be used if prescribed, but close monitoring of blood gases must be observed since it may aggravate CO_2 retention.
- Prolonged nebulization causes solution to become more concentrated impeding drug delivery. Therefore, after three-quarters of initial volume has been nebulized, the remainder may be diluted with an approximately equal volume of sterile water for injection.
- Cleanse nebulizing equipment immediately after use to prevent occluded openings and corrosion of metal parts. Wash face and mask and have patient rinse mouth with water. The drug leaves a sticky coating.
- Acetylcysteine is a reducing agent and therefore it is incompatible with oxidizing agents such as hydrogen peroxide. Solutions of acetylcysteine are incompatible with ampicillin, amphotericin B (Fungizone), tetracyclines, erythromycin lactobionate, iodinized oil, and trypsin.
- Collaborate with physiotherapist in constructing a teaching plan for the patient with chronic pulmonary insufficiency. *See Index: Nursing Interventions: chronic pulmonary insufficiency.*
- Once opened, vial should be stored in refrigerator to retard oxidation, and used within 96 hours. A light purple colour apparently does not significantly impair its mucolytic effectiveness.
- Unopened vial should be stored at room temperature, preferably between 15° and 30°C (59° and 86°F), unless otherwise directed by manufacturer.

Actinomycin D ────────────────────

(Cosmegen, Lyovac)   *Antineoplastic*

ACTIONS AND USES   Potent cytotoxic antibiotic derived from mixture of actinomycins produced by *Streptomyces parvullus*. Toxic properties precludes its use as antibiotic. Complexes with DNA, thereby inhibiting DNA, RNA, and protein synthesis. Causes delayed myelosuppression; is strongly tissue corrosive and has a low therapeutic index. Potentiates effects of radiotherapy; the converse also appears likely. Recent reports indicate increased potential for secondary primary tumours following treatment with radiotherapy and actinomycin.

Used as single agent or in combination with other antineoplastics and/or radiation to treat Wilms' tumour, rhabdomyosarcoma, carcinoma of testes and uterus, Ewing's sarcoma, and sarcoma botroides.

ACTINOMYCIN D (continued)
ROUTE AND DOSAGE   Highly individualized. **Intravenous.**

ABSORPTION AND FATE   Very little active drug is detected in plasma 2 to 5 minutes after IV injection. Concentrates in liver, spleen, and kidneys but does not cross blood–brain barrier. **Plasma half-life**: 36 hours. About 50% of dose is excreted unchanged in bile and 10% in urine.

CONTRAINDICATIONS AND PRECAUTIONS   Chicken pox, herpes zoster, and other viral infections; patients of childbearing age, pregnancy, lactation, infants under 6 months of age. **Cautious Use**: previous therapy with antineoplastics or radiation within 3 to 6 weeks, bone marrow depression, infections, history of gout, impairment of kidney or liver function, obesity.

ADVERSE/SIDE EFFECTS   Acne, hyperpigmentation and reactivation of erythema especially over previously irradiated areas, alopecia (reversible), other adverse/side effects include: cheilitis, ulcerative stomatitis, oesophagitis, dysphagia, pharyngitis, hepatomegaly, proctitis, anorexia, nausea, vomiting, abdominal pain, diarrhoea, GI ulceration. Anaemia (including aplastic anaemia), agranulocytosis, leucopenia, thrombocytopenia, pancytopenia, reticulopenia can also occur. Malaise, fatigue, lethargy, fever, myalgia, anaphylaxis, gonadal suppression, hypocalcaemia, hyperuricaemia, thrombophlebitis; necrosis, sloughing and contractures at site of extravasation. *Following isolation-perfusion administration*: haematopoietic depression, increased susceptibility to infection, impaired wound healing, oedema of extremity involved, damage to soft tissues, venous thrombosis.

NURSING IMPLICATIONS
- Actinomycin is reconstituted by adding 1.1 ml sterile water for injection (without preservative); the resulting solution will contain approximately 0.5 mg/ml. Other solvents may cause precipitation.
- Once reconstituted, actinomycin may be added directly to infusion solutions of 5% dextrose injection or sodium chloride injection, or into tubing or side arm of a running IV infusion, and administered over a 10- to 15-minute period. Because there is no preservative in the solution, discard unused portion.
- If direct IV injection is given the needle used to withdraw dose from vial after reconstitution is discarded; a fresh sterile needle is used for direct injection into vein.
- Following IV injection, some clinicians recommend injecting 5 to 10 ml IV solution into the side arm or flushing the vein with running IV infusion for 2 to 5 minutes to remove any remaining drug from tubing.
- Drug handling precautions: manufacturer advises use of gloves and eye shield to protect the person making the solution. If skin is contaminated, rinse with running water for 10 minutes; then rinse with buffered phosphate solution. If solution gets into the eyes, wash with water immediately, then irrigate with water or isotonic saline for 10 minutes.
- Particular care should be taken to avoid extravasation. Palpate injection site frequently; if extravasation occurs, stop infusion immediately.
- Follow hospital protocol for precautions to be taken if there is spillage, and for pro-

A

ACTINOMYCIN D (continued)

tection of personnel during cleanup of spilled drug. There should be specific directions about:

☐ Protective covering for face, hands, eyes

☐ What to do when eyes are contaminated

☐ How and in what container to dispose of spilled drug

☐ Where to take container for disposal

☐ How to prevent further spillage

- Nausea and vomiting usually occur a few hours after drug administration and are generally controlled by an antiemetic drug. Vomiting may be severe enough to require intermittent therapy. Observe patient daily for signs of drug toxicity.

- Frequent determinations of renal, hepatic, and bone marrow function are advised. White blood cell counts should be performed daily and platelet counts every 3 days to detect hematopoietic depression. Check laboratory values for indicated adaptations to nursing care.

- Monitor temperature and inspect oral membranes daily. *See Mustine for nursing care of stomatitis, xerostomia.*

- The combination of stomatitis, diarrhoea, and severe haematopoietic depression (leucopenia or thrombocytopenia) usually requires prompt interruption of therapy until drug toxicity subsides (leucocyte and platelet recovery and improved clinical condition).

- Be alert for signs of agranulocytosis (which may develop abruptly, especially when dactinomycin and radiation are combined): extreme weakness and fatigue, sore throat, stomatitis, fever, chills. Report to physician. Antibiotic therapy, reverse precautions, and discontinuation of the antineoplastic are indicated.

- Actinomycin is usually given no later than the first 5 to 7 days of radiation therapy because of risk of severe drug-induced skin reactions (erythema, desquamation, pigmentation).

- Radiation therapy is generally continued despite the occurrence of drug-induced skin reactions and the side effects of radiation (gastric distress, and severe mucositis near site of radiation).

- Discuss possibility of gonadal suppression (amenorrhoea or azoospermia) with patient before therapy is instituted. This may be an irreversible side effect.

- The obese or oedematous patient is given a lower dose of actinomycin (*see Route and Dosage*). Monitor daily for symptoms of toxicity from overdosage.

- Observe and report symptoms of hyperuricaemia: swelling of lower legs and feet, flank, stomach, and joint pain. Urge patient to increase fluid intake up to 3,000 ml/day if allowed. Treatment with allopurinol and alkalinization of urine may be instituted.

- Report onset of unexplained bleeding (ecchymosis, melaena, epistaxis, petechiae or easy bruising), jaundice, and wheezing.

- Store drug at temperature between 15° and 30°C (59° and 86°F), unless otherwise advised by manufacturer. Protect from heat and light.

Diagnostic test interferences   Actinomycin may increase serum and urine uric acid levels.

ACTINOMYCIN D (continued)
DRUG INTERACTIONS *Actinomycin*

PLUS	INTERACTIONS
Antigout agent	Elevated uric acid level produced by actinomycin may necessitate dose adjustment of the antigout agent
Myelosuppressants, other	Potentiation of effects of both actinomycin and other myelosuppressant
Radiation	Potentiated effects of both. Actinomycin may reactivate erythema from previous radiation therapy
Vitamin K	Decreased vitamin K effects (antihaemorrhagic) leading to prolonged clotting time and potential haemorrhage

Acyclovir

(Acycloguanosine, Zovirax)   *Antiinfective, antiviral agent*

Acyclovir sodium

ACTIONS AND USES Synthetic acyclic purine nucleoside analogue, derived from guanine. Selectively absorbed by virus infected cells. Drug activity depends chiefly on its phosphorylation to acyclovir triphosphate by virus-coded enzymes in cells infected with herpes virus. Acyclovir's virostatic action interferes with DNA synthesis of herpes simplex virus types 1 and 2 (HSV-1 and HSV-2) and varicella-zoster virus, thereby inhibiting viral replication. Demonstrates antiviral activity against herpes virus simiae (B virus), Epstein-Barr (infectious mononucleosis) and cytomegalovirus. Does not eradicate the latent herpes virus.

Used systemically for treatment of initial and recurrent mucosal and cutaneous herpes simplex (HSV-1 and HSV-2) infections in immunocompromised adults and children and for severe initial episodes of herpes genitalis in immunocompetent (normal immune system) patients. Used topically for initial episodes of herpes genitalis and in limited non life-threatening mucocutaneous herpes simplex virus infections in immuno-compromised patients.

Also used in immunocompromised patients to treat herpes zoster (shingles), varicella (pox), and other herpetic infections.

ROUTE AND DOSAGE **Intravenous:** 5–10 mg/kg every 8 hrs by slow infusion over 1 hour. **Ophthalmic:** ointment applied to lesions 4 hrly five times a day. **Oral:** Herpes simplex 200 mg 5 times a day for 5 days (400 mg if immunocompromised), herpes zoster 800 mg 5 times a day for 5 days.

ACYCLOVIR SODIUM (continued)

ABSORPTION AND FATE   Peak serum levels in about 1 hour following IV administration with maximal renal concentration within 2 hours. Minimal systemic absorption follows topical application. Widely distributed to most body tissues including brain, kidneys, lungs, liver, and to body fluids and secretions, including vesicular fluids, CSF, and saliva. About 9 to 30% protein-binding. Biphasic decline in plasma concentration: **initial half-life**: ≃0.34 hour; **terminal half-life**: ≃3 hours (in patients with renal impairment up to 20 hours). Probably metabolized by liver. More than 95% of IV dose excreted in urine as unchanged drug within 24 hours; less than 2% eliminated in faeces. Crosses placenta; distribution into breast milk not known.

CONTRAINDICATIONS AND PRECAUTIONS   History of acyclovir hypersensitivity; rapid or bolus injection of acyclovir; pregnancy; herpes zoster, labialis, or simplex in immunocompromised patient. **Cautious Use**: nursing mother, neurological renal, hepatic or electrolyte abnormalities; hypoxia, dehydration, history of neurological reactions to cytotoxic drugs; concomitant administration of nephrotoxic drugs or intrathecal methotrexate or interferon.

ADVERSE/SIDE EFFECTS   (Generally minimal and infrequent.) Lethargy, obtundation, tremors, confusion, hallucinations, agitation, seizures, light-headedness, dizziness, headache, jitteriness, delirium, coma. Hypotension. Nausea, vomiting, abdominal or epigastric pain. Thrombocytosis, thrombocytopenia, transient elevations of: BUN, serum creatinine, AST (SGOT), ALT (SGPT), alkaline phosphatase; leucopenia, lymphopenia, megaloblastic haematopoiesis, bone marrow hypoplasia. Haematuria, renal tubular damage, acute renal failure. Rash, urticaria, pruritus, burning, stinging sensation, irritation, sensitization. Inflammation or phlebitis at IV injection site, sloughing (with extravasation); diaphoresis, unusual thirst, substernal burning sensation, vulvitis.

NURSING IMPLICATIONS

Parenteral administration
- Acyclovir sodium is reconstituted first by adding 10 ml sterile water for injection to 500 mg vial (provides concentration of 50 mg/ml). Shake well to assure complete dissolution of drug. This solution should be used within 12 hours.
- For infusion, withdraw appropriate dose of reconstituted solution from vial and add to designated compatible IV infusion solution. To reduce risk of renal injury and phlebitis, final concentration should be 7 mg/ml or less. Once prepared for infusion, solution should be used within 24 hours.
- Manufacturer approves use of standard commercially available electrolyte and glucose solutions for the infusion solution. Acyclovir sodium is reportedly incompatible with biologicals and colloidal solutions, e.g., blood products and protein containing solutions.
- Acyclovir sodium is intended **for IV infusion only** and it must be administered over a period of at least 1 hour to prevent renal tubular damage. Rapid or bolus IV, and IM or SC administration must be avoided.

ACYCLOVIR SODIUM (continued)

- Monitor IV flow rate and observe infusion site during and for a few days following infusion.
- Maximum drug concentration in urine occurs within the first 2 hours following infusion. Keep patient adequately hydrated during this time to maintain sufficient urinary flow and thus prevent precipitation of drug in renal tubules.
- Consult physician about amount and length of time oral fluids need to be encouraged after IV drug treatment.
- Monitor intake and output ratio and pattern. *Note*: unusual tiredness and weakness are suggestive symptoms of early renal failure.
- Refrigeration may cause precipitation; however, crystals will redissolve at room temperature.
- Store acyclovir powder and reconstituted solutions at controlled room temperature preferably between 15° and 30°C (59° and 86°F) unless otherwise directed by manufacturer.

Topical administration

- Teach patient to be thorough in hand washing before and after treatment of lesions and after cautious handling and disposition of secretions. Virus is killed by thorough washing with soap and water. Reportedly it cannot be spread by dry towels or sheets or by baths and swimming pools.
- Cleanse area with soap and water three or four times daily; dry well. Hair dryer may be helpful. Advise patient to wear loose fitting clothing and absorbent (e.g., cotton) underclothing.
- Instruct patient to apply topical preparation with finger cot or surgical glove to prevent further self-infection as well as spread of virus to others. Use sufficient ointment to completely cover lesions.
- Avoid drug contact in or around the eyes. Any unexplained eye symptoms (e.g., redness, pain) should be reported immediately. Untreated infection can lead to corneal keratitis and blindness.
- Warn patient to avoid use of self-prescribed emollient creams or ointments unless specifically prescribed by physician. These agents tend to delay healing and may even spread the lesions.
- Notify physician if local reactions are pronounced or annoying, and if no improvement is noted within 1 week.
- Store topical preparation in dry placed, preferably at 15° and 25°C (59° and 78°F) unless otherwise directed by manufacturer.

General

- The incidence of genital herpes has increased 10-fold from 1966 to 1980.
- Acyclovir therapy is most effective when started as soon as possible after onset of signs and symptoms.
- Diagnosis of HSV-1 and HSV-2 virus infection is based on presence of characteristic lesions and on finding multinucleated giant cells in exudate and scrapings of lesions, and by positive cultures. Possibility of other sexually-transmitted diseases should be ruled out.

ACYCLOVIR SODIUM (continued)

- Risk of virus transfer is negligible. If sheets, underclothing, toilet seats, etc., are dry, contact is safe. If moisture is present handle with surgical gloves.
- When virus is on plastic or other hard surfaces, life span is only several minutes.
- Caution patient to refrain from sexual intercourse if either partner has signs and symptoms of herpes infection. It is generally true that asymptomatic persons cannot transmit the disease, however, transmission can occur even when signs and symptoms are so mild that person is not aware of them. (Symptoms of initial genital herpes occur within 2 to 10 days after exposure through sexual contact.)
- Pregnant patients should be followed closely to detect reinfection.
- Women with genital herpes reportedly are at a high risk level for developing cervical cancer. Urge patient to have a Papanicolaou (Pap) smear at least annually to detect early cervical changes.
- Acyclovir is not a cure for herpetic infections. HSV-1 virus (cold sore or fever blister) remains latent in the trigeminal ganglia for life and may emerge periodically to cause symptoms. In some instances it attacks new sites such as the brain or eyes. HSV-2 virus, responsible for most genital herpes, lodges in sacral ganglia and can cause repeated infections.
- Be aware that symptoms of genital herpes caused by either HSV-1 or HSV-2 may appear to be similar but the rate and frequency of occurrence is much lower in HSV-1 infections.
- Children are unlikely to contract genital herpes except by incest or sexual assault.
- The patient should be aware that even after the HSV infection is controlled by acyclovir, the latent virus can be activated by such stimuli as: stress, exposure to sunlight, sexual intercourse, treatment with immunosuppressive drugs.
- Before the patient is discharged from medical supervision he or she should understand how long acyclovir is to be used, and when a return visit is scheduled. Urge compliance with treatment and assessment schedules.

DRUG INTERACTIONS   Acyclovir

PLUS	INTERACTIONS
Agents that decrease renal function or compete for renal excretion (e.g., aminoglycocides, amphotericin B)	Increased risk of nephrotoxicity. Used with caution
Interferon Methotrexate }	Possibility of neurological abnormalities with occurrent use. Used with caution
Probenecid	Decreases real clearance of acyclovir

Adrenaline

(Medihaler-epi, Min-i-jet adrenaline)   *α-Adrenergic agonist (direct); bronchodilator*

ADRENALINE (continued)

ACTIONS AND USES   Naturally occurring catecholamine obtained from animal adrenal glands; also prepared synthetically. Acts directly on both alpha and beta receptors; the most potent activator of alpha receptors. Imitates all actions of sympathetic nervous system except those on arteries of the face and sweat glands. Strengthens myocardial contraction; increases blood pressure, cardiac rate, and cardiac output. In common with other adrenergic antagonists, stimulates the enzyme adenyl cyclase and consequently enhances synthesis of cyclic AMP (cAMP), which mediates bronchial muscle relaxation. Also constricts bronchial arterioles and inhibits histamine release; thus reduces congestion and oedema and increases tidal volume and vital capacity. Constricts arterioles, particularly in skin, mucous membranes, and kidneys, but dilates skeletal muscle blood vessels. Raises blood sugar by promoting conversion of glycogen reserves in liver to glucose and inhibits insulin release in pancreas. Relaxes uterine musculature and inhibits uterine contractions. CNS stimulation believed to result from peripheral effects. Topical applications to the eye lowers intraocular pressure possibly by decreasing aqueous humour formation and by increasing facility of aqueous outflow; produces brief mydriasis, and slight relaxation of ciliary muscle. Has only slight effect on normal eye, and reportedly is more effective in light-coloured eyes than in dark eyes.

Used for temporary relief of bronchospasm, acute asthmatic attack, mucosal congestion, hypersensitivity, and anaphylactic reactions, syncope due to heart block or carotid sinus hypersensitivity, and to restore cardiac rhythm in cardiac arrest. Ophthalmic preparation is used in management of simple (open-angle) glaucoma, generally as an adjunct to topical miotics and oral carbonic anhydrase inhibitors; also used as ophthalmic decongestant. Used to prolong action and delay systemic absorption of local and intraspinal anaesthetics, and topically to control superficial bleeding.

ROUTE AND DOSAGE   **Parenteral: Adults:** *Anaphylaxis*: 0.5 to 1 ml of 1:1,000 SC or IM. SC doses may be repeated at 10 to 15 minute intervals as necessary. **Child:** 10 mcg/kg. *Airway obstruction*: 200–500 mcg repeated after 15–20 min as required. **Child:** 10 mcg/kg maximum 500 mcg as a single dose. **Inhalation:** 280–840 mcg (1–3 puffs) repeated after 30 min as required. No more than 8 times a day. *Ophthalmic*: drops 1% or cream 1% as required for examination.

ABSORPTION AND FATE   Rapid onset but brief duration of action. (Inactive when swallowed.) **Subcutaneous injection**: bronchodilation occurs within 3 to 5 minutes following administration of 1:1,000 solution, with maximal effects in 20 minutes. **Oral inhalation**: bronchodilation occurs within 1 minute. **Topical application**: to conjunctiva reduces intraocular pressure within 1 hour; maximal effects in 4 to 8 hours; action may persist 12 to 24 hours or more. Mydriasis usually occurs within a few minutes and may last several hours. Crosses placenta but not blood–brain barrier; enters breast milk.

CONTRAINDICATIONS AND PRECAUTIONS   Hypersensitivity to sympathomimetic amines or to any ingredient in the formulation; narrow-angle glaucoma; haemorrhagic, traumatic, or cardiogenic shock; cardiac dilatation, cerebral arteriosclerosis, coronary

ADRENALINE (continued)

insufficiency, arrhythmias, organic heart or brain disease; during second stage of labour; for local anaesthesia of fingers, toes, ears, nose, genitalia. Safe use during pregnancy, in nursing women, and in children not established. *Cautious Use*: elderly or debilitated patients, prostatic hypertrophy; hypertension; diabetes mellitus; hyperthyroidism; Parkinson's disease; tuberculosis; psychoneurosis; during pregnancy; in patients with long-standing bronchial asthma and emphysema with degenerative heart disease, in children under 6 years of age.

ADVERSE/SIDE EFFECTS   **Nasal use**: burning, stinging, dryness of nasal mucosa, sneezing, rebound congestion. **Ophthalmic use**: transient stinging or burning of eyes, lacrimation, browache, headache, rebound conjunctival hyperaemia, allergy, iritis; with prolonged use: melaninlike deposits on lids, conjunctiva, and cornea; corneal oedema; loss of lashes (reversible); maculopathy with central scotoma in aphakic patients (reversible). **Systemic reactions**: nervousness, restlessness, sleeplessness, fear, anxiety, tremors, severe headache, cerebrovascular accident, weakness, dizziness, syncope, pallor, nausea, vomiting, sweating, dyspnoea, precordial pain, palpitation, hypertension, myocardial infarction, tachyarrhythmias including atrial fibrillation; bronchial and pulmonary oedema, urinary retention, tissue necrosis, metabolic acidosis, elevated serum lactic acid, transient elevations of blood glucose, altered state of perception and thought, psychosis.

NURSING IMPLICATIONS

Parenteral

- A tuberculin syringe may assure greater accuracy in measurement of parenteral doses.
- Adrenaline injection should be protected from exposure to light at all times. Do not remove ampoule from carton until ready to use.
- Before withdrawing adrenaline suspension into syringe, shake ampoule thoroughly to disperse particles; then inject promptly.
- Carefully aspirate before injecting adrenaline. Inadvertent IV injection of usual subcutaneous or IM doses can result in sudden hypertension and possibly cerebral haemorrhage.
- Drug absorption (and action) can be hastened by massaging the injection site.
- Repeated injections may cause tissue necrosis due to vascular constriction. Rotate injection sites and observe for signs of blanching.
- If IM route is prescribed, injection into buttocks should be avoided. Adrenaline induced vasoconstriction reduces oxygen tension of tissues and thus favours growth of anaerobic *Clostridium welchii* (gas gangrene), which may be present in faeces and on buttocks.
- Monitor blood pressure, pulse, respirations, urinary output, and observe patient closely.
- Patients receiving adrenaline IV would have cardiac monitor. Have resuscitation and defibrillation equipment available.
- When administered IV, blood pressure should be checked repeatedly during first 5 minutes then checked every 3 to 5 minutes until stabilized.

ADRENALINE (continued)

Inhalation

- Treatment should start with first symptoms of bronchospasm. The least number of inhalations that provide relief should be used. Caution patient that overuse or too frequent use can result in severe adverse effects.

- Adrenaline reduces bronchial secretions and thus may make mucus plugs more difficult to dislodge. Use postural drainage, breathing exercises, and adequate hydration (3,000 to 4,000 ml) to facilitate expectoration. Spirometric measurements may be used to assess response to therapy.

- Describe sputum colour, consistency, and estimate amount.

- Advise patient to report difficulty in voiding or urinary retention (especially male patients). It may be advisable to have patient void before taking drug.

- Adrenaline may increase blood glucose levels. Patients with diabetes should be observed closely for loss of diabetes control.

- Instruct patient to take medication only as prescribed and to report the onset of systemic effects of adrenaline. A decrease in frequency of administration or concentration of drug or temporary discontinuation of therapy may be indicated.

- Adrenaline is destroyed by oxidizing agents, alkalies (including sodium bicarbonate), halogens, permanganates, chromates, nitrates, and salts of easily reducible metals such as iron, copper, and zinc.

- Oxidation of adrenaline imparts a colour ranging from pink to brown. Discard discoloured or precipitated solutions.

- Preserved in tight, light-resistant containers. Commercial preparations vary in stability; therefore, follow manufacturer's directions with respect to expiration date and storage requirements for each product.

DRUG INTERACTIONS   *Adrenaline and other adrenergics*_____

PLUS	INTERACTIONS
Anaesthetics, general, e.g., cyclopropane, halothane and other halogenated anaesthetics	Possibility of additive arrhythmic effects. These agents may sensitize heart to catecholamines. Concurrent use with cyclopropane avoided. Used with caution if at all with other agents
Antidiabetic agents	Adrenaline may increase blood glucose levels. Used concomitantly with caution
Digitalis glycosides (high doses)	May sensitize heart to adrenaline effects. Concurrent use generally avoided.
Guanethedine	Antihypertensive effects of guanethidine may be reversed resulting in severe hypertension and arrhythmias. Guanethidine may prolong mydriatic effects of adrenaline. Concurrent use generally avoided
Phentolamine, Phenothiazines and other alpha-adrenergic blocking agents	Antagonize adrenaline pressor effects with possibility of additive hypotension. Used concurrently with caution
Propranolol and other beta-adrenergic blocking agents	Blockade of adrenaline beta effects causes domination of alpha effects with resulting hypertension and reflex bradycardia

ADRENALINE (continued)
PLUS
(continued)

INTERACTIONS

Tricyclic antidepressants

Potentiation of adrenaline pressor response with possibility of severe hypertension. Concurrent use generally avoided

Allopurinol

(Aloral, Aluline, Caplenal, Cosuric, Hamarin, Zyloric)

Antigout agent; antilithic, enzyme inhibitor

ACTIONS AND USES   In contrast to uricosuric agents, which act by increasing renal excretion of uric acid, allopurinol reduces endogenous uric acid by selectively inhibiting action of xanthine oxidase, enzyme responsible for converting hypoxanthine to xanthine and xanthine to uric acid (end product of purine metabolism). Unlike uricosuric agents, action is not antagonized by salicylates.

Used to control primary hyperuricaemia that accompanies severe tophaceous gout complicated by advanced renal insufficiency or uric renal calculi. Has been used to prevent other types of recurrent renal calculi. Also used prophylactically for secondary hyperuricaemia, a potential of antineoplastic and radiation therapies.

ROUTE AND DOSAGE   Highly individualized; dosage adjusted on basis of serum uric acid levels and renal function. Manufacturer recommends dividing doses greater than 300 mg. **Oral: Adult:** *Gout*: initially 100 mg for 3 or 4 days, increased to a maintenance dose of 300–400 mg a day. *Secondary hyperuricaemia*, 200 mg three times a day prior to treatment, maintenance as required 300 mg a day. **Children** 20 mg/kg a day.

ABSORPTION AND FATE   Approximately 80% of oral dose is absorbed. Plasma level peaks in 2 to 4 hours. Widely distributed to all extracellular fluid; less concentration in brain. Not bound to plasma proteins. Rapidly cleared from plasma (probable **half-life** 2 to 3 hours). About 5 to 7% of dose excreted unchanged in urine within 6 hours; 20% eliminated unchanged in faeces within 48 to 72 hours. Remainder rapidly metabolized to active metabolites, chiefly oxypurinol (**half-life** of 18 to 30 hours) thought to be primarily responsible for xanthine oxidase inhibition. Metabolite is excreted slowly; therefore, it may accumulate with chronic administration of allopurinol.

CONTRAINDICATIONS AND PRECAUTIONS   Hypersensitivity to allopurinol as initial treatment for acute gouty attacks, idiopathic haemochromatosis (or those with family history), children (except those with hyperuricaemia secondary to neoplastic disease and chemotherapy). Safe use during pregnancy or in fertile women and nursing mothers not established. **Cautious Use**: impaired hepatic or renal function, history of peptic ulcer, lower GI tract disease, bone marrow depression.

ADVERSE/SIDE EFFECTS   Nausea, vomiting, metallic taste, diarrhoea, abdominal discomfort, precipitation of peptic ulcer. Agranulocytosis (fever, sore throat, unusual fatigue, malaise), anaemia, aplastic anaemia, transient leucopenia or leucocytosis, bone

A

ALLOPURINOL (continued)

marrow depression, pancytopenia, thrombocytopenia. Drowsiness, headache, vertigo, peripheral neuritis (numbness, tingling, pain, weakness of hands and feet). Retinopathy, macular degeneration, cataracts (may accompany severe dermatitis). Pruritic maculopapular rash (common); exfoliative, urticarial, and purpural dermatitis; erythema multiforme including Stevens–Johnson syndrome; toxic epidermal necrolysis, alopecia (rare); severe furunculosis of nose, ichthyosis. Lymphadenopathy, lymphoedema, tachycardia, xanthine renal calculi, especially in children with Lesch–Nyhan syndrome; pancreatitis, hepatotoxicity, hyperlipaemia, adrenal insufficiency; precipitation of acute gout.

NURSING IMPLICATIONS

- Generally the drug is best tolerated when taken following meals. If necessary, tablet may be crushed before administration and taken with fluid or mixed with food.
- When used to prevent secondary hyperuricaemia associated with antineoplastic therapy, allopurinol should be prescribed 1 or 2 days before chemotherapy begins.
- Instruct patient to report promptly the onset of itching or rash especially if ampicillin is prescribed concurrently, or any other unusual sign or symptom (*See Adverse/Side Effects*).
- A skin rash, which may appear after after 1 to 5 weeks (and reportedly even after 2 years) of therapy, is the most common adverse reaction and is an indication to stop drug therapy.
- Hypersensitivity reaction (sometimes fatal) has followed the onset of a skin rash. It commonly occurs in patients with impaired renal function and is generally accompanied by malaise, fever, and aching.
- Patients with renal disorders should be closely monitored for any further deterioration of kidney function. These patients tend to have a higher than usual incidence of renal stones and dermatological (hypersensitivity) problems.
- Advise patient to minimize exposure and to shield eyes from ultraviolet or sunlight. Ultraviolet light may stimulate the development of cataracts. Patients should be examined periodically for lens changes.
- Aim of therapy is to lower serum urate level gradually to about 2 mmol/L. Serum uric acid levels should be evaluated at least every 1 to 2 weeks to check adequacy of dosage. A sudden decrease in serum uric acid can precipitate an acute gouty attack.
- Baseline complete blood counts and liver and kidney function tests should be performed before initiating therapy and monthly, particularly during first few months of therapy.
- Acute gouty attacks are most likely to occur during first 6 weeks of allopurinol therapy, possibly because of mobilization of urates from tissue deposits. Concurrent maintenance therapy with colchicine may be prescribed, as prophylaxis, for the first 3 to 6 months of allopurinol therapy.
- When allopurinol is prescribed for patient who has been taking a uricosuric, dose of the latter should be reduced slowly over several weeks while allopurinol is being increased gradually to desired dose.
- Allopurinol may cause drowsiness and vertigo. Caution patient to avoid driving or performing other complex tasks until reaction to drug has been evaluated.

ALLOPURINOL (continued)

- It is advisable to maintain fluid intake sufficient to produce urinary output of at least 2,000 ml daily (fluid intake of at least 3,000 ml daily) and to keep urine neutral or slightly alkaline by oral administration of sodium bicarbonate or potassium citrate. These measures are prescribed to reduce risk of xanthine stone formation.
- Fluid intake–output ratio and pattern should be monitored. Since allopurinol and metabolites are excreted chiefly by kidneys, decreased renal function causes drug accumulation. Instruct patient to report diminishing urinary output, cloudy urine, unusual colour or odour to urine, pain or discomfort on urination.
- A rigid low purine diet is not usually prescribed for patients with gout. However, physician may advise patient to omit or limit certain of these high purine foods: offal (e.g., kidney, liver, sweetbreads, brains), anchovies, sardines, salmon, meat soups, gravies, lentils, dried peas and beans.
- Weight reduction may be prescribed and should be undertaken slowly and during quiescent phase of the disease to avoid precipitating a gouty attack (*see Colchicine*).
- **Food–drug interaction** Excessive alcohol or coffee consumption can cause secondary hyperuricaemia and therefore should be avoided.
- Allopurinol is generally continued indefinitely. Advise patient to remain under medical supervision. The drug can cause severe adverse reactions.
- Therapeutic response to allopurinol is indicated by normal serum and urinary uric acid levels (usually by 1 to 3 weeks), gradual decrease in size of tophi, absence of new tophaceous deposits (after approximately 6 months), with consequent relief of joint pain and increased joint mobility.
- Store at room temperature preferably between 15° and 30°C (59° and 86°F) in a well-closed container.

Teaching plan for patient with chronic gout *See Colchicine.*

Diagnostic test interferences Possibility of elevated blood levels of **alkaline phosphatase** and **serum transaminases**, and decreased blood **Hct, Hgb, leukocytes**.

DRUG INTERACTIONS *Allopurinol*_____

PLUS	INTERACTIONS
Alcohol (Ethanol)	Excessive alcohol promotes formation of lactic acid and ketone bodies which inhibit renal excretion of uric acid
Amoxicillin } Ampicillin	Increased risk of skin rash
Anticoagulants, oral	Enhanced anticoagulant effects. (Allopurinol inhibits hepatic drug metabolizing enzymes.) May require lower anticoagulant dosage
Azathioprine	Increased toxicity. (Azathioprine metabolism depends on xanthine oxidase.) Generally prescribe lower initial azathioprine dosage
Chlorpropamide	Hypoglycaemic effects increased (chlorpropamide excretion decreased). Monitor for excessive hypoglycaemia
Cyclophosphamide	Potentiates cyclophosphamide. Monitor closely for bone marrow depression

ALLOPURINOL *(continued)*

PLUS (continued)	INTERACTIONS
Diuretics	May interfere with renal excretion of uric acid
Iron preparations	Increased hepatic deposition of iron (based on animal studies)
Mercaptopurine	Increased risk of mercaptopurine toxicity (metabolism depends on xanthine oxidase)
Phenytoin, and other hydantoins	Possibility of increased phenytoin effects. (Allopurinol inhibits hepatic drug metabolism.)
Probenecid	Allopurinol inhibits probenecid metabolism. Probenecid reduces allopurinol effect by enhancing urinary excretion of its active metabolite
Pyrazinamide	May interfere with renal excretion of uric acid
Theophylline	Theophylline toxicity increases with high allopurinol dosages. (Allopurinol inhibits hepatic drug metabolism.)
Thiazides (and possibly other diuretics)	Increased risk of allopurinol toxicity and hypersensitivity (especially with impaired renal function). Monitor renal and hepatic function
Tamoxifen	Possibility of hepatotoxicity
Vitamin C (Ascorbic acid) in large doses, and other urinary acidifiers	May increase possibility of renal calculi
Vidarabine	Increased vidarabine toxicity (reduced drug metabolism). Concurrent use generally avoided

Alfacalcidol

(One-alpha)   *Calcium regulator*

ACTIONS AND USES   Vitamin D preparation used to treat hypocalcaemia in patients undergoing renal dialysis.

For further information *see* Calcitriol.

ROUTE AND DOSAGE   Oral: **Adult** and **child** over 20 kg initial 1 mcg/day, increased according to response. Child under 20 kg, 50 nanograms/kg/day.

Alprazolam

(Xanax)   *Psychotropic; anxiolytic; benzodiazepine*

ACTIONS AND USES   Shares CNS depressant actions of other benzodiazepines, but compared to most drugs of this group, duration of activity is relatively short and

ALPRAZOLAM (continued)

associated with significantly less drowsiness. Has antidepressant as well as anxiolytic actions.

Used in management of anxiety disorders or for short-term relief of anxiety symptoms. Also used as adjunct in management of anxiety associated with depression, and for panic disorders, such as agoraphobia.

ROUTE AND DOSAGE   Oral: *Initial*, 0.25 to 0.5 mg three times daily. Total dose not to exceed 3 mg/day in divided doses. Highly individualized. **Elderly and debilitated patients, patients with liver disease or low serum albumin**: *Initial*: 0.25 mg two or three times daily; gradually increased if necessary and tolerated.

ABSORPTION AND FATE   Rapidly and well absorbed following oral administration. Peak blood levels in 1 to 2 hours. Protein binding about 80%. **Half-life**: 12 to 15 hours (in elderly males may be 19 to 20 hours).

ADVERSE/SIDE EFFECTS   Nasal congestion, weight gain or loss, blurred vision. *See Chlordiazepoxide for additional adverse/side effects.*

NURSING IMPLICATIONS

- Alprazolam is not intended for management of anxieties and minor distresses associated with everyday life. Ideally, diagnosis of underlying difficulties should be attempted before drug is prescribed.
- Oversedation, drowsiness, unsteadiness, light-headedness, and other adverse reactions, which may occur during early high dose therapy, usually disappear with continuing therapy. Advise patient to keep physician informed; dosage adjustments may be indicated. Note implications especially for elderly and debilitated patients (bedsides; supervise ambulation).
- Following continuous use, dosage should be tapered off before drug is stopped. Abrupt discontinuation of drug may cause withdrawal symptoms (nausea, vomiting, abdominal and muscle cramps, sweating, confusion, tremors, convulsions).
- Psychological and physical dependence may occur with large doses given over prolonged periods of time.
- Store in tightly-covered, light-resistant containers preferably between 15° and 30°C (59° and 86°F), unless otherwise directed by manufacturer.
- For further information *see* also Chlordiazepoxide.

Aluminium acetate solution ━━━━━━━━━━━━━━━

Antipruritic (topical); astringent

ACTIONS AND USES   Prepared from aluminium subacetate and glacial acetic acid. Has antiinflammatory, antipruritic, mild astringent, and antiseptic properties. Reportedly maintains protective acidity of skin.

Used in treatment of mildly irritated or inflamed skin.

ALUMINIUM ACETATE SOLUTION (continued)

ROUTE AND DOSAGE   Topical (wet dressings): 1:10 to 1:40 solution. Applied for 15 to 30 minutes at 4- to 8-hour intervals. **Ear drops:** 4 to 6 drops instilled slowly along wall of external ear. Repeat every 2 or 3 hours. Cream, lotion, and solution preparations available.

NURSING IMPLICATIONS

- Following instillation of ear drops the patient's position should be maintained with affected ear uppermost for about 2 minutes. If physician prescribes an ear wick, solution may be added to wick as often as directed.
- For wet dressings, warm or cold solution (as ordered) may be carefully poured on dressing at prescribed intervals. May be bandaged lightly and loosely, but do not cover with plastic or other occlusive material without consulting the physician.
- Protect eyes from solution.
- Use should be discontinued if irritation or extension of inflammatory condition occurs.
- Store drug below 30°C (86°F). Avoid freezing.

Aluminium chloride hexahydrate ————————————

(Anhydrol forte, Driclor)   *Astringent*

ACTIONS AND USES   The antiperspirant contains 20% aluminium chloride hexahydrate in absolute alcohol. Controls sweating by astringent action which coagulates protein in sweat glands and causes temporary reduction in duct size or closure. Also has mild antibacterial action. An ingredient in several OTC preparations. Used to control hyperhidrosis of palms, soles, and axillae.

ROUTE AND DOSAGE   *Hyperhidrosis* (20%): Apply to affected area once daily, only at bedtime. When excessive sweating is controlled, applied once or twice weekly or as needed.

NURSING IMPLICATIONS

- Inform patient that medication may produce a burning, prickly sensation.
- Avoid contact with eyes. Advise patient to wash hands thoroughly with soap and water after each application.
- Treated areas should be washed and dried thoroughly each day.
- Dry area completely before applying medication.
- Preparation should not be applied to broken, irritated, or recently shaved or depilated skin.
- Instruct patient to discontinue drug if irritation or sensitization occurs, and to report to physician.
- Inform patient that medication may damage certain fabrics.
- Store in airtight container.

A

Aluminium hydroxide ————————————————————

(Alu-Cap, Aludrox)   *Antacid; antilithic*

ACTIONS AND USES Nonsystemic antacid with limited neutralizing action. Reacts with gastric acid to form aluminium chloride, believed to be responsible for astringent and constipating effects. Chloride is reabsorbed in small intestines, thus preserving systemic acid—base balance. Neutralizing capacity of liquid suspension is reported to surpass that of dried gel because particle size is much smaller. Decreases rate of gastric emptying and has demulcent, adsorbent, and mild astringent properties. Lowers serum phosphate by binding dietary phosphorus to form insoluble aluminium phosphate, which is excreted in faeces. This prevents formation of urinary phosphatic calculi by decreasing excretion of phosphates in urine. Phosphate-binding capacity not as great as that of aluminium carbonate. Used for symptomatic relief of gastric hyperacidity associated with gastritis oesophageal reflux, and hiatus hernia; used as adjunct in treatment of gastric and duodenal ulcer. Also has been used in management of hyperphosphatemia of renal failure and in treatment of phosphatic urinary calculi. More commonly used in combination with other antacids. Available in fixed-dose combination with magnesium hydroxide: e.g., Aludrox, Maalox.

ROUTE AND DOSAGE Oral: 10 ml, or 1 or 2 tablets or capsules, four to six times a day if necessary, between meals and at bedtime.

ABSORPTION AND FATE Slow onset of action; duration about 20 to 40 minutes if drug is taken on empty stomach, and approximately 2 hours with food in stomach. Excreted in faeces, primarily as insoluble phosphates. Minimal amounts of aluminium may be absorbed; traces excreted in urine.

CONTRAINDICATIONS AND PRECAUTIONS Sensitivity to aluminium; prolonged use of high doses in presence of low serum phosphate, or in patients on sodium restriction. **Cautious Use**: renal impairment, gastric outlet obstruction, elderly patients, decreased bowel activity (e.g., patients receiving anticholinergic, antidiarrhoeal, or antispasmodic agents), patients who are dehydrated or on fluid restriction.

ADVERSE/SIDE EFFECTS Constipation (common), nausea, vomiting, faecal impaction, intestinal concretions, and obstruction. *Phosphorus deficiency syndrome*: (malaise, anorexia, profound muscle weakness, tremors, absent deep tendon reflexes, mental depression, bone pain, negative Ca balance: hypercalciuria, urinary calculi, osteoporosis, osteomalacia); hypomagnesaemia.

NURSING IMPLICATIONS
■ Shake liquid well before pouring.
■ If administered in tablet form, instruct patient to chew the tablet until thoroughly wetted before swallowing (swallowing undissolved particles increases risk of developing intestinal concretions). *For antacid use*: follow tablet with one-half glass of water or milk; follow liquid preparation (suspension) with sip of water to assure passage into stomach.

ALUMINIUM HYDROXIDE (continued)

- Drug is sometimes left at the bedside if it is to be given frequently, but only if the patient is able to assume responsibility for following a prescribed schedule.
- During the 4- to 6-week period required for healing an active peptic ulcer, some physicians prescribe antacid 1 and 3 hours after meals, and at bedtime. Others alternate antacid and meals on a 2-hour schedule and advise patients to take an extra antacid dose when discomfort is felt.
- The objective of therapy for an active ulcer is to ensure that the stomach is not left empty, i.e., without food or antacid, for more than 2 hours. Food itself has considerable buffering capacity. For example, if antacid is given 1 hour after a meal, buffering action will persist an additional 2 hours; administration 3 hours after a meal extends buffering action another hour.
- The value of a milk diet is not supported by objective evidence; this adjunct of therapy has largely been abandoned. The neutralizing effect of milk is slight; large amounts may actually stimulate gastric acid secretion for at least 3 hours after ingestion. *Note*: the traditional bedtime milk snack is particularly to be avoided to prevent an excess of unbuffered gastric acid during sleep.
- Since frequency of meals may vary in the elderly particularly, explain specifically the best time to take an antacid.
- Pain is used as a clinical guide for adjusting dosage. Advise patient to keep physician informed. Pain that persists beyond 72 hours may signify serious complications such as perforation or malignancy.
- *Food–drug interactions* Patients receiving large doses of antacids for prolonged periods and who eat a diet low in phosphorus (e.g., avoiding milk, milk products, poultry, whole grain cereals) and low in protein can develop phosphorus deficiency syndrome (*see Adverse/Side Effects*). It has occurred within 2 weeks of continuous antacid use. The elderly patient in poor nutritional state is at high risk. Both vitamin A and thiamine deficiencies also can occur in some patients because of reduced absorption.
- Note number and consistency of stools. Constipation occurs commonly and is dose-related. Intestinal obstruction from faecal concretions has been reported. If constipation is a problem, physician may prescribe alternate or combination therapy with an antacid with laxative action, such as magnesium hydroxide, magnesium oxide, or magnesium trisilicate.
- Explain to patient that antacid may cause stools to appear speckled or whitish in colour.
- Length of antacid therapy for patients with duodenal ulcer is usually 4 to 6 weeks, and for gastric ulcers until healing has taken place.
- Serum calcium and phosphorus levels should be determined at periodic intervals in patients receiving prolonged high dose therapy or who have impaired renal function.
- Patients with *gastro-oesophangeal reflux* associated with hiatus hernia are generally advised to (1) avoid possible causes of heartburn (a prominent symptom) such as overeating, fatty foods (which also delay gastric emptying), foods known to cause heartburn or gas (based on individual intolerance), concentrated fruit juices, chocolate, coffee, alcohol; (2) limit fluid intake during meals; (3) eat meals at regular intervals in a relaxed atmosphere. Eat and drink slowly to avoid gulping air; (4) avoid

ALUMINIUM HYDROXIDE (continued)

lying down sooner than 1 hour after a meal; (5) elevate head of bed 6 to 8 inches on bed blocks (use of pillows alone tends to 'jackknife' abdomen); (6) avoid straining and heavy lifting; (7) avoid tight abdominal garments; (8) maintain ideal weight, if possible.

- Now not commonly prescribed.
- Caution individuals who self-medicate with antacids to seek medical help if indigestion is accompanied by shortness of breath, sweating, or chest pain, if stools are very dark or tarry, or if symptoms are recurrent.
- Self-prescribed antacid use should not exceed 2 weeks before seeking medical advice and supervision.
- Store preferably between 15° and 30°C (59° and 86°F) in tightly closed container, unless otherwise directed by manufacturer.

DRUG INTERACTIONS

An increase in pH (as with antacid therapy) delays gastric emptying time leading to variation and unpredictability in drug absorption. Therefore, in general, it is best to avoid taking an antacid any sooner than 1 hour before or until 2 to 3 hours after another oral medication, unless otherwise advised. **Digoxin, indomethacin, iron salts**, and **tetracycline** particularly should be spaced as far from an antacid as possible. Also note that antacid-induced elevations in gastric pH may increase rate of absorption of buffered or enteric coated preparations by causing premature dissolution.

Concurrent use of aluminium-hydroxide or other aluminium-containing antacids inhibits absorption of:

- ☐ Anticholinergic agents
- ☐ Chlordiazepoxide
- ☐ Chloroquine
- ☐ Cimetidine
- ☐ Corticosteroids
- ☐ Diazepam
- ☐ Digoxin
- ☐ Indomethacin

- ☐ Iron salts
- ☐ Isoniazid (INH)
- ☐ Penicillamine
- ☐ Phenothiazines
- ☐ Phenytoin
- ☐ Tetracyclines
- ☐ Vitamin A and possibly other fat soluble vitamins

PLUS	INTERACTIONS
Pseudoephedrine	Concurrent use of antacid may increase drug absorption (by decreasing drug excretion)
Sodium polystyrene sulphonate	Coadministration with nonsystemic antacid can cause significant rise in blood bicarbonate level, and may impair potassium lowering ability of sodium polystyrene sulphonate

Amantadine hydrochloride ——————————————

(Symmetrel)

Anticholinergic (antimuscarinic); antiparkinson agent; antiviral; parasympatholytic

ACTIONS AND USES Synthetic tricyclic amine with virostatic action. Believed to act by inhibiting penetration of host cell by virus, or by preventing uncoating of viral

AMANTADINE HYDROCHLORIDE (continued)

nucleic acid. Because it does not suppress antibody formation it can be administered for interim protection in combination with influenza A virus vaccine until antibody titre is adequate, or to augment prophylaxis in a previously vaccinated individual. Active against several strains of influenza A virus; not effective against influenza B infections. Has mild anticholinergic activity. Mechanism of action in Parkinson's disease not understood, but may be related to release of dopamine and other catecholamines from neuronal storage sites. Reportedly less effective than levodopa, but produces more rapid clinical response and causes fewer adverse reactions.

Used in initial therapy or as adjunct with anticholinergic drugs or levodopa in treatment of all forms of parkinsonism (arteriosclerotic, idiopathic, postencephalitic) and for relief of drug-induced extrapyramidal reactions, and symptomatic parkinsonism caused by carbon monoxide poisoning. Also used for prophylaxis and symptomatic treatment of influenza A infections.

ROUTE AND DOSAGE   Oral: *Parkinsonism*: Adults: 100 mg twice daily. *Influenza* and *herpes zoster* 100 mg twice daily.

ABSORPTION AND FATE   Readily and almost completely absorbed from GI tract. **Maximal blood concentrations** after 1 to 4 hours. **Onset of action** within 48 hours. **Half-life** about 24 hours (range 9 to 37 hours), prolonged in patients with impaired renal function. Not metabolized. Distributed to saliva, nasal secretions, breast milk; crosses blood–brain barrier. Approximately 90% of dose excreted unchanged in urine. Acidification of urine increases rate of elimination. Crosses placenta. Excreted in breast milk.

CONTRAINDICATIONS AND PRECAUTIONS   Known hypersensitivity to amantadine, nursing mothers. Safe use during pregnancy, in women of childbearing potential, and in children under 1 year not established. **Cautious Use:** history of epilepsy or other types of seizures; congestive heart failure, peripheraloedema, orthostatic hypotension, recurrent eczematoid dermatitis, psychoses, severe psychoneuroses, hepatic disease, renal impairment; elderly patients with cerebral arteriosclerosis.

ADVERSE/SIDE EFFECTS   Usually dose related: dizziness, light-headedness, headache, ataxia, drowsiness, fatigue, weakness, irritability, anxiety, nervousness, difficulty in concentrating, depression, psychosis, confusion, slurred speech, visual and auditory hallucinations, insomnia, nightmares, tremor, convulsions. Orthostatic hypotension, peripheraloedema, dyspnoea, congestive heart failure. Dermatitis, livedo reticularis, photosensitization. Anorexia, nausea, vomiting, constipation, dry mouth. Urinary retention, frequency. Leucopenia, neutropenia (rare). Blurring or loss of vision, oculogyric episodes.

NURSING IMPLICATIONS
- Capsule may be emptied and contents swallowed with water or mixed with food.
- To be effective in treatment of influenza, amantadine must be administered preferably within 24 hours but no later than 48 hours after onset of symptoms and should be continued for 24 to 48 hours after symptoms disappear.
- Administration of last daily dose too close to retiring may produce insomnia. If

AMANTADINE HYDROCHLORIDE (continued)

insomnia is a problem, medication should be scheduled several hours before bedtime. Suggest that patient limit number of daytime naps.

- CNS and psychic disturbances are most likely to appear within 1 day to a few days after initiation of drug therapy, or after dosage has been increased. Symptoms tend to subside when drug is given in two divided doses.
- Solicit help of family members to establish a baseline profile of the patient's disabilities. This information is essential for accurate differentiation between disease symptoms (e.g., dementia) and drug-induced neuropsychiatric adverse reactions. A quantitative scoring system may be of help.
- Patients receiving doses above 200 mg daily should be closely observed for amantadine toxicity. Monitor vital signs for at least 3 or 4 days following increases in dosage.
- Elderly patients with cerebrovascular disease or impaired renal function are more prone to develop symptoms of toxicity.
- Because orthostatic hypotension may be a problem, caution patient not to go to sleep in a sitting position, and advise elderly male patients particularly to sit down to urinate, especially at night.
- Advise patient to make all position changes slowly, particularly from recumbent to upright position, and to dangle legs a few minutes before standing. Caution patient to lie down immediately if faint or dizzy.
- Instruct patient and responsible family members to report to physician onset of shortness of breath, peripheral oedema, significant weight gain, dizziness, inability to concentrate, and other changes in mental status, dysuria.
- Activities requiring mental alertness such as driving a car should be avoided until patient's response to the drug has been evaluated.
- Patients with parkinsonism may show reduction of salivation, akinesia, and rigidity within 4 to 48 hours after initiation of therapy. Generally, drug has little effect on tremors. If significant improvement is not noted within 1 or 2 weeks, drug is usually discontinued.
- Patient should remain under close medical supervision while receiving amantadine therapy. Maximum therapeutic response generally occurs within 2 weeks to 3 months. Effectiveness sometimes wanes after 6 to 8 weeks of treatment. Report to physician. Decision may be made to increase dosage or to discontinue drug temporarily or to use another antiparkinsonian agent.
- Abrupt discontinuation of amantadine therapy in patients with parkinsonism may precipitate *parkinsonian crisis* within 24 hours to 3 days (severe akinesia, rigidity, tremor). Warn patient to adhere to established dosage regimen.
- **Treatment of overdosage** Immediate gastric lavage or induction of emesis. Physostigmine and chlorpromazine must be available for neurological manifestations. General supportive measures: maintenance of airway, administration of oxygen, fluids, urinary acidifier. Monitor urinary output and pH, serum electrolytes, vital signs. Observe for seizures.
- *Care plan* should address problems that frequently accompany parkinsonism: (1) Mental depression. (2) Sleep disturbances. (3) Constipation. (4) Urinary retention especially in elderly males with enlarged prostate. (5) Complications related to

AMANTADINE HYDROCHLORIDE (continued)

inactivity (pressure sores, contractures, postural deformities). Patients should have medical follow-up at regular intervals.

- Store in tightly closed container preferably between 15° and 30°C (59° and 86°F) unless otherwise directed by manufacturer. Avoid freezing.

DRUG INTERACTIONS *Amantadine*

PLUS	INTERACTIONS
Alcohol, and other CNS depressants	Additive CNS effects
Anticholinergics	Amantadine may potentiate CNS effects of large doses of anticholinergic drugs. Dosage of either should be reduced.

Amikacin sulphate

(Amikin)   *Aminoglycoside; antibiotic; antiinfective*

ACTIONS AND USES   Semisynthetic derivative of kanamycin with broadest range of antimicrobial activity of the aminoglycosides. Pharmacological properties essentially the same as those of gentamicin (q.v.). Unlike other aminoglycosides, resists destruction by bacterial enzymes, (except acetyltransferase and an adenylating enzyme). Like other aminoglycosides, inhibits protein synthesis in bacterial cell and is bactericidal. Effective against a wide variety of gram-negative bacilli including *Escherichia coli*, *Enterobacter*, *Klebsiella pneumoniae*, most strains of *Pseudomonas aeruginosa*, and many strains of *Proteus* species, *Serratia*, *Providencia sturatii*, *Citrobacter freundii*, *Acinetobacter*. Also effective against penicillinase and non-penicillinase-producing staphylococci. Active against *Mycobacterium tuberculosis* and atypical mycobacteria, but not against majority of other gram-positive anaerobic bacteria, or rickettsiae, fungi, and viruses.

Used primarily for treatment of serious nosocomial gram-negative bacillary infections resistant to gentamicin and tobramycin. Has been used in combination with carbenicillin or ticarcillin for severe pseudomonas infections.

ROUTE AND DOSAGE   Dosage calculations should be based on estimate of ideal body weight (IBW). **Intramuscular, intravenous infusion: Adults, children, and older infants**: 15 mg/kg daily in 2 divided doses.

ABSORPTION AND FATE   Serum levels peak in 45 minutes to 2 hours following IM administration and within 30 minutes following IV. **Half-life**: about 2 to 3 hours in adults and 4 to 8 hours in neonates; 28 to 86 hours in anephric patients. Small amounts (4 to 8%) protein bound. Primarily distributed to extracellular fluid; progressively accumulates in renal cortex and fluid of inner ear over course of therapy. Penetrates CSF particularly when meninges are inflamed. Excreted unchanged in urine; 94 to 98% of dose excreted within 24 hours. Crosses placenta. Excretion into breast milk not known.

AMIKACIN SULPHATE (continued)

CONTRAINDICATIONS AND PRECAUTIONS   History of hypersentivity or toxic reaction with aminoglycosides. Safe use during pregnancy or breast feeding not determined. **Cautious Use**: impaired renal function, eighth cranial nerve impairment, dehydration, fever, the elderly, neonates and infants, myasthenia gravis, parkinsonism, hypocalcaemia.

ADVERSE/SIDE EFFECTS   Drowsiness, headache, unsteady gait, weakness, clumsiness, paraesthesias, tremors, neuromuscular blockade with respiratory depression. Hypotension, tachycardia. Nausea, vomiting, stomatitis. Infrequent: anaemia, leucopenia, granulocytopenia, thrombocytopenia. Skin rash, urticaria, pruritis, generalized burning sensation, drug fever, arthralgia, eosinophilia. *Auditory*: high frequency hearing loss, complete hearing loss (occasionally permanent); tinnitus; fullness, ringing, or buzzing in ears; *vestibular*: dizziness, vertigo, ataxia, nausea, vomiting, nystagmus. Oliguria, urinary frequency, red and white blood cells in urine, frank haematuria, casts, albuminuria, azotaemia, increase in BUN and serum creatinine, decrease in creatinine clearance, specific gravity; renal damage and failure. Unusual thirst, difficult breathing, superinfections, peripheral neuritis; rare: hypocalcaemia with symptoms of tetany; weakness, lethargy, and associated with hypokalaemia and hypomagnesaemia. *See also Gentamicin*.

NURSING IMPLICATIONS

■ Culture and susceptibility tests should be performed before initial dose, but therapy may begin pending test results. Most infections respond to amikacin therapy in 24 to 48 hours. If therapeutic response does not occur in 3 to 5 days, susceptibility tests should be repeated and therapy reevaluated.

■ Baseline weight, vital signs, and tests of renal function and eighth cranial (vestibulocochlear) nerve function should be performed before therapy and at regular intervals during therapy.

■ Renal function and eighth cranial nerve function should be closely monitored in the elderly, in patients with history of ear problems, patients with renal impairment, or during high dose or prolonged therapy.

■ Ototoxicity is primarily cochlear (auditory); however, vestibular toxicity can also occur (*see Adverse/Side Effects*). High frequency deafness usually appears first and can be detected only by audiometer.

■ Patient should be questioned periodically about hearing, and symptoms related to vestibular disturbances.

■ Tinnitus is not a reliable index of ototoxicity in the very old who may already have hearing problems, or in the very young who cannot talk. In these patients blood drug levels must be monitored to follow therapy.

■ Monitor fluid intake and output. Report any change in intake–output ratio or pattern, oliguria, haematuria, or cloudy urine. Keeping patient well hydrated reduces chemical irritation of renal tubules (nephrotoxicity). Consult physician regarding optimum fluid intake.

■ Be aware of renal function test results. Decreasing urine specific gravity and creatin-

AMIKACIN SULPHATE (continued)

ine clearance, and increasing creatinine, BUN, and white and red blood cells in urine are significant indicators of declining renal function.

- Usual duration of treatment is 7 to 10 days. If treatment is continued for more than 10 days, daily tests of renal function and weekly audiograms and vestibular tests are advised.
- To reduce risk of nephrotoxicity and ototoxicity, periodic measurements of serum amikacin levels in addition to serum creatinine, and creatinine clearance (generally preferred) are recommended. These values are used as guidelines for determining dosage adjustments needed to maintain desired serum concentrations.
- Blood for determining peak amikacin level is drawn 1 hour after IM administration and 1 hour after IV infusion begins.
- Therapeutic peak serum amikacin concentrations range from 20 to 25 mcg/ml; therapeutic trough levels are 5 to 10 mcg/ml. High trough or peak levels are associated with toxicity.
- Monitor vital signs. Amikacin serum levels are reportedly lower in patients with fever.
- Be on the alert for symptoms of respiratory tract infections and other symptoms indicative of superinfections. Notify physician should they occur.
- To prepare IV solution, dilute calculated dose in 100 or 200 ml sterile diluent recommended by manufacturer and administer over 30- to 60-minute period for adults. In paediatric patients, volume of diluent depends on patient need. Infants should be given a 1- to 2-hour infusion. Monitor drip rate prescribed by physician. A rapid rise in serum level can cause respiratory depression and other signs of toxicity.
- Manufacturer recommends that no other drug be combined with amikacin; that is, it should be administered separately.
- Colour of solution may vary from colourless to light straw colour or very pale yellow. Discard dark coloured solutions.
- Stored preferably between 15° and 30°C (59° and 86°F) unless otherwise directed by manufacturer. Protect from freezing. *See also Gentamicin.*

DRUG INTERACTIONS *Amikacin*

PLUS	INTERACTIONS
Concurrent or sequential administration of drugs with potential for nephrotoxicity, ototoxicity, or neurotoxicity is generally avoided, e.g.:	
☐ Aminoglycosides, other amphotericin B ☐ Bacitracin ☐ Capreomycin	☐ Cephalothin ☐ Cisplatin ☐ Diuretics (potent): e.g., bumetanide, ethacrynic acid, frusemide ☐ Polymyxin B
Anaesthetics (general) skeletal muscle relaxants (nondepolarizing), e.g., succinyl choline	Additive neuromuscular blocking action; used with caution
Dimenhydrinate and other antiemetics	May mask symptoms of ototoxicity
Penicillins	Possibility of aminoglycoside inactivation. Also, administered separately, because of physical incompatibility

A

Amiloride hydrochloride————————————————

(Midamor)   *Diuretic (potassium-sparing)*

ACTIONS AND USES   Potassium-sparing diuretic, structurally similar to triamterene, with mild diuretic and antihypertensive actions. Induces urinary excretion of sodium, e.g., bicarbonates, and calcium and reduces excretion of potassium and hydrogen ions by direct action on distal renal tubules. Potassium-sparing action results in rise of total body concentration of potassium; reduction in hydrogen ions causes moderate increase in urinary pH.

Used for its potassium-sparing effect in prevention or treatment of diuretic-induced hypokalaemia in patients with congestive heart failure, hepatic cirrhosis, or hypertension. Also used in management of primary hyperaldosteronism. Usually combined with a potassium-wasting diuretic such as a thiazide or loop diuretic. Commercially available in fixed-dose combination with hydrochlorothiazide (Moduretic). The combination is more effective than either drug alone, and risk of hyperkalaemia is reduced.

ROUTE AND DOSAGE   Oral: *Initial*: 5 mg/day. Increased to 10 mg/day, if necessary; up to 20 mg/day.

ABSORPTION AND FATE   Approximately 50% absorbed from GI tract following oral administration. **Onset of diuretic action** within 2 hours, peaks at 6 to 10 hours, and is completed in 24 hours. Approximately 23% protein bound; **half-life**: 6 to 9 hours (longer in patients with impaired renal function). Excreted unchanged 20 to 50% via kidneys, 40% in faeces. In animals, crosses placenta and enters breast milk. Human studies incomplete.

CONTRAINDICATIONS AND PRECAUTIONS   Elevated serum potassium (>5.5 mEq/ L), concomitant use of other potassium-sparing diuretics; anuria, acute or chronic renal insufficiency, evidence of diabetic nephropathy; type I (insulin-dependent) diabetes mellitus, metabolic or respiratory acidosis, hepatic function impairment. Safe use in pregnancy, nursing mothers, and children not established. **Cautious Use**: debilitated patients, diet-controlled or uncontrolled diabetes mellitus, cardiopulmonary disease, elderly.

ADVERSE/SIDE EFFECTS   Generally well tolerated. Headache, dizziness, tremors, nervousness, insomnia, somnolence, confusion, depression, paraesthesias. Orthostatic hypotension, angina, palpitation, cardiac arrhythmias. Hyperkalaemia, hyponatraemia, metabolic acidosis; rare (causal relationship not established): eosinophilia, leucopenia, neutropenia, aplastic anaemia, elevated Hct, positive Coombs' test. Tinnitus, nasal congestion. Diarrhoea or constipation, anorexia, nausea, vomiting, abdominal cramps, abdominal bloating, flatulence, heartburn; dry mouth, alterations of taste, thirst, jaundice; reactivation of peptic ulcer (causal relationship not established). Polyuria, dysuria, bladder spasms, urinary frequency. Visual disturbances, increased intraocular pressure. Cough, dyspnoea, shortness of breath. Erythematous rash, pruritus, alopecia, photosensitivity reactions. Weakness, fatigue, muscle cramps and musculoskeletal discomfort, impotence, decreased libido, minor psychiatric symptoms.

AMILORIDE HYDROCHLORIDE (continued)
NURSING IMPLICATIONS

- Administered preferably with food to reduce possibility of gastric distress.
- Generally taken in the morning to avoid interrupting nocturnal sleep. Advise patient to take amiloride at the same time each day.
- Serum K levels (record fluid intake and output) should be monitored for all patients particularly when therapy is initiated, whenever dosage adjustments are made, and during any illness that may affect kidney function.
- Hyperkalaemia occurs in about 10% of patients receiving amiloride. Even with concurrent thiazide therapy (a combination designed to decrease K retention) serum K can rise suddenly and without warning. *Symptoms of hyperkalaemia* life-threatening cardiac arrhythmias, unusual fatigue, weakness or heaviness of limbs, general muscle weakness, muscle cramps, paraesthaesias, flaccid paralysis of extremities, shortness of breath, nervousness, confusion.
- Hyperkalaemia frequency is higher in the elderly, and in patients with diabetes or renal disease (fosters potassium retention).
- In addition to periodic serum K concentrations, intermittent evaluations of BUN, creatinine, and ECG are advised for patients with renal or hepatic dysfunction, diabetes mellitus, or who are elderly or debilitated.
- Potassium supplements, salt substitutes, high intake of dietary K (*see Index: Food sources*) are all contraindicated. Exception: these measures may be prescribed by physician for patients with severe or refractory hypokalaemia, along with close monitoring of serum K levels.
- Because amiloride can cause visual disturbances and dizziness particularly during early therapy, advise patient to be cautious when driving or performing other potentially hazardous tasks.
- Instruct patient to consult physician before self-medicating with OTC products. Many preparations contain adrenergic agents that may aggravate high blood pressure (e.g. nasal decongestants, cough, cold or asthma remedies, and appetite suppressants).
- *For other teaching points for patients with hypertension, see Reserpine.*
- Store preferably between 15° and 30°C (59° and 86°F) in a well-closed container, unless otherwise directed by manufacturer.

Diagnostic test interferences   Manufacturer advises discontinuing amiloride in patients with diabetes mellitus at least 3 days prior to glucose tolerance tests.

DRUG INTERACTIONS   *Amiloride*

PLUS	INTERACTIONS
Antihypertensives	Potentiation of antihypertensive effects. Used concomitantly with caution
Blood from blood banks (plasma content: plasma may contain up to 30 mEq/L; whole blood may contain up to 65 mEq/L when stored over 10 days)	
Captopril	

AMILORIDE HYDROCHLORIDE (continued)

PLUS (continued)	INTERACTIONS
Diuretics, potassium-sparing: spironolactone, triamterene	⎫ Possibility of hyperkalaemia
Potassium-containing medications, e.g., parenteral penicillin G potassium, potassium supplements	⎬
Salt substitutes (high in potassium chloride)	⎭
Digoxin	Possibility of altered digoxin response and reduced inotropic effect
Glucose-insulin infusion Sodium bicarbonate	Reduces serum K levels by promoting shift of K ions into cells
Lithium	Amiloride reduces lithium renal excretion with possibility of toxicity. Concurrent use not recommended

Aminoglutethimide —————————————————————

(Orimeten)

*Adrenal suppressant;
enzyme inhibitor*

ACTIONS AND USES   Analogue of glutethimide. Blocks adrenal corticosteroid bio-synthesis (i.e., mineralocorticoids, glucocorticoids, and other steroids) by inhibiting enzymatic conversion of cholesterol to pregnenolone precursors of cortisol and aldosterone. Goitre and mild hypothyroidism can develop with prolonged use because drug may block iodination of tyrosine. Aminoglutethimide has weak anticonvulsant properties.

Used for temporary treatment of selected patients with Cushing's syndrome associated with adrenal carcinoma, ectopic ACTH-producing tumours, or adrenal hyperplasia. Produces medical adrenalectomy in postmenopausal women with positive oestrogen receptor test, metastatic breast cancer, or who fail or relapse with tamoxifen, and for patients with prostatic carcinoma. Former use as an anticonvulsant supplement has been abandoned, because of its adrenal suppressant activity.

ROUTE AND DOSAGE   Oral: *metastatic breast cancer*: *Initial*: 250 mg two or three times daily for approximately 2 weeks (usually combined with hydrocortisone). *Maintenance*: 250 mg four times daily, preferably every 6 hours. *Cushing's syndrome*: *Initial*: 250 mg every 6 hours; increased in increments of 250 mg daily every 1 or 2 weeks, if necessary, up to 2 g daily.

ABSORPTION AND FATE   Onset of adrenal suppression: 3 to 5 days. Approximately 20 to 25% protein bound. *Half-life*: 13 hours (decreases to about 7 hours with prolonged use because aminoglutethimide accelerates its own metabolism by inducing hepatic enzymes). Recovery of adrenal responsiveness to stress usually occurs in 36 to 72 hours, following discontinuation of aminoglutethimide. Metabolized in liver.

AMINOGLUTETHIMIDE (continued)

Excreted by kidneys: 50% of dose as unchanged drug and 20 to 50% as mildly active metabolites. Crosses placenta. Distribution into breast milk not known.

CONTRAINDICATIONS AND PRECAUTIONS   Hypersensitivity to aminoglutethimide or to glutethiamide; hypothyroidism; infection. Safe use in pregnancy, nursing mothers, and in children not established. Use with caution in the elderly.

ADVERSE/SIDE EFFECTS   Lethargy, drowsiness, orthostatic dizziness or light-headedness, uncontrolled eye movements (dose related); clumsiness, ataxia, fever, headache, mental depression, confusion, respiratory depression, coma (overdosage). Orthostatic or persistent hypotension, tachycardia. Masculinization including hirsutism, adrenal insufficiency. Nausea, vomiting, anorexia, elevation of liver enzymes (SGOT, alkaline phosphatase), cholestatic jaundice (possibly hypersensitivity). Neutropenia, leucopenia, thrombocytopenia, pancytopenia, agranulocytosis, decreased Hgb and Hct, anaemia, Coombs' negative haemolytic anaemia. Measles-like (morbilliform) rash, pruritis, urticaria, darkening of skin. Myalgia, arthralgia, hypothyroidism, goitre (with prolonged use).

NURSING IMPLICATIONS

- Therapy is generally initiated in the hospital until dosage is stabilized.
- Baseline and periodic determinations should be made of 0800 hrs fasting *plasma cortisol* levels, full blood count, serum alkaline phosphatase (clue for early bone recurrence); AST (SGOT); bilirubin; thyroid function tests; *urinary aldosterone* (normal: 2 to 26 mcg/24 hours); serum electrolytes; CO_2.
- Baseline and regularly scheduled blood pressure readings indicate the effect of reduced aldosterone levels on BP. Orthostatic and persistent hypotension (subjectively experienced as dizziness, light-headedness, weakness) results from reduced aldosterone production. Some patients require mineralocorticoid replacement, e.g., fludrocortisone.
- Advise patient to make position changes gradually, pausing between each change. Also warn patient not to stand still for prolonged periods. Support tights may be helpful. Consult physician.
- The elderly are particularly sensitive to the CNS effects of aminoglutethimide (e.g., lethargy, ataxia, orthostatic dizziness, lightheadedness). Note implications for ambulation.
- Drowsiness, nausea, and anorexia often disappear spontaneously within 1 to 2 weeks of continuing therapy. Caution patient not to stop taking drug but to inform physician if symptoms persist or become pronounced.
- Report skin rash that persists beyond 5 to 8 days. Physician may discontinue drug and possibly restart it after rash disappears.
- Tolerance to lethargy and ataxia usually develops after 4 weeks of therapy (metabolism of aminoglutethimide accelerates with continuing use). If symptoms are severe, however, drug discontinuation may be necessary.
- Emphasize importance of contacting physician immediately at times of stress such as surgery, dental work, acute illness, acute emotional situations. Steroid supplements, i.e., glucocorticoids (cortisone) and mineralocorticoids (fludrocortisone)

A

AMINOGLUTETHIMIDE (continued)

may be indicated because normal body response to stress including infection and inflammation is impeded by adrenal suppression. Physician may temporarily stop aminoglutethimide.

- Patients with Cushing's syndrome may show reduced effect (increasing cortisol levels) with continuing therapy possibly because ACTH rises reflexly in response to declining glucocorticoid levels. These patients are generally not treated beyond 3 months with aminoglutethimide.
- *Adrenal insufficiency* (hypoadrenalism) symptoms include: anorexia, nausea, vomiting, weight loss, weakness, hypotension, dizziness, hypoglycaemia, oliguria, low serum sodium, elevated K and BUN, arthralgia, myalgia, hyperpigmentation.
- Because *hypothyroidism* may be induced, make appropriate observations. Report: cool, pale, dry skin; puffiness of hand and face (especially periorbitaloedema); constipation; sensitivity to cold; fatigue; slow relaxation phase in deep tendon reflexes, enlarged thyroid. Some patients require supplementary thyroid hormone therapy.
- If patient becomes pregnant or must take aminoglutethimide during pregnancy she should be apprised of potential foetal deformities. Advise patient to notify physician immediately if pregnancy is suspected.
- When aminoglutethimide is to be discontinued, dosage tapering is not necessary because the adrenal cortex returns to pretreatment level rather rapidly after drug is withdrawn.
- Because of the possibility of drowsiness and dizziness, warn patient to avoid driving and other potentially hazardous activities until the reaction to drug is known.
- Advise patient to carry card or jewellery (Medic Alert) indicating medical diagnosis, medication(s), physician's name, address, and telephone number.
- Reenforce importance of continuous medical follow-up.
- Store preferably between 15° and 30°C (59° and 86°F) in well-closed containers, unless otherwise directed by manufacturer.

DRUG INTERACTIONS *Aminoglutethimide*

PLUS	INTERACTIONS
Dexamethasone	Acceleration of dexamethasone metabolism

Aminophylline

(Theodrox, Phyllocontin continus)   *Smooth muscle relaxant;*
bronchodilator; xanthine

ACTIONS AND USES   Ethylenediamide salt of theophylline with effects similar to those of other xanthines, e.g., caffeine and theobromine. Action is dependent on theophylline content (approximately 79%). Only xanthine derivative given IV for acute bronchial asthma attack. *See theophylline.*

AMINOPHYLLINE (continued)

Used to prevent and relieve symptoms of acute bronchial asthma, and treatment of bronchospasm associated with chronic bronchitis and emphysema. Also used as a respiratory stimulant in Cheyne-Stokes respiration and for treatment of apnoea and bradycardia in prematures. Use as cardiac stimulant and diuretic, in treatment of congestive heart failure, and as antispasmodic for acute biliary attack, has largely been replaced by more effective drugs.

ROUTE AND DOSAGE *Individualized*: Oral: Adult: 100–300 mg 3–4 times a day. **Slow release preparations: Adult**: 225–350 mg every 12 hrs increased to 450–700 mg after 1 week if required, for nocturnal attacks 225–700 mg at night. **Paediatric**: 6 mg/kg every 12 hrs increased to 12 mg/kg after one week if required. **Intravenous**: Adult: 5 mg/kg when necessary by slow injection (over 20 min); *maintenance* when required 500 mcg/kg/hr by slow IV infusion. **Child**: 5 mg/kg by slow IV injection (over 20 min) *maintenance* 6 months–9 yrs 1 mg/kg/hr, 10–16 yrs 800 mcg/kg/hr all by slow IV infusion. **Rectal: Adult**: 360 mg once or twice a day. Child up to 1 yr 12.5–25 mg, 1–5 yrs 50–100 mg, 6–12 yrs 100–200 mg all once or twice a day.

ABSORPTION AND FATE **Time to peak serum concentrations: IV** administration: within 30 minutes; **uncoated tablet**: 2 hours. **Suppository form** is absorbed erratically. Metabolized in liver and excreted by kidneys, primarily as metabolites. Crosses placenta; excreted in breast milk.

CONTRAINDICATIONS AND PRECAUTIONS Hypersensitivity to xanthine derivatives or to ethylenediamine component. **Cautious Use**: severe hypertension, cardiac disease, arrhythmias, impaired hepatic or renal function, diabetes mellitus, hyperthyroidism, glaucoma, prostatic hypertrophy, fibrocystic breast disease, history of peptic ulcer, neonates and young children, patients over 55, COPD, acute influenza or patients receiving influenza immunization. *See theophylline.*

ADVERSE/SIDE EFFECTS Nervousness, restlessness, severe depression, insomnia, irritability, headache, dizziness, light-headedness, hyperactive reflexes, muscle twitching, convulsions. Flushing, palpitation, tachycardia, PVCs; with rapid IV: hyperventilation, precordial pain, severe hypotension, cardiac arrest. Nausea, vomiting, anorexia, bitter aftertaste, haematemesis, diarrhoea, epigastric pain. Urticaria, contact dermatitis, exfoliative dermatitis, pruritus, angioneuroticoedema. Rectal burning or irritation (suppository form), local pain and tissue sloughing (IM use), dehydration (from diuresis), hyperglycaemia, tinnitus, flashes of light (toxicity).

NURSING IMPLICATIONS
- Some patients may require a round-the-clock dosage schedule.
- Toxic effects are generally related to theophylline serum levels over 20 mcg/ml (therapeutic range 10 to 20 mcg/ml).
- Dosages are based on ideal body weight because aminophylline (theophylline) is not distributed to fatty tissue.
- **Smoking–drug interaction** Smoking (tobacco or marijuana) tends to increase aminophylline elimination (shortens half-life) and therefore dosage requirements may be higher and dosage intervals shorter than in nonsmokers. Reportedly, 3

AMINOPHYLLINE (continued)

months to 2 years of no smoking may be required to attain normal theophylline utilization.

- Absorption may be delayed but is not reduced by presence of food in stomach.
- Oral drug is absorbed faster if taken with a full glass of water on an empty stomach (½ to 1 hour before or 2 hours after meals).
- GI symptoms may be minimized by administering oral drug with or immediately following a meal or food. It may be necessary to lower dosage or discontinue therapy if GI symptoms persist.
- Slow release preparations should not be chewed or crushed before swallowing; however, some tablets are scored and can be broken in half, then swallowed.
- To avoid overdosing, patient should be questioned whether he or she has received any aminophylline or theophylline preparation during previous 12 to 24 hours, before aminophylline regimen is started.
- Rectally administered preparations are generally ordered when the patient must fast or cannot tolerate the drug orally. Drug absorption is enhanced if rectum is empty; give drug in relation to patient's evacuation time.
- Because peristaltic activity is stimulated reflexly by presence of food in stomach, patient may experience less difficulty in retaining rectal medication if it can be given before a meal. Also advise patient to remain recumbent for 15 to 20 minutes or until defaecation reflex subsides.
- High incidence of toxicity is associated with rectal suppository use because of erratic rate of absorption. Children in contrast to adults absorb drug more quickly by rectum.
- Administered IV aminophylline solution should be at room temperature.
- Patients receiving parenteral aminophylline should be closely observed for signs of hypotension, arrhythmias, and convulsions until serum theophylline stabilizes within the therapeutic range.
- Monitor vital signs; measure and record fluid intake and output. Improvements in quality and rate of pulse and respiration, as well as diuresis, are expected clinical effects. A sudden, sharp, unexplained rise in heart rate is a useful clinical indicator of toxicity.
- The elderly, acutely ill, and patients with severe respiratory problems, liver dysfunction, or pulmonary oedema are at greater risk of toxicity because of reduced drug clearance.
- Dizziness is a relatively common side effect, particularly in the elderly. Take necessary safety precautions and forewarn patient of this possibility.
- Children appear to be more susceptible than adults to the CNS stimulating effects of xanthines (nervousness, restlessness, insomnia, hyperactive reflexes, twitching, convulsions). Dosage reduction may be indicated.
- When a change is made from one administration route to another, observe patient closely until dosage is regulated. Changes in brands or dosage forms must be prescribed by physician.
- Many popular OTC remedies for treatment of asthma or cough contain ephedrine in combination with various salts of theophylline. Caution patient to take only those medications approved by physician.

AMINOPHYLLINE (continued)

- Aminophylline should not be mixed in a syringe with other drugs. Because aminophylline solutions are strongly alkaline, they are incompatible with alkali-labile drugs such as adrenalin (noradrenaline, isoprenaline or penicillin G potassium. Aminophylline solutions are also incompatible with strong acid solutions, e.g., ascorbic acid. Consult pharmacist for specific compatibility information.
- Do not use aminophylline solutions if discoloured or if crystals are present.
- Stored preferably between 15° and 30°C (59° and 86°F) in tightly closed containers unless otherwise directed by manufacturer.
- Follow manufacturer's directions regarding storage of suppositories. Some are stored at room temperature, others must be refrigerated.
- *See Theophylline for patient teaching, food–drug interactions, diagnostic test interferences, and drug interactions.*

Amiodarone _____

(Cordarone X)   *Antiarrhythmic*

ACTIONS AND USES   Iodinated benzofuran derivative structurally related to thyroxine. Exhibits antiarrhythmic, antianginal, and antiadrenergic properties (antagonizes both alpha and beta responses to catecholamines). Totally unrelated to other antiarrhythmics. By direct action on cardiac tissue, increases SA node conduction and recovery time, and thus depresses sinus, atrial, and AV nodal function. Other haemodynamic effects: increased cardiac output, decreased peripheral and coronary vascular resistance, and bradycardia. During early treatment period (first 3 months) thyroid hormone metabolism is altered as evidenced by elevated serum T_4 and lowered T_3 concentrations. Usually normal levels are restored (unknown reason) after this period even with continuation of therapy.

Used to treat refractory supraventricular and ventricular tachyarrhythmias, particularly in patients with atrial fibrillation complicated by Wolff–Parkinson–White syndrome.

ROUTE AND DOSAGE   Oral: (dosages vary widely): *Dose range*: 200 to 800 mg/day; in divided doses. **Intravenous**: 5 to 10 mg/kg/day. Smallest effective dose is advised regardless of route.

ABSORPTION AND FATE   Serum concentration peaks in 2 to 10 hours, but onset of clinical effect is slow (*see Nursing Implications*). **Half-life**: 13 to 107 days (with chronic therapy). Extensively metabolized in liver releasing 6 mg iodine/200 mg dose daily. Eliminated in urine.

CONTRAINDICATIONS AND PRECAUTIONS   Severe sinus bradycardia, advanced AV block, severe liver disease. **Cautious Use**: Hashimoto's thyroiditis or goitre.

AMIODARONE (continued)

ADVERSE/SIDE EFFECTS   These include: tremor, abnormal gait, ataxia, peripheral neuropathy (proximal muscle weakness, numbness, tingling), headache, depression, insomnia, nightmares, hallucinations. Other side effects are as follows: bradycardia, myocardial depression, hypotension, sinoatrial block, sinus arrest, cardiogenic shock, anorexia, nausea, vomiting, abdominal pain, constipation, blurred vision, coloured halos around lights, yellow-brown corneal microdeposits, photophobia, alveolitis, pulmonary fibrosis, hypersensitivity pneumonitis, necrotizing pneumonitis, slate-blue discolouration (slowly reversible), photosensitivity, high frequency of drug-induced hyperthyroidism and hypothyroidism; hepatic toxicity, significant elevations in AST, ALT; bone marrow depression, transient ischaemic attacks.

NURSING IMPLICATIONS

- Onset of pharmacological effects range from 5 to 30 days. Full clinical effects may not be apparent for 1½ to 3 months.
- Neurological symptoms may develop within a week after therapy with amiodarone begins.
- Amiodarone-induced thyroid dysfunction depends on environmental factors: i.e., if patient is in a geographical area of iodine deficiency, hyperthyroidism is common; but if iodine intake is normal, hypothyroidism can occur.
- During early treatment period, especially, watch for and report symptoms of drug-induced thyroid dysfunction: *hypothyroidism*: periorbitaloedema, lethargy, puffy hands and feet; cool, pale skin; vertigo, nocturnal cramps, decreased GI motility, enlarged thyroid gland. *Hyperthyroidism* (thyrotoxicosis): warm, flushed, moist skin; tachycardia, exophthalmos, infrequent lid blinking, lid oedema, weight loss in spite of increased appetite, frequent urination, menstrual irregularity, breathlessness, hypoventilation, congestive heart failure.
- Baseline and periodic assessments should be made of liver, lung, thyroid, and neurological function.
- Skin and corneal discoloration (*lipofuscinosis*) seen in most patients who receive drug for 2 months or more, is reportedly reversible but may take several months to fade completely. Generally, corneal deposits do not interfere with vision. After drug steady state is established, regular drug holidays may minimize or interrupt development of corneal deposits.
- Photophobia may be eased by wearing dark glasses but some patients are unable to go outdoors at all in the daytime even with such protection.
- Alert patient to the possibility of a photosensitivity reaction; advise use of sun screen lotion (SPF above 15) and protective clothing to reduce reaction in exposed skin areas.
- Be alert to symptoms of *pulmonary toxicity*: progressive dyspnoea, fatigue, cough, pleuritic pain, fever. Drug will be stopped pending diagnosis.
- Monitor heart rate and rhythm until drug response has stabilized. Report promptly symptomatic bradycardia (light-headedness, syncope, fatigue) and onset of worsening arrhythmia. After patient is stabilized, cardiac rhythm should be checked by patient or primary caregiver.
- Proximal muscle weakness, a common side effect, intensified by tremors present a

AMIODARONE (continued)

great hazard to the ambulating patient. Assess severity of these drug-induced effects and protect patient from falling if he or she walks, or restrict ambulation if necessary.

■ Noncardiac side effects of this drug (especially lipofuscinosis, photophobia, insomnia) are major factors in noncompliance even though reversible. Check periodically to reenforce importance of adhering to the established drug regimen.

■ Report adverse reactions promptly. Bear in mind that long elimination half-life means that drug effects will persist long after regimen adjustment or discontinuation, and that it serves, too, as a camouflage for noncompliance.

DRUG INTERACTIONS *Amiodarone*

PLUS	INTERACTIONS
β-blockers, e.g., propranolol Calcium channel blockers, e.g., verapamil	Possibility of additive bradycardia; used with caution
Digoxin	Possibility of elevated serum digoxin levels; used with caution
Disopyramide Quinidine	Pharmacological effects of disopyramide and quinidine may be increased with development of atypical ventricular tachycardia. Used with caution, if at all
Lignocaine	Severe bradycardia and sinoatrial arrest can occur. Monitor closely
Warfarin	Enhanced anticoagulant effect. Initial anticoagulant doses reduced by 32 to 50%

Amitriptyline hydrochloride

(Domical, Lentizol, Tryptizol)

Psychotropic; antidepressant; tricyclic

ACTIONS AND USES Dibenzocycloheptene tricyclic antidepressant with greater anticholinergic and sedative actions than imipramine. May suppress alpha rhythm in EEG; most active of the tricyclic antidepressants in inhibition of serotonin uptake from synaptic gap. Has H_2-receptor blocking activity (inhibits gastric acid secretion). Antimigraine effect appears to be independent of antidepressant action. Actions, uses, contraindications, precautions, adverse effect similar to those of *imipramine*. Used to treat endogenous depression, anxiety and nocturnal enuresis in children.

ROUTE AND DOSAGE Highly individualized. **Oral: Adults**: *Initial*: 50 to 100 mg/day; gradually increased to 200 to 300 mg/day, if necessary. *Alternate regimen*: *Initial*: 50 to 100 mg at bedtime, increased gradually to 150 mg/day, if necessary. **Adolescents, elderly**: 10 mg three times daily with 20 mg at bedtime. *Maintenance*: 25 to 100 mg/day in single dose at bedtime. *Enuresis*: 7 to 10 yrs/10 to 20 mg and

AMITRIPTYLINE HYDROCHLORIDE (continued)

11 to 16 yrs/50 mg at bedtime for up to 3 months then gradually withdrawn. **Intramuscular**: 10 to 20 mg four times daily (until patient can or will take tablet form).

ABSORPTION AND FATE   Rapidly absorbed from GI tract and injection sites. **Peak plasma concentrations (for oral and IM routes)** occur within 2 to 12 hours. Steady state attained in 4 to 10 days. **Half-life**: 10 to 50 hours; 96% protein bound. Metabolized in liver; intermediate active metabolite is nortriptyline. About 25 to 50% of dose excreted in urine as inactive metabolites within 24 hours. Small amounts eliminated in faeces via bile. Crosses placenta and enters breast milk.

CONTRAINDICATIONS AND PRECAUTIONS   Acute recovery period following myocardial infarction; pregnancy, nursing mothers, children under 12. **Cautious Use**: prostatic hypertrophy, history of urinary retention or obstruction, angle-closure glaucoma, history of seizures, diabetes mellitus, hyperthyroidism, patient with cardiovascular, hepatic, or renal dysfunction; patient with suicidal tendency or on electroschock therapy; schizophrenia, respiratory disorders; elderly, adolescent age groups. *See also imipramine.*

ADVERSE/SIDE EFFECTS   These include: drowsiness, dizziness, nervousness, restlessness, fatigue, headache, disorientation, confusion, insomnia, nightmares, paraesthesias, ataxia, tremors, orthostatic hypotension, hypertension, palpitation, tachycardia, ECG changes, tinnitus, nasal congestion, increased appetite, weight gain or loss, epigastric distress, dry mouth, sour or metallic taste, constipation, nausea, vomiting, rash, pruritus, urticaria, photosensitivity, blurred vision, ophthalmoplegia, urinary retention, leucopenia. *See also imipramine.*

NURSING IMPLICATIONS
- Oral drug may be taken with or immediately after food to reduce possibility of gastric irritation.
- Tablet may be crushed if patient is unwilling to take it whole; administer with food or fluid, or use oral suspension.
- Dose increases by 25 to 50 mg are preferably made in late afternoon and/or at bedtime because sedative action precedes antidepressant effect.
- Because amitriptyline is long-acting, physician may prescribe entire oral dose at one time. A single dose at bedtime is useful for patients who complain of insomnia or dizziness or when daytime sedation interferes with work productivity. Drug effect on depression is not affected by time of day dose is taken.
- ***Smoking–drug interaction***   Smoking increases metabolism of tricyclics. A higher dose of amitriptyline may be required for heavy smokers than for non- or moderate smokers. Urge patient to stop or at least reduce cigarette smoking.
- Monitor blood pressure and pulse rate in patients with cardiovascular disease. Withhold drug if there is a significant fall in systolic BP (10 to 20 mm Hg) or a sudden increase in pulse rate. Notify physician.
- Desired therapeutic effects for depression may not be evident until after 3 to 4 weeks of therapy, because of long serum half-life. Dosage should then be reduced gradually to lowest effective level.

AMITRIPTYLINE HYDROCHLORIDE (continued)

- Maintenance regimen is usually continued for at least 3 months to prevent relapse. Typical length of therapy for depression is 6 months to 1 year. Patient should be evaluated at regular intervals to determine need for continued drug therapy.
- Parenteral preparation is for IM use only.
- Baseline and periodic leucocyte and differential counts, BP, cardiac and hepatic function tests are recommended in patients receiving high doses or prolonged therapy.
- Plasma levels (therapeutic range: 125 to 250 ng/ml) do not always correlate with clinical effectiveness and therefore are not done routinely.
- The actions of both alcohol and amitriptyline are potentiated when used concurrently during therapy and for up to 2 weeks after drug is discontinued. Consult physician about safe amount of alcohol, if any, that can be taken.
- If a patient uses excessive amounts of alcohol it should be borne in mind that the potentiation of amitriptyline effects may increase the dangers of overdosage or suicide attempt.
- Suicide is an inherent risk with any depressed patient and may remain until there is significant improvement. Supervise patient closely during early phase of therapy. The amount of amitriptyline dispensed to the patient should be strictly controlled.
- Tolerance or adaptation to distressing anticholinergic actions (dry mouth, constipation, blurred vision, urinary retention) usually develops after patient goes on maintenance regimen.
- During initial therapy be alert to orthostatic hypotensive and sedative effects, and confusional episodes, especially in the elderly. Institute measures to prevent falling. Instruct patient to change from recumbency to upright position slowly and in stages. Support tights may help. Consult physician.
- Caution patient to avoid potentially hazardous activities such as driving until response to the drug is known.
- Monitor weight. Amitriptyline may increase the appetite for carbohydrate foods.
- Withdrawal symptoms (headache, nausea, malaise, musculoskeletal pain, weakness) can be avoided by tapering dosage over a 2-week period.
- When used for migraine prophylaxis, therapeutic effect may occur in 1 to 6 weeks. Drug is usually discontinued after patient has been headache-free for 1 to 2 months. If headache recurs, physician may prescribe another course of treatment.
- Amitriptyline may impart blue-green colour to urine.
- Store drug at 15° to 30°C (59° to 86°F) unless otherwise instructed by manufacturer. Protect from light. *See imipramine.*

DRUG INTERACTIONS   *Amitriptyline*

PLUS	INTERACTIONS
Anticoagulants, oral	Decreased hypoprothrombinaemic effects. Monitor closely
Antihypertensives: clonidine guanethidine methyldopa	Antihypertensive action may be decreased. Combination avoided, when possible

AMITRIPTYLINE HYDROCHLORIDE (continued)

PLUS	INTERACTIONS
(continued)	
CNS depressants, e.g., alcohol (Ethanol), barbiturates, sedatives, hypnotics	Potentiation of CNS depression. Also, barbiturates reduce TCA blood levels. Used with caution
Disulphiram	Possibility of acute organic brain syndrome: confusion, psychosis. Described for amitriptyline only. Used with caution
MAO inhibitors	Possibility of severe reactions (toxic psychosis, hyperpyrexia, tachycardia, seizures). Used with extreme caution
Levodopa ⎫ Sympathomimetics ⎭	Possibility of sympathetic hyperactivity with hypertension and hyperpyrexia. Used with caution

See also imipramine

Amoxycillin

(Amoxil, Augmentin)

Antiinfective, antibiotic (Beta lactam); penicillin

ACTIONS AND USES   Broad spectrum, acid-stable, semisynthetic aminopenicillin and analogue of ampicillin. Like ampicillin, it is bactericidal, has essentially the same antibacterial spectrum, and is inactivated by penicillinase. Reportedly, rash and diarrhoea occur less frequently than with ampicillin, and at equal doses produces higher serum levels because it is more completely absorbed. Less effective in treatment of shigellosis than ampicillin and is more expensive.

Used in infections of ear, nose, and throat, GU tract, skin and soft tissue caused by susceptible strains of *E. coli*, *P. mirabilis*, *H. influenzae*, streptococci (including *S. faecalis* and *S. pneumoniae*), and nonpenicillinase-producing staphylococci. Also used in uncomplicated gonorrhoea. Available in combination with potassium clavulanate (Augmentin), which extends antibacterial spectrum of amoxycillin.

ROUTE AND DOSAGE   Oral: **Adults**: 250–500 mg every 8 hours for severe infections. **Child** up to 10 yrs 125 mg every 8 hours. *Dental prophylaxis*: 3 g one hour before treatment. **IV: Adult**: 1g/6 hourly. **Child**: 50–100 mg/kg daily in divided doses.

ABSORPTION AND FATE   Absorption is rapid and nearly complete following oral administration. Resists inactivation by gastric acid. **Serum levels peak** in about 2 hours after administration of capsule and in 1 hour following oral suspension. Measurable serum levels still present after 8 hours. Diffuses into most tissues and body fluids except synovial fluid and CSF (unless meninges are inflamed). Approximately 20% bound to plasma proteins. **Half-life**: 1 to 1.3 hours. About 60% of dose excreted in urine in 6 to 8 hours, as intact amoxycillin and penicillinoic acid. Crosses placenta. Excreted in breast milk in very small amounts.

AMOXYCILLIN (continued)

CONTRAINDICATIONS AND PRECAUTIONS Hypersensitivity to penicillins or cephalosporins; infectious mononucleosis. Safe use during pregnancy not established. **Cautious Use**: history of or suspected atopy or allergy (hives, eczema, hay fever, asthma); history of GI disease; severely impaired renal function.

ADVERSE/SIDE EFFECTS As with other penicillins: Side effects include: abdominal cramps, diarrhoea, nausea, vomiting. **Hypersensitivity**: pruritus, erythema, urticaria, or other skin eruptions, severe morbilliform rash (patients with infectious mononucleosis), fever, wheezing; anaphylaxis, serum sickness (rare); haemolytic anaemia, thrombocytopenia, purpura, eosinophilia, leucopenia, agranulocytosis, pseudomembranous colitis (rare). **Other**: superinfections, conjunctival ecchymosis, numbness and tingling of extremities. *See penicillin G*.

NURSING IMPLICATIONS

- If necessary, capsule may be emptied and contents swallowed with water.
- Chewable tablet should be chewed or crushed before swallowing with a liquid.
- Serum levels are not significantly affected by food; therefore, amoxicillin may be given without regard to meals.
- Oral suspension reconstituted when dispensed from pharmacy. Date and time of reconstitution, and discard date, should appear on container. Stable for 7 days at room temperature, i.e., around 25°C (77°F) or 14 days if refrigerated, depending on product. (Refrigeration is preferable, but not required.) Shake well before using.
- For children, reconstituted suspension may be added to milk, fruit juice, water, ginger ale, or other soft drink. Administer all of the prepared dose promptly.
- Instruct patient to take medication around the clock, not to miss a dose, and to continue therapy until all medication is taken, unless otherwise directed by physician.
- Before therapy is initiated, careful history should be obtained of patient's previous exposure and sensitivity to penicillins and cephalosporins, and other allergic reactions of any kind.
- Therapy may be instituted prior to obtaining results of bacteriological and sensitivity tests.
- Periodic assessments of renal, hepatic, and haematological functions should be made during prolonged therapy.
- When amoxicillin is used to treat urinary tract infections, frequent bacteriological and clinical evaluations are recommended.
- Patients being treated for gonorrhoea and suspected of having syphilis should have darkfield examination before receiving amoxicillin as well as monthly serological tests, for a minimum of 4 months.
- For most infections, treatment is continued for a minimum of 48 to 72 hours beyond the time that patient is asymptomatic or cultures are negative.
- Patients with haemolytic streptococcal infections should receive at least 10 days of treatment to prevent occurrence of acute rheumatic fever.
- Advise patient to report to physician the onset of itching, skin rash or hives, wheezing, diarrhoea, and symptoms of superinfection (sore mouth, malodorous vaginal discharge, rectal or vaginal itching, cough, return of fever).

A

AMOXYCILLIN (continued)

- Store tablets, capsules in tightly-covered containers preferably between 15° and 30°C (59° and 86°F), unless otherwise directed by manufacturer.
- *See penicillin G.*

Diagnostic test interferences   Elevations of SGOT (AST) and SGPT (ALT).

DRUG INTERACTIONS   *Amoxycillin*

PLUS	INTERACTIONS
Chloramphenicol Erythromycins Tetracyclines }	May inhibit bactericidal activity of amoxycillin. Concurrent therapy generally avoided

Amphotericin

(Fungizone, Fungilin)

Antiinfective; antibiotic (macrolide); antifungal

ACTIONS AND USES   Polyene fungistatic antibiotic produced by *Streptomyces nodosus*. Fungicidal at higher concentrations, depending on sensitivity of fungus. Exerts antifungal action on both resting and growing cells. Because it may also interfere with function of human cell membrane, it can produce severe adverse effects. Not effective against bacteria, rickettsiae, or viruses.

Used intravenously for a wide spectrum of potentially fatal systemic fungal (mycotic) infections including aspergillosis, blastomycosis, coccidioidomycosis, cryptococcosis, disseminated candidiasis, histoplasmosis, sporotrichosis, and others. Has been used to potentiate antifungal effects of flucytosine (Al cobon), and to provide anticandidal prophylaxis in certain susceptible patients receiving rifampicin or tetracycline therapy. Used topically for cutaneous and mucocutaneous infections caused by *Candida* (Monilia).

ROUTE AND DOSAGE   Adult and pediatric: Intravenous infusion: *Initial*, 0.25 mg/kg daily infused over 6 hours. Dosage increased gradually to 1 mg/kg/day as tolerance permits. Not to exceed 1.5 mg/kg/day. If therapy is interrupted for longer than 1 week, restarted at initial dosage and again increased gradually. **Oral: tablets**: 100 to 200 mg/6 hrly, suspension: 100 mg/ml, lozenges: 10 mg dissolved in the mouth 4 times a day to max of 8 daily. **Topical**: (3% cream, lotion, ointment): apply enough to cover affected area and rub in gently two to four times a day.

ABSORPTION AND FATE   Topical applications poorly absorbed. **Peak blood levels** in 1 to 2 hours after IV injection. Approximately 90 to 95% bound to serum proteins; **plasma half-life** about 24 hours. Minimal amounts enter CSF, aqueous humour, pleural, pericardial, and synovial fluid. Serum and urine concentrations similar. Metabolic pathways and distribution unknown. Approximately 40% excreted by kidneys

AMPHOTERICIN (continued)

over 7-day period. Can be detected in blood and urine for at least 7 to 8 weeks after discontinuation of therapy. Excretion increased in alkaline urine. Crosses placenta.

CONTRAINDICATIONS AND PRECAUTIONS   Hypersensitivity to amphotericin; severe bone marrow depression or renal function impairment. Safe use during pregnancy and in nursing mothers not established.

ADVERSE/SIDE EFFECTS   These include: headache, sedation, muscle or nerve pain, arthralgia, weakness, paraesthesias; peripheral neuropathy, footdrop (rare), convulsions, flushing, arrhythmias, hypertension, hypotension; ventricular fibrillation and cardiac arrest (rapid IV). Other side effects include: tinnitus, vertigo, loss of hearing, nausea (especially during IV infusion): vomiting, diarrhoea, epigastric cramps, haemorrhagic gastroenteritis, anorexia, weight loss, leucopenia, coagulation defects, thrombocytopenia, agranulocytosis, eosinophilia, anaemia (normochromic, normocytic), Coombs' positive haemolytic anaemia (rare), hypokalaemia, hypomagnesaemia, hyponatraemia, pruritus, urticaria, skin rashes, fever, shaking chills, anaphylaxis, blurred vision, diplopia, difficult micturition; nephrotoxicity, (oliguria, haematuria, granular and hyaline casts in urine, renal tubular acidosis, renal damage); nephrocalcinosis, dry skin, erythema, pruritus, burning sensation; allergic contact dermatitis, exacerbation of lesions, pain, tissue irritation (with extravasation); thrombi; thrombophlebitis (IV site); chemical meningitis, acute liver failure, superinfections, severe pulmonary reaction in patients receiving leucocyte transfusions.

NURSING IMPLICATIONS
Intravenous administration

- Amphotericin is administered IV only to hospitalized patients or to those under close clinical supervision who have a confirmed diagnosis of progressive, potentially fatal mycotic infection susceptible to the drug.
- Prior to systemic therapy, diagnosis is confirmed by positive cultures or histological studies.
- Check with physician regarding IV flow rate. Generally the drug is administered slowly over a 6-hour period. If a reaction occurs, interrupt therapy and report promptly to physician.
- During initial IV therapy, monitor vital signs every 30 minutes for at least 4 hours and observe patient closely for adverse effects. Febrile reactions (fever and chills) usually occur in 1 to 2 hours after onset of therapy and subside within 4 hours after drug is discontinued.
- Severity of adverse reactions may be reduced by prophylactic use of aspirin or paracetamol antiemetics, antihistamines, and corticosteroids.
- Renal and haematologic status should be determined before therapy.
- Nephrotoxicity is a predictable complication in patients receiving intensive therapy. Monitor intake and output. Report immediately oliguria, any change in intake and output ratio and pattern, or appearance of urine, e.g., sediment, pink or cloudy urine (haematuria), or abnormal renal function tests. Renal damage is usually reversible if drug is discontinued when first signs of renal dysfunction appear.

A

AMPHOTERICIN (continued)

- If serum creatinine rises above 3 mg/dl, withhold drug and report to physician. Dosage should be reduced or drug discontinued until renal function improves.
- Amphotericin may cause local inflammatory reaction or thrombosis at injection site, particularly if extravasation occurs. Risk of thrombophlebitis associated with IV infusion may be reduced by using paediatric scalp vein needle in the most distal vein possible, by alternating veins, by addition of heparin to the infusion, and by alternate day dosage schedule.
- Frequently check IV site for leakage. It is more apt to occur in the elderly patient because loss of tissue elasticity with ageing may promote extravasation around the needle.
- Hypokalaemia occurs commonly and occasionally can be life-threatening. Report immediately the onset of these possible signs of hypokalaemia: anorexia, drowsiness, profound muscle weakness, hypoactive reflexes, paraestheias, polyuria, polydypsia, dizziness.
- The drug is potentially ototoxic. Report promptly any evidence of hearing loss or complaints of tinnitus, vertigo, or unsteady gait.
- Check weight at weekly intervals, or more frequently if patient has anorexia.
- A flow chart may be useful for organizing significant observations.
- Several weeks of therapy (approximately 6 to 12 weeks) are usually required to assure adequate response and to prevent relapse. Some infections require 9 to 12 months of therapy, e.g., sporotrichosis, aspergillosis.

Preparation and administration

- Keep dry powder refrigerated and protected from exposure to light. Avoid freezing.
- Amphotericin is reconstituted with sterile water for injection without preservatives or bacteriostatic agent. Follow manufacturer's directions. Diluents containing a preservative or bacteriostatic agent such as benzyl alcohol, or acidic solutions, sodium chloride or other electrolyte solutions should not be used because they may cause precipitation.
- Following reconstitution with sterile water for injection, solution is stable for 24 hours at room temperature and for 1 week under refrigeration. Discard any solution before this time if it is cloudy or contains a precipitate.
- For IV infusion, the reconstituted amphotericin is added to dextrose 5% in water, with pH above 4.2. If pH is less, a sterile buffer must be added, using strict aseptic technique. See package insert. Solutions prepared for IV infusion must be used promptly.
- An in-line membrane filter can be used during IV infusion. If used, the mean pore diameter should be no less than 1 micron, to avoid reducing concentration of amphotericin delivered.
- Although manufacturer recommends protecting aqueous solutions of amphotericin from light during IV infusion, short-term exposure (e.g., less than 8 hours) does not appreciably affect potency.

Topical applications

- Do not cover with plastic wrap or other occlusive dressings.
- Request physician to specify when and how lesions are to be washed.

AMPHOTERICIN (continued)

- Cream is preferred for intertriginous areas such as creases of neck, groin, armpit. Some clinicians advise exposure of skin to air.
- Topical treatment should be discontinued promptly if signs of hypersensitivity, irritation, or worsening of lesions occurs.
- The appearance of mild erythema surrounding lesions may be an indication to reduce frequency of application. Consult physician about applying a protective circle of petroleum jelly on normal skin surrounding easily accessible lesions.
- Advise patient to notify physician if improvement does not occur within 1 to 2 weeks, or if lesions appear to worsen.
- Most skin lesions require about 1 to 3 weeks of drug therapy. Paronychia and inter-digital lesions may not respond before 2 to 4 weeks of treatment. Nail infections (onychomycoses) usually require several months or longer.
- Towels and clothing in contact with affected areas should be washed after each treatment.
- Topical cream slightly discolours the skin. Generally, lotion and ointment do not stain skin when rubbed into lesion, but nail lesions may be stained.
- To remove cream or lotion from fabric, wash with soap and water. Ointment may be removed from fabric with a standard cleaning fluid.

Patient-teaching points to prevent spread and recurrence of lesions (relevance depends on location of lesions)

- ☐ Careful handwashing technique before and after application of medication. Dry hands well.
- ☐ Avoid pulling hangnails.
- ☐ Avoid squeezing pimples or picking at scabs. In general, keep hands off skin.
- ☐ Wear nonconstricting, absorbent underclothing.
- ☐ Anything that contacts skin should be kept separate, e.g., face-cloths, towels, bed linen.
- ☐ Use freshly laundered clothing and bedding every day.
- ☐ Keep affected areas dry and exposed to air, if possible.
- ☐ Follow prescribed treatment as directed.
- ☐ Keep follow-up appointments.

- Store topical forms in well-closed containers at room temperature, preferably 15° to 30°C (59° to 86°F), unless otherwise directed by manufacturer.
- Hold suspension in mouth after food close to lesions four times a day.
- For further advice on mouthcare see mustine.

DRUG INTERACTIONS Amphotericin

PLUS	INTERACTIONS
Drugs with nephrotoxic potential, e.g., aminoglycosides	Synergistic nephrotoxicity and ototoxicity. Concurrent and sequential use generally avoided, if possible
Corticosteroids	Potentiate amphotericin-induced hypokalaemia. Used only when necessary to counteract adverse reactions

AMPHOTERICIN (continued)

PLUS (continued)	INTERACTIONS
Digitalis glycosides	Amphotericin-induced hypokalaemia may increase potential for digitalis toxicity. Used with caution
Flucytosine	Effects of either may be increased. Used with caution
Miconazole	Antagonistic antifungal effects. Concurrent use generally avoided
Skeletal muscle relaxants (nondepolarizing)	Amphotericin-induced hypokalaemia may potentiate effects of curariform drugs. Used with caution
Urinary alkalizers, e.g., acetazolamide	May increase excretion of amphotericin b

Ampicillin ▬▬▬▬▬▬▬▬▬▬▬▬▬▬▬▬▬▬▬▬▬▬▬▬▬

(Amfipen, Ampilar, Britcin, Penbritin, Vidopen, Ampiclox Flu-Amp, Magnapen)

Antiinfective; antibiotic (beta lactam); penicillin

ACTIONS AND USES   Broad spectrum semisynthetic aminopenicillin derived from 6-aminopenicillanic acid, the basic penicillin nucleus. Relatively stable in gastric acid. Highly bactericidal even at low concentrations, but is inactivated by penicillinase (beta-lactamase). Resembles penicillin G (qv) in its activity against gram-positive microorganisms such as alpha- and beta-haemolytic streptococci, *Diplococcus pneumoniae*, and non-penicillinase-producing staphylococci. Major advantage over penicillin G is enhanced action against most strains of enterococci, and several gram-negative strains including *Escherichia coli*, *Neisseria gonorrhoea*, *N. meningitidis*, *Haemophilus influenzae*, *Proteus mirabilis*, *Salmonella* (including typhosa), and *Shigella*.

Used in infections of urinary, respiratory, and gastrointestinal tracts, and skin and soft tissues. Also used in the treatment of gonococcal infections, bacterial meningitis, and otitis media, septicaemia, and for prophylaxis of bacterial endocarditis. Used parenterally only for moderately severe to severe infections. Commercially available in combination with flucloxacillin (Magapen).

ROUTE AND DOSAGE   Oral: Adults: 250 mg–1 g every 6 hrs. **Intravenous, intramuscular: Adults:** 500 mg 4–6 hrly, **children** half the adult dose. *Gonorrhoea*: **Adults** 2 g with probenecid 1 g as a single dose (repeat for women). *Urinary infection*: 500 mg/8 hrly. Bacampicillin: 400 mg/2–3 times a day.

ABSORPTION AND FATE   Approximately 30 to 60% of oral dose absorbed from GI tract. **Serum levels peak** within 2 hours (oral route), within 1 hour (IM route), and within 5 minutes (IV route). Equivalent oral and parenteral doses produce higher blood concentrations by parenteral route. Diffuses into most body tissues and fluids; high concentrations in CSF only when meninges are inflamed. About 20 to 25% bound to

AMPICILLIN (continued)

plasma proteins. **Half-life**: 50 to 110 minutes; higher in infants and prematures (due to immature kidney function). Appears to be partially inactivated by liver; enters enterohepatic circulation. Excreted unchanged; high concentrations in urine and bile (through faeces). Crosses placenta. Eliminated in breast milk.

CONTRAINDICATIONS AND PRECAUTIONS   Hypersensitivity to penicillin derivatives or cephalosporins. Safe use during pregnancy not established. **Cautious Use**: history of or suspected atopy or allergy (hay fever, asthma, hives, eczema); renal, liver, or GI disease; infectious mononucleosis, hyperuricaemia, lymphatic leukaemia, prematures and neonates.

ADVERSE/SIDE EFFECTS   (Similar to penicillin G). Side effects include: headache, convulsive seizures, diarrhoea, abdominal pain, nausea, vomiting, pseudomembranous colitis (rare), drug fever, pruritus, urticaria, and other skin eruptions, eosinophilia, haemolytic anaemia, thrombocytopenia, leucopenia, agranulocytosis, delayed respiratory distress syndrome, interstitial nephritis, anaphylactoid reaction, serum sickness, severe pain (following IM); phlebitis (following IV); hypokalaemia (large IV doses), morbilliform rash (ampicillin rash), superinfections. *See penicillin G*.

NURSING IMPLICATIONS

- A careful history should be taken before therapy begins, to determine previous hypersensitivity reactions to penicillins, cephalosporins, and other allergens.
- As a guide to therapy, culture and sensitivity tests should be done prior to and periodically during therapy. Therapy may be initiated before results are known.
- Although ampicillin is comparatively acid-stable, food hampers its absorption. Maximum absorption is achieved if it is taken with a glass of water on an empty stomach (at least 1 hour before or 2 hours after meals).
- Following reconstitution of oral suspension or paediatric drops (by pharmacist), solutions are stable for 14 days under refrigeration. Date and time or reconstitution, and discard date, should appear on container; medication should be dispensed with a calibrated measuring device. Shake well before using.
- Ampicillin sodium (for parenteral use) may be reconstituted with sterile water for injection. Follow manufacturer's directions for amount of diluent to use. Solutions for IM or direct IV should be administered within 1 hour after preparation.
- Administration of drug by direct IV should be done slowly, over at least 10 to 15 minutes. Rapid administration can result in seizures (neurotoxicity).
- For administration by IV infusion, the reconstituted solution (see above) must be added to suitable IV fluid. Consult product information for list of acceptable diluents, concentration to use, and stability period.
- Note that the sodium content must be taken into consideration in patients on sodium restriction.
- Contact dermatitis occurs frequently in sensitized individuals. Those who must handle ampicillin repeatedly are advised to wear disposable gloves.
- Inspect skin daily and instruct patient to do the same. The appearance of a rash

A

AMPICILLIN (continued)

should be carefully evaluated to differentiate an ampicillin rash (nonallergic) from a hypersensitivity reaction. Report promptly to physician if it appears.

- *Ampicillin rash* is characteristically dull red, macular or maculopapular, and mildly pruritic. It generally begins on light-exposed or pressure areas such as knees, elbows, palms, soles, and may spread in a symmetric pattern over most of body. The rash usually develops after 5 to 14 days of treatment, but occasionally appears on first day of therapy or after therapy has stopped. It disappears within a week after discontinuation of drug therapy.
- The incidence of ampicillin rash is higher in patients with infectious mononucleosis or other viral infections, *Salmonella infections*, lymphocytic leukaemia, and in patients taking allopurinol or who have hyperuricaemia.
- Since ampicillin rash is believed to be nonallergic in origin, its appearance is not an absolute contraindication to future therapy with ampicillin or other penicillins.
- Advise patient to report diarrhoea and not to self-medicate. A detailed report should be given to the physician regarding onset, duration, character of stools, associated symptoms, and patient's temperature and weight to help rule out the possibility of drug-induced, potentially fatal pseudomembranous colitis.
- Baseline and periodic assessments of renal, hepatic, and haematological functions are advised particularly during prolonged or high-dose therapy.
- Frequent bacteriological and clinical evaluations are essential in the treatment of urinary tract and intestinal infections. Follow-up for several months after cessation of therapy may be indicated.
- Female patients receiving ampicillin for treatment of gonorrhoea should have cultures of endocervical and anal canal to determine cure.
- Superinfections are more likely to occur with broad spectrum derivatives of penicillin, such as ampicillin. Instruct patient to report the onset of black, hairy tongue; oral lesions (stomatitis, glossitis); rectal or vaginal itching; vaginal discharge; loose, foul-smelling stools; unusual odour to urine.
- Instruct patient to take medication around the clock, not to miss a dose, and to continue taking medication until it is all gone, unless otherwise directed by physician or pharmacist.
- If no improvement is noted within a few days after therapy is started, physician should be notified.
- Treatment for most infections is continued 48 to 72 hours beyond the time that patient becomes asymptomatic or negative cultures are obtained. A minimum of 10 days is recommended for group A beta-haemolytic streptococci to help prevent rheumatic fever.
- Capsules and unopened vials are stored preferably between 15° and 30°C (59° and 86°F) unless otherwise directed by manufacturer.
- *See also penicillin G.*

Diagnostic test interferences   Elevated CPK levels may result from local skeletal muscle injury following IM injection. Urine glucose: high urine drug concentrations can result in false-positive test results with Clinitest. SGOT(AST) may be elevated (significance not known). *See also penicillin G.*

AMPICILLIN (continued)
DRUG INTERACTIONS *Ampicillin*_____

PLUS	INTERACTIONS
Allopurinol	Allopurinol may predispose patient to 'ampicillin rash'
Bacteriostatic antibiotics e.g., chloramphenicol; erythromycins, tetracyclines	Bactericidal effects of ampicillin may be reduced. Concurrent administration generally avoided
Contraceptives, oral	Ampicillin may interfere with contraceptive action (by decreasing urinary excretion of endogenous oestrogens). Female patients should be advised to consider use of a nonhormonal contraceptive

See also penicillin G.

Ascorbic acid ━━━━━━━━━━━━━━━━━━━━━━━━━━━━━━

(Redoxon)

Antiscorbutic; antioxidant;
vitamin C; acidifier; urinary

ACTIONS AND USES   Water-soluble vitamin essential for synthesis and maintenance of collagen. Necessary for wound healing. Powerful antioxidant and reducing agent essential for many cellular enzymatic activities. Functions in carbohydrate metabolism, the conversion of folic acid to folinic acid, metabolism of phenylalanine and tyrosine, reduction of plasma transferrin to liver ferritin, the formation of serotonin, and in maintenance of vascular tone and integrity.

Used for prophylaxis and treatment of scurvy, to facilitate intestinal absorption of nonhaeme iron, for treatment of methemoglobinaemia, to promote tissue healing, and in a wide variety of malnutrition, deficiency, and haemorrhagic states. Ascorbic acid (not the ascorbates) has been used with limited success with methenamine to acidify urine when ammonium chloride is contraindicated or not tolerated.

ROUTE AND DOSAGE   Oral, intramuscular, intravenous. **Therapeutic**: at least 250 mg/day in divided doses. **Prophylactic**: 25–75 mg/day.

ABSORPTION AND FATE   Readily absorbed following oral or parenteral administration; widely distributed to body tissues, with highest concentrations in glandular tissue, leucocytes, platelets, and lens. Reportedly better utilized following IM rather than IV administration. Limited body storage. Rapidly excreted from body when plasma level exceeds renal threshold of 1.4 mg/dl. Metabolized in liver. Excess amounts excreted chiefly in urine as unchanged drug, oxalic acid, and other metabolites. Crosses placenta. Excreted in breast milk. Removed by haemodialysis.

CONTRAINDICATIONS AND PRECAUTIONS   Use of sodium ascorbate in patients on sodium restriction, use of calcium ascorbate in patients receiving digitalis. **Cautious**

A

ASCORBIC ACID (continued)

Use: excessive doses in patients with G6PD deficiency, iron overload associated with repeated blood transfusions, haemochromatosis, thalassaemia, sideroblastic anaemia; sickle cell anaemia; patients prone to gout or renal calculi. Safe use during pregnancy and in nursing mothers not established.

ADVERSE/SIDE EFFECTS   Acute haemolytic anaemia (patients with deficiency of G6PD); sickle cell crisis (patients with sickle cell anemia); decreased urine urobilinogen excretion. **With excessive doses**: nausea, vomiting, heartburn, diarrhoea, abdominal cramps, fatigue, flushing, headache; insomnia or sleepiness, increase in urination, urine acidification, and possibly crystalluria, (oxalate, cystine, or urate stones); dental erosion with high doses and prolonged use of chewable tablets. Parenteral administration: mild soreness at IV injection site; dizziness and temporary faintness with rapid administration, deep venous thrombosis; tissue necrosis following IM calcium ascorbate in infants.

NURSING IMPLICATIONS

- Ampoules containing ascorbic acid injection should be opened with caution. After prolonged storage, decomposition may occur with release of carbon dioxide and resulting increase in pressure within ampoules.
- Parenteral vitamin C is incompatible with many drugs. Consult pharmacist for compatibility information.
- Large doses of vitamin C (i.e., 1,000 mg/day) are given in divided amounts because the body utilizes only what is needed at a particular time and excretes the rest in urine. Megadoses may increase pH of the small intestine leading to interference with absorption of vitamin B_{12}.
- Oral solutions of vitamin C may be dropped directly in mouth or mixed with food.
- Effervescent tablet form should be dissolved in a glass of water immediately before ingestion.
- Minimum daily requirement of vitamin C to prevent scurvy is 10 mg. Recommended daily dietary allowance for adults is 60 mg (equivalent to about 4 ounces of orange juice); during pregnancy, 80 mg; during lactation, 100 mg; for infants, 35 mg; and for children, 45 mg.
- High doses of vitamin C are not recommended during pregnancy. Foetus can adapt to high levels by developing the capacity to inactivate vitamin C. Rebound scurvy can result when vitamin C intake is reduced to normal.
- Infants fed on cow's milk alone require supplemental vitamin C. A daily dose of 35 mg has been recommended during first week of life if feed contains two to three times the amount of protein found in human milk.
- *Normal plasma concentration of ascorbic acid*: approximately 0.4 to 1.5 mcg/dl.
- Vitamin C requirements are significantly increased in conditions that elevate metabolic rate, e.g., hyperthyroidism, fever, infection, burns and other severe trauma, postoperative states, neoplastic disease, chronic alcoholism. Reportedly, patients taking oral contraceptives also require vitamin C supplements.
- Subclinical vitamin C deficiency may exist in persons who subsist on diets low in fruits and vegetables. Particularly vulnerable are the indigent, the elderly, food faddists, drug addicts, alcoholics, patients on restricted therapeutic diets, and those

ASCORBIC ACID (continued)

receiving prolonged IV fluids, parenteral hyperalimentation, or chronic haemodialysis without adequate supplementation.

- Symptoms of vitamin C deficiency usually become objectively evident after 3 to 5 months of inadequate intake: irritability, emotional disturbances, general debility, pallor, anorexia, sensitivity to touch; limb and joint pain, follicular hyperkeratosis (particularly on thighs and buttocks), easy bruising, petechiae, bloody diarrhaea, delayed wound healing, loosening of teeth, sensitive, swollen, bleeding gums, anaemia.
- **Smoking–drug interaction** Smokers appear to have increased requirements for ascorbic acid because the vitamin is oxidized and excreted more rapidly than in nonsmokers. Advise patient with vitamin C deficiency to modify or stop smoking. Replacement dosages will be greater for the smoker.
- Most fruits and vegetables contain vitamin C, with highest levels in citrus fruits, strawberries, rose hips, guava, cantaloupe, leafy vegetables, tomatoes, potatoes, cabbage, green peppers, and parsley.
- Further studies are needed to determine the value of ascorbic acid in the prevention of atherosclerosis and in the prophylaxis or treatment of the common cold.
- Vitamin C is rapidly oxidized when exposed to air (deterioration is accelerated by light and heat). Slight darkening of tablets may occur without loss of potency.
- **Food–drug interaction**   Vitamin C increases the absorption of iron when taken at the same time as iron-rich foods.
- Large losses of vitamin C may result from: (1) Prolonged exposure to light and air (e.g., storage of foods and fruit juices in uncovered containers; early precutting). (2) Prolonged cooking. (3) Prolonged soaking. (4) Addition of sodium bicarbonate to foods. (5) Contact with copper and iron utensils.
- Stored in airtight, light-resistant, nonmetallic containers, away from heat and sunlight, preferably between 15° and 30°C (59° and 86°F), unless otherwise directed by manufacturer.

Diagnostic test interferences   High doses of vitamin C can produce false-negative results for **urine glucose** with glucose oxidase methods (Clinitest); false-positive results with copper reduction methods (Benedict's solution, Clinitest); and false increases in **serum uric acid** determination (by enzymatic methods). Interferes with **urinary steroid** (17-OHCS) determinations (by modified Reddy, Jenkins, Thorn procedure), and decreases in **serum bilirubin**. May cause false-negative tests for occult blood in stools.

DRUG INTERACTIONS *Ascorbic acid in megadoses (high enough to increase urine acidity)*_____

PLUS	INTERACTIONS
Aminosalicylic acid (PAS)	Increases risk of crystalluria
Amphetamines } Antidepressants, tricyclics }	Effects of these drugs may be decreased
Contraceptives, oral	May enhance effect of oral contraceptive, but contraceptive failure may result with abrupt discontinuation of vitamin C

A

ASCORBIC ACID (continued)

PLUS (continued)	INTERACTIONS
Disulphiram	May reduce disulphiram reaction
Digitalis	Calcium ascorbate may precipitate arrhythmias in patients taking digitalis
Phenothiazines	Decreases phenothiazine blood levels
Salicylates	Potentiates salicylate effects (vitamin C decreases salicylate excretion). Salicylates may inhibit uptake of vitamin C
Sulphonamides	Increases risk of crystalluria

Asparaginase

(Erwinase)   *Antineoplastic enzyme*

ACTIONS AND USES   A highly toxic drug with a low therapeutic index. This enzyme, isolated from *Escherichia coli* is active in solution at pH 6.5 to 8.0 and functions chiefly during postmitotic G_1 phase of cell division. Catalyzes hydrolysis (breakdown) of asparagine to ammonia and aspartic acid, thus depleting extracellular supply of an amino acid essential to synthesis of DNA and other nucleoproteins. Reduced availability of asparagine has little effect on most normal cells but tumour cells unable to synthesize their own supply are destroyed. Because some normal cells have high rates of protein synthesis, they also depend on an extracellular source of asparagine; thus drug-induced deficiency interferes with synthesis of important proteins by cells in, e.g., liver (clotting factors), pancreas (insulin), lymphocytes (antibodies). Bone marrow depression or cytotoxic effects on cells of GI tract, oral mucosa, hair follicles rarely occurs. Resistance to cytotoxic action develops rapidly; therefore asparaginase is not effective in treatment of solid tumours and is not recommended for maintenance therapy. No cross-resistance to other antineoplastic agents has been demonstrated.

Used primarily in combination regimens with other antineoplastic agents to treat acute lymphocyte leukaemia. Has been used investigationally alone or in combination regimens in treatment of other leukaemias, lymphosarcoma, and (intra-arterially) in treatment of hypoglycaemia due to pancreatic islet cell tumor.

ROUTE AND DOSAGE   Highly individualized regimens. Intravenous.

ABSORPTION AND FATE   Distribution is primarily within the intravascular space (80%). About 3 hours after IV dose, remaining drug (20%) is distributed in lymph and (low levels) in CSF, pleural and peritoneal fluids. **Plasma half-life,** 8 to 30 hours, is unaffected by age, hepatic or renal function, or by diagnosis or extent of disease. **Metabolic fate** unknown; small amounts of the enzyme are found in urine; presence in milk has not been demonstrated.

ASPARAGINASE (continued)

CONTRAINDICATIONS AND PRECAUTIONS   History of previous hypersensitivity to asparaginase; history of or existing pancreatitis. Safe use during pregnancy and in nursing mothers not established. **Cautious Use:** liver impairment, diabetes mellitus, infections, history of urate calculi or of gout, patients who have had previous antineoplastic and/or radiation therapy.

ADVERSE/SIDE EFFECTS   These include: depression, headache, irritability, personality disorders, fatigue, lethargy, confusion, agitation, hallucinations, coma, seizures (rare), organic brain syndrome, Parkinson-like syndrome with tremor and progressive increase in muscle tone, severe vomiting, nausea, anorexia, abdominal cramps, diarrhoea, oral and intestinal ulcerations, malabsorption syndrome (rare), acute pancreatitis, uric acid nephropathy, azotaemia, renal shutdown or insufficiency, proteinuria, hypofibrino ginaemia, reduced clotting factors (especially V, VII, VIII, IX), decreased circulating platelets, marked leucopenia. Further side effects include: liver function abnormalities: jaundice, fluctuations in total serum lipids, increases in: blood ammonia, alkaline phosphatase, SGOT (AST), SGPT (ALT), BUN, bilirubin, cholesterol, skin rashes, urticaria, arthralgia; anaphylaxis, chills, fever, perspiration, weight loss, fatal hyperthermia, hyperglycaemia, glycosuria, polyuria, hypoalbuminaemia associated with peripheraloedema, hypocalcaemia, hyperuricaemia, infections.

NURSING IMPLICATIONS

- Patient should be informed before treatment is initiated of the positive and negative effects of drug therapy. Some degree of toxicity generally occurs.
- Caution is warranted in handling, administering and disposing of antineoplastic drugs because of their carcinogenic, mutagenic, and teratogenic potential. Follow agency policy.
- *Have immediately available*: personnel, drugs, antihistamine, diphenhydramine, IV corticosteroid), oxygen, and equipment for treatment anaphylactic reaction, whenever drug is administered.
- Because of the possibility of allergic reactions, an intradermal skin test is performed before the initial dose of asparaginase and when the drug is readministered after an interval of a week or more.
- Observe test site for at least 1 hour for evidence of positive reaction (wheal, erythema). A negative skin test, however, does not preclude possibility of an allergic reaction.
- Positive reactors can be desensitized with increasing IV doses at 10-minute intervals (provided no allergic reaction occurs) until patient's total dose for that day is reached. Be aware that desensitization itself can be hazardous because asparaginase is a large foreign protein and is antigenic.
- Unlike many other desensitization regimens, asparaginase desensitization does not eliminate risk of subsequent allergic reactions with retreatments.
- During asparaginase administration, monitor vital signs and be alert to evidence of hypersensitivity reactions or anaphylaxis: hypotension, irregular pulse, feeling of lump in throat or hoarseness (laryngealoedema), bronchospasm (wheezing), dyspnoea,

ASPARAGINASE (continued)

cyanosis, chest constriction. Anaphylaxis usually occurs within ½ to 1 hour after dose has been given. It is more apt to happen with intermittent administrations and when IM route is used.

- When given concurrently with or immediately before a course of prednisone and vincristine, toxicity potential is increased.
- Maintenance of adequate fluid intake, alkalinization of urine and/or administration of allopurinol may accompany treatment as prophylaxis against uric acid stones.
- Tests for glycosuria should be done regularly. Report polyuria, polydipsia, or positive urine test to the physician.
- Surveillance of body weight is important. Instruct patient to notify physician of continued loss of weight or onset of foot and ankle swelling.
- Serum amylase, blood glucose, plasma coagulation factor determinations, ammonia and uric acid levels, hepatic and renal function tests, peripheral blood counts, and bone marrow function are monitored regularly during treatment. Liver function tests are done at least twice weekly during therapy.
- Circulating lymphoblasts decrease markedly in the first several days of treatment and leucocyte counts may fall below normal. Protection from infection during this period is crucial. Dressings and treatments should be done with sterile technique and health personnel, and visitors with respiratory or other infections should be restricted. Reverse precautions may be ordered. Signs of infection in the patient (chill, fever, aches, sore throat) should be reported promptly.
- Report sudden severe abdominal pain with nausea and vomiting, particularly if these symptoms occur after medication is discontinued (may indicate pancreatitis).
- Elevations of BUN and serum ammonia are expected findings because of enzymatic action. Blood ammonia levels are elevated in most patients as high as 700 to 900 mcg/dl (normal 80 to 110 mcg/dl). Watch for signs of *hyperammonaemia*: anorexia, vomiting, lethargy, weak pulse, depressed temperature, irritability, asterixis, seizures, coma. The treatment is usually *low-protein diet* (i.e., low protein breads, most vegetables and fruits, avoidance of meat, sea food, legumes) with ample amounts of simple carbohydrate e.g., jellies, syrups, honey, sugar, candy, to increase calorific intake. Collaborate with dietitian and physician.
- Because of potential serious hepatic dysfunction, enzymatic detoxification of other drugs may be reduced, therefore anticipate possibility of prolonged or exaggerated effects of concurrently given drugs and/or their toxicity; report incidence promptly.
- Asparaginase toxicity is reportedly less in children than in adults. In general, because of the low therapeutic index characteristic of this agent, a therapeutic response will most likely be accompanied by some toxicity in all patients.
- Nausea, vomiting, and anorexia can interrupt scheduled doses at first, but lessen with continued treatment. Instruct patient to try to continue all prescribed medications if at all possible but if not possible, the physician should be notified without delay.
- Urge patient to report the onset of unusual bleeding, bruising, petechiae, skin rash or itching, yellowed skin and sclera, joint pain, puffy face, or dyspnoea.
- CNS function (general behaviour, emotional status, level of consciousness, thought content, motor function) should be evaluated before and during therapy.
- Drowsiness, decreased alertness, and shakiness are symptoms that can accompany

ASPARAGINASE (continued)

treatment with this drug. Driving or operating equipment that requires alertness and skill can be hazardous. Urge caution and inform patient that these effects can continue several weeks after last dose of the drug.

- Reenforce necessity to keep scheduled appointments for evaluation of therapy.
- The lyophilized powder is reconstituted with sterile water for injection for IV administration or with NaCl for injection for IV and IM administration. Shake vial well to promote dissolution of powder. Avoid vigorous shaking: ordinary shaking does not inactivate the enzyme or cause foaming of content.
- For IV infusion, the reconstituted solution should be further diluted with NaCl or 5% dextrose injection and administered into tubing of an already running infusion, in not less than 30 minutes. If a filter is used it should be a 5-micron filter. Use of a 0.2-micron filter can reduce potency of asparaginase solution.
- Limit the IM injection volume to 2 ml in one site. Select a second site if volume exceeds 2 ml.
- Unless otherwise directed by manufacturer, store sealed vial of lyophilized powder below 8°C (46°F); reconstituted solutions can be stored at 2° to 8°C (36° to 46°F) for up to 8 hours, then discard. Do not use cloudy solution.

Diagnostic test interferences Asparaginase may interfere with interpretation of thyroid function tests (pretreatment values return within 4 weeks after drug is discontinued).

DRUG INTERACTIONS *Asparaginase*

PLUS	INTERACTIONS
Antigout agents	Since asparaginase raises blood uric acid levels adjustment of antigout drug dose may be necessary
Corticosteroids (glucocosteroids) especially prednisone	Increase hyperglycaemic effect of asparaginase and may increase risk of neuropathy and erythropoietric pathology
Hypoglycaemics	Hypoglycaemic effect reduced; dose adjustment required during and after asparaginase treatment
Immunosuppressives or radiation therapy	Effects enhanced by asparaginase
Methotrexate	Antineoplastic effect of methotrexate blocked when administered immediately before or with asparaginase
Vincristine	*See corticosteroids (above)*

Aspirin

(Acetylsalisylic Acid, Aspergum, Breoprin, Caprin, Claradin, Laproprin, Levius, Nusaels asprin, Palaprin forte, Paynocil, Solprin)

NSAID; analgesic/antipyretic; antiplatelet; enzyme inhibitor; antirheumatic; salicylate

ASPIRIN (continued)

ACTIONS AND USES   A salicylic ester of acetic acid; each gram contains about 760 mg salicylate. Major actions, i.e., analgesic, antiinflammatory, and antipyretic appear to be associated with inhibition of synthesis and release of prostaglandins. *Analgesic action*: principally peripheral with limited action in the CNS possibly on the hypothalamus, and results in relief of mild to moderate pain. *Antiinflammatory action: aspirin and other salicylates inhibit* prostaglandin synthesis. Prostaglandins directly mediate many of the signs of inflammation, e.g., release of lysosomal substance, increased lymphocyte activation, formation of autoantibodies. As an antiinflammatory agent, aspirin appears to be involved in increased antigen removal, reduction of spread of inflammation in ground substances, and depression of the total inflammatory process. These antiinflammatory effects also contribute to analgesic effects. As an *antipyretic*, aspirin lowers body temperature in fever by inhibiting prostaglandin synthesis and release, and by indirectly causing centrally mediated peripheral vasodilation and sweating. Aspirin (but not other salicylates) is a powerful inhibitor of platelet aggregation and prolongs bleeding time (measurable *antiplatelet effect* may persist 3 to 7 days).

Urate excretion (*uricosuric effect*) is enhanced by high doses of aspirin (over 5 g/day) and suppressed by usual analgesic doses (less than 2 g/day). Has hypocholesterolaemic and hypoglycaemic effects in large doses.

Used to relieve pain of low to moderate intensity, such as headache, dysmenorrhoea, neuralgia, discomforts of common cold, cancer pain, postoperative (after second or third day), and postpartum pain. Also used for various inflammatory conditions, such as acute rheumatic fever, systemic lupus erythematosus, rheumatoid arthritis, osteoarthritis, bursitis, calcific tendonitis, and to reduce fever in selected febrile conditions.

Buffered aspirins generally contain aspirin with sodium bicarbonate or calcium carbonate.

Unbuffered products containing aspirin in combination with caffeine alone (Anadin, Antoin) or with paracetamol (Powerin).

ROUTE AND DOSAGE   Oral. **Adult**: 300-900 mg/4–6 hrly as necessary, maximum 4 g daily.

ABSORPTION AND FATE   Rapidly and completely absorbed from stomach and upper bowel. Administration with food retards absorption rate, but does not reduce total amount absorbed. Erratic absorption times reported for enteric-coated, rectal suppository, and extended release forms. Readily absorbed by most body fluids and all tissues. **Peak plasma levels** in 1 to 2 hours. Extensively bound to plasma proteins. **Half-life** is dose dependent (about 2 to 3 hours with low or single doses and 5 to 18 hours with moderate doses). Rapidly hydrolyzed in GI tract, plasma, and liver to salicylate. Additional metabolism by liver microsomal system. Individual differences in metabolism and excretion rates reported. At low doses, 50% of dose excreted in urine in 2 to 4 hours, and in 15 to 30 hours at high doses. Eliminated as salicyluric acid and conjugates; about 1% excreted unhydrolyzed. Urinary excretion rate is pH dependent. Alkaline salts increase absorption rate and renal clearance; urinary acidification promotes retention. Readily crosses placenta; excreted in breast milk.

CONTRAINDICATIONS AND PRECAUTIONS   Hypersensitivity to salicylates including methyl salicylate (oil of wintergreen), to other NSAIDs or to tartrazine; patients with

ASPIRIN (continued)

'aspirin traid' (rhinitis, nasal polyps, asthma); chronic rhinitis, history of GI ulceration or bleeding; haemophilia or other bleeding disorders, carditis; use during pregnancy especially in third trimester, in nursing mothers, except under advice and supervision of physician. **Cautious Use**: otic diseases, allergies, gout, children with fever accompanied by dehydration; cardiac disease, renal or hepatic impairment, vitamin K deficiency, G6PD deficiency, anaemia, preoperatively, Hodgkin's disease. Not used for children under 12 yrs because of the association with Reye's disease.

ADVERSE/SIDE EFFECTS With large doses: pulmonary oedema (increase in plasma volume), rapid pulse; gastric irritation (nausea, vomiting, heartburn, anorexia, stomach pain, GI ulceration and bleeding); easy bruising, ecchymoses, increased bleeding before and after delivery, hypoglycaemia (especially in diabetics), iron-deficiency anaemia, thrombocytopenia, purpura, leukopenia, agranulocytosis, haemolytic anaemia (G6PD deficiency). **Hypersensitivity**: bronchospasm (wheezing), tightness in chest, severe rhinitis, skin eruptions, angiooedema, urticaria, anaphylaxis. *Marked intoxication*: (symptoms as for mild intoxication, but more pronounced and occur more rapidly): haemorrhage, tachycardia, pulmonary oedema, hypoglycaemia or hyperglycaemia, hyponatraemia, hypokalaemia, disturbances in acid–base balance, hyperpyrexia, nephropathy, hepatotoxicity, acute pancreatitis, dehydration, 'salicylic jag' (CNS stimulation: restlessness, incoherent speech, hallucinations resembling alcoholic inebriation but without euphoria, convulsions); CNS depression, delirium, coma, respiratory failure. **Otic**: (dose related and usually reversible): tinnitus, decreased hearing, deafness. **Salicylism**: *mild intoxication*: rapid and deep breathing (hyperpnoea), tinnitus, diminished hearing, dizziness, severe or continuing headache, dimmed vision, mental confusion, lassitude, drowsiness, fever, flushing, sweating, thirst, nausea, vomiting, diarrhoea, anorexia, rapid pulse. **Other**: prolonged pregnancy, labour.

Benorylate-aspirin/paracetamol ester is converted to the original compounds in the body used for patients who cannot tolerate the gastrointestinal effects of aspirin.

NURSING IMPLICATIONS

- GI side effects may be minimized by administering with a full glass of water (240 ml, preferably warm), milk, food, or an antacid. Exception: enteric-coated tablet; may dissolve too quickly if administered with milk. Also enteric-coated tablet should not be crushed or chewed. The aim is to prevent direct contact of drug particles with gastric mucosa.
- If patient has difficulty in swallowing tablets, plain aspirin can be crushed to a fine powder and mixed with apple sauce or other food that patient likes.
- Buffered aspirin or aspirin administered with an antacid may be better tolerated; however, large doses or repeated use can contribute to alkalinization of urine which enhances salicylate excretion.
- Buffered aspirin preparations in an effervescent vehicle, are more rapidly absorbed than plain aspirin, and cause less GI irritation and bleeding, but do have a high sodium content, they should not be used on a scheduled basis or in patients on sodium restriction.
- Because aspirin lacks topical anaesthetic action there is no logical basis for applying it locally for toothache or for using aspirin gargle or gum for sore throat. Any relief gained is due to systemic absorption, not local action.

ASPIRIN (continued)

- When prescribed for dysmenorrhea, explain to patient that for best results aspirin should be taken 1 or 2 days before menses (to reduce prostaglandin-induced uterine contractions). Patients having heavy menstrual blood loss should be advised to take another analgesic, such as paracetamol instead of aspirin.
- For treatment of rheumatic diseases, physician may prescribe daily dose increase of 1 or 2 tablets/day on basis of serum salicylate concentrations, or until therapeutic response occurs (usually within 3 to 5 days after beginning regular dosing), or symptoms of toxicity (salicylism) intervene. Symptoms of toxicity are often eliminated after dosage reduction of as little as 325 mg (5 grains).
- Schedule aspirin administration at least 30 minutes before physiotherapy or other planned exercise to keep discomfort at a minimum.
- To reduce risk of bleeding, generally, aspirin therapy is discontinued about 1 week before surgery. Patients undergoing oral surgery should be advised not to take aspirin-containing gargles and not to chew aspirin products for at least 1 week following surgery. Prolonged contact with aspirin can cause haemorrhage and injury to oral tissues.
- Chronic administration of high-dose aspirin during the last 3 months of pregnancy may prolong pregnancy and labour, increase maternal bleeding before and after delivery, and cause weight increase and haemorrhage in the neonate.
- Therapeutic range for rheumatic diseases: 20 to 30 mg/dl. Symptoms of toxicity generally occur when serum salicylate level are over 30 mg/dl.
- Previous nonreaction to salicylates does not guarantee future safety. Subsequent sensitivity especially to aspirin is not uncommon.
- Patients with asthma, nasal polyps, perennial vasomotor rhinitis, or hay fever demonstrate a high frequency of salicylate hypersensitivity.
- Advise patient to discontinue use with onset of ringing in the ears, impaired hearing, dizziness, GI discomfort or bleeding. Hearing impairment resulting from salicylate toxicity is generally reversible.
- Tinnitus and decreased hearing are not always reliable indicators of toxicity because these changes may pass unnoticed in the hearing impaired, the elderly, and in children.
- Potential for toxicity is high in the elderly who are chronic aspirin users because they have less serum proteins to bind salicylates and also are less able to excrete it.
- Accidental ingestion of salicylates is one of the most common causes of poisoning and death in young children. Caution patients to keep drug out of the reach of children.
- Caution patient to avoid aspirin products if he or she has been drinking alcohol (*see Drug Interactions*).
- **Food–drug interaction**   Chronic ingestion of aspirin may be associated with depressed plasma ascorbic acid (vitamin C) and folate levels in some patients. Supplemental therapy may be indicated.
- Prolonged use of high salicylate doses can lead to iron-deficiency anaemia, especially in women. Average blood loss with daily use of several aspirin tablets is reportedly 2 to 6 ml; 10% of patients on chronic high doses may loss as much as 80 ml/day.
- **Instructions for patients receiving repeated or large doses of salicylates:**
  - ☐ Observe and report symptoms of salicylism (*see Adverse/Side Effects*): petechiae, ecchymoses, bleeding gums, bloody or black stools.

ASPIRIN (continued)

- ☐ Maintain adequate fluid intake (consult physician) to prevent salicylate crystalluria.
- ☐ Report for periodic haematocrit, prothrombin time, and blood and urine salicylate determinations as directed by physician. Hepatic and renal function tests are also recommended at regular intervals, particularly for patients with systemic lupus erythematosus and juvenile rheumatoid arthritis. Diabetic patients should be closely monitored (*see Drug Interactions*).
- ☐ Avoid other medications containing aspirin unless directed by physician, because of danger of overdosing. (There are more than 500 aspirin-containing compounds.)
- ☐ Supplemental ascorbic acid and folates, if prescribed.
- ■ **Treatment of overdosage** Acute salicylate toxicity requires immediate emesis or gastric lavage and activated charcoal. Further treatment is designed to maintain hydration, electrolyte and acid–base balance, and to reduce hyperthermia (IV fluids); to reduce excitement or convulsions (diazepam or barbiturates); and to force diuresis by alkalinizing urine. Haemodialysis in adults, peritoneal dialysis in children, and exchange transfusion in infants may be required. Patients who have ingested sustained-release aspirin must be observed for at least 3 days after toxicity treatment.
- ■ Most aspirin tablets develop a hard shell with age, a change that lengthens disintegration time, increases risk of GI irritation, and delays onset of therapeutic action. Advise patient not to buy aspirin in large quantities.
- ■ Aspirin tablets rapidly hydrolyze on exposure to heat, moisture, and air. Instruct patient to smell tablet before taking it. If a vinegar like (acetic acid) odour is detected discard all tablets.
- ■ Store preferably between 15° and 30°C (59° and 86°F) in airtight container, unless otherwise directed by manufacturer.

Diagnostic test interferences Bleeding time is prolonged 4 to 7 days (life or exposed platelets) following a single 325 mg dose of aspirin. Large doses of aspirin (5 g or more/day) may cause prolonged **prothrombin time**, interference with **pregnancy tests** (using mouse or rabbit), decrease in **serum cholesterol, potassium**, and **PBI. Serum uric acid** may increase when plasma salicylate levels are below 10 and decrease when above 15 mg/dl. **Urine 5-HIAA**: test interference by fluorescent methods. **Urine ketones**: interference with Gerhardt test (reaction with ferric chloride produces a reddish colour that persists after boiling). **Urine glucose**: moderate to large doses of aspirin (2.4 g or more per day) may produce false-negative results with glucose oxidase methods (e.g., Clinistix, and false-positive results with copper reduction methods (Benedict's solution, Clinitest). Urinary **PSP excretion** may be reduced. **Urine VMA** falsely elevated (by most tests), or reduced (by Pisano method).

DRUG INTERACTIONS *Aspirin (and other salicylates)*

PLUS	INTERACTIONS
Alcohol (Ethanol)	Potentiation of ulcerogenic effects. Concomitant ingestion not advised
Aminosalicylic acid (PAS)	Increased PAS toxicity (salicylates decrease renal excretion of PAS)

ASPIRIN *(continued)*

PLUS (continued)	INTERACTIONS
Ammonium chloride and other acidifying agents	Elevate serum salicylate levels (increases renal tubular reabsorption of salicylates by lowering urine pH)
Antacids, including sodium bicarbonate and other urinary alkalinizing agents.	Reduce serum salicylate levels (alkalinization of urine, decreases renal tubular reabsorption of salicylate)
Anticoagulants	Additive hypoprothrombinaemic effect (by decreasing plasma protein binding). Combination avoided, if possible
Antidiabetic agents	Increased hypoglycaemic activity with moderate to large salicylate doses, i.e., >2 g/day (by decreased plasma protein binding). Concurrent use generally avoided. If used, dosage reduction of both drugs may be necessary
Carbonic anhydrase inhibitors, e.g., acetazolamide	May induce metabolic acidosis and thus enhance salicylate intoxication in patients receiving high salicylate doses
Corticosteroids	Decrease serum salicylate levels (possibly by increasing renal excretion); additive ulcerogenic effects. Concurrent use generally avoided
Indomethacin and other NSAIDs	Decreased serum indomethacin levels possibly by decreasing GI absorption; additive ulcerogenic effects. Concurrent use generally avoided
Methotrexate	Increased methotrexate levels (by decreasing renal clearance and decreasing plasma protein binding of methotrexate). Concurrent use generally avoided, if possible
Niacin	Aspirin blocks high dose niacin-induced flushing
Phenylbutazone Probenecid Sulphinpyrazone	Salicylates in small to moderate doses may antagonize uricosuric action of these drugs. Concurrent use generally avoided during uricosuric therapy
Sulphonamides	Salicylates reportedly increase serum sulphonamide levels, possibly by displacing them from serum protein binding sites
Tetracyclines	May form complex with aluminium- or magnesium-containing antacids in buffered aspirins. Salicylates should be administered at least 1 hour before or after tetracyclines

Atenolol

(Tenormin)   *Adrenergic blocking agent (beta$_1$-selective); antihypertensive*

ACTIONS AND USES   In therapeutic doses this drug selectively blocks beta$_1$-adrenergic receptors located chiefly in cardiac muscle. With large doses preferential effect is lost

ATENOLOL (continued)

and inhibition of beta$_2$-adrenergic receptors (especially in bronchial and vascular musculature) may lead to increased airway resistance, especially in patients with asthma or COPD. Unlike propranolol (a nonselective beta-blocker), atenolol lacks membrane-stabilizing and intrinsic sympathomimetic (partial agonist) activities. Mechanisms for antihypertensive action include central effect leading to decreased sympathetic outflow to periphery, reduction in renin activity with consequent suppression of the renin–aldosterone–angiotensin system, and competitive inhibition of catecholamine binding at beta adrenergic receptor sites. Cardiac output is reduced, as is diastolic blood pressure. Atenolol increases peripheral vascular resistance both at rest and with exercise.

Used for the management of hypertension as a single agent or concomitantly with other antihypertensive agents, especially a diuretic. Also has been used in treatment of stable angina pectoris.

ROUTE AND DOSAGE   Oral: *Initial*: 50 mg daily alone or added to diuretic therapy. If full effect is not achieved within 1 or 2 weeks, dose should be increased to 100 mg given as single daily dose. Higher dosages unlikely to produce further benefit. Dosage adjustment necessary in patients with creatinine clearance below 35 ml/min/1:73 m^2.

ABSORPTION AND FATE   About 50% oral dose rapidly absorbed from GI tract. **Peak blood levels** within 2 to 4 hours after ingestion. **Minimal protein binding** (6 to 16%); thus plasma blood levels are relatively consistent (with about a fourfold inter-patient variation). Does not readily cross blood–brain barrier. **Half-life**: 6 to 7 hours; longer in patients with impaired renal function. Both beta blocking and resultant antihypertensive effects persist at least 24 hours. Little or no hepatic metabolism. Approximately 40 to 50% of dose eliminated unchanged in urine; remainder excreted unchanged in faeces.

CONTRAINDICATIONS AND PRECAUTIONS   Sinus bradycardia, greater than first-degree heart block, overt cardiac failure, cardiogenic shock. Safe use during pregnancy, in nursing women, and in children not established. **Cautious Use**: hypertensive patients with congestive heart failure controlled by digitalis and diuretics, asthma and chronic obstructive disease (COPD), diabetes mellitus, impaired renal function, hyperthyroidism.

ADVERSE/SIDE EFFECTS   (Usually well tolerated.) Side effects include: dizziness, vertigo, light-headedness, fatigue, lethargy, drowsiness, headache, vivid dreams, bradycardia, hypotension, congestive heart failure, cold extremities, leg pains, nausea, vomiting, diarrhoea, dry eyes, visual disturbances, wheezing, dyspnoea, bronchospasm, rash, increase in serum triglycerides. *See also propranolol for potential adverse/side effects.*

NURSING IMPLICATIONS
- If necessary, tablet may be crushed before administration and taken with fluid of patient's choice.
- Check apical pulse before administration of drug, especially in patients receiving digitalis (both drugs slow AV conduction). If below 60 bpm withhold dose and consult physician.

ATENOLOL (continued)

- Monitor apical pulse, blood pressure, respirations, and peripheral circulation throughout dosage adjustment period. Consult physician for acceptable parameters.
- Bradycardia and severe hypotension are treated with atropine. Isoprenaline or cardiac pacemaker may be required if AV block occurs.
- If patient on atenolol therapy requires haemodialysis, patient shoud be hospitalized because marked drop in blood pressure can occur. Atenolol, 50 mg, is given after each dialysis.
- Advise patient to adhere rigidly to dose regimen. Sudden discontinuation of drug can exacerbate angina and precipitate tachycardia or myocardial infarction in patients with coronary artery disease, and thyroid storm in patients with hyperthyroidism.
- Caution patient to make position changes slowly and in stages, particularly from recumbent to upright posture.
- Expected therapeutic effects in patients receiving atenolol for angina include the reduction in frequency of anginal attacks and in the amount of glycerol trinitrate required, and increase in exercise tolerance.
- As with other beta-blockers, the decision to discontinue therapy before surgery remains controversial. If atenolol is to be withdrawn, it should be done 48 hours before surgery. If treatment is to be continued, anaesthetic agents that depress the myocardium (e.g., cyclopropane, ether, trichlorethylene) must be used with extreme caution.
- Store in well-closed, light-resistant container between 15° and 30°C (59° and 86°F), unless otherwise directed by manufacturer.
- See also propranolol for Nursing Implications, Diagnostic Test Interferences, Drug Interactions.

DRUG INTERACTIONS   Atenolol

PLUS	INTERACTIONS
Atropine and other anticholinergics	Atenolol effects may be increased (anticholinergics enhance GI absorption of atenolol)
Indomethacin	Indomethacin decreases hypotensive effect of beta-blockers. Combination generally avoided
	Possibility of increased lignocaine plasma levels and toxicity. Used concurrently with caution
Prazosin	Hypotensive effect of first prazosin dose may be more severe and of longer duration
See also propranolol.	

Atropine sulphate

(Isopto Atropine)

Anticholinergic
(parasympatholytic);
antimuscarinic;
antispasmodic; mydriatic

ATROPINE SULPHATE (continued)

ACTIONS AND USES   Naturally occurring alkaloid and tertiary amine derived from *Atropa belladonna* (deadly nightshade). Selectively blocks all muscarinic responses (*antimuscarinic action*) to acetylcholine (ACh) whether excitatory or inhibitory. Forms strong drug-receptor complex at postganglionic parasympathetic neuroeffector sites in smooth muscle, cardiac muscle, and exocrine glands, thereby blocking action of ACh and antagonizes action of 5-hydroxytryptamine (serotonin) and histamine. Blocks vagal impulses to heart with resulting increased heart rate and cardiac output, and shortened PR interval. Causes vasodilation of small blood vessels usually with little effect on blood pressure. Selective depression of CNS relieves rigidity and tremor of Parkinson's syndrome. Reduces amplitude, tone, and frequency of smooth muscle contractions in stomach, intestinal tract, ureters, and urinary bladder; effect on gall-bladder and bile ducts is not consistent. Antisecretory action causes suppression of sweating, lacrimation and salivation, as well as bronchial mucus and gastric secretions. Produces mydriasis and cycloplegia by blocking response of iris sphincter muscle and ciliary muscle of lens to cholinergic stimulation; effects occur with both systemic and local administration.

Used as adjunct in symptomatic treatment of GI disorders, e.g., peptic ulcer, pylorospasm, hypermotility, irritable bowel syndrome. **Ophthalmic Use**: to produce mydriasis, and cycloplegia prior to refraction and for treatment of anterior uveitis and iritis. **Preoperative Use**: to suppress salivation, perspiration, and respiratory tract secretions and for its bronchodilating effect during surgery. **Cardiac and Other Uses**: to abolish vagal reflexes in cardiac arrest and to counteract bradycardia induced by propranolol and other drugs with cholinergic effects, organophosphorous insecticides, and *Amanita* mushroom poisoning, and in selected patients with early myocardial infarction for relief of sinus bradycardia associated with hypotension and increased ventricular irritability. Also used to diagnose sinus node dysfunction and to evaluate coronary artery disease during pacing. Available in fixed combination with diphenoxylate (Lomotil), and phenobarbital, e.g., Donnatal.

ROUTE AND DOSAGE   **Oral**: 0.25–2 mg daily. **Intravenous**: 0.3–1 mg, Maximum 3 mg in 24 hrs.

ABSORPTION AND FATE   Well absorbed from all administration sites and widely distributed in body. Peak plasma concentrations within 1 hour following oral ingestion, 30 minutes following IM injection, and 1.5 to 4 hours after inhalation. Peak increase in heart rate following IV occurs in 2 to 4 minutes. Inhibition of salivation may last up to 4 hours. Mydriatic action following topical instillation peaks in 30 to 40 minutes, and may persist 7 to 12 days; effect on accommodation may last up to 14 days or longer. Crosses blood–brain barrier. About 18% bound to plasma proteins; **plasma half-life**: 2 to 3 hours. Metabolized in liver. Most (77 to 94% of dose) is excreted in urine within 24 hours as unchanged drug (30 to 50%) and metabolites. Crosses placenta. Traces appear in breast milk.

CONTRAINDICATIONS AND PRECAUTIONS   Hypersensitivity to belladonna alkaloids or to any ingredients in the formulation; synechia, angle-closure glaucoma, parotitis, obstructure uropathy, e.g., bladder neck obstruction caused by prostatic hypertrophy;

A

ATROPINE SULPHATE (continued)

intestinal atony, paralytic ileus, obstructive diseases of GI tract, severe ulcerative colitis, toxic megacolon, tachycardia secondary to cardiac insufficiency or thyrotoxicosis; acute haemorrhage, myasthenia gravis. Safe use during pregnancy and in nursing women not established. **Cautious Use:** myocardial infarction, hypotension; coronary artery disease, congestive heart failure, tachyarrythmias, gastric ulcer, GI infections, hiatal hernia with reflux oesophagitis, hyperthyroidism, chronic lung disease, hepatic or renal disease, the elderly, debilitated patients, children under 6 years of age, Down's syndrome, autonomic neuropathy, spastic paralysis, brain damage in children.

ADVERSE/SIDE EFFECTS   These include: headache, drowsiness, ataxia, dizziness, restlessness, excitement, mental depression, confusion, disorientation, insomnia, hallucinations, delirium, toxic psychosis, hyperpyrexia, respiratory depression, coma, hypertension or hypotension, tachycardia, palpitation, angina, ectopic ventricular beats, paradoxical bradycardia, AV dissociation, ventricular or atrial fibrillation. Other side effects are: flushed, dry skin; anhidrosis, skin rash (face and upper trunk), urticaria, contact dermatitis, allergic conjunctivitis, fixed-drug eruption, dry mouth (xerostomia) with thirst, dysphagia, loss of taste; nausea, vomiting, constipation, paralytic ileus, abdominal distention, urinary hesitancy and retention, dysuria, impotence, mydriasis, blurred vision, photophobia, increased intraocular pressure, cycloplegia, eye pain, oedema of eyelids, eye dryness, chronic conjunctivitis (with continued use), leucocytosis, bronchial plugging, suppression of lactation, nasal dryness or congestion.

NURSING IMPLICATIONS

- Oral atropine is usually given 30 minutes before meals and at bedtime.
- Smaller doses of atropine are indicated for the elderly because of the possibility of atropine-induced tachycardia, mydriasis, and increased intraocular pressure in this glaucoma-prone age group. Intraocular pressure should be determined before atropine is prescribed.
- Monitor vital signs. Pulse is a sensitive indicator of patient's response to atropine. Be alert to changes in quality and rate of pulse and respiration and changes in blood pressure and temperature.
- Initial paradoxic bradycardia following IV atropine usually lasts only 1 to 2 minutes. It is most likely to occur when IV is administered very slowly or when small doses (less than 0.5 mg) are used. Following parenteral administration, postural hypotension may occur if the patient ambulates too soon.
- Atropine may contribute to the problem of urinary retention. On initiation of therapy, establish a baseline of 24-hour urinary output, and monitor daily output thereafter; especially important in older patients and in patients who have had surgery. Have patient void before giving atropine.
- If constipation is a problem, check for abdominal distention and auscultate for bowel sounds. (Symptoms of paralytic ileus include abdominal distention, constipation, absent bowel sounds usually associated with nausea, vomiting, and epigastric pain.)
- Increased fluid intake and increased bulk in the diet may help to overcome constipating effects of atropine.
- The following measures may help to relieve dry mouth: small, frequent mouth rinses

ATROPINE SULPHATE (continued)

with tepid water; meticulous mouth and dental care; gum chewing or sucking hard sweets, (sugarless); humidification of air; use of saliva substitute. Avoid overuse of commercial mouthwashes because of the possibility of changing the normal oral flora. Additionally, most contain alcohol which enhances drying. Reduction of dosage may be necessary.

■ The elderly patient is especially prone to develop 'atropine fever' (hyperpyrexia due to suppression of perspiration and heat loss) lending to the risk of heatstroke. Warn patient to avoid excessive heat. Initial symptoms may include dizziness, weakness, headache, sudden loss of consciousness, hot, red dry skin. Treatment consists of rapid cooling (temperatures sometimes rise above 41°C (106°F) by wetting skin with tap water and fanning (evaporative cooling), and ice packs to neck, axillae, groin, and abdomen.

■ Intraocular tension should be determined before and during therapy with ophthalmic preparations. Note that ophthalmic solutions and ointments are available in various strengths.

■ Instruct patient to prepare for impaired visual acuity of several days duration (*see Absorption and Fate*) and to protect eyes by wearing dark glasses during drug action period.

■ Caution patient that in addition to causing sensitivity to light and blurring of near vision, atropine will temporarily impair ability to judge distance. Advise patient to avoid driving and other activities requiring visual acuity while vision is affected.

■ Ophthalmic preparations should be discontinued if eye pain, conjunctivitis, palpitation, rapid pulse, or dizziness occurs. Report symptoms promptly to physician.

■ Frequent and continued use of eye preparations, as well as overdosage, can produce systemic effects of atropine. Studies reveal that over one-half of atropine deaths have resulted from systemic absorption following ocular administration and have been in infants and children.

■ Ointment dosage form is preferred by some clinicians for use in children because it is less likely to be absorbed systemically than solution formulations.

■ Onset of mydriatic action may be slower and duration longer in persons with dark eyes.

■ Infants and children with spastic paralysis, brain damage, or Down's syndrome, and blonde, blue-eyed individuals appear to be highly sensitive to the effects of atropine.

■ Patients receiving atropine via inhalation sometimes manifest mild CNS stimulation with doses in excess of 5 mg and mental depression and other mental disturbances with larger doses.

■ **Treatment of overdosage** If swallowed, remove drug from stomach by gastric lavage or emesis. Have available antidote physostigmine, diazepam to control CNS stimulation, oxygen, measures to treat respiratory depression and hyperpyrexia.

■ Protected in light-resistant containers at room temperature, preferably between 15° and 30°C (59° and 86°F) unless otherwise directed by manufacturer.

Diagnostic test interferences Upper GI series findings may require qualification because of anticholinergic effects of atropine (reduced gastric motility).

A

ATROPINE SULPHATE (continued)
DRUG INTERACTIONS   *Atropine (and other anticholinergic drugs)*_____

PLUS	INTERACTIONS
Amantadine	Enhanced anticholinergic effects (especially with high doses)
Antidepressants; tricyclics	Additive anticholinergic effects
Levodopa	Decreased levodopa effect; (delayed gastric emptying by anticholinergic drugs increases gastric degradation of levodopa). Used concurrently with caution
Methotrimeprazine	Possibility of precipitating extrapyramidal symptoms. Used concurrently with caution
MAO inhibitors	Action of anticholinergic drugs may be potentiated
Nitrofurantoin	Increased nitrofurantoin effect (decreased GI motility by anticholinergics results in increased nitrofurantoin absorption)
Phenothiazines	Decreased antipsychotic effect of phenothiazines. (Anticholinergics may reduce GI absorption of phenothiazines.) Used concurrently with caution

Azatadine maleate ▬▬▬▬▬▬▬▬▬▬▬▬▬▬▬▬▬▬▬▬▬▬▬▬▬

(Optimine)   *Antihistamine; H_1-receptor antagonist*

ACTIONS AND USES   Long-acting antihistamine acts by competitively antagonizing the effects of histamine at H_1-receptor sites on smooth muscle of blood vessels, bronchioles, and GI tract. This action blocks or reduces intensity of allergic responses and cell tissue injury associated with histamine release. In common with other antihistamines, has anticholinergic and sedative actions. Also reported to have antiserotonin activity.

Used for symptomatic relief of hay fever, allergic rhinitis, and chronic urticaria.

ROUTE AND DOSAGE   Oral: 1 or 2 mg twice a day, usually in the morning and evening. **Child**: 1–5 yr 250 mcg, 6–12 yrs 0.5–1 mg both twice daily.

ABSORPTION AND FATE   Readily absorbed from GI tract. **Plasma levels peak** in about 4 hours. Probably crosses blood–brain barrier since it causes CNS effects. Minimally bound to plasma proteins. **Half-life**: 9 to 12 hours. About 50% of dose excreted in urine within 5 days, 20% as unchanged drug. Appears to cross placenta. Distribution into breast milk not known.

CONTRAINDICATIONS AND PRECAUTIONS   Hypersensitivity to other H_1-receptor antagonists; MAO inhibitor therapy, lower respiratory tract disease including asthma.

AZATADINE MALEATE (continued)

Safe use during pregnancy in nursing women, and in children under age 12 not established. **Cautious Use:** increased intraocular pressure, narrow-angle glaucoma, pyloroduodenal obstruction, stenosing peptic ulcer, prostatic hypertrophy, bladder neck obstruction; history of bronchial asthma, hyperthyroidism, hypertension, cardiovascular disease, patients with convulsive disorders.

ADVERSE/SIDE EFFECTS   These include: drowsiness (common); dizziness, disturbed coordination, fatigue, confusion, paraesthesias, neuritis; excitation, nervousness, euphoria. **CNS stimulation:** restlessness, hysteria, insomnia, tremor, irritability, convulsions. Other side effects include: hypotension, palpitation, tachycardia, extrasystoles, nasal stuffiness; dryness of nose, mouth and throat; tinnitus, labyrinthitis (vertigo), epigastric distress, nausea, vomiting, anorexia, diarrhoea or constipation, urinary frequency, dysuria, urinary retention, early menses. Some rare adverse effects are: haemolytic anaemia, thrombocytopenia, agranulocytosis. Finally, urticaria, rash, photosensitivity, anaphylactic shock, blurred vision, diplopia, dilated pupils, thickening of bronchial secretions, chest tightness and wheezing can occur in some people. **Other:** excessive perspiration, chills, headache.

NURSING IMPLICATIONS

- GI side effects may be minimized by administering drug with food or milk.
- Because drug commonly causes drowsiness, sedation, and dizziness, caution patient not to drive a car or engage in other potentially hazardous activities until reaction to drug is known.
- Azatadine is most likely to cause sedation, dizziness, hypotension, and confusion in the elderly. Advise patient to report these effects. Reduction in dosage may be indicated.
- Patient should be informed that azatadine may produce additive CNS depression with alcohol and other CNS depressants (e.g., sedatives, anxiolytics, sleep medications).
- Dry mouth (xerostomia) may be relieved by the following measures: (1) frequent rinses with tepid water. Preferred to commercial mouth washes, overuse of which can change oral flora, also many contain alcohol which enhances drying; (2) increase fluid intake (if allowed) or at least maintain normal intake; (3) brush with soft tooth brush after every meal; (4) floss teeth daily with waxed floss or ribbon; (5) sugarless gum or sugarless lemon drops; (6) use of artificial saliva.
- **Treatment of overdosage**   is symptomatic and supportive. Vomiting is induced by ipecacuanha syrup. Following emesis, activated charcoal slurry and if necessary gastric lavage is given. Have on hand vasopressors, short-acting barbiturates, diazepam or paraldehyde, and equipment for respiratory assistance.
- Stored in tightly closed container at room temperature, preferably between 2° and 30°C (36° and 86°F), unless otherwise directed by manufacturer.

Diagnostic test interferences   As a general rule, H_1-receptor antagonists are discontinued about 4 days before skin testing procedures are to be performed since they may produce false-negative results.

AZATADINE MALEATE (continued)
DRUG INTERACTIONS   *Azatadine*

PLUS	INTERACTIONS
Alcohol (Ethanol) and other CNS depressants	Possibility of additive CNS depression
Anticoagulants, oral	Action may be reduced by azatadine
MAO inhibitors	May prolong and intensify anticholinergic effects of azatadine
Tricyclic antidepressants	Possibility of additive CNS and anticholinergic effects

Azathioprine

(Imuran, Azamune)   *Immunosuppressant*

ACTIONS AND USES   Imidazolyl derivative of mercaptopurine (6-mercaptopurine) to which it is metabolized in body. Precise mechanism of action not determined. Antagonizes purine metabolism and appears to inhibit DNA, RNA, and normal protein synthesis in rapidly growing cells. Suppresses T-cell effects before transplant rejection, i.e., during induction phase of antibody response.

Used as adjunctive agent to prevent rejection of kidney allografts, usually with other immunosuppressants. Also used in selective patients with severe, active rheumatoid arthritis unresponsive to conventional therapy, in patients with myasthenia gravis refractory to other therapy, and in treatment of systemic lupus erythematosus, Crohn's disease, polymyositis, idiopathic thrombocytopenia, and other systemic inflammatory and autoimmune diseases.

ROUTE AND DOSAGE   Highly individualized on basis of clinical response and haematopoietic toxicity. **Oral:** 1–5 mg/kg daily.

ABSORPTION AND FATE   Readily absorbed following oral or IV administration. Well distributed throughout body. Metabolized primarily by xanthine oxidase in liver to active metabolite mercaptopurine. About 30% bound to plasma proteins. Approximately 50% of dose eliminated in urine within 24 hours; small amount excreted as unchanged azathioprine and mercaptopurine. **Half-life** of active metabolite and azathioprine approximately 3 hours. Crosses placenta.

CONTRAINDICATIONS AND PRECAUTIONS   Hypersensitivity to drug; clinically active infection, anuria, pancreatitis, patients receiving alkylating agents (increased risk of neoplasms). Safe use during pregnancy and in women of childbearing potential not established. **Cautious Use:** impaired kidney and liver function, patients receiving cadaveric kidney.

ADVERSE/SIDE EFFECTS   These include: nausea, vomiting, anorexia, ulcerations of lips and mouth, oesophagitis, diarrhoea, steatorrhoea, (bone marrow depression):

AZATHIOPRINE (continued)

leucopenia, acute leukaemia, macrocytic anaemia, aplastic anaemia, agranulocytosis, pancytopaenia, thrombocytopenia, hepatitis with elevations in bilirubin, alkaline phosphatase, SGOT, SGPT; biliary stasis. **Hypersensitivity**: skin eruptions, formication (sensation of crawling ants), serum sickness, polyarthritis, polyneuritis, allergic hepatitis, interstitial pneumonitis. **Other**: secondary infection (immunosuppression); acute pancreatitis, dysphagia, dysarthria, alopecia, muscle wasting (negative nitrogen balance), drug fever, Raynaud's phenomenon, pulmonary oedema, arthralgia retinopathy. Carcinogenic and teratogenic potential reported.

NURSING IMPLICATIONS

- Gastric disturbances may be minimized by administering oral drug in divided doses (prescribed), or with or immediately after meals.
- Azathioprine sodium for IV injection is reconstituted by adding 5 ml sterile water for injection into vial. Swirl vial until drug is dissolved.
- For IV infusion, reconstituted solution may be further diluted with sodium chloride injection or 5% dextrose in sodium chloride injection.
- Azathioprine therapy is usually instituted 1 to 5 days before kidney transplantation and restarted within 24 hours post transplantation.
- Azathioprine carries warning that chronic immunosuppression may increase risk of neoplasia and haematologic toxicity, and that it has mutagenic potential in both men and women.
- Close medical supervision both in and out of hospital is necessary during therapy. The patient should understand toxicity potential, as well as expected benefits. Clinical effects of azathioprine appear within 2 to 4 days of administration.
- Complete blood counts, including platelets, and liver and kidney function tests should be performed prior to and at least weekly during first month of therapy, twice monthly during second and third months, and monthly, or more frequently if indicated, thereafter.
- Kidney function is monitored to prevent drug accumulation (urine protein, urine electrolytes, creatinine clearance, serum creatinine, BUN).
- Surveillance of fluid intake and output ratio is crucial. Up to a twofold increase in toxicity is possible in anephric or anuric patients. Note colour, character, and specific gravity of urine. Report an abrupt decrease in urinary output or any change in intake and output ratio.
- Azathioprine has a high toxic potential. Because it may have delayed action, dosage should be reduced or drug withdrawn at the first indication of a decreasing leucocyte or platelet count to avoid irreversible bone marrow depression.
- Thrombocytopenia occurs less commonly than leucopenia; however, be alert to signs of abnormal bleeding (easy bruising, bleeding gums, petechiae, purpura, melaena, epistaxis, haemoptysis, haematemesis).
- If *hepatic dysfunction* develops (pruritus, abdominal pain, and distention, clay-coloured stools, dark urine, yellow skin, and sclera) report promptly.
- Intercurrent infection is a constant hazard of immunosuppressive therapy. Monitor vital signs. Warn patient to avoid contact with persons who have colds or other infections and to report signs of impending infection (coryza, fever, chills, sore throat, malaise) which are also possible symptoms of agranulocytosis. Personal

AZATHIOPRINE (continued)

hygiene should be scrupulous. Azathioprine dosage may be reduced until the infection is controlled by appropriate therapy.

- Hospitalized patient may be in isolation for protection. Explain significance to patient and family.
- Patients should be advised to practice birth control during azathioprine therapy and for 4 months after discontinuation.
- Patient should be informed that vaccinations or other immunity conferring agents may cause unusually severe reactions because of the immunosuppressive effects of azathioprine.
- Preserved in tightly closed, light-resistant containers at room temperature, preferably between 15° and 30°C (59° and 86°F), unless otherwise directed by manufacturer.

Diagnostic test interferences   Azathioprine may decrease plasma and urinary uric acid in patients with gout.

DRUG INTERACTIONS   *Azothioprine*

PLUS	INTERACTIONS
Allopurinol	Increased pharmacological effect and toxicity of azothioprine (inhibition of xanthine oxidase by allopurinol interferes with degradation of active metabolite [mercaptopurine] to inactive products). Dosage of azothioprine should be reduced by one-third to one fourth
Anticoagulants, oral	Possibility of reduced anticoagulant effect
Tubocurarine, and other nondepolarizing skeletal relaxants	Neuromuscular blocking effect may be reversed or inhibited by azathioprine

Azlocillin

(Securopen)

*Antiinfective; antibiotic
(beta lactam); penicillin*

ACTIONS AND USES   Semisynthetic, extended spectrum, bactericidal acylureido-penicillin. Antibacterial spectrum similar to that of mezlocillin, but azlocillin is more active against *Pseudomonas aeruginosa* and less active against *Klebsiella*. Believed to act by interfering with bacterial cell wall synthesis.

Used primarily for treatment of serious infections caused by *Pseudomonas aeruginosa* in lower respiratory tract, urinary tract, skin and skin structures, bone and joints, and for bacterial septicaemia. Most often used concurrently with an aminoglycoside, e.g., amikacin for synergistic effects against *Pseudomonas* strains.

ROUTE AND DOSAGE   Intravenous (direct slow IV injection or intermittent IV infusion): by bolus injection up to 2 g every 8 hours, by infusion doses 2−5 g over 20−30 min every 8 hours.

AZLOCILLIN (continued)

ABSORPTION AND FATE   Following IV administration, distributed in active form to bile, serum, urine, bronchial and wound secretions, bone, and other tissues. Poor CSF penetration unless meninges are inflamed. Bile levels approximately 15 times higher than serum levels. **Elimination half-life**: 55 to 70 minutes (longer with impaired renal function); 25 to 45% **protein bound**. Less than 10% metabolized by liver. About 50 to 70% of dose eliminated unchanged in urine within 24 hours; 20 to 25% excreted unchanged in bile. Crosses placenta. Low concentrations in breast milk.

CONTRAINDICATIONS AND PRECAUTIONS   Hypersensitivity to any of the penicillins or cephalosporins; common bile duct obstruction. Safe use during pregnancy not established. **Cautious Use**: impaired renal or hepatic function, history of drug allergy or hypersensitivity to multiple allergens; nursing mothers, history of bleeding disorders, GI disease; patients on restricted sodium intake, hypokalaemia and other electrolyte imbalances, dehydration.

ADVERSE/SIDE EFFECTS   These include: headache, dizziness, overdosage: neuromuscular hyperirritability, convulsive seizures, disturbances of taste and smell, stomatitis, flatulence, nausea, vomiting, diarrhoea, epigastric pain, eosinophilia, leucopenia, neutropenia, thrombocytopenia; decreased: Hgb and Hct, and serum uric acid; prolonged prothrombin and bleeding times, hypokalaemia; increased: serum alkaline phosphatases, LDH, bilirubin, creatinine, BUN, SGPT (ALT), and SGOT (AST); hypernatraemia, rash, pruritus, urticaria, arthralgia, myalgia, drug fever, chills, chest discomfort, anaphylactic reactions, superinfections, transient chest discomfort with rapid IV injection: pain and thrombophlebitis at IV site.

NURSING IMPLICATIONS

- Culture and sensitivity tests should be performed before initiation of drug therapy and periodically thereafter to detect possible emergence of bacterial resistance. Treatment may begin pending test results.
- Azlocillin is administered either by direct slow IV injection over 5 minutes or longer, or by IV infusion over 30 minutes. Rapid IV injection can cause transient chest pains.
- A careful drug history should be obtained before initiation of therapy to determine patient's previous exposure and sensitivity to penicillin, cephalosporin, and other allergens.
- When other antibiotics are prescribed concomitantly with azlocillin, it is advisable to administer each drug separately because mutual inactivation may occur when mixed together.
- Baseline and periodic evaluation of renal, hepatic, and haematopoietic functions, and serum electrolytes, especially K and Na, is advisable during prolonged therapy.
- Monitor fluid intake and output ratio and pattern, particularly in patients with impaired renal function. Serum drug and creatinine levels and creatinine clearance are recommended to determine appropriate dosages.
- Although rare, azlocillin can cause abnormalities in coagulation tests (thrombocytopenia), particularly in patients with renal impairment. Check values of clotting time, platelet aggregation, prothrombin, and partial prothrombin times. Instruct

AZLOCILLIN (continued)

patient to report any unexplained bleeding or bruising (haematomas, petechiae, ecchymoses).

- Superinfections occur commonly during prolonged use of extended spectrum antibiotics. Be alert to symptoms and report their onset immediately to physician, e.g., fever, cough, sore mouth or throat (oral thrush), vaginitis, diarrhoea.
- For treatment of anaphylactoid reactions, have on hand epinephrine, IV steroids, oxygen, equipment for intubation and for maintaining airway.
- Therapy is generally continued for at least 2 days after signs and symptoms have disappeared. Usual duration of therapy is 10 to 14 days, but may be longer in complicated infections.
- If Y-type or 'piggyback' method of administration is used, infusion of any other solution should be temporarily discontinued during administration of azlocillin.
- Reconstituted solutions should be clear, colourless to pale yellow, and free of particulate matter. Solutions are stable at room temperature for 24 hours (potency loss less than 10%) in suitable diluents (see above). Concentrations up to 100 mg/ml are stable for 24 hours when refrigerated below 8°C (46.4°F).
- Prior to reconstitution, store vial containing azlocillin below 30°C (86°F), unless otherwise directed by manufacturer.

Diagnostic test interferences   Transient lowering of **serum uric acid** levels. False-positive **urinary protein** reactions (pseudoproteinuria) with many methods; bromphenol blue (multi-stix) method reportedly reliable. **Platelet abnormalities** may persist for as long as 2 weeks following drug discontinuation.

DRUG INTERACTIONS *Azlocillin*

PLUS	INTERACTIONS
Aminoglycosides	Synergistic effect; however, physiochemical inactivation can occur depending on contact time. Scheduling 1 hour apart may help
Anticoagulants, oral	Increased risk of bleeding (by platelet function impairment)
Chloramphenicol Erythromycins Sulphonamides Tetracyclines	Possibility of azlocillin antagonism. Concurrent use generally avoided
Contraceptives, oral	Effectiveness of oral contraceptives may be reduced because of increased (unsubstantiated report) oestrogen metabolism
Probenecid	Increased azlocillin serum levels and half-life (by decreasing renal tubular secretion of azlocillin)

Aztreonam

(Azactam)   *Antiinfective; beta-lactam*

AZTREONAM (continued)

ACTIONS AND USES Recently introduced monocyclic beta-lactam antibiotic active against gram-negative aerobic bacteria including *Neisseria gonorrhoea*, *Pseudomonas aeruginosa* and *Haemophillus influenzae*. Used to treat sensitive infections.

ROUTE AND DOSAGE IM infection, IV injection or infusion: 1 g/8 hourly or 2 g/12 hourly increased to 2 g every 6–8 hours in severe infections. *Urinary tract infection*: 0.5–1 g/8–12 hourly. *Gonorrhoea*: single dose of 1 g by IM route.

CONTRAINDICATIONS, ADVERSE, AND SIDE EFFECTS Not recommended for children. *See gentamicin.*

NURSING IMPLICATIONS
- Single doses over 1 g should be given by the IM route.
- Adverse reactions should be reported to the Committee on Safety of Medicines.

Bacampicillin Hydrochloride

(Ambaxin)

For further information *see ampicillin*

Baclofen

(Lioresal)   *Skeletal muscle relaxant*

ACTIONS AND USES Centrally acting skeletal muscle relaxant. Depresses polysynaptic afferent reflex activity at spinal cord level thereby reducing skeletal muscle spasm caused by upper motor neuron lesions. Relaxes external sphincter of the hyperreflexic urinary bladder and appears to have an anticholinergic-like effect on involuntary bladder contractions.

Used to provide symptomatic relief of painful spasms in multiple sclerosis and in the management of detrusor sphincter dyssynergia in spinal cord injury or disease.

ROUTE AND DOSAGE Oral: 5 mg three times a day; increased gradually until optimum response obtained. Total daily dosage should not exceed 100 mg.

ABSORPTION AND FATE Rapidly absorbed from GI tract and widely distributed in body. Absorption thought to be dose-dependent; reduced absorption occurs at high dosage levels. Wide individual variations in extent of absorption and elimination. **Peak serum levels** appear in 2 to 3 hours; significant levels persist about 8 hours. Approximately 30% protein bound. **Half-life:** 3 to 4 hours. About 15% of dose metabolized in liver. Primarily eliminated in urine within 72 hours, mostly as unchanged drug (70 to 85%); remainder excreted in faeces. Crosses placenta.

BACLOFEN (continued)

CONTRAINDICATIONS AND PRECAUTIONS Hypersensitivity to baclofen. Safe use during pregnancy, in nursing mothers, and in children under 12 years not established. **Cautious Use**: impaired renal and hepatic function, epilepsy, diabetes mellitus, patients with psychiatric or brain disorders, peptic ulcer.

ADVERSE/SIDE EFFECTS These include: hypotension, nausea, vomiting, transient drowsiness, vertigo, dizziness, weakness, fatigue; ataxia, headache, confusion, insomnia; rarely: paraesthesias, tremors, dysarthria (slurred speech), muscle pain and rigidity, hypotonia, euphoria, excitement, depression, hallucinations, loss of seizure control in epileptic patients; respiratory depression, seizures, coma (overdosage).

NURSING IMPLICATIONS

- If patient complains of GI distress, drug may be administered with food.
- Supervise ambulation. In common with other skeletal muscle relaxants, initially, the loss of spasticity induced by baclofen may affect patient's ability to stand or walk. (In some patients, spasticity associated with multiple sclerosis and spinal cord disease helps patient to maintain upright posture and balance.)
- Advise patient to report adverse reactions to physician. Most can be reduced by decreasing dosage. Incidence of CNS symptoms (drowsiness, dizziness, ataxia) reportedly high in patients over 40 years of age. Dose increases should be made with caution.
- Caution patient that CNS depressant effects of baclofen will be additive to other CNS depressants, including alcohol.
- Patients with epilepsy should be closely monitored by EEG, clinical observation and interview at regular intervals for possible loss of seizure control.
- Inform diabetic patients that baclofen may raise blood glucose levels. Urge patient to report promptly changes in urine or blood tests to the physician. Dose adjustment of insulin may be indicated during and after baclofen treatment is stopped for a short period.
- Warn patient to avoid driving and other potentially hazardous activities until the reaction to baclofen is determined.
- Observe for and record patient's response to drug. Therapeutic effectiveness may be noted in a few hours to weeks by: decrease in frequency of spasms and in severity of knee and ankle clonus, increase in ease and range of joint motion and in performance of activities of daily living. If therapeutic effectiveness is not observed within a reasonable trial period (1 to 2 months), drug should be withdrawn.
- Caution patient not to self-dose with OTC drugs without physician's approval.
- The elderly are especially sensitive to this drug. Observe carefully for side effects: mental confusion, depression, hallucinations.
- Inform patient that drug withdrawal should be accomplished gradually over a 1- to 2-week period. Abrupt withdrawal following prolonged administration may cause anxiety, agitated behaviour, auditory and visual hallucinations, severe tachycardia, and acute exacerbation of spasticity.
- **_Treatment of overdosage_** If patient is alert, emesis is induced, followed by gastric lavage. If patient is obtunded: maintain adequate respiratory exchanges, without

BACLOFEN (continued)

use of respiratory stimulants, and maintain high urinary output. Dialysis may be indicated in renal failure.

■ Store at room temperature, preferably between 15° and 30°C (59° and 86°F) in tightly closed container, unless otherwise directed by manufacturer.

B

Diagnostic test interferences   Possibility of increased blood glucose, serum alkaline phosphatase, and SGOT (AST) levels.

DRUG INTERACTIONS *Baclofen*

PLUS	INTERACTIONS
CNS depressants, e.g., alcohol, antihistamines, general anaesthetics, tricyclic antidepressants, barbiturates and other sedatives,and skeletal muscle relaxants	Additive CNS depression

Beclomethasone diproprionate

(Becloforte, Beclotide, Beconase, Ventide)   *Corticosteroid*

ACTIONS AND USES   Synthetic corticosteroid with potent antiinflammatory activity. When applied topically (by oral and nasal inhalation) about 10 to 15% dose reaches mucous membranes of the bronchioles and bronchi; the remainder deposits in the oropharynx to be swallowed. Due to metabolic inactivation by first-pass metabolism, beclomethasone produces little or no glucocorticoid action usually associated with oral and parenteral corticosteroids. Action mechanism on lung tissue unknown, but its effect is to suppress signs and symptoms of bronchial asthma in patients not responding to bronchodilators or nonsteroid treatment. Unlike hydrocortisone (q.v.), this corticosteroid does not suppress the hypothalamus–pituitary–adrenal function.

Used to treat chronic steroid-dependent bronchial asthma adjunctively with other therapy (sympathomimetics, xanthines), and for treatment of seasonal and perennial rhinitis. Beclomethasone is prophylactic and fails to provide immediate benefit in acute asthma. Has been used for symptomatic treatment of nasal polyposis.

ROUTE AND DOSAGE   Oral inhalation: 100 mcg (2 puffs Becotide) 3–4 times a day or 200 mcg (4 puffs) twice a day; in severe asthma dose may be increased to 500 mcg (2 puffs Becloforte) twice a day or 250–500 mcg (1–2 puffs) 3–4 times a day. Child 50–100 mcg (1–2 puffs Beclotide) 2–4 times a day. In combination with salbutamol (Ventide) 2 puffs 3–4 times a day. Child 1–2 puffs 2–4 times a day.

ABSORPTION AND FATE   Systemic absorption occurs promptly following inhalation. Rapidly metabolized in lung and GI tissues, and in liver; 87% bound to plasma protein. Half-life of inhaled dose: first phase, 3 hours; second phase, about 15 hours. Drug

BECLOMETHASONE DIPROPRIONATE (continued)

and its metabolites are excreted principally in faeces (over 90%); remainder excreted in urine. Possibly crosses placenta, and secreted in breast milk.

CONTRAINDICATIONS AND PRECAUTIONS   Hypersensitivity to beclomethasone or to any ingredient in the formulation, e.g., oleic acid, fluorocarbons, asthma adequately controlled by bronchodilators or nonsteroidal medication; nonasthmatic bronchitis, primary treatment of status asthmaticus, acute attack of asthma, bronchopulmonary mycoses, or other untreated infections of mouth, throat or lungs. Safe use during pregnancy; in the nursing mother, in women of childbearing potential and in children younger than 6 years not established. **Cautious Use**: patients receiving systemic corticosteroids; nasal septal ulcers, nasal trauma, or surgery. *See also hydrocortisone.*

ADVERSE/SIDE EFFECTS   Candidal infection of oropharynx and occasionally larynx especially with oral inhalation (75% of patients, especially females); unmasking of previously suppressed allergic conditions; hoarseness, dry mouth, sore throat, sore mouth; rarely, bronchospasm; rash. With use of nasal inhaler: epistaxis, bloody mucus, nasopharyngeal itching, dryness, crusting, and ulceration; transient irritation, burning, sneezing. *See also hydrocortisone.*

NURSING IMPLICATIONS

- Instructions for inhaler use are included with package. Review information with patient to assure complete understanding.
- If patient is also receiving bronchodilators by inhalation isoprenaline, adrenaline, etc.), bronchodilator should be used several minutes before beclomethasone aerosol to enhance penetration of the steroid into the bronchial tree and to reduce the potential toxicity of fluorocarbon propellants.
- Improvement in pulmonary function may require as long as 3 weeks when beclomethasone is given to patient not receiving systemic steroids.
- Rinsing mouth and gargling with warm water after each inhalation removes residual medication thereby preventing further drug absorption. Mouth care may also delay or prevent onset of oral dryness, hoarseness, and candidiasis.
- Oral membranes should be inspected frequently for indications of candida infection (white patches, red, sore membranes) and patient should be questioned about symptoms, e.g., cough, sore mouth or throat. If present, antifungal therapy (e.g., Nystatin) will be instituted.
- Warn patient not to use higher than recommended doses or regular doses at shorter intervals. If response is not adequate, notify physician.
- Clean inhaler daily: remove cap and nosepiece from canister, rinse with warm water, and dry thoroughly.
- When patient dependent on systemic steroids is transferred to beclomethasone, management may be troublesome because recovery from suppressed adrenal function may require as long as 12 months.
- Monitor blood pressure and weight during withdrawal–transfer period. Hypotension and weight loss (signs of adrenal insufficiency) indicate need for temporary boost in systemic steroid and slower withdrawal schedule.
- During period of steroid withdrawal, symptoms of adrenal insufficiency (joint and/or

BECLOMETHASONE DIPROPRIONATE (continued)

muscular pain, depression, lassitude, fatigue, weakness, dizziness, light-headedness (hypotension]) may occur in spite of maintenance and even improvement of respiratory function.

- During transfer from systemic steroid therapy to aerosol administration, conditions previously suppressed (rhinitis, conjunctivitis, eczema) may be unmasked. Instruct patient to report to physician promptly.
- Caution patient/significant other to report to the physician if stress (e.g., infection, trauma, surgery, gastroenteritis, emotional crisis) or a severe asthma attack occurs during transfer period. Supplemental treatment with large doses of systemic steroid will be required.
- Patient should have a reserve supply of oral corticosteroid and be instructed to use it during time of extreme stress or a severe asthma attack.
- Patient should carry a card indicating need for supplementary systemic steroid during a severe asthma attack or periods of stress.
- Long-term effects of beclomethasone have not been determined. Specifically, local effects of drug deposits on oropharyngeal membranes and lung tissue as well as long-term systemic effects, are unknown.
- When symptoms for which beclomethasone was prescribed are relieved, dosage should be reduced gradually to lowest effective level. Keep physician informed.
- Urge patient to keep follow-up appointments. Periodic evaluation of therapy is essential.
- Store inhaler and aerosol dispenser out of reach of children.
- Keep inhaler away from open flame or heat above 120°F (may cause bursting). Do not puncture container and do not discard into fire or incinerator.
- Store between 15° and 30°C (59° and 86°F), unless otherwise directed by manufacturer.
- *See hydrocortisone.*
- Similar drug budesonide (Pulmicort).

Belladonna alkaloids

(Alka-Donna, Aluhyde, Bellocarb, Carbellon, Neutradonna, Peptard)

Anticholinergic (parasympatholytic); antispasmodic; belladonna alkaloid

ACTIONS AND USES Prepared from *Atropa belladonna* (deadly nightshade). Shares same actions, precautions, and adverse reactions as other tertiary amine antimuscarinics; *see atropine.*

Used as adjunct to suppress gastric secretions in gastric and duodenal ulcers, and to inhibit spasms and motility in spastic or irritable colon, mucous colitis, diarrhoea, diverticulitis, and pancreatitis. Usually in combination with an antacid. Paediatric mixture contains 45 mcg/5 ml.

BELLADONNA ALKALOIDS (continued)

ROUTE AND DOSAGE   Oral: variable depends on the preparation. **Paediatric mixture:** up to 1 yr/5 ml, 1–5 yrs/10 ml give dose 30 min before food.

CONTRAINDICATIONS AND PRECAUTIONS   Obstructive uropathy, atony of urinary bladder, oesophageal reflux, obstructive disease of GI tract, severe ulcerative colitis, toxic megacolon, myasthenia gravis, narrow-angle glaucoma, cardiovascular disease. *See also atropine.*

ADVERSE/SIDE EFFECTS   Dry mouth, choking sensation, mydriasis, blurred vision, acute glaucoma, urinary hesitancy or retention (especially older males), constipation, headache, drowsiness, excitement/palpitation, mental confusion, tachycardia. *See also atropine.*

NURSING IMPLICATIONS

■ When given for GI problems, usually administered 30 to 60 minutes before meals and at bedtime.

■ Dosage should be reduced if flushing or other signs of toxicity appear.

■ Because of the possibility of heat intolerance, caution patient to avoid hot baths, saunas, strenuous work or exercise during hot and humid weather.

■ Advise patient to refrain from driving and other potentially hazardous activities until reaction to drug is determined.

■ If mouth dryness is a problem instruct patient to practise meticulous oral hygiene. Sugarless gum or lemon drops may help. *See atropine.*

■ Store preferably at 15° to 30°C (59° to 86°F) in tightly covered, light-resistant containers, unless otherwise directed by manufacturer.

■ *See also atropine.*

Bendrofluazide————————————————

Diuretic; thiazide

ACTIONS AND USES   Benzothiadazine (thiazide) derivative. Similar to chlorothiazide (q.v.) in pharmacological actions, uses, contraindications, precautions, adverse effects, and interactions. Reportedly does not alter serum electrolyte concentrations appreciably at recommended doses.

ROUTE AND DOSAGE   Oral: Adult: *Diuretic*: *Initial* 5–10 mg in the morning each, day or on 3–5 days of the week. *Maintenance* 2.5–15 mg 1–3 times a week. *Antihypertensive*: 2.5–5 mg/day as a single dose in the morning.

ABSORPTION AND FATE   Onset of diuretic effect in 1 to 2 hours; peaks between 6 to 12 hours and lasts 18 to 24 hours. Highly protein bound. Excreted unchanged in urine within 24 hours. *See chlorothiazide.*

BENDROFLUAZIDE (continued)
CONTRAINDICATIONS AND PRECAUTIONS   Anuria, hypersensitivity to thiazides, sulphonamides, pregnancy, lactation. **Cautious Use**: history of allergy, renal and hepatic disease, gout, diabetes mellitus, sympathectomy. *See also chlorothiazide.*

ADVERSE/SIDE EFFECTS   Xerostomia, sialadenitis, anorexia, unusual fatigue, paraesthesias, photosensitivity, vasculitis, orthostatic hypotension, agranulocytosis, electrolyte imbalance, hyperglycaemia, impaired glucose tolerance, hyperuricaemia, exacerbation of gout, systemic lupus erythematosis. *See also chlorothiazide.*

B

NURSING IMPLICATIONS
- Diuretic action lasts more than 18 hours permitting longer intervals between doses and therefore fewer problems with electrolyte balance.
- Administer drug early in AM after eating (to reduce gastric irritation) to prevent possibility of interrupted sleep because of diuresis.
- Antihypertensive effects may be noted in 3 to 4 days; maximal effects may require 3 to 4 weeks.
- Monitor blood pressure, fluid intake and output ratio and pattern, and weight particularly during first phase of antihypertensive therapy. Report a sudden fall in BP which may initiate severe postural hypotension and potentially dangerous perfusion problems of the extremities, especially in older patients.
- Older patients may be sensitive to average doses. Orthostatic hypotension and hypokalaemia may be the most distressing side effects.
- Monitor patient for hypokalaemia: dry mouth, anorexia, thirst, paraesthesias, muscle cramps, cardiac arrhythmias. Report promptly. Physician may change dose and institute supplement therapy.
- Hypokalaemia is rarely severe in most patients even on long-term therapy with thiazides. To prevent onset, urge patient to eat a normal diet (usually includes K-rich foods such as fruit juices, potatoes, cereals, skimmed milk) and to include a banana (about 370 mg K) and at least 6 ounces orange juice (about 330 mg K) every day.
- If hypokalaemia develops, dietary K supplement of 1,000 to 2,000 mg (25 to 50 mEq) is usually an adequate treatment.
- Dietary management is important in thiazide treatment for hypertension. The physician will specifically order the goal of diet, i.e., electrolyte, weight, or fluid control. Collaborate with dietitian and arrange for patient–dietitian planning for an individualized diet.
- Asymptomatic hyperuricaemia can be produced because of interference with uric acid excretion although thiazides rarely precipitate acute gout. Report onset of joint pain and limitation of motion. Patient with history of gout may be continued on a thiazide with adjusted dosage of uricosuric agent.
- Counsel patient to avoid use of OTC drugs unless approved by physician. Many preparations contain both potassium and sodium and if misused, or if patient overdoses, could induce electrolyte side effects.
- Notify the anaesthetist that patient is on thiazide therapy.
- Store tablets in tightly closed container, preferably at 15° to 30°C (59°C to 86°F), unless otherwise specified by the manufacturer.
- *See chlorothiazide.*

BENDROFLUAZIDE (continued)
DRUG INTERACTIONS *Bendrofluazide*

PLUS	INTERACTIONS
Cholestyramine Colestipol	Pharmacological effects of thiazide may be reduced. Separate administration as far apart as possible
Diazoxide	Additive pharmacological effects of both drugs. Monitor for hyperglycaemia, hyperuricaemia, hypotension
Digitalis glycosides	Thiazide induced hypokalaemia can sensitize myocardium to digitalis toxicity. Monitor serum potassium
Lithium	Possibility of lithium toxicity (renal lithium excretion reduced). Monitor serum lithium levels
Tolbutamide and other sulphonylureas	Decreased hypoglycaemic effects. Higher sulphonylureas doses may be necessary

See chlorothiazide for other possible interactions

Benperidol

(Anquil)   *Neuroleptic*

For further information *see Haloperidol*

ROUTE AND DOSAGE   Oral: 0.25 – 1.5 mg/day in divided doses.

Benzoyl peroxide

(Acetoxyl, Acnegel Benoxyl, Benzagel, Clearasil   *Keratolytic*
  Nericur, Quinoderm, Theraderm)

ACTIONS AND USES   Slowly releases oxygen that exerts bactericidal action on *Propionibacterium* (*Corynebacterium*) *acnes*, anaerobic rods found in sebaceous follicles and comedones responsible for formation of irritating free fatty acids in sebum. In addition to being an oxidizing agent, it also has antiseborrhoeic (drying) and keratolytic (peeling) actions which help to keep pilosebaceous orifices open and draining properly. Reportedly not as effective as retinoic acid in comedolytic activity.

Used in local treatment of mild to moderate acne vulgaris and acne rosacea.

ROUTE AND DOSAGE   Topical: Apply one or two times a day. Fair-skinned individuals are advised to initiate treatment with one application of lower concentration at bedtime.

BENZOYL PEROXIDE (continued)

ABSORPTION AND FATE   Approximately 50% of dose may be absorbed through skin. Major metabolite is benzoic acid. Excreted in urine as benzoate.

CONTRAINDICATIONS AND PRECAUTIONS   Hypersensitivity to benzoyl peroxide and to benzoic acid derivatives. Use on inflamed, denuded, thin, or highly sensitive skin.

ADVERSE/SIDE EFFECTS   Local skin irritation, feeling of warmth, stinging; excessive scaling, erythema, oedema (especially with gel preparation), allergic contact dermatitis.

NURSING IMPLICATIONS

- Avoid contact of medication with eyes, eyelids, lips, inside of nose, and sensitive skin areas of neck.
- It is usually advisable to initiate acne therapy with a single application of a small amount of medication until patient's reaction to drug is known. Some clinicians recommend the following conservative approach which may be modified for individual patients: apply medication for 15 minutes the first evening then wash off with soap and water, and dry well. Increase length of exposure by 15 minutes every evening until tolerated for 2 hours, then leave on overnight and wash off in the morning. Morning applications may be started when indicated.
- Inform patient that mild peeling and dryness are anticipated therapeutic actions. If these effects are not observed within 3 or 4 days, application should be increased to twice daily.
- Because benzoyl peroxide is an oxidizing agent, it may bleach coloured fabrics. Lotion and cleansing lotion formulations, particularly may also bleach hair.
- Some forms of benzoyl peroxide may be purchased OTC. The gels are reportedly more penetrating but also tend to be more drying and irritating.
- Forewarn patient that medication may cause transitory redness and feeling of warmth or slight smarting. If symptoms are excessive, advise patient to remove medication with mild soap and water, dry skin well. Application may be attempted cautiously the following day using less medication at reduced frequency.
- Advise patient that skin irritation caused by benzoyl peroxide may be further aggravated by harsh soap, vigorous scrubbing of skin, and by other acne medications.
- Benzoyl peroxide may be worn under makeup, if desired.
- Inform patient that if improvement does not occur within 2 weeks, consult a physician.
- Some patients develop a delayed hypersensitivity reaction to benzoyl peroxide. If allergic sensitization is suspected, it may be confirmed by a patch test with 5% benzoyl perozide in petrolatum.

Patient-teaching points for acne

- ☐ There is no single cause or treatment for acne. Therapy may control but does not cure it.
- ☐ Acne is not caused by inadequate washing. However, careful washing does help remove surface oil. If skin is oily, wash face several times a day with toilet soap; otherwise wash once or twice daily.
- ☐ Do not pick, squeeze, or finger lesions since infection and scarring may result.

BENZOYL PEROXIDE (continued)

☐ Use water based cosmetics.

☐ If skin is not irritated a *controlled* amount of sunlight may help to dry lesions.

☐ Shampoo frequently if hair is oily.

☐ Avoid greasy hair dressings and keep hair away from face.

☐ Based on present evidence, many clinicians are convinced that dietary restrictions are not warranted. However, if patient believes that certain foods cause flare-up of lesions he or she should be advised to omit these foods. Encourage patient to eat a well-balanced diet.

☐ Psychological support is needed and should be provided. Patient should be encouraged to ask questions and to express concerns.

☐ Some physicians teach responsible family member to remove large comedones using a loop extractor.

■ Preferably stored between 15° and 30°C (59° and 86°F), unless otherwise directed by manufacturer.

Benzhexol

(Artane, Bentex, Brofen)

Anticholinergic; antiparkinsonian agent

ACTIONS AND USES   Used to treat parkinsonism and related extrapyramidal symptoms of neuroleptic drugs such as chlorpromazine and haloperidol.

ROUTE AND DOSAGE   Oral: Adult: *initial* dose 1 mg/day increased to a *maintenance* dose of 5–15 mg/day in 3–4 divided doses.

For further information *see benztropine mesylate.*

Benztropine mesylate

(Cogentin)

Anticholinergic; (parasympatholytic); antiparkinsonian agent

ACTIONS AND USES   Synthetic centrally acting anticholinergic (antimuscarinic) agent, chemically similar to atropine and diphenhydramine. Also exhibits antihistaminic, and local anaesthetic activity. Acts by diminishing excess cholinergic effect associated with dopamine deficiency. (Normal motor activity relies upon a balance between cholinergic and dopaminergic activity in corpus striatum.) Suppresses tremor and rigidity; does not alleviate tardive dyskinesia.

B

BENZTROPINE MESYLATE (continued)

Used in symptomatic treatment of all forms of parkinsonism (arteriosclerotic, idiopathic, postencephalitic), and to relieve extrapyramidal symptoms associated with neuroleptic drugs e.g., haloperidol, phenothiazines, thiothixene. Commonly used as supplement to levodopa therapy.

ROUTE AND DOSAGE   *Parkinsonism*: **Oral**: *Initial*: 0.5 to 1 mg, gradually increased up to 6 mg/day if required and tolerated. (Generally low doses are given to patients with arteriosclerotic parkinsonism, the elderly, thin patients, and older children.) *Extrapyramidal reactions*: **Oral, intramuscular, intravenous**: 1 to 4 mg one or two times daily.

ABSORPTION AND FATE   Onset of action following IM and IV injections occurs within 15 minutes; onset occurs about 1 hour following oral administration. Effects may persist 6 to 10 hours or more.

CONTRAINDICATIONS AND PRECAUTIONS   Hypersensitivity to benztropine or to any ingredients in the formulation; narrow angle glaucoma, myasthenia gravis, obstructive diseases of GU and GI tracts, tendency to tachycardia, patients with tardive dyskinesia, children under 3 years of age. Safe use during childbearing potential, pregnancy and in nursing women not established. **Cautious Use**: older children, elderly or debilitated patients, patients with poor mental outlook, mental disorders. *See also atropine.*

ADVERSE/SIDE EFFECTS   These include: sedation, dizziness, nervousness, paraesthesias; in high doses: depression, preceded or followed by stimulation, agitation, hallucinations, delirium, mental confusion, toxic psychosis, muscular weakness, ataxia. Other adverse effects could include: palpitation, tachycardia, nausea, vomiting, xerostomia, constipation, paralytic ileus, dysuria, urinary retention. **Ophthalmic**: blurred vision, mydriasis, photophobia, anhidrosis. *See atropine for other possible adverse effects.*

NURSING IMPLICATIONS

- Administration of drug immediately after meals or with food may help to prevent gastric irritation. If patient cannot swallow tablet, it may be crushed prior to administration and sprinkled on or mixed with food.
- Patients with arteriosclerotic or idiopathic parkinsonism generally experience greatest relief by taking benztropine at bedtime. Younger patients with postencephalitic parkinsonism usually require more frequent doses.
- Physician will rely on accurate observations and reporting to establish patient's optimum dosage level and frequency of doses and to determine appropriateness of therapy. For example, if extrapyramidal (acute dystonic) reactions are not relieved, causes other than drug-induced must be investigated, e.g., hypocalcaemia.
- Patients with mental illness should be closely observed for intensification of mental symptoms, particularly during early therapy.
- When used as an adjunct to antipsychotic drugs, generally benztropine is not continued beyond 3 months because prolonged use may predispose patient to tardive dyskinesia.

B

BENZTROPINE MESYLATE (continued)

- Effects of benztropine are cumulative: therefore, clinical improvement may not be evident until 2 or 3 days after oral drug is started. Drug therapy is usually initiated at low doses, with subsequent increments of 0.5 mg made at 5- or 6-day intervals, if necessary.
- Elderly patients should not kept under close surveillance especially at beginning of drug therapy or whenever dosage increases are made.
- Monitor intake and output ratio and pattern. Advise patient to report difficulty in urination or infrequent voiding. Dosage reduction may be indicated.
- Appearance of intermittent constipation, abdominal pain, and distention may herald onset of paralytic ileus. Patients receiving combination drugs with anticholinergic action should be closely monitored for these symptoms.
- Therapeutic effect in the patient with parkinsonism is evidenced by lessening of rigidity, drooling (sialorrhoea) and oculogyric crises, and by improvement in gait, balance, and posture. Usually, tremors are not appreciably relieved. Note that muscle weakness is an adverse side effect and requires dosage reduction.
- Most of the atropine-like side effects of benztropine are controlled by adjustment of dosage. However, severe reactions, such as signs and symptoms of CNS depression or excitement, generally require interruption of drug therapy.
- Caution patient about possibility of drowsiness and blurred vision, and advise against operating vehicles or machinery or other activities requiring alertness until reaction to the drug is known. Supervision of ambulation and bedsides may be indicated.
- Inform patient that alcohol and other CNS depressants may cause additive drowsiness and therefore should be avoided. Also advise patient not to take OTC cold, cough, or hay fever remedies unless approved by physician because they commonly contain anticholinergic and antihistaminic agents.
- Mouth dryness may be relieved by frequent rinsing of mouth with tepid water, or by sugarless gum or boiled sweets, diligent dental hygiene such as brushing with soft tooth brush after meals and at bedtime, use of fluoride toothpaste, and daily flossing. If symptom persists, and particularly if associated with difficulty in swallowing, anorexia, and weight loss, benztropine dosage should be reduced or drug should be discontinued temporarily.
- Anhidrosis (diminished sweating) especially in hot weather, may require dose adjustments because of possibility of heat stroke. This condition is particularly apt to occur in the elderly patient. Check temperature daily in this age group. Caution patient to avoid doing manual labour or strenuous exercise in a hot environment.
- Benztropine has drug abuse potential and has been misused by narcotic addicts for its hallucinogenic effects.
- Preserved in tightly covered, light-resistant container at room temperature preferably between 15° and 30°C (59° and 86°F), unless otherwise directed by manufacturer.

DRUG INTERACTIONS   *Benztropine*

PLUS	INTERACTIONS
Alcohol and other CNS depressants	Potentiation of sedative and other CNS depressant effects

B

BENZTROPINE MESYLATE (continued)

PLUS	INTERACTIONS
(continued)	

Amantadine
Antidepressants, tricyclic
Antihistamines
MAO inhibitors
Phenothiazines
Procainamide
Quinidine

Additive anticholinergic (atropinelike) side effects: confusion, hallucinations, paralytic ileus. Used concomitantly with caution

---

Betahistine

(Serc)   *Antihistamine*

ACTION AND USES   Histamine agonist used for the treatment of vertigo and nausea due to Meniere's disease.

For further information *see chlorpromazine.*

ROUTE AND DOSAGE   8–16 mg/3 times a day after food maximum 48 mg/day.

CONTRAINDICATIONS AND PRECAUTIONS   Phaeochromocytoma, **cautious use** in asthma and peptic ulcer.

ADVERSE/SIDE EFFECTS   Nausea, rashes, sometimes headache.

Betamethasone

(Betnean, Betnesol, Diprosalic, Bextasol [inhalation],   *Corticosteroid*
    Betnovate and Fucibet [cream])

ACTIONS AND USES   Synthetic long-acting glucocorticoid with minor mineralocorticoid properties but strong immunosuppressive, antiinflammatory, and metabolic actions. Topical use provides relief of inflammatory manifestations of corticosteroid-responsive dermatoses.

With the exception of use as replacement therapy in adrenocortical insufficiency and salt-losing forms of adrenogenital syndromes, betamethasone has the same indications for use, absorption and fate, limitations of use, and adverse/side effects as hydrocortisone (q.v.).

ROUTE AND DOSAGE   Doses highly individualized on basis of response of patient and disease being treated. **Oral:** 0.5–5 mg/day. **Intramuscular/intravenous:** 4–20 mg up

B

BETAMETHASONE (continued)

to 4 times in 24 hrs. **Topical**: (valerate) apply a thin film to the affected part 1–3 times a day. **Inhalation**: (valerate) Adult, 200 mcg (2 puffs) 3–4 times a day. **Child:** 100 mcg (1 puff) 3–4 times a day reduce to the minimum effective dose.

NURSING IMPLICATIONS

- **Topical preparations**: *Lotions* are generally better for use on weeping lesions or on areas subject to friction (e.g., axilla, groin), and also for hairy areas. *Aerosols and gels* are appropriate for use on hairy areas, especially scalp. Ointments are mostly suitable for dry scaly lesions. They are the most occlusive of all topical forms. *Creams* are good for general use.
- Consult physician regarding cleansing skin before treatments. Some clinicians recommend thorough washing with mild soap and water before each application. Others prefer that area not be disturbed. *See hydrocortisone for special points about topical application.*
- Percutaneous absorption is enhanced by occlusion of the medication by means of plastic wrap or occlusive dressing. Adverse systemic steroid effects are most apt to occur if the skin is abraded or otherwise altered.
- Advise patient to avoid exposing areas treated with topical corticosteroid to sunlight. Severe burns have been reported, especially when occlusive dressing is used.
- Carefully and routinely note condition of skin to which topical betamethasone has been applied. Report evidence of limited response or intercurrent infection which may necessitate adjunctive treatment with an appropriate antifungal or antibacterial agent.
- See manufacturer's directions for stability and storage.
- *See hydrocortisone.*

Betaxolol hydrochloride

(Kerlone)   *Beta-adrenergic blocker*

ACTIONS AND USES   Hypertension.

ROUTE AND DOSAGE   Oral: 20 mg/day reduced to 10 mg for elderly patients, maximum 40 mg/day.

For further information *see propranolol.*

Bethanechol chloride

(Myotonine)   *Cholinergic*
                                                                      (parasympathomimetic)

BETHANECHOL CHLORIDE *(continued)*

ACTIONS AND USES   Synthetic choline ester with effects similar to those of acetyl-choline acts directly on postsynaptic receptors and, since it is not hydrolyzed by cholinesterase, its action is prolonged. Produces muscarinic effects primarily on GI tract and urinary bladder with minimal effects on CV system, autonomic ganglia, neuromuscular junction, sweat glands, salivary glands, and eyes. Increases tone and peristaltic activity of oesophagus, stomach, and intestines; contracts detrusor muscle of urinary bladder, usually enough to initiate micturition.

Used in treatment of acute postoperative and postpartum nonobstructive (functional) urinary retention, and for neurogenic atony of urinary bladder with retention.

ROUTE AND DOSAGE   Oral: Adults: 10 to 30 mg three to four times daily

ABSORPTION AND FATE   Onset of action occurs within 30 to 90 minutes following oral administration. Effects persist about 1 hour after oral administration (reportedly up to 6 hours with large doses). Excreted via kidneys.

CONTRAINDICATIONS AND PRECAUTIONS   Hypersensitivity to bethanechol; obstructive pulmonary disease, history of or active bronchial asthma, hyperthyroidism, recent urinary bladder surgery, cystitis, bacteriuria, urinary bladder neck or intestinal obstruction, peptic ulcer, recent GI surgery, peritonitis, marked vagotonia, pronounced vasomotor instability, AV conduction defects, severe bradycardia, hypotension or hypertension, coronary artery disease, recent myocardial infarction, epilepsy, parkinsonism.

ADVERSE/SIDE EFFECTS   Side effects include: hypotension with dizziness, faintness; orthostatic hypotension (large doses); mild reflex tachycardia, atrial fibrillation (hyperthyroid patients), transient complete heart block, transient syncope with cardiac arrest. In addition the following can occur: nausea, vomiting, abdominal cramps, bloody diarrhoea, borborygmi, belching, faecal incontinence (large doses), urge to defecate (or urinate) acute asthmatic attack, dyspnoea (large doses) flushing of skin, increased sweating, salivation and lacrimation, malaise, headache, blurred vision, miosis, substernal pain or pressure (possibly due to bronchoconstriction or oesophageal spasm), hypothermia. *Cholinergic overstimulation*: may occur with overdosage, hypersensitivity, fall in blood pressure, bradycardia, reflex tachycardia, severe abdominal cramps, bloody diarrhoea, shock, sudden cardiac arrest, circulatory collapse.

NURSING IMPLICATIONS
- Bethanechol should be given on an empty stomach ½ hour after or at least 2 hours after meals) to lessen possibility of nausea and vomiting, unless otherwise advised by physician.
- *To determine minimum effective oral dose*: physician may prescribe an initial test dose of 5 to 10 mg and a repeat of same dose at hourly intervals to a maximum of 30 mg, unless satisfactory response or disturbing side effects intervene. Alternatively, 10 mg followed at 6-hour intervals by 25 mg then 50 mg until desired response obtained.
- Adverse effects are most commonly associated with subcutaneous administration, and high oral doses. Monitor blood pressure and pulse in these patients. Report early signs of overdosage: salivation, sweating, flushing, abdominal cramps, nausea.
- Syringe containing atropine sulpate (specific antidote) should be ready for

B

BETHANECHOL CHLORIDE (continued)

instantaneous use to abolish severe side effects, 0.6 to 1.2 mg for adults administered IM, slow IV, or SC; and 0.01 mg/kg for infants and children repeated every 2 hours, if necessary. Specific directions for administering antidote should be prescribed by physician.

- Because orthostatic hypotension is a possible side effect, caution patient to make position changes slowly and in stages, particularly from recumbent to upright posture, not to stand still, to avoid hot baths or showers, and to lie down at first indication of faintness or light-headedness.

- When bethanechol is administered to relieve urinary retention or abdominal distention, a bedpan or urinal should be readily available to the patient. It may be necessary to insert a rectal tube to facilitate passage of flatus.

- Monitor fluid intake and output. Observe and record patient's response to bethanechol, and report any failure of the drug to relieve the particular condition for which it was prescribed.

- Bear in mind that reflux infection can occur in patients with preexisting bacteriuria when urine is forced up into ureters and kidney by bethanechol-induced bladder contractions.

- Store at room temperature, preferably between 15° and 30°C (59° and 86°F), unless otherwise directed by manufacturer.

Diagnostic test interferences   Bethanechol may cause increases in **serum amylase** and **serum lipase**, by stimulating pancreatic secretions, and may increase **SGOT**, **serum bilirubin**, and **BSP retention** by causing spasms in sphincter of Oddi.

DRUG INTERACTIONS   *Bethanechol*

PLUS	INTERACTIONS
Cholinergics, especially cholinesterase inhibitors, e.g., ambenonium neostigmine	Additive cholinergic effects
Ganglionic blocking agents, e.g., mecamylamine	Concurrent use may cause severe abdominal symptoms and precipitous fall in blood pressure
Procainamide ⎫ Quinidine ⎬	Antagonize cholinergic effects of bethanechol

Bethanidine

(Bendogen, Esbatal)   *Adrenergic blocking agent*

ACTIONS AND USES   Used to treat moderate to severe hypertension.

ROUTE AND DOSAGE   Oral: 10 mg three times a day after food. Increased as required to maximum of 200 mg/day.

For further information *see guanethidine*.

Bisacodyl ▬▬▬▬▬▬▬▬▬▬▬▬▬▬▬▬▬▬

(Dulcodos, Dulcolax.) *Laxative; stimulant*

B

ACTIONS AND USES Diphenylmethane laxative structurally related to phenolphthalein. On contact, sensory nerve endings in the colonic wall are stimulated and by reflex parasympathetic action, widespread colonic peristaltic contractions produce evacuation.

Used for temporary relief of constipation and for evacuation of colon before surgery, proctoscopy sigmoidoscopy and radiographic examinations. Also used to cleanse colon and to relieve constipation in patients with spinal cord damage. Available as one component of bowel evacuant kits with a saline laxative.

ROUTE AND DOSAGE Oral: **Adults:** 10 mg, at night **Rectal suppository** (at the time a bowel movement is required): **Adults** 10 mg; **Children (under 10 years):** 5 mg.

ABSORPTION AND FATE Acts within 6 to 12 hours following oral administration; acts 15 to 60 minutes after insertion of rectal suppository. Approximately 5% may be absorbed from GI tract metabolized in liver, and excreted in urine, bile, and milk in conjugated form.

CONTRAINDICATIONS AND PRECAUTIONS Hypersensitivity to bisacodyl or to ingredients in formulation; acute surgical abdomen, nausea, vomiting, abdominal cramps, intestinal obstruction, faecal impaction: use of rectal suppository in presence of anal or rectal fissures, ulcerated haemorrhoids, proctitis.

ADVERSE/SIDE EFFECTS Systemic effects not reported. Rarely: mild cramping, nausea, vertigo, diarrhoea, fluid and electrolyte disturbances (especially potassium and calcium). Rectal burning, irritation, and proctitis following use of suppositories for several weeks.

NURSING IMPLICATIONS
- In view of action time, administer oral drug in the evening. Suppository may be inserted at time bowel movement is desired.
- Tablets are enteric coated to avoid gastric irritation. Therefore, they should be swallowed whole and not cut, crushed, or chewed. Preferably taken with a full glass (240 ml) of water or other liquid.
- Advise patient not to take tablets within 1 hour of antacids or milk. These substances may cause premature dissolution of enteric coating, with release of drug in stomach resulting in gastric irritation and loss of cathartic action.
- Bisacodyl usually produces 1 or 2 soft formed stools. Periodically evaluate patient's need for continued use of bisacodyl.
- Patients with hypertension and cardiovascular disease should be cautioned to avoid excessive straining (*Valsalva manoeuvre*) during defaecation. Straining causes concurrent rises in intrathoracic and venous pressures, momentarily interfering with free flow of blood out of heart. When patient stops straining, blood is quickly rushed through heart; this may result in tachycardia and even cardiac arrest in the susceptible patient.
- Because of OTC availability, laxative abuse, especially among the elderly, is

BISACODYL (continued)

widespread. Recognize that the elderly patient who is preoccupied with bowel function may erroneously believe that failure to have a daily bowel movement can lead to 'autointoxication'.

- Inform the habitual laxative user that a normal pattern for elimination varies from three bowel movements a day to three a week, depending on a self-established functionally effective schedule.

Food–drug interactions

- *High fibre* in the diet is frequently prescribed as a supplement and eventual substitute for laxative use. Examples of high fibre foods: fruits (don't peel), blackberries, vegetables, baked beans, broccoli, artichoke, bran, wheat cereals and breads, coconut, nuts, and seeds.
- Dietary fibre absorbs water, increases stool volume, decreases intracolonic pressure, and reduces faecal transit time.
- Indiscriminate use of laxatives or dietary fibre can lead to changes in intestinal bacterial flora; some high fibre cereals (containing phytates) bind and reduce absorption of calcium, iron, zinc, and other trace minerals.
- Both selection and amounts of high fibre foods to supplement diet should be part of the teaching aimed at reducing laxative dependence. Some physicians recommend a supplement of 6 to 12 teaspoons of unprocessed bran a day. Consult physician and dietitian.
- Overuse or misuse of bisacodyl or other laxatives can lead to decreased absorption of vitamin K and oral anticoagulants because of decreased transit time in the intestine.
- A teaching plan designed to interrupt an older person's dependency on laxatives should take into account several age-related phenomena which influence gut motility:
  - Heavy reliance on processed foods.
  - Decreased salivary flow.
  - Decreased thirst and hunger perceptions.
  - Inadequate food and fluid intake.
  - Dental problems.
  - Inactivity.

Teaching points regarding prevention of constipation

- Adequate fluid intake (7 to 10 glasses if allowed).
- Regular meal times.
- High fibre foods (increase gradually to reduce intestinal flatus).
- Daily exercise programme e.g., brisk walking (if allowed).
- Unhurried and regular defaecation time (duodenocolic and defaecation reflexes are most active after meals, especially breakfast).
- Control of emotional factors, such as anxiety and depression.

- Bisacodyl tablets and suppositories are preserved in tight containers at temperatures not exceeding 30°C (86°F).

Drug interactions   In general it is best not to take a laxative within 2 hours of taking other medications.

Bleomycin ▬▬▬▬▬▬▬▬▬▬▬▬▬▬▬▬▬▬▬▬

Antineoplastic; antibiotic

B

ACTIONS AND USES   Mixture of cytotoxic glycopeptide antibiotics from a strain of *Streptomyces verticillus*. A toxic drug with low therapeutic index; intensely cytotoxic. By unclear mechanism, blocks DNA, RNA, and protein synthesis. A cell cycle-phase nonspecific. Causes minimal immunosuppression and has capacity to release intracellular pyrogens leading to promal hyperpyrexia. Weak antibiotic activity is overshadowed by potent cytotoxic effects. Has strong affinity for skin and lung tumour cells, in contrast to its low affinity for cells in haematopoietic tissue (perhaps due to the high levels of bleomycin degrading enzymes found in bone marrow).

Used as single agent or in combination with other chemotherapeutic agents as adjunct to surgery and radiation therapy. Used in treatment of squamous cell carcinomas of head, neck, penis, cervix, and vulva; also lymphomas (including reticular cell sarcoma, lymphosarcoma, Hodgkin's), and testicular carcinoma. Intrapleural administration: to prevent pleural fluid accumulation.

ROUTE AND DOSAGE   Dosage regimen highly individualized based on published protocols.

ABSORPTION AND FATE   Absorbed systemically following subcutaneous, IV, IM, intrapleural, intraperitoneal, or intraperiocardial administration. Concentrates mainly in skin, lungs, kidneys, lymphocytes, peritoneum. **Metabolic fate** poorly understood; **protein binding** about 1%. In patient with creatinine clearance of more than 35 ml/minute, half-life is about 2 hours; in patient with clearance less than 35 ml/minute, **half-life** increases exponentially as creatinine clearance decreases. 60 to 70% of dose recovered in urine as active bleomycin.

CONTRAINDICATIONS AND PRECAUTIONS   Hypersensitivity to bleomycin, pregnancy, women of childbearing age. **Cautious Use:** compromised hepatic, renal, or pulmonary function, patients who have had previous cytotoxic drug or radiation therapy.

ADVERSE/SIDE EFFECTS   These include: (over 50% of patients): stomatitis, oral ulcerations, alopecia, hyperpigmentation, patchy hyperkeratosis, peeling of skin, rash, striae, pruritic erythema, vesiculation, peeling, bleeding, acne, pigmented banding of nails and thickening of nail bed, angioedema, radiation recall, nausea, vomiting, anorexia, diarrhoea, weight loss, thrombocytopenia, leucopenia, mild anaemia. Other side effects (dose- and age-related include): interstitial pneumonitis, pneumonia, or fibrosis. Anaphylactoid reaction: fever, chills, severe hyperpyrexia, hypotension, mental confusion, wheezing; headache, cystitis, pain at tumour site, phlebitis; renal, hepatic, and CNS toxicity; Raynaud's phenomenon, necrosis at injection site.

NURSING IMPLICATIONS
- Reconstituted solutions are stable at room temperature use on discard within 24 hrs.
- IV and intrarterial injections should be administered slowly over a 1−2 minute period.

BLEOMYCIN (continued)

- Inject IM bleomycin deeply into upper outer quadrant of buttock; change sites with each injection, 2 ml 1% lignocaine used as diluent.
- Favourable response, if any is to occur, is expected within 2 weeks for treatment of Hodgkin's or testicular tumour, and within 3 weeks for squamous cell cancers.
- Profound hyperthermia (chills and fever) especially after a large single dose may occur 4 to 6 hours after administration and lasts 4 to 12 hours. This reaction can be fatal. It is most apt to appear in patients with lymphoma. Reactions become less frequent with continued use of the drug, but may recur sporadically. Tepid sponge baths may provide relief.
- Anaphylactoid reactions, sometimes fatal, may occur several hours after first or second dose, especially in lymphoma patients (10%). Hydrocortisone cover on prescription.
- Usually a test dose of 2 units of bleomycin is given to these patients for the first 2 doses. Patient is closely observed for at least 24 hours. If there is no acute reaction (hypotension, fever, chills, confusion, wheezing), regular dosage schedule is resumed.
- If the treatment regimen includes concomitant therapy with an oral antineoplastic (such as vinblastine), plan with the patient the most feasible schedule for taking medication. Stress complete adherence to the established regimen.
- Counsel patient to avoid using OTC drugs during antineoplastic treatment period unless such drugs are approved by physician.
- Although bone marrow toxicity is rare, unexplained bleeding or bruising should be promptly reported to the physician.
- Monitor patient for evidence of deterioration of renal function, i.e., changed fluid intake and output ratio and pattern, weight gain (oedema), decreasing creatinine clearance. Bleomycin will be discontinued if kidney function diminishes, because of increased danger of toxicity. Reference limits for creatinine clearance: 90 to 120 ml/minute.
- Pulmonary toxicity occurs in about 10% of all patients and most frequently in patients over 70 years of age or when the total of all doses approaches 400 units. It may also occur in young people, however, and with lower doses.
- Monitor, by interrogation of patient, for nonproductive cough, chest pain, dyspnoea; by auscultation for fine rales; and by serial chest radiographs for structural signs of pulmonary toxicity. If pulmonary fibrosis is present, drug will be discontinued.
- Skin toxicity usually develops in second or third week of treatment and after 150 to 200 units of bleomycin have been administered. Report symptoms (hypoesthaesias, urticaria, tender swollen hands) promptly; therapy may be discontinued.
- Be alert to evidence of *radiation recall*, i.e., erythema that develops in a previously irradiated field. Most frequently occurs when chemotherapy is started during or shortly after radiation therapy, but it also may be observed several years after the treatment. Protect such an area or a pressure area by frequent observation, gentle, soapless skin care, and programmed mobility.
- Inform patient that hyperpigmentation may occur in areas subject to friction and pressure, skin folds, nail cuticles, scars, and intramuscular sites.
- Stomatitis may be a dose-limiting factor because oral ulcerations can interfere with adequate nutrient intake leading to severe debilitation. Consult physician if an oral

BLEOMYCIN (continued)

local anaesthetic seems to be indicated. It may help patient to eat if agent is applied about 10 minutes before eating.

■ Check weight at regular intervals under standard conditions. Weight loss and anorexia may persist a long time after therapy has been discontinued. Arrange for a conference between the dietitian and patient to allow joint planning for strategies to maintain oral intake.

■ Although this drug causes nausea and vomiting, it is important that the established administration schedule for injections be maintained. Antiemetic drugs may be prescribed.

■ If patient is receiving bleomycin for testicular carcinoma, advise him to observe and report early signs of Raynaud's phenomenon: hands and feet constantly cold especially when exposed; intermittent blanching and cyanosis in finger and toe tips; swelling of fingers and toes. Signs can occur during or after therapy has been discontinued.

■ Store unopened ampoules between 15° and 30°C (59° and 85°F), unless otherwise specified by manufacturer.

■ Nurse caution. Allergies have been reported; avoid contact with drug by use of mask, gloves and goggles during reconstitution. In case of accidents wash with water.

Patient-Teaching Points for Mouth Care

☐ Inspect oral membranes regularly for oral bleeding, pain, or ulceration. Report if present.

☐ Caries following radiation or chemotherapy must be controlled if teeth are to be retained. Mechanical removal of plaque is the best preventive measure.

☐ Initiate prophylactic and comfort measures: frequent rinses with warm water, saline, or diluted hydrogen peroxide solution; use a soft toothbrush or cotton-covered finger, flossing with waxed floss at least once daily, avoid overuse of commercial mouth rinses, avoid highly acid food and drink, and coarse physically 'scratchy' foods.

☐ *See mustine for additional points about mouth care.*

Drug interactions   Antineoplastics, other **radiation therapy** may lead to increased bleomycin toxicity including bone marrow depression. Pharmacological effects of phenytoin may be reduced. Monitor phenytoin plasma levels.

Bretylium tosylate ▬▬▬▬▬▬▬▬▬▬▬▬▬▬▬▬

(Bretylate)   *Adrenergic blocking agent*
                                                             (sympatholytic)

ACTIONS AND USES   Quaternary ammonium compound; mechanism of action is complex and not fully understood. Suppresses ventricular fibrillation by direct action on the myocardium and ventricular tachycardia by adrenergic blockade. Has no apparent CNS or cholinergic blockade effect, and effect on GI motility is less than with other

BRETYLIUM TOSYLATE (continued)

adrenergic blockers. Has weak local anaesthetic properties. Because onset of desired action is delayed, bretylium is not a first-line antiarrhythmic agent.

Used for short-term treatment of life-threatening ventricular tachycardia in patients who have not responded to conventional therapy such as lignocaine procainamide, direct current countershock (cardioversion). Formerly used orally for treatment of hypertension, but found to be unsuitable for long-term therapy because of tolerance and troublesome side effects (orthostatic hypotension, parotid pain).

ROUTE AND DOSAGE   **Intravenous**: 5–10 mg/kg over 8–10 min, *maintenance* 1–2 mg/min. **Intramuscular**: 5 mg/kg repeated after 6–8 hrs as required, *maintenance* 5–10 mg/kg 6–8 hrly.

ABSORPTION AND FATE   Antifibrillatory effect begins within minutes following IV administration. Suppression of ventricular tachycardia, PVCs, and other arrhythmias may require 20 minutes to 2 hours (delay is longer after IM than IV); **maximal effect** in 6 to 9 hours; **duration** up to 24 hours. **Half-life**: 4 to 17 hours (longer in patients with impaired renal function). Does not pass blood–brain barrier. Not metabolized. Eliminated unchanged by kidneys; 70 to 80% of dose excreted during first 24 hours, and an additional 10% over the following 3 days. Distribution to placenta and breast milk not known.

CONTRAINDICATIONS AND PRECAUTIONS   No contraindications for use in life-threatening ventricular fibrillation or arrhythmias. Contraindications for less serious arrhythmia: digitalis-induced arrythmias, patients with fixed cardiac output such as severe aortic stenosis, severe pulmonary hypertension (profound hypotension can result without compensatory increase in cardiac output). Safe use during pregnancy, in nursing mothers, and in children not established. **Cautious Use**: impaired renal function, sinus bradycardia, patients on digitalis maintenance. Do not give concurrently with noradrenaline type drugs.

ADVERSE/SIDE EFFECTS   These include: both supine and postural hypotension with dizziness, vertigo, light-headedness, faintness, syncope, transitory hypertension, bradycardia, increased frequency of PVCs, exacerbation of digitalis-induced arrhythmias, precipitation of angina, sensation of substernal pressure, nausea, vomiting (particularly with rapid IV), loose stools, diarrhoea, abdominal pain, anorexia, involuntary head movements, headache, muscle weakness, aching sensation in legs, generalized tenderness; confusion, paranoid psychosis, emotional lability, lethargy, anxiety, erythematous macular rash, flushing, sweating, nasal stuffiness, mild conjunctivitis, hiccoughs, renal dysfunction, injection site reactions, shortness of breath, respiratory depression, hyperthermia.

NURSING IMPLICATIONS

- Use of bretylium should be limited to patients in facilities adequately equipped and staffed for constant monitoring of ECG and blood pressure, and for cardiopulmonary resuscitation, and cardioversion, if necessary.
- Administer no more than 5 ml in any one IM site. Avoid injecting into or near a

BRETYLIUM TOSYLATE (continued)

major nerve. Keep a record of injection sites. Injection into same site can cause muscle atrophy, necrosis and fibrosis.

- Monitor patient closely for initial transient rise in blood pressure, increased heart rate, PVCs and other arrhythmias, or worsening of existing arrhythmias which may occur within a few minutes to 1 hour after drug administration. Usually patients eventually stabilize to these effects.

- Initial effect of hypertension is usually followed within 1 hour by a fall in supine blood pressure and by orthostatic hypotension.

- The supine position is recommended until patient develops tolerance to the hypotensive effect of bretylium (generally in several days). Hypotension can occur in the supine position, particularly in patients with severely compromised cardiac function. It may not readily respond to therapy (e.g., vasopressors, fluids), therefore, early reporting is essential.

- A systolic blood pressure greater than 75 mm Hg usually need not be treated unless associated with symptoms of hypotension: faintness, light-headedness, dizziness. If systolic blood pressure drops to 75 mm Hg or below, it is cautiously treated with dopamine or low doses of diluted noradrenaline. Plasma or blood may be required for plasma volume expansion.

- To prevent orthostatic hypotension, raise or lower head of bed slowly and advise patient to make position changes slowly. If patient is allowed to be out of bed caution to dangle legs for a few minutes before standing and not to stand still for prolonged periods. Advise male patient to sit on toilet to urinate.

- IV administration is associated with a high incidence of nausea and vomiting. These side effects can be minimized by slow administration of drug (over 10 or more minutes).

- Bretylium dosage should be reduced gradually and discontinued after 3 to 5 days under close ECG monitoring. Another antiarrhythmic agent may be substituted if indicated.

- Unopened vials stored preferably between 15° and 30°C (59° and 86°F), unless otherwise directed by manufacturer.

Diagnostic test interferences Urinary VMA, adrenaline and nonadrenaline levels may be decreased during bretylium therapy.

DRUG INTERACTIONS *Bretylium*

PLUS	INTERACTIONS
Antiarrhythmics, other e.g., lignocaine, procainamide, propranolol, quinidine	Cardiac effects may be antagonistic or additive; toxic effects may be additive when administered concomitantly with bretylium
Antihypertensive agents	Potentiation of hypotensive effect (during early bretylium therapy)
Digitalis glycosides	May worsen arrhythmias caused by digitalis toxicity. Bretylium and digitalis should not be given simultaneously as initial treatments

Bromazepam

(Leoxtan)   *Anxiolytic; benzodiazepine*

ROUTE AND DOSAGE   Oral 3–18 mg a day in divided doses, reduce dose to half in elderly patients. Maximum dose 60 mg in one day for hospitalized patients.
For further information *see diazepam*.

Bromocriptine

(Parlodel)   *Dopamine receptor agonist;*
antiparkinsonian agent

ACTIONS AND USES   Semisynthetic ergot alkaloid derivative, but devoid of oxytocic activity generally attributed to drugs of this class. Reduces elevated serum prolactin levels in men and women by activating postsynaptic dopaminergic receptors in hypothalamus to stimulate release of prolactin inhibiting factor and possibly luteinizing hormone release factor. Ovulation and ovarian function in amenorrhoeic women are restored (by direct action on ovary), thus correcting female infertility secondary to elevated prolactin levels. (Correction of male infertility has not been documented.) Growth hormone secretion is increased transiently in patient with normal concentrations but parodoxically is suppressed in some patients with acromegaly. Pretreatment levels are restored 2 to 4 weeks after bromocriptine is discontinued. Activates dopaminergic receptors in neostriatum of CNS, which may explain action in parkinsonian syndrome: improvement in symptoms 30 to 90 minutes after administration of the drug with maximum effects experienced in 2 hours. Bromocriptine also reduces blood pressure in the hypertensive and normotensive individual and may cause peripheral vasoconstriction (large doses) and increased sodium excretion.

Used for short-term management of amenorrhoea/galactorrhoea or female infertility associated with hyperprolactaemia (when there is no indication of pituitary tumour) and to prevent physiological lactation.

ROUTE AND DOSAGE   Oral: *Amenorrhoea/galactorrhoea*; *female infertility*: Initial: 1.25 to 2.5 mg daily; *maintenance*: 2.5 mg two or three times daily. *Suppression of puerperal lactation*: 2.5 mg on the day of delivery, followed by 2.5 mg twice a day for 14 days. *Cyclical breast or menstrual disorders*: 1.25 mg at bedtime increased gradually to 2.5 mg twice a day. *Acromegaly*: *initial* 1–1.25 mg daily increased to 60 mg/day. Most patients respond to a dose between 20 and 60 mg a day.

ABSORPTION AND FATE   Approximately 28% of oral dose absorbed from GI tract. Plasma levels peak in about 1 to 2 hours; **duration of action** 4 to 8 hours. About 90 to 96% bound to serum albumin. **Half-life**: 3 to 8 hours. Completely metabolized in liver to inactive metabolites. Eighty-five per cent of dose excreted within 5 days in faeces via bile; about 3 to 6% eliminated in urine.

BROMOCRIPTINE (continued)

CONTRAINDICATIONS AND PRECAUTIONS Sensitivity to ergot alkaloids: severe ischaemic heart disease or peripheral vascular disease; patients with pituitary tumour; patients with normal prolactin levels, nursing women. Safe use during pregnancy and in children under 15 years not established. **Cautious Use:** hepatic and renal dysfunction, history of psychiatric disorder, history of myocardial infarction with residual arrhythmia.

ADVERSE/SIDE EFFECTS   (Mostly dose-related.) These include: transient decrease in blood pressure, orthostatic hypotension, shock, palpitation, extrasystoles, digitospasm in response to cold (Raynaud's phenomenon), red, tender, hot oedematous extremities (erythromelalgia), exacerbation of angina, arrhythmias, urticaria, rash, mottling, livedo reticularis, nausea, vomiting, epigastric pain, abdominal cramps, constipation (long-term use) or diarrhoea; metallic taste, dry mouth, dysphagia, anorexia, peptic ulcers, GI tract haemorrhage, diuresis, urinary frequency, urinary incontinence, urinary retention, headache, dizziness, vertigo, light-headedness, fainting, sedation, nightmares, insomnia, dyskinesia, confusion, ataxia; visual and auditory hallucinations, paranoid delusions (particularly in patients with Parkinson's disease or those receiving high dosages); 'on–off' phenomenon, mania, nervousness, anxiety, depression, seizures, blurred vision, burning sensation in eyes, blepharospasm, diplopia, fatigue, asthenia, nasal congestion, ergotism (tingling and numbness of fingers, cramps in feet and legs, cold extremities), pulmonary infiltration, pleural effusion and thickening with long-term therapy (6 to 36 months), severe postpartum hypertension (causal relationship not established), hepatotoxicity (rare).

NURSING IMPLICATIONS

General information for all patients

- Administer with meals, milk, or other food to reduce incidence of GI side effects.
- Establish data regarding baseline vital signs. Therapy should not be initiated until vital signs are stable.
- Since hypotension with dizziness and fainting may occur, particularly following first dose in sensitive patients, initial dose is usually prescribed for evening administration.
- Blood pressure should be monitored closely during the first few days of therapy and periodically throughout therapy, for all patients. Compare readings with baseline data.
- Instruct patient to make position changes slowly and in stages, especially from recumbent to upright posture, and to dangle legs over bed for a few minutes before ambulating. Caution patient to lie down immediately if lightheadedness or dizziness occurs.
- Inform patient that a mild diuresis may occur due to vasodilating action of bromocriptine on renal arteries.
- Side effects occur commonly but they are usually mild to moderate in degree and respond to dosage reduction or discontinuation of drug.
- Since bromocriptine is associated with dose-related lightheadedness, dizziness, and

BROMOCRIPTINE (continued)

syncope, caution patient to avoid driving and other potentially hazardous activites until reaction to drug has been determined.

- Bromocriptine can cause digital vasospasm, particularly in patients with acromegaly and patients receiving high dosages. Advise patient to avoid exposure to cold and to report the onset of pallor of fingers or toes.
- Patients should be advised that bromocriptine may make them more sensitive to the effects of alcohol.
- Periodic evaluations should be made of hepatic, haematological, cardiovascular, and renal function in patients on prolonged therapy.
- Store in well-closed, light-resistant containers, preferably between 15° and 30°C (59° and 86°F), unless otherwise directed by manufacturer.

Suppression of puerperal lactation

- Because hypotension occurs most commonly in the postpartum patient, it is recommended that therapy not be started any sooner than 4 hours after delivery and then only if vital signs have stabilized.
- Severe postpartum hypertension (including cerebrovascular accidents and seizures) have occurred 6 to 9 days after delivery. Causal relationship not established. Monitor blood pressure at regular intervals.
- Patients receiving bromocriptine to suppress postpartum lactation may have temporary rebound breast enlargement and pain following drug withdrawal.

Amenorrhea/galactorrhea; infertility

- In patients with hyperprolactinaemia, a complete evaluation of the sella turcica is recommended before initiation of therapy, including x-rays, posterior, anterior, and lateral tomography, to rule out pituitary tumour.
- Patients being treated for amenorrhoea/galactorrhoea should be informed that restoration of regular menses occurs in 6 to 8 weeks (range: a few days to 24 weeks). (If patient has been amenorrhoeic more than 4 years, restoration of menses may require considerable time.) Galactorrhoea suppression is usually seen after 7 to 12 weeks of therapy, but may not occur for more than 24 weeks. Maximum reduction of prolactin level generally occurs within the first 4 weeks of therapy. Normal plasma prolactin concentration is approximately 5 to 10 ng/ml.
- Because long-term drug effects are not known, it is recommended that duration of therapy for amenorrhoea and galactorrhoea not exceed 6 months.
- Recurrence rates of amenorrhoea and galactorrhoea are high (70 to 80%) following withdrawal of bromocriptine. Amenorrhoea usually returns within 4 to 24 weeks; galactorrhoea within 2 to 12 weeks; serum prolactin increases to pretreatment levels within 1 to 6 weeks.
- Since restoration of fertility may result during therapy, patients being treated for amenorrhoea and galactorrhoea should be advised to use barrier type contraceptive measures until normal ovulating cycle is restored. Oral contraceptives are contraindicated because they may cause amenorrhoea and galactorrhoea.
- Advise patient to inform physician immediately if pregnancy occurs during therapy. Bromocriptine should be discontinued without delay. These patients should be carefully observed throughout pregnancy. Because of the possible presence of a

BROMOCRIPTINE (continued)

previously undetected prolactin-secreting pituitary tumour, which could cause optic nerve compression, visual fields should be checked monthly.

- A pregnancy test is recommended at least every 4 months during the period of amenorrhoea. Once menstruation is reestablished, a pregnancy test should be performed every time patient misses a menstrual period.

Diagnostic test interferences   Transient increases in **serum growth hormone** may occur in patients with normal levels, and paradoxical decreases in patients with acromegaly. **SGOT (AST), SGPT (ALT), alkaline phosphatase, GGPT, CPK, BUN, uric acid** may be transiently increased (generally not significant at therapeutic doses).

DRUG INTERACTIONS   *Bromocriptine*

PLUS	INTERACTIONS
Alcohol	Possibility of decreased tolerance to alcohol particularly patients with acromegaly
Antihypertensives	Additive hypotensive effects
Contraceptives, oral	May interfere with effect of bromocriptine by causing amenorrhoea and galactorrhoea
Amitriptyline Droperidol Haloperidol Imipramine Methyldopa Phenothiazines Reserpine	Increases in serum prolactin levels induced by these drugs may interfere with bromocriptine action and require higher bromocriptine dosage
Levodopa	Possibility of additive effects allows reduction of levodopa dosage when given concomitantly with bromocriptine

Brompheniramine maleate

(Dimotane)   *Antihistamine; (H₁-receptor antagonist)*

ACTIONS AND USES   Propylamine (alkylamine) antihistaminic similar to chlorpheniramine (q.v.) in actions, uses, pharmacokinetics, contraindications, and adverse effects. Produces less sedative effect than chlorpheniramine.

Used for symptomatic treatment of allergic manifestations. Also used in various cough mixtures and antihistamine-decongestant cold formulations.

ROUTE AND DOSAGE   Oral: Adults: 4−8 mg every 4−6 hrs as required. Child: 0−3 yrs 0.4−1 mg/kg/day in 4 divided doses, 4−5 yrs 2 mg/3−4 times a day, 6−12 yrs 2−4 mg/3−4 times a day.

ABSORPTION AND FATE   Serum levels peak in 2 to 5 hours following oral administration. **Maximal antihistaminic effect** with 3 to 9 hours; **duration** up to 48

BROMPHENIRAMINE MALEATE (continued)

hours. **Half-life:** 12 to 34 hours. About 40% of oral dose excreted in urine within 72 hours (5–10% as unchanged drug); 2% faecal elimination.

CONTRAINDICATIONS AND PRECAUTIONS   Hypersensitivity to antihistamines, use in newborns, nursing mothers, acute asthma, patients receiving MAO inhibitors. **Cautious Use:** prostatic hypertrophy, narrow angle glaucoma. *See also chlorpheniramine.*

ADVERSE/SIDE EFFECTS   Sedation, drowsiness, dry mouth, dizziness, headache, disturbed coordination, urticaria, rash, agranulocytosis, thrombocytopenia. *See chlorpheniramine.*

NURSING IMPLICATIONS

- If gastric distress occurs advise patient to take medication with meals or a snack.
- Acute hypersensitivity reaction with sudden severe agranulocytosis reportedly can occur within minutes to hours after drug ingestion. The reaction is manifested by high fever, chills, and possible development of gangrenous ulcerations of mouth and throat, pneumonia, and prostration. Patient should seek medical attention immediately.
- Elderly patients tend to be particularly susceptible to sedative effect, dizziness, and hypotension. Most symptoms respond to reduction in dosage.
- Bear in mind that brompheniramine has an atropine-like effect (thickens bronchial secretions) that may make expectoration difficult.
- Thickened bronchial secretions and dry mouth, nose, and throat may be relieved by increasing fluid intake. Relief of dry mouth may be provided by sugarless gum or lemon drops, frequent rinses with warm water, diligent mouth care.
- Blood counts should be performed in patients receiving long-term therapy, in order to preclude possibility of blood dyscrasias.
- Caution patient to avoid driving a car or other potentially hazardous activities until reaction to drug is known.
- Advise patient not to take alcoholic beverages and other CNS depressants, e.g., tranquilizers, sedatives, pain or sleeping medicines, without consulting physician.
- In common with other antihistamines, brompheniramine may cause false-negative allergy skin tests. The drug should be discontinued about 4 days before such tests are done.
- Store in tightly covered container, preferably between 15° and 30°C (59° and 86°F) unless otherwise directed by manufacturer. Elixir and parenteral form should be protected from light.
- *See chlorpheniramine for Nursing Implications and Drug Interactions.*

Budesonide ————————————————————

(Pulmicort, Nebuhaler)   *Corticosteroid; antiasthmatic*

For further information *see beclomethasone*

BUDESONIDE (continued)
ROUTE AND DOSAGE Adult: **Inhalation** by aerosol *initial* 200 mcg (1 puff of Pulmicort) twice a day, used according to response at the minimal effective dose. **Child:** 50–200 mcg (1–4 puffs Pulmicort Paediatric) up to twice a day.

B

Bumetanide

(Burinex)

Diuretic (loop); sulphonamide derivative

ACTIONS AND USES Sulphonamide derivatives structurally related to frusemide and with similar pharmacological effects. Diuretic activity is 40 times greater, however, and duration of action is shorter than that of frusemide. Inhibits sodium and chloride reabsorption by direct action on ascending limit of the loop of Henle. Also appears to inhibit phosphate and bicarbonate reabsorption in proximal renal tubule. Produces only mild hypotensive effects at usual diuretic doses.

Used for oedema associated with congestive heart failure, and hepatic or renal disease, including nephrotic syndrome. Has been used in management of postoperative and premenstrual oedema and oedema accompanying disseminated carcinoma, and for mild hypertension. May be used concomitantly with a potassium-sparing diuretic to prevent hypokalaemia.

ROUTE AND DOSAGE Oral: 1 mg once a day, increased in oliguria to maximum of 5 mg/day. **Intravenous/intramuscular:** 1–2 mg (slowly IV over 1–2 min) repeat dose if necessary after 20 min.

ABSORPTION AND FATE Rapidly and almost completely absorbed following oral administration; completely absorbed following IM or IV injection. **Onset of diuretic effect:** 30 to 60 minutes after oral, about 40 minutes after IM, and within a few minutes following IV administration. With usual doses, diuresis is usually completed within 4 hours after oral or IM administration and 2 to 3 hours after IV. About 95% protein bound; **half-life** 60 to 90 minutes. Partially metabolized in liver. About 80% of dose excreted in urine within 48 hours (50% as unchanged drug); 10 to 20% eliminated in faeces via bile. Excreted in breast milk.

CONTRAINDICATIONS AND PRECAUTIONS Hypersensitivity to bumetanide or to other sulphonamides; anuria, markedly elevated BUN; hepatic coma, severe electrolyte deficiency. Safe use during pregnancy, in nursing mothers, and in children under 18 years not established. **Cautious Use:** hepatic cirrhosis, ascites.

ADVERSE/SIDE EFFECTS These include: dizziness, headache, weakness, fatigue, hypotension, ECG changes, chest pain, hypovolaemia, circulatory collapse with thromboses and emboli, nausea, vomiting, abdominal or stomach pain, GI distress, diarrhoea, dry mouth, dehydration; increases or decreases Hgb, Hct, platelets, leucocytes; changes in differential count; hypokalaemia, hyponatraemia, hyperuricaemia, hyperglycaemia; decreases in blood magnesium, calcium, chloride, ammonium,

BUMETANIDE (continued)

bicarbonate, phosphorus; increased serum creatinine; azotaemia, increased or decreased serum cholesterol, increased LDH, AST (SGOT), ALT (SGPT), alkaline phosphatase, muscle cramps, muscle stiffness or tenderness, arthritic pain, ear discomfort, impaired hearing, breast or nipple tenderness, gynaecomastia, premature ejaculation, difficulty maintaining erection, pruritis, urticaria, rash, purpura, Stevens-Johnson syndrome, sweating, hyperventilation, renal failure (rare), glycosuria.

NURSING IMPLICATIONS

- Usually administered in the morning as a single dose, either daily or by intermittent schedule. For some patients, diuresis is reportedly more effective when administered in two divided doses, morning and evening.
- Monitor fluid intake and output, BUN, and serum creatinine. Report promptly the onset of oliguria or other changes in intake and output ratio and pattern.
- Monitor weight, blood pressure, and pulse rate.
- High doses or frequent administration, particularly in the elderly, can cause profound diuresis, hypovolaemia, and resulting circulatory collapse with development of thrombi and emboli. Careful monitoring is essential.
- Hypokalaemia is a constant threat in all patients and particularly in those receiving digitalis, or who have congestive heart failure, hepatic cirrhosis, ascites, diarrhoea, or potassium-losing nephropathy. Careful monitoring and hospitalization during initial therapy and dosage adjustment periods are advised in these patients.
- Advise patient to report symptoms of electrolyte imbalance promptly to physician: weakness, dizziness, fatigue, faintness, confusion, muscle cramps, headache, paraesthesias.
- It is important for patient to maintain an adequate daily intake of potassium while taking bumetanide. *See Index: Food Sources.*
- Patients with hepatic disease should be carefully observed. Alterations in fluid and electrolyte balance can precipitate encephalopathy (inappropriate behaviour, altered mood, impaired judgment, confusion, drowsiness, coma).
- Be alert to complaints about hearing difficulty or ear discomfort. Patients at risk of bumetanide-induced ototoxic effects include: patients receiving the drug IV, especially at high doses; rapid IV administration; patients with severely impaired renal function and those receiving other potentially ototoxic or nephrotoxic drugs.
- Serum electrolytes, blood studies, liver and kidney function tests, and blood sugar (particularly diabetics) should be monitored at regular intervals especially in patients receiving prolonged treatment, high doses, or who are on Na restriction.
- Note therapeutic effectiveness in patients being treated for oedema: reductions in body weight, abdominal girth, ankle oedema, blood pressure, and heart rate.
- Instruct patient to keep scheduled appointments for medical evaluation.
- For IV infusion, parenteral bumetanide is compatible with 5% dextrose, 0.9% sodium chloride, and lactated Ringer's. Infusion should be used within 24 hours after preparation.
- Drug will discolour on exposure to light. Inspect parenteral bumetanide before administration. Discard if it contains particles or is discoloured.
- Store in tight, light-resistant containers preferably at 15° to 30°C (59° to 86°F), unless otherwise directed by manufacturer.

Buprenorphine

(Temgesic) *Synthetic narcotic; analgesic*

ACTIONS AND USES   Synthetic opiate with partial agonist/antagonist action and of longer duration of effect morphine: Buprenorphine is a partial agonist, and for this reason in combination with an opiate agonist will not enhance analgesia, but will diminish it. Used to treat moderate to severe pain.

ROUTE AND DOSAGE   **Sublingual:** *initial* 200 mcg every 8 hrs increased to 200–400 mcg every 6–8 hrs if required. **Intramuscular/intravenous** (slow injection): 300–600 mcg every 6–8 hrs.

NURSING IMPLICATIONS
- Lower risk of dependence, less side effects than morphine.
- May precipitate withdrawal symptoms in narcotic-dependent patients. Effects only partially reversed by naloxone, doxapram will reverse severe respiratory depression.
- Not subject to controlled drug regulations.
- *For Adverse/side effects and additional nursing implications see morphine sulphate.*

Busulphan

(Myleran) *Antineoplastic, alkylating agent; nitrosurea*

ACTIONS AND USES   Potent cytotoxic alkylating agent that may be a carcinogen in itself. Cell cycle nonspecific. Acts predominantly on slowly proliferating stem cells by inducing cross linkage in DNA thus blocking replication and causing cell death. Reduces total granulocyte mass but has little effect on lymphocytes and platelets except in large doses. May cause widespread epithelial cellular dysplasia severe enough to make it difficult to interpret exfoliative cytoglogic examinations from lung, breast, bladder, and uterine cervix. May be mutagenic and carcinogenic. Acquired resistance may develop and is thought due to intracellular inactivation of busulphan before it reaches nuclear DNA.

Used in palliative treatment of chronic myelogenous (myeloid, granulocytic, myelocytic) leukaemia for patients no longer responsive to radiation therapy or to previously tried antineoplastics. Does not appreciably extend survival time.

ROUTE AND DOSAGE   Dosage highly individualized. **Oral: Adults:** 60 mcg daily until maximal clinical and haematologic improvement is obtained. *Maintenance* 0.5–2 mg daily (individualized).

ABSORPTION AND FATE   Within 4 hours after oral dose, a constant blood level of 1 to 3% of the dose is reached and maintained for about 4 hours. Metabolized in the liver. About 10 to 50% of dose excreted in urine as metabolites within 48 hours.

BUSULPHAN (continued)

CONTRAINDICATIONS AND PRECAUTIONS Prior irradiation or chemotherapy, therapy-resistant chronic myelocytic leukaemia, neutrophilia, thrombocytopenia, infection, pregnancy. Safe use during lactation not established. **Cautious Use**: men and women in childbearing years, history of gout or urate renal stones.

ADVERSE/SIDE EFFECTS (Major toxic effects are related to bone marrow failure.) Side effects include: alopecia, hyperpigmentation (especially if dark complexioned), cheilosis, urticaria, erythema multiforme and nodosum, porphyria cutanea tarda, excessive dryness and fragility, of skin with anhydrosis, nausea, vomiting, diarrhoea, glossitis, stomatitis, anorexia, renal calculi, uric acid nephropathy, (hyperuricaemia, hyperuricosuria), acute renal failure, gynaecomastia, testicular atrophy, azoospermia, impotence, sterility in males, ovarian suppression, amenorrhoea (potentially irreversible), menopausal symptoms. Other side effects (usually dose-related) include: agranulocytosis (rare), pancytopenia, thrombocytopenia, leucopenia, anaemia. In addition the following can occur: irreversible pulmonary fibrosis ('busulphan lung'), endocardial fibrosis, dizziness, cholestatic jaundice, cataracts, myasthenia gravis, Addison-like syndrome: (weakness, severe fatigue, confusion, anorexia, nausea, vomiting, diarrhoea, weight loss, melanoderma), cellular dysplasia, superinfections, haemorrhagic complications. Potentially mutagenic and carcinogenic.

NURSING IMPLICATIONS

- Advise patient to take busulphan as directed, at the same time each day.
- Hgb, Hct, total WBC, differential and quantitative platelet counts, liver and kidney function tests are obtained initially and at least weekly during therapy with busulphan.
- Patients sensitive to busulphan may manifest abrupt onset of haematotoxicity. Recovery from busulphan-induced pancytopenia may take 1 month to 2 years. It may be irreversible in some patients.
- Usually the leucocyte count does not start to decrease for about 10 to 15 days after therapy begins; it may actually increase during this period.
- With recommended dosage of busulphan, the normal leucocyte count is usually achieved in about 2 months.
- Remissions are characterized by increased appetite and sense of well-being within a few days after therapy begins.
- Monitor fluid intake and output ratio and pattern. Urge patient to increase fluid intake to 10 to 12 glasses (240 mls each) daily to assure adequate urinary output. Allopurinol and urine alkalinization are prescribed prophylactic measures with hydration to reduce incidence of hyperuricaemia and/or hyperuricuria.
- Weigh patient at least weekly. A slow but steady change in weight should be communicated to physician.
- Make daily inspection of skin, oral membranes, and sites used for blood specimens for abnormal bleeding due to thrombocytopenia. Ecchymotic or petechial bleeding, epistaxis, or bleeding gums should be reported promptly.
- Because of hyperpigmentation, signs of cholestatic jaundice may be overlooked. Caution patient to report yellow sclera, dark urine, or light-coloured stools.

BUSULPHAN (continued)

- Advise patient to report immediately the onset of cough, low grade fever, dyspnoea, possible symptoms of pulmonary fibrosis (busulphan lung), easy bruising or bleeding, sore mouth or throat, unusual fatigue (agranulocytosis), blurred vision (cataract), flank or joint pain, swelling of lower legs and feet (hyperuricaemia).
- Be alert to symptoms suggestive of superinfection: fever, white patches in mouth, black hairy tongue, foul smelling vaginal discharge or stools, anogenital itching, diarrhoea.
- Ovarian suppression and amenorrhoea with menopausal symptoms commonly occur in premenopausal women. Effects are not apparent for 4 to 6 months. Amenorrhoea may be irreversible.
- Contraceptive measures should be used during busulphan therapy and for at least 3 months after drug is withdrawn.
- Discuss possibility of alopecia with patient so that wigs may be ordered if desired. Advise patient to brush hair gently and not more than is necessary.
- Busulphan is a highly toxic drug and additionally some patients eventually develop resistance to it. Urge patient to keep follow-up appointments.
- Instruct patient that it is critically important to report promptly symptoms of bone marrow suppression: i.e., fever, sore throat, bleeding from any site, symptoms suggestive of anaemia, signs of local infection. Any of these symptoms may indicate either busulphan toxicity or transformation of the disease to an acute 'blastic' form.
- *See mustine for nursing care of oral side effects.*
- Store drug in tightly capped, light-resistant container at temperature between 15° and 30°C (59° and 86°F), unless otherwise specified by the manufacturer.

Diagnostic test interferences   Busulphan may decrease *urinary 17-CS excretion*, and may increase **blood and urine uric acid** levels. Drug-induced cellular dysplasia may interfere with interpretation of **cytologic studies.**

DRUG INTERACTIONS   *Busulphan*

PLUS	INTERACTIONS
Antigout medication (e.g., probenecid)	Busulphan increases uric acid levels; dose of antigout agent may require adjustment

Butriptyline

(Evadyne)   *Tricyclic antidepressant*

ACTIONS AND USES   Used to treat depression.

ROUTE AND DOSAGE   Oral: 25 mg three times a day increased to maximum of 150 mg/day if necessary.

For further information *see amytryptyline.*

Calciferol

(Calciferol, Ergocalcifercl, Chocovite,   *(Serum) calcium regulator;*
                                                                      vitamin D

ACTIONS AND USES   Vitamin D analogue and major transport form of cholecalciferol (D$_3$); fat soluble. It is affected by the activity of other vitamin D analogues (e.g., ergocalciferol, qv), parathyroid hormone, and calcitonin. Pharmacological effects are related to intrinsic properties as well as to the properties of active metabolites which result from renal metabolism.

   Used in management of metabolic bone disease and hypocalcaemia associated with chronic renal failure in patients undergoing renal dialysis. Has been used for treatment of osteopenia caused by prolonged glucocorticoid therapy and for osteomalacia secondary to hepatic disease.

ROUTE AND DOSAGE   Oral: Variable, depending on indication.

ABSORPTION AND FATE   Rapidly absorbed from intestines. Peak serum concentrations reached after about 4 hours. **Half-life:** varies from 12 to 22 days, duration of action 15 to 20 days.

CONTRAINDICATIONS AND PRECAUTIONS   Hypersensitivity to vitamin D, vitamin D toxicity, hypercalcaemia. Safe use of doses in excess of RDA during pregnancy, in nursing women, and in children not established. **Cautious Use:** patients receiving digitalis glycosides.

ADVERSE/SIDE EFFECTS   Vitamin D intoxication and hypercalcaemia: drowsiness, lethargy, headache, weakness, vertigo, anorexia, nausea, vomiting, dry mouth, thirst, constipation, abdominal cramps, metallic taste, muscle or bone pain, polyuria, hypercalciuria, hyperphosphataemia. Idiosyncratic reaction: headache, nausea, vomiting, diarrhoea, fever. *See calciferol.*

NURSING IMPLICATIONS
- Baseline and periodic determinations should be made of serum calcium, phosphorus, magnesium, and alkaline phosphatase, and 24-hour urinary calcium and phosphorus levels.
- Serum calcium levels particularly should be monitored at least once weekly, or whenever dosage adjustments are made, and at periodic intervals thereafter.
- Effectiveness of therapy depends on an adequate daily intake of calcium. Since dietary calcium and phosphate are difficult to control, the physician may prescribe a calcium supplement as needed.
- Patients undergoing dialysis may require aluminium carbonate or hydroxide gels to bind intestinal phosphate and thus lower serum phosphate levels. Magnesium-containing antacids should not be used because of the possibility of hypermagnesaemia.
- Since calcitriol is a metabolite of vitamin D$_3$, all sources of vitamin D are usually withheld during therapy.
- Patients receiving digitalis glycosides will require close monitoring. Elevated serum calcium in these patients may precipitate arrhythmias.

CALCIFEROL (continued)

- Instruct patient to withhold drug and report immediately signs and symptoms of hypercalcaemia (*see Adverse/Side Effects*).
- Advise patient to consult physician before taking an OTC medication. Magnesium-containing laxatives and antacids, mineral oil, and vitamin D preparations should be avoided.
- Store preferably between 15° and 30°C (59° and 86°F) in tightly covered, light-resistant container unless otherwise directed by manufacturer.

DRUG INTERACTIONS *Calciferol*

PLUS	INTERACTIONS
Thiazide diuretics	Concurrent administration may result in hypercalcaemia
Verapamil and possibly other calcium channel blockers	Calciferol induced hypercalcaemia may result in decreased verapamil effectiveness (antagonist action). Monitor closely
Digitalis glycosides	Calciferol-induced hyperglycaemia may precipitate arrhythmias

Calcitonin

Hormone; (serum) calcium regulator

ACTIONS AND USES   Synthetic polypeptide derived from salmon or porcine calcitonin. Inhibits bone resorption, lowers serum calcium concentration, and appears to accelerate bone formation and mineral deposition. Inhibition of bone resorption decreases both mineral release and collagen breakdown. Promotes renal excretion of calcium and phosphorus and causes transient sodium and water loss. Decreased volume and acidity of gastric juice and decreased volume of pancreatic trypsin and amylase are also transient effects. Increases small bowel secretion of potassium, chlorides, sodium, and water but not calcium. In Paget's disease, slows rate of bone turnover, with resultant decreases in serum alkaline phosphatase and urinary hydroxyproline, biochemical changes that seem to correspond with more normal bone formation. In some patients, long-term use initiates drug resistance due to formation of neutralizing antibodies. Transient hypocalcaemia that follows therapeutic doses is asymptomatic and mild.

Used in treatment of symptomatic Paget's disease of bone (porcine only), as short-term adjunctive treatment of severe hypercalcaemia of cancer (with or without metastasis), immobilization, or hyperparathyroidism, particularly when renal, hepatic, or cardiac disease limits use of other forms of treatment.

ROUTE AND DOSAGE   Subcutaneous, intramuscular: *Paget's disease Initial*: 4–8 units/kg/day increased according to biochemical results. *Paget's disease of the bone*:

CALCITONIN (continued)

80–60 units 3 times a week increased to daily in patients with bone pain or nerve compression. *Hypercalcaemia*: 200 units according to biochemical results.

ABSORPTION AND FATE   Following IM or SC injection, action begins within 15 minutes, peaks in 4 hours, and persists 8 to 24 hours. Rapidly metabolized, primarily by kidneys. Excreted as inactive metabolites in urine. Does not cross placenta barrier; passage to CSF or to breast milk not established.

CONTRAINDICATIONS AND PRECAUTIONS   Hypersensitivity to fish and calcitonin; history of allergy; children, pregnancy, nursing mothers. **Cautious Use**: renal impairment, osteoporosis, pernicious anaemia, Zollinger–Ellison syndrome.

ADVERSE/SIDE EFFECTS   Transient nausea, vomiting, local inflammatory reaction at injection site, swelling, tingling, and tenderness of hands, facial flushing, unusual taste sensation, headache, diarrhoea, skin rash (rare), diuresis, calcitonin antibody formation, hypersensitivity (systemic) reaction, hypocalcaemic tetany (rare).

NURSING IMPLICATIONS
- If patient is being taught to self-administer calcitonin, the SC route is preferred.
- Teach patient to recognize and seek advice about local inflammatory reactions at site of injection. Careful avoidance of consecutive use of same area is as important as the required sterile technique.
- When the volume of calcitonin to be injected exceeds 2 ml, the IM route is employed, and multiple sites should be used. Rotate injection sites.
- Compliance with daily injections of calcitonin is based on complete understanding of rationale for treatment and a technique that is as free from discomfort as possible.
- Since calcitonin is a protein, systemic allergic reaction is a possibility. A skin test is usually done prior to initiation of therapy. The appearance of more than mild erythema or wheal 15 minutes after intracutaneous injection of calcitonin constitutes a positive response and indicates that the drug should not be given.
- Have on hand adrenaline antihistamines, oxygen in the event of a reaction. Also have readily available parenteral calcium, particularly during early therapy. Hypocalcaemic tetany is a theoretical possibility.
- Periodic laboratory examination of urine specimens for sediment is recommended when patient is on long-term therapy.

Paget's disease
- Diuresis that occurs during early therapy is thought to be related to improvement in circulation.
- Drug effect is monitored by evaluation of symptoms and periodic measurement of serum alkaline phosphatase, 24-hour urinary hydroxyproline and serum calcium.
- Clinical response to calcitonin therapy in Paget's disease may not occur until after several months of therapy. It is evidenced by reduced bone pain, lowered skin temperature over involved bone, slight improvement or at least no further loss of hearing (hearing loss is due to compression of temporal bone on eighth cranial nerve), possible reversal of neurological symptoms related to compression of spinal cord and

CALCITONIN (continued)

nerves, measurable decreases in cardiac output, and decreases in serum alkaline phosphatase and urinary hydroxyproline values.

- Therapeutic effectiveness of long-term calcitonin treatment generally persists months after drug is withdrawn; pretreatment status usually returns after 1 to 2 years therapy.
- If biochemical (hypercalcaemia) or clinical relapse (return of painful symptoms of Paget's disease) occurs, calcitonin antibody title and patient compliance should be evaluated.
- Test for high antibody title. After overnight fasting, a sample of blood is drawn for determination of serum calcium prior to IM administration of calcitonin. Patient then eats usual breakfast. At 3 and 6 hours postinjection, additional blood samples are drawn. Findings: decrease from fasting serum calcium levels of 0.5 mg% or more is seen in the responsive patient. A decrease of 0.3 mg% or less constitutes inadequate hypocalcaemic response. Further use of calcitonin will be ineffective.
- Circulating antibodies to salmon calcitonin may occur in 30 to 50% of patients after 2 to 18 months of treatment. A relapse after good initial response suggests probable treatment failure.

Hypercalcaemia

- Many patients have a return to the original elevated serum calcium after but a few days of emergency use of calcitonin. Hypercalcaemia is suspected if the following symptom are present: deep bone and flank pain, renal calculi, polyuria, anorexia, nausea, vomiting, thirst, constipation, muscle hypotonicity, pathological fracture, bradycardia, lethargy, psychosis.
- Teach patient the importance of maintaining drug regimen even though symptoms have been ameliorated, to prevent early relapses.
- Theoretically, calcitonin can lead to hypocalcaemic tetany (increased neuromuscular excitability).
- If calcitonin is being used as an antihypercalcaemic, the physician may prescribe reduced dietary calcium intake. High-calcium foods include greens, milk, and dairy products. Coordinate dietary planning with dietitian, patient, and family.
- Advise patient to consult physician before using OTC preparations. Some supervitamins, haematinics, and antacids contain calcium.
- Store calcitonin in refrigerator preferably at 2° to 8°C (36° to 46°F) unless otherwise directed by manufacturer.

Calcitriol

(Rocaltrol)   (Serum) Calcium regulator

ACTIONS AND USES Synthetic form of 1,25-dihydroxycholecalciferol, an active metabolite of ergocalciferol (q.v.). In the liver, cholecalciferol (vitamin D_3) and

CALCITRIOL *(continued)*

ergocalciferol (vitamin D_2) are enzymatically metabolized to calciferol an activated form of vitamin D_3.

Used in management of hypocalcaemia in patients undergoing chronic renal dialysis, and in patients with hypoparathyroidism or pseudohypoparathyroidism.

ROUTE AND DOSAGE   Oral: *Initial*: 1−2 mcg/day. May be increased by 0.25 mcg/day at 4- to 8-week intervals for dialysis patients, and 2- to 4-week intervals for hypoparathyroid patients if necessary, to a maximum of 2−3 mcg/day.

ABSORPTION AND FATE   Rapidly and completely absorbed from the intestine. **Onset of action** in about 2 to 6 hours. **Peak hypercalcaemic effect** in 10 to 12 hours; **duration of action** 3 to 5 days. **Half-life**: 3 to 6 hours. Metabolized in liver. Elimination is mainly faecal, being excreted with bile; about 4 to 6% excreted in urine. Approximately 65% of dose eliminated within 6 days.

CONTRAINDICATIONS AND PRECAUTIONS   Hypercalcaemia or vitamin D toxicity. Safe use during pregnancy in nursing women, and in children not established. **Cautious Use**: hyperphosphataemia, patients receiving digitalis glycosides.

ADVERSE/SIDE EFFECTS   Vitamin D intoxication and *hypercalcaemia* (drowsiness, headache, weakness, anorexia, nausea, vomiting, dry mouth, thirst, constipation, abdominal cramps, muscle or bone pain, metallic taste); hypercalciuria, hyperphosphataemia. *See also ergocalciferol.*

NURSING IMPLICATIONS

- Baseline and periodic determinations should be made of serum calcium, phosphorus, magnesium, alkaline phosphatase, creatinine, and 24-hour urinary calcium and phosphorus levels.
- To guard against metastatic calcification, the product of serum calcium multiplied by phosphate (Ca × P) should not be allowed to exceed 70. A fall in serum alkaline phosphatase frequently signals the onset of hypercalcaemia.
- During early therapy, serum calcium levels particularly should be monitored twice weekly. Some clinicians prescribe weekly serum calcium levels for the first 12 weeks of therapy, and monthly after dosage is stabilized.
- Effectiveness of therapy depends on an adequate daily intake of calcium and phosphate. Since dietary calcium and phosphate are difficult to control, the physician may prescribe a calcium supplement on an as needed basis.
- Excessive intake of calcium and phosphate can cause hypercalcaemia, hypercalciuria, and hyperphosphataemia.
- Review symptoms of hypercalcaemia with patient and advise him or her to withhold drug and contact physician if they occur.
- If hypercalcaemia develops, calcium supplements (if being taken) should be discontinued until serum calcium returns to normal. Reduction of dietary calcium intake should also be considered. (*See Index: Food sources.*)
- Since calcitriol is the most potent form of vitamin D_3 all sources of vitamin D should be withheld during therapy, to avoid possibility of hypercalcaemia.
- Patients undergoing dialysis may require aluminium carbonate or hydroxide gels to

CALCITRIOL (continued)

bind intestinal phosphate and thus lower serum phosphate levels. Magnesium-containing antacids are not to be used, to avoid possibility of hypermagnesaemia.

- Advise patient to consult physician before taking an OTC medication.
- **Treatment of overdosage**   Induction of emesis or gastric lavage. General supportive therapy.
- Monitor serial serum electrolytes (especially calcium), urinary calcium, and ECG. Discontinue supplemental calcium, and institute low calcium diet.
- Capsules should be protected from heat, light, and moisture. Store in well-closed container preferably between 15° and 30°C (59° and 86°F), unless otherwise directed by manufacturer.
- See also calciferol.

DRUG INTERACTIONS   *Calcitriol*

PLUS	INTERACTIONS
Digitalis glycosides	Calcitriol-induced hypercalcaemia may precipitate arrhythmias. Close monitoring indicated
Thiazide diuretics	Pharmacological effects of calcitriol may be increased with possibility of hypercalcaemia. Monitor closely
Verapamil, and possibly other calcium channel blockers	Calcitriol-induced hypercalcaemia may antagonize antiarrhythmic properties of verapamil. Monitor closely

Calcium carbonate

(Nulacin, Titralac)   *Antacid*

ACTIONS AND USES   Antacid with rapid action, high neutralizing capacity, relatively prolonged duration of action, and low cost. Although classified as a nonsystemic antacid, a slight to moderate alkalosis usually develops with prolonged therapy.

Used for symptomatic relief of hyperacidity associated with peptic ulcer and for relief of transient symptoms of acid indigestion, heartburn, sour stomach, peptic oesophagitis, and hiatus hernia.

ROUTE AND DOSAGE   Oral: *Antacid*: 0.5 to 2 g four to six times daily, if necessary.

NURSING IMPLICATIONS

- When used as antacid, taken between meals (e.g., 1 hour after meals) and at bedtime. When used as calcium supplement, taken with meals.
- Available in tablet and powder form. For maximum effectiveness, tablet should be chewed well before swallowing, or allowed to dissolve completely in mouth; followed with water. Powder form is dispersed in water or may be sprinkled on food if taken as calcium supplement.

CALCIUM CARBONATE (continued)

- Because of acid rebound, which generally occurs after repeated use for 1 or 2 weeks, one can quickly become a chronic user of calcium carbonate. Explain to patient the potential dangers of self-medication.
- Now mostly replaced by H_2 receptor antagonists such as Cimetidine.

Calcium gluconate

Replenisher; Calcium

ACTIONS AND USES   Calcium is an essential element for regulating the excitation threshold of nerves and muscles, for blood clotting mechanisms, cardiac function (rhythm, tonicity, contractility), maintenance of renal function, for body skeleton and teeth. Also plays a role in regulating storage and release of neurotransmitters and hormones; regulating amino acid uptake and absorption of cyanocobalamin (vitamin B_{12}); gastrin secretion, and in maintaining structural and functional integrity of cell membranes and capillaries. Calcium gluconate acts like digitalis on heart, increasing cardiac muscle tone and force of systolic contractions (positive inotropic effect).

Used to treat negative calcium balance (as in neonatal tetany, hypoparathyroidism, vitamin D deficiency, alkalosis, and intestinal malabsorption states). Also used to overcome cardiac toxicity of hyperkalaemia, for cardiopulmonary resuscitation, to prevent hypocalcaemia during transfusion of citrated blood, used as antidote for magnesium sulphate, for acute symptoms of lead colic, to decrease capillary permeability in sensitivity reactions, and to relieve muscle cramps in treatment of insect bites or stings, e.g., black widow spider. Oral calcium may be used to maintain normal calcium balance during pregnancy, lactation, and childhood growth period and to prevent primary osteoporosis. Effervescent preparation in combination with calcium lactate (Sandocal).

ROUTE AND DOSAGE   **Adults: Oral:** 1 to 2 g two to four times a day. *Supplement in osteoporosis:* 1 to 1.5 g daily. **Intravenous:** 0.5 to 2 g (5 to 20 ml) 10% solution given slowly at rate not exceeding 0.5 ml/minute. **Children:** 500 mg/kg/day in divided doses, orally or well diluted and given slowly by IV.

ABSORPTION AND FATE   Cardiac response to IV injection is immediate and lasts ½ to 2 hours. Following oral administration, approximately one-third of dose is absorbed, primarily from proximal segments of small bowel. Vitamin D probably increases active transport of calcium from gut lumen. About 45% bound to plasma proteins. Largely excreted unchanged in faeces; small amounts also excreted in urine, pancreatic juice, saliva, and breast milk. Crosses placenta.

CONTRAINDICATIONS AND PRECAUTIONS   Ventricular fibrillation, metastatic bone disease, injection into myocardium; administration by SC or IM routes; renal calculi, hypercalcaemia. **Cautious Use:** digitalized patients, renal or cardiac insufficiency, sarcoidosis, history of lithiasis, immobilized patients.

CALCIUM GLUCONATE (continued)

ADVERSE/SIDE EFFECTS   Hypercalcaemia: anorexia, nausea, thirst, vomiting, abdominal pain, constipation, ileus, somnolence, fatigue, headache, decreased excitability of muscles and nerves, pathological fractures, muscle and joint pain, excessive thirst, nocturia, polyuria, azotemia, mental confusion, psychosis, renal calculi, acute pancreatitis, bradycardia and other arrhythmias. **IV injection**: tingling sensations, calcium (chalky) taste; Rapid IV: sense of oppression or 'heat waves' (vasodilation), hypotension, bradycardia and other arrhythmias, syncope, cardiac arrest. Local reaction: tissue irritation, burning, cellulitis, soft tissue calcification, necrosis and sloughing (following IV extravasation). Oral preparations: constipation.

NURSING IMPLICATIONS

- IV calcium should be administered slowly through a small bore needle into a large vein, to avoid possibility of extravasation and resultant necrosis. If administered to children, scalp veins should be avoided.
- Physician will prescribe specific IV flow rate. High concentrations of calcium suddenly reaching the heart can cause fatal cardiac arrest.
- During IV administration, ECG is monitored to detect evidence of hypercalcaemia: decreased QT interval associated with inverted T wave.
- Direct IV injection may be accompanied by cutaneous burning sensations and peripheral vasodilation, with moderate fall in blood pressure. Injection should be stopped if patient complains of any discomfort. Patient should be advised to remain in bed for ½ to 1 hour or more following injection, depending on response.
- Observe IV site closely. Extravasation may result in tissue irritation and necrosis.
- Although sometimes prescribed for the adult, the IM route is not recommended. It is specifically contraindicated in children because it may result in abscess formation.
- Oral calcium preparations are best utilized when administered 2 to 3 hours after meals. Calcium gluconate is reported to be nonirritating to GI mucosa.
- Therapeutic effects in treatment of tetany (hypocalcaemia) are evaluated by amelioration of neuromuscular hyperexcitability: paraesthesias (numbness and tingling of fingers, toes, and lips), skeletal muscle spasms, twitching of facial muscles, intestinal hypermotility and colic, carpopedal spasm, laryngospasm, convulsions, and cardiac arrhythmias.
- If patient has hypocalcaemia or if it is suspected, padded side rails are advisable. Also, have on hand mouth gag, airway, and suction apparatus in the event of laryngeal spasm. Control environmental stimuli, e.g., noise level.
- Recommended daily intake of calcium for infants younger than 6 months: 360 mg; for infants ½ to 1 year: 540 mg; for children 1 to 10 years and adults: 800 mg/day; for pregnant and lactating women and during adolescence (10 to 18 years): 1200 mg/day.

Food–drug interactions

- Vitamin D is required for absorption of Ca; therefore it is used to fortify milk and calcium supplements.
- Milk products are best sources of calcium (and phosphorus); other sources include: green leafy vegetables (see below) as well as sardines, clams, and oysters.

CALCIUM GLUCONATE (continued)

■ Avoid taking drug with cereals. Phytic acid (phytates) in outer hulls of many grains (especially wheat and bran) combine with Ca to form insoluble nonabsorbable compounds.

■ Ca absorption is blocked when its compounds are ingested with oxalate-rich foods: spinach, rhubarb, greens, almonds, cashews, chocolate, cocoa.

■ If diet is low in Ca and high in oxylate foods, calcium deficiency is enhanced.

■ Ca absorption may be inhibited by zinc-rich foods: nuts, seeds, sprouts, legumes, soy products (tofu).

■ Calcium should be taken 2 hours before or 3 hours after meals. This may be particularly important to the total vegetarian who often has marginal Ca intake.

■ To facilitate intestinal absorption of calcium gluconate, physician may prescribe reduced phosphate intake (milk and other dairy products) or simultaneous administration of aluminium hydroxide, which forms insoluble phosphate salts.

Diagnostic test interferences IV calcium may cause false decreases in **serum and urine magnetism** (by Titan yellow method) and transient elevations of **plasma 11-OHCS** levels by Glenn-Nelson technique. Values usually return to control levels after 60 minutes; **urinary steroid** values may be decreased.

Drug interactions Calcium gluconate and other Ca containing drugs enhance the inotropic and toxic effects of **digitalis glycosides** and may precipitate cardiac arrhythmias; may compete with **magnesium** for absorption with resulting magnesium deficiency (note that calcium can also produce false decrease in tests for serum Mg). Oral calcium forms a complex with **tetracyclines** and thus decreases their effect; do not administer within 3 hours of each other. (The two drugs are also incompatible in parenteral solutions.) Calcium gluconate-induced hypercalcaemia may antagonize effectiveness of verapamil and possibly other calcium channel blockers.

Calcium lactate

Replenisher; calcium

ACTIONS AND USES Oral calcium preparation reportedly well tolerated. Contains approximately 13% calcium. Similar to calcium gluconate (q.v.) in actions, uses, contraindications, and adverse reactions.

Used to treat mild hypocalcaemia and for maintenance calcium therapy.

ROUTE AND DOSAGE Oral: Adults: 325 mg to 1.3 g three times a day with meals. Children: 500 mg/kg/24 hours in divided doses.

NURSING IMPLICATIONS

■ Tablets or powder can be dissolved in hot water; then add cool water to patient's taste.

CALCIUM LACTATE (continued)

- May be administered with lactose (amount prescribed) to increase solubility.
- Hospital pharmacy may prepare calcium lactate solution on request.
- Blood calcium levels should be checked periodically. Hypercalcaemia may occur during prolonged administration particularly if patient is also taking vitamin D.
- Bear in mind that an increase in serum calcium in digitalized patients increases risk of digitalis toxicity.
- Store in airtight containers.
- *See calcium gluconate.*

Capreomycin

(Capastat)

Antiinfective; antibiotic (polypeptide); antituberculosis

ACTIONS AND USES   Polypeptide antibiotic derived from *Streptomyces capreolus*. Bacteriostatic in action; mechanism not clear. Active against human strains of *Mycobacterium tuberculosis* and other strains of *Mycobacterium*. Cross-resistance between capreomycin and both kanamycin and neomycin has been reported. Produces neuromuscular blockade in large doses.

Used in treatment of pulmonary tuberculosis when causative organism has become resistant.

ROUTE AND DOSAGE   Intramuscular: 1 g daily (not to exceed 20 mg/kg body weight per day) given for 60 to 120 days, followed by 1 g two or three times weekly.

ABSORPTION AND FATE   Peak drug serum levels in 1 to 2 hours. Serum concentrations fall to low levels by 24 hours. Half-life: 4 to 6 hours. Approximately 52% is excreted in urine within 12 hours (if renal function is normal) essentially unchanged. Distribution to placenta and breast milk not known.

CONTRAINDICATIONS AND PRECAUTIONS   Hypersensitivity to capreomycin. Safe use during pregnancy, in nursing women and in infants and children not established. **Cautious Use:** extreme caution, if used at all in patients with renal insufficiency, auditory impairment, history of allergies (especially to drugs), preexisting liver disease, myasthenia gravis, parkinsonism.

ADVERSE/SIDE EFFECTS   These include: leukocytosis, leukopenia, eosinophilia. urticaria, maculopapular rash may be associated with febrile reaction, photosensitivity. **Nephrotoxicity:** (long-term therapy): elevated BUN and NPN, abnormal urine sediment, haematuria, pyuria, albuminuria, depressed creatinine clearance and PSP excretion, tubular necrosis. Other side effects include: eighth nerve (auditory and vestibular) damage: hearing loss, tinnitus, headache, vertigo. Others: hypokalaemia, and other electrolyte imbalances (associated with disturbed renal function; impaired

CAPREOMYCIN (continued)

hepatic function (decreased BSP excretion); neuromuscular blockade (large doses): skeletal muscle weakness, respiratory depression or arrest; IM site reactions: pain, induration, excessive bleeding, sterile abscesses.

NURSING IMPLICATIONS

- The following determinations are used as guidelines for therapy and should be performed before drug is started and at regular intervals during therapy: (1) appropriate bacterial susceptibility tests; (2) audiometric measurements and tests of vestibular function; (3) complete blood counts; (4) function studies (BUN, NPN, creatinine clearance, sediment); (5) liver function tests; (6) serum potassium levels.
- IM injections should be made deep into large muscle mass. Superficial injections are more painful and are associated with sterile abscess. Aspirate carefully before injecting drug to avoid inadvertent entry into blood vessel (IV injection can cause neuromuscular blockade). Rotate injection sites.
- Observe injection sites for signs of excessive bleeding and inflammation.
- Monitor fluid intake and output. Report immediately to physician any change in fluid output or intake and output ratio, any unusual appearance of urine.
- Instruct patient to report any change in hearing or disturbance of balance. Capreomycin can cause injury to both auditory and vestibular portions of cranial nerve VIII. These effects are sometimes reversible if drug is withdrawn promptly when first symptoms appear.
- Hypokalaemia is a significant side effect. Observe for and report muscle weakness, paraesthesias, depressed reflexes, polyuria, polydipsia, gastric distention, unexplained anxiety.
- Patient and responsible family members should be completely informed about adverse reactions. They should be urged to report immediately the appearance of any unusual symptom, regardless how vague it may seem.
- Capreomycin is reconstituted by adding isotonic sodium chloride injection or sterile water for infection to vial; allow 2 to 3 minutes for drug to dissolve completely. *See manufacturer's directions for volume of diluent.*
- Solution may become pale straw colour and darken with time, but this does not indicate loss of potency or toxicity.
- After reconstitution, solution may be stored 48 hours at room temperature and up to 14 days under refrigeration, unless otherwise directed by manufacturer.
- Store preferably between 15° and 30°C (59° and 86°F), unless otherwise directed by manufacturer.

DRUG INTERACTIONS *Capreomycin*

PLUS	INTERACTIONS
Drugs with high nephrotoxic or ototoxic potential, e.g., aminoglycoside antibiotics, colistin, polymyxin B, vancomycin	Increased risk of nephrotoxicity and ototoxicity. Concurrent or sequential use generally avoided
Aminoglycoside antibiotics Phenothiazines Tubocurarine and other nondepolarizing skeletal muscle relaxants	Possibility of additive neuromuscular blocking actions. Monitor for respiratory depression

Captopril

(Acepril Capoten)   *Antihypertensive*

ACTIONS AND USES   Lowers blood pressure (renovascular and essential) by specific inhibition of the angiotensin-converting enzyme. Additionally, captopril is associated with interference with degradation of bradykinin (a potent vasodilator), increased plasma levels of a prostaglandin E_2 metabolite with vasodilator properties and a K-sparing effect (due to reduced aldosterone level). In heart failure, captopril administration is followed by a fall in CVP and pulmonary wedge pressure. Hypertensive action in essential hypertension appears to be unrelated to plasma renin levels. Available in fixed combination with hydrochlorothiazide.

Used in treatment of mild to moderate hypertension; in severe hypertension resistant to conventional multidrug regimen and in conjunction with digitalis and diuretics in treatment of intractable oedema or congestive heart failure.

ROUTE AND DOSAGE   Oral: *Initial* 12.5 mg, increased to maximum of 150 mg/day. *Usual maintenance dose* 25 mg twice a day.

ABSORPTION AND FATE   About 60 to 75% of dose absorbed rapidly following oral administration. Hypotensive effect of a single dose begins within 15 minutes, is maximal in 1 to 2 hours, and continues for 6 hours with small doses and up to 12 hours with larger doses. Rapid distribution to all tissues except CNS. Approximately 25 to 30% bound to plasma proteins. **Half-life**: less than 2 hours; increases to 20 to 40 hours when creatinine clearance is less than 20 ml/min. Over 95% of an absorbed dose excreted in urine as unchanged drug (40 to 50%) and metabolites. Removed by haemodialysis. It is not known if it crosses placenta, but it is distributed to breast milk.

CONTRAINDICATIONS AND PRECAUTIONS   Pregnancy: safe use in nursing mothers and children not established. **Cautious Use**: impaired renal function; patient with solitary kidney; autoimmune diseases (particularly systemic lupus erythematosus), patient receiving immunosuppressants or other drugs that cause leukopenia or agranulocytosis; coronary or cerebrovascular disease; severe salt/volume depletion.

ADVERSE/SIDE EFFECTS   These include: slight increase in heart rate, hypotension, dizziness, fainting; rare: tachycardia, palpitation, angina pectoris, myocardial infarction, Raynaud's syndrome. Other adverse effects include: oncholysis, maculopapular rash (especially on upper extremities and trunk), urticaria, pruritus, angio-oedema, photosensitivity, severe anorexia, GI distress, neutropenia, agranulocytosis, pancytopenia, proteinuria, urinary frequency, oliguria, impaired renal function, nephrotic syndrome, membranous glomerulonephritis, reversible 'scalded mouth sensation' (loss of taste perception, persistent salt or metallic taste); weight loss, cholestatic jaundice (rare), positive antinuclear antibody titres, hyperkalaemia.

NURSING IMPLICATIONS
- If necessary, tablet may be crushed and taken with fluid. Best administered 1 hour before meals. Food reduces absorption by 30 to 40%.

CAPTOPRIL (continued)

■ Hyponatraemia is a good predictor of potential first-dose phenomenon. Liberalized salt intake and termination of diuretic therapy are usual preparations 7 to 10 days before captopril treatment.

■ Bed rest and blood pressure monitoring are advised for the first 3 hours after the initial dose.

■ First dose phenomenon (hypotensive effect) (i.e., a precipitous drop in blood pressure) may occur within 1 to 3 hours of first dose, especially in the patient with very high blood pressure or one on a diuretic and controlled salt intake regimen. An IV infusion of normal saline for volume expansion will counteract the hypotensive response. (This initial response is not usually considered an indication to stop therapy with captopril.)

■ If patient is advised to restrict salt intake, emphasize that a salt substitute should be used only if prescribed. The abuse of a substitute (principal ingredient: K) can reinforce susceptibility to drug-induced hyperkalaemia. (*See Index: Salt substitutes*.)

■ At least 2 weeks of therapy may be required before full therapeutic effects are achieved. If patient has impaired renal function, doses must be smaller and attainment of steadystate captopril levels will require more time.

■ Baseline urinary protein levels should be established prior to initiation of therapy and checked at monthly intervals for the first 8 months of treatment and then periodically thereafter.

■ WBC and differential counts are recommended before starting therapy and at approximately 2-week intervals for the first 3 months of therapy and then periodically thereafter.

■ Urge patient to report to physician without delay the onset of unexplained fever, unusual fatigue, sore mouth or throat, easy bruising or bleeding (pathognomonic of agranulocytosis).

■ Since excessive vomiting, diarrhoea, and perspiration can lead to depleted fluids with consequent drop in blood pressure, advise patient to consult physician if these symptoms occur.

■ Mild skin eruptions are most likely to appear during the first 4 weeks of therapy and may be accompanied by fever and eosinophilia. Advise patient to report to physician. Dosage reduction or discontinuation may be indicated.

■ Darkening, separating, or crumbling of nailbeds (onycholysis) has been reported. These changes usually disappearing with dose reduction or termination.

■ Taste impairment (dysgeusia) occurs in 5 to 10% of patients and generally reverses in 2 to 3 months even with continued therapy. In some patients, it may be associated with anorexia and weight loss and may necessitate discontinuation of drug. If therapy is stopped, symptoms usually disappear within 3 to 4 weeks.

■ *Treatment of overdosage* involves correction of hypotension by blood volume expansion with IV infusions and possibly by haemodialysis.

■ See *guanethidine* for teaching summary related to pharmacotherapy in hypertension.

■ Store in light-resistant containers at no more than 30°C (86°F) unless otherwise directed by manufacturer.

CAPTOPRIL (continued)

Diagnostic test interferences   In some patients elevated **urine protein levels** may persist even after captopril has been discontinued. Possibility of transient elevations of BUN and **serum creatinine**, slight increase in **serum potassium**, and **serum prolactin**, increases in **liver enzymes**, and false-positive **urine acetone**.

DRUG INTERACTIONS   *Captopril*

PLUS	INTERACTIONS
Antihypertensives that cause renin release [e.g., minoxidil]	Additive hypotensive action of captopril
Ganglionic blocking agents [e.g., mecamylamine] and other nitrates	Possible enhancement of hypotensive action of captopril (by reducing CNS support of blood pressure)
	Possibility of enhanced hypotensive effect (by vasodilation) of captopril
Indomethacin } Salicylates }	Antihypertensive effectiveness of captopril may be decreased. Dosage adjustments may be indicated
Potassium-sparing diuretics [e.g., amiloride] K supplements (e.g., potassium chloride) }	Possibility of hyperkalaemia
Probenecid	Pharmacological effects of captopril may be increased

Carbachol

(Isopto carbachol)

Cholinergic; direct (parasympathomimetic); miotic

ACTIONS AND USES   Potent synthetic choline ester similar to acetylcholine in pharmacological properties. Inactivation by cholinesterase is slow; therefore its actions are more prolonged than those of acetylcholine; also more potent and longer-acting than pilocarpine. Acts directly on neuroeffectors of circular pupillary constrictor and ciliary muscles, producing miosis and spasms of accommodation, thus facilitating drainage from anterior chamber with consequent lowering of intraocular pressure.

Used intraocularly to produce pupillary miosis during ocular surgery. Used topically to reduce intraocular pressure in open-angle or narrow-angle glaucoma, particularly when patient has become intolerant of or resistant to pilocarpine. Also used to treat urinary retention.

ROUTE AND DOSAGE   Topical ophthalmic: 1 or 2 drops of 0.75 to 3% solution instilled into lower conjunctival sac two or four times daily.

CARBACHOL (continued)

Acute urinary   Retention: Oral 2 mg/3 times a day half an hour before food. Subcutaneous: 250 mcg repeated twice after 30 minute intervals if necessary.

ABSORPTION AND FATE   Poor penetration of intact cornea. **Miotic action** occurs in 10 to 20 minutes following topical application and lasts 4 to 8 hours. Miotic action occurs in 2 to 5 minutes following intraocular administration and persists about 24 hours.

CONTRAINDICATIONS AND PRECAUTIONS   Known hypersensitivity to any of the components; corneal abrasions, acute iritis. Safe use during pregnancy, in nursing women and in children not established. **Cautious Use**: acute cardiac failure, bronchial asthma, peptic ulcer, GI spasms, obstructive ileus, hyperthyroidism, urinary tract obstruction, Parkinson's disease; use following topical anaesthetics or tonometry.

ADVERSE/SIDE EFFECTS   Headache, brow and eye pain, conjunctival hyperaemia, ciliary spasm with temporary reduction in visual acuity, iritis. **Systemic absorption**: sweating, flushing, ciliary spasm, abdominal cramps, increased peristalsis, diarrhoea, contractions of urinary bladder, transient fall in blood pressure with reflex tachycardia, asthma. Hypersensitivity reactions (infrequent).

NURSING IMPLICATIONS

- Eye drops are sterile and therefore should be handled so as to avoid contamination.
- Frequent administration of potent eye preparations presents the danger of systemic absorption if drug is allowed to drain into lacrimal system. Application of gentle pressure to nasolacrimal duct for 1 minute immediately after drop is instilled and before patient closes eyes prevents entry of drug into nasopharynx and general circulation. (For more complete description of administration technique, *See Index: Drug Administration: Eye drops.*)
- Patient may blot lid with clean tissue, but advise patient not to rub or squeeze lids together.
- Frequency and strength of drops are determined by patient's response and tolerance. Resistance may develop suddenly in some patients.
- The patient with glaucoma should remain under medical supervision for periodic tonometer measurements, since patient usually will require miotics for the rest of his or her life. The patient must understand that even in the absence of symptoms progressive ocular damage can occur unless appropriate treatment is received.
- Caution patient that drug may temporarily impair visual acuity particularly adaptation to dark and therefore to observe necessary safety precautions.
- Store preferably between 15° and 30°C (59° and 86°F), unless otherwise directed by manufacturer.
- Relieves urinary retention problems postoperatively or in neurological conditions.
- Following catheterization for acute retention, assess patients ability to void urine normally at regular intervals.
- Avoid the use of drugs with anticholinergic or sympathomimetic actions, these may cause retention by action on the bladder.
- Now rarely used in the UK.

Carbamazepine

(Tegretol) *Anticonvulsant*

ACTIONS AND USES Structurally related to tricyclic antidepressants but lacks anti-depressant properties. Anticonvulsant actions appear qualitatively similar to those of phenytoin. Like phenytoin, provides relief in trigeminal neuralgia by reducing synaptic transmission within trigeminal nucleus.

Used alone or concomitantly with other anticonvulsants in treatment of grand mal and psychomotor or temporal lobe epilepsy and mixed seizures in patients who have not responded satisfactorily to other agents. Also used for symptomatic treatment of trigeminal and glossopharyngeal neuralgias and for pain and paroxysmal symptoms associated with multiple sclerosis, and other neurological disorders and for antidiuretic effect in diabetes insipidus.

ROUTE AND DOSAGE **Oral:** 100−200 mg, 1−2 times a day initially increased slowly to 0.8−1.2 g daily according to need.

ABSORPTION AND FATE Slowly absorbed from GI tract; unpredictable absorption rate. **Peak serum levels** in 2 to 8 hours (variable). Widely distributed in body, especially in saliva, duodenal fluid, and bile; high concentrations in CSF. **Half-life:** 14 to 16 hours. Induces liver microsomal enzymes and thus may accelerate its own metabolism and that of drugs metabolized in liver. Highly bound (75 to 90%) to plasma proteins. Metabolites and less than 1% of unchanged drug excreted in urine and faeces. Crosses placenta and appears in breast milk in high concentrations.

CONTRAINDICATIONS AND PRECAUTIONS Hypersensitivity to carbamazepine and to tricyclic compounds; history of myelosuppression or haematological reaction to other drugs; increased intraocular pressure; systemic lupus erythematosus cardiac, hepatic, renal, or urinary tract disease; coronary artery disease; hypertension. Safe use in women of childbearing potential and during pregnancy, in nursing women, and in children younger than 6 years of age not established. **Cautious Use:** the elderly; history of cardiac disease.

ADVERSE/SIDE EFFECTS These include: dizziness, vertigo, drowsiness, disturbances of coordination, ataxia, confusion, headache, fatigue, tinnitus, abnormal hearing acuity, speech difficulty, development of minor motor seizures, hyperreflexia, involuntary movements, tremors, peripheral neuritis, paraesthesias, visual hallucinations, activation of latent psychosis, mental depression with agitation and talkativeness, oedema, congestive heart failure, aggravation of coronary artery disease, hypertension, hypotension, syncope, arrhythmias, heart block, thrombophlebitis, circulatory collapse. Other adverse reactions are as follows: skin rashes, urticaria, petechiae, Stevens-Johnson syndrome, photosensitivity reactions, altered skin pigmentation, exfoliative dermatitis, alopecia, wheezing nausea, vomiting, anorexia, abdominal pain, diarrhoea, constipation, dry mouth and pharynx, glossitis, stomatitis, urinary frequency and retention, oliguria, impotence, albuminuria, glycosuria, elevated blood urea nitrogen, acute renal

CARBAMAZEPINE (continued)

failure (rare), aplastic anaemia, reticulocytosis, leucopenia, leucocytosis, agranulo-cytosis, eosinophilia, thrombocytopenia, purpura, hyponatraemia, abnormal liver function tests, granulomatous hepatitis, cholestatic and hepatocellular jaundice, lens opacities, conjunctivitis, blurred vision, transient diplopia, oculomotor disturbances, nystagmus, mydriasis, idiosyncratic virus-like infection (fever, chills, lymphadeno-pathy), diaphoresis, pneumonitis, myalgia, arthralgia, leg cramps, hypothyroidism.

NURSING IMPLICATIONS

- Absorption of drug is enhanced by administration with meals.
- Physician will rely on accurate observation and early reporting to determine lowest effective dosage level.
- The following reactions occur commonly during early therapy: drowsiness, dizziness, lightheadedness, ataxia, gastric upset. If these symptoms do not subside within a few days, dosage adjustments may be indicated.
- In general, therapy should be discontinued if any signs of myelosuppression occur.
- Therapeutic serum levels reported to be 4 to 12 mcg/ml. Steady-state is generally reached in 2 to 4 days. Bear in mind that serum levels do not always reflect daily dosage requirements.
- Home patients and responsible family members should be instructed to withhold drug and notify physician immediately if early signs of a possible haematological problem appear, e.g., fever, sore throat or mouth, malaise, unusual fatigue, tendency to bruise or bleed, petechiae, ecchymoses, bleeding gums, nose bleeds.
- Monitor fluid intake and output ratio and vital signs during period of dosage adjustment. Report oliguria, signs of fluid retention (oedema, night coughing, dyspnoea), changes in intake and output ratio, and changes in blood pressure or pulse patterns.
- Doses higher than 600 mg/day may precipitate arrhythmias in patients with heart disease.
- The pain of trigeminal neuralgia is so excruciating that it has driven some patients to suicide. Learn from the patient what provokes attacks. Common triggering stimuli include drafts, shaving, washing face, talking, chewing, hot or cold fluids or foods, and jarring the bed.
- Because dizziness, drowsiness, and ataxia are common side effects, warn patient to avoid hazardous tasks requiring mental alertness and physical coordination.
- Impress on the patient and family the importance of remaining under close medical supervision throughout therapy.
- Confusion and agitation may be aggravated in the elderly; therefore side rails and supervision of ambulation may be indicated.
- Because photosensitivity reactions have been reported, caution patient to avoid excessive sunlight. Suggest application of a sunscreen (if allowed) with sun protection factor of 12 or above to exposed skin areas when outdoors.
- Patients taking oral contraceptives should be informed that carbamazepine may cause breakthrough bleeding and may also affect the reliability of oral contraceptives.
- At least every 3 months throughout therapy it is recommended that physician

CARBAMAZEPINE (continued)

attempt dosage reduction or termination of drug therapy, if possible, in patients with trigeminal neuralgia. Some patients develop tolerance to the effects of carbamazepine.

- In patients with epilepsy, abrupt withdrawal of any anticonvulsant drug may precipitate seizures or even status epilepticus.
- Store preferably between 15° and 30°C (59° and 86°F), unless otherwise directed by manufacturer.

DRUG INTERACTIONS *Carbamazepine*

PLUS	INTERACTIONS
Anticoagulants, oral Doxycycline Oral contraceptives Phenytoin Theophyllines	Carbamazepine appears to enhance metabolism of these drugs by inducing hepatic microsomal enzymes. Monitor closely for altered drug effectiveness when carbamazepine is initiated or discontinued
Erythromycins Isoniazid (INH) Niacinamide Propoxyphene	Carbamazepine actions may be increased (metabolism may be inhibited by these drugs). Monitor for carbamazepine toxicity
Lithium	Possibility of increased lithium effects and toxicity (may not be reflected in plasma lithium levels). Used concomitantly with caution
MAO inhibitors	Possibility of additive pharmacological actions. Concomitant use avoided

Carbenicillin disodium

(Pyopen)

Antibiotic (beta lactam); penicillin

ACTIONS AND USES Extended spectrum, penicillinase-sensitive, semisynthetic penicillin derived from penicillin G (benzylpenicillin). Similar to penicillin G (q.v.) in actions and adverse effects, but differs in having a broader range of antibacterial activity. Bactericidal against a variety of gram-negative and gram-positive microorganisms. Particularly effective against gram-negative infections caused by *Pseudomonas aeruginosa*, *Proteus*, susceptible strains of *Escherichia coli*, *Enterobacter*, *Haemophilus influenzae*, and *Neisseria gonorrhoeae*.

Used in the treatment of bacterial pneumonia, infection following burns, infections in patients with impaired immunological defenses, and urinary tract infections caused by microorganisms resistant to penicillin G and ampicillin. May be used concurrently with gentamycin and tobramycin pending results of culture and susceptibility test and with probenicid to attain higher and more prolonged serum levels.

ROUTE AND DOSAGE Highly individualized according to severity of infection and

CARBENICILLIN DISODIUM (continued)

status of renal function. **Intramuscular**: **Adult** 2 g every 6 hrs, **child**: 50–100 mg/kg/day in divided doses. **Intravenous**: by slow injection or rapid infusion; **adult**: 5 g every 4–6 hrs, **child**: 250–400 mg/kg/day in divided doses.

ABSORPTION AND FATE   **Serum concentrations peak** in 1 to 2 hours following IM injection, decline considerably by 3 hours, and are very low or absent by 6 hours. **Blood levels** are higher (in 15 to 30 minutes) following IV, but decrease more rapidly. **Serum half-life** about 67 minutes; prolonged to 10 to 15 hours in hepatic dysfunction and in renal impairment. Widely distributed in body tissues and fluids; low concentrations in CSF unless meninges are inflamed. Approximately 50% bound to plasma proteins. About 80 to 99% of single dose excreted unchanged in urine within 24 hours, most excreted in first 6 hours. Crosses placenta. Excreted in breast milk in small amounts.

CONTRAINDICATIONS AND PRECAUTIONS   Hypersensitivity to pencillins or cephalosporins. **Cautious Use**: history of or suspected atopy or allergies (asthma, hay fever, hives, eczema), renal or hepatic disease; coagulation disorders, patients on sodium restriction (cardiac patients; hypertensives). Safe use during pregnancy not established.

ADVERSE/SIDE EFFECTS   As for penicillin G (q.v.):

NURSING IMPLICATIONS
- Culture and sensitivity tests are performed initially and at regular intervals throughout therapy in order to monitor drug effectiveness.
- Careful inquiry should be made concerning hypersensitivity reactions to penicillin, cephalosporins, and other allergens.
- Check expiration date.
- IM injections should not exceed 2 g per individual injection site. Administer IM well into body of large muscle. Gluteus maximus and midlateral thigh are preferred sites for adults; midlateral thigh is the preferred site for children. Rotate injection sites.
- Pain and other local reactions associated with IM injections may be minimized by reconstituting drug with 0.5% lignocaine hydrochloride without adrenaline or bacteriostatic water for injection containing 0.9% benzyl alcohol. The latter must *not* be used in neonates.
- Follow manufacturer's directions explicitly regarding diluent and amount to use for initial reconstitution and for further dilution, to avoid tissue irritation and phlebitis.
- After reconstitution, IM solutions retain their stability for 24 hours at room temperature, and for 72 hours if refrigerated. Indicate time and date of reconstitution on container. Follow manufacturer's recommendations for stability, storage, and compatibility information.
- Monitor fluid intake and output. Report any change in intake and output ratio, pattern, and unusual appearance of urine. Consult physician regarding advisable fluid intake.
- Patients with impaired renal function are particularly susceptible to nephrotoxicity, neurotoxicity, and haemorrhagic manifestations and therefore must be closely monitored.

CARBENICILLIN DISODIUM (continued)

- Bleeding tendency is most likely to occur 12 to 24 hours after initiation of therapy, in patients receiving high dose therapy and in those with impaired renal function. Observe patient for frank bleeding, nose bleed, bleeding gums, haematuria, purpura, petechiae, easy bruising or ecchymoses. If bleeding manifestations appear, drug should be stopped. Report promptly to physician.
- Serum electrolytes, renal, hepatic, cardiac status and haematopoietic functions, and bleeding time assessments should be made prior to and at regular intervals during prolonged therapy, and in patients receiving high doses or who have impaired renal or hepatic function.
- Serum electrolytes (particularly potassium and sodium) should be closely monitored in patients on sodium restriction.
- Observe patients for symptoms of hypernatraemia (confusion, neuromuscular excitability, muscle weakness, seizures); congestive heart failure (paroxysmal nocturnal dyspnoea, cough, fatigue or dyspnoea on exertion, tachycardia, oedema, weight gain); and hypokalaemia (paraesthesias, muscle weakness, depressed reflexes, polyuria, disturbances in cardiac rhythm, gastric distention, ileus).
- Report immediately signs and symptoms of hypersensitivity reaction. (*See penicillin G, Adverse/Side Effects.*) Have on hand: epinephrine, IV corticosteroids, oxygen, suction, endotracheal tube, tracheostomy equipment.
- Bear in mind that superinfections are particularly likely to occur in patients receiving extended spectrum penicillins. Report black, furry overgrowth on tongue, sore mouth, rectal or vaginal itching, vaginal discharge, loose foul-smelling stools, unusual odour to urine, cough, sudden fever.
- Store preferably between 15° and 30°C (59° and 86°F), unless otherwise directed by manufacturer.
- *See Penicillin G.*

Diagnostic test interferences   Elevated **serum sodium** levels with large carbenicillin doses due to high sodium content.

DRUG INTERACTIONS *Carbenicillin* _____

PLUS	INTERACTIONS
Aminoglycoside antibiotics	Synergistic action when administered concurrently. However, carbenicillin activity may be impaired (1) if patient has severe renal impairment, (2) during aminoglycoside assay procedures, (3) if either is mixed in same infusion fluid. Combination generally avoided
Anticoagulants, oral; heparin	Possibility of increased risk of bleeding with high carbenicillin doses. Monitor prothrombin time closely
Tetracyclines	Bactericidal activity of carbenicillin may be reduced. Combination generally avoided

Note: Similar drug carfecillin (Uticillin) converted to carbenicillin in the body.

Carbenoxolone───────────────────

(Biogastrone, Duogastrone, Pyrogastrone, Bioral gel)   *Antiinflamatory*

ACTION AND USES   Carbenoxolone is a synthetic derivative of glycyrrhizic acid which is a constituent of liquorice. It is mainly used in the treatment of gastric ulceration. Method of action is thought to be by the stimulation of mucus synthesis and by the prolongation of the life of epithelial cells. Also used in the treatment of mouth ulcers.

ROUTE AND DOSAGE   Oral: *gastric ulceration*: 50–100 mg three times a day after meals. Available as tablet, chewable tablet or liquid. *Duodenal ulceration*: 50 mg capsule (Duogastrone) 15–30 min before meals with liquid 4 times a day. *Mouth ulcers*: apply gel to lesions after meals and at bedtime. *Oesophagitis*: 10 ml or 1 tablet (Pyogastrone) three times a day after meals.

ABSORPTION AND FATE   Absorbed in the gastrointestinal tract; the main site being the stomach. In the circulation, it is carried bound to proteins. Excretion of the pure compound or derivatives is mainly in the bile.

CONTRAINDICATIONS AND PRECAUTIONS   Use with spironolactone or amiloride should be avoided. **Cautious use**: in elderly patients, impaired renal or hepatic function, cardiac disease and hypertension. **Cautious use** in pregnancy.

ADVERSE/SIDE EFFECTS   Sodium/water retention, oedema, alkalosis, hypokalaemia and hypertension particularly in the elderly. Heartburn on swallowing the tablets. Headache and nausea. Reduced glucose tolerance.

NURSING IMPLICATIONS
- Not recommended for elderly patients as side effects are more severe.
- Weigh before commencing treatment and monitor weekly. Advise physician of weight gain.
- Check for oedema.
- Advise on salt reduced diet, encourage potassium rich foods (bananas, tomatoes, oranges).
- Potassium supplements may be given to those at risk of hypokalaemia.
- Monitor blood pressure regularly.
- Patients prescribed digitalis glycosides should have weekly checks of serum electrolytes.
- If patient suffers heartburn on swallowing tablets, he or she should be advised to take them with milk.
- Thiazide diuretics should be given to combat oedema.
- The gel should remain in contact with the lesion for as long as possible, to ensure successful treatment of mouth ulcers.

Drug interactions   The use of spironolactone or amiloride will reduce the therapeutic effects of carbenoxolone.

Carbimazole

(Neo-Mercazole) *Antithyroid agent*

For further information *see Propylthiouracil*

ROUTE AND DOSAGE Adult: highly individualized, usual 30–60 mg a day in divided doses for the first month then reduce to maintain the patient euthyroid. Child: usual initial dose 5 mg three times a day reduced to maintain the patient euthyroid.

CONTRAINDICATIONS AND PRECAUTIONS Cautious use: in pregnancy use the smallest effective dose.

Carboplatin

(Paraplatin) *Antineoplastic*

ACTIONS AND USES Derivative of cisplatin with similar antineoplastic properties. Used for the treatment of advanced ovarian cancer and small cell carcinoma of the lung.

ROUTE AND DOSAGE Intravenous: individualized.

ABSORPTION AND FATE After intravenous administration the terminal half life for the total platinum content is 24 hrs. Excretion is mostly via the urine, the majority of the drug being excreted in 6 hrs.

CONTRAINDICATIONS AND PRECAUTIONS Should not be used in patients with severe renal impairment, severely myelosuppressed or with a history of severe allergic reactions to platinum-containing compounds (carboplatin, cisplatin) or to mannitol.

ADVERSE/SIDE EFFECTS Nephrotoxicity, ototoxicity, neurotoxicity, myelosuppression, abnormal liver function. Allergic reactions similar to other platinum compounds. Nausea and vomiting reported in 25% of patients, generally less severe than with cisplatin.

NURSING IMPLICATIONS
- Toxic effects similar to, but less severe than, cisplatin.
- Myelosuppressive effects may be severe, doses should not be given at less than 4 week intervals. Nadir occurs between 14 and 21 days after treatment. At this time the patient may require hospitalization until blood counts return to an acceptable level.
- For further information *see cisplatin.*

Carmustine———————————————————————

(BiCNU)   *Antineoplastic; alkylating*
                                                 agent; nitrosurea

ACTIONS AND USES   Highly lipid-soluble nitrosurea derivative with cell cycle non-specific activity against rapidly proliferating cell populations. Produces cross-linkage of DNA strands, thereby blocking DNA, RNA, and protein synthesis. Drug metabolites thought to be responsible for antineoplastic and toxic activities. Major toxic effect is bone marrow suppression.

Used as single or in combination with other antineoplastics in treatment of Hodgkin's disease and other lymphomas.

ROUTE AND DOSAGE   **Intravenous**: individualized.

ABSORPTION AND FATE   Rapid absorption and hepatic degradation. Intact drug leaves plasma within 15 minutes. **Half-life**: 5 to 15 minutes (active metabolites may persist in plasma for days). About 60 to 70% excreted in urine in 96 hours; 6 to 10% excreted as CO_2 by lungs, and about 1% via faeces. Effectively crosses blood–brain barrier. Distributed into breast milk.

CONTRAINDICATIONS AND PRECAUTIONS   Previous sensitivity to carmustine; infection, decreased circulating platelets, leucocytes, or erythrocytes. Safe use during pregnancy and in nursing women not established. **Cautious Use**: hepatic and renal insufficiency; patient with previous cytotoxic medication, or radiation therapy.

ADVERSE/SIDE EFFECTS   These include: dizziness, ataxia, stomatitis, dysphagia, nausea, vomiting, diarrhoea, anorexia, delayed myelosuppression (dose-related). Further side effects (high doses) include: increases in transaminases, alkaline phosphatase, bilirubin, jaundice, encephalopathy. Ophthalmic problems (with high doses) can result in: infarctions, retinal haemorrhage, suffusion of conjunctiva. In addition: pulmonary infiltration and/or fibrosis, decrease in kidney size, progressive azotemia, renal failure, skin flushing, burning pain at injection site, hyperpigmentation of skin (from contact), thrombosis (rare) can occur.

NURSING IMPLICATIONS
- Wear disposable gloves when preparing carmustine. Contact of drug with skin can cause burning, dermatitis, and hyperpigmentation.
- If possible avoid starting infusion into dorsum of hand, wrist, or the antecubital veins; extravasation in these areas can damage underlying tendons and nerves leading to loss of mobility of entire limb.
- Slow infusion over a 1- to 2-hour period (by IV drip) and adequate dilution will reduce pain of administration. Frequently check rate of flow and blood return; palpate injection site for extravasation. If there is any question about patency, line should be restarted.
- Carmustine is not a vesicant, but can cause burning discomfort even in the absence of extravasation. Instruct patient to report burning sensation immediately. Infusion will

CARMUSTINE (continued)

be discontinued and restarted in another site. Ice application over the area may decrease the discomfort.

- Inform patient that intense flushing of skin may occur during IV infusion. This side effect usually disappears in 2 to 4 hours.
- Nausea and vomiting (dose related) may occur within 2 hours after drug administration and persist for up to 6 hours. Prior administration of an antiemetic may help to decrease or prevent these side effects.
- Platelet nadir usually occurs within 4 to 5 weeks, and leucocyte nadir within 5 to 6 weeks after therapy is terminated. Thrombocytopenia may be more severe than leucopenia; anaemia is less severe. Blood studies are continued following infusion, at weekly intervals, for at least 6 weeks.
- Because carmustine causes myelosuppression, patient will be highly susceptible to infection and to haemorrhagic disorders. Be alert to hazardous periods of drug-induced lowered defence mechanisms that occur 4 to 6 weeks after a dose of carmustine. If possible, invasive procedures (e.g., IM injections, enemas, rectal temperatures) should be avoided during this period.
- Check temperature daily. Avoid use of rectal thermometer to prevent injury to mucosa. An elevation of 0.6°F or more above usual temperature warrants reporting.
- Infection prevention in all patient-related activities during period of leucopenia is imperative. Screen contacts to prevent exposure of patient to upper respiratory or other infections.
- Antibiotics and red cell and platelet transfusions may be given to control infections during periods of drug-induced leucopenia and thrombocytopenia.
- In addition to haematopoietic studies, baseline and periodic tests of hepatic, pulmonary, and renal function are recommended throughout therapy. Most patients receiving carmustine inevitably show some signs of toxicity.
- Symptoms of lung toxicity (cough, shortness of breath, fever) should be reported to the physician immediately.
- Be alert to signs of hepatic toxicity (jaundice, dark urine, pruritus, light coloured stools) and renal insufficiency (dysuria, oliguria, haematuria, swelling, of lower legs and feet).
- Instruct patient to report promptly the onset of sore throat, weakness, fever, chills, infection of any kind, or abnormal bleeding (ecchymosis, petechiae, epistaxis, bleeding gums, haematemesis, melaena).
- Reconstituted solutions of carmustine are clear and colourless and may be stored at 2° to 8°C (36° to 46°F) for 24 hours protected from sunlight.
- Reconstituted solutions, which are further diluted with NaCl for injection or 5% dextrose for injection, are stable for 48 hours when refrigerated and protected from light.
- Note that carmustine powder contains no preservative, therefore storage requirements must be carefully observed. Signs of decomposition of carmustine in unopened vial: liquifaction and appearance of oil film at bottom of vial. Discard drug in this condition.
- *See mustine.*

CARMUSTINE (continued)
DRUG INTERACTIONS   *Carmustine*

PLUS	INTERACTIONS
Cimetidine	Carmustine-induced bone marrow toxicity may increase. Concurrent use generally avoided
Phenytoin	Possibility of reduced phenytoin absorption. Monitor phenytoin plasma levels

Cascara

Laxative; anthraquinone

ACTIONS AND USES   Anthraquinone derivative obtained from bark of buckhorn tree (*Rhamnus purshiana*). Acts principally in large intestine. Causes propulsive movements of colon by direct chemical irritation.

Used for temporary relief of constipation and to prevent straining at stool in various disease conditions. Rarely given on prescription.

ROUTE AND DOSAGE   Oral: **Adult**: 1–2 tablets at bedtime.

ABSORPTION AND FATE   Hydrolyzed in colon to active principles which are conveyed to colonic mucosa, bile, and saliva, and possibly other body tissues and fluids. Acts in 6 to 12 hours. Metabolized in liver. Excreted in faeces and in urine. Also eliminated in breast milk. Following partial absorption, reaches large intestine indirectly via bloodstream and partly by direct passage through small intestine.

CONTRAINDICATIONS AND PRECAUTIONS   Nausea, vomiting, abdominal pain, faecal impaction; GI bleeding, ulcerations; appendicitis, gastroenteritis, intestinal obstruction, nursing mothers, congestive heart failure.

ADVERSE/SIDE EFFECTS   *Large doses*: anorexia, nausea, griping, abnormally loose stools, hypokalaemia, impaired glucose tolerance, calcium deficiency, discolouration of urine. *Chronic Use*: constipation rebound, melanosis of colon.

NURSING IMPLICATIONS
- A single dose taken before retiring usually results in evacuation of soft stool 6 to 12 hours later.
- For best results administer with a full glass of water on an empty stomach. Results may be delayed somewhat by food.
- An increase in fluid intake will enhance laxative action. Unless contraindicated advise patient to drink a minimum of 6 to 8 full (240 ml) glasses a day.
- Frequent or prolonged use of irritant cathartics disrupts normal reflex activity of colon and rectum and can lead to drug dependence for evacuation.
- Constipation, which is especially common in the elderly, may be caused by poor eating habits, inadequate fluid intake, lack of exercise, or habitual use of cathartics

CASCARA (continued)

based on the erroneous notion that autointoxication will result if bowels are not evacuated daily.

■ Evaluate patient's need that autointoxication will result if bowels are not evacuated daily.

■ Evaluate patient's need for continued use of drug.

■ Stored preferably between 15° and 30°C (59° and 86°F), in tightly covered, light-resistant containers, unless otherwise directed by manufacturer.

■ *See bisacodyl: for other patient teaching points.*

Diagnostic test interferences Possibility of interference with **PSP excretion test** because of urine discoloration.

Drug interactions Cathartics in large doses may result in decreased absorption of **vitamin K**, **oral anticoagulants**, and possibly other drugs by decreasing transit time in intestinal tract.

Castor oil

Laxative (stimulant)

ACTIONS AND USES Obtained from the seeds of *Ricinus communis*. Hydrolyzed in small intestine to glycerol and ricinoleic acid, a local irritant. Stimulates motor activity in small intestine and inhibits antiperistalsis in colon, thus preventing normal fluid absorption from intestinal contents. Rapid evacuation of copious liquid or semiliquid stools follows, with little or no colic.

Used to prepare abdomen for radiographic examination of colon and kidneys and to evacuate irritants and poisons from intestinal tract. Rarely used to relieve constipation. Also applied locally to skin as emollient and protectant and to conjunctiva (sterile) to alleviate irritation caused by the presence of a foreign body. Rarely given on prescription.

ROUTE AND DOSAGE Oral: Adults: 5 to 20 ml.

ABSORPTION AND FATE Poorly absorbed. Acts in 2 to 3 hours. Appears in breast milk.

CONTRAINDICATIONS AND PRECAUTIONS Hypersensitivity to castor bean; dehydration, faecal impaction, abdominal pain, nausea, vomiting, appendicitis, GI bleeding, ulcerations, perforation, obstruction, use in conjunction with fat-soluble vermifuges; pregnancy, nursing women, menstruation.

ADVERSE/SIDE EFFECTS Severe purgation, nausea, vomiting, abdominal cramps, flatus, rebound constipation, irritation of colon, pelvic congestion (rare); dehydration, electrolyte imbalance, elevation of blood glucose levels (extended use).

CASTOR OIL (continued)
NURSING IMPLICATIONS

- More active if taken on empty stomach. Because castor oil is a fat, it may retard gastric emptying time.
- In general it is best not to schedule a laxative within 2 hours of taking other medications.
- Action begins in 2 to 3 hours, depending on dose. Time the administration so as not to interfere with patient's sleep.
- For visualization or surgical procedures, patient is generally given a residue free diet the day before and a cleansing enema on the day of the procedure. Some physicians prescribe standardized senna fluid extract to be taken 4 hours after castor oil.
- Castor oil has objectionable odour, taste, and consistency. It may be made somewhat more palatable by chilling it and administering it with cold fruit juice or milk.
- Emulsified forms are reported to be less disagreeable to taste. Shake emulsion well before pouring. Mix with ½ to 1 glass (120 to 240 ml) of liquid (water, soft drink, fruit juice, milk).
- Inform patient that castor oil causes complete emptying of intestinal contents, and therefore normal evacuation may be delayed for 2 days or more.
- Long-term use may result in laxative dependence.
- Preserved in tightly covered containers preferably between 15° and 30°C (59° and 86°F), unless otherwise directed by manufacturer. Avoid exposure to excessive light.

Cefaclor

(Distaclor)

Antibiotic (beta-lactam); cephalosporin

ACTIONS AND USES   Semisynthetic, second generation oral cephalosporin antibiotic similar to other drugs of this group. Possibly more active than other oral cephalosporins against gram-negative bacilli, especially beta-lactamase-producing *Haemophilus influenzae*, including ampicillin-resistant strains. Also active against *Escherichia coli*, *Proteus mirabilis*, *Klebsiella*, and certain gram-positive strains, e.g., *Streptococcus pneumoniae*, *S. pyogenes*, and *Staphylococcus aureus*.

Used in treatment of infections of upper and lower respiratory tract, urinary tract, skin and skin structures, and mainly for otitis media.

ROUTE AND DOSAGE   Oral: **Adults:** 250 to 500 mg every 8 hours. Not to exceed 4 g daily. **Children (1 month or older):** 20 to 40 mg/kg daily in divided doses every 8 hours. Not to exceed 1 g daily. Available in capsules and oral suspension.

ABSORPTION AND FATE   Acid stable. Well absorbed following oral administration. Peak serum levels in 30 to 60 minutes when taken on an empty stomach. **Half-life:** 36 to 54 minutes (prolonged in impaired renal function). About 22 to 25% **protein bound.** Approximately 50 to 85% of dose eliminated within 8 hours unchanged in

CEFACLOR *(continued)*

urine, with most of dose being excreted within first two hours. Crosses placenta; appears in breast milk.

CONTRAINDICATIONS AND PRECAUTIONS   Hypersensitivity to cephalosporins. Safe use during pregnancy, in nursing mothers, and infants younger than 1 month not established. **Cautious Use**: history of sensitivity to penicillins or other allergies; markedly impaired renal function.

ADVERSE/SIDE EFFECTS   These include: (common): diarrhoea; nausea, vomiting, anorexia, transient leucopenia, transient leucocytosis, slight elevations of AST (SGOT), ALT (SGPT), alkaline phosphatase, BUN, serum creatinine; positive direct Coombs' test, serum sickness-like reaction: urticaria, pruritus, morbilliform eruptions, eosinophilia, joint pain or swelling, fever: superinfections. *See also cephalothin.*

NURSING IMPLICATIONS

- Cefaclor may be administered without regard to meals. Although peak blood levels may be slightly lower and delayed when drug is administered with food, total amount absorbed is unchanged. Administration with food may help to reduce incidence of nausea and vomiting.
- Before therapy is initiated, a careful inquiry should be made concerning previous hypersensitivity to cephalosporins, penicillins, and other drug allergies.
- Culture and susceptibility tests recommended prior to and periodically during therapy.
- Be on the alert for signs and symptoms of superinfections (black tongue, sore mouth, perianal irritation and itching, foul-smelling vaginal discharge, loose stools, sudden fever, cough).
- Diarrhoea, the most frequent adverse effect, may be due to a pharmacological effect or to associated change in intestinal flora. If it persists, interruption of therapy may be necessary.
- Yogurt or buttermilk (if allowed) may serve as a prophylactic against intestinal superinfections by helping to maintain normal intestinal flora.
- Instruct patient to take medication for the full course of therapy as directed by physician. Drug therapy for beta-haemolytic streptococcal infections should continue for at least 10 days to reduce risk of rheumatic fever.
- After stock oral suspension is prepared, it should be kept refrigerated. Expiration date should appear on label. Discard unused portion after 14 days. Shake well before pouring. A calibrated liquid measuring device for home use should be included when dispensed by pharmacist.
- Store capsules preferably between 15° and 30°C (59° and 86°F) in tightly closed container, unless otherwise directed by manufacturer.
- *See cephalothin sodium.*

Diagnostic test interferences   Cefaclor may produce positive direct Coombs' test, which can complicate **cross-matching procedures** and **haematological studies**. False-positive urine glucose determinations, using copper sulphate reduction methods.

CEFACLOR (continued)
DRUG INTERACTIONS *Cefaclor* _____

PLUS	INTERACTIONS
Aminoglycosides, colistimethate and other potentially nephrotoxic drugs	Possibility of additive nephrotoxic effects. Monitor renal function
Probenecid	May result in higher and more prolonged serum cefaclor levels (probenecid inhibits cefaclor excretion). Used concomitantly with caution

Note: Similar drugs, cephalexin (Ceporex), cephradine (Velosef), and cefadroxil (Baxan)

C

Cefadroxil _____

(Baxan)   *Antibiotic (beta-lactam);*
                                                                         cephalosporin

ACTIONS AND USES Semisynthetic, first generation cephalosporin antibiotic with antibacterial spectrum similar to that of other members of this group. At equivalent doses, reportedly has longer duration in serum and urine than attained by other oral cephalosporins. Active against organisms that liberate cephalosporinase and penicillinase.

Used primarily in treatment of urinary tract infections caused by *Escherichia coli*, *Proteus mirabilis*, and *Klebsiella* species; infections of skin and skin structures caused by staphylococci and streptococci; and for treatment of Group A beta-haemolytic streptococcal pharyngitis.

ROUTE AND DOSAGE Oral: **Adult:** 0.5–1 g twice a day. **Child:** under 1 yr 25 mg/kg/day in divided doses, 1–6 yrs 250 mg twice a day, over 6 yrs 500 mg twice a day.

ABSORPTION AND FATE Acid stable. Rapidly and almost completely absorbed from GI tract. **Peak serum levels** in 1.2 to 1.5 hours. Measurable levels persist in serum 12 hours after administration. Approximately 20% protein bound. **Half–life:** 1 to 2 hours. More than 90% of a single dose is excreted unchanged in urine within 8 hours; appreciable bacterial inhibitory levels persist for 20 to 22 hours. Crosses placenta; appears in breast milk.

CONTRAINDICATIONS AND PRECAUTIONS Hypersensitivity to cephalosporins. Safe use during pregnancy, in nursing mothers, and in children not established. **Cautious Use:** sensitivity to penicillins or other drug allergies; impaired renal function, history of GI disease, particularly colitis.

ADVERSE/SIDE EFFECTS These include: nausea, vomiting, gastritis, bloating, cramps, diarrhoea, pseudomembranous colitis (rare), rash, swollen eyelids (angio-edema), pruritus, chills, dysuria, dizziness, headache, positive direct Coombs' test; increased SGOT, SGPT, alkaline phosphatase; transient neutropenia, superinfections.

CEFADROXIL (continued)
NURSING IMPLICATIONS

- The incidence of nausea (most frequent side effect) may be reduced by administration of drug with food. Rate of absorption and serum levels not affected by presence of food. If nausea persists, cessation of therapy may be necessary.
- Before therapy is initiated a careful inquiry should be made concerning previous hypersensitivity to cephalosporins, penicillins, and other drug allergies.
- Culture and testing recommended prior to and periodically during therapy.
- Baseline and periodic renal function studies should be performed in patients with renal function impairment, and fluid intake and output ratio and pattern should be monitored.
- Instruct patient to take medication for the full course of therapy as directed by the physician.
- Drug therapy for beta-haemolytic streptococcal infections should continue for at least 10 days to guard against risk of rheumatic fever.
- Be on the alert for signs and symptoms of superinfections (furry, black tongue; sore mouth; perianal itching or irritation; foul-smelling vaginal discharge; loose stools; and sudden fever; cough).
- Store in tight container, preferably between 15° and 30°C (59° and 86°F), unless otherwise directed by manufacturer. Oral suspensions are stable for 14 days under refrigeration at 2° to 8°C (36° to 46°F). Avoid freezing. Note expiration date on label.

Diagnostic test interferences   Cefadroxil-induced positive direct Coombs' test may interfere with **cross-matching procedures** and **haematological studies**.

DRUG INTERACTIONS   *Cefadroxil*

PLUS	INTERACTIONS
Aminoglycosides, and other potentially nephrotoxic drugs	Possibility of additive nephrotoxic effects. Monitor renal function
Probenecid	May result in higher and more prolonged serum cefadroxil levels (probenecid inhibits excretion). Used concomitantly with caution

Cefotaxime

(Claforan)

Antibiotic (beta-lactam); cephalosporin

ACTIONS AND USES   Semisynthetic third generation cephalosporin antibiotic. In common with other cephalosporins, acts by inhibiting bacterial cell wall synthesis. Less active against gram-positive bacteria, e.g., *Staphylococcus aureus*, group A and B Streptococci, and *Streptococcus pneumoniae* than first and second generation

CEFOTAXIME (continued)

cephalosporins. Effective against a variety of gram-negative organisms resistant to first and second generation drugs, but not generally preferred over an aminoglycoside for this purpose. Reportedly, resistant strains of *Enterobacter*, *Pseudomonas aeruginosa*, and *Serratia* have developed during cefotaxime therapy. More resistant to inactivation of beta-lactamase (both penicillinases and cephalosporinases) than first and second generation cephalosporins except cefoxitin. Therefore, effective against many beta-lactamase-producing organisms including *Neisseria gonorrhoeae*, *Haemophilus influenzae*, and a wide variety of *Enterobacteriaceae*.

Used for serious infections of lower respiratory tract, skin and skin structures, bones and joints, CNS including meningitis and ventriculitis, for gynaecological and genitorurinary tract infections, including uncomplicated and disseminated gonococcal infections caused by penicillinase-producing *Neisseria gonorrhoeae*. Also used to treat, bacteraemia/septicaemia, intraabdominal infections, and perioperative prophylaxis.

ROUTE AND DOSAGE   Intramuscular, intravenous: **Adults:** 1 g every 12 hours. *Life-threatening infections*: 2 g **IV** every 8 hours, *Gonorrhea*: 1 g **IM** in single dose. **Neonate:** 50 mg/kg/day in 2–4 divided doses. *Child*: 100–150 mg/kg/day in 2–4 divided doses.

ABSORPTION AND FATE   Peak serum levels within 30 minutes following IM, and in about 5 minutes after IV injection. Widely distributed to body tissues and fluids, particularly bile. Penetrates CSF when meninges are inflamed. **Half-life** about 1 hour; 35 to 64% protein bound. Partially metabolized in liver in active metabolites. About 40 to 62% of dose excreted unchanged in urine within 24 hours (most excreted within first 2 hours). Approximately 24% eliminated as active metabolites and about 10% excreted in faeces via bile. Crosses placenta. Small amounts excreted in breast milk.

CONTRAINDICATIONS AND PRECAUTIONS   Hypersensitivity to cephalosporins. Safe use during pregnancy not established. **Cautious Use:** history of hypersensitivity to penicillins, history of allergy particularly to drugs, renal impairment, history of colitis or other GI disease, nursing mothers.

ADVERSE/SIDE EFFECTS   These include: diarrhoea, abdominal pain, colitis, pseudomembranous colitis (rare); anorexia, nausea, vomiting, transient leucopenia, granulocytopenia, thrombocytopenia, neutropenia, eosinophilia, positive direct Coombs' test, transient increases in BUN and serum creatinine, rash, pruritus, fever, inflammatory reaction, phlebitis, thrombophlebitis (IV site); pain, induration, and tenderness (IM site), superinfections: moniliasis, vaginitis.

NURSING IMPLICATIONS
- Culture and sensitivity tests should be performed prior to initiation of therapy and periodically during therapy, if indicated. Therapy may be instituted pending test results.
- Before therapy is initiated, a careful inquiry should be made to determine previous hypersensitivity reactions to cephalosporins, penicillins, and history of other allergies, particularly to drugs.

CEFOTAXIME (continued)

- IM injections are prepared by adding 2, 3, or 5 ml of sterile water for injection or bacteriostatic water for injection to each 500 mg, 1 g, or 2 g vial, respectively.
- Following reconstitution, shake well to dissolve drug, and inspect for particulate matter and discolouration. Solutions may range in colour from light yellow to amber depending on drug concentration, diluent used, and storage conditions. Manufacturer states that this does not adversely affect product potency.
- IM injections should be made deeply into large muscle mass such as upper outer quadrant of gluteus maximus. Aspirate carefully to avoid inadvertent entry of drug into blood vessel. Rotate injection sites.
- Manufacturer recommends administration of no more than 1 g into a single IM site. Large doses may be extremely painful and can cause local tissue reactions.
- For IV use, reconstitute all strengths with at least 10 ml of sterile water for injection. For infusion bottles add 50 or 100 ml of 0.9% sodium chloride injection, 5% dextrose injection or other diluents recommended by manufacturer.
- Reconstituted solutions may be further diluted to 50 to 1,000 ml with IV fluids recommended by manufacturer. These solutions maintain potency for 24 hours at room temperature.
- After reconstitution cefotaxime may be stored in disposable glass or plastic syringes for same time periods as for reconstituted solutions, i.e., 24 hours at room temperature.
- For direct intermittent IV administration, injection is made over a 3- to 5-minute period. Drug may also be administered more slowly into tubing of a freshly flowing IV of compatible solution. See manufacturer's directions for details.
- Report onset of loose stools or diarrhoea. Most patients respond to replacement of fluids, electrolytes, and proteins (see Index: Nursing Interventions: Rehydration). Discontinuation of drug may be required for some patients. Although pseudomembranous colitis occurs rarely, this potentially life-threatening complication should be considered a possible cause of diarrhoea during or after antibiotic therapy.
- Monitor fluid input and output ratio and pattern in patients with impaired renal function, or who are receiving high dosages, or an aminoglycoside concomitantly. Renal status (serum creatinine, creatinine clearance, BUN) should be evaluated at regular intervals.
- Patients with impaired renal function do not usually need dosage adjustments until creatinine clearance falls below 20 ml/minute. Dosage is then usually halved.
- Chronic urinary tract infections may require frequent clinical and bacteriological follow-up for several months after drug has been discontinued.
- Observe and report onset of superinfections: fever, sore mouth or throat, white patches in mouth, black hairy tongue, diarrhoea, foul-smelling stools or vaginal discharge, vaginitis, anogenital itching, moniliasis (fungal infection of skin, vagina, bronchi, lungs).
- Disulphiram-type reaction upon ingestion of alcohol not reported with cefotaxime, but since it has occurred with other cephalosporins, caution is warranted.
- Cefotaxime therapy should continue for a least 48 to 72 hours after patient becomes afebrile or other signs of infection have disappeared.
- Therapy for group A beta-haemolytic streptococci should be continued for a

CEFOTAXIME (continued)

minimum of 10 days to reduce risk of glomerulonephritis and rheumatic fever.

- If an aminoglycoside is prescribed, it must be administered separately and not mixed with cefotaxime. Also do not mix with sodium bicarbonate or any fluid with a pH above 7.5.
- Store dry powder preferably between between 15° and 30°C (59° and 86°F), unless otherwise directed by manufacturer. Protect from excessive light.

Diagnostic test interferences   False-positive reactions for **urine glucose** have not been reported using copper solphate reduction methods, e.g., Benedict's, Fehling's, Clinitest. Because it has occurred with other cephalosporins, however, it may be advisable to use glucose oxidase tests (Clinistix). Positive direct Coombs' test results may interfere with **haematological studies** and **crossmatching** procedures.

DRUG INTERACTIONS   *Cefotaxime*

PLUS	INTERACTIONS
Aminoglycosides	Concomitant use may increase risk of nephrotoxicity and ototoxicity
Probenecid	May prolong cefotaxime plasma levels with possible toxicity

Cefoxitin

(Mefoxin)

Antibiotic (beta-lactam); cephalosporin-like

ACTIONS AND USES   Semisynthetic broad-spectrum antibiotic, derivative of cephamycin C (produced by *Streptomyces lactamdurans*). Generally classified as second generation cephalosporin. Structurally and pharmacologically related to cephalosporins and penicillins, and like them exerts bactericidal action by inhibition of cell wall synthesis. Antimicrobial spectrum broader than that of cephalothin; more active against many gram-negative bacteria, e.g., strains of *Escherichia coli*, *Klebsiella*, *Proteus mirabilis*, and *Bacteroides fragilis*. Highly resistant to beta-lactamases (cephalosporinases and penicillinases) produced by gram-negative aerobic and anaerobic bacteria. Reportedly has only moderate activity against *Haemophilus influenzae*.

Used in treatment of serious infections of lower respiratory tract, genitourinary tract, skin and soft tissue, bones and joints, and in gynaecological infections, septicaemia, peritonitis, and other intra-abdominal infections. Used as alternative to spectinomycin in treatment of penicillinase-producing *Neisseria gonorrhoeae* and gonococcal infections unresponsive to penicillin or tetracycline therapy. Also used for perioperative prophylaxis in patients undergoing surgery with high risk of infection.

ROUTE AND DOSAGE   Intramuscular, intravenous: Adults: *Infections*: 1 to 2 g

CEFOXITIN (continued)

every 6 to 8 hours, depending on severity of infection. Up to 12 g daily in life-threatening infections.

For Nursing Implication see cefotaximine.

ABSORPTION AND FATE   Peak serum levels within 20 to 30 minutes following IM and within 5 minutes or less after IV administration. Widely distributed to body tissues and fluids including pleural, synovial, ascitic fluid, and bile. About 50 to 60% bound to serum proteins. Half-life: 45 minutes to 1 hour, considerably longer with impaired renal function. Poor diffusion into CSF even when meninges are inflamed. Rapidly excreted in urine (approximately 85% of single dose excreted within 6 hours), mostly unchanged. Readily crosses placenta; small amounts appear in breast milk.

CONTRAINDICATIONS AND PRECAUTIONS   Hypersensitivity to cefoxitin or to cephalosporins. Safe use in women of childbearing potential, during pregnancy, in nursing mothers, and in children under 3 months not established. Cautious Use: history of sensitivity to penicillin or other allergies, particularly to drugs, impaired renal function.

ADVERSE/SIDE EFFECTS   These include: rash, exfoliative dermatitis, pruritus, urticaria, drug fever, eosinophilia, superinfections, local reactions (common): pain, tenderness, and induration (with IM), thrombophlebitis (with IV); nephrotoxicity and oliguria (rare).

Cefsulodin

(Monaspor)

ACTIONS AND USES   Cephalosporin used to treat Psendomonas aeruginosa.

ROUTE AND DOSAGE   IM, IV: 1–4 g/day in 2–4 divided doses.

For further information see cephalothin.

Ceftazidime

(Fortum)

ACTIONS AND USES   Cephalosporin used to treat gram-positive and gram-negative infections.

ROUTE AND DOSAGE   IM, IV, IV infusion: 1–6 g/day in divided doses. Child (up to 2 mths): 25–60 mg/kg/day; (over 2 mths): 30–100 mg/kg/day in divided doses.

Cetizoxime

(Cefizox)

ACTIONS AND USES   Cephalosporin used to treat sensitive infections.

ROUTE AND DOSAGE   **IM, IV; Adult:** up to 8 g/day in divided doses. Child over 3 months 30–60 mg/kg/day in divided doses. *Gonorrhoea*: **IM:** 1g as a single dose.
    For further information *see Cephalothin*

Cefuroxime

(Zinacef)   *Antibiotic (beta-lactam);*
                                                                   cephalosporin

ACTIONS AND USES   Semi-synthetic second generation cephalosporin antibiotic. Resistance against beta-lactamase producing strains exceeds that of first generation cephalosporins. Has broader spectrum of activity against anaerobes and gram-negative microorganisms than most other second generation cephalosporins.
    Used in treatment of serious infections of lower respiratory tract, urinary tract, skin and skin structures, and for septicaemia, meningitis, uncomplicated and disseminated gonococcal infections. Also used for preoperative prophylaxis.

ROUTE AND DOSAGE   **Intramuscular, intravenous: Adults:** 750 mg to 1.5 g every 8 hours for 5 to 10 days depending on severity of infection. *Uncomplicated gonococcal infections*: 1.5 g IM as single dose (but divided and given at two different sites), together with 1 g oral probenecid. *Preoperative prophylaxis*: 1.5 g IV on induction of anaesthesia. **Children (over 3 months):** 30 to 100 mg/kg/day in equally divided doses every 6 to 8 hours.
    For further information *see cefotaximine*.

ABSORPTION AND FATE   Peak serum levels in 15 to 60 minutes after IM injection and in about 3 minutes after IV administration. Widely distributed in body tissues and fluids. Crosses blood–brain barrier; therapeutic concentrations achieved in CSF even when meninges are not inflamed. **Protein binding:** 33 to 50%; **half-life:** 1 to 2 hours (prolonged in patients with impaired renal function). Very little if any is metabolized. About 90 to 100% eliminated unchanged in urine within 24 hours (mostly excreted within first 6 hours after drug administration). Excreted in breast milk.

CONTRAINDICATIONS AND PRECAUTIONS   Hypersensitivity to cephalosporins. Safe use during pregnancy and in children under 3 months not established. **Cautious Use:** history of allergy, particularly to drugs; penicillin sensitivity, renal insufficiency, history of colitis or other GI disease, nursing women.

ADVERSE/SIDE EFFECTS   **GI:** diarrhoea, nausea, colitis, pseudomembranous colitis

CEFUROXIME (continued)

(rare). Other side effects include: decreased Hgb and Hct, transient eosinophilia, neutropenia, leucopenia, transient increases in AST (SGOT), ALT (SGPT), alkaline phosphatase, LDH, and bilirubin, rash, pruritus, urticaria, positive Coombs' test, increased serum creatinine and BUN, decreased creatinine clearance (causal relationship not established), local reactions: thrombophlebitis (IV site); pain, burning, cellulitis (IM site).

Cephalexin

(Keflex, Ceporex)

Antibiotic (beta-lactam); cephalosporin

ACTIONS AND USES   Semisynthetic derivative of cephalosporin C. Broad-spectrum, first generation cephalosporin, antibiotic similar to cephalothin (q.v.), but reportedly less potent. In common with other cephalosporins, generally not effective against methicillin-resistant staphylococci.

Used as follow-up oral therapy in patients initially treated with parenteral cephalosporins. Has been used to treat infections caused by susceptible pathogens in respiratory and urinary tracts, middle ear, skin, soft tissue, and bone. Some clinicians recommend that it be reserved for treatment of urinary tract infections due to susceptible *Klebsiella* organisms resistant to other oral antibacterials.

ROUTE AND DOSAGE   Oral: Adults: 250 mg every 6 hours or 500 mg/8 hrly. Children: 25 to 50 mg/kg/day in 4 equally divided doses. In severe infections, dosage may be doubled. Available in capsules, oral suspension.

ABSORPTION AND FATE   Stable in stomach acid; rapidly and almost completely absorbed from GI tract. (Absorption is delayed in young children and may be reduced in patients with pernicious anaemia or obstructive jaundice.) Peak serum level in 1 hour. Measurable levels persist for 6 hours. Higher and more prolonged blood levels in patients with renal insufficiency and in neonates. Widely distributed in body fluids, with highest concentrations in kidney. About 6 to 15% bound to **plasma proteins.** **Half-life**: 0.6 to 1.2 hours. Over 90% of dose excreted in urine as unchanged drug within 8 hours. May cross placenta; appears in breast milk.

CONTRAINDICATIONS AND PRECAUTIONS   Hypersensitivity to cephalosporins. Safe use during pregnancy not established. **Cautious Use**: history of hypersensitivity to penicillin or other drug allergy; severely impaired renal function. *See cephalothin.*

ADVERSE/SIDE EFFECTS   These include: toxic paranoid reactions (high doses in patients with renal impairment); dizziness, headache, fatigue, diarrhoea (generally mild), nausea, vomiting, anorexia, abdominal pain, slightly elevated SGPT, SGOT, alkaline phosphatase; eosinophilia, positive direct Coombs' test *Hypersensitivity*: angioedema, rash, urticaria, anaphylaxis.

CEPHALEXIN (continued)
NURSING IMPLICATIONS

- Cephalexin is not destroyed by gastric acid, but peak blood levels are slightly lower and delayed when administered with food. Total amount absorbed is unchanged however.
- Before therapy is initiated, careful inquiry should be made concerning history of sensitivity to cephalosporins, penicillins, and other allergies particularly to drugs.
- Culture and susceptibility testing is recommended prior to and periodically during therapy.
- Physician should specify dosage interval. For example, four times a day may signify every 6 hours around the clock or it may mean to take the drug at evenly spaced intervals during waking hours, e.g., 7.00 hrs, 12.00 hrs, 17.00 hrs, 22.00 hrs.
- Instruct patient to take medication for the full course of therapy as directed by physician.
- Drug therapy for beta-haemolytic streptococcal infections should continue for at least 10 days to prevent risk of rheumatic fever.
- Advise patient to keep physician informed if adverse reactions appear.
- Periodic evaluations of renal and hepatic function should be made in patients receiving prolonged therapy.
- Be alert to signs and symptoms of superinfections: furry, black tongue, sore mouth, anogenital irritation or itching, foul-smelling vaginal discharge, loose stools, sudden fever, cough.
- After reconstitution cephalexin oral suspension should be refrigerated; discard unused portions 14 days after preparation. Label should indicate expiry date. Keep tightly covered. Shake suspension well before pouring.
- Store capsules and tablets preferably between 15° and 30°C (59° and 86°F) unless otherwise specified by manufacturer.

Diagnostic test interferences   False-positive **urine glucose** determinations using copper sulphate reduction tests such as Benedict's reagent, or Fehling's solution, but not with glucose oxidase (enzymatic) tests, e.g., Clinistix. Positive Coombs' test may complicate transfusion **cross-matching procedures** and **haematological studies**.

DRUG INTERACTIONS *Cephalexin*

PLUS	INTERACTIONS
Aminoglycosides, colistimethate and other drugs with nephrotoxic potential	Possibility of additive nephrotoxic effects. Monitor renal function

Cephalothin

(Ceporacin, Keflin, Seffin)

Antibiotic (beta-lactam); cephalosporin

CEPHALOTHIN (continued)

ACTIONS AND USES   Semisynthetic, broad spectrum, first generation cephalosporin derived from cephalosporin C, a substance produced by the fungus *Cephalosporium acremonium*. Structurally and pharmacologically related to penicillins. Inhibits synthesis of bacterial cell wall; has broad antibacterial spectrum. Primarily bactericidal but also bacteriostatic against most gram-positive organisms including nonpenicillinase and penicillinase-producing staphylococci, beta-haemolytic Streptococci, *S. pneumoniae*, and *S. viridans*; and some gram-negative strains, particularly *Escherichia coli*, *Klebsiella*, *Haemophilus influenzae*, *P. mirabilis*, *Salmonella*, and *Shigella*. Most indole-positive *Proteus*, *Bacteroides*, *Serratia*, *Pseudomonas*, and motile *Enterobacter* species are resistant. Ineffective as prophylaxia against *Clostridium perfringens* (gas gangrene). Cephalothin is highly resistant to cephalosporinases (inactivating enzyme produced by certain bacteria).

Used in treatment of severe infections of respiratory, GI, and urinary tracts, bones, joints, soft tissue, and skin, and for septicaemia, endocarditis, meningitis. Also used for perioperative prophylaxis in patients undergoing surgery with high risk of infection. Used intraperitoneally for bacterial peritonitis and has been used as systemic treatment for intraocular infections.

ROUTE AND DOSAGE   **Intravenous: Adults:** *Infections*: 1 g every 4 to 6 hours; up to 12 g/day for life-threatening infections. **Paediatric:** *Infections*: 80 to 160 mg/kg/day in divided doses.

ABSORPTION AND FATE   Peak serum levels in 30 minutes after IM and 15 minutes after IV injection. Widely distributed in body tissues and fluids, including aqueous humour. Does not readily penetrate brain or CSF unless inflammation is present. **Serum half-life** is 30 to 60 minutes; 65 to 79% bound to **plasma proteins**. Partly deacetylated in liver and kidney. About 60 to 95% of dose excreted by kidneys within 6 hours, largely as unchanged drug and relatively active desacetyl metabolites. Readily crosses placenta; low concentrations in breast milk.

CONTRAINDICATIONS AND PRECAUTIONS   Hypersensitivity to cephalosporin antibiotics. Safe use during pregnancy not determined. **Cautious Use:** history of allergies, particularly to drugs, hypersensitivity to penicillins, impaired renal or hepatic function, patients on sodium restriction.

ADVERSE/SIDE EFFECTS   These include: dizziness, vertigo, headache, fatigue, malaise, toxic paranoid reactions (patients with renal impairment), nausea, vomiting, diarrhoea, anorexia, abdominal cramps, pseudomembranous colitis (rare), neutropenia, leucopenia, pancytopenia (bone marrow toxicity), agranulocytosis, thrombocytopenia, hypoprothrombinaemia, haemolytic anaemia, direct positive Coombs' test (particularly patients with azotaemia), transient rise in SGOT, SGPT, and alkaline phosphatase; increased plasma thymol turbidity and increased serum bilirubin, maculopapular, morbilliform, or pruritic rash, urticaria, serum sickness-like reactions (arthralgia, myalgia, lymphadenopathy, fever), anaphylactic shock, eosinophilia, drug fever, nephrotoxicity (with high dose therapy): elevated BUN, decreased creatinine clearance, oliguria, renal failure, superinfections; especially *Pseudomonas* or *Candida*; local reactions: pain, induration, slough, abscess (IM site); thrombophlebitis (IV site).

CEPHALOTHIN (continued)
NURSING IMPLICATIONS
- Observe IV sites for evidence of inflammatory reaction. IV infusions of doses large than 6 g/day for more than 3 days can result in thrombophlebitis.
- For further information *see cephamandole.*

DRUG INTERACTIONS   *Cephalothin*_____

PLUS	INTERACTIONS
Aminoglycoside antibiotics, colistimethate, and other drugs with nephrotoxic potential	Possibility of additive nephrotoxic effect. Monitor renal function

Cephamandole nafate

(Kefadol)   *Antibiotic (beta-lactam);*
                                                              cephalosporin

ACTIONS AND USES   Semisynthetic, second generation cephalosporin antibiotic similar to other drugs of this class. Reported to have a wider spectrum of antibacterial activity than other cephalosporins and to be effective against more strains of cephalosporinase- and penicillinase-producing gram-negative organisms (e.g., *E. coli, Enterobacter* species, indole-positive *Proteus,* and *H. influenzae*). In common with other cephalosporins, most strains of *Bacteroides fragilis, Serratia, Pseudomonas,* and *Acinetobacter calcoaceticus* are generally resistant to cephamadole.

Used in treatment of serious infections of respiratory, urinary, and biliary tracts, skin and soft tissue, bones and joints, and septicaemia and peritonitis.

ROUTE AND DOSAGE   **Intramuscular, intravenous: Adults:** 500 mg to 2 g every 4 to 8 hours. Up to 2 g IV every 4 hours for life-threatening infections. **Paediatric (1 month and over):** 50 to 100 mg/kg/day in divided doses every 4 to 8 hours; up to 150 mg/kg/day, but not to exceed maximum adult dose.

ABSORPTION AND FATE   **Peak serum levels** in ½ to 2 hours after IM and in 10 minutes following IV administration. **Serum half-life** after IM: 60 to 120 minutes; after IV dose: 32 minutes. About 65 to 75% bound to serum proteins. Rapidly hydrolyzed in plasma to compound that is more active than parent drug. Poor penetration into CSF even when meninges are inflamed. Extensive enterohepatic circulation; high concentrations in bile. Excreted unchanged in urine; 60 to 95% eliminated within 6 to 8 hours.

CONTRAINDICATIONS AND PRECAUTIONS   Hypersensitivity to cephalosporins. Safe use during pregnancy, in nursing mothers, and in children between 1 and 6 months not

CEPHAMANDOLE NAFATE (continued)

established. **Cautious Use**: history of sensitivity to penicillins, or other drug allergies, renal function impairment, history of GI disease, particularly colitis.

ADVERSE/SIDE EFFECTS These include: nausea, vomiting, abdominal cramps, diarrhoea, pseudomembranous colitis. Additional adverse effects (rare): neutropenia, thrombocytopenia, hypoprothrombinaemia (vitamin K deficiency), positive Coombs' test, transient elevations in SGOT, SGPT, alkaline phosphatase, BUN, decreased creatinine clearance. Others: rash, urticaria, drug fever, eosinophilia, pain, redness and induration at IM site, thrombophlebitis (following IV), superinfections.

NURSING IMPLICATIONS
- Culture and susceptibility testing recommended prior to and periodically during therapy.
- Cepthamandole therapy may be instituted pending test results.
- Before therapy is initiated, careful inquiry should be made concerning previous hypersensitivity to cephalosporins, penicillins, and other drugs.
- Administer IM deep into a large muscle mass such as gluteus maximus or lateral thigh. Reportedly, cephamandole IM produces less pain than cephalothin.
- Baseline and periodic studies of renal function and prothrombin time determinations should be performed.
- Monitor fluid intake and output ratio and pattern particularly in patients with impaired renal function, patients over 50 years, or who are receiving high doses. Note number and consistency of stools.
- Be on the alert for signs and symptoms of superinfection (ulceration or white patches in mouth, glossitis, black hairy tongue, anogenital itching, foul-smelling vaginal discharge, and diarrhoea, sudden fever, cough).
- Report the onset of diarrhoea, which may or may not be dose-related and is seen specially in patients with history of drug-associated GI disturbances. Bear in mind that pseudomembranous colitis, a potentially life-threatening condition, starts with diarrhoea. It is caused by overgrowth of resistant toxic-producing clostridia.
- Cephamandole may inhibit production of vitamin K by normal bacterial flora. Although rare, hypoprothrombinaemia with or without haemorrhage has been reported in patients with impaired renal function receiving high doses, patients who have had intestinal resection, the elderly or debilitated, and patients being maintained on IV fluids with no oral intake. Observe these patients for bleeding manifestation. Prophylactic administration of vitamin K may be necessary.
- Drug therapy for beta-haemolytic streptococcal infections should continue for at least 10 days to reduce risk of rheumatic fever and glomerulonephritis.
- Prior to reconstitution store cephamandole powder preferably between 15° and 30°C (59° and 86°F), unless otherwise directed by manufacturer. The power must be protected from prolonged exposure to light to prevent discolouration. Once reconstituted, cephamandole is no longer light sensitive. Solutions appear light yellow to amber in colour. Do not use if otherwise coloured or if a precipitate is present.

CEPHAMANDOLE NAFATE (continued)

- Clumping may be avoided by tapping powder to stopper end of vial, introducing diluent away from powder, and then quickly shaking vial vigorously for even dispersion. This prevents the insoluble lump that occurs when only the powder surface is wetted.
- Following reconstitution, cephamandole is stable for 24 hours at room temperature (25°C or 77°F) and for 96 hours under refrigeration (5°C or 41°F).
- After reconstitution, cephamandole may liberate carbon dioxide (CO_2) whether stored at room temperature or refrigerated. Pressure exerted by CO_2 allows medication to be withdrawn without injecting air. Manufacturer cautions not to store medication in syringes as pressure build-up from CO_2 may force plunger out of barrel. Gas production is apparently of little consequence when drug is stored in its original container or is added to IV solutions.
- For direct IV administration, each gram of cephamadole should be reconstituted with 10 ml sterile water for injection, 5% dextrose injection, or 0.9% sodium chloride injection. Appropriate dose is administered slowly over 3 to 5 minutes.
- Cephamandole may also be given by intermittent IV infusion via a Y-type administration set or volume control set, or by continuous IV in compatible IV infusion solutions. Consult package insert.
- Because cephamandole is formulated with sodium carbonate, it is incompatible with fluids containing magnesium or calcium ions. Consult package insert for compatible IV infusion fluids and stability and storage times.

Diagnostic test interferences   Cephamandole induced positive direct Coombs' test may interfere with **cross-matching procedures** and **haematological studies**.

DRUG INTERACTIONS   *Cephamandole*

PLUS	INTERACTIONS
Alcohol	Ingestion of alcoholic beverages within 48 to 72 hours after cephamandole administation may produce a disulphiram reaction (flushing, throbbing headache, tachycardia). Concurrent use avoided
Aminoglycosides, colistimethate, and other potentially nephrotoxic drugs	Possibility of additive nephrotoxic effects. Monitor renal function

Cephazolin sodium

(Kefzol)

Antibiotic (beta-lactam);
cephalosporin

ACTIONS AND USES   Semisynthetic, first generation derivative of cephalosporin C. Broad-spectrum antibiotic similar to cephalothin (q.v.). Reported to be less irritating to

CEPHAZOLIN SODIUM (continued)

tissue and less nephrotoxic than cephalothin, and to produce higher and more sustained serum levels at equivalent dosages. Appears to be less resistant to bacterial beta-lactamases (cephalosporinases and penicillinases) than other cephalosporins.

Used for treatment of severe infections of urinary and biliary tracts, skin, soft tissue, and bone, and for bacteraemia and endocarditis caused by susceptible organisms. Also used for preoperative prophylaxis in patients undergoing procedures associated with high risk of infection such as open heart surgery.

ROUTE AND DOSAGE   **Intramuscular, intravenous: Adults:** 500 mg to 1 g every 6–12 hours. **Children and infants (over 1 month):** 25 to 50 mg/kg/day divided into three or four equal doses; total daily dose not to exceed 100 mg/kg even for severe infections.

ABSORPTION AND FATE   **Peak serum concentrations** in 1 to 2 hours following IM and in 5 minutes following IV injection. Average **half-life**: 69 to 130 minutes. Concentrations in gall-bladder and bile may exceed those in serum; high concentrations in diseased bones also. Approximately 74 to 86% bound to plasma proteins. Excreted unchanged in urine, about 56 to 89% excreted within 6 hours, and 80 to 100% within 24 hours (slower excretion in patients with renal impairment). Readily crosses placenta. Excreted in small amounts in breast milk.

CONTRAINDICATIONS AND PRECAUTIONS   Hypersensitivity to any cephalosporin. Safe use during pregnancy, in nursing mothers, and in infants under 1 month not established. **Cautious Use**: history of penicillin sensitivity, impaired renal function, patients on sodium restriction.

ADVERSE/SIDE EFFECTS   These include: nausea, vomiting, anorexia, abdominal cramps, diarrhoea, pseudomembranous colitis (rare), neutropenia, leucopenia, thrombo-cytopenia, positive direct and indirect Coombs' test, transient rise in BUN, AST (SGOT), ALT (SGPT), alkaline phosphatase. **Hypersensitivity**: anaphylaxis, maculopa-pular rash, urticaria, fever, eosinophilia. **Other**: pain and induration at IM site, phle-bitis (IV site), superinfections seizure (high doses in patients with renal insufficiency).

Diagnostic test interferences   Because of cephazolin effect on the Coombs' test, trans-fusion **cross-matching procedures** and **haematological studies** may be complicated.

DRUG INTERACTIONS   *Cephazolin*

PLUS	INTERACTIONS
Alcohol	Ingestion of alcoholic beverages within 48 to 72 hours after cephazolin administration may produce a disulphiram reaction (flushing, throbbing headache, tachycardia). Concurrent use avoided
Aminoglycosides, colistimethate, and other potentially nephrotic drugs	Possibility of additive nephrotoxic effects. Monitor renal function

Note: for further information *see cephradine*

Cephradine

(Velosef)   *Antibiotic (beta-lactam);*
                                                              cephalosporin

ACTIONS AND USES Semisynthetic acid-stable, first generation, board-spectrum cephalosporin similar to cephalothin (q.v.). Powder for parenteral use contains 3.5 mg anhydrous sodium carbonate (to increase solubility) per gram.

Used for serious infections of respiratory and urinary tracts, skin, and soft tissues, and for otitis media caused by susceptible pathogens. Has been used for perioperative prophylaxis in patients undergoing vaginal hysterectomy. Oral preparation is used primarily as follow-up to parenteral cephalosporin therapy and in treatment of urinary tract infections due to susceptible *Klebsiella* organisms resistant to other antibacterials.

ROUTE AND DOSAGE **Adults: Oral:** 250 to 500 mg every 6 hours or 500 mg to 1 g every 12 hours, depending on severity of infection. Not to exceed 4 g/day. **Intramuscular, intravenous:** 500 mg to 1 g every 6 to 12 hours; not to exceed 8 g/day. **Children (9 months or older): Oral:** 25 to 50 mg/kg daily in equally divided doses every 6 to 12 hours, up to 4 g daily. **Intramuscular, intravenous: Children (over 1 year):** 50 to 100 mg/kg/day in equally divided doses every 6 hours. Not to exceed 8 g daily. Dosages modified for patients with renal function impairment.

ABSORPTION AND FATE Well-absorbed from all routes. Peak serum levels obtained within 1 hour following oral administration, in 1 to 2 hours after IM, and in 5 minutes after IV administration. **Half-life:** 1 to 2 hours. Up to 20% bound to plasma proteins. Approximately 60 to 90% or more excreted unchanged in urine within 6 hours. Crosses placenta; excreted in breast milk.

CONTRAINDICATIONS AND PRECAUTIONS Hypersensitivity to cephalosporins. Safe use during pregnancy, in nursing mothers, and children under 1 year not established. **Cautious Use:** history of penicillin or other allergies, particularly to drugs; renal function impairment, patients on sodium restriction (use of parenteral cephradine).

ADVERSE/SIDE EFFECTS These include: nausea, vomiting, diarrhoea or loose stools, abdominal pain, heartburn, pseudomembranous colitis (rare), neutropenia, leucopenia, positive direct Coombs' test, elevations of SGOT, SGPT, alkaline phosphatase, serum bilirubin, lactic dehydrogenase (following parenteral use), elevated BUN, urticaria, rash, pruritus, joint pains, eosinophilia. **Other:** dizziness, tightness in chest, pain and induration at IM injection site; thrombophlebitis at IV injection site; paraesthesias, superinfections, hepatomegaly (rare).

NURSING IMPLICATIONS
- Before therapy is initiated, a careful inquiry should be made concerning previous hypersensitivity to cephalosporins, penicillins, and other drug allergies.
- Culture and susceptibility tests and renal function studies should be performed prior to and periodically during drug therapy.

CEPHRADINE *(continued)*

- Recommended dosage schedule in patients with reduced renal function is lower than usual and is based on creatinine clearance determinations and severity of infection. Dosage recommendations vary widely.
- Oral cephradine may be given without regard to meals, as it is not destroyed by gastric acid; however, the presence of food may delay absorption.
- To minimize pain and induration of IM site, inject deep into large muscle mass such as gluteus maximus or lateral aspect of thigh. Sterile abscess has been reported with SC injection.
- Following reconstitution, IM or direct IV solutions should be used within 2 hours at room temperature. With refrigeration (5°C), potency is retained 24 hours. Reconstituted solutions may vary in colour from light straw to yellow; this does not affect potency.
- Consult package insert for specific directions concerning types and amount of fluids used for reconstitution of cephradine for parenteral administration and for information on stability, storage, and compatible IV infusion fluids.
- The risk of thrombophlebitis may be reduced by proper dilution of IV fluid, use of small IV needles and large veins, and by alternating injection sites.
- Physician should specify dosage interval for patient taking cephradine at home. For example, four times a day may signify every 6 hours around the clock or it may indicate that drug should be taken at evenly spaced intervals during waking hours, e.g., 7.00, 12.00, 17.00, 22.00 hrs.
- Instruct patient to take medication for the full course of therapy as directed by physician. Therapy is usually continued for at least 48 to 72 hours after patient becomes asymptomatic.
- Drug therapy for beta-haemolytic streptococcal infections should continue for at least 10 days to reduce risk of rheumatic fever.
- Be on the alert for symptoms of superinfections (furry, black tongue, sore mouth, anogenital irritation or itching, foul-smelling vaginal discharge, and loose stools, sudden fever, cough).
- Report onset of diarrhoea. Bear in mind that pseudomembranous colitis, a potentially life-threatening condition may occur during or after cephalosporin therapy. It is a superinfection caused by clostridia.
- Following reconstitution, oral suspension may be stored at room temperature up to 7 days or in refrigerator for up to 14 days. Shake well before pouring. A calibrated liquid measuring device should be included when dispensed. Expiration date should be indicated on label.
- All forms of cephradine, i.e., capsules, tablets, powder for oral suspension, and powder for injection are stored preferably between 15° and 30°C (59° and 86°F) unless otherwise directed by manufacturer. Protect drug from concentrated light or direct sunlight.

Diagnostic test interferences   Note that cephradine may produce positive Coombs' test and therefore may complicate **cross-matching procedures** and **haematological studies**.

CEPHRADINE (continued)
DRUG INTERACTIONS   *Cephradine*

PLUS	INTERACTIONS
Aminoglycosides, colistimethate and other drugs with nephrotoxic potential	Possibility of additive nephrotoxic effects. Monitor renal function

Chenodeoxycholic acid

(Chendol, Chenofalk)   *Antilithic*

ACTIONS AND USES   One of the major naturally occuring human bile acids synthesized by liver. Following administration total chenodeoxycholic acid in bile acid pool increases. Biliary cholesterol saturation decreases, perhaps due to drug-induced suppression of hepatic synthesis of cholesterol and decreased biliary cholesterol secretion. By decreasing cholesterol saturation in bile, chenodeoxycholic acid promotes dissolution of uncalcified cholesterol gallstones. (Pathogenesis of cholesterol gallstone formation: bile acids, e.g., chenodeoxycholic and cholic acids, form micellar aggregates with cholesterol and phospholipids, primarily lecithin. Cholesterol crystals form in excess; unsolubilized cholesterol and stones precipitate.) Has no effect on calcified stones or on radiolucent bile pigment stones. Absorption of fluid in colon tends to be inhibited by chenodeoxycholic acid and therefore may cause loose stools or diarrhoea. Increases in low-density lipoproteins by about 10% may pose a potential risk to patients with atherosclerosis. Does not affect serum or urinary bile acid levels with drug discontinuation cholesterol supersaturation of bile returns. Prophylactic use of low doses in preventing stone recurrence is ineffective.

Used to dissolve small or floating radiolucent cholesterol gallstones in carefully selected patients with radiographically well-visualized gall-bladders and who are high surgical risks because of systemic disease or age.

ROUTE AND DOSAGE   Oral: 10–15 mg/kg/day as a single dose at bedtime or in divided doses for 3–24 months.

ABSORPTION AND FATE   Rapidly absorbed from small intestine. Partially metabolized in intestines by anaerobic bacteria to form lithocholic acid (major metabolite). Distributed mainly into bile. **Half-life** following IV administration (biphasic): 3.1 minutes; 16.4 minutes. Approximately 96% protein bound; 60 to 80% of dose metabolized in liver on first pass; enters enterohepatic circulation. About 80% excreted in faeces via bile, along with metabolite and unmetabolized chenodeoxycholic acid. Probably crosses placenta; distribution into breast milk not confirmed.

CONTRAINDICATIONS AND PRECAUTIONS   Hepatocellular dysfunction, bile duct abnormalities, nonvisualized gall-bladder following two consecutive single doses, oral cholecystographic agent, patients with radiopaque stones, gallstone complications,

CHENODEOXYCHOLIC ACID *(continued)*

compelling reasons for gall-bladder surgery (e.g., unremitting acute cholecystitis, biliary obstruction, biliary GI fistula). Safe use during pregnancy or in fertile women, nursing mothers, children, and use beyond 6 months not established. **Cautious Use:** atherosclerosis.

ADVERSE/SIDE EFFECTS   These include: mild diarrhoea (dose related), severe diarrhoea (overdosage), faecal urgency, nausea, vomiting, dyspepsia, epigastric distress, anorexia, heartburn, flatulence, abdominal cramps, constipation (rare), elevated serum total cholesterol, transient elevations of SGPT (ALT), especially and/or SGOT (AST), slight reduction of serum triglycerides, potential for hepatotoxicity leucopenia.

NURSING IMPLICATIONS

- Chenodeoxycholic acid should be taken with meals or milk. Food generally decreases rate but not extent of absorption.
- Not recommended for fertile women unless effective contraception is practised.
- Women who become pregnant while taking chenodeoxycholic acid should be advised to notify physician as soon as possible. They should be informed of potential hazards to foetus.
- Cholecystograms and/or ultrasonograms are recommended before initiation of therapy to determine presence of functioning gall-bladder and radiolucent stones. Studies are repeated at 6- and 9-month intervals during therapy to monitor response to therapy, i.e., stone dissolution, and also to rule out recurrence. (Gallstones can be expected to recur in up to 50% of patients within 5 years.)
- Diarrhoea, usually mild and transient, occurs in about 30 to 40% of patients, more frequently at beginning of therapy, but may occur at any time during therapy. Treatment generally consists of temporary dosage reduction (by about ½) until diarrhoea is controlled; dosage is then gradually increased to original level. Antidiarrhoeal agents may also be prescribed.
- Patient should be informed that the crampy abdominal pain that sometimes accompanies bouts of diarrhoea is to be distinguished from the pain of biliary colic. The latter pain occurs in right upper quadrant or epigastric region, is frequently associated with nausea and vomiting, and should be reported to physician immediately.
- To reduce risk of stone recurrence, encourage patient to attain and maintain ideal body weight, to include high-fibre foods in diet, and to reduce cholesterol and carbohydrate intake. Collaborate with physician, dietitian, patient, and significant family members in design of a therapeutic diet plan.
- Patient should be well informed about the requirements of the therapeutic regimen, and motivated to accept long-term therapy.
- Safe use depends on careful monitoring of liver function.
- Dissolution of gallstones by chenodeoxycholic acid (confirmed by cholecystogram and/or ultrasonogram) may require 6 to 24 months. When complete dissolution has occurred, repeat studies should be performed after 1 to 3 months of continued chenodeoxycholic acid administration for verification.
- If partial stone dissolution does not occur by 9 to 12 months, it is unlikely that

CHENODEOXYCHOLIC ACID (continued)

further treatment will be effective. Therapy should be discontinued if no response has occurred by 18 months.

■ Store preferably between 15° and 30°C (59° and 86°F) in well-closed container, unless otherwise directed by manufacturer.

DRUG INTERACTIONS   *Chenodeoxycholic acid*_____

PLUS	INTERACTIONS
Cholestyramine colestipol and other anion-exchange resins Aluminium-containing antacids	Cause binding of chenodiol, reducing its absorption Simultaneous administration not advised
Oestrogens, oestrogen—progesterone combinations, clofibrate	May counteract chenodeoxycholic acid effectiveness by increasing biliary cholesterol secretion

Chloral hydrate _____

(Noctec)   *Sedative, hypnotic*

ACTIONS AND USES   Produces 'physiological sleep' by mild cerebral depression with little effect on respirations or blood pressure and little or no hangover. Principal action thought to be due in part to trichloroethanol, its reduction product. Does not affect sleep physiology (e.g., REM sleep) in low doses. The oldest chloral derivative and still regarded as a relatively safe, effective, and inexpensive sedative—hypnotic. Has little or no analgesic action. May cause enzyme induction and displace certain drugs from protein binding sites.

Used in short-term management of insomnia, for general sedation (especially in the young and the elderly), for sedation before and after surgery,

ROUTE AND DOSAGE   Oral: **Adults:** *sedative*: 250 mg 3 times a day after meals; *hypnotic*: 500 mg to 1 g 15 to 30 minutes before bedtime. Single dose should not exceed 2 g. **Children:** 30–50 mg/kg with maximum single dose of 1 g.

ABSORPTION AND FATE   Readily absorbed following oral or rectal administration. Hypnotic dose produces sleep within 30 minutes to 1 hour, lasting 4 to 8 hours. Rapidly reduced in body to active metabolite, trichloroethanol 70 to 80% of which is protein bound. Well distributed to body fluids and to all tissues. **Plasma half-life:** about 8 to 11 hours. Active and inactive metabolites excreted in urine in 24 to 48 hours. Small portion excreted in faeces via bile. Crosses placenta; appears in breast milk in negligible amounts.

CONTRAINDICATIONS AND PRECAUTIONS   Known hypersensitivity to drug; severe hepatic, renal, or cardiac disease; rectal dosage form in patients with proctitis; oral use in patients with oesophagitis, gastritis, gastric or duodenal ulcers. Safe use during pregnancy and in nursing women not established.

CHLORAL HYDRATE (continued)

ADVERSE/SIDE EFFECTS (Generally well tolerated). Side effects include: light-headedness, dizziness, ataxia, drowsiness, headache, hangover (infrequent), nightmares; rarely: paradoxical excitement, somnambulistic reaction with disorientation and incoherence, paranoid behavior, nausea, vomiting, diarrhoea, flatulence, unpleasant taste. **Hypersensitivity:** fever, purpura, urticaria, erythematous rash, eczema, erythema multiforme, angioedema, eosinophilia. **Overdose:** hypotension, hypothermia; respiratory depression, cardiac arrhythmias, miosis, areflexia, oesophageal stricture, gastric necrosis. **Other:** breath odour, leucopenia, ketonuria, precipitation of acute intermittent porphyria. **Chronic Use:** fixed drug eruptions, severe gastritis, renal, and hepatic damage, sudden death.

NURSING IMPLICATIONS

- Chloral hydrate is not intended for relief of pain. When used in the presence of pain it may cause excitement and delirium.
- Corrosive to skin and mucous membranes unless well diluted. Has an aromatic, pungent odour and bitter, pungent taste; these may be minimized by use of the capsule form or by dilution of liquid preparations in chilled fluids.
- To minimize gastric irritation, administer drug after meals. Capsules should be swallowed whole and taken with a full glass of water, fruit juice, or ginger ale. Syrups or elixirs may be administered in half a glass of the same liquids.
- When used as an hypnotic, prepare patient for sleep by providing maximum comfort measures and reducing environmental stimuli.
- Because hypnotic doses may cause dizziness, caution patient not to ambulate without assistance and remove matches, cigarettes, etc., if patient is a smoker. Bed rails may be advisable for the elderly patient.
- Prolonged use can lead to tolerance, physical dependence, and addiction. Sudden withdrawal from dependent patients may produce delirium, mania, or convulsions.
- Allergic skin reactions may occur within several hours or as long as 10 days after drug administration.
- Caution patient to avoid concomitant use of alcoholic beverages. The acute poisoning that occurs from the combination of chloral hydrate and alcohol (Mickey Finn) produces vasodilation, with flushing, headache, tachycardia, and hypotension.
- Inform patient that driving and other potentially hazardous activities should be avoided while under the influence of chloral hydrate.
- Evaluate patient's response to chloral hydrate and continued need for the drug.
- Habituation may be minimized by evaluating and treating the underlying cause or causes of the symptom of insomnia.
- Solutions are preserved in tightly covered, light-resistant containers. All forms preferably stored at between 15° and 30°C (59° and 86°F), unless otherwise directed by manufacturer.

DRUG INTERACTIONS   Chloral hydrate

PLUS	INTERACTIONS
Alcohol, barbiturates, paraldehyde, tranquilizers, and other CNS depressants	Potentiation of CNS depression. Tachycardia, facial flushing may occur with alcohol. Combination generally avoided or used with great caution

CHLORAL HYDRATE (continued)

PLUS	INTERACTIONS
(continued)	
Anticoagulants, oral	Increased anticoagulant effects. Monitor prothrombin activity
Frusemide by IV route	Possibility of flushing, diaphoresis and blood pressure changes. Combination generally avoided

Chlorambucil

(Leukeran)

Antineoplastic; alkylating agent; nitrogen mustard

ACTIONS AND USES   Potent aromatic derivative of the alkylating agent, mechlorethamine (nitrogen mustard) and slowest acting and least toxic of the nitrogen mustards. A cell cycle nonspecific (kills both resting and dividing cells), it causes cytotoxic cross linkage in DNA thus preventing synthesis of DNA, RNA, and proteins. Myelosuppression in therapeutic doses is moderate and rapidly reversible. Lymphocytic effect is marked. Has mutagenic and embryotoxic properties.

Used as single agent or in combination with other antineoplastics in treatment of chronic lymphocytic leukaemia, malignant lymphomas including lymphosarcoma, Hodgkin's disease and giant follicular lymphoma, and in treatment of carcinoma of the ovary, breast, and testes. Also has been used in rheumatoid arthritis.

ROUTE AND DOSAGE   Oral: Adults: individualized.

ABSORPTION AND FATE   Well-absorbed following oral administration. **Plasma half-life**: 90 minutes; fat storage may occur because of lipophilic properties. Believed to be highly bound to plasma and tissue proteins. Metabolized in liver. About 60% excreted in urine 24 hours after administration mostly as metabolites. Probably crosses placenta.

CONTRAINDICATIONS AND PRECAUTIONS   Hypersensitivity to chlorambucil or to other alkylating agents; administration within 4 weeks of a full course of radiation or chemotherapy; full dosage if bone marrow is infiltrated with lymphomatous tissue or is hypoplastic; small pox and other vaccines. Safe use during pregnancy and in nursing women not established. **Cautious Use**: excessive or prolonged dosage, pneumococcus vaccination.

ADVERSE/SIDE EFFECTS   Bone marrow depression: leucopenia, thrombocytopenia, anaemia; sterility; hyperuricaemia. Low incidence of gastric discomfort (high doses), drug fever, skin rashes, alopecia, peripheral neuropathy, sterile cystitis, pulmonary complications, hepatotoxicity, seizures (high doses). Suspect mutagenic, teratogenic, and carcinogenic potential.

CHLORAMBUCIL *(continued)*
NURSING IMPLICATIONS

- Nausea and vomiting may be controlled by giving entire daily dose at one time, 1 hour before breakfast or 2 hours after evening meal, or at bedtime. Consult physician.
- If patient has difficulty swallowing tablet, ask pharmacist about the possibility of preparing an oral suspension.
- CBC, haemoglobin, total and differential leucocyte counts, and serum uric acid should be checked initially and at least once weekly during treatment.
- Body weight, size of spleen, and temperature charted before initiation of therapy and at the time of blood counts provide a useful profile for determining degree of bone marrow suppression.
- Leucopenia usually develops after the third week of treatment; it may continue for up to 10 days after last dose then rapidly return to normal.
- About one quarter of the patients receiving a total dose of approximately 450 mg and one-half those receiving this dosage 8 weeks or less may develop severe neutropenia.
- With confirmation of bone marrow depression (low platelet and neutrophil counts or peripheral lymphocytosis), it is recommended that dosage not exceed 0.1 mg/kg.
- If possible, avoid or reduce to minimum injections and other invasive procedures (e.g., rectal temperatures, enemas) when platelet count is low because of danger of bleeding.
- Clinical improvement is usually apparent by third week. Produces remission in a substantial number of patients.
- During treatment with chlorambucil it is dangerous for the patient to go longer than 2 weeks without a clinical examination and blood studies. Reinforce importance of keeping appointments with the physician.
- Advise patient to notify physician if the following symptoms occur: unusual bleeding or bruising, sores on lips or in mouth; flank, stomach or joint pain; fever, chills, or other signs of infection, sore throat, cough, dyspnoea.
- Skin reactions are rare, but all appear to show a consistent pattern: pustular eruption on mouth, chin, cheeks; urticarial erythema on trunk that spreads to legs. The rash occurs early in treatment period and lasts about 10 days after last dose. Responses become more and more severe with repeated challenges. Urge the patient to report immediately the onset of cutaneous reaction.
- Urine alkalinization and allopurinol may be prescribed to prevent elevated serum uric acid levels (can lead to nephrotoxicity). If physician agrees, urge patient to drink at least 10 to 12 glasses (240 mls each) of fluid/day and to report to physician if urine output decreases below normal amounts.
- Because of drug-impaired immune response, pneumococcus vaccine effectiveness is reduced therefore it is not generally given during chlorambucil therapy.
- Advise patient to report to physician immediately if she becomes pregnant. She should be informed of the potential hazard to the foetus.
- Discuss possibility of gonadal suppression with patient (amenorrhoea or azoospermia may be irreversible), which occurs especially with high doses.
- During maintenance therapy, physician may occasionally interrupt drug schedule in order to determine if patient is in remission.

CHLORAMBUCIL (continued)

- Store preferably at 15° to 30°C (59° to 86°F) in well-closed, light-resistant container.
- *See Mustine for nursing implications of neoplastic therapy.*

DRUG INTERACTIONS *Chlorambucil*——————————————————————

PLUS	INTERACTIONS
Antigout agent	Dosage of antigout agent may have to be adjusted because chlorambucil causes hyperuricaemia

C

Chloramphenicol ————————————————————————————————

(Chloromycetin, Kemicetine)   *Antibiotic; antirickettsial*

ACTIONS AND USES Synthetic broad-spectrum antibiotic formerly derived from *Streptomyces venezuelae*. Principally bacteriostatic but may be bactericidal in certain species (e.g., *H. influenzae*) or when given in higher concentrations. Effective against a wide variety of gram-negative and gram-positive bacteria and most anaerobic microorganisms. Believed to act by interfering with synthesis of bacterial ribosomes.

Used only in severe infections when other antibiotics are ineffective or are contraindicated. Particularly effective against *Salmonella typhi* and other Salmonella species, *S. pneumoniae*, *Neisseria*, meningeal infections caused by *H. influenzae*.

ROUTE AND DOSAGE Oral: Adult: 500 mg/6 hrly. **Intramuscular/intravenous**: injection or infusion 50 mg/kg/day in divided doses. **Child**: 50–100 mg/kg/day; **infant (less than two weeks of age)** and **children with immature metabolic function**: 25 mg/kg/day in divided doses. **Topical cream (1%)**: gently rub into affected area 3 or 4 times daily after cleansing. **Ophthalmic ointment (1%)**: apply small strip of ointment to lower conjunctival sac every 3 to 4 hours. **Ophthalmic solution (0.5%)**: instill 1 or 2 drops every 1 to 6 hours. **Ear drops: (5%)**: Instill 2 or 3 drops into affected ear 3 times daily, at 6- to 8-hour intervals.

NURSING IMPLICATIONS
- Oral drug is taken preferably with a full glass of water on an empty stomach, at least 1 hour before or 2 hours after a meal, to achieve optimum blood levels.
- Generally patient is hospitalized during systemic chloramphenicol therapy to facilitate laboratory tests and close observation.
- Bacterial culture and sensitivity tests are essential and may be performed concurrently with initiation of therapy and periodically thereafter.
- Baseline CBC, platelets, serum iron, and reticulocyte cell counts are recommended prior to initiation of therapy, at 48-hour intervals during therapy, and periodically during follow-up period.
- Inform patient that bitter taste may occur 15 to 20 seconds following IV injection

CHLORAMPHENICOL *(continued)*

and that it usually lasts only 2 to 3 minutes. Oral form is substituted as soon as feasible.

- Chloramphenicol blood levels should be closely monitored (desired concentration between 5 and 20 mcg/ml).
- Close observation of the patient is also crucial, because blood studies are not always reliable predictors of irreversible bone marrow depression.
- Non-dose-related irreversible bone marrow depression may appear weeks or months after drug therapy is terminated. The potential for this side effect is greatest in patients with impaired hepatic or renal function, infants, children, and premenopausal women.
- Tell patient to report immediately sore throat, fever, fatigue, petechiae, nose bleeds, bleeding gums, or other unusual bleeding or bruising, or any other suspicious sign or symptom. Drug therapy should be discontinued if abnormal bleeding occurs.
- Check temperature at least every 4 hours. Usually chloramphenicol is discontinued if temperature remains normal for 48 hours. Some clinicians recommend that treatment for typhoid be continued 8 to 10 days after patient becomes afebrile to lessen the possibility of relapse.
- Up to 10% of patients treated with chloramphenicol for typhoid reportedly become temporary or permanent carriers and therefore require further therapy with either ampicillin or amoxicillin. Chloramphenicol is not recommended for treatment of carriers.
- Report any appreciable change in fluid intake and output ratio or pattern.
- Watch for signs and symptoms of superinfection by nonsusceptible organisms; stomatitis, glossitis with or without black tongue, anogenital irritation or itching, vaginal discharge, elevated temperature, diarrhoea (enterocolitis), cough.
- More frequent determinations of serum glucose are recommended in patients receiving oral antidiabetic agents (*see Drug Interactions*).
- Gray syndrome has occurred 2 to 9 days after initiation of high dose chloramphenicol therapy in prematures and newborns, and in children up to 2 years of age. Report early signs: abdominal distention, failure to feed, pallor, changes in vital signs.
- Chloramphenicol solution for injection may form crystals or a second layer when stored at low temperatures. Solution will clarify by shaking vials. Do not use cloudy solutions.
- Follow manufacturer's directions for dilution and storage of IV preparation.
- ***Topical use***   Systemic absorption and toxicity can occur with prolonged or frequent intermittent use of topical preparations.
- Topical preparations are *not* interchangeable. Use only as designated.
- Advise patient to follow dosage and duration of therapy as prescribed by physician.
- Instruct patient to stop medication immediately if signs of hypersensitivity, superinfection, or other adverse reactions appear.
- Instillation of eye drops: apply light pressure to lacrimal duct for 1 minute to prevent drainage into nasopharynx and systemic absorption. *See Index: Drug administration: eye drops for more complete description.*
- Applications to skin are generally preceded by a soap and water cleansing and thorough drying of part before reapplication of medication. Consult physician.

CHLORAMPHENICOL (continued)

- Avoid warming chloramphenicol solutions (e.g., otic solution) above body temperature, to prevent loss of potency.
- Ophthalmic solution should be protected from light.
- Store topical and oral forms, and unopened vials, preferably between 15° and 30°C (59° and 86°F), unless otherwise directed by manufacturer.

Diagnostic test interferences   Possibility of false-positive results for **urine glucose** by copper reduction methods (e.g., Clinitest). Chloramphenicol may interfere with urinary steroid determinations with **urobilinogen excretion**, and with responses to **tetanus toxoid** and possibly other active immunizing agents.

DRUG INTERACTIONS   *Chloramphenicol*

PLUS	INTERACTIONS
Anticoagulants, oral	
Chlorpropamide, tolbutamide and possibly other sulphonylureas (oral antidiabetic agents)	By inhibiting hepatic microsomal enzyme activity, chloramphenicol may prolong half-life and potentiate action of drugs metabolized by this system. Used concurrently with caution
Cyclophosphamide	
Phenytoin and other hydantoins	
Phenobarbitone and other barbiturates	Phenobarbitone may reduce chloramphenicol plasma levels and phenobarbitone effects may increase. Dosage adjustments may be indicated
Penicillins	Chloramphenicol may antagonize action of bactericidal antibiotics (theoretical possibility). Combination used with caution
Cyanocobalamin (vitamin B_{12}) Folic acid Iron preparations	By interfering with erythrocyte maturation, chloramphenicol may reduce response of these substances
Paracetomol	Half–life of chloramphenicol increased

Chlordiazepoxide hydrochloride

(Librium, Tropium)   *Psychotropic anxiolytic;*
                                                           benzodiazepine

ACTIONS AND USES   Benzodiazepine derivative, prototype of the anxiolytic agents. Exerts depressant effects on subcortical levels of CNS, and in high doses, on the cortex. Calming effect thought to be due to action on the limbic system. Produces mild sedative, anticonvulsant, and skeletal muscle relaxant effect. Has long-acting hypnotic properties. Causes mild suppression of REM sleep and of deeper phases, particularly stage 4, while increasing total sleep time. Usually does not result in withdrawal insomnia even with prolonged use.

Used for relief of various anxiety and tension states, preoperative apprehension and

CHLORDIAZEPOXIDE HYDROCHLORIDE (continued)

anxiety, and for management of withdrawal symptoms of acute alcoholism. Also used as an antidyskinetic.

ROUTE AND DOSAGE   *Anxiety states*: **Oral**: **Adults**: 10 mg three times a day to a maximum of 100 mg/day, debilitated and elderly patients reduce the dose. **Child**: 5–20 mg/day in divided doses. *Acute panic attacks and alcohol withdrawal symptoms*: **Intramuscular**: by slow deep injection 50–100 mg, repeated as required by 25–100 mg 3–4 times a day.

ABSORPTION AND FATE   Well-absorbed from GI tract. Peak plasma levels reached in 1 to 4 hours after oral administration, 15 to 30 minutes after IM administration. **Half-life**: 5 to 30 hours. Metabolized in liver. Active and inactive metabolites slowly excreted, primarily in urine and small amount in faeces. Urinary excretion continues for several days after last dose. Crosses placenta; excreted in breast milk.

CONTRAINDICATIONS AND PRECAUTIONS   Hypersensitivity to chlordiazepoxide and other benzodiazepines; narrow-angle glaucoma, prostatic hypertrophy, shock, comatose states, primary depressive disorder or psychoses, pregnancy, lactation, oral use in children under 6 years of age, parenteral use in children under 12 years. **Cautious Use**: anxiety states associated with impending depression, history of impaired hepatic or renal function; addiction-prone individuals, allergic dermatoses, blood dyscrasias; in the elderly, debilitated patients, children; hyperkinesis, chronic obstructive pulmonary disease.

ADVERSE/SIDE EFFECTS   These include: drowsiness, dizziness, lethargy (common), changes in EEG pattern (low-voltage fast activity); blurred vision, nystagmus, diplopia, vivid dreams, nightmares, headache, extrapyramidal symptoms, vertigo, syncope, tinnitus, confusion, hallucinations, parodoxic rage, depression, delirium, ataxia, orthostatic hypotension, tachycardia, changes in ECG patterns, xerostomia, nausea, constipation, increased appetite, urinary frequency, menstrual irregularities, anovulation, increased or decreased libido, oedema, weight gain, pain in injection site, photosensitivity, skin rash, blood dyscrasias (including agranulocytosis), jaundice, acute intermittent porphyria, hiccoughs, elevation of LDG. **Overdosage**: somnolence, confusion, diminished reflexes, paradoxical excitation, depressed respirations, coma.

NURSING IMPLICATIONS
- Patients who complain of gastric distress may obtain relief by taking the drug with or immediately after meals or with milk. If an antacid is prescribed, it should be taken at least 1 hour before or after chlordiazepoxide to prevent delay in drug absorption.
- Tablet may be crushed before swallowing if patient cannot take it whole, or capsule may be emptied and contents swallowed with fluid or mixed with foods.
- If patient is known to be addiction-prone, observe for signs of developing physical and/or psychological dependency such as requests for change in drug regimen (dose and dose interval), diminishing favourable response (e.g., disturbed sleep pattern, increase in psychomotor activity), manipulative behaviour, withdrawal symptoms. Investigate the symptoms of ataxia, vertigo, slurred speech; the patient may be taking more than the prescribed dose.

CHLORDIAZEPOXIDE HYDROCHLORIDE (continued)

- Advise patient to take drug specifically as prescribed: not to skip, increase, or decrease doses, change intervals, or terminate therapy without physician's advice. Emphasize that patient should not lend or offer any of drug to another person.
- Benzodiazepines are not intended for management of episodic minor anxieties and tensions associated with everyday living.
- OTC drugs should not be taken unless prescribed. Check patient's self-medication habits. Sometimes a patient does not consider that a self-prescribed drug for minor pains and aches or for gastric distress or a cold is a 'medication.'
- Prepare parenteral solution immediately before use; discard unused portion. Drug is unstable in light and when in solution.
- Use special diluent provided by manufacturer to make the IM solution. Add diluent carefully to avoid bubble formation; gently agitate until solution is clear. Resulting solution: 50 mg/ml. Discard diluent if it is not clear.
- Do not mix any other drug with chlordiazepoxide solution.
- In early part of therapy, check blood pressure and pulse before giving benzodiazepine. If blood pressure falls 20 mm Hg or more or if pulse rate is above 120 beats/minute, delay medication and consult physician.
- Orthostatic hypotension and tachycardia occur more frequently with parenteral administration. Patient should stay recumbent 2 to 3 hours after IM or IV injection; observe closely and monitor vital signs.
- Instruct patient to change position from recumbency to standing slowly and in stages. Support lights may be helpful. Discuss with physician.
- Until drug dosage is stabilized monitor fluid intake and output. Report changes in fluid intake and output ratio and dysuria to physician. Cumulative (overdosage) effects can result with renal dysfunction. The elderly are especially vulnerable (normal ageing changes compromise kidney efficiency).
- Observe intake of patient who is seriously agitated or depressed; willful reduction of fluids can be hazardous.
- Paradoxic reactions (excitement, stimulation, disturbed sleep patterns, acute rage) may occur during first few weeks of therapy in psychiatric patients and in hyperactive and aggressive children receiving chlordiazepoxide. Withhold drug and report to physician.
- Suicidal tendencies may be manifested in anxiety states accompanied by depression. Observe necessary protective precautions.
- Long-term use of this drug may cause xerostomia. Good oral hygiene can alleviate the discomfort: frequent rinses with warm water, daily flossing with waxed floss, brushing with small soft toothbrush and fluoride toothpaste, use of saliva substitute, sugarfree gum, or lemon drops. For more complete description, *see Index: Nursing interventions: dry mouth.*
- Observe patient's sleep pattern and quality. If dreams or nightmares (which usually occur during REM sleep) interfere with rest, notify physician. A change in the dosing schedule, dose, or an alternate drug may be prescribed.
- If drug has been prescribed for anxiety-induced insomnia and is used every day, its effect begins in 2 or 3 nights; however, usefulness for this problem lasts only a few weeks.

CHLORDIAZEPOXIDE HYDROCHLORIDE (continued)

- Periodic blood cell counts and liver function tests are recommended during prolonged therapy.
- Sore throat or mouth, upper respiratory infection, fever, and malaise should alert one to the possibility of agranulocytosis. Total and differential WBC counts should be ordered immediately, and protective isolation instituted.
- Most signs and symptoms associated with chlordiazepoxide therapy are dose-related. Physicians will rely on accurate observations and reporting of patient's response to drug to determine lowest effective maintenance dose.
- Adverse reactions, such as drowsiness, dizziness, lethargy, syncope, ataxia, confusion, constipation, and urinary retention, are dose-related but even at lower ranges may occur in elderly and debilitated patients. Supervision of ambulation is indicated, and possibly side rails.
- Warn ambulatory patient that sedation may occur during early therapy. Activities requiring mental alertness and precision should be avoided until reaction to the drug has been evaluated.
- Caution patient against drinking alcoholic beverages. When combined with chlordiazepoxide, effects of both are potentiated.
- **Smoking–drug interaction**   Some studies suggest that smoking increases clearance rate of chlordiazepoxide. The heavy smoker may require higher dosage of the drug for therapeutic effectiveness than the nonsmoker.
- If patient becomes pregnant during therapy or intends to become pregnant advise her to communicate with physician about continuing therapy.
- Advise patient to avoid excessive sunlight. Photosensitivity has been reported. A sun screen lotion (SPF 12 or above) should be used (if allowed).
- Effectiveness of chlordiazepoxide in long-term use for more than 6 months is not established. Periodic evaluations should be made of patient's response before continuing therapy.
- Because drug is excreted slowly and is converted to active metabolites, habituation can occur. Incidence of physical dependency, however, is low.
- Abrupt discontinuation of drug in patients receiving high doses for long periods has precipitated withdrawal symptoms, but not for at least 5 to 7 days because of slow elimination. Symptoms may include restlessness, unreal or distant feeling paraesthesias, abdominal and muscle cramps, tremors, insomnia, vomiting, anorexia, profuse sweating, psychomotor activity including convulsions and delirium. In most cases, after usual doses there is no withdrawal syndrome.
- **Management of overdosage**   Induce vomiting, monitor vital functions, provide general support measures (avoid use of barbiturates).
- Store in tight, light-resistant containers at temperature between 15° and 30°C (50° and 86°F), unless otherwise specified by manufacturer. The special diluent supplied by manufacturer for IM preparation should be kept refrigerated, preferably between 2° and 8°C (36° and 46°F), until ready for use.

Diagnostic test interferences   Chlordiazepoxide increases **serum bilirubin**. SGOT and **SGPT**; decreases **radioactive iodine uptake**; and may falsely increase readings for urinary **17-OHCS**.

C

CHLORDIAZEPOXIDE HYDROCHLORIDE (continued)
DRUG INTERACTIONS   *Chlordiazepoxide*_____

PLUS	INTERACTIONS
Alcohol (ethanol), and other CNS depressants	Potentiation of CNS depressant effects. (Reaction with alcohol may occur up to 10 hours after last dose of benzodiazepine)
Cimetidine	Increased chlordiazepoxide plasma levels. (Cimetidine inhibits chlordiazepoxide metabolism.) Lower chlordiazepoxide doses may be indicated
Disulphiram	Pharmacological effects of chlordiazepoxide may be increased. Lower chlordiazepoxide doses may be necessary
Levodopa	Monitor for possibility of reduced antiparkinsonian effect (based on limited evidence)
MAO inhibitors	Enhanced benzodiazepine effects. Concurrent use generally avoided
Oral contraceptives	Pharmacological effects of benzodiazepines may be increased or decreased. Dosage adjustments may be indicated
Phenytoin	Serum levels of phenytoin may be increased with potentiation of pharmacological effects. Monitor serum phenytoin levels

Chlormethiazole ▬▬▬▬▬▬▬▬▬▬▬▬▬▬▬▬▬▬▬

(Heminevrin)   *Hypnotic; anticonvulsant*

ACTIONS AND USES   Chemically related to part of the vitamin B_1 complex, animal studies have shown high sedative, hypnotic and anticonvulsant activity. Mode of action is uncertain but anticonvulsant effects may be due to activity in the GABA systems within the central nervous system. Sedative action may also effect catecholamine activity.

Used as a general sedative, particularly in the elderly. Relieves restlessness and anxiety including that due to delirium tremens (alcohol withdrawal). Induces sleep. Administered intravenously to control convulsive states in pre-eclampsia and status epilepticus. Sedative during regional anaesthesia.

ROUTE AND DOSAGE   Oral: Adult: sedation, 1 capsule or 5 ml syrup three times a day; hypnotic, 2 capsules or 10 ml syrup at night; delirium tremens, up to 12 capsules a day in divided doses. **Intravenous**: *Alcohol withdrawal*: **Adult**: (0.8% solution of chlormethiazole edisylate) 40–100 ml over 5–10 min (initial dose 320–800 mg) then titrated to effect required. *Status epilepticus*: by **IV infusion**: 0.8% solution 40–100 ml (320–800 mg) at rate of 60–150 drops/min.

CHLORMETHIAZOLE (continued)

ABSORPTION AND FATE   Readily absorbed by mouth, chlormethiazole has a short plasma **half-life** of 3–5 hours. **Binding to plasma protein** is 63%. Liver metabolism may be reduced when given concurrently with diazepines or cimetidine. Capsule containing 192 mg base is equipotent to 5 ml syrup containing 250 mg edisylate.

CONTRAINDICATIONS AND PRECAUTIONS   Not recommended as a sedative in children. Concomitant use with other sedatives or alcohol should be avoided. Deep sleep induced by intravenous administration may lapse into unconsciousness. Drug is adsorbed to PVC with some loss of drug during continuous infusion. **Cautious use** in alcoholics, drug abusers and individuals with marked personality disorders or those with obstructive pulmonary disease.

ADVERSE/SIDE EFFECTS   Tingling in the nose, sneezing, stuffiness (particularly with intravenous infusion). CNS depression. Conjunctival irritation. Drop in blood pressure. Confusion. Gastrointestinal disturbance. Local thrombophlebitis at intravenous injection site.

NURSING IMPLICATIONS

- One capsule is equipotent to 5 ml syrup.
- Used as a sedative in the elderly because of its short action in the body.
- As with any sedative, use should be reviewed regularly.
- Hangover effect may occur in the elderly but is uncommon.
- Should excessive sedation occur when used in the daytime, dose should be adjusted.
- Patient should be cautioned not to drive or operate machinery.
- Check that alcoholic patients do not take alcohol during treatment as this will increase the sedative effect.
- Observe for signs of conjunctival irritation.
- Observe for possible nasal congestion and respiratory depression.
- During intravenous use: monitor blood pressure; have airway and suction ready; observe IV site for thrombophlebitis; use a teflon catheter.
- Drug absorbs to PVC with some loss in potency, dose should therefore be titrated to effect during IV infusion.
- Use a glass syringe in an infusion control pump for children.
- Store capsules/syrup at room temperature, if syrup is diluted with water discard after 14 days. Store IV preparation at 5–8° C.

DRUG INTERACTIONS   Chlormethiazole

PLUS	INTERACTIONS
Cimetidine	Enhanced effect possibly due to decreased hepatic metabolism
Alcohol	Increased sedation
Benzodiazepines } CNS depressants }	Increased sedation
Reduced effect PVC giving sets	Loss of potency

Chlormezanone ━━━━━━━━━━━━━━━━━━━━━━━━━━━━━━━━━

(Trancopal)   *Psychotropic; anxiolytic*

ACTIONS AND USES   A nonhypnotic anxiolytic with CNS depressant effects similar to those of meprobamate (q.v.). Believed to act on subcortical levels of CNS to produce mild sedation and skeletal muscle relaxant effects.

Used in symptomatic treatment of mild anxiety and tension states. Has been used as adjunct to rest, analgesics, and physical therapy for relief of painful musculoskeletal conditions.

ROUTE AND DOSAGE   Oral: **Adults**: 100 to 200 mg 3 or 4 times/day, or 400 mg at bedtime. Reduced dosages in elderly and debilitated patients.

ABSORPTION AND FATE   Rapidly absorbed from GI tract. Action begins in 15 to 30 minutes and may last up to 6 hours or longer. Plasma **half-life**: 24 hours. Widely distributed in most tissues, especially kidneys, heart, liver. Metabolized in liver. Excreted in urine as unchanged drug and metabolites. Passage across placenta or into breast milk unknown.

CONTRAINDICATIONS AND PRECAUTIONS   Hypersensitivity to chlormezanone; children less than 5 years of age. Safe use during pregnancy and in nursing women not established. **Cautious Use**: renal or hepatic disease, history of drug abuse.

ADVERSE/SIDE EFFECTS   CNS: drowsiness, dizziness, slurred speech, headache, weakness, ataxia, lethargy, mental depression, tremor, excitement, confusion, increased anxiety. **GI**: drug mouth, impaired sense of taste (ageusia), nausea, anorexia. *Hypersensitivity*: skin rash, fever, chills. **Other**: flushing, inability to void, cholestatic jaundice (rare), oedema, tightness in throat.

For further information *see diazepam*.

Chloroquine hydrochloride ━━━━━━━━━━━━━━━━━━━━━━━━━━

(Avlocor, Malarivon, Nivaquine)   *Antimalarial; 4-aminoquinoline*

ACTIONS AND USES   Synthetic 4-aminoquinoline derivative. Antimalarial activity is believed to be based on ability to form complexes with DNA of parasite, thereby inhibiting replication and transcription to RNA and nucleic acid synthesis. Highly active against erythrocytic forms of plasmodia, providing suppressive prophylaxis and clinical cure. Not effective against exoerythrocytic tissue stages and therefore does not provide causal prophylaxis. Also has amoebicidal activity, antiinflammatory action, quinidine-like effect on heart, antihistamine and antiserotonin properties, and inhibits prostaglandin effects on cells. Certain adverse effects are related to affinity of chloroquine for melanin-bearing cells particularly in ear and eyes.

CHLOROQUINE HYDROCHLORIDE (continued)

Used for suppression and treatment of malaria caused by *P. malariae*, *P. ovale*, *P. vivax*, and susceptible forms of *P. falciparum* and in treatment of extraintestinal amoebiasis. Concomitant therapy with primaquine (an 8-aminoquinoline) is necessary for radical cure of vivax and malariae malarias. Has been used in treatment of giardiasis, discoid and systemic lupus erythematosus, porphyria cutanea tarda, solar urticaria, polymorphous light eruptions, and in rheumatoid arthritis not controlled by other less toxic drugs.

ROUTE AND DOSAGE   Dosage is often expressed or calculated in terms of chloroquine base. Each 250 mg tablet (phosphate) = 150 mg (base) = 200 mg (sulphate). *Acute malaria*: Oral: **Adult**: 600 mg followed by 300 mg after 6−8 hrs then 300 mg for two days. **Child(1−4 yrs)**: 150 mg (base) followed by 75 mg after 6 hrs then 75 mg a day for two days; **(5−8 yrs)**: 300 mg (base) followed by 150 mg after 6 hrs then 150 mg a day for two days, **(8−12 yrs)** 450 mg (base) followed by 225 mg after 6 hrs then 225 mg a day for 2 days. *Suppression of malaria*: Oral: **Adult**: 600 mg weekly when at risk continued for 4−6 weeks after exposure. **Child**: 5 mg/kg per week during risk continued for 4−6 weeks after exposure. *Hepatic amoebiasis*: Oral: **Adult**: 300 mg twice a day for two days then 300 mg daily for 2−3 weeks. **Child**: 6 mg/kg twice a day then 6 mg/kg daily for 2−3 weeks. *Rheumatoid arthritis*: 75−300 mg/day for 2−3 months.

ABSORPTION AND FATE   Rapidly absorbed following oral administration. **Maximum plasma concentration** in 1 to 2 hours. Approximately 55% **bound to plasma proteins. Plasma half-life** after 3 to 5 days. High concentrations in liver, kidney, lung, brain, spinal cord, eyes, and erythrocytes. Partially metabolized in liver. Excreted slowly in urine as metabolites (25% of dose) and free drug (70% of dose); about 8% excreted unchanges in faeces. Urinary excretion increased by acidification and decreased by alkalinization of urine. Small amounts of drug detectable in urine for months and sometimes for years following discontinuation of therapy. Crosses placenta. Excreted in breast milk.

CONTRAINDICATIONS AND PRECAUTIONS   Hypersensitivity to 4-aminoquinolines, psoriatic arthritis, porphyria, renal disease, 4-aminoquinoline-induced retinal or visual field changes; long-term therapy in children. Safe use during pregnancy, in nursing women, and women of childbearing potential not established. **Cautious Use**: impaired hepatic function, alcoholism, psoriasis, eczema, patients with G6PD deficiency, infants and children, haematological, GI, and neurological disorders.

ADVERSE/SIDE EFFECTS   These include: mild transient headache, fatigue, irritability, confusion, psychic stimulation, psychoses, nightmares, skeletal muscle weakness, paraesthesias, reduced reflexes, quinidinelike effect (heart block, asystole with syncope, hypotension), pruritus, lichen planus-like eruptions, eczema, exfoliative dermatitis, exacerbation of psoriasis, grey pigmentation of skin, nails, mucous membranes; bleaching of hair, patchy alopecia (reversible), tinnitus, vertigo, reduced hearing, auditory nerve damage. **GI**: diarrhoea, abdominal cramps, nausea, vomiting, anorexia. **Others**: anaemia, leucopenia, thrombocytopenia, agranulocytosis, haemolytic anaemia

CHLOROQUINE HYDROCHLORIDE (continued)

(patients with G6PD deficiency), visual disturbances, retinal artery constriction, extraocular muscle palsies, photophobia, night blindness, scotomata, visual field defects, optic atrophy, photophobia, corneal oedema, opacity, or deposits; retinal changes, slight weight loss, myalgia, lymphoedema of hands and arms, acute inter-mittent porphyria. **Overdosage**: shock, cardiac arrhythmias, convulsions, respiratory and cardiac arrest, sudden death (infants and children).

NURSING IMPLICATIONS

- GI side effects may be minimized by administering oral drug immediately before or after meals.
- Aspirate carefully before injecting drug IM to avoid inadvertent intravascular injection. IV injection may produce quinidinelike effects of heart (hypotension, depressed myocardial excitability, asystole with syncope). Rotate injection sites.
- Children are susceptible to the effects of chloroquine (especially the parenteral drug) and other 4-aminoquinoline compounds. Oral administration should substitute parenteral drug as soon as possible. Long-term therapy is not recommended in children.
- Complete blood cell counts and ECG are advised prior to initiation of therapy and periodically thereafter in patients on long-term therapy.
- A test for G6PD deficiency is recommended for American blacks and individuals of Mediterranean ancestry, prior to therapy.
- Baseline and regularly scheduled audiometric and ophthalmoscopic examinations, including slit lamp, fundus, and visual fields, should be performed.
- Retinopathy (generally irreversible) can be progressive even after termination of therapy. Patient may be asymptomatic or complain of night blindness, scotomata, visual field changes, blurred vision, or difficulty in focusing. Chloroquine should be discontinued immediately.
- Advise patient to report promptly visual or hearing disturbances, muscle weakness, or loss of balance, symptoms of blood dyscrasia (fever, sore mouth or throat, unexplained fatigue, easy bruising or bleeding).
- Use of dark glasses in sunlight or bright light may reduce risk of ocular damage.
- Patients on long-term therapy should be questioned regularly about skeletal muscle weakness, and periodic tests should be made of muscle strength and deep tendon reflexes. Positive signs are indications to terminate therapy.
- If possible, suppressive therapy should begin 2 weeks before exposure and should be continued for 8 weeks after leaving endemic area.
- Therapeutic effects in rheumatoid arthritis do not generally occur until after several weeks of therapy, and maximal benefit may not occur until 6 months to 1 year of therapy. Chloroquine is usually discontinued if no objective improvement occurs within 6 months.
- Inform patient that chloroquine may cause rusty yellow or brown discolouration of urine.
- Caution patient to keep chloroquine out of reach of children; a number of fatalities have been reported following accidental ingestion.
- **Treatment of overdosage**   is symptomatic and must be promptly administered.

CHLOROQUINE HYDROCHLORIDE (continued)

Stomach is immediately evacuated by emesis or gastric lavage; finely powdered activated charcoal in slurry is given after lavage. Have on hand ultra-short-acting barbiturate, vasopressors, equipment for tracheal intubation, tracheostomy. Monitor patient closely for at least 6 hours. Follow-up therapy: force fluids, acidification of urine to pH 4.5 or lower with ammonium chloride (8 g daily in divided doses for a few days), monitor urine pH.

■ Store in well-closed container preferably between 15° and 30°C (59° and 86°F), unless otherwise directed by manufacturer.

DRUG INTERACTIONS *Chloroquine*

PLUS	INTERACTIONS
Aluminium (e.g., Kaolin) or magnesium compounds (e.g., magnesium trisilicate)	Pharmacological effects of chloroquine may be increased (aluminium and magnesium reduce GI absorption of chloroquine). Separate administration by at least 4 hours, if possible

Chlorothiazide

(Saluric)

Diuretic; antihypertensive; thiazide; pregnancy category B

ACTIONS AND USES   Chemically related to sulphonamides. Primary action is production of diuresis by reducing sodium reabsorption and by increasing potassium secretion by the distal convoluted tubules. Promotes renal excretion of sodium, bicarbonate, and potassium; decreases renal calcium excretion and supports uric acid retention. Antihypertensive mechanism is unclear but correlates with contraction of extracellular and intravascular fluid volumes, and direct vasodilation effect on vascular wall. This initially reduces cardiac output with subsequent decrease in peripheral resistance through autoregulatory mechanisms. Thiazide-induced hypokalaemia may promote hyperglycaemia by suppressing release of endogenous insulin. Has paradoxic antidiuretic effect in diabetes insipidus, and increases total serum cholesterol and triglyceride levels. Cross-allergy reported among chemically related drugs, e.g., frusemide sulphonylureas, acetazolamide and other sulphonamides.

Used adjunctively to manage oedema associated with congestive heart failure, hepatic cirrhosis, renal dysfunction, corticosteroid, or oestrogen therapy. Used alone as step 1 agent in stepped care approach, or in combination with other agents for treatment of hypertension. Also used to reduce polyuria of central diabetes insipidus, and to prevent calcium-containing renal stones.

ROUTE AND DOSAGE   Oral: intravenous: **Adults:** *Oedema*: 500 mg to 1 g once or twice daily. ***Antihypertensive*** (oral only): **Adults:** *Initial*: 500 mg to 1 g twice daily, increased or decreased according to response.

CHLOROTHIAZIDE (continued)

ABSORPTION AND FATE   Diuretic response following oral administration: onset within 2 hours, peak effect, 4 hours; duration, 6 to 12 hours. **Half-life**: 1 to 3 hours. Following IV injection: **onset of diuresis**, in 15 minutes with maximal effect in 30 minutes that lasts 2 to 4 hours. Distributed throughout extracellular fluid; concentrates in renal tissues. Does not appear to be metabolized. About 35 to 60% of oral dose is excreted unchanged in the urine within 24 hours. Readily crosses placenta and appears in breast milk.

CONTRAINDICATIONS AND PRECAUTIONS   Hypersensitivity to thiazides or sulphonamides; anuria, oliguria, renal decompensation; hypokalaemia; IV use in infants and children. Hazardous potential in women of childbearing age, during pregnancy and in nursing mothers. **Cautious Use**: history of allergy, bronchial asthma, impaired renal or hepatic function, or gout; hypercalcaemia, diabetes mellitus, lupus erythematosus, advanced arteriosclerosis; elderly or debilitated patients, pancreatitis, sympathectomy, jaundiced children.

ADVERSE/SIDE EFFECTS   These include: unusual fatigue, dizziness, mental changes, vertigo, headache, paraesthesias, yellow vision, irregular heart beat, weak pulse, orthostatic hypotension. **GI**: nausea, xerostomia, sialadenitis, vomiting, anorexia, heartburn, acute pancreatitis, diarrhoea, constipation, abdominal cramps. Further adverse effects include: urticaria, purpura, photosensitivity, skin rash, fever, necrotizing vasculitis with haematuria (rare), respiratory distress, anaphylactic reaction. **Other**: dehydration, transient blurred vision, gout, jaundice, vascular thrombosis.

NURSING IMPLICATIONS

- Tablets may be crushed, if necessary, to facilitate swallowing and taken with fluid of patient's choice.
- Oral drug may be administered with or after food to prevent gastric irritation.
- Schedule daily doses to avoid nocturia and interrupted sleep.
- When used to promote diuresis, drug-free days (administration on alternate days or on 3 to 5 days each week) may reduce electrolyte imbalance or hyperuricaemia.
- Explain to patient that he or she will be passing greater amounts of urine and more frequently than usual, and that there will be an unusual sense of tiredness. With continued therapy, diuretic action decreases; hypotensive effects usually are maintained, and sense of tiredness diminishes.
- Missed dose: If patient forgets to take AM dose, he or she should take it when remembered, so long as it is no later than 18.00 hrs in order not to disturb sleep with diuresis. Warn patient not to double or skip a dose of chlorothiazide.
- Antihypertensive action of a thiazide diuretic requires several days before effects are observed, usually optimum therapeutic effect is not established for 3 to 4 weeks.
- Stepped-care approach in treatment of hypertension starts with a thiazide diuretic. (If hypokalaemia develops, a K-sparing diuretic or K supplement is added.) Failure to produce desired clinical effects is an indication for the next steps: beta-adrenergic blocker, vasodilator, another antihypertensive (added or substituted). As other antihypertensive agents are added to thiazide therapy, their dosage is reduced to prevent excessive hypotension.

CHLOROTHIAZIDE (continued)

- Baseline and periodic determinations are indicated for blood count, serum electrolytes, CO_2, BUN, creatinine, uric acid, and blood sugar. For patients on maintenance doses, some physicians suggest repeat determinations every 6 to 8 weeks until stable and at least every 6 months thereafter.

- Thiazide therapy can cause hyperglycaemia and glycosuria in diabetic and diabetic-prone individuals. Dosage adjustment of hypoglycaemic drugs may be required. Correction of hypokalaemia (see *Actions and Uses*) sometimes resolves problem of hyperglycaemia.

- Asymptomatic hyperuricaemia can be produced because of interference with uric acid excretion, although thiazides rarely precipitate acute gout. Report onset of joint pain and limitation of motion. Patient with history of gout may be continued on a thiazide with adjusted doses of uricosuric agent.

- Monitor fluid intake and output ratio. Excessive diuresis (with consequent dehydration), or oliguria may cause electrolyte imbalance and necessitate prompt dosage adjustment. To prevent dehydration, urge patient to report GI illness accompanied by protracted vomiting or prolonged period of diarrhoea.

- Establish baseline weight prior to initiation of therapy. Weigh patient at the same time in the morning under standard conditions. Consult physician about acceptable range of weight change. Usually a gain of more than 2 pounds within 2 or 3 days and a gradual weight gain over the week's period is reportable. Tell patient to check for signs of oedema (hands, ankles, pretibial areas).

- Blood pressure should be closely monitored during early drug therapy. Physician may want initial measurements for patients with hypertension taken in standing, sitting, and lying positions to evaluate drug effects.

- If orthostatic hypotension is a troublesome symptom (and it may be, especially in the elderly), inform patient of measures that may help tolerate the effect, and to prevent falling: (1) change from sitting or lying down positions slowly and in stages; (2) suggest that men sit down to urinate, especially if they need to void at night; (3) use a commode or urinal; (4) avoid hot showers or baths, sunbathing extremes of environmental heat, unaccustomed physical activity; (5) when on a long air flight, walk about when it is permissible to do so; (6) when travelling by road, stop every hour or so to stretch and walk about; (7) consult physician about wearing support stockings; (8) lie down immediately if sensation of light-headedness, faintness, or dizziness occurs.

- Skin and mucous membranes should be inspected daily for evidence of petechiae in patients receiving large doses and those on prolonged therapy.

- Xerostomia and sialadenitis require fastidious oral hygiene because decreases in salivary lubrication of oral membranes and teeth promotes demineralization of tooth surfaces and membrane erosion. Urge patient to floss teeth daily and to use a soft tooth brush for frequent brushing especially after eating. Frequent rinses with clear water is preferred to use of commercial mouth rinses (overuse of which may change oral flora and cause irritation to tissues).

- In an attempt to relieve dry mouth, patient may significantly increase fluid intake. Consult physician about permissible intake volume. Because of the possibility of dehydration, caution patient against drinking large quantities of coffee or other

C

CHLOROTHIAZIDE (continued)

caffeine drinks (sometimes the major type of self-selected fluid). Caffeine is a CNS stimulant with diuretic effects.

■ Patients on digitalis therapy should be observed closely for signs and symptoms of hypokalaemia. Even moderate reduction in serum K can precipitate digitalis intoxication in these patients.

■ Hypokalaemia is not clinically significant in many patients, but those most apt to develop electrolyte imbalance are the elderly or debilitated, or those with oedema. Imbalance may occur after pathophysiological loss of body fluids (e.g., vomiting) or after iatrogenic fluid loss (e.g., parencentesis, GI drainage).

■ Signs of hypokalaemia include: dry mouth, anorexia, nausea, vomiting, thirst, paraesthesias, mental confusion, irritability, drowsiness, muscle cramps and weakness, paralytic ileus, abdominal distention, hypoactive reflexes, dyspnoea, hypotension, cardiac arrhythmias, polyuria.

Food–drug interactions

■ Hypokalaemia may be prevented if the daily diet contains K-rich foods (e.g., banana, fruit juices, apricots, potatoes, beef, chicken, whole grain cereals, skimmed milk). Urge patient to eat a banana (about 370 mg K) and drink at least 180 mls orange juice (about 330 mg K) every day. Collaborate with dietitian.

■ The patient should be aware that some K-rich foods are also high in Na, e.g., pressed cheese, canned spinach, tomato juice, carrots, sardines, frozen peas.

■ Rigid sodium restriction is not usually prescribed; however, foods high in sodium content should be avoided when thiazides are in use (e.g., luncheon meats, instant or quick cooked foods, bouillon, beer, pretzels, snack foods, ham, bacon, Chinese foods).

■ The physician may advise the patient not to add salt to food. Use of a salt substitute must be prescribed by the physician. Most substitutes are high in potassium, contain some sodium, and are contraindicated in renal pathology.

■ If hypokalaemia develops, dietary K supplement of 1,000 to 2,000 mg (25 to 50 mEq) is usually adequate treatment.

■ Weight control is an important adjunct to hypertension therapy. Some patients may require a diet tailored to correct lipid abnormalities and to prevent electrolyte imbalance problems.

■ Provide opportunity for the patient/family to work with the dietitian in planning an individualized diet based on patient's food preferences, life-style, customs, and habits.

■ The patient should be advised to avoid or at least to greatly reduce smoking. (Smoking raises blood pressure.)

■ Discuss self-medication habits with patient. Some frequently used OTC drugs contain liberal amounts of sodium (Alka-Seltzer, BiSoDol) and potassium (Alka-Seltzer). Advise patient to consult physician before dosing with any nonprescribed medication.

■ Warn patient about the possibility of photosensitivity reaction and to notify physician if it occurs. Thiazide-related photosensitivity is considered a photoallergy (radiation changes drug structure and makes it allergenic for some individuals) and

CHLOROTHIAZIDE *(continued)*

occurs 1½ to 2 weeks after initial sun exposure. Avoid use of PABA sunscreen products. (*See Drug Interactions.*)

■ Thiazide therapy need not be interrupted because of surgery, but the anaesthetist should be made aware of such therapy.

■ Although the syndrome of inappropriate secretion of antidiuretic hormone is uncommon, it can occur in susceptible individuals even with a brief exposure to a thiazide. Be suspicious if the following clinical findings are present: low urine output (less than 500 ml/24 hours) and low specific gravity, weight gain, pitting oedema in ankles and pretibial areas, elevated BP and pulse, nausea, vomiting, watery diarrhoea, venous congestion, muscle cramps, twitching, and drowsiness, weakness, lethargy, confusion, disorientation, signs of pulmonary oedema, low serum Na, K, Cl. Treatment is restoration of potassium and restricted water intake.

Patient instructions related to antihypertensive therapy should include the following:

☐ Dosage regimen, drug action, reportable signs and symptoms.

☐ Importance of compliance in preventing complications of hypertension.

☐ Maintenance of weight.

☐ Diet restrictions, if any; stop smoking.

☐ Moderate exercise plan.

☐ Dates for follow-up at clinic.

■ **Overdosage** is treated by evacuation of gastric contents, and supportive measures to maintain hydration, electrolyte balance, respiratory and cardiovascular–renal function.

■ Store tablets, oral solutions, and parenteral dosage forms at temperature between 15° and 30°C (59° and 86°F), unless otherwise directed by manufacturer.

Diagnostic test interferences Chlorothiazide (thiazides) cause marked increases in **serum amylase** values, decrease in **PBI** determinations, may increase excretion of **PSP**, and increase **BSP retention**, and possibly cause false-negative **phentolamine** and **tyramine** tests, and interfere with **urine steroid** determinations. Thiazides should be discontinued before **parathyroid function tests** because they alter (decrease) calcium excretion.

DRUG INTERACTIONS *Chlorothiazide (thiazides)*

PLUS	INTERACTIONS
Amphotericin B, corticosteroids, and other drugs with hypokalaemic effect	Intensification of hypokalaemia effect. Monitor serum potassium
Antidiabetic agents (insulins, sulphonylureas)	Hypoglycaemic effects antagonized by hyperglycaemic action of thiazides. Monitor for decreased diabetic control
Cholestyramine	Decreased thiazide effects (due to formation of complex). Administer thiazides at least 2 hours before these drugs
Diazoxide	Hyperglycaemic, hypotensive, hyperuricaemic effects of both drugs intensified. Used concomitantly with caution

CHLOROTHIAZIDE (continued)

PLUS (continued)	INTERACTIONS
Digitalis glycosides	Increased potassium and magnesium loss may lead to digitalis toxicity. Monitor serum potassium and magnesium levels
Lithium	Possibility of lithium toxicity (renal clearance suppressed by thiazides). Monitor serum lithium levels
Skeletal muscle relaxants (nondepolarizing), e.g., tubocurarine	Prolonged neuromuscular blocking effects. Used concomitantly with caution
PABA sunscreen products	Exaggerate thiazide-induced photosensitivity

C

Chlorpheniramine maleate————————————

(Alunex, Piriton)

Antihistamine; H_2-receptor antagonist

ACTIONS AND USES Propylamine antihistamine, derivative of pheniramine. Generally produces less drowsiness than other antihistamines, but side effects involving CNS stimulation may be more common. Competes with histamine for H_1-receptor sites on effector cells, thus blocking the histamine action that promotes capillary permeability and oedema formation and the constrictive action on respiratory, gastrointestinal, and vascular smooth muscles. Has antiemetic, antitussive, anticholinergic, and local anaesthetic actions.

Used for symptomatic relief of various uncomplicated allergic conditions; to prevent transfusion and drug reactions in susceptible patients, and used as adjunct to adrenaline and other standard measures in anaphylactic reactions.

ROUTE AND DOSAGE **Adults**: **Oral**: 4 mg three or four times daily. **Subcutaneous, intramuscular, and intravenous**: 5 to 20 mg as single dose. *Maximum* 40 mg/daily. IV injection should be made over period of 1 minute. **Children (under one year)**: 1 mg twice a day, **(1–5 yrs)**: 1–2 mg three times a day; **(6–12 yrs)**: 2–4 mg 2–4 times a day.

ABSORPTION AND FATE **Onset of action following oral administration** occurs in 20 to 60 minutes; **duration** 8 to 12 hours. **Half-life**: 20 to 24 hours; 69 to 72% bound to plasma proteins. Detoxified in liver. Metabolites and some free drug excreted primarily in urine; 19% of dose excreted in 24 hours and 34% in 48 hours.

CONTRAINDICATIONS AND PRECAUTIONS Hypersensitivity to antihistamines of similar structure; lower respiratory tract symptoms (including asthma), narrow-angle glaucoma, obstructive prostatic hypertrophy or other bladder neck obstruction, GI obstruction or stenosis, pregnancy, nursing mothers, premature and newborn infants, during or within 14 days of MAO inhibitor therapy. **Cautious Use**: convulsive dis-

CHLORPHENIRAMINE MALEATE *(continued)*

orders, increased intraocular pressure, hyperthyroidism, cardiovascular disease, hypertension, diabetes, mellitus, history of bronchial asthma, elderly patients, patients with G6PD deficiency.

ADVERSE/SIDE EFFECTS   Low incidence of side effects. These include: drowsiness, sedation, headache, dizziness, vertigo, tinnitus, fatigue, disturbed coordination, tingling, heaviness, weakness of hands, tremors, euphoria, nervousness, restlessness, insomnia, palpitation, tachycardia, mild hypotension or hypertension, dryness of mouth, nose, and throat, tinnitus, vertigo, acute labyrinthitis, thickened bronchial secretions, wheezing, sensation of chest tightness, epigastric distress, anorexia, nausea, vomiting, constipation or diarrhoea, urinary frequency or retention, dysuria. **Hypersensitivity**: skin rash, urticaria, photosensitivity, anaphylactic shock, **Other** (following parenteral administration): transitory stinging or burning at injection site, sweating, pallor, transient hypotension, early menses. **Overdosage** (especially in children): hallucinations, excitement, agitation, feeling of terror, fever, ataxia, athetosis, convulsions, coma, cardiovascular collapse.

NURSING IMPLICATIONS

- Sustained release tablets should be swallowed whole and not crushed or chewed.
- In patients receiving antihistamines for allergic manifestations, a careful history should be taken to discover the allergen involved, if possible. Some common precipitating factors of allergy include: changes in dietary habits, contact with animals, a new drug, changes in home environment (e.g., new rug, curtains, pillows), emotional upsets.
- Solutions for injection should not be given intradermally.
- If patient manifests any reaction following parenteral administration, drug should be discontinued. (Exception: patient may experience transitory stinging sensation that rarely lasts longer than a few minutes.)
- Caution patient to avoid driving a car or other potentially hazardous activities until drug response has been determined.
- Warn patient that antihistamines have additive effects with alcohol and other CNS depressants (e.g., hypnotics, sedatives, tranquilizers).
- Patients on prolonged therapy should have periodic blood cell counts.
- Antihistamines have no therapeutic effect on the common cold. Their continued popularity, as cold cures, apparently stems from the comfort afforded by their drying effects. Patients with cough should be advised that this drying action may cause thickened bronchial secretions, thus making expectoration difficult.
- Dry mouth may be relieved by sugarless gum or lemon drops, frequent rinses with water, increasing (noncaloric) fluid intake (if allowed), use of a saliva substitute.
- Caution patient to store antihistamines out of reach of children. Fatalities have been reported.
- Patients with allergies should be advised to carry at all times medical identification jewellery or card indicating specific allergy, name, and physician's name, address, and telephone number.
- Store preferably between 15° and 30°C (59° and 86°F) unless otherwise directed by

CHLORPHENIRAMINE MALEATE (continued)

manufacturer. Syrup and injection forms should be protected from light to prevent discolouration.

Diagnostic test interferences   Antihistamines should be discontinued 4 days prior to skin testing procedures for allergy because they may obscure otherwise positive reactions.

DRUG INTERACTIONS   *Chlorpheniramine*

PLUS	INTERACTIONS
Alcohol (Ethanol) and other CNS depressants	Additive CNS depression (especially drowsiness and impaired psychomotor ability). Used with caution if at all
MAO inhibitors	Anticholinergic effects of antihistamines may be prolonged and intensified. Concomitant use avoided
Phenytoin and possibly other hydantoins	Possibility of increased pharmacological effects of phenytoin. Monitor phenytoin plasma levels

Chlorpromazine hydrochloride

(Chloractil, Dozine, Largactil)

Psychotropic; antipsychotic (neuroleptic); antiemetic; phenothiazine

ACTIONS AND USES   Derivative of phenothiazine with actions at all levels of CNS. Mechanism that produces strong antipsychotic effects is unclear, but thought to be related to blockade of postsynaptic dopamine receptors in the brain. Actions on hypothalamus and reticular formation produce strong sedation, depressed vasomotor reflexes leading to centrally mediated hypotension, inhibition of hypothalamic and pituitary hormone release, and depressed temperature regulation. Has strong alpha-adrenergic blocking action and weak anticholinergic effects. Directly depresses the heart; may increase coronary blood flow. Exerts quinidine-like antiarrhythmic action. Recent reports suggest an inhibitory effect on dopamine reuptake, possibly the basis for moderate extrapyramidal symptoms.

Used to control manic phase of manic-depressive illness, in management of severe nausea and vomiting, to control excessive anxiety and agitation prior to surgery and for treatment of severe behaviour problems in children, e.g., attention deficit disorder. Also used to relieve acute intermittent porphyria, hiccoughs and as adjunct in treatment of tetanus.

ROUTE AND DOSAGE   **Adults: Oral:** 75 to 300 mg in divided doses. **Elderly, emaciated, debilitated:** 25 mg three times daily. **Intramuscular:** 25 to 50 mg one to four times daily. **Rectal suppository:** 50 to 100 mg three or four times daily as needed.

CHLORPROMAZINE HYDROCHLORIDE (continued)

ABSORPTION AND FATE   Erratic absorption following oral administration: rapid absorption after IM injection. Widely distributed; accumulates in brain and other tissues with a rich blood supply. Wide intraindividual variation (perhaps genetic) in plasma concentrations. Average peak levels 2 to 4 hours after oral intake, 15 to 20 minutes after IM administration. Metabolized in liver. Approximately 95% bound to plasma proteins. **Biphasic elimination half-lives**: 2 hours, and 30 hours. Excreted in urine mostly as metabolites; less than 1% excreted unchanged within 72 hours. Crosses placenta and appears in breast milk.

CONTRAINDICATIONS AND PRECAUTIONS   Hypersensitivity to phenothiazine derivatives; withdrawal states from alcohol, barbiturates, and other nonbarbiturate sedatives; comatose states, brain damage, bone marrow depression, myasthenia gravis, Reye's syndrome; children younger than 6 months. Safe use during pregnancy and in nursing mothers not established. **Cautious Use**: agitated states accompanied by depression, seizure disorders, respiratory impairment, glaucoma, diabetes, hypertensive disease, peptic ulcer, prostatic hypertrophy; thyroid, cardiovascular, and hepatic disorders; patients exposed to extreme heat or organophosphate insecticides; previously detected breast cancer.

ADVERSE/SIDE EFFECTS   (Usually dose-related.) These include: sedation, drowsiness, dizziness, syncope, insomnia, reduced REM sleep, bizarre dreams, cerebral oedema, convulsive seizures, hyperpyrexia, inability to sweat, depressed cough reflex, catatonic-like states, psychotic symptoms, adverse behaviour effects, extrapyramidal symptoms (*see Nursing Implications*), EEG changes, orthostatic hypotension, hypertension, palpitation, tachycardia, bradycardia, ECG changes (usually reversible): prolonged QT and PR intervals, blunting of T-waves, ST depression, fixed-drug eruption, urticaria, contact dermatitis, exfoliative dermatitis, photosensitivity reaction with cutaneous pigmentation producing blue-grey colouration of exposed skin surfaces; hirsutism (long-term therapy), oral syndrome (xerostomia, loosened dentures, vesicular lesions on tongue and mucous membranes, cheilitis, white or black furry tongue, glossitis); constipation, adynamic ileus, cholestatic jaundice, aggravation of peptic ulcer, dyspepsia, increased appetite, agranulocytosis, thrombocytopenic purpura, pancytopenia (rare), blurred vision, increased intraocular pressure, lenticular opacities, mydriasis or miosis, photophobia, anovulation, infertility, pseudopregnancy, menstrual irregularity, gynaecomastia, galactorrhoea, inhibition of ejaculation, reduced libido, urinary retention and frequency, nasal congestion, laryngospasm, bronchospasm, respiratory depression, hypoglycaemia, hyperglycaemia, glycosuria (high doses), enlargement of parotid glands, peripheral oedema, muscle necrosis (following IM), anaphylactoid reactions, sudden unexplained death.

NURSING IMPLICATIONS
- Before initiating treatment with phenothiazine derivatives, establish baseline blood pressure in standing and recumbent positions, pulse, and respiratory capacity values.
- Metabolic and elimination rates of antipsychotic medication decrease with advancing age. Smaller doses are used for the elderly; side effects (especially hypotensive neuromuscular) in this age group may be more pronounced.

CHLORPROMAZINE HYDROCHLORIDE (continued)

- Maintenance therapy is usually administered as a single dose at bedtime.
- Hypotensive reactions, dizziness, and sedation are common during early therapy particularly in patients on high doses or in the elderly receiving parenteral doses. Patients usually develop tolerance to these side effects; however, lower doses or longer intervals between doses may be required.
- Inform and reassure the patient that side effects are reversible with prompt dosage adjustment or discontinuation of drug; therefore urge patient to report unusual signs or symptoms without delay: dark-coloured urine, pale stools, jaundice, impaired vision, unusual bleeding or bruising, skin rash, weakness, tremors, sore throat, fever.
- Tablet may be crushed before administration and taken with fluid or mixed with food. Capsules should not be opened.
- Watch to see that oral drug is swallowed and not hoarded. Suicide attempt is a constant possibility in the depressed patient, particularly when improving.
- Chlorpromazine concentrate should be mixed just before administration in at least ½ glass juice, milk, water, coffee, tea, carbonated beverage, or with semi-solid food.
- **Smoking–drug interaction**   Smoking increases metabolism of phenothiazines resulting in shortened half-life, and more rapid clearance of drug. Higher dosage in smokers may be required. Advise patient to stop smoking, if possible.
- Avoid drug contact with skin, eyes, and clothing because of its potential for causing contact dermatitis. Personnel who frequently handle injectable and liquid forms should use rubber gloves. Patient on maintenance doses of concentrate at home should be warned to flush spilled solution off skin promptly.
- While titrating initial dosages, marked changes from established baseline data should be reported.
- Inject IM preparations slowly and deep into upper outer quadrant of buttock; massage site well. Avoid SC injection; it may cause tissue irritation and nodule formation. If irritation is a problem consult physician about diluting medication with normal saline or 2% procaine. Rotate injection sites.
- The patient should remain recumbent for at least ½ hour after parenteral administration. Observe closely. Hypotensive reactions may require head-low position and pressor drugs, e.g., phenylephrine, adrenaline and other pressor agents are contraindicated since they may cause sudden paradoxic drop in BP.
- Phenothiazine derivatives form incompatible admixtures with many drugs; consult pharmacist before mixing with other drugs.
- Avoid injecting undiluted chlorpromazine into a vein.
- Lemon yellow colour of parenteral preparation does not alter potency; if otherwise coloured or markedly discoloured, solution should be discarded.
- Therapeutic effects of phenothiazine therapy include: emotional and psychomotor quieting in excited, hyperactive patients; reduction of paranoidal symptoms, hallucinations, delusions, fears, and hostility; stimulation of withdrawn patients and productive organization of thought and behaviour.
- Some patients fail to experience improvement for as long as 7 or 8 weeks of therapy; thus, they may not realize the importance of medication compliance. Stress necessity of keeping appointments for follow-up evaluation of dosage regimen.

CHLORPROMAZINE HYDROCHLORIDE (continued)

- Urge patient on home therapy not to alter dosing regimen; tell patient not to give the drug to another person.
- Warn patient not to take any other drugs, especially OTC medications, without physician's approval.
- Monitor dietary intake and bowel pattern. Increased fluid intake and a gradual increase in high-fibre foods may help to prevent GI complications (faecal impaction, constipation).
- Monitor fluid intake and output ratio and pattern. Urinary retention due to depression and compromised renal function may occur. If serum creatinine becomes elevated, therapy should be discontinued.
- Inform patient that phenothiazines may cause pink to red-brown discolouration of urine (due to a metabolite).
- Note that chlorpromazine may suppress cough reflex. Be alert to danger of bronchopneumonia which may occur in the severely depressed patient, especially if elderly. Depressed thirst and lethargy can lead to dehydration, haemoconcentration, and reduced pulmonary ventilation.
- Patients on home therapy should be advised which laxative to take, if needed. Many OTC drugs contain anticholinergic components that can precipitate adynamic ileus. Support stockings and elevation of legs when sitting may minimize drug induced hypotension (discuss with physician). Supervise ambulation. Instruct patient to make gradual position changes from recumbent to upright posture, and to dangle legs over bed a few minutes before ambulation. Caution against standing still for prolonged periods and advise against hot showers or baths, long exposure to environmental heat.
- Since chlorpromazine may affect the temperature regulating mechanism; report patient's complaint of feeling cold. Applying a blanket next to the body may help. Hotwater bottles and other heating devices are not recommended because phenothiazines tend to depress conditioned avoidance responses.
- Chlorpromazine (phenothiazine) use is accompanied by loss of thermoregulation, and inability to sweat. Patient exposed to extremes in environmental temperature, or high fever due to illness may develop heat stroke (red, dry hot skin; headache, dizziness, dilated pupils, dyspnoea; full, bounding, strong pulse; temperature above 40.6°C (105°F), mental confusion, sudden loss of consciousness). Inform physician and prepare to institute measures to rapidly lower body temperature, e.g., move patient into shade; evaporative cooling (application of tap water with simultaneous fanning).
- Antiemetic effect of chlorpromazine may obscure signs of overdosage of other drugs or other causes of nausea and vomiting.
- Be alert to complaints of diminished visual acuity, reduced night vision, photophobia, and a perceived brownish discolouration of objects. Patient may be more comfortable with dark glasses. Facilitate periodic ophthalmic examination for patients on long-term therapy.
- Photosensitivity associated with chlorpromazine therapy is a phototoxic reaction involving photoactivated changes in cell structure. Severity of response depends on amount of ultraviolet ray exposure and drug dose. Exposed skin areas have appearance

C

CHLORPROMAZINE HYDROCHLORIDE (continued)

of an exaggerated sunburn. If reaction occurs, patient should wear protective clothing and sun screen lotion (SPF above 12) when outdoors, even on dark days.

- Xerostomia may be relieved by frequent sips of water, by rinsing mouth with warm water, or by increasing noncalorie fluid intake. Sugarfree sweets or chewing gum may also help to stimulate salivary flow. If these measures fail, a saliva substitute may help.
- Oral candidiasis occurs frequently in patients receiving chlorpromazine. Emphasize meticulous oral hygiene: daily flossing with waxed dental floss, brushing teeth with soft, small brush after eating, and use of a fluoride toothpaste. Overuse of antiseptic mouth rinses can change oral flora and should be discouraged. Inspect oral cavity of severely depressed patient; assist with oral hygiene if necessary.
- Since chlorpromazine reduces REM sleep it is usually not used for night-time sedation in patients with auditory or visual hallucinations.
- Extrapyramidal symptoms associated with antipsychotic drug use: *pseudoparkinsonism*: (slowing of volitional movement [akinesia], mask facies, rigidity and tremor at rest, especially upper extremities, pill rolling motion) occurs most frequently in women, the elderly of both sexes, and dehydrated patients; may be mistaken for depression. *Acute dystonia*: (abnormal posturing, grimacing, spastic torticollis and oculogyric crisis) occurs most frequently in men and patients under 25 years of age; may be misdiagnosed as hysteria or seizures. *Akathisia*: (compelling need to move without specific pattern; inability to sit still) occurs most frequently in women and is often misdiagnosed as agitation. *Tardive dyskinesia* (generally irreversible): involuntary rhythmic, bizarre movements of face, jaw, mouth, tongue, and sometimes extremities. Usual first sign of *tardive dyskinesia*: vermicular movements of the tongue. It is critical that this sign be noticed as soon as it appears and that the drug be withdrawn. Prompt action may prevent irreversibility.
- Observe patient closely to recognize early indications of extrapyramidal symptoms. Maximal risk times following start of therapy for: pseudoparkinsonism and acute dystonia: 1 to 5 days; akathisia: 50 to 60 days; tardive dyskinesia: after months or years of treatment. (All patients on long-term phenothiazine treatment are at high risk for development of tardive dyskinesia.)
- Diabetics or prediabetics on long-term, high-dose therapy should be monitored for reduced glucose tolerance and loss of diabetes control. Urine and blood glucose should be checked regularly. Drug therapy may have to be discontinued or substituted by another agent.
- If an antipsychotic must be used during pregnancy, drug treatment should be discontinued 1 to 2 weeks prior to delivery to avoid neonatal distress. The newborn may display hyperreflexia, jaundice, and prolonged extrapyramidal symptoms.
- Close supervision of the infant is critical if the nursing mother must be on phenothiazine therapy.
- Elevated temperature, sore mouth, gums, or throat, upper respiratory infection, fatigue and weakness (early manifestations of agranulcoytosis) are most likely to occur within first 4 to 10 weeks of therapy, particularly in women and the elderly. Blood studies should be instituted promptly.
- Cholestatic jaundice occurs more frequently in women, usually between second and

CHLORPROMAZINE HYDROCHLORIDE (continued)

fourth weeks, and is reversed by drug withdrawal. May begin with abrupt fever, flu-like symptoms, and abdominal discomfort, followed in about 1 week by jaundice. Pruritus, usually an early symptom of jaundice, may not be present because of the antipruritic effects of phenothiazines.

- Complete blood counts, liver function tests, urinalysis, ocular examinations, EEG (in patients over 50 years of age) are recommended before and periodically during prolonged therapy.
- Chlorpromazine may impair mental and physical abilities, especially during early therapy. Caution patient against driving a car or undertaking activities requiring precision and mental alertness until drug response is known.
- **Overdosage** with chlorpromazine leads to CNS depression to the point of somnolence and coma. Treatment: early gastric lavage, close observation of patient, maintenance of open airway. Vomiting should not be induced because possible occurrence of dystonic reaction of head and neck coupled with drug-depressed cough reflex could lead to aspiration of vomitus.
- Abrupt withdrawal of drug or deliberate dose skipping, especially after prolonged therapy with large doses, can cause onset of extrapyramidal symptoms and severe GI disturbances. Urge patient to adhere to dosage regimen without changes. When treatment is to be discontinued, dosage must be reduced gradually over a period of several weeks.
- Brand interchange of oral and suppository forms is not recommended.
- Store preferably between 15° and 30°C (59° and 86°F) protected from light, unless otherwise specified by the manufacturer. Avoid freezing.

Diagnostic test interferences   Chlorpromazine may increase **cephalin flocculation**, and possibly other **liver function tests**; also may increase **PBI**. False-positive results may occur for **amylase, 5-hydroxyindole acetic acid, porphobilinogens, urobilinogen** (Ehrlich's reagent), **urine bilirubin** and **pregnancy tests** possibly caused by a metabolite of phenothiazines which discolors urine.

DRUG INTERACTIONS *Chloropromazine (phenothiazines)*_____

PLUS	INTERACTIONS
Alcohol (Ethanol), and other CNS depressants	Enhanced CNS depression (hypotension, respiratory depression). Used concomitantly with caution if at all
Anorexigenic agents	Inhibition of anorexiant effect. Avoid combination, if possible
Antacids, antidiarrhoeals	Decreased absorption of oral phenothiazines. Space administration at least 2 hours apart
Amphetamines	Decreased amphetamine effects. Concurrent use generally avoided
Anticholinergics	Additive anticholinergic action, and reduced antipsychotic effect of phenothiazines. Used concomitantly with caution
Barbiturates	Possibility of increased metabolism of phenothiazines, (by induction of hepatic enzymes). Observe for reduced phenothiazine effects

CHLORPROMAZINE HYDROCHLORIDE (continued)

PLUS (continued)	INTERACTIONS
Barbiturate anaesthetics	Increase in excitation (tremor, involuntary muscle movements), and hypotension. Combination generally avoided
Beta-adrenergic blockers, e.g., propranolol	Additive hypotensive effects. Mutual inhibition of metabolism. Used concomitantly with caution. Dosage adjustment may be indicated
Guanethidine	Phenothiazines may block antihypertensive action (inhibit neuronal uptake of guanethidine). Monitor patient closely
Lithium	Lowers plasma level of phenothiazines. Observe for reduced phenothiazine effects
Ototoxic medications	Phenothiazines may mask symptoms of ototoxicity
Phenytoin	Inhibits phenytoin metabolism thus increased potential for its toxicity. Monitor phenytoin serum levels
Sympathomimetics, e.g., phenylpropanolamine	Possibility of sudden death. Mechanism not established. Used concurrently with caution
Tricyclic antidepressants	Mutual intensification of sedative and anticholinergic actions. Used concomitantly with caution

Chlorpropamide ━━━━━━━━━━━━━━━━━

(Diabinese, Glymese)

Antidiabetic; sulphonylurea; sulphonamide derivative

ACTIONS AND USES Longest-acting first generation sulphonylurea compound structurally and pharmacologically related to tolbutamide (q.v.). Although a sulphonamide derivative, it has no antiinfective activity. Lowers blood glucose by stimulating beta cells in pancreas to release endogenous insulin. May potentiate available antidiuretic hormone, a property not shared by other sulphonylureas. Has longer duration of action and about six times the potency of tolbutamide, as well as a higher incidence of side effects. Reported to be associated with fewer primary and secondary failures. Not effective as sole therapy of diabetes.

Used in the management of mild to moderately severe, stable non-insulin-dependent diabetes mellitus in patients who cannot be controlled by diet alone, and who do not have complications of diabetes. Treatment of neurogenic diabetes insipidus.

ROUTE AND DOSAGE Oral: *Antidiabetic*: *Initial*: 250 mg daily (**elderly** patient: 100 to 125 mg daily). Dosage may be increased by 50 to 125 mg at 3- to 5-day intervals, as necessary. *Maintenance*: 100 to 500 mg daily; not to exceed 750 mg daily. *Antidiuretic*: 100 to 250 mg daily; dosage adjusted at 2- or 3-day intervals if necessary, up to 500 mg daily.

CHLORPROPAMIDE (continued)

ABSORPTION AND FATE   Promptly and completely absorbed from GI tract after oral ingestion. Wide distribution in extracellular fluid compartment. Action begins in 1 hour: peaks in 3 to 6 hours, with duration of 60 to 72 hours. Approximately 88 to 96% bound to plasma proteins. **Half-life**: 30 to 40 hours. Plasma levels become stabilized 5 to 7 days after initiation of therapy; therefore, undue accumulation in blood does not occur during prolonged therapy. As much as 80% may be metabolized in liver with formation of metabolites that may also have antidiabetic activity. Renal excretion is slow: 80 to 90% of a single dose excreted as unchanged drug and metabolites within 96 hours. Rate of excretion is accelerated in alkaline urine and is decreased in acidic urine. Excreted in milk.

CONTRAINDICATIONS AND PRECAUTIONS   Known hypersensitivity to sulphonylureas and to sulphonamides; insulin-dependent diabetes, diabetes complicated by severe infection; acidosis; severe renal, hepatic, or thyroid insufficiency; pregnancy; safe use in lactating women and in children not established. **Cautious Use**: elderly patients, Addison's disease, congestive heart failure. *See also tolbutamide.*

ADVERSE/SIDE EFFECTS   Hypoglycaemia; GI distress, skin reactions, drowsiness, muscle cramps, weakness, paraesthesias, photosensitivity; cholestatic jaundice hypersensitivity reactions, leucopenia, thrombocytopenia, anaemia (rare); agranulocytosis; disulphiram reaction; antidiuretic effect, hyponatraemia, hyposthenuria. *See also tolbutamide.*

NURSING IMPLICATIONS

- Chlorpropamide may be prescribed as a single morning dose with breakfast or divided into two or three doses and taken with meals to minimize GI side effects and to achieve maximum diabetes control.
- Tablet may be crushed if patient is unable to swallow it whole. Be sure it is not swallowed dry, but with an allowable liquid.
- With long-acting hypoglycaemic agents, mild CNS symptoms of hypoglycaemia predominate, whereas other symptoms may go unnoticed or simply may be tolerated (e.g., abnormalities in sleep pattern, frequent nightmares, night sweats, morning headache). The patient and responsible family members should be alerted to the necessity of reporting all symptoms promptly to the physician.
- Patient should be examined and evaluated during first 6 weeks of chlorpropamide therapy to determine drug effectiveness.
- Ordinarily transfer from another antidiabetic medication to chlorpropamide does not require a conversion period.
- *Food–drug interactions*   The individually planned diet for the non-insulin-dependent patient is less rigid than for the insulin-dependent patient. In general it stresses: (1) 3 meals with or without a snack in the afternoon or evening; (2) avoiding excessive intake of carbohydrates at a single meal or large amounts between meals particularly as liquids and unaccompanied by other food types; (3) fibre rich diet. Modifications are not required for moderate exercise, missed meals, or mild intercurrent illness.
- *See also tolbutamide.*

Chlorprothixene

(Taractan)   *Psychotropic; antipsychotic*
                                                              (neuroleptic)

ACTIONS AND USES   Thioxanthene derivative structurally and pharmacologically similar to the phenothiazines. Has strong antiemetic, sedative, and hypotensive actions but less anticholinergic and antihistaminic activity. Incidence of extrapyramidal symptoms is low. *See chlorpromazine.*

Used for management of manifestations of psychotic disorders.

ROUTE AND DOSAGE   Individually adjusted: **Oral: Adults:** 25 to 50 mg three or four times daily; increased as necessary and tolerated. Maximum dose usually no higher than 600 mg daily. **Elderly, debilitated, and children (over 6 years of age):** 10 to 25 mg three or four times daily. **Intramuscular:** 25 to 50 mg three or four times daily. Oral concentrate contains 100 mg/5 ml.

ABSORPTION AND FATE   Onset of effects occurs 10 to 30 minutes following IM administration. Presumably metabolized in liver and excreted in urine and faeces as unchanged drug and sulphoxide metabolite.

CONTRAINDICATIONS AND PRECAUTIONS   Hypersensitivity to phenothiazine derivatives; adrenaline use, circulatory collapse, congestive heart failure, coronary artery disease, cerebral vascular disorders, comatose states. Safe use not established: during pregnancy, lactation, in women of childbearing potential, oral use in children under age 6 or parenteral use in those under age 12. **Cautious Use:** persons exposed to extreme heat or organophosphate insecticides, persons with suicide tendency; history of drug abuse, peptic ulcer, cardiovascular or respiratory disease, previously detected breast cancer, persons receiving ototoxic medications (especially aminoglycoside antibiotics).

ADVERSE/SIDE EFFECTS   Drowsiness, lethargy, dizziness, orthostatic hypotension, tachycardia, dry mouth, constipation, ocular disturbances, inability to sweat, contact dermatitis, photosensitivity, uricosuria, urinary retention, extrapyramidal symptoms, transient leucopenia, agranulocytosis pain and induration IM site (usually minimal). Shares toxic potential of phenothiazines. *See chlorpromazine.*

NURSING IMPLICATIONS
- Oral concentrate may be given alone or diluted in water, milk, fruit juice, coffee, or carbonated beverage just before administration. Warn patient not to spill oral liquid on skin or clothing because drug can cause contact dermatitis.
- If necessary, tablet may be crushed before administration and taken with fluid of patient's choice.
- Administer IM in upper outer quadrant of buttock or midlateral thigh. Aspirate carefully to avoid inadvertent entry into blood vessel. Rotate injection sites.
- Monitor fluid intake and output ratio and bowel elimination pattern. Patient should

CHLORPROTHIXENE (continued)

know what laxative may be used if necessary. Consult physician about prescribing a high-fibre diet.

■ Since postural hypotension may occur in some patients, IM injection should be given with patient recumbent or seated. Observe patient until weakness or, dizziness, if present, passes.

■ Chlorprothixene may discolour urine pink to red, or red brown.

■ Store in light-resistant, tightly covered container between 15° and 30°C (59° and 86°F) unless otherwise specific by manufacture.

■ *See chlorpromazine.*

C

Chlortetracycline hydrochloride ━━━━━━━━━━

(Aureomycin)   *Antibiotic; tetracycline*

ACTIONS AND USES   Broad-spectrum antibiotic derived from *Streptomyces aureofaciens*. Closely related chemically and in actions to other tetracyclines. Primarily bacteriostatic in action. Effective against a variety of gram-negative and gram-positive pathogens.

Ophthalmic ointment is used as adjunct with oral therapy in the treatment of trachoma inclusion, conjunctivitis, chlamydial infections, and for superfical ocular infections caused by susceptible organisms. Skin ointment is used for treatment of superficial pyogenic skin infections.

ROUTE AND DOSAGE   **Ophthalmic ointment (1%):** apply small amount to infected eye every 2 hours, as condition and response indicate. **Skin ointment (3%):** apply directly to involved area, preferably on sterile gauze, one or more times daily.

CONTRAINDICATIONS AND PRECAUTIONS   Hypersensitivity to tetracyclines, or to any ingredients in the formulation. Safe use during pregnancy, in nursing women, and in children not established.

ADVERSE/SIDE EFFECTS   **Hypersensitivity:** itching, burning, urticaria, dermatitis, angioneurotic oedema; superinfection.

NURSING IMPLICATIONS
■ The ophthalmic ointment and skin ointment are *not* interchangeable.

■ Use ophthalmic ointment only for eyes. Inform patient that vision will be temporarily blurred following administration. *See Index: Drug administration: eye ointment.*

■ Consult physician regarding procedure for cleansing infected skin area prior to reapplications of skin ointment.

■ Caution patient with skin problem to avoid prolonged exposure to sunlight unless otherwise advised by physician.

■ Advise patient to apply medication as directed by physician and not to exceed

CHLORTETRACYCLINE HYDROCHLORIDE (continued)

prescribed duration of therapy. Prolonged or frequent intermittent use of an anti-biotic should be avoided because of danger of hypersensitization.

- Instruct patient to discontinue medication and notify physician if an adverse reaction occurs.
- Review personal hygiene practices.
- Store in tightly closed container preferably between 15° and 30°C (59° and 86°F) unless otherwise directed by manufacturer.

C

Chlorthalidone _____

(Hygroton)

Diuretic; antihypertensive; thiazide; sulphonamide derivative

ACTIONS AND USES   Phthalimidine derivative of benzenesulphonamide. Structurally and pharmacologically related to thiazides, with similar actions, uses, contraindications, adverse reactions and interactions. Reportedly causes elevations in total cholesterol, LDL cholesterol, and triglycerides, in some patients. *See chlorothiazide.*

ROUTE AND DOSAGE   Oral: **Adults**: *Oedema*: 50 mg once daily, or 100 to 200 mg once every other day, *Antihypertensive*: *Initial*: 25 mg daily. If poor response, dosage may be increased to 60 mg once daily.

NURSING IMPLICATIONS

- If necessary, tablet may be crushed and administered with fluid of patient's choice.
- When used as a diuretic, an intermittent dose schedule may reduce incidence of adverse reactions.
- *See chlorothiazide.*

DRUG INTERACTIONS   *Chlorthalidone* _____

PLUS	INTERACTIONS
Cholestyramine Colestipol	Pharmacological effects of chlorthalidone may be reduced (decreased absorption). Separate administration as far apart as possible
Corticosteroids Digitalis glycosides	Increased risk of hypokalaemia (with resultant predisposition of patient to digitalis toxicity). Monitor serum potassium
Diazoxide	Action of both drugs potentiated, with resultant hyperglycaemia, hyperuricaemia and hypotension. Used concomitantly with caution
Hypoglycaemic agents, oral (sulphonylureas) and insulin	Chlorthalidone-induced elevation of blood sugar antagonizes hypoglycaemic effect of antidiabetic drugs. Dosage adjustments may be required

Cholestyramine resin

(Questran)

Resin exchange agent (anion);
bile acid sequestrant;
antilipemic

ACTIONS AND USES Quaternary ammonium anion-exchange resin used for its cholesterol-lowering effect. Adsorbs and combines with intestinal bile acids in exchange for chloride ions to form an insoluble, nonabsorbable complex that is excreted in the faeces. As a result, bile salts are continually (but not entirely) prevented from reentry to the enterohepatic circulation. Increased faecal loss of bile acids leads to lowered serum total cholesterol by decrease in low density lipoprotein (LDL) cholesterol and in reduction of bile acid deposit in dermal tissues. Effectiveness of cholestyramine in patients with cholestatic pruritus is based on the assumption that it is the result of bile acid deposits in the skin. Sequestration of bile acids may interfere with absorption of calcium, dietary fat, and fat soluble vitamins A, D, and K. As an anion-exchange resin, cholestyramine may have a strong affinity for selected drugs given concomitantly.

Used primarily for relief of pruritus associated with partial biliary stasis, chronic renal failure, and polycythaemia vera; as adjunct to diet therapy in management of primary hypercholesterolaemia and to reduce the risk of atherosclerotic coronary artery disease and myocardial infarction. Also used in treatment of medication overdoses (particularly digitalis toxicity). To control diarrhoea caused by excess bile acids in colon, as in hyperoxaluria, pseudomembranous colitis, erythroprotoporphyria; and for reducing half-life of the pesticide chlordecone in cases of poisoning and as adjunct in treatment of cardiac glycoside toxicity.

ROUTE AND DOSAGE **Oral: Adult: Initial:** 4 g three or four times daily before meals and at bedtime. *Maintenance*: 4 g daily in one dose or divided in three to four doses. *Pruritus*: up to 16 g/day. *Hyperlipoproteinaemia*: up to 36 g/day. **Children (6 to 12 years):** 80 mg/kg 3 times/day; **(12 years and older):** adult dose. Each 9 g-packet or scoopful contains 4 g of anhydrous cholestyramine.

ABSORPTION AND FATE Not absorbed from GI tract. Excreted in faeces as insoluble complex.

CONTRAINDICATIONS AND PRECAUTIONS Complete biliary obstruction, hypersensitivity to bile acid sequestrants. Safe use by pregnant women, nursing mothers, and children not established. **Cautious Use:** osteoporosis, impaired renal function, bleeding disorders, coronary artery disease, haemorrhoids, impaired GI function, peptic ulcer malabsorption states (e.g., steatorrhoea), the elderly.

ADVERSE/SIDE EFFECTS These include: headache, anxiety, dizziness, fatigue, tinnitus, syncope, drowsiness, femoral nerve pain, paraesthesia, claudication, arteritis, thrombophlebitis, myocardial infarction, angina, constipation (may be severe); faecal impaction, haemorrhoids, abdominal pain and distention, flatulence, bloating sensation, belching, nausea, vomiting, heartburn, anorexia, diarrhoea, steatorrhoea. The following have been reported but causal relationship not established: dysphagia, hiccoughs, sour taste, pancreatitis, diverticulitis, peptic ulcer, cholecystitis, cholelithiasis, black stools,

CHOLESTYRAMINE RESIN (continued)

rectal pain, haemorrhoidal bleeding, urticaria, dermatitis, asthma, shortness of breath, backache, muscle and joint pains, arthritis, osteoporosis, arcus juvenitis, uveitis, haematuria, dysuria, burnt odour to urine, diuresis, xanthoma of hands and fingers, weight loss or gain, increased libido, swollen glands, oedema, gingival bleeding, vitamin A, D, and K deficiencies, hypoprothrombinaemia, hyperchloraemic acidosis, decreased erythrocyte folate levels, rash, irritations of skin, tongue, and perianal areas.

NURSING IMPLICATIONS

- A trial of diet therapy, exercise, and weight reduction is usually instituted before starting resin treatment.
- Place contents of one packet or one level scoopful (60–180 mls) on surface of the preferred liquid. Permit drug to hydrate by standing without stirring 1 to 2 minutes, twirling glass occasionally; then stir until suspension is uniform. A shaker may help. After ingestion of preparation, rinse glass with small amount liquid and drink to ensure taking entire dose. Administer before meals.
- Water, highly flavoured liquids, or other noncarbonated drinks, thin soups, pulpy fruits with high moisture content (crushed pineapple) disguise the taste somewhat.
- Always dissolve cholestyramine before administration; it is irritating to mucous membranes and may cause oesophageal impaction if administered in dry form.
- Cholestyramine colour may vary with different batches but this does not affect drug action. Has a slight aminelike odour and a disagreeable taste; in solution its consistency is sandy or gritty.
- Baseline serum cholesterol and triglyceride levels will be established at beginning of therapy and periodically evaluated to insure that desired levels are maintained.
- Serum cholesterol levels in hyperlipoproteinaemia are reduced within 24 to 48 hours after treatment starts and may continue to decline for a year. After withdrawal of cholestyramine, cholesterol levels usually return to baseline level in about 2 to 4 weeks.
- If response is unsatisfactory after 3 months of treatment, drug is usually withdrawn. (Exception: treatment of xanthoma tuberosum which is continued as long as size and number of xanthomata decrease.)
- Periodic erythrocyte folate levels are recommended, particularly in children.
- Hyperchloraemic acidosis (result of chloride liberation by cholestyramine) occurs most frequently in children and in adults receiving high doses. Serum levels should be monitored.
- Supplemental water-miscible or parenteral vitamins A and D and folic acid may be required by patient on long-term therapy with cholestyramine.
- Adjunctives to drug therapy for pruritus include: adequate fluid intake, use of mild soaps, and soft absorbent clothing, high ambient humidity, even room temperature. Relief of pruritus is an individual response, but therapy is usually continued at least 3 weeks before final evaluation. With improvement, dosage is lowered. Withdrawal of drug may result in return of pruritus within 1 to 2 weeks. (Cholestyramine effect on serum cholesterol of these patients varies considerably.)
- With daily dosage higher than 24 g, side effects increase.
- Preexisting constipation should be evaluated before starting treatment since it may be

CHOLESTYRAMINE RESIN (continued)

worsened by the drug, particularly in elderly patients, women, and when dose is high (more than 24 g/day). Instruct patient to report change in normal bowel elimination pattern promptly to physician.

- If constipation becomes a problem, dosage may be lowered or temporarily interrupted. A stool softener is frequently ordered, especially if patient has heart disease or if haemorrhoids develop. Occasionally this side effect necessitates withdrawal of the drug.

- High bulk diet (bran and other grains, fruit, raw vegetables) with adequate fluid intake is an essential adjunct to cholestyramine treatment and generally resolves the problems of constipation and bloating sensation. Collaborate with physician and dietitian.

- Chronic use can cause increased bleeding tendency. Patient should be alert to early symptoms of hypoprothrombinaemia (petechiae, ecchymoses, abnormal bleeding from mucous membranes, tarry stools) and report their occurrence promptly. Usually, parenteral vitamin K will reverse the symptoms. Oral vitamin K may be administered subsequently as a prophylactic.

- The patient should completely understand the dose and drug schedule established for him or her when leaving direct medical supervision.

- Warn patient not to omit doses. Sudden withdrawal of cholestyramine can promote uninhibited absorption of other drugs taken concomitantly leading to toxicity or overdosage.

- Warn patient not to change dosage or dose intervals, or to stop taking medication even though it may be distasteful, without the physician's approval. Usually GI side effects subside after the first month of drug therapy. Distress following fat ingestion is apt to occur especially when the patient is on large cholestyramine doses.

Food–drug interactions

- Diets for hyperlipoproteinaemia usually low in cholesterol, high in polyunsaturated fat and low in saturated fat. Collaborate with dietitian in making out a dietary teaching plan.

- Foods with high cholesterol content include: egg yolk, turkey (dark meat and skin), gravies, offal, crab meat, shrimp, sardines, caviar, cream, butter, cakes, pies, waffles. There is no cholesterol in plant foods such as fruits, vegetables, nuts, grains, cereals.

- Many foods high in cholesterol are also high in saturated fats: most animal products (including meats, dairy products, eggs, ice cream, cheese), solid and hydrogenated shortenings (lard, coconut oil, cocoa butter, palm oil, non-dairy cream substitutes).

- A controlled amount of polyunsaturated fats are usually allowed because they help to eliminate newly-formed cholesterol. Polyunsaturated fats are found in liquid vegetable oils e.g., sunflowers, corn, soyabean, cottonseed, (olive oil and peanut oil are rich in monounsaturated fats. They neither raise nor lower serum cholesterol).

- Patients with hypercholesterolaemia should attempt to eliminate or at least alter risk factors such as smoking, obesity, faulty dietary habits, excessive alcohol intake, and sedentary lifestyle.

- Warn patient to avoid self-medication with OTC drugs unless physician approves.

CHOLESTYRAMINE RESIN (continued)

Consult physician about use of alcohol; it may be restricted because it increases triglycerides.

- The following symptoms may be drug-induced and should be reported promptly: severe gastric distress with nausea and vomiting (pancreatitis); unusual weight loss (steatorrhoea, malabsorption); black stools, haemorrhoids; sudden back pain (osteoporosis — especially in postmenopausal women not on oestrogens); sore throat, fever (agranulocytosis).
- Questran contains tartrazine which can cause an allergic reaction (including bronchial asthma) in susceptible individuals. Frequently such persons are also sensitive to aspirin.
- Store in tightly closed container at temperature between 15° and 30°C (59° and 86°F) unless otherwise specified by manufacturer.

Diagnostic test interferences   Cholestyramine therapy may be accompanied by increased serum **SGOT, phosphorus, chloride,** and **alkaline phosphatase** levels; decreased **serum calcium, sodium,** and **potassium** levels.

Drug interactions   Cholestyramine may delay or decrease absorption of other oral drugs and thus reduce their effects. Therefore, as a general rule, other medications should be administered at least 1 hour before or 4 to 6 hours after cholestyramine. When cholestyramine is to be discontinued in patients taking potentially toxic drugs, monitor for toxicity. If possible concomitant administration with warfarin and other oral anticoagulants is avoided. If not, administer at least 6 hours apart and closely monitor anticoagulant response. Patients receiving digitalis glycosides should be monitored for underdigitalization; when cholestyramine is to be discontinued, monitor for digitalis toxicity.

Cimetidine _____

(Tagamet)   *Antihistamine; H₂-receptor antagonist*

ACTIONS AND USES   An imidazole derivative structurally similar to histamine. Belongs chemically to antihistamine group, but unlike classical antihistamines, e.g., chorpheniramine, which block histamine at H_1 receptors, cimetidine competitively inhibits histamine at H_2 receptor sites on parietal cells. Reduces volume and hydrogen ion concentration of gastric acid secretion in the nocturnal basal (fasting) state and also when stimulated by food, caffeine, histamine, insulin, pentagastrin, and bethanechol. Demonstrates weak antiandrogenic action and some antiviral activity.

Used for short-term treatment of active duodenal ulcer, prophylaxis against duodenal ulcer recurrence, and in treatment of pathological hypersecretory conditions (Zollinger–Ellison syndrome, systemic mastocytosis, and multiple endocrine adenomas). Treatment of gastric ulcer, stress ulcers, upper GI bleeding.

CIMETIDINE *(continued)*

ROUTE AND DOSAGE   Adults: **Oral:** 400 mg twice a day or going at bedtime. **Intramuscular, intravenous:** (cimetidine hydrochloride 200–400 mg 6 hourly. (No dilution necessary for IM.) **Intermittent intravenous infusion:** 400 mg in 100 ml 0.9% sodium chloride for infusion given over 30 to 60 min, repeat at 4–6 hour intervals. Continuous infusion rate 50–100 ml/hr over 24 hrs. **Child:** By oral or parenteral routes 20–30 mg/kg/day in divided doses.

ABSORPTION AND FATE   About 70% absorbed from GI tract following oral administration. Blood concentrations peak in 1 to 1.5 hours. In fasting state gastric output is reduced about 90% for 4 hours; with food, output is reduced 66% for around 3 hours. Distributed widely to most tissues; passes blood–brain barrier in high doses. About 15 to 23% **bound to plasma proteins. Half-life** ranges from 1.5 to 2 hours (longer in patients with impaired renal function). Metabolized in liver. Most of drug eliminated within 24 hours, primarily in urine; approximately 40 to 60% of oral drug and 77% of parenteral drug excreted unchanged. Some excretion in bile and faeces. Crosses placenta. Excreted in breast milk.

CONTRAINDICATIONS AND PRECAUTIONS   Safe use in women with childbearing potential, in nursing mothers, or during pregnancy, or in children younger than 16 years not determined. **Cautious Use:** elderly or critically ill patients; impaired renal or hepatic function; organic brain syndrome.

ADVERSE/SIDE EFFECTS   Most frequently reported: headache, tiredness, diarrhoea, constipation, dizziness, rash, muscle pain, mild gynaecomastia. Others: bradycardia and other arrhythmias, dizziness, lightheadedness, headache, confusion, restlessness, disorientation, paranoid psychosis, focal twitching or tremor, ataxia, diplopia, transient apnoea, seizures, diarrhoea or constipation, abdominal discomfort, paralytic ileus, facial oedema, rash, urticaria, Stevens-Johnson syndrome, exfoliative dermatitis, dyspnoea, laryngospasm, gynaecomastia (males), galactorrhoea (females), impotence, alopecia, profuse sweating, flushing, fever, interstitial nephritis (rare), slight increase in serum uric acid, transient pain at IM site. Increased prothrombin time; rare: neutropenia, leucopenia, agranulocytosis, thrombocytopenia, autoimmune haemolytic or aplastic anaemia. **Over-dosage:** tachycardia, respiratory failure.

NURSING IMPLICATIONS

- Taken with or immediately after meals. Food delays absorption and thus prolongs drug effect; also peak blood level of cimetidine will coincide with peak food-induced gastric acid secretion.
- Concurrent administration of antacid may be prescribed to control acute ulcer pain. Administer at least 1 hour before or 1 hour after cimetidine.
- Oral administration is substituted for IV therapy when bleeding has been controlled for at least 48 hours.
- Gastric pH may be determined periodically during therapy. Ideally dosage is adjusted to maintain an intragastric pH greater than 5.
- Monitor intake and output particularly in the elderly, severely ill, and in patients with impaired renal function.

CIMETIDINE (continued)

- Paralytic ileus has been reported in patients who are receiving cimetidine to prevent stress ulcers. Report loss of bowel sounds, absence of bowel movement or flatus, vomiting, crampy pain, abdominal distention.
- Periodic evaluations of blood count, renal and hepatic function are advised during therapy.
- Therapy for active duodenal ulcer is continued until healing is demonstrated by endoscopy (usually 4 to 6 weeks, but not to exceed 8 weeks).
- Advise patient to keep clinican informed of any unusual symptoms and the effect of drug therapy.
- Relapse of duodenal ulcer occurs commonly following discontinuation of therapy. Frequency of recurrence is apparently reduced if cimetidine withdrawal is gradual and if a prophylactic bedtime dose is given. Instruct patient undergoing withdrawal to report promptly the recurrence of abdominal pain, black stools, or any other suspicious symptom.
- Gynaecomastia may occur after a month or more of therapy. It may disappear spontaneously or remain throughout therapy. Instruct patient to report this symptom to physician. Adverse reproductive symptoms are most commonly seen in males with Zollinger–Ellison syndrome or other pathological hypersecretory disorders that require prolonged high dose therapy.
- Mental confusion, dizziness, focal twitching, and other CNS symptoms (*See Adverse/Side Effects*), are most likely to occur in the elderly (even with recommended doses), the severely ill, and in patients with impaired renal function. Report immediately; drug should be withdrawn.
- Since dizziness, light-headedness, and mental confusion are possible side effects, caution patient to avoid driving and other potentially hazardous activities until reaction to drug is known.
- **Smoking–drug interactions**   Research studies show that ulcer recurrence is greater in smokers than in nonsmokers. If abstinence is not possible, advise patient to at least refrain from smoking after taking evening dose of cimetidine to prevent interfering with drug control of nocturnal gastric acid secretion (contributes to more rapid ulcer healing).
- **Food–drug interactions**   Although strict dietary control is no longer considered a necessary therapeutic adjunct to the antiulcer drug regimen, the patient should avoid:
  - ☐ Known food intolerance.
  - ☐ Dietary stimulants of gastric acid secretion (gastric irritants): e.g., caffeine beverages, alcohol, black pepper, harsh spices, excessive intake of high calcium foods and beverages (e.g., milk and milk products), extremely hot/cold foods or liquids, pattern of frequent eating.
  - ☐ Overeating and not chewing food thoroughly before swallowing.
- Urge patient not to self-dose with OTC antacids, aspirin or aspirin products (ulcerogenic) or other analgesics unless advised to do so by physician.
- Parenteral solutions are stable for 48 hours at room temperature when added to commonly used IV solutions for dilution: 0.9% sodium chloride injection, 5% or 10% dextrose injection, lactated Ringer's solution, 5% sodium bicarbonate injection. Follow manufacturer's directions.

CIMETIDINE (continued)
Pertinent patient-teaching points

☐ Impress on patient and responsible family member(s) that duodenal or gastric ulcer is a chronic recurrent condition that requires long-term therapy to avoid relapses.

☐ The patient and responsible family members should receive advice about management of life style in general: e.g., (1) create a relaxed atmosphere at mealtimes; (2) control or avoid anxiety-provoking situations; (3) emphasize the benefits of adequate rest and relaxation and advise curtailment of unnecessary activities during ulcer healing stages; (4) inform patient that ulcers tend to recur in the spring and the autumn and therefore particular caution about ulcerogenic factors at these times is prudent.

■ Store all forms of cimetidine preferably between 15° and 30°C (59° and 86°F) and protected from light unless otherwise directed by manufacturer.

Diagnostic test interferences Cimetidine may cause transient increases in **alkaline phosphatase, serum transaminase levels,** and **plasma creatinine.** False-positive **test for gastric bleeding** reported with haemoccult if test is performed within 15 minutes of oral cimetidine administration.

DRUG INTERACTIONS *Cimetidine*

PLUS	INTERACTIONS
Alcohol	Ethanol effects may be increased. Patient should be informed of possible reaction
Antacids	Antacids may reduce GI absorption of cimetidine. Administer antacids one hour before or after cimetidine
Antidepressants, tricyclics	Pharmacological effects of tricyclics may be increased with possibility of toxicity (cimetidine decreases clearance of tricyclics). Dosage adjustments of tricyclics may be required
Anticoagulants, oral	Increased action (hypoprothrombinaemia) of anticoagulant. Cimetidine inhibits hepatic metabolism of oral anticoagulants. Concurrent use generally avoided
Carmustine	Cimetidine may increase carmustine toxicity (bone marrow suppression). Combination avoided if possible
Lignocaine	Increased lignocaine effects with possibility of toxicity (cimetidine reduces renal clearance of lignocaine
Procainamide	Increased procainamide effects with possibility of toxicity (cimetidine reduces renal clearance of procainamide. Monitor plasma levels of procainamide and NAPA (its active metabolite)
Benzodiazepines: alprazolam, chlordiazepoxide, diazepam, flurazepam, triazolam. Exceptions: lorazepam, oxazepam, temazepam (inactivated by glucuronidation) are not affected	

CIMETIDINE (continued)

PLUS (continued)	INTERACTIONS
Metoprolol, propranolol and possibly other beta-adrenergic blockers metabolized by liver Phenytoin and other hydantoins Quinidine Theophyllines	By inhibiting hepatic microsomal enzymes, cimetidine impairs metabolism and may lead to toxic accumulation of these drugs. Monitor plasma levels and clinical response when cimetidine is added to, discontinued, or dosage is altered

Cinoxacin

(Cinobac)   *Antiinfective (urinary tract)*

ACTIONS AND USES   Bactericidal agent with properties similar to those of nalidixic acid (q.v.). but with fewer side effects. Used to treat urinary tract infections caused by susceptible microorganisms.

ROUTE AND DOSAGE   Oral: 1 g/day divided into 2 to 4 doses, for 7 to 14 days. For patients with impaired renal function: *initial*: 500 mg; *maintenance* doses based on creatinine clearance values.

NURSING IMPLICATIONS
- Since cinoxacin may cause dizziness, caution patient to avoid driving and other potentially hazardous tasks until reaction to drug is known.
- Photophobia may be relieved by wearing dark glasses.
- *See naladixic acid.*

Ciprofloxacin

(Ciproxin)   *4-quinolone; antiinfective*

ACTIONS AND USES   Recently introduced 4-quinolone derivative active against gram-negative and gram-positive bacteria.

Used to treat sensitive infections in the respiratory and urinary tracts, gonorrhoea, gastrointestinal system and septicaemia.

ROUTE AND DOSAGE   Oral: **Adults**: 250–750 mg twice a day. *Gonorrhoea*: 250 mg as a single dose. **Intravenous infusion**: 200 mg twice a day over 30–60 minutes; *urinary tract infection*: 100 mg twice a day. *Gonorrhoea*: 100 mg as a single dose.

CONTRAINDICATIONS AND PRECAUTIONS   Safe use during pregnancy and lactation

CIPROFLOXACIN (continued)

not established. Not recommended for children. **Cautious use** in epilepsy, excessive urinary alkalinity, low fluid intake, renal impairment.

ADVERSE/SIDE EFFECTS   Nausea, vomiting, diarrhoea, abdominal pain and dyspepsia. Dizziness, headache, fatigue, rash.

NURSING IMPLICATIONS
- Monitor fluid intake and output ratio.
- Be alert for side effects and report them promptly.
- Adverse reactions should be reported to the Committee on Safety of Medicines.

Cisplatin

(Neoplatin, Platinex, Platosin)   *Antineoplastic*

ACTIONS AND USES   Inorganic complex with platinum as central atom surrounded by 2 chloride atoms and 2 ammonia molecules in the *cis* position. Biochemical properties similar to those of bifunctional alkylating agents. Produces interstrand and intrastrand crosslinkage in DNA of rapidly dividing cells, thus preventing DNA, RNA, and protein synthesis. Cell cycle nonspecific, i.e., effective throughout the entire cell life cycle. Carcinogenicity has not been fully studied, but other compounds with similar action mechanisms and mutagenicity have been reported to be carcinogenic.

Used in established combination therapy (cisplatin, vinblastine, bleomycin) in patient with metastatic testicular tumours and with doxorubicin for metastatic ovarian tumours following appropriate surgical and/or radiation therapy. Has been used in treatment of carcinoma of endometrium, bladder, head, and neck.

ROUTE AND DOSAGE   **Intravenous**: Individualized.

ABSORPTION AND FATE   Following IV dose, widely distributed in body with highest concentrations in liver, large and small intestines, and kidneys. Poor penetration into CNS. Plasma levels decline in biphasic pattern: **initial phase half-life**: 25 to 49 minutes; **later phase**: 58 to 73 hours up to 10 days. More than 90% bound to plasma proteins. Partly excreted in urine (27 to 43% in 5 days). Platinum may be detected in tissues for 4 months or more after administration.

CONTRAINDICATIONS AND PRECAUTIONS   History of hypersensitivity to cisplatin or other platinum-containing compounds, impaired renal function, myelosuppression, impaired hearing, use of other ototoxic and nephrotoxic drugs, history of gout and urate renal stones. **Cautious Use**: previous cytoxic drug or radiation therapy.

ADVERSE/SIDE EFFECTS   *Anaphylactoid reaction*: facial oedema, wheezing, tachycardia, hypotension, bronchoconstriction. Other side effects include: ototoxicity (may be irreversible): tinnitus, bilateral or unilateral hearing loss in high frequency range

CISPLATIN (continued)

(4,000 to 8,000 Hz) deafness; seizures, headache; peripheral neuropathies (may be irreversible): numbness or tingling of fingers, toes, or face; loss of taste, marked nausea, vomiting, anorexia, stomatitis, xerostomia, diarrhoea, constipation, myelosuppression (25 to 30% patients): leucopenia, thrombocytopenia; haemolytic anaemia, haemolysis, (dose-related cumulative): nephrotoxicity, cardiac abnormalities, hyperuricaemia, elevated SGOT.

NURSING IMPLICATIONS

- Administered only under supervision of a qualified physician experienced in the use of antineoplastics and where adequate diagnostic and treatment facilities are available.
- Patient should be closely monitored for dose-related adverse reactions. Since drug action is cumulative, severity of most adverse effects increases with repeated doses.
- A single course of therapy is given no more frequently than once every 3 or 4 weeks.
- A pretreatment ECG and cardiac monitoring during induction therapy are indicated because of possible myocarditis or focal irritability.
- Hydration is started with 1 to 2 litres IV infusion fluid to reduce risk of nephrotoxicity and ototoxicity. Drug is then diluted in 5% dextrose saline or normal saline. Mannitol (an osmotic diuretic) is infused to aid diuresis. Hydration and forced diuresis are continued for at least 24 hours following drug administration to ensure adequate urinary output.
- Monitor urine output and specific gravity for 4 consecutive hours before treatment and for 24 hours after therapy. Report if output is less than 100 ml/hour or if specific gravity is more than 1.030. A urine output of less than 75 ml/hour necessitates medical intervention to avert a renal emergency.
- Advise patient to continue maintenance of adequate hydration (at least 3,000 ml/24 hours oral fluid if physician agrees) and to report promptly the symptoms of nephrotoxicity: reduced urinary output, flank pain, anorexia, nausea, vomiting, dry mucosae, itching skin, urine odour on breath, fluid retention (oedema of extremities and sacral area).
- Intractable nausea and vomiting severe enough to warrant discontinuation of drug usually begin 1 to 4 hours after treatment and may last 24 hours or persist for up to 1 week after treatment is ended.
- Usually a parenteral antiemetic agent is administered ½ hour before cisplatin therapy is instituted and given on a scheduled basis throughout day and night as long as necessary.
- Although psychological support is always important, do not give false reassurance that vomiting will not occur. Assist the patient to maintain nutrient intake if possible by offering frequent light meals or clear liquids (cold foods are better tolerated than hot foods) and foods of particular interest.
- The following tests should be done before initiating every course of therapy and repeated each week during treatment period: serum uric acid and creatinine, BUN, urinary creatinine clearance. A decline in creatinine clearance and elevation of other values is indicative of nephrotoxicity.
- Liver function should also be checked periodically.
- Complete blood and platelet counts are performed weekly for 2 weeks following each course of treatment. The nadirs in platelet and leucocyte counts occur between days

CISPLATIN (continued)

18 and 23 with most patients recovering in 13 to 62 days. A decrease in haemoglobin (more than 2 g/dl) occurs at approximately the same time and with the same frequency.

- Check blood pressure, mental status, pupils, and fundi every hour during therapy. Hydration and mannitol may increase blood pressure which, combined with vomiting, increases the danger of elevated intracranial pressure.

- Tingling, numbness, and tremors of extremities; loss of position sense and taste; and constipation are early signs of neurotoxicity associated with both cisplatin and vincristine. Warn patient to report their occurrence promptly to prevent irreversibility. Pain with heel walking and difficulty in getting out of bed or chair are late indicators of nerve damage.

- Monitor and report abnormal bowel elimination pattern. Constipation and the possibility of faecal impaction may be caused by neurotoxicity; diarrhoea may be the response to GI irritation. A laxative for constipation or an antispasmodic for diarrhoea may be prescribed.

- Audiometric testing should be performed prior to the first dose of cisplatin and before each subsequent dose. Children who receive repeated doses are especially susceptible.

- Inspect oral membranes daily for xerostomia, white patches and ulcerations, and tongue for signs of fungal overgrowth (black, furry appearance). Frequent rinses with warm water and avoidance of highly acid fluids and rough foods will decrease irritation.

- It is important to allerviate dryness of mouth if possible. Deprivation of saliva hastens demineralization of tooth surfaces and mucosal erosion. Advise patient to carefully clean teeth (with fluoride toothpaste) with soft toothbrush or with moistened gauze over finger to avoid gingival trauma. Daily flossing with waxed floss is also important.

- Keep vestibular stimulation to the minimum to avoid dizziness or falling: avoid unnecessary turning of patient in bed, and warn ambulating patient to change position gradually and slowly.

- Monitor needle puncture wounds and other areas of minor trauma, skin and body excretions for bleeding. Instruct patient to report promptly evidence of unexplained bleeding and easy bruising.

- Advise patient to report unexplained fatigue, fever, sore mouth and throat, abnormal body discharges. Because of haematological side effects of combination therapy, patient is highly susceptible to bacterial infection.

- Infection precautions should be instituted promptly if a temperature increase of 1°C over the previous reading is noted. Use strict aseptic technique when caring for the patient to prevent superimposed infections.

- The patient should be weighed under standard conditions (same time, clothing, scale) every day. A gradual ascending weight profile occurring over a period of several days should be reported.

- Anaphylactoid reactions particularly in patient previously exposed to cisplatin may occur within minutes of drug administration. IV adrenaline, antihistamines, corticosteroids, and equipment to maintain respiratory function should be immediately available.

CISPLATIN (continued)

- Hyperuricaemia may occur 3 to 5 days after doses of cisplatin greater than 50 mg/m^2. Allopurinol is prescribed to reduce uric acid levels.
- Use disposable gloves when preparing cisplatin solutions. If drug accidentally contacts skin or mucosa, wash immediately and thoroughly with soap and water.
- Reconstituted drug with sterile water for injection should be clear and colourless. Keep at room temperature; refrigeration will cause a precipitate to form. Since it lacks bacterial preservatives it should be used within 20 hours.
- Unless otherwise specified by manufacturer, store unopened vial in refrigerator at 2° to 8°C (36° to 46°F). Stability with proper storage is 2 years. Check expiration date.

Drug interactions **Aminoglycoside antibiotics** increase risk of ototoxicity and nephrotoxicity; concurrent use not recommended. **Antigout agents** may require dosage adjustment since cisplatin raises blood uric acid levels. Pharmacological effects of **phenytoin** may be decreased.

Clemastine

(Tavegil)   *Antihistamine; H$_1$-receptor*
                                                                              antagonist

ACTIONS AND USES   An ethanolamine derivative antihistamine (H$_1$-receptor antagonist) with prominent antipruritic activity and low incidence of unpleasant side effects. Anticholinergic effects are weak, and central sedative effects generally mild. Reportedly no more effective than chlorpheniramine for treatment of allergic disorders, but transient drowsiness occurs more frequently with clemastine.

Used for symptomatic relief of allergic rhinitis (sneezing, rhinorrhoea, pruritus) and mild uncomplicated allergic skin manifestations such as urticaria and angioedema.

ROUTE AND DOSAGE   Oral: **Adults and children (over 12 years):** 1 mg twice daily. **Child (under 12 yrs):** 0.5–1 mg twice a day.

ABSORPTION AND FATE   Rapidly and almost completely absorbed from GI tract. Peak antihistaminic effect in 5 to 7 hours; duration of activity 10 to 12 hours or longer. Excreted chiefly in urine.

CONTRAINDICATIONS AND PRECAUTIONS   Hypersensitivity to clemastine or to other antihistamines of similar chemical structure; lower respiratory tract symptoms, including acute asthma; concomitant MAO inhibitor therapy; in children younger than 12 years. Safe use during pregnancy and in nursing mothers not established. **Cautious Use:** history of bronchial asthma, increased intraocular pressure, GI or GU obstruction, hyperthyroidism, cardiovascular disease, hypertension, elderly patients.

ADVERSE/SIDE EFFECTS   These include: sedation, transient drowsiness (most common side effects), headache, dizziness, weakness, fatigue, disturbed coordination; less fre-

CLEMASTINE (continued)

quent: confusion, restlessness, nervousness, hysteria, convulsions, tremors, irritability, euphoria, insomnia, paraesthesias, neuritis, hypotension, palpitation, tachycardia, extrasystoles, dry mouth, epigastric distress, anorexia, nausea, vomiting, diarrhoea, constipation, urinary frequency, difficult urination, urinary retention, early menses, haemolytic anaemia, thrombocytopenia, agranulocytosis, urticaria, rash, photosensitivity, anaphylaxis, others: dry nose and throat, thickening of bronchial secretions, tightness of chest, wheezing, nasal stuffiness, excess perspiration, chills.

NURSING IMPLICATIONS

- May be administered with food, water, or milk to reduce possibility of gastric irritation.
- Advise patient to check with physician before taking alcohol or another CNS depressant, since effects may be additive.
- Elderly patients usually require less than average adult dose. Inform the patient that clemastine may make him or her feel sleepy.
- Advise elderly patients to make position changes slowly and in stages, particularly from recumbent to upright posture since they are more likely to experience dizziness and hypotension than younger patients.
- Caution patient not to drive and to avoid other potentially hazardous activities until response to the drug has been established.
- Inform patient that clemastine should be discontinued about 4 days before skin testing procedures since it may prevent otherwise positive reactions.
- Store preferably between 15° and 30°C (59° and 86°F) unless otherwise directed by manufacturer.
- See also *diphenhydramine*.

Clindamycin

(Dalacin C)   *Antibiotic (macrolide)*

ACTIONS AND USES   Semisynthetic derivative of lincomycin. Reported to have greater degree of antibacterial activity *in vitro*, better absorption, and lower incidence of GI side effects than lincomycin. Like lincomycin, suppresses protein synthesis by binding to 50 S subunits of bacterial ribosomes, and therefore inhibits other antibiotics (e.g., erythromycin) that act at this site.

Used for treatment of serious infections when less toxic alternatives are inappropriate. Particularly effective against susceptible strains of anaerobic streptococci, *Bacteroides* (especially *B. fragilis*), *Fusobacterium*, *Actinomyces israelii*, *Peptococcus* and *Clostridium* species. Also effective against aerobic gram-positive cocci, including *Staphylococcus aureus*, *S. epidermidis*, *Streptococci* (except *S. faecalis*), and *Pneumococci*. Topical applications used in treatment of acne vulgaris.

ROUTE AND DOSAGE   Adults: Oral: 150 to 450 mg every 6 hours. Intramuscular,

CLINDAMYCIN (continued)

intravenous (clindamycin phosphate): 300 to 600 mg every 6 to 8 hours, up to 2400 mg daily, if necessary. **Paediatric (over 1 month): Oral:** 8 to 25 mg/kg/day divided into three or four equal doses. **Intramuscular, intravenous:** 15 to 40 mg/kg/day divided into three or four equal doses or 350 to 450 mg/m^2/day. All dosages individualized according to severity of infection and renal status. **Topical solution:** apply to affected area twice daily.

ABSORPTION AND FATE   Almost complete (90%) absorption following oral administration. Peak plasma concentrations within 45 minutes following 150-mg oral dose; effective levels persist 6 hours. Following IM injection, peak levels within 3 hours; effective levels persist 8 to 12 hours. Steady state attained after third dose. Approximately 10% of topical application absorbed into skin. Widely distributed to body fluids and tissues, including saliva and bone. No significant concentrations in cerebrospinal fluid, even when meninges are inflamed. About 90% protein-bound. **Average half-life** 2.4 hours. Most of drug is inactivated by hepatic metabolism; metabolized more rapidly in children than in adults. Excreted in urine, bile, and faeces as bioactive and inactive metabolites and about 10% unchanged drug. Not cleared from blood by haemodialysis or peritoneal dialysis. Readily crosses placenta and may appear in breast milk.

CONTRAINDICATIONS AND PRECAUTIONS   History of hypersensitivity to clindamycin or lincomycin; history of regional enteritis, ulcerative colitis, or antibiotic-associated colitis. Safe use during pregnancy and in nursing mothers not established. Not recommended for infants younger than 1 month of age. **Cautious Use:** history of GI disease, renal or hepatic disease, atopic individuals (history of eczema, asthma, hay fever), history of drug or other allergies; older patients.

ADVERSE/SIDE EFFECTS   These include: diarrhoea, abdominal pain, flatulence, bloating, nausea, vomiting, pseudomembranous colitis (potentially fatal): oesophageal irritation, loss of taste, medicinal taste (high IV doses), leucopenia (chiefly neutropenia), eosinophilia, agranulocytosis, thrombocytopenia, jaundice, abnormal liver function tests. *Hypersensitivity*: skin rashes, urticaria, pruritus, fever, erythema multiforme resembling Stevens-Johnson syndrome (rare), anaphylactoid reactions, serum sickness. **Local reactions**: pain, induration, sterile abscess (following IM injections); thrombophlebitis (IV infusion). **Other**: sensitization, swelling of face (following topical use); dizziness, headache, hypotension (following IM), cardiac arrest (rapid IV), generalized myalgia, superinfections, proctitis, vaginitis, urinary frequency.

NURSING IMPLICATIONS
- Advise patient to take clindamycin capsules with a full (240 mls) glass of water to prevent oesophagitis. Absorption of oral clindamycin is not significantly affected by food, or gastric acid although peak serum levels may be somewhat delayed.
- Instruct patient to take drug for the full course of therapy as prescribed.
- Store in tight containers, preferably between 15° and 30°C (59° and 86°F) unless otherwise directed by manufacturer.

CLINDAMYCIN (continued)

Diagnostic test interferences   Clindamycin may cause increases in: **serum alkaline phosphatase, bilirubin, creatine phosphokinase (CPK)** from muscle irritation following IM injection; **SGOT**, and **SGPT**.

DRUG INTERACTIONS   *Clindamycin*

PLUS	INTERACTIONS
Chloramphenicol ⎫ Erythromycin ⎭	Possibility of mutual antagonism (*See Actions and Uses*)
Antiperistaltic compounds, e.g., diphenoxylate and opiates	Reduces rate but not extent of GI absorption of oral clindamycin. May prolong diarrhoea
Neuromuscular blocking agents (nondepolarizing muscle relaxants), e.g., ether, tubocurarine, pancuronium	Enhanced neuromuscular blocking action. Used with caution
For further information *see lincomycin*	

Clobazam

(Frisium)   *Anxiolytic; anticonvulsant*

ACTIONS AND USES   Long-acting benzodiazepine used to treat anxiety and as an adjunctive drug in epilepsy.

ROUTE AND DOSAGE   **Oral: Adult:** 20–30 mg/day in divided doses or as a single dose at bedtime. *Maximum* 60 mg. Reduced dose in elderly patients. **Child (over 3 yrs)** up to half the adult dose. **Child (under 3 yrs):** not recommended *Epilepsy*: **Adult:** initial 1 mg at night increased to 4–8 mg. **Child: (up to 1 yr)** *initial* 250 mg increased to 0.5–1 mg; **1–5 yrs** 250 mg increased to 1–3 mg: **6–12 yrs** 500 mg increased to 3–6 mg.
    For further information *see diazepam*

Clofibrate

(Atromid-S)   *Antilipemic*

ACTIONS AND USES   Aryloxisobutyric acid derivative structurally unrelated to other antilipemic agents. Reduces very low density lipoproteins rich in triglycerides to a greater extent than low density lipoproteins rich in cholesterol. Mechanism of action is unclear. Effects of drug-induced lowering of serum cholesterol and other lipids on morbidity and mortality due to atherosclerosis or coronary heart disease have not been

CLOFIBRATE (continued)

determined. Use of drug reportedly increases risk of cholelithiasis and cholecystitis requiring surgery to twice nonusers.

Used as adjunct to appropriate dietary regulation and other measures for reduction of serum lipids in patients with hypercholesterolaemia and/or hypertriglyceridaemia. Drug of choice for treatment of hyperlipoproteinaemia.

ROUTE AND DOSAGE.   Oral: **Adult**: 2g/day in 2 to 4 divided doses.

ABSORPTION AND FATE   Intestinal biotransformation to active form *p*-chlorophenoxyisobutyric acid occurs before absorption which is slow but complete. **Peak plasma levels**: 2 to 6 hours. **Elimination half-life**: 6 to 25 hours (in presence of renal impairment: 30 to 110 hours). Plasma clearance of unbound drug is reduced in renal failure, and cirrhosis. About 40 to 60% drug eliminated as metabolites of CPIB; remainder as unchanged CPIB.

CONTRAINDICATIONS AND PRECAUTIONS   Impaired renal or hepatic function, primary biliary cirrhosis, pregnancy, nursing mothers. Safe use in children younger than 14 years not established. **Cautious Use**: history of jaundice or hepatic disease, peptic ulcer, gout, patients receiving frusemide or oral anticoagulants: existing or suspected coronary artery disease.

ADVERSE/SIDE EFFECTS   These include: thrombophlebitis, pulmonary embolus, intermittent claudication, increase or decrease in angina, congestive failure, arrhythmias, swelling and phlebitis at xanthoma sites, skin rash, dry skin, dry brittle hair, alopecia, allergy, urticaria, pruritus, nausea (common), vomiting, loose stools, diarrhoea, flatulence, bloating, abdominal distress, gastritis, polyphagia, weight gain or loss, stomatitis, hepatomegaly, cholelithiasis, pancreatitis, impotence, decreased libido, renal dysfunction (dysuria, haematuria, proteinuria, decreased urinary output), leucopenia, anaemia, eosinophilia, agranulocytosis, potentiation of anticoagulant effect, flu-like symptoms: myalgia, myositis, arthralgia. **Others**: fatigue, weakness, drowsiness, dizziness, headache, (direct relationship to drug action not known): peptic ulcer, GI haemorrhage, tremor, diaphoresis, systemic lupus erythematosus, rheumatoid arthritis, thrombocytopenic purpura, gynaecomastia, malignancy, blurred vision, altered taste sensation (hypogensia).

NURSING IMPLICATIONS
- If gastric distress is a problem, administer drug with meals.
- Before initiation of therapy a complete health history should be obtained, including physical examination, appropriate laboratory determinations, and personal family and dietary history.
- Serum cholesterol and triglyceride levels should be determined initially and evaluated every 2 weeks during first few months of therapy, and then at monthly intervals. If tests show a steady rise or are otherwise abnormal, clofibrate should be withdrawn.
- Since hyperlipoproteinaemia is frequently genetically determined, family members especially children, should be screened for abnormal lipid levels.
- Clofibrate is not generally prescribed until every effort is made to lower serum cholesterol and triglycerides by dietary regulations, weight control, and exercise.
- Reduction to ideal weight, correction of sedentary habits, and control of smoking are

CLOFIBRATE (continued)

applicable to all patients with hyperlipoproteinaemia. Collaborate with dietitian in planning with the patient how to coordinate new adjustments to life-style and diet. Stress importance of adhering to diet.

- Therapeutic response is indicated by reduction of lipid levels; this generally occurs during the first or second month of therapy. Rebound may occur in second or third month, followed by a further decrease; and may also occur with sudden withdrawal of drug.
- Clofibrate therapy for increased serum cholesterol and triglycerides is generally withdrawn after 3 months if the response is not adequate. When used for xanthoma, therapy may be continued even up to 1 years, provided there is some reduction in size of lesions.
- Flulike symptoms (malaise, muscle soreness, aching, weakness) should be reported promptly to the physician. Other reportable symptoms include: fever, chills, sore throat (leucopenia); gastric pain, nausea, vomiting (pancreatitis, cholecystitis); chest pain, dysnoea (pulmonary oedema); dysuria, haematuria, lower legoedema (renal toxicity).
- Since alcohol is a source of carbohydrate, its use may be restricted. Check with physician.
- Women of childbearing years should be on a birth control regimen. If pregnancy is desired, clofibrate therapy should be discontinued at least 2 months before conception (discuss with physician). If patient becomes pregnant while on clofibrate treatment, the risk to the foetus: should be fully understood.
- Advise patient to adhere to drug regimen as established. Instruct patient not to alter the dose or dose intervals and to not stop taking the drug without consulting the physician.
- Caution patient about self-dosing with OTC drugs without the approval of the physician.
- Frequent serum transaminase and other liver tests are advocated, as well as periodic complete blood counts, renal function tests, and determinations of plasma and urine steroid levels, serum electrolyte levels, and blood sugar.
- Preserved in closed, light-resistant containers at temperature between 15° and 30°C (59° and 86°F), unless otherwise directed by manufacturer.
- *See cholestyramine.*

Diagnostic test interferences   Clofibrate therapy may lead to increased **BSP** retention, thymol turbidity; increased **serum creatine phosphokinase (CPK), SGOT, SGPT** levels; **proteinuria**, parodoxical increase in **LDL** or **cholesterol** levels (if there is a large decrease in VLDL level); decreased **plasma fibrinogen** levels. Lower fasting **blood glucose** and **serum insulin** levels in patients with diabetes mellitus.

Drug interactions   Clofibrate increases effects of **oral anticoagulants** by decreasing plasma protein binding. Concomitant use of **clofibrate** and **frusemide** may result in enhanced effect of both drugs. Clofibrate may enhance hypoglycaemia effect of **tolbutamide** and other **sulphonylureas**. **Oral contraceptives** may antagonize the actions of clofibrate.

Note: *Similar drug BEZAFIBRATE (Bezalip)*

Clomiphene citrate

(Clomid, Serophene)   *Ovulation stimulant;*
                                                       antioestrogenic

ACTIONS AND USES   Nonsteroidal compound related to chlorotrianisene. Used to induce ovulation in anovulatory women. Increased gonadotropins lead to formation of large cystic ovaries, maturation of ovarian follicle, ovulation, and development and function of corpus luteum. Increases plasma progesterone levels in the luteal phase. A single ovulation is induced, by a single course of therapy; normal ovulatory function dose not usually resume after treatment or after pregnancy.

   Used for treating infertility in appropriately selected women desiring pregnancy and in the management of idiopathic post-pill amenorrhoea.

ROUTE AND DOSAGE   Oral: **First course of therapy**: 50 mg/day for 5 days beginning on 5th day of cycle or at any time if cycles are absent. Dose may be increased to a maximum of 200 mg if no ovulation occurs.

ABSORPTION AND FATE   Readily absorbed from GI tract. Detoxified in liver; 50% of dose is excreted in faeces after 5 days; the remaining metabolites and drug are excreted from enterohepatic pool or are stored in body fat for later release.

CONTRAINDICATIONS AND PRECAUTIONS   Pregnancy, fibroid tumour, ovarian cyst, hepatic disease or dysfunction, abnormal and unexplained bleeding, visual abnormalities, mental depression, thrombophlebitis. **Cautious Use**: enlarged ovaries, pelvic discomfort, sensitivity to pituitary gonadotropins.

ADVERSE/SIDE EFFECTS   (Dose related). These include: skin rash, urticaria, allergic dermatitis, nausea, vomiting, increased appetite, constipation, urinary frequency, polyria. **Others**: (reversible and of short duration): transient blurring, diplopia, scintillating scotomata, photophobia, floaters, photopsia, decreased visual acuity (rare). Additional adverse effects: spontaneous abortion, multiple ovulations, birth defects, ovarian failure, acute (irreversible) transition to menopause (rare). *Hyperstimulation of ovaries*: (mild) ovarian enlargement, abdominal distention, weight gain; (severe) ascites, pleural effusion, electrolyte imbalance, hypovolaemia with hypotension and oliguria, tremendously enlarged ovaries with multiple follicular cysts. Also, hot flushes, breast discomfort, abdominal pain, pain of mittelschmerz, heavy menses, unfavourable cervical mucus, exacerbation of endometriosis, dryness and loss of hair, nervous tension, depression, headache, fatigue, restlessness, insomnia, dizziness, vertigo, cholestatic jaundice. The following have been reported but causal relationships have not been established: detachment of posterior vitreous, posterior capsular cataract, thrombosis of temporal arteries of retina; hydatidiform mole.

NURSING IMPLICATIONS
- The importance of properly timed coitus must be understood by the patient and her partner. Each course of therapy should start on or about the fifth cycle day once ovulation has been established.

CLOMIPHENE CITRATE (continued)

- A complete history, physical examination, thyroid, adrenal and pituitary disorders, diagnosed endometrial biopsy and liver function tests are checked before therapy begins.
- Determine level of understanding of patient and her partner; reinforce teaching already begun. They should have a full understanding of frequency and potential hazards of multiple pregnancy before treatment is started.
- Incidence of multiple pregnancy with clomiphene use is as high as 20% and appears to increase with dose increases.
- A pelvic examination should be performed before initiation of each cycle of therapy and immediately, if abdominal pain occurs.
- Patient who is going to respond usually ovulates after the first course of therapy (within 5 to 14 days).
- The likelihood of conception diminishes with each succeeding course of therapy. If pregnancy is not achieved after 3 or 4 ovulatory responses, further treatment with clomiphene is not recommended.
- The matching of times for apparent ovulation, viability of sperm, and fertilizability of the ovum is crucial. If timing is off it can take months for a woman to become pregnant. Review treatment regimen with patient to test understanding.
- Symptoms that should be reported if they continue and are distressing: hot flushes resembling those associated with menopause; nausea, vomiting, headache. Appropriate drug therapy may be prescribed. Symptoms disappear after drug is discontinued.
- Yellowing of eyes, light-coloured stools, yellow, itchy skin and fever symptomatic of jaundice should be reported promptly.
- If abnormal bleeding occurs, full diagnostic measures are crucial.
- Instruct patient to stop taking clomiphene if she suspects pregnancy and to contact physician for a confirmatory examination.
- Visual symptoms due to intensification and prolongation of after images are accentuated on exposure to a more brightly lit environment. If patient needs to wear dark glasses even, or if she has blurred or decreased vision or scotomatas (signs of ocular toxicity), she should promptly report for a complete ophthalmic examination. Drug will be stopped until symptoms subside (usually in a few weeks).
- Because of the possibility of lightheadedness, dizziness, and visual disturbances, caution the patient against performing hazardous tasks requiring skill and coordination in an environment with variable lighting.
- Warn patient to report excessive weight gain, signs of oedema, bloating, decreased urinary output (signs of ovarian overstimulation). Hospital care is necessary to prevent ovarian rupture and to restore electrolyte balance.
- Maximum enlargement of the ovary does not occur until several days after clomiphene is discontinued; enlargement and cyst formation then regress spontaneously within a month.
- Pelvic pain indicates the need for immediate pelvic examination for diagnostic purposes. If pain is due to abnormal enlargement of the ovary or to polycystic ovary syndrome, medication will be stopped until pretreatment size is attained—usually in a few days. During next course of treatment, dosing regimen will be reduced.
- Many monitoring procedures are important during clomiphene therapy. Help patient

CLOMIPHENE CITRATE (continued)

to understand importance of her cooperation and strict adherence to the therapeutic plan.

■ Advise patient to take the medicine at same time every day. This helps to maintain drug levels and prevents forgetting a dose.

■ Missed dose: instruct patient to take drug as soon as possible. If not remembered until time for next dose, take both doses together, then resume regular dosing schedule. If more than one dose is missed, patient should check with physician.

■ Store at temperature between 15° and 30°C (59° and 86°F) in tightly capped, light-resistant container.

Diagnostic test interferences Clomiphene may increase **BSP** retention; **plasma transcortin, thyroxine, and sex hormone binding globulin (TBG)** levels. Also increases **follicular-stimulating** and **luteinizing hormone** secretion in most patients.

Clomipramine hydrochloride —————————————

(Anafranil)   *Antidepressant; tricyclic*

ROUTE AND DOSAGE   Oral: *Initial* 10 mg daily increased to 30−150 mg. Reduce dose in the elderly. **Intramuscular:** up to 150 mg/day. **Intravenous:** *initial* dose of 20−25 mg to test tolerance and then 100 mg/day for 7−10 days. *See amitriptyline.*

Clonazepam ————————————————————

(Rivotril)   *Anticonvulsant;*
                                                                          benzodiazepine derivative

ACTIONS AND USES   Benzodiazepine derivative with strong anticonvulsant activity and several other pharmacological properties characteristic of the drug class. Used alone or with other drugs in absence, myoclonic, and akinetic seizures.

ROUTE AND DOSAGE   Highly individualized. **Oral: Adults:** *Initial*: 1 mg at night for 4 nights increased to 4−8 mg/day gradually over 2−4 weeks. **Child (under one year):** 250 mcg increased to 0.5−1 mg; **(1−5 yrs):** 250 mcg increasing to 1−3 mg; **(6−12 yrs):** 500 mcg increasing to 3−6 mg. **Intravenous:** in status epilepticus **Adult:** 1 mg over 30 seconds. **Child:** 500 mcg by slow injection or infusion.

ABSORPTION AND FATE   Maximal plasma levels reached in 1 to 2 hours after oral administration. Therapeutic serum concentrations: 20 to 80 ng/ml. **Plasma protein**

CLONAZEPAM *(continued)*

binding: 82%. **Half-life**: 18 to 50 hours. Excreted in urine as metabolites (less than 2% excreted unchanged).

CONTRAINDICATIONS AND PRECAUTIONS   Hypersensitivity to benzodiazepines, liver disease, acute narrow-angle glaucoma, breast feeding. Safe use in pregnancy and in women of childbearing potential not established. **Cautious Use**: renal disease, drug-controlled open-angle glaucoma, addiction-prone individuals; children (because of unknown consequences of long-term use on growth and development); patient with several coexisting seizure disorders, chronic obstructive airways disease.

ADVERSE/SIDE EFFECTS   These include: palpitations, bradycardia, hirsutism, hair loss, skin rash, ankle and facial oedema, xerostomia, sore gums, anorexia, increased salivation, increased appetite, nausea, constipation, diarrhoea, dysuria, enuresis, nocturia, urinary retention, agranulocytosis, anaemia, leucopenia, thrombocytopenia, eosinophilia, drowsiness (common), ataxia, insomnia, nystagmus, abnormal eye movements, aphasia, choreiform movements, coma, dysarthria, dysdiadochokinesia, 'glassy-eyed' appearance, headache, hemiparesis, hypotonia, slurred speech, tremor, vertigo, confusion, depression, hallucinations, aggressive behaviour, hysteria, increased libido, suicide attempt, chest congestion, respiratory depression, rhinorrhoea, dyspnoea, hypersecretion in upper respiratory passages.

NURSING IMPLICATIONS

- Anticonvulsant activity is often lost after 3 months of therapy; dosage adjustment may reestablish efficacy. Patient should be aware of necessity to report loss of seizure control promptly.
- Counsel patient to take drug as prescribed and not to alter dosing regimen or stop medication without consulting physician. Additionally the patient should not give any of it to another person.
- If a new anticonvulsant is to be substituted, it is usually added to the drug regimen as the former medication is gradually withdrawn. Slow tapering of dose over several days time is imperative. Abrupt withdrawal in patient on high doses and long-term therapy can precipitate status epilepticus. Other withdrawal symptoms: convulsion, tremor, abdominal and muscle cramps, vomiting, sweating.
- Caution patient not to self-medicate with OTC drugs before consulting the physician.
- Monitor fluid intake–output ratio and other indicators of renal function. Excess accumulation of metabolites because of impaired excretion leads to toxicity.
- If multiple anticonvulsants are being given, watch patient carefully for signs of overdosage and/or drug interaction, i.e., increased depressant adverse effects.
- If used as treatment for restless legs, suggest the following supportive measures (with physician approval):
    - □ Avoid use of caffeine beverages at dinner and during evening.
    - □ Bed cradle to keep bedding off legs.
    - □ Support stockings.
    - □ Stretch exercises for calf muscles.
    - □ Silk pyjamas.

CLONAZEPAM (continued)

☐ Ice bag or heat; aspirin.

- Alcohol and CNS depressants should be avoided during therapy with clonazepam.
- Advise patient not to drive a car or engage in other activities requiring mental alertness and physical coordination until reaction to the drug is known. Drowsiness occurs in approximately 50% of patients.
- Liver function tests, platelet counts, blood counts, and clinical evaluation of drug efficacy should be a part of the follow-up care of the patient on clonazepam.
- Patient should carry identification ('Medic Alert') bearing information about medication in use and the diagnosis.
- **Overdosage symptoms** Somnolence, confusion, diminished reflexes, coma. Treatment includes: monitoring of vital signs, immediate gastric lavage, IV fluids, maintenance of open airway, vasopressors, CNS antidepressants.
- Both psychological and physical dependence may occur in the patient on long-term, high-dose therapy.
- Store in tightly closed container protected from light, at temperature between 15° and 30°C (59° and 86°F) unless otherwise specified by the manufacturer.

Diagnostic test interferences Clonazepam causes transient elevation of **serum** transaminase and alkaline phosphatase.

DRUG INTERACTIONS   *Clonazepam*

PLUS	INTERACTIONS
Alcohol, barbiturates, antianxiety agents, antipsychotics, MAO inhibitors, tricyclic antidepressants, other anticonvulsants	Potentiate CNS depressant effect of clonazepam
Carbamazepine	Increases metabolism, and therefore reduces effects of clonazepam
Valproic acid	May produce absence (petit mal) status

Clonidine hydrochloride

(Catapres, Dixarit)

Alpha-adrenergic agonist (centrally-acting); antihypertensive

ACTIONS AND USES Centrally acting sympatholytic imidazoline derivative chemically related to tolazoline. Stimulates α_2-adrenergic receptors in CNS to produce inhibition of sympathetic vasomotor centres. Central actions result in reduced peripheral sympathetic nervous system activity, reduction in systolic and diastolic blood pressure, and decrease in heart rate. Other possible effects: inhibition of centrally induced salivation, decreased GI secretions and motility, decreased intraocular pressure, prolonged circulation time and inhibition of renin release from kidneys. Reportedly minimizes or eliminates many of the common clinical signs and symptoms associated

CLONIDINE HYDROCHLORIDE (continued)

with withdrawal of heroin, methadone, or other opiates. This action is believed to be related to stimulation of inhibitory receptors in locus coeruleus, a major noradrenergic nucleus in brain.

Used in treatment of hypertension, either alone or with diuretic or other antihypertensive agents. Also used to reduce menopausal flushing.

ROUTE AND DOSAGE   Oral: 50–100 mcg three times a day increased every second or third day to a maximum (average) dose of 1.2 mg. *Migraine*: 50 mcg twice a day, increased to 75 mcg twice a day after 2 weeks if necessary.

ABSORPTION AND FATE   Well absorbed from GI tract. Plasma drug level peaks in 3 to 5 hours; **plasma half-life**: 12 to 14 hours (25 to 37 hours in patients with impaired renal function). **Duration of hypotensive effect** is 8 hours in normotensive individuals and 4 to 24 hours or more in hypertensive patients. Believed to be widely distributed in body tissues. Metabolized in liver; 65% of dose is excreted by kidneys as unchanged drug (about 32%) and metabolites; about 20% is excreted through enterohepatic route in faeces. Approximately 85% of single dose is eliminated within 72 hours; excretion completed after 5 days. Crosses blood–brain barrier.

CONTRAINDICATIONS AND PRECAUTIONS   Safe use during pregnancy and in women of childbearing potential and children not established. **Cautious Use**: severe coronary insufficiency, recent myocardial infarction, cerebrovascular disease, chronic renal failure, Raynaud's disease, thromboangiitis obliterans, history of mental depression.

ADVERSE/SIDE EFFECTS   Most frequent: dry mouth, drowsiness, sedation, constipation, dizziness, headache, weakness, sluggishness, fatigue, slight transient bradycardia. Other side effects include: postural hypotension (mild), Raynaud's phenomenon, congestive heart failure, ECG changes, bradycardia, palpitation, flushes, paradoxical increase in blood pressure (gross overdosage), vivid dreams, nightmares, insomnia, behaviour changes, nervousness, restlessness, anxiety, mental depression, rash, angioneurotic oedema, urticaria, pruritus, thinning of hair, anorexia, nausea, vomiting, parotid pain, hepatitis, hyperbilirubinaemia, weight gain (sodium retention), impotence, urinary retention, dry, itchy, and burning eyes, retinal degeneration (animal studies); constricted pupils (overdosage), dry nasal mucosa, pallor, increased sensitivity to alcohol, gynaecomastia, bone pain.

NURSING IMPLICATIONS

- Hypotensive response begins within 30 to 60 minutes after drug administration. Maximum decrease in blood pressure usually occurs in 2 to 4 hours. Antihypertensive effect lasts approximately 6 to 8 hours.
- Last dose is commonly administered immediately before retiring to ensure overnight blood pressure control and to minimize daytime drowsiness.
- Dosage is increased gradually over a period of weeks so as not to lower blood pressure abruptly (especially important in the elderly). Follow-up visits should be scheduled every 2 to 4 weeks until BP stabilizes, then every 2 to 4 months.
- For patients undergoing surgery, clonidine is usually given 4 to 6 hours before scheduled surgery. Patient may be given a parenteral antihypertensive until oral medication can be resumed.

C

CLONIDINE HYDROCHLORIDE (continued)

- Dry mouth may be relieved by frequent rinses with clear water, increase in (noncaloric) fluid intake, or by sugarless gum, lemon drops or saliva substitutes.
- Side effects that occur most frequently (*see Adverse/Side Effects*) tend to diminish with continued therapy, or they may be relieved by dosage reduction.
- Although postural hypotension occurs infrequently, advise patient to make position changes slowly, and in stages, particularly from recumbent to upright position, and to dangle legs a few minutes before standing. Caution patient to lie down immediately if he or she feels faint.
- Monitor fluid intake and output during period of dosage adjustment. Report change in intake−output ratio or change in voiding pattern.
- Determine weight daily. Patients not receiving a concomitant diuretic agent may gain weight, particularly during first 3 or 4 days of therapy, because of marked sodium and water retention. Consult physician regarding allowable sodium intake.
- Patients with history of mental depression require close supervision, as they may be subject to further depressive episodes.
- Tolerance sometimes develops in some patients. Physician may increase dosage or prescribe concomitant administration of a diuretic to enhance antihypertensive response.
- Inform patient of the possible sedative effect of clonidine and caution against potentially hazardous activities such as operating machinery or driving until reaction to drug has been determined.
- Blood pressure should be closely monitored whenever a drug is added to or withdrawn from therapeutic regimen.
- If drug is to be discontinued, it is withdrawn over a period of 2 to 4 days. Abrupt withdrawal, particularly after long-term therapy, may result in restlessness and headache 2 to 3 hours after a missed dose and hypertensive crisis within 8 to 24 hours. Other symptoms associated with sudden withdrawal include anxiety, sweating, palpitation, increased heart rate, insomnia, tremors, muscle and stomach pain, and salivation; rarely, hypertensive encephalopathy and death may ensue.
- It is recommended that patient be monitored for at least one month after clonidine is withdrawn.
- Warn patient of the danger of omitting doses or stopping the drug without consulting the physician.
- Periodic eye examination is advised (based on animal studies).
- Advise patient to carry appropriate medical identification card or jewellery.
- Caution patient not to take OTC medications without prior approval of physician.
- Symptoms of clonidine overdosage usually respond to supportive treatment. Severe poisoning can be reversed by administration of tolazoline hydrochloride.
- Store in well-closed container, preferably between 15° and 30°C (59° and 86°F) unless otherwise directed by manufacturer.

Diagnostic test interferences   Possibility of decreased urinary excretion of **aldosterone**, **catecholamines**, and **VMA** (however, sudden withdrawal of clonidine may cause increases in these values); transient increases in blood glucose; weakly positive direct antiglobulin (Coombs') tests.

CLONIDINE HYDROCHLORIDE (continued)
DRUG INTERACTIONS   *Clonidine*_____

PLUS	INTERACTIONS
Beta adrenergic blocking agents e.g., propranolol	Paradoxical hypertension with combination therapy and following clonidine withdrawal. If withdrawal hypertension occurs discontinued drug is reinstituted. Withdrawal of beta adrenergic before clonidine suggested
CNS depressants (e.g., alcohol, barbiturates, sedatives, tranquillzers)	Enhanced CNS depression
Digitalis glycosides, guanethidine, propranolol, and other drugs that may decrease heart rate	Possibility of additive bradycardic effect
Levodopa	Clonidine may inhibit antiparkinson action
Tricyclic antidepressants	Possibility of rise in blood pressure. Concomitant use generally avoided

Clorazepate dipotassium ━━━━━━━━━━━━━━━━━━━━

(Tranxene)   *Psychotropic; anxiolytic; anticonvulsant; benzodiazepine*

ACTIONS AND USES   Psychotherapeutic agent with actions, uses, and interactions qualitatively similar to those of chlordiazepoxide (q.v.) but with less unwanted side effects, e.g., sedation.

Used for the management of anxiety disorders, for short-term relief of anxiety symptoms, as adjunct in management of partial seizures, and for symptomatic relief of acute alcohol withdrawal.

ROUTE AND DOSAGE   Oral: Adult: 7.5−22.5 mg at bedtime or in 2−3 divided doses. Reduce dose in the elderly.

For further information *see diazepam.*

ABSORPTION AND FATE   Decarboxylated in stomach; absorbed as active metabolite, desmethydiazepan **Peak serum levels** in about 1 hour; **duration of action** about 24 hours. **Half–life** approximately 48 hours. Metabolized in liver; excreted primarily in urine. Crosses placenta; excreted in breast milk.

Clotrimazole ━━━━━━━━━━━━━━━━━━━━━━━━━━━

(Canesten)   *Antibiotic; antifungal*

ACTIONS AND USES   Imidazole derivative closely related chemically to miconazole. Broad spectrum of antifungal activity essentially identical to that of miconazole, but is

CLOTRIMAZOLE (continued)

reportedly less effective than miconazole for epidermophytoses and for candidiasis. Acts by damaging fungal cell membrane thereby altering its permeability which permits loss of potassium and other cellular constituents. Also active against some gram-negative bacteria.

Used topically in treatment of tinea pedis, cruris, and corporis due to *Trichophyton rubrum*, *T. mentagrophytes*, *Epidermophyton floccosum*, and *Microsporum canis*, and for tinea versicolour due to *Malassezia furfur*, a vulvovaginal and oropharyngeal candidiasis (moniliasis) caused by *Candida albicans*.

ROUTE AND DOSAGE   Topical (skin): cream 1%; solution 1%; gently massage small amount (of cream or solution) into affected and surrounding skin areas twice daily (morning and evening). **Vaginal**: Vaginal tablet 100 mg: using applicator supplied, insert 2 tablet intravaginally daily for 3 consecutive days, preferably at bedtime. Alternatively, one 100 mg tablet inserted daily for six days, or one 500 mg tablet at night as a single dose. Vaginal cream (2%) 5 g inserted twice daily for 3 days or once at night for 6 days.

ABSORPTION AND FATE   Negligible amounts appear to be absorbed systemically following topical or intravaginal administration.

CONTRAINDICATIONS AND PRECAUTIONS   History of hypersensitivity to clotrimazole; use for systemic mycoses. Safe use during pregnancy, in nursing mothers, and in children under 3 years not established.

ADVERSE/SIDE EFFECTS   Skin: stinging, erythema, oedema, vesication, desquamation, pruritus, urticaria. **Vaginal**: mild burning sensation, lower abdominal cramps, bloating, cystitis, urethritis, mild urinary frequency, vulval erythema and itching and skin rash, abnormal liver function tests; occasional nausea and vomiting (with oral troche).

NURSING IMPLICATIONS
- Skin cream and solution preparations should be applied sparingly. Protect hands with plastic gloves when applying medication.
- Avoid contact of clotrimazole preparations with the eyes.
- Occlusive dressings should not be applied unless otherwise directed by physician.
- Consult physician for procedure to use for cleansing skin before applying medication. Some physicians recommend just plain tap water, others prefer use of a mild soap with thorough rinsing. Regardless of procedure used, dry skin thoroughly.
- Diagnosis of superficial fungal infections can be determined by potassium hydroxide (KOH) smears and/or cultures. Since vaginal preparations have been shown to be effective only for candidiasis (moniliasis), diagnosis should be confirmed before initiation of therapy.
- Advise patient to use clotrimazole as directed and for the length of time prescribed by physician.
- Generally, clinical improvement is apparent during first week of therapy. Keep physician informed.

CLOTRIMAZOLE (continued)

- Urine and blood glucose studies and microbacteriological analysis are indicated in patients who show no response to therapy.
- Resistant candidiasis may be a presenting sign of unrecognized diabetes mellitus.
- Inform patient receiving the drug vaginally that sexual partner may experience burning and irritation of penis or urethritis and therefore to refrain from sexual intercourse during therapy, or advise sexual partner to wear a condom.
- Advise patient to report to physician if condition worsens or if signs of irritation or sensitivity develop, or if no improvement is noted after 4 weeks of therapy.
- Review patient's hygienic practices for possible sources of infection.
- Recurrence of vulvovaginal candidiasis occurs frequently. Discontinuation of systemic antibiotics and oral contraceptives have helped some patients.

General patient-teaching points for tinea corporis (ringworm of body)

- □ Advise patient to keep linen, clothing, towels, face-cloths, and other toilet articles separate.
- □ Wash anything that contacts affected areas, after each treatment.
- □ Launder clothing daily in hot water and nonirritating soap or detergent.
- □ Wear light clothing (or footwear) that will allow ventilation.
- □ Loose-fitting cotton underwear (and socks) are ideal.
- □ Keep skin and dry.
- □ For patients with tinea pedis (athlete's foot), leather shoes or sandals are best; avoid plastic footwear. Advise patient to put on socks before underwear.

- Store cream and solution formulations preferably between 2° and 30°C (35° and 86°F); do not store troches or vaginal tablets above 35°C (95°F) unless otherwise directed by manufacturer.

Cloxacillin, sodium ━━━━━━━━━━━━━━━━━━━━━━━━

(Orbenin)   *Antibiotic (beta-lactam);*
                                                          penicillin

ACTIONS AND USES Semisynthetic, acid-stable, penicillinase-resistant, isoxazolyl penicillin. Mechanism of bactericidal action, contraindications, precautions, and adverse reactions as for penicillin G (q.v.). In common with other isoxazolyl penicillins (dicloxacillin, oxacillin) is highly active against most penicillinase-producing staphylococci, but less potent than penicillin G against penicillin-sensitive microorganisms, and is generally ineffective against gram-negative bacteria and methicillin-resistant staphylococci.

Used primarily in treatment of infections caused by penicillinase-producing staphylococci and penicillin-resistant staphylococci. May be used to initiate therapy in suspected staphylococcal infections pending culture and susceptibility test results. As with other penicillins, serum concentrations are enhanced by concurrent use of probenecid.

CLOXACILLIN, SODIUM (continued)

ROUTE AND DOSAGE   Oral: Adults and children (weighing 20 kg or more): 250 to 500 mg or more every 6 hours. Infants and children (up to 20 kg): 12.5 mg/kg every 6 hours. **Intramuscular: Adults:** 250 mg 4–6 hrly. **Intravenous: Adults:** 500 mg every 4–6 hrs.

ABSORPTION AND FATE   Peak serum levels within 1 hour; effective levels maintained 4 to 6 hours after single dose. Distributed throughout body with highest concentrations in kidney and liver; cerebrospinal fluid penetration is low. Almost 90 to 98% protein bound. **Half-life:** 30 to 60 minutes. Excreted primarily in urine as active metabolite and intact drug; significant hepatic elimination through bile. Crosses placenta. Excreted in breast milk.

CONTRAINDICATIONS AND PRECAUTIONS   Sensitivity to penicillins or cephalosporins. Safe use during pregnancy and in neonates not established. **Cautious Use:** history of or suspected atopy or allergy (asthma, eczema, hives, hay fever), renal or hepatic function impairment.

ADVERSE/SIDE EFFECTS   Nausea, vomiting, flatulence, diarrhoea. **Hypersensitivity reactions** (*see penicillin G*): pruritus, urticaria, wheezing, sneezing, chills, drug fever, anaphylaxis; eosinophilia, leucopenia, agranulocytosis (malaise, elevated temperature, sore throat, adenopathy); elevated SGOT, SGPT, jaundice (rare), superinfections. *See also penicillin G*.

NURSING IMPLICATIONS
- Before treatment is initiated, a careful inquiry should be made concerning patient's previous exposure and sensitivity to penicillins and cephalosporins, and other allergic reactions of any kind.
- Best taken on an empty stomach (at least 1 hour before or 2 hours after meals), unless otherwise advised by physician. Food reduces rate and extent of drug absorption.
- For further information *see pencillin G*.

Codeine ——————————————————————————

Codeine phosphate

Narcotic analgesic; opiate agonist; antitussive

ACTIONS AND USES   Phenathrene derivative of opium made by methylation of morphine. Similar to morphine (q.v.) in actions, uses, contraindications, precautions, and adverse reactions. Not as potent as morphine and has shorter duration of action, thus produces less severe adverse reactions. In contrast to morphine, orally administered codeine is about 60% as potent as the parenteral form. Histamine-releasing action appears to be more potent than that of morphine and may result in hypotension, flushing and rarely, bronchoconstriction. Analgesic potency is about one-sixth that of morphine; antitussive activity is also a little less than that of morphine. Oral codeine

CODEINE PHOSPHATE (continued)

65 mg is approximately equivalent to aspirin 650 mg (analgesic property). Reportedly not as effective for uterine or dental pain as are prostaglandin inhibitors such as aspirin.

Used for symptomatic relief of mild to moderately severe pain, when control cannot be obtained by nonnarcotic analgesics, and to suppress hyperactive or nonproductive cough.

ROUTE AND DOSAGE   Oral, subcutaneous, intramuscular: **Adults: Analgesic:** 15 to 60 mg four times a day. *Antitussive*: 10 to 20 mg orally every 4 to 6 hours, if necessary. Not to exceed 120 mg/24 hours. **Intramuscular:** up to 30 mg as required. *Diarrhoea*: 10–60 mg 4–6 hrly; **Child (over 4 yrs):** 1–3 mg/kg in divided doses.

ABSORPTION AND FATE   Following oral or parenteral administration, **onset of action** occurs in 15 to 30 minutes and peaks in 1 to 1½ hours; **duration of action** 4 to 6 hours. **Half-life:** 2.5 to 4 hours. About 7% protein bound. Metabolized primarily in liver. Excreted chiefly in urine as norcodeine and free and conjugated morphine. Negligible amounts of codeine and metabolites excreted in faeces. Crosses placenta and appears in breast milk.

CONTRAINDICATIONS AND PRECAUTIONS   Hypersensitivity to codeine or other morphine derivatives, acute asthma, chronic obstructive lung disease, increased intracranial pressure, head injury, acute alcoholism, hepatic or renal dysfunction, hypothyroidism. **Cautious Use:** prostatic hypertrophy, debilitated patients, very young and very old patients; *see also morphine sulphate.*

ADVERSE/SIDE EFFECTS   These include: dizziness, lightheadedness, drowsiness, sedation, lethargy, euphoria, agitation, palpitation, orthostatic hypotension, bradycardia, nausea, vomiting, constipation, urinary retention, difficult urination, fixed-drug eruption; histamine-releasing effects: urticaria, pruritus, excessive perspiration (hyperhidrosis), facial flushing, shortness of breath, bronchoconstriction (rare). **Overdosage:** restlessness, exhilaration, convulsions, tachycardia, bradycardia, hypotension, miosis, narcosis, respiratory paralysis, circulatory collapse. *See also morphine sulphate.*

NURSING IMPLICATIONS
- Administer oral codeine with milk or other food to reduce possibility of GI distress.
- Record relief of pain and duration of analgesia.
- Since orthostatic hypotension is a possible side effect, instruct patient to make position changes slowly and in stages particularly from recumbent to upright posture. Also advise patient to lie down immediately if lightheadedness or dizziness occurs.
- Nausea appears to be aggravated by ambulation. Advise patient to lie down when feeling nauseated and to notify physician if this symptom persists.
- Inform patient that codeine may impair ability to perform tasks requiring mental alertness and therefore to avoid driving and other potentially hazardous activities until reaction to drug is known.
- Advise patient not to take alcohol or other CNS depressant unless approved by physician.
- Treatment of cough is directed toward decreasing frequency and intensity of cough

CODEINE PHOSPHATE (continued)

without abolishing protective cough reflex, which serves the important function of removing bronchial secretions.

- Excessive nonproductive cough tends to be self-perpetuating because it causes irritation of pharyngeal and tracheal mucosa.
- Inform patient that hyperactive cough may be lessened by voluntary restraint and by avoiding irritants such as smoking, dust, fumes, and other air pollutants. Humidification of ambient air may provide some relief. *See Nursing Interventions: Inhalation therapy.*
- Preserved in tight, light-resistant containers preferably between 15° and 30°C (59° and 86°F) unless otherwise directed by manufacturer.
- *See morphine sulphate* (opiate agonist).

DRUG INTERACTIONS   *Codeine*

PLUS	INTERACTIONS
Alcohol (ethanol), barbiturates and other CNS depressants	Additive CNS depression. Used concomitantly with caution if at all

Colchicine

Antigout agent

ACTIONS AND USES   Alkaloid of the autumn crocus *Colchicum autumnale* with antimitotic and indirect antiinflammatory properties. Selective action in gouty arthritis believed to be related to inhibition of microtubule formation in leucocytes thus interfering with their migration and phagocytosis in gouty joints. Lactic acid produced by phagocytosis is reduced, and crystal deposition fostered by acid pH is decreased. The net effect is inhibition of inflammation and reduction of pain and swelling. Colchicine is nonanalgesic and nonuricosuric. Direct action on bone marrow produces temporary leucopenia later replaced by leucocytosis. Stimulates prostaglandin synthesis which may be one of the reasons for GI side effects. Tends to increase faecal excretion of Na, K, fat, nitrogen, and carotene and in large doses may reduce serum cholesterol and interfere with absorption of vitamin B_{12} (cyanocobalamin). Tolerance to colchicine does not develop.

Used prophylactically for recurrent gouty arthritis and as specific for acute gout, either as single agent or in combination with a uricosuric such as probenecid, allopurinol, or sulphinpyrazone.

ROUTE AND DOSAGE   Oral: Acute gouty attack: *Initial*: 1 mg, then 500 mcg every 2–3 hrs until pain is relieved or until GI symptoms (nausea, vomiting, abdominal pain) occur or a total of 10 mg is reached. Repeat only after 3 days. **Prophylaxis**: 500 mcg 2–3 times a day.

COLCHICINE (continued)

ABSORPTION AND FATE   Following oral administration, rapidly absorbed from GI tract and partially metabolized in liver. Metabolites and active drug recycled to intestinal tract via biliary and intestinal secretions. **Plasma levels peak** in 0.5 to 2 hours then decline for 1 to 2 hours before increasing again because of recycling. High concentrations appear in leucocytes, kidney, liver, spleen, and intestinal tract. **Plasma half-life** is 20 minutes; **half-life in leucocytes** is about 60 minutes. Partly deacetylated in liver. Metabolites and active drug excreted primarily in faeces; 10 to 20% (variable) excreted in urine.

CONTRAINDICATIONS AND PRECAUTIONS   Hypersensitivity to colchicine; blood dyscrasias; severe GI, renal, hepatic, or cardiac disease. Safe use during pregnancy, and in nursing mothers and children not established. **Cautious Use**: elderly and debilitated patients, early manifestations of GI, renal, hepatic, or cardiac impairment.

ADVERSE/SIDE EFFECTS   Dose-related: These include: mental confusion, peripheral neuritis (numbness, tingling, pain, or weakness of hands or feet); loss of deep tendon reflexes, ascending CNS paralysis, respiratory failure, fever, delirium, convulsions, nausea, vomiting, diarrhoea, abdominal pain, anorexia, haemorrhagic gastroenteritis, steatorrhoea, hepatotoxicity, pancreatitis, paralytic ileus (overdosage), severe neutropenia (with IV use), bone marrow depression (leucopenia followed by leucocytosis), thrombocytopenia, agranulocytosis, aplastic anaemia, azotemia, proteinuria, haematuria; oliguria, burning sensations of throat, stomach, skin (overdosage), malabsorption syndrome, alopecia, bladder spasms, muscular weakness, hypothyroidism; arrhythmias, hypotension (large doses).

NURSING IMPLICATIONS

- Administer oral drug with milk or food to reduce possibility of GI upset.
- Baseline and periodic determinations of serum uric acid are advised, as well as complete blood count, including haemoglobin.
- Side effects (dose-related) are most likely to occur during the initial course of treatment. A latent period of several hours between drug administration and onset of toxic symptoms is usual.
- Early signs of colchicine toxicity include weakness, abdominal discomfort, anorexia, nausea, vomiting, and diarrhoea, regardless of administration route. Report to physician. To avoid more serious toxicity, drug should be discontinued promptly until symptoms subside. Diarrhoea may require treatment with an antidiarrhoeal agent.
- Monitor fluid intake and output (during acute gouty attack). High fluid intake promotes urate excretion and reduces danger of crystal formation in kidneys and ureters; intake is usually prescribed to maintain urinary output of at least 2,000 ml/day.
- Since acute gout can be precipitated by even minor surgical procedures, the patient is usually given colchicine before and after surgery.
- To avoid cumulative toxicity, a given course of colchicine therapy for acute gout is generally not repeated within 3 days.
- During an acute attack, weight-bearing and heat to involved joint should be avoided.

COLCHICINE (continued)

Bed cradle to keep off weight of bedclothes and elevation of gouty foot may provide relief. Mobilization is permitted when joint is no longer painful. Physical therapy and self-help devices may be indicated for patients with residual disability.

- Gout commonly occurs in the great toe; however, the instep, ankle, and knee are also common sites. Wrist, finger, or elbow may be affected with recurrent attacks.
- Keep physician informed of patient's progress. Drug should be stopped when pain of acute gout is relieved. Therapeutic response: articular pain and swelling generally subside within 8 to 12 hours and usually disappear in 24 to 72 hours after oral therapy.
- Patients taking colchicine at home should be advised to withhold drug and report to the physician the onset of GI symptoms or signs of bone marrow depression (nausea, sore throat, bleeding gums, sore mouth, fever, fatigue, malaise, unusual bleeding or bruising).
- Patients with gout should be instructed to keep colchicine at hand at all times so that they can start therapy or increase dosage, as prescribed by physician, at the first suggestion of an acute attack. An attack can be aborted or reduced in severity by early recognition of prodromal signs: local pruritus or discomfort in joint, mood changes, diuresis.

Food–drug interactions

- Long-term dietary management for patients with gout includes gradual weight reduction for obese patients (no more than 2 to 2½ lb/week, 1–1.5 kgs a week). Sudden weight loss can precipitate a gouty attack. Physician may prescribe a diet high in carbohydrate, with moderate protein and low fat. To potentiate action of colchicine, some physicians advise increased intake of alkaline ash foods: milk, most fruits and vegetables, with the exception of corn, lentils, plums, prunes, cranberries. (Marked urinary acidity tends to occur during acute gout.)
- A low-purine diet contains almost no meat and therefore is unpleasant for most patients (seldom prescribed today since the use of a gout suppressant obviates the need for strict diet therapy). Some physicians merely advise patient to limit intake of high purine foods such as liver, kidney, sweetbreads. Other foods high in purine content include wild game, goose, pork, caviar, anchovies, herring, sardines, mackerel, scallops, broth, meat extracts, gravy. Foods containing moderate amounts of purines include other meats, fish, seafood, fowl, asparagus, spinach, peas, and dried legumes.

- Physician may prescribe sodium bicarbonate, or sodium or potassium citrate, to maintain alkaline urine and thus prevent formation of urate stones.
- In addition to diet prescription:

Teaching plan for patients with chronic gout

- ☐ Nature and volume of fluid intake.
- ☐ How to test urine pH with reagent strip.
- ☐ Importance of early recognition of prodromal symptoms of an acute attack.
- ☐ Importance of keeping drug at hand at all times and of initiating prescribed drug regimen when prodromal symptoms appear.

COLCHICINE (continued)

☐ Adverse drug reactions that should be reported.

☐ Medical follow-up appointment schedule.

☐ Atiological factors in acute gout: (a) trauma, e.g., poor-fitting shoes and socks, (b) overindulgence of food or alcohol, (c) fatigue, (d) emotional or physical stress, (e) infections, (f) surgery.

☐ Confer with physician for specific guidelines.

■ Fermented beverages such as beer, ale, and wine may precipitate gouty attack and therefore should be avoided. The physician may allow distilled alcoholic beverages in moderation. Large amounts of alcohol reportedly can reduce the effects of colchicine.

■ Preserved in tight, light-resistant containers preferably between 15° and 30°C (59° and 86°F) unless otherwise directed by manufacturer.

Diagnostic test interferences   Colchicine tends to reduce **serum cholesterol**, and **serum carotene** and may elevate **alkaline phosphatase**, **SGOT**, and **SGPT**. False-positive **urine tests for RBC's** and **haemoglobin** reported.

DRUG INTERACTIONS   *Colchicine*

PLUS	INTERACTIONS
Alcohol, ethyl	Large amounts may decrease effects of colchicine
CNS depressants	Colchicine may sensitize patients to these drugs
Sympathomimetic agents	Enhanced response to these drugs (based on animal studies)
Vitamin B$_{12}$ (cyanocobalamin)	Colchicine can cause malabsorption of vitamin B$_{12}$
Acidifying agents; alkalinizing agents	Colchicine action is inhibited by acidifying agents and potentiated by alkalinizing agents

Colestipol hydrochloride

(Colestid)

ACTIONS AND USES   Resin exchange agent used to lower cholesterol levels.

ROUTE AND DOSAGE   5–10 g/day in divided doses before meals.
For further information *see cholestyramine.*

Colistin sulphate

(Colomycin)   *Antibiotic (polypeptide);*
                                                          polymyxin

COLISTIN SULPHATE (continued)
ACTIONS AND USES   Polymyxin antibiotic derived from *Bacillus polymyxa var. colistinus*. Similar to polymyxin B (q.v.) in actions, contraindications, precautions, and adverse reactions. Antibacterial potency appears to be equal to that of polymyxin B. Bactericidal against most gram-negative enteric pathogens especially *Escherichia coli*, *Shigella*, *Pseudomonas aeruginosa*, *Klebsiella pneumoniae*, and *Aerobacter aerogenes*. Not effective against *Proteus* or gram-positive microorganisms.

Used to treat diarrhoea in infants and children, caused by susceptible organisms, and to minimise bowel flora, in neutropenic patients.

ROUTE AND DOSAGE   Oral: 1.5–3 million units/8 hrly. **Intramuscular and intravenous**: 2 million units/8 hrly.

For further information *see polymyxin B*.

Corticotropin

(ACTH, Acthar)   *Hormone; glucocorticoid*

ACTIONS AND USES   Adrenocorticotropic hormone extracted from pituitary of domestic animals (usually pigs). Stimulates functioning adrenal cortex to produce and secrete corticosterone, cortisol (hydrocortisone), several weak androgens and limited amounts of aldosterone. Therapeutic effects appear more rapidly than do those of hydrocortisone (q.v.). Suppresses further release of corticotropin by negative feedback mechanism. Chronic administration of exogenous cortico steroids decreases ACTH store and causes structural changes in pituitary. Lack of ACTH stimulation can lead to adrenal cortex atrophy.

Used for diagnostic test of adrenocortical function and to treat adrenal insufficiency produced by cortisone, hydrocortisone, prednisone, and other corticosteroids by direct stimulation of atrophic adrenal gland. Used for its antiinflammatory and immunosuppressant properties and its effect on blood and lymphatic systems. Also used in the symptomatic treatment of acute exacerbation of multiple sclerosis and to increase muscle strength in patients with severe myasthenia gravis that is refractory to treatment with anticholinesterases. *See also hydrocortisone*.

ROUTE AND DOSAGE   **Subcutaneous and intramuscular** (depot preparations): *initially* 40–80 units/day, reduced according to response.

ABSORPTION AND FATE   Rapid absorption with **onset of action** within 6 hours following injection. **Duration of action** about 2 to 4 hours; **half-life** less than 20 minutes. (Repository preparations: absorption over an 8- to 16-hour period; duration of effect: 18 to 72 hours.) Binds to plasma proteins and concentrates in many tissues. Excreted in urine. Probably does not cross placenta.

CONTRAINDICATIONS AND PRECAUTIONS   Ocular herpes simplex, recent surgery,

CORTICOTROPIN (continued)

congestive heart failure, scleroderma, osteoporosis, systemic fungoid infections, hypertension, sensitivity to porcine proteins, conditions accompanied by primary adrenocortical insufficiency or hyperfunction. Use during pregnancy, in lactating women or women in childbearing years requires evaluation of expected benefits against possible hazards to mother and child. **Cautious Use**: patients with latent tuberculosis or those reacting to tuberculin; hypothyroiditis, impaired hepatic function. *See also hydrocortisone.*

ADVERSE/SIDE EFFECTS   (Usually reversible with discontinuation of treatment.) Hypersensitivity, Na and water retention, increased K excretion, calcium loss, impaired wound healing, reactivation of tuberculosis. With prolonged use: antibody production, loss of stimulating effect of ACTH, post-subcapsular cataracts, glaucoma, possible damage to optic nerve, pancreatitis. *See also hydrocortisone.*

NURSING IMPLICATIONS

- Verification tests (for adrenal responsiveness to corticotropin) are recommended prior to treatment using the route of administration proposed for treatment (IM or SC).
- Before giving corticotropin to patient with suspected sensitivity to porcine proteins, hypersensitivity skin testing should be performed.
- Dosage is individualized according to disease being treated and medical condition of patient. Changes in dosage regimen are gradual and only after full drug effects have become apparent.
- Observe patient closely for 15 minutes for hypersensitivity reactions during IV administration or immediately after SC or IM injections. Adrenaline 1:1,000 should be readily available for emergency treatment.
- Adrenal response to corticotropin is measured against a baseline plasma cortisol level 1 hour before the 8-hour test.
- Before, during, and after an unusual stressful event, rapidly acting corticosteroids may be given to supplement activity of corticotropin.
- Corticotropin does not alter natural course of disease but may only suppress signs and symptoms of chronic disease.
- Prolonged use increases risk of hypersensitivity reaction (skin reactions, dizziness, nausea, vomiting, mild fever, anaphylactic shock, wheezing, circulatory failure, death).
- New infections, e.g., fungal or virus infection of eye, can appear during treatment. Because of decreased resistance and inability to localize the infection, it may be severe. Report immediately. Antiinfective therapy is indicated.
- Eye examinations should be done before expected long-term therapy and periodically during treatment. Instruct patient to report to physician if blurred vision occurs.
- Growth and development of a child receiving this drug should be carefully monitored.
- Dietary salt restriction and K supplementation may be necessary to minimize oedema caused by overstimulation of the adrenal cortex by corticotropin. Facilitate information-exchange conferences related to patient's diet-drug therapies with nutritionist, physician, patient, and responsible family member.
- Patient should not be vaccinated while receiving corticotropin.

CORTICOTROPIN (continued)

■ Adminstration of the hormone at high dosage levels is tapered rather than withdrawn suddenly. A 2- to 5-day period of adrenocortical hypofunction follows discontinuation of corticotropin.

■ *See also hydrocortisone.*

Cortisone acetate ────────────────────

(Cortelan, Cortistab, Cortisyl)   *Corticosteriod; glucocorticoid;*
                                               mineralocorticoid

ACTIONS AND USES   Short-acting synthetic steroid with prominent glucocorticoid actions and in high doses, mineralocorticoid properties. Therapeutic activity depends on *in vivo* conversion to hydrocortisone (q.v.), with which it shares uses, absorption, fate, contraindications, adverse/side effects, and interactions.

ROUTE AND DOSAGE   Highly individualized. **Adults: Oral, Intramuscular:** *Initial*: 25 to 3 mg daily, as single or divided doses.

ABSORPTION AND FATE   Rapid onset after oral administration but slow (24 to 48 hours) after IM administration. **Peak effect** (oral): 2 hours; (IM), 20 to 48 hours. **Duration of action**: 1.25 to 1.5 days. **Half-life (plasma)**: 0.5 hours. **HPA** (hypothalamic–pituitary–adrenal). Axis suppression: 8 to 12 hours.

CONTRAINDICATIONS AND PRECAUTIONS   Safe use in pregnancy, during lactation, or by children not established. *See hydrocortisone.*

NURSING IMPLICATIONS

■ Sodium chloride and a mineralocorticoid are usually given with cortisone as part of replacement therapy.

■ Store at temperature between 15° and 30°C (59° and 86°F) in well-closed container, unless otherwise directed by manufacturer.

■ *See hydrocortisone for additional Nursing Implications and Drug Interactions.*

Co–trimoxazole ────────────────────

(Batrim, Chemotrim, Comox, Fectrim, Laratrim,   *Antiinfective*
    Septrin)

ACTIONS AND USES   A combination of 5 parts sulphamethoxazole and 1 part trimethoprim which act synergistically to prevent folate synthesis in bacteria. By

CO-TRIMOXAZOLE (continued)

inhibiting chemical reactions at sequential points in the same pathway, maximum potentiation of each drug occurs and the possibility of adaptive resistance is reduced.

Used to treat infections due to *H. Influenzae*, urinary tract infections, sinusitis, chronic bronchitis, typhoid fever and invasive salmonellosis. Also used for brucellosis and *Pneumocystis carnii* infections, pyoderma and wound infections.

ROUTE AND DOSAGE   Oral: adult: 960 mg/12 hourly up to 1.44 g may be given in severe infections, dose reduced to 480 mg/12 hourly when treatment continues for more than 14 days. **Child (6 weeks to 5 months):** 120 mg/12 hourly; **(6 months to 5 years):** 240 mg/12 hourly; **(6–12 years):** 480 mg/12 hourly. *Gonorrhoea*: 1.92 g every 12 hours for 2 days. **IM injection/IV infusion: adult:** 960 mg/12 hourly.

CONTRAINDICATIONS AND PRECAUTIONS   Use should be avoided in patients with a history of sulphonamide or trimethoprim hypersensitivity, pregnancy, infants under six weeks, renal or hepatic failure or haematological disorders.

ADVERSE/SIDE EFFECTS   Nausea, vomiting, glossitis, diarrhoea, rashes, erythema multiforme, purpura, agranulocytopenia, agranulocytosis, megaloblastic anaemia.

NURSING IMPLICATIONS
- Monitor fluid intake and output; an adequate fluid intake is required to prevent crystalluria.
- Be alert for signs of hypoglycaemia in patients taking oral antidiabetic drugs.
- Prepare intravenous drug by dilution according to manufacturers instructions immediately before administration, ensure thorough mixing.
- Discard turbid or crystallized infusion.
- Do not confuse intramuscular and intravenous preparations; they are *not* interchangeable.
- *See also sulphadiazine and trimethoprim.*
- Store at room temperature.

Cyanocobalamin ——————————————

(Cytacon, Cytamen, Heptacon)   *Vitamin B$_{12}$; antianaemic*

ACTIONS AND USES   Vitamin B$_{12}$ is a cobalt-containing substance produced by *Streptomyces griseus*. Essential for normal growth, cell reproduction, maturation of RBC's, nucleoprotein synthesis, maintanance of nervous system (myelin synthesis), and believed to be involved in protein and carbohydrate metabolism. Now, most often used for vitamin B$_{12}$ absorption (Schilling) test.

ROUTE AND DOSAGE   Intramuscular: *initial* 1 mg every 2–3 days for 10 doses then *maintenance* of 1 mg/month.

Cyclandelate ▬▬▬▬▬▬▬▬▬▬▬▬▬▬▬▬▬▬▬▬▬▬▬▬▬▬

(Cyclobral, Cyclospasmol)   *Vasodilator; peripheral*

ACTIONS AND USES   Produces vasodilation by exerting papaverinelike relaxation of peripheral vascular smooth muscle by direct action. Principle effect is on vascular smooth muscle. Has no significant adrenergic stimulating or blocking actions.

Used as adjunctive therapy in arteriosclerosis obliterans, intermittent claudication, thrombophlebitis (to control associated vasospasm and muscular ischaemia), nocturnal leg cramps, Raynaud's phenomenon, and in selected cases of ischaemic cerebrovascular disease. Clinical effectiveness not confirmed.

ROUTE AND DOSAGE   Oral: 1.2–1.6 g/day in divided doses.

ABSORPTION AND FATE   Readily absorbed from GI tract. Effects appear in 15 minutes, with maximum response in about 1 to 1½ hours. Duration of action approximately 3 to 4 hours. Metabolic fate unknown.

CONTRAINDICATIONS AND PRECAUTIONS   Known hypersensitivity to cyclandelate. Safe use during pregnancy and in nursing mothers not established. **Cautious Use**: severe obliterative coronary artery or cerebrovascular disease, recent myocardial infarction, bleeding tendencies, active bleeding, glaucoma, hypertension.

ADVERSE/SIDE EFFECTS   Reported to be relatively nontoxic. Infrequent: dizziness, facial flushing, sweating, tingling sensation in face, fingers, toes; tachycardia, weakness, headache; GI disturbances: heartburn (pyrosis), eructation, stomach pain, possible prolongation of bleeding time (high doses).

NURSING IMPLICATIONS
- GI distress may be relieved by taking medication with meals, milk, or an antacid (if prescribed).
- Some patients experience mild flushing, headaches, weakness, and tachycardia during the first week of therapy, requiring dosage reduction.
- Cyclandelate can cause dizziness in some patients. Caution patient to make position changes slowly particularly from recumbent to upright posture and to dangle legs over bed for a few minutes before ambulating. Also instruct patient to lie down if feels faint or dizzy, and to notify physician if these symptoms persist.
- Patient should be informed that improvement usually occurs gradually and that prolonged therapy may be necessary.
- Therapeutic effect on peripheral circulation may be manifested by: slight rise in skin temperature, increased pulse volume, the ability to walk longer distances without discomfort, and lessened pain.
- Meticulous hygiene is an important adjunct in treatment of peripheral vascular problems.
- *See isoxuprine hydrochloride for additional patient teaching points.*
- Since nicotine constricts blood vessels, patient should be advised to stop smoking.

CYCLANDELATE (continued)
■ Store in well-closed container preferably between 15° and 30°C (59° and 86°F) unless otherwise directed by manufacturer.

Cyclizine

(Valoid)

Antihistamine; antiemetic

ACTIONS AND USES   Piperazine derivative antihistamine (H_1-receptor blocking agent) structurally and pharmacologically related to other cyclizine compounds (e.g., buclizine, hydroxyzine, meclizine). In common with these agents, it exhibits CNS depression and anticholinergic, antispasmodic, local anaesthetic, and antihistaminic activity. Has prominent depressant action on labyrinthine excitability and on conduction in vestibular-cerebellar pathways, thus producing marked antimotion and antiemetic effects. Precise mechanism of action not known.

Used chiefly for prevention and treatment of motion sickness and postoperative nausea and vomiting.

ROUTE AND DOSAGE   **Adults: Oral/IM/IV:** 50 mg every 4 to 6 hours as needed; not to exceed 200 mg daily. **Children (up to 10 years):** 25 mg three times a day.

ABSORPTION AND FATE   Rapid onset of action, with duration of 4 to 6 hours. Metabolic fate unknown.

CONTRAINDICATIONS AND PRECAUTIONS   Hypersensitivity to cyclizine; pregnancy, women of childbearing potential, nursing mothers, children under 6 years of age. **Cautious Use:** narrow-angle glaucoma, prostatic hypertrophy, obstructive disease of GU and GI tracts; postoperative patients. Epilepsy, liver disease, prostatic hypertrophy.

ADVERSE/SIDE EFFECTS   Usually dose-related: hypotension, palpitation, tachycardia, drowsiness, vertigo, dizziness, restlessness, excitement, insomnia, euphoria, auditory and visual hallucinations, hyperexcitability alternating with drowsiness, convulsions, respiratory paralysis, dry mouth, nose and throat; blurred vision, diplopia, tinnitus, anorexia, nausea, vomiting, diarrhoea or constipation, difficult or painful urination, urinary retention or frequency. **Hypersensitivity:** urticaria, rash, cholestatic jaundice, anaphylaxis (inadvertent IV administration).

NURSING IMPLICATIONS
■ Advise patient to take cyclizine with food or a glass of milk or water to minimize GI irritation.
■ Aspirate carefully before injecting IM to avoid entry into a blood vessel. Anaphylactic reactions following inadvertent IV have been reported.
■ Forewarn patient about side effects of drowsiness and dizziness and advise not to drive

CYCLIZINE (continued)
a car or engage in other potentially hazardous activities until reaction to the drug is known.
- Caution patient that sedative action may be additive to that of alcohol, barbiturates, narcotic analgesic, and other CNS depressants.
- Recommended dosage when used to prevent motion sickness: 1 tablet (50 mg) ½ hour before anticipated departure, repeated in 4 to 6 hours if required. No more than 4 tablets should be taken in 1 day. For succeeding days of travel, 50 mg 3 times daily before meals. Continued administration after first 2 or 3 days of extended travel may be unnecessary.
- Advise patient taking cyclizine to relieve motion sickness by positioning him- or herself during travel where there is least motion (e.g., over wing of plane, or amidships), to avoid reading, and to refrain from excessive eating or drinking while travelling.
- For prophylaxis of postoperative nausea and vomiting, cyclizine is usually prescribed with preoperative medication or is administered 20 to 30 minutes before expected termination of surgery.
- Since cyclizine can cause hypotension, the postoperative patient receiving the drug will require close monitoring of vital signs.
- Dry mouth may be relieved by rinsing mouth with clear water or by sugarless gum or lemon drops.
- Store tablets in tight, light-resistant container, preferably between 15° and 30°C (59° and 86°F) unless otherwise directed by manufacturer. Store parenteral form in a cold place preferably between 5° and 10°C (41° and 50°F). When parenteral solution is stored at room temperature for prolonged periods it may become slightly yellow, but this does not indicate loss of potency.

Diagnostic test interferences   Since cyclizine is an antihistamine, inform patient that **skin testing** procedures should not be scheduled for about 4 days after drug is discontinued or false-negative reactions may result.

Drug interactions   Cyclizine may have additive effects with **alcohol, barbiturates, CNS depressants** (i.e., hypnotics, sedatives, tranquilizers, and anxiolytic agents), and it may mask signs of ototoxicity produced by **aminoglycoside antibiotics, aspirin,** or other **salicylates.**

Cyclopenthiazide ▬▬▬▬▬▬▬▬▬▬▬▬▬▬▬▬

(Navidrex)

For further information *see bendrofluazide*

ROUTE AND DOSAGE   *Oedema*: *initial* 0.5 – 1 mg in the morning, then 500 mcg on alternate days. *Hypertension*: 250 – 500 mcg in the morning, *maximum* 1.5 mg/day.

Cyclophosphamide ━━━━━━━━━━━━━━━━━━━━━━

(Endoxana)

Antineoplastic; alkylating agent; immunosuppressant; nitrogen mustard

C

ACTIONS AND USES   Cell cycle nonspecific alkylating agent chemically related to the nitrogen mustards. Has pronounced immunosuppressive activity and is a highly toxic drug; thus therapeutic effects are usually accompanied by evidence of toxicity. Associated with increased risk of development of secondary malignancies, including urinary bladder, myeloproliferative and lymphoproliferative malignancies. These may be detected several years after cyclophosphamide has been discontinued. Paternal use of drug in combination therapy prior to conception has been associated with cardiac and lymph abnormalities in the infant. Advantages over other nitrogen mustards include oral effectiveness and the possibility of giving fractional doses over long periods of time.

Used as single agent or in combination with other chemotherapeutic agents in treatment of malignant lymphoma, multiple myeloma, leukaemias, mycosis fungoides (advanced disease), neuroblastoma, adenocarcinoma of ovary. Carcinoma of breast or malignant neoplasms of lung are infrequently responsive.

ROUTE AND DOSAGE   **Intravenous or oral**: Individualized.

ABSORPTION AND FATE   Completely absorbed from GI tract and parenteral sites. Disappears rapidly from plasma, with peak concentration 1 hour after oral dose. Hepatic metabolism. Following IV administration, **half-life** is 4 to 6 hours, but drug and metabolites may be detected in plasma up to 72 hours. Distributed throughout body including brain and CSF. **Protein binding**: 10 to 56%. Excreted in urine as metabolites; less than 25% as unchanged drug. Crosses blood–brain barrier and is excreted in breast milk.

CONTRAINDICATIONS AND PRECAUTIONS   Men and women in childbearing years, serious infections (including chicken pox, herpes zoster); myelosuppression, pregnancy, lactation. **Cautious Use**: history of radiation or cytotoxic drug therapy, hepatic and renal impairment, recent history of steroid therapy, varicella-zoster and other infections, bone marrow infiltration with tumour cells, history of urate calculi and gout, patient with leucopenia, thrombocytopenia.

ADVERSE/SIDE EFFECTS   These include: alopecia, transverse ridging and darkening of nails and skin, nonspecific dermatitis, nausea, vomiting, mucositis, anorexia, hepatotoxicity, diarrhoea, sterile haemorrhagic and nonhaemorrhagic cystitis, bladder fibrosis, nephrotoxicity, gonadal suppression (amenorrhoea, azoospermia, oligospermia possibly irreversible). Severe hyperkalaemia, hyponatraemia, weight gain (but without oedema) or weight loss, hyperuricaemia. Leucopenia, thrombocytopenia, anaemia, thrombophlebitis, suppression of positive reactions to skin tests, interference with normal healing, pulmonary emboli and oedema, interstitial pulmonary fibrosis, transient dizziness, fatigue, facial flushing, diaphoresis, fever, anaphylaxis, cardiotoxicity.

CYCLOPHOSPHAMIDE (continued)
NURSING IMPLICATIONS

- Administer oral drug on empty stomach. If nausea and vomiting are severe, however, take drug with food. An antiemetic medication given before this drug may control GI reactions.
- **IV solution**: To reconstitute add sterile water for injection to vial and shake vigorously to dissolve (5 ml to 100 mg vial). Should be used within 24 hours.
- Usually extravasation does not cause local irritation, unlike other nitrogen mustards.
- Total WBC and thrombocyte counts are determined at least twice a week during maintenance period. Periodic determinations of liver and kidney function and serum electroytes should be made.
- Marked leucopenia is the most serious side effect. Nadir may occur in 2 to 8 days after first dose, but may be as late as 1 month after a series of several daily doses.
- Leucopenia usually reverses 7 to 10 days after therapy is discontinued. Has been fatal.
- Check leucocyte count. During severe leucopenic period, protect the patient from infection and trauma, and from visitors and medical personnel who have colds or other infections.
- Report onset of unexplained fever, chills, sore throat, tachycardia.
- During period of neutropenia, purulent drainage may become serosanguinous because there are not enough WBC to result in pus. Monitor temperature carefully and report elevation of 38°C or higher. Observe and report character of wound drainage.
- The immunosuppressive property of cyclophosphamide makes the patient particularly susceptible to varicella-zoster infections (chicken pox, herpes zoster).
- Because of suppressed immune mechanisms wound healing may be prolonged or incomplete.
- Untreated stomatitis is not only uncomfortable, it also interferes with drinking and eating.
- Anorexia should not be ignored. Plan with patient, dietitian, and physician a nutritional regimen, especially for leucopenic period.
- Report any sign of overgrowth with opportunistic organisms (black furry or white, patchy appearance of tongue and oral membranes; diarrhoea, foul-smelling stools; vulvar itching and vaginal discharge, cough) especially if patient is also receiving corticosteroids or has recently been on steroid therapy.
- Maintenance of nutrition may depend as much on taste as on any other one factor. Discuss changing preferences for foods with patient and family member. When the patient experiences decreased (but not absent) taste (hypogeusia), cold foods high in protein with added flavourings may be liked best (e.g., ice cream, gelatin salad with cream or cottage cheese, fruit stuffed with peanut butter, puddings, custards). Increased sugar added to foods, and highly seasoned foods also seem to be tolerated and preferred. Meat is frequently rejected, but alternative protein sources (eggs, fish, milk) may be accepted. Consult dietitian for suggestions.
- If a pattern to nausea and vomiting can be detected, an attempt should be made to plan the treatment/meals/antiemetic so as not to confront patient with food or start therapy when nausea is at its peak.

CYCLOPHOSPHAMIDE (continued)

- If a strong anti emetic is given only once a day, administering it late in the evening with a sedative may help the patient tolerate nausea.

- Nausea has a strong suggestive component; the public is becoming increasingly aware that nausea and vomiting often accompany cancer chemotherapy. The patient needs to believe that antiemetic therapy will help. Listen, however, to patient's or family's suggestions about what might also help and if possible implement these suggestions. Vomiting can be the strongest reason for refusing further treatment. *See estramustine for additional notes.*

- Diarrhoea may signal onset of hyperkalaemia, particularly if accompanied by colicky pain, nausea, bradycardia, and skeletal muscle weakness. These symptoms warrant prompt reporting to physician.

- Promptly report haematuria or dysuria. Drug schedule is usually interrupted and fluids are forced. Alert patient to the fact that haematuria may resolve spontaneously, or it may persist several months. In some cases, it has been serious enough to require transfusions.

- Hyperuricaemia occurs commonly during early treatment period in patients with leukaemias or lymphoma. Report oedema of lower legs and feet, joint flank, or stomach pain. Alkalinization of urine, hydration, and allopurinol may prevent this side effect.

- Fluid intake and output ratio should be monitored. Since drug is a chemical irritant, fluid intake is generally increased to prevent renal irritation.

- When high doses are used mesna is used to reduce the MSK of haemorrhagic cystitis.

- Encourage the patient to start increased fluid intake early in the day to reduce night voiding when extra fluids are required.

- Since patients are usually well hydrated as part of the therapy, watch for symptoms of dilutional hyponatraemia (excess body Na with low serum Na): lethargy, confusion, headache, decreased skin turgor, tremors, convulsions. Should this condition occur, fluid intake may be reduced.

- Report fever, dyspnoea, and nonproductive cough. Pulmonary toxicity is not usual but the already debilitated patient is particularly susceptible.

- Record body weight at least twice weekly (basis for dose determination). Alert physician to sudden change or slow, steady weight gain or loss over a period of time that appears inconsistent with caloric intake.

- Observe and report signs of hepatotoxicity (frothy dark urine, light-coloured stools, jaundice, pruritus) most apt to appear in the patient with liver impairment prior to institution of cyclophosphamide therapy.

- Because of mutagenic potential, adequate means of contraception should be employed during and for at least 4 months after termination of drug treatment. Breast feeding should be discontinued before cyclophosphamide therapy is initiated.

- Skin and nails may become darker during therapy and nonspecific dermatitis has been reported. These side effects are usually reversible.

- Alopecia occurs in about 33% of patients on cyclophosphamide therapy. Discuss the possibility with the patient early in therapy. Hair loss may be noted 3 weeks after therapy begins; regrowth (may differ in texture and colour) usually starts 5 to 6 weeks

CYCLOPHOSPHAMIDE (continued)

after drug is withheld and may occur while patient is on maintenance doses. This side effect, related as it is to sexuality and self-image, requires much understanding. Help the patient to plan for cosmetic substitution if desired.

- Amenorrhoea may last up to 1 year after cessation of therapy in 10 to 30% of women receiving cyclophosphamide (due to lack of follicular maturation).
- Urge patient to adhere to dosage regimen: he or she should not omit, increase, decrease, or delay doses; if for any reason the drug cannot be taken, notify the physician.
- Cyclophosphamide may be carcinogenic; therefore, prolonged follow-up of patient following cyclophosphamide treatment is important; reportedly many years may elapse between treatment and development of bladder cancer.
- Consult physician about plans for disclosure of diagnosis, prognosis and particulars about treatment so that discussions with patient and family are supportive and nonconflicting.
- Store at temperature between 2° and 30°C (36° and 90°F) unless otherwise recommended by the manufacturer.

Diagnostic test interferences Cyclophosphamide increases **blood** and **urine uric acid**, decreases **serum pseudocholinesterase**, and suppresses positive reactions to **Candida, mumps, trichophyta, tuberculin PPD**. May cause a false-positive **Papanicolaou (PAP) test.**

DRUG INTERACTIONS *Cyclophosphamide* _____

PLUS	INTERACTIONS
Allopurinol	May inhibit hepatic microsomal enzyme activity, leading to enhanced pharmacological effects of cyclophosphamide and bone marrow toxicity
Antigout agents	Elevates serum and urine uric acid levels necessitating dose adjustment of antigout agent
Chloramphenicol Chloroquine Corticosteroids	*See allopurinol (above)*
Daunorubicin Doxorubicin	May increase potential for cardiotoxicity
Imipramine	*See Allopurinol (above)*
Phenobarbitone	Increases rate of drug metabolism and leucopenic activity of cyclophosphamide
Phenothiazines Postassium chloride Sex hormones	*See allopurinol (above)*
Succinylcholine	Inhibits metabolism of succinylcholine leading to prolonged neuromuscular blocking activity (apnoea). Used with caution
Vitamin A	*See allopurinol (above)*
Oral antidiabetics	A change in hypoglycaemic therapy may be required

Cycloserine

*Antiinfective; antituberculosis
agent*

ACTIONS AND USES   Broad-spectrum antiinfective derived from strains of *Streptomyces orchidaceus* or *S. garyphalus*; also produced synthetically. Structural analogue of the amino acid D-alanine. Inhibits cell wall synthesis in susceptible strains of gram-positive and gram-negative bacteria and in *Mycobacterium tuberculosis* by competitively inhibiting the incorporation of D-alanine into the bacterial cell wall. May be bacteriostatic or bactericidal depending on concentration at site of infection and susceptibility of organism.

Used in treatment of tuberculosis unresponsive to conventional treatment.

ROUTE AND DOSAGE   **Oral**: Usual dose 250 mg 12 hrly. Daily dosage should not exceed 1 g.

ABSORPTION AND FATE   About 70 to 90% of dose readily absorbed from GI tract. **Serum levels peak** within 3 to 4 hours. Not bound to plasma proteins. Concentrations in lung, ascitic, pleural, synovial fluids approximately equal to plasma drug levels. Cerebrospinal fluid levels are about 50 to 80% of plasma levels when meninges are normal and 80 to 100% when meninges are inflamed. About 60 to 70% of drug is eliminated unchanged in urine within 72 hours. Small amounts excreted in faeces. Readily crosses placenta and may appear in breast milk.

CONTRAINDICATIONS AND PRECAUTIONS   Hypersensitivity to cycloserine; epilepsy, depression, severe anxiety, history of psychoses; severe renal insufficiency, chronic alcoholism. Safe use during pregnancy and safe paediatric use not established.

ADVERSE/SIDE EFFECTS   These include: dermatitis; photosensitivity, arrhythmias, congestive heart failure, vitamin B_{12} and/or folic acid deficiency, megaloblastic or sideroblastic anaemia, drowsiness, anxiety, headache, tremors, myoclonic jerking, convulsions, vertigo, visual disturbances, speech difficulties (dysarthria), lethargy, depression, disorientation with loss of memory; confusion, nervousness, psychoses (possibly with suicidal tendencies), character changes, hyperirritability, aggression, hyperreflexia, peripheral neuropathy, paraesthesias, paresis, dyskinesias, blurred vision, loss of vision, eye pain (optic neuritis), photophobia, abnormal liver function tests, jaundice, superinfections.

NURSING IMPLICATIONS
- Advise patient to take cycloserine after meals to prevent GI irritation.
- Culture and bacterial sensitivity tests should be performed prior to initiation of therapy and periodically thereafter to detect possible bacterial resistance.
- Monitoring of blood–drug levels, haematological, renal, and hepatic function at regular intervals is advised.
- Stress importance of compliance in following medication regimen as prescribed and in keeping follow-up appointments.

CYCLOSERINE (continued)

- Neurotoxic effects generally appear within first 2 weeks of therapy and disappear after drug is discontinued.
- Advise patient/responsible family member to notify physician immediately about onset of skin rash and early signs of neurotoxicity: drowsiness, confusion, headache, vertigo, anxiety, tremors, paraesthesias, behaviour changes.
- Drug should be discontinued or dosage reduced if symptoms of neurotoxicity or allergy develop.
- Advise patient to avoid potentially hazardous tasks such as driving until reaction to cycloserine has been determined.
- Caution patient to avoid alcoholic beverages. Ingestion of alcohol increases the risk of convulsive seizures.
- **Cycloserine overdosage** is treated with pyridoxine (vitamin B_6), anticonvulsants for seizure control, tranquilizers or sedative to control anxiety and tremors, and symptomatic and supportive therapy such as gastric lavage, oxygen, artificial respiration, measures for shock, and maintenance of body temperature.
- Store in well-closed container preferably between 15° and 30°C (59° and 86°F) unless otherwise directed by manufacturer.

Diagnostic test interferences   SGOT and SGPT levels may be increased.

DRUG INTERACTIONS   *Cycloserine*

PLUS	INTERACTIONS
Alcohol, ethyl	Increased risk of seizures especially with chronic alcohol abuse
Ethionamide ⎱ Isoniazid ⎰	Potentiate neurotoxic effects of cycloserine
Phenytoin	Possibility of phenytoin toxicity (cycloserine inhibits hepatic metabolism of phenytoin)

Cyclosporin

(Sandimmune)   *Immunosuppressant*

ACTIONS AND USES   Immunosuppressant agent derived from an extract of soil fungi. Action appears to be due to selective and reversible inhibition of helper-T lymphocytes (which normally stimulate antibody function), creating an imbalance in favour of suppressor T-lymphocytes (which inhibit antibody production), thus immune response is subdued. Does not cause significant bone marrow depression. Believed to have antimalarial, antischistosomal, as well as antifungal activity.

Used in conjunction with adrenal corticosteroids to prevent organ rejection after kidney, liver, and heart transplants (allografts). Has had limited use in pancreas, bone marrow, and heart/lung transplantations. Also used for treatment of chronic transplant

CYCLOSPORIN *(continued)*

rejection in patients previously treated with other immunosuppressants. Used prophylactically in selected patients to reduce severity of graft-vs-host reaction after bone marrow transplantation.

ROUTE AND DOSAGE   Highly individualized.

ABSORPTION AND FATE   Following oral administration, GI absorption is variable and incomplete (about 40% of dose is absorbed). Bioavailability may increase with dosage increments and longer duration of therapy. **Peak plasma concentrations** in 3 to 4 hours. Widely distributed to body tissues and fluids. Approximately 90% bound, primarily to lipoproteins. **Biphasic half-life**: 1.2 hours; 19 to 27 hours. Extensively metabolized in liver on first pass. Primarily eliminated in bile via faeces. About 6% excreted in urine (0.1% as unchanged drug). Crosses placenta. Excreted in breast milk.

CONTRAINDICATIONS AND PRECAUTIONS   Hypersensitivity to cyclosporin or to ingredients in commercially available formulations, e.g., Cremophor (polyoxyl 35 castor oil) in parenteral preparation. Safe use during pregnancy, in nursing women, and in children not established. **Cautious Use**: renal and hepatic function impairment, hypertension, infection, malabsorption problems.

ADVERSE/SIDE EFFECTS   These include: hypertension, myocardial infarction (rare), hirsutism, oily skin, acne, brittle fingernails, hair breaking, pruritus, ecchymoses or bruises (due to increased capillary permeability), sinusitis, tinnitus, hearing loss, sore throat, visual disturbances, conjunctivitis (rare), gum hyperplasia, diarrhoea, nausea, vomiting, abdominal discomfort, hepatotoxicity; infrequent: anorexia, gastritis, peptic ulcer, hiccoughs, mouth sores, swallowing difficulty, upper GI bleeding, pancreatitis, constipation, leucopenia, anaemia, thrombocytopenia, elevated hepatic functions tests (hepatotoxicity), abnormal renal function tests (nephrotoxicity), hyperkalaemia, hyperuricaemia, decreased serum bicarbonate, hyperglycaemia, anaphylaxis associated with polyoxyl 35 castor oil in IV formulation (flushing, dyspnoea, wheezing, hypotension, tachycardia, respiratory arrest), tremor, convulsions, headache, paraesthesias, hyperaesthesia, flushing, night sweats, confusion, anxiety, flat affect, depression, lethargy, weakness, quadriparesis, paraparesis ataxia, amnesia, urinary retention, frequency, haematuria, nephrotoxicity, haemolytic–uraemic syndrome (microangiopathic haemolytic anaemia, thrombocytopenia, hypertension, renal failure), benign fibroadenoma of breasts, lymphoma (causal relationships not established); gynaecomastia, chest pain, muscle and joint pain, leg cramps, oedema, fever, chills, weight loss, infections possibly due to concomitant corticosteroid therapy.

NURSING IMPLICATIONS
- Patient should be informed of the potential benefits and risks associated with the use of cyclosporin.
- Patients receiving the drug parenterally should be observed continuously for at least 30 minutes after start of IV infusion and at frequent intervals thereafter to detect allergic or other adverse reactions. Equipment for maintaining airway, epinephrine, and oxygen should be immediately available.

CYCLOSPORIN *(continued)*

- Hypersensitivity reactions have been associated with Cremophor emulsifying agent in the parenteral formulation, but not with the oral solution, which does not contain this ingredient. (Cremophor can cause phthalate stripping from PVC tubing.)

- Monitor fluid intake and output ratio and pattern. Nephrotoxicity has been reported in about ⅓ of transplant patients. It has occurred in mild forms as late as 2 to 3 months after transplantation. In severe form it can be irreversible and therefore early recognition is critically important.

- *Signs and symptoms suggestive of nephrotoxicity*: oliguria, urinary frequency, haematuria, cloudy urine, elevated BUN and serum creatinine associated with high trough drug levels. Laboratory values respond to dosage reduction.

- Signs of rejection in patients with renal transplant can be almost indistinguishable from nephrotoxicity. Indicators of graft rejection include low blood or plasma cyclosporin concentrations occurring with rapid rise in serum creatinine, fever, graft tenderness or enlargement. Laboratory values do not respond to dosage reduction.

- Monitor vital signs. Be alert to indicators of local or systemic infection which can be fungal, viral, or bacterial. Also report significant rise in blood pressure.

- Immunosuppression can occur with cyclosporin alone or in combination with corticosteroids. Although no causal relationship has been established, it appears that patients receiving cyclosporin may be more susceptible to infection and to development of lymphoma.

- Lymph glands and breasts should be gently palpated at periodic intervals (consult physician) to detect abnormalities. Patients who have received T-cell globulin appear to be particularly prone to develop these complications.

- Periodic tests should be made of neurological function. Neurotoxic effects generally occur over 13 to 195 days after initiation of cyclosporin therapy. Signs and symptoms are reportedly fully reversible with dosage reduction or discontinuation of drug. Symptoms appear to occur most commonly in cancer patients who have received prior intrathecal methotrexate, cyclophosphamide, or total body irradiation.

- Baseline and periodic tests are advised for (1) renal function (BUN, serum creatinine), (2) liver function (SGOT, SGPT, serum amylase, bilirubin, and alkaline phosphatase), and (3) serum potassium.

- Blood or plasma drug concentrations should be monitored at regular intervals particularly in patients receiving the drug orally for prolonged periods since drug absorption is erratic. Patients with hepatic transplants should also be closely monitored because they tend to absorb drug with difficulty.

- Advise patient to practise good oral hygiene: use soft tooth brush; brush gently (teeth and tongue); floss at least once daily; rinse or brush after food or sweet drinks; keep dental appointments. Some patients require gingivectomy for gingival hyperplasia.

- Reassure patient that hirsutism is reversible with discontinuation of drug.

- Before use, inspect concentrate for injection and diluted parenteral preparations for particulate matter and discolouration. Cyclosporin concentrate must be diluted immediately before administration: dilute each ml in 20 to 100 ml of 0.9% sodium chloride or 5% dextrose injection. Administered by slow infusion over approximately 2 to 6 hours, as prescribed by physician. Rapid IV can result in nephrotoxicity.

CYCLOSPORIN (continued)

Patient instructions regarding taking oral cyclosporin

☐ Take medication at same time each day to maintain therapeutic blood levels.

☐ Use the specially calibrated pipette provided to measure dose.

☐ Palatability of oral solution may be enhanced by mixing it with milk, flavoured milk or orange juice, preferably at room temperature. Mix in glass rather than plastic container (minimal sticking to sides of container). Stir well, drink immediately, and rinse glass with small quantity of diluent to assure getting entire dose.

☐ Medication may be taken with meals or milk to reduce nausea or GI irritation.

☐ Keep scheduled follow-up appointments.

■ Store preferably between 15° and 30°C (59° and 86°F) in well-closed containers. Do not refrigerate. Protect ampoules from light. Once opened, oral solution should be dated and contents used within 2 months.

Diagnostic test interferences Hyperlipidaemia and abnormalities in electrophoresis reported; believed to be due to polyoxyl 35 castor oil (Cremophor) in IV cyclosporin.

DRUG INTERACTIONS *Cyclosporin*

PLUS	INTERACTIONS
Acyclovir Aminoglycosides	Additive nephrotoxic effects. Concurrent use generally avoided
Amphotericin B Ketoconazole	May increase plasma or blood cyclosporin levels, with possibility of additive nehrotoxicity. Used concomitantly only with great caution
Cimetidine	Possibility of increased plasma or blood cyclosporin levels (by decreasing hepatic metabolism). Close monitoring advised
Immunosuppressants, other (e.g., corticosteroids	Increased risk of infection and lymphoproliferative diseases. With exception of corticosteroids, concurrent use generally avoided
Phenobarbitone Phenytoin and possibly other hydantoins Rifampicin	May cause decrease in blood or plasma cyclosporin concentrations (possibly by increasing hepatic metabolism). Monitor cyclosporin levels

Cyproheptadine hydrochloride

(Periactin)

Antihistamine; H_2-receptor antagonist

ACTIONS AND USES Potent antihistamine with pharmacological actions similar to those of azatadine (q.v.). Also stimulates appetite, perhaps by activation of hypothalamic appetite-regulating centre.

Used for symptomatic relief of various allergic conditions, including hay fever,

CYPROHEPTADINE HYDROCHLORIDE (continued)

vasomotor rhinitis, allergic conjunctivitis, urticaria caused by cold sensitivity, pruritus of allergic dermatoses, migraine; and to ameliorate drug, blood, and plasma reactions. Effective in treatment of anaphylactoid reactions as adjunct to adrenaline and other standard measures, after acute symptoms have been controlled and for migraine. Use as appetite stimulant in children has been questioned.

ROUTE AND DOSAGE   Adult: Oral: *Allergy*: 4–20 mg/day in divided doses. **Child (2–6 yrs):** 2 mg/3 times a day; **(7–14 yrs):** 4 mg/3 times a day. *Migraine*: 4 mg initially with 4 mg after 30 mins if required. *Appetite stimulant*: **Adult:** 4 mg/3 times a day. **Child (2–6 yrs):** 8 mg/day; **(7–14 yrs):** 12 mg/day in divided doses.

ABSORPTION AND FATE   Duration of action approximately 4 to 6 hours. Small amount appears in breast milk.

NURSING IMPLICATIONS

- Cyproheptadine is most likely to cause sedation, dizziness, and hypotension in the elderly. Advise patient to report these symptoms. Children are more apt to manifest CNS stimulation, e.g., confusion, agitation, tremors, hallucinations. Reduction in dosage may be indicated.
- In some patients, the sedative effect disappears spontaneously after 3 or 4 days of drug administration.
- Patient should know that cyproheptadine may increase and prolong the effects of alcohol, barbiturates, narcotic analgesics, tranquillizers, and other CNS depressants.
- Monitor weight and keep physician informed of any significant weight gain.
- For treatment of dry mouth (xerostomia), *see azatadine.*
- Store in tightly covered containers at room temperature, preferably between 15° and 30°C (59° and 86°F) unless otherwise directed by manufacturer.

Diagnostic test interferences   As a general rule, antihistamines are discontinued about 4 days before skin testing procedures are to be performed since they may produce false-negative results.

For further information *see azatadine.*

Cytarabine ━━━━━━━━━━━━━━━━━━━━━━━━━━━━

(Alexan, Cytosar, Cytosine)   *Antineoplastic; antimetabolite*

ACTIONS AND USES   Pyrimidine analogue with cell phase specificity affecting rapidly dividing cells in S-phase (DNA synthesis). Has strong myelosuppressant activity. Immunosuppressant properties are exhibited by obliterated cell-mediated immune responses, such as delayed hypersensitivity skin reactions.

Used primarily to induce and maintain remission in acute myelocytic leukaemia, acute lymphocytic leukaemia, and meningeal leukaemia in adults and children. Also

CYTARABINE (continued)

used in combination with other antineoplastics in established chemotherapeutic protocols.

ROUTE AND DOSAGE   **Intravenous or intrathecal**: All doses highly individualized.

ABSORPTION AND FATE   Incompletely (less than 20%) absorbed from GI tract. After IV dose, drug is rapidly cleared from blood. **Half-life**: distribution phase, 10 minutes; elimination phase, 1⅓ hours. With intrathecal administration, half-life: 2 hours. Metabolized in liver, excreted in urine (about 80% total dose in 24 hours). Crosses blood–brain barrier.

CONTRAINDICATIONS AND PRECAUTIONS   Known hypersensitivity to cytarabine, drug-induced myelosuppression, infants; during pregnancy (particularly during first trimester), women of childbearing age. **Cautious Use**: impaired renal or hepatic function, gout, drug-induced myelosuppression.

ADVERSE/SIDE EFFECTS   These include: nausea, vomiting, stomatitis, oesophagitis, anorexia, diarrhoea, anal inflammation or ulceration, abdominal pain, haemorrhage, myelosuppression (reversible): leucopenia, thrombocytopenia, anaemia, megaloblastosis, reduced reticulocytes (rare), freckling, rash, keratitis, alopecia (rare), skin ulcerations, weight loss, sore throat, fever, dizziness, cellulitis, thrombophlebitis and pain at injection site; pericarditis, hepatic and renal dysfunction, jaundice, urinary retention, transient hyperuricaemia, bleeding (any site), chest pain, pneumonia, conjunctivitis, photophobia, headache, neurotoxicity, neuritis, lethargy, confusion, anaphylaxis; 'flu'-like syndrome (infrequent): fever, malaise, myalgia, bone pain, chest pain, maculopapular rash. Potentially carcinogenic and mutagenic.

NURSING IMPLICATIONS

- Toxicity necessitating dosage alterations almost always occurs.
- Report adverse reactions immediately.
- Leucocyte and platelet counts should be evaluated daily during initial therapy. Blood uric acid and hepatic function tests should be performed at regular intervals throughout treatment period.
- Monitor blood reports for indicated adaptations of drug regimen and nursing intervention.
- Nausea and vomiting of several hours' duration complicate rapid IV injection. Effects are less severe with IV infusion. Administration of cytarabine one hour before meals, or giving an antiemetic prior to cytarabine may reduce these side effects.
- Noncontinuous dosage schedules may permit the patient to tolerate larger amounts of drug.
- To reduce potential for urate stone formation, fluids are forced in excess of 2 L if tolerated. Consult physician.
- 'Flu'-like syndrome occurs usually within 6 to 12 weeks after drug administration and may recur with successive therapy.
- Monitor fluid intake–output ratio and pattern. Advise patient to report promptly protracted vomiting or signs of nephrotoxicity.
- During the granulocytic periods, development of usual signs of inflammation may be

CYTARABINE (continued)

inhibited. Monitor body temperature. Be alert to the most subtle signs of infection especially low-grade fever and report promptly. WBC nadir is usually reached in 5 to 7 days after therapy has been stopped. Therapy is restarted with appearance of bone marrow recovery and when above cell counts are reached.

- Inspect injection sites for signs of cellulitis.
- Provide good oral hygiene to diminish side effects and chance of superinfection. Stomatitis and cheilosis usually appear 5 to 10 days into therapy (*see mustine for nursing implications*).
- Store cytarabine in refrigerator until reconstituted. The 100-mg and 500-mg vials are reconstituted with 5 ml and 10 ml, respectively, of bacteriostatic water for injection with benzyl alcohol 0.9%. Reconstituted solutions may be stored at room temperature preferably between 15 and 30°C (59° and 86°F) for 48 hours. Solutions with a slight haze should be discarded.
- For intrathecal injection, reconstitute with an isotonic, buffered diluent without preservatives. Follow manufacturer's recommendations. Solution should be administered as soon as possible after preparation.
- *See mustine for nursing implications of antineoplastic therapy.*

Dacarbazine

(DTIC)   *Antineoplastic; alkylating agent*

ACTION AND USES   Cytotoxic triazine with alkylating properties. Cell cycle nonspecific. Has minimal immunosuppressive activity; reportedly carcinogenic, mutagenic, and teratogenic.

Used as single agent or in combination with other antineoplastics in treatment of metastatic malignant melanoma, Hodgkin's disease, various sarcomas, and neuroblastoma.

ROUTE AND DOSAGE   **Intravenous**: individualized.

ABSORPTION AND FATE   Only slightly (approximately 5%) protein-bound. **Biphasic half-life**: initial phase about 20 minutes: terminal phase: 5 hours. Localizes primarily in liver; concentration in CSF about 14% of that in plasma. 35 to 50% of dose eliminated by renal tubule secretion within 6 hours as unchanged drug and metabolite in approximately equal amounts.

CONTRAINDICATIONS AND PRECAUTIONS   Hypersensitivity to dacarbazine. Safe use in pregnancy; not established.

ADVERSE/SIDE EFFECTS   These include: confusion, headache, seizures, blurred vision, erythematosus, urticarial rashes; hepatotoxicity, photosensitivity, anorexia, nausea,

DACARBAZINE (continued)

vomiting, diarrhoea (rare), severe leucopenia and thrombocytopenia, mild anaemia, alopecia, facial paraesthesia and flushing, 'flu'-like syndrome, myalgia, malaise, anaphylaxis, pain along injected vein.

NURSING IMPLICATIONS

- Should be administered to hospitalized patients because close observation and frequent laboratory studies are required during and after therapy.
- Monitor injection site. Subcutaneous extravasation causes severe pain and tissue damage. Treat infiltrated area with ice compresses.
- During platelet nadir avoid if possible all tests and treatments (e.g., IM) requiring needle punctures. Observe carefully and report evidence of unexplained bleeding: ecchymosis, petechiae, epistaxis, melaena, or bruising.
- Protect patient from excess expenditure of energy, and from infection, especially during leucocyte nadir (screen visitors and personnel that may enter patient's room).
- Severe nausea and vomiting (over 90% of patients) begins within 1 hour after drug administration and may last for as long as 12 hours.
- Restriction of oral fluids and food for 4 to 6 hours prior to treatment may prevent vomiting. Palliation and prevention of vomiting may be provided also by administration of an antiemetic (e.g., dexamethasone, prochloperazone). *See Index: Nursing Interventions: nausea and vomiting.*
- Most patients develop tolerance to vomiting and diarrhoea after the first 1 or 2 days. If vomiting persists, discontinuation of therapy with dacarbazine may be necessary.
- Monitor fluid intake–output ratio and pattern and daily temperature. Renal impairment extends the half-life and increases danger of toxicity. Report symptoms of renal dysfunction and even a slight elevation of temperature.
- 'Flu'-like syndrome (fever, myalgia, malaise) may occur during or even a week after treatment is terminated and last 7 to 21 days. Symptoms frequently recur with successive treatments.
- Caution patient to avoid prolonged exposure to sunlight or to ultraviolet light during treatment period and for at least 2 weeks after last dose. Protect exposed skin with sun screen lotion (SPF 15 or higher) and avoid exposure in midday.
- Warn patient to report promptly if blurred vision or paraesthesia (sensation of prickling, tingling, heightened sensitivity, or numbness) occurs.
- Follow agency protocol for handling antineoplastic drug, for precautions to be taken if there is spillage, and for protection of personnel during preparation of solutions or during cleanup of spilled drug.
- All handlers of dacarbazine should wear gloves. If solution gets into the eyes, wash with soap and water immediately then irrigate with water or isotonic saline.
- Reconstitute drug with sterile water for injection to make a solution containing 10 mg/ml dacarbazine (pH 3.0 to 4.0). Resulting solution is administered IV with 5% dextrose injection or sodium chloride injection for administration by IV infusion. The reconstituted solution may be further diluted.
- **Extravasation** Monitor injection site frequently (instruct patient to do so if able):
  - □ Give prompt attention to patient's complaint of swelling, stinging and burning sensation around injection site. Perivenous extravasation can occur painlessly and

DACARBAZINE (continued)

without visual signs. Sometimes demonstrated blood return is from a leak around the venepuncture site; this is a particular possibility in the elderly.

- □ Full skin damage by dacarbazine can lead to deep necrosis requiring surgical debridement, skin grafting and even amputation. At risk are the elderly, very young (who cannot communicate the associated pain), comatose, and debilitated patients. Other risk factors include establishing an IV line in a vein previously punctured several times and non-plastic catheters.
- □ *Danger areas for extravasation*: dorsum of hand or ankle (especially if peripheral arteriosclerosis is present), joint spaces and previously irradiated areas. If possible avoid using antecubital vein or veins on dorsum of hand or wrist where extravasation could damage underlying tendons and nerves leading to loss of mobility of entire limb. Avoid veins in extremity with compromised venous or lymphatic drainage and veins near joint spaces.
- □ If extravasation is suspected, stop infusion immediately and restart in another vein. Report to the physician, Prompt institution of local treatment is imperative: infiltration of the area with SC hydrocortisone and application of ice compresses. (Aspiration of extravasated drug may be attempted by physician.)
- □ Continue to apply hydrocortisone to the whole area twice a day while redness remains.
- □ Store reconstituted solution up to 72 hrs at $4°C$ or at room temperature for up to 8 hrs. Store diluted reconstituted solution at room temperature for up to 8 hrs or for 24 hrs at $4°C$.

Danazol ━━━━━━━━━━━━━━━━━━━━━━━━━━━━━━

(Danol)   *Androgen*

ACTIONS AND USES   Synthetic androgen steroid; derivative of alpha-ethinyl testosterone with dose-related mild androgenic effects but no oestrogenic or progestational activity. Suppresses pituitary output of follicle-stimulating hormone and luteinizing hormone, resulting in anovulation and associated amenorrhoea. Interrupts progress and pain of endometriosis by causing atrophy and involution of both normal and ectopic endometrial tissue. Has no effect on large endometriomas or on anatomic deformities associated with pain of dysmenorrhoea.

Used for treatment of endometriosis. Also used to treat fibrocystic breast disease gynaecomastia, menorrhagia and hereditary angioedema.

ROUTE AND DOSAGE   Oral: *Endometriosis*: 400 mg twice daily for 3 to 6 months. Started during menstruation or if pregnancy test is negative. Therapy may be extended 9 months if necessary. If symptoms recur after termination of therapy, drug regimen can be reinstituted. *Fibrocystic breast disease*: 100 to 400 mg in 2 doses daily as tolerated (regimen started as with endometrosis).

DANAZOL (continued)

ABSORPTION AND FATE   Metabolized to 2-hydroxymethylethisterone, which attains plasma levels 5 to 10 times higher than that of parent drug. Distribution and elimination data not available.

CONTRAINDICATIONS AND PRECAUTIONS   Pregnancy, nursing mothers, undiagnosed abnormal genital bleeding; impaired renal, cardiac, or hepatic function. **Cautious Use**: migraine headache, epilepsy. *See also testosterone.*

ADVERSE/SIDE EFFECTS   These include: skin rashes, nasal congestion, acneiform lesions, oily skin and hair oedema, weight gain, clitoral enlargement, mild hirsutism, deepening of voice, increased hoarseness, decrease in breast size, dizziness, headache, sleep disorders, fatigue, tremor, paraesthesias in extremities (rare), irritability, visual disturbances, changes in appetite, chills, gastroenteritis; rarely, nausea, vomiting, constipation, haematuria (rare), flushing; sweating; emotional lability; nervousness; vaginitis with itching, drying, burning, or bleeding; amenorrhoea. Causal relationship of danazol to the following reactions has been neither confirmed nor refuted: muscle cramps or spasms in back, neck, or legs, hair loss, decreased libido, elevated blood pressure, pelvic pain, conjunctival oedema, possibility of cholestatic jaundice, acne vulgaris; carpal tunnel syndrome.

D

NURSING IMPLICATIONS

- Inform patient that drug-induced amenorrhoea (due to anovulation) is reversible. Ovulation and cyclic bleeding usually return within 60 to 90 days after therapeutic regimen is discontinued. Advise patient that potential for conception may also be restored at that time.
- A nonhormonal contraceptive should be used during danazol treatment (if the patient wishes birth control) because ovulation may not be suppressed.
- Routine breast examinations should be carried out during therapy. Advise patient to report to physician if any nodule enlarges or becomes tender or hard during therapy.
- In fibrocystic breast disease, inform patient that pain and discomfort may be relieved in 2 to 3 months; the nodularity in 4 to 6 months. Menses may be regular or irregular in pattern during therapy.
- Because danazol may cause fluid retention, patients with cardiac or renal problems, epilepsy, or migraine should be observed closely during therapy. Also, drug-induced oedema may cause compression on median nerve producing symptoms of carpal tunnel syndrome. If patient complains of wrist pain that worsens at night, paraesthesias in radial palmer aspect of the hand and fingers, consult physician. Condition is reversible within a few weeks with discontinuation of the drug.
- Baseline and periodic liver function tests should be performed in all patients.
- Advise patient to report voice changes promptly. Drug should be stopped to avoid permanent damage to voice. Although the side effects usually disappear when drug therapy is terminated, continue to observe patient for signs of virilization (sometimes irreversible).
- Danazol is very expensive.
- Store capsules between 15° and 30°C (59° and 86°F) in a well-closed container.
- *See testosterone.*

Danthron with Docusate

(Normax)

Laxative (stimulant);
anthraquinone

ACTIONS AND USES   Laxative combination of anthroquinone group.

Used for temporary management of constipation particularly in geriatric, cardiac, and surgical patients.

ROUTE AND DOSAGE   Oral: 25 to 75 mg usually at bedtime.

ABSORPTION AND FATE   Acts in about 6 to 12 hours following oral administration. Metabolized in liver. Excreted in urine. Appears in breast milk.

CONTRAINDICATIONS AND PRECAUTIONS   Nausea, vomiting, abdominal pain, or other symptoms of acute surgical abdomen; faecal impaction; intestinal obstruction or perforation; rectal bleeding; nursing mothers.

ADVERSE/SIDE EFFECTS   Usually dose-related: nausea, vomiting, diarrhoea, abdominal cramps, perianal irritation. With prolonged use: discolouration of rectal mucosa (melanosis coli), hypokalaemia, dehydration, elevation of blood glucose, hepatic injury (when used repeatedly with an emollient laxative).

NURSING IMPLICATIONS
- Administration of danthron with the evening meal usually produces evacuation of a soft stool the next morning.
- Prolonged use may lead to laxative dependence.
- Pink to red colouration of urine is harmless and usually indicates that urine is alkaline.
- Melanosis coli is a benign pigmentation of the colonic mucosa that occurs with prolonged use. It is usually reversible within 4 to 12 months after danthron is discontinued.
- Store in tightly-closed container preferably between 15° and 30°C (59°C and 86°F), unless otherwise directed by manufacturer.
- *See cascara for patient-teaching points.*

Diagnostic test interferences   Danthron may cause an apparent increase in urinary excretion of **PSP** due to urine discoloration.

Dantrolene sodium

(Dantrium)

Skeletal muscle relaxant;
hydantoin

ACTIONS AND USES   Hydantoin derivative, structurally related to phenytoin, with peripheral skeletal muscle relaxant action. Directly relaxes the spastic muscle by inter-

DANTROLENE SODIUM (continued)

fering with Ca ion (contraction activator) release from sarcoplasmic reticulum. Clinical doses produce about a 50% decrease in contractility of skeletal muscles but no effect on smooth or cardiac muscles. Relief of spasticity may be accompanied by muscle weakness, sufficient to affect overall functional capacity of the patient. Reduces spastic or reflex contractions more than voluntary activity.

Used orally for the symptomatic treatment of skeletal muscle spasms secondary to spinal cord injury, stroke, cerebral palsy, multiple sclerosis. Also used in malignant hyperthermia.

ROUTE AND DOSAGE   Oral: *Relief of spasticity*: **Adults**: *Initial*: 25 mg once daily; increased to 25 mg two to four times daily, then by increments of 25 mg up to 100 mg two to four times daily, if necessary. Each dosage level should be maintained for 4 to 7 days to determine patient's response. **Intravenous**: *in malignant hyperthermia*: 1mg/kg by rapid injection repeated if required after 5–10 min to a maximum of 10 mg/kg.

ABSORPTION AND FATE   Absorption from GI tract is slow and incomplete, but rate is consistent. Significant amounts bound to plasma proteins, mostly albumin; binding is readily reversible. **Mean half-life**: 8.7 hours after 100 mg oral dose, and about 5 hours following IV administration. Slowly metabolized by liver. About 25% excreted in urine chiefly as metabolites and small smount of unchanged drug. About 45 to 50% eliminated in bile.

CONTRAINDICATIONS AND PRECAUTIONS   Active hepatic disease; when spasticity is necessary to sustain upright posture and balance in locomotion or to maintain increased body function; spasticity due to rheumatic disorders. Safe use during pregnancy, in women of childbearing potential, in nursing mothers and in children under 5 years not established. **Cautious Use**: impaired cardiac or pulmonary function, patients over 35 years, females.

ADVERSE/SIDE EFFECTS   These include: drowsiness, muscle weakness, dizziness, light-headedness, unusual fatigue, speech disturbances, headache, confusion, nervousness, mental depression, insomnia, euphoria, seizures, tachycardia, erratic blood pressure, phlebitis (IV extravasation), diarrhoea, constipation, nausea, vomiting, anorexia, swallowing difficulty, alterations of taste, gastric irritation, abdominal cramps, GI bleeding, haematuria or dark urine, crystalluria with pain or burning with urination, urinary frequency, urinary retention, nocturia, enuresis, difficult erection, hepatitis, jaundice, hepatomegaly, pruritus, urticaria, eczematoid skin eruption, photosensitivity, pleural effusion (with shortness of breath, dry cough, fever, chest pains, eosinophilia), blurred vision, diplopia, changes in vision, photophobia, general malaise, myalgia, backache, pulmonary effusion, feeling of suffocation, increased salivation, lacrimation, or sweating; chills, fever, acne-like rash, abnormal hair growth.

NURSING IMPLICATIONS

■ If necessary, an oral suspension for a single dose may be made by emptying contents of capsule(s) into fruit juice or other liquid. Pharmacist can prepare a multiple dose suspension on request. Suspension should be shaken well before pouring. Since it will

DANTROLENE SODIUM (continued)

not contain a preservative, avoid contamination, keep refrigerated, and use within several days.

- Prior to initiation of therapy, an assessment should be made of patient's neuromuscular function as a baseline for comparison.
- Supervise ambulation until patient's reaction to drug is known. Relief of spasticity may be accompanied by some loss of voluntary strength, which may impede patient's ability to maintain balance and an upright posture.
- The most common side effects of dantrolene are drowsiness, dizziness, fatigue, muscular weakness (which may be manifested by slurred speech, drooling, and enuresis), general malaise, headache, diarrhoea. Symptoms are generally transient, lasting up to 14 days after initiation of therapy. Keep physician informed. Reduction in dosage or discontinuation of dantrolene may be necessary if symptoms persist.
- Patients with impaired cardiac or pulmonary function should be closely monitored for cardiovascular or respiratory symptoms such as tachycardia, blood pressure changes, feeling of suffocation.
- Because of the possibility of hepatic injury, it is recommended that drug be discontinued if improvement is not evident within 45 days.
- Keep physician informed of therapeutic effectiveness. Improvement may not be apparent until a week or more of drug therapy.
- Baseline and regularly scheduled hepatic function tests (alkaline phosphatase, SGOT (AST), SGPT (ALT), total bilirubin), blood cell counts, and renal function tests should be performed.
- Risk of hepatotoxicity appears to be greater in females, patients over 35 years, patients taking other medications in addition to dantrolene, and in patients taking high dantrolene doses (400 mg or more daily) for prolonged periods.
- Instruct patient to report promptly the onset of jaundice: yellow skin or sclerae, dark urine, clay-coloured stools; itching, abdominal discomfort. Hepatotoxicity more frequently occurs between third and twelfth months of therapy.
- Advise patient to report symptoms of allergy (rash, erythema, pruritus, urticaria) and allergic pleural effusion (shortness of breath, pleuritic pain, dry cough).
- Monitor bowel function. Persistent diarrhoea may necessitate drug withdrawal. Severe constipation with abdominal distention and signs of intestinal obstruction have been reported.
- Forewarn patient of the possibility of dizziness and drowsiness and advise to avoid driving and other potentially hazardous activities until reaction to drug is known.
- Since hepatotoxicity occurs more commonly when other drugs are taken concurrently with dantrolene, advise patient not to take OTC medications, alcoholic beverages, or other CNS depressants unless otherwise advised by physician.
- Because of the possibility of photosensitivity reactions, advise patient to avoid unnecessary exposure to sunlight and to use physical protection such as a hat, protective clothing, and a sunscreen agent (SPF 12 or above).
- **Treatment of overdosage** Immediate gastric lavage. General supportive measures include maintaining airway, monitoring cardiac and renal function. Large quantities of fluids are given to prevent crystalluria.
- Store capsules in tightly-closed light-resistant container. Contents of vial (for IV use)

DANTROLENE SODIUM (continued)

must be protected from direct light and used within 6 hours after reconstitution, since it does not contain a preservative. Both oral and parenteral forms are stored perferably between 15° and 30°C (59° and 86°F), unless otherwise directed by manufacturer.

Drug Interactions   Alcohol and other **CNS depressants** may cause additive CNS depression. Concurrent use of **oestrogens** in females over 35 years reportedly associated with a relatively higher frequency of hepatotoxicity.

Dapsone

Antiinfective

ACTIONS AND USES   Sulphone derivative chemically related to sulphonamides, with bacteriostatic rather than bactericidal action. Spectrum of activity includes *Mycobacterium leprae, M. tuberculosis*, and non-acid-fast organisms such as *Streptococci*. Mechanism of anti-bacterial action thought to be competitive inhibition of bacterial synthesis of folic acid from para-aminobenzoic acid (PABA). Also causes fragmentation of bacilli in lesions by unknown mechanism and is thought to increase host resistance.

Used in treatment of all types of leprosy (Hansen's disease) and to control symptoms of dermatitis herpetiformis.

ROUTE AND DOSAGE   Oral: Adult: *Leprosy*: 1 to 2 mg/kg daily. *Dermatitis herpetiformis*: 50 mg daily. May be increased by 50 mg/day up to 300 mg daily or higher if necessary.

ABSORPTION AND FATE   Almost completely absorbed from GI tract, mainly from upper part of small intestines. **Peak plasma levels** in 4 to 8 hours. Distributed to all body tissues, with high concentrations in kidney, liver, muscle, and skin. About 50% **bound to plasma proteins. Half-life**: 10–50 hours (with mean of 28 hours). Acetylated in liver (degree of acetylation is genetically determined). Enters enterohepatic circulation following biliary excretion. Approximately 70 to 80% of dose is excreted slowly in urine, primarily as water soluble metabolites, with some free drug; a small percentage is excreted in faeces. Traces may be found in blood 8 to 12 days after single 200-mg dose and for 35 days following discontinuation of repeated doses. Small amounts excreted in sweat, tears, saliva, sputum, and breast milk.

CONTRAINDICATIONS AND PRECAUTIONS   Hypersensitivity to sulphones or its derivatives; advanced renal amyloidosis, severe anaemia, methaemoglobin reductase deficiency. Safe use during pregnancy not established. **Cautious Use**: chronic renal, hepatic, pulmonary, or cardiovascular disease, refractory anaemias, albuminuria, G6PD deficiency.

ADVERSE/SIDE EFFECTS   These include: headache, giddiness, dizziness, lethargy,

DAPSONE (continued)

malaise, nervousness, insomnia, tinnitus, blurred vision, reversible peripheral neuropathy (especially thenar muscles of thumbs), paraesthesias, motor neuropathy (muscle weakness), neuralgic pain, psychosis, methaemoglobinaemia (common); haemolytic-type anaemia, macrocytic anaemia, aplastic anaemia, leucopenia, agranulocytosis, pancytopenia (infrequent), hypermelanotic macules (fixed eruptions), pruritus, erythema multiforme (erythematous, oedematous, or bullous lesions of skin or mucous membranes), exfoliative dermatitis (dry, itchy, red, scaly skin), loss of hair, toxic epidermal necrolysis ('scalded skin syndrome'), drug fever, allergic rhinitis, hepatitis, hepatic necrosis anorexia, nausea, vomiting, abdominal colic, tachycardia, haematuria, proteinuria.

NURSING IMPLICATIONS

- Administer with food to reduce possibility of GI distress.
- Patients with lepromatous leprosy tend to be sensitive to dapsone and therefore may require dosage reduction to control adverse reactions.
- Complete blood counts are performed prior to initiation of therapy, weekly during the first month of therapy, at monthly intervals for at least 6 months, and semi-annually thereafter. Periodic determinations of dapsone blood levels are also recommended. Dapsone blood levels of 0.1 to 7 mcg/dl reflect safe dosage.
- Mild decrease in haemoglobin level may occur during the first few weeks of therapy. If haemoglobin falls below 9 g/dl, dosage should be reduced or drug temporarily discontinued. Drug therapy is usually terminated if RBC count falls below 2.5 million/mm^3 or remains persistently low after 6 weeks of therapy, or if leucocyte count falls below 5,000/mm^3.
- Monitor temperature during first few weeks of therapy. If fever is frequent or severe, dosage should be reduced or therapy interrupted.
- Instruct patient to report to physician if symptoms of leprosy do not improve within 3 months or if they get worse. Bacterial resistance to dapsone has been reported.
- Suspect methaemoglobinaemia if patient appears cyanotic and mucous membranes have a brownish hue. Report to physician. Usually, discontinuation of therapy is not required unless anoxaemia is present.
- The appearance of a skin rash should be reported promptly because if may signify developing sensitization which can lead to potentially fatal complications. Allergic skin reactions occur most frequently before the tenth week of therapy and indicate that drug should be discontinued. Interruption of therapy is usually not necessary for hypermelanotic, macular-type localized lesions which may develop 1 week to 1 year after treatment begins.
- Because of cumulative effects patient should be carefully taught to report the onset of adverse reactions.
- Therapeutic effects in leprosy may not appear until after 3 to 6 months of therapy. Skin lesions respond well; recovery from nerve involvement is usually limited.
- Deformities such as contractures may be prevented by physical therapy, careful positioning of anaesthetic limbs or application of casts. Other disfigurements may necessitate reconstructive surgery.
- Lepromatous eye lesions sometimes develop or progress during treatment, since the drug does not appreciably penetrate ocular tissues.

DAPSONE (continued)

- Optimum duration of therapy has not been determined. Some authorities recommend continuing treatment for lepromatous leprosy at least 10 years or more; current thinking seems to favour maintenance therapy for life. For the indeterminate and tuberculoid types, treatment may be continued for at least 3 years after disease is clinically quiescent. Leprosy is considered inactive when skin scrapings and/or biopsy are negative for bacteria, and there is no evidence of clinical activity for at least a year.
- Hospitalization is advised during initial therapy for leprosy, but thereafter ambulatory treatment is sufficient. No special isolation procedures are necessary when patient is hospitalized but nasal discharge and discharge from lesions must be carefully disinfected.
- Leprosy is transmitted by active skin lesions or nasal discharge of infected persons, but only susceptible people develop the disease. According to recent evidence most people have partial or complete resistance to leprosy.
- Scheduled follow-up is critical to detection of possible relapse. Examination of close contacts at 6- to 12-month intervals for at least 10 years is recommended.
- Many clinicians believe that infants should not be separated from leprous mothers receiving therapy and that breast feeding should be encouraged as a means of providing chemopro-phylaxis for the infant.
- Infants fed breast milk containing dapsone may develop methaemoglobinaemia. This is reversible and reportedly is not serious except in infants with G6PD deficiency.

Food–drug interactions

- Physician may prescribe a gluten-controlled diet in patients with dermatitis herpetiformis because the disease is usually accompanied by gluten sensitive lesions of the jejunum. Gluten control may improve intestinal inflammation and skin lesions to some extent and thus allow for reduction in dapsone dosage.
- Foods rich in gluten include the cereal grains, such as wheat, barley, oats, rye, bran, millet, wheat germ, and malt. (Corn and rice cereals are allowed.) Foods that may contain cereals should also be avoided, e.g., certain coffees, root beer, meat loaf, pasta and macaroni products. Advise patient to read product labels carefully and to avoid commercially prepared foods containing gluten.

- Preserved in tightly covered, light-resistant containers at 15° to 30°C (59° to 86°F). Drug discoloration apparently does not indicate a chemical change.

Drug interactions   **Probenecid** may cause elevated dapsone blood levels (by inhibiting renal excretion of dapsone).

Daunorubicin hydrochloride

(Cerubidine)   *Antineoplastic; antibiotic*

DAUNORUBICIN HYDROCHLORIDE (continued)

ACTIONS AND USES Cytotoxic and antimitotic anthracycline glycoside antibiotic; cell cycle specific for S-phase of cell division. Toxic properties preclude its use as an antibiotic. A potent bone marrow suppressant, with immunosuppressive properties. Induces cardiac toxicity and may be mutagenic carcinogenic (development of secondary carcinomas).

Used as single agent or in combination with cytarabine to induce remission in acute nonlymphocytic leukaemia (myelogenous, monocytic, erythroid) in adults. Also used to treat solid tumours of childhood and non-Hodgkin's lymphoma.

ROUTE AND DOSAGE Intravenous: individualized. Dosage modifications are based on serum bilirubin and creatinine values.

ABSORPTION AND FATE Rapid disappearance from plasma following IV administration indicates rapid distribution to tissues. Thereafter, plasma levels slowly decline with a half-life of 18.5 hours. Hepatic metabolism within 1 hour. Active metabolite, daunorubicinol, predominates in plasma and maintains a half-life of 26.7 hours. About 25% administered dose excreted as metabolite in urine; 40% excreted in bile. Does not cross blood–brain barrier. Probably crosses placenta. Distribution to breast milk not known.

CONTRAINDICATIONS AND PRECAUTIONS Severe myelosuppression, pregnancy (especially in first trimester), and preexisting cardiac disease unless risk-benefit is evaluated; lactation, uncontrolled systemic infection. **Cautious Use**: history of gout, urate calculi, hepatic or renal function impairment, elderly patients with inadequate bone reserve due to age or previous cytotoxic drug therapy, cell infiltration of bone marrow, patient who has received potentially cardiotoxic drugs or related antineoplastics.

ADVERSE/SIDE EFFECTS These include: generalized alopecia (reversible), rash (rare), pericarditis, myocarditis, arrhythmias, congestive heart failure, acute nausea and vomiting (mild), anorexia, mucositis, diarrhoea (occasionally), thrombocytopenia, leucocytopenia, anaemia, hyperuricaemia, fever, chills (rare), gonadal suppression, severe cellulitis or tissue sloughing at site of drug extravasation.

NURSING IMPLICATIONS
- Not to be confused with doxorubicin.
- Use of gloves during preparation of the solution for infusion is recommended to prevent skin contact with the drug. If this occurs, decontaminate with copious amounts of water with soap. (*See Index: Antineoplastics: handling drug solutions.*)
- Reconstitute vial contents with 10 to 20 ml sterile water for injection, 5% glucose or normal saline solution.
- Extravasation can cause severe tissue necrosis and therefore must be avoided.
- Daunorubicin should never be administered IM or SC, and it should never be mixed with heparin or other drugs.
- Hepatic and renal function tests should be performed prior to and during each course of treatment. If function is impaired therapeutic dosage levels are reduced to prevent toxicity.
- Prior to each course of therapy an ECG and/or determination of systolic ejection

DAUNORUBICIN HYDROCHLORIDE (continued)

fraction is performed to recognize patients at greatest risk for development of acute congestive heart failure.

- Monitor blood pressure, temperature, pulse and respiratory function during daunorubicin treatment.
- Report immediately breathlessness, orthopnoea, change in pulse and blood pressure parameters.
- A profound suppression of bone marrow is required to induce a complete remission. Peripheral blood and bone marrow studies are essential to treatment plans.
- Nadirs for thrombocytes and leucocytes usually reached in 10 to 14 days after drug administration.
- Myelosuppression imposes risk of superimposed infection. Promptly report elevation of temperature, chills, symptoms of upper respiratory tract infection, tachycardia, symptoms of overgrowth with opportunistic organisms (red or furry tongue, sore mouth, diarrhoea with foul-smelling stools, vaginal itching, and discharge, sudden fever, cough).
- Be alert to significance of immunosuppressive activity: reduced capacity to resist and overcome inflammatory conditions, slower wound healing, long periods of low-grade chronic infections. Protect patient from contact with persons with infections. The most hazardous period is during nadirs of thrombocytes and leucocytes.
- Drug-induced hyperuricaemia may occur because of rapid lysis of leukaemic cells. Monitor *serum uric acid levels* (normal: 178.5 to 416.4 mmol/L).
- The attainment of a normal bone marrow after daunorubicin administration may require as may as three courses of induction therapy.
- A regimen of encouraged increase in oral fluid intake, alkalinization of urine, and allopurinol may reduce incidence of hyperuricaemia. Report pain in flank, stomach, or joints, and changes in fluid intake and output ratio and pattern.
- Nausea and vomiting are usually mild and may be controlled by antiemetic therapy.
- Inspect oral membranes daily. Mucositis may occur 3 to 7 days after drug is administered. Institute appropriate nursing measures to reduce interference with adequate nutritional intake because of oral discomfort. *See Mustine for nursing care of stomatitis, xerostomia.*
- Discuss probability of onset of alopecia with patient but inform patient that recovery is usual in 6 to 10 weeks.
- Discuss possibility of gonadal suppression (amenorrhoea or azoospermia) with patient before treatment begins. Patient should understand that usually it is an irreversible side effect.
- Advise against conception during daunorubicin treatment period because of teratogenic properties of the drug. Advise patient to report to the physician should she become pregnant.
- Daunorubicin may impart a red colour to urine (a transient effect).
- Reconstituted solution is stable 24 hours at room temperature and 48 hours under refrigeration between 2° and 8°C (36° and 46°F) protected from light.

Diagnostic test interferences   Daunorubicin may elevate serum and urine uric acid levels.

DAUNORUBICIN HYDROCHLORIDE (continued)
DRUG INTERACTIONS *Daunorubicin*_____

PLUS	INTERACTIONS
Antigout agent	Increases uric acid level; dose adjustment of antigout agent may be necessary
Cyclophosphamide, doxorubicin radiation	Prior treatment with any of these modalities increases cardiac toxicity potential from daunorubicin therapy
Hepatotoxic drugs	Concurrent use increases risk of toxicity

Debrisoquine _____

(Declinax)

For further information: *see guanethidine*

ROUTE AND DOSAGE   10 mg 1–2 times a day, increased by 10 mg every three days, maximum 120 mg/day.

Demeclocycline hydrochloride _____

(Ledermycin)   *Antibiotic; tetracycline*

ACTIONS AND USES   Used to treat sensitive infections and hypenatraemia due to inappropriate antidiuretic hormone secretion.

ROUTE AND DOSAGE   Oral: Adults: *Antiinfective*: 150 mg every 6 hours or 300 mg every 12 hours. *Hyponatraemia*: *initial* 0.9–1.2 g/day in divided doses, *maintenance* 600–900 mg/day in divided doses.
  For further information: *see tetracycline*.

Desipramine hydrochloride _____

(Pertofran)   *Antidepressant; tricyclic*

ACTIONS AND USES   Dibenzazipine tricyclic antidepressant. Active metabolite of imipramine (q.v.) with similar pharmacological actions, uses, limitations, and interactions. Onset of action is more rapid than that of imipramine; has mild sedative and anticholinergic actions.

DESIPRAMINE HYDROCHLORIDE (continued)

Used to treat endogenous depression and various depression syndromes.

ROUTE AND DOSAGE   Oral: **Adults:** 75 to 150 mg/day in divided doses or as a single dose. **Elderly, Adolescents:** 25 to 50 mg/day (doses above 100 mg not recommended). *Maintenance:* lowest effective dose once a day continued for at least 2 months after a satisfactory response has been achieved.

ABSORPTION AND FATE   Well-absorbed from GI tract. Hepatic metabolism. **Half-life:** 12 to 76 hours; effective therapeutic plasma levels: 150 to 300 ng/ml. Steady state reached in 2 to 11 days. Excreted in urine; crosses placenta.

For further information: *see imipramine.*

Desmopressin acetate

(DDAVP)   *Antidiuretic agent; antienuretic*

ACTIONS AND USES   Synthetic analogue of the natural human posterior pituitary (antidiuretic) hormone, arginine vasopressin. Has more specific and longer duration of action than antidiuretic hormone and lower incidence of allergic reactions. Also, oxytoccic and vasopressor actions are not apparent at therapeutic dosages. Unlike vasopressin, it does not stimulate release of adrenocorticotropic hormone nor does it increase plasma cortisol, growth hormone, prolactin, or luteinizing hormone levels. Reduces urine volume and osmolality in patients with central diabetes insipidus by increasing reabsorption of water by kidney collecting tubules. Produces a dose-related increase in factor VIII levels. Not effective in treatment of nephrogenic diabetes insipidus. Tolerance to drug effect rarely develops during prolonged therapy.

Used to control and prevent symptoms and complications of central (neurohypophyseal) diabetes insipidus.

ROUTE AND DOSAGE   Intranasally: IV/IM: according to individual requirements.

ABSORPTION AND FATE   Slowly absorbed from nasal mucosa. Onset of antidiuretic effect occurs within 1 hour, peaks in 1 to 5 hours, and persists 8 to 20 hours. **Biphasic half-life:** 8 and 76 minutes. Drug is excreted in milk, otherwise distribution and metabolic fate unknown.

CONTRAINDICATIONS AND PRECAUTIONS   Hypersensitivity to desmopressin acetate; nephrogenic diabetes insipidus; safe use during pregnancy and in nursing mothers not established. **Cautious Use:** coronary artery insufficiency, hypertensive cardiovascular disease.

ADVERSE/SIDE EFFECTS   Dose-related: transient headache, drowsiness, listlessness nasal congestion, rhinitis, nasal irritation, nausea, heartburn, mild abdominal cramps, vulval pain, shortness of breath, slight rise in blood pressure, flushing.

DESMOPRESSIN ACETATE (continued)
NURSING IMPLICATIONS
- Check expiration date on label.
- Initial dose usually administered in the evening and antidiuretic effect observed. Dose is increased each evening until uninterrupted sleep (free of nocturia) is obtained.
- Monitor fluid intake and output ratio and pattern (timing). Fluid intake must be carefully controlled particularly in the elderly and in the very young to avoid water retention and sodium depletion. Symptoms suggestive of water intoxication; subtle changes in mental status, confusion, lethargy, neuromuscular excitability.
- Weigh patient daily and observe for oedema.
- Monitor vital signs during dosage regulating period and whenever drug is administered parenterally.
- Severe water retention may require reduction in dosage and use of a diuretic such as frusemide.
- Therapeutic effectiveness is judged by adequacy of urine volume (control of polyuria and nocturia), relief of polydipisia, increased urine osmolality (concentration).
- Report upper respiratory tract infection or nasal congestion when in tranasal solution used. Although manufacturer states that drug effectiveness should not be affected some patients may require increased dosage.
- Demonstrate administration technique to patient. Follow manufacturer's instructions to ensure delivery of drug high into nasal cavity and not down throat. A flexible calibrated plastic tube (rhingle) is provided.
- Nasal solution has an expiry date of 1 year following date of manufacture.
- Store desmopressin parenteral solution and nasal spray in refrigerator preferably at 4°C (39.2°F) unless otherwise directed by manufacturer. Discard solutions that are discoloured or contain particulate matter.

DRUG INTERACTIONS *Desmopressin*

PLUS	INTERACTIONS
Alcohol Demeclocycline Adrenaline Heparin Lithium carbonate	May decrease antidiuretic response. Used with caution
Carbamazepine Chlorpropamide Clofibrate Fludrocortisone Urea	May potentiate antidiuretic response. Used with caution

Desonide

(Tridesilon)   *Corticosteroid; glucocorticoid*

DESONIDE (continued)

ACTIONS AND USES Synthetic nonfluorinated corticosteroid with antiinflammatory, antipruritic, and vasoconstrictive activity.

Used to relieve inflammatory symptoms of a variety of skin disorders responsive to corticosteroids. *See hydrocortisone for absorption, fate, contraindications, and interactions.*

ROUTE AND DOSAGE Topical: Apply thin layer of cream or ointment (0.05%) two or three times daily.

ADVERSE/SIDE EFFECTS Dermatological burning sensation, pruritus, acneiform eruptions, hypopigmentation, hypertrichosis, folliculitis. With occlusive dressing: maceration of skin, atrophy, striae, secondary infection, miliaria. *See also hydrocortisone for systemic effects.*

NURSING IMPLICATIONS

- Avoid putting medication in or near eyes.
- Before application of topical medication, cleanse skin area, dry thoroughly, then gently rub in a thin layer of the drug.
- If signs of systemic absorption, skin irritation or ulceration, hypersensitivity, or infection occurs, patient should notify the physician.
- Caution patient to apply medication as scheduled and not to change intervals or amount. Inform patient not to use the preparation for any other skin disorder, and not to share the topical drug with anyone else.
- Bandage or wrap treated area only if prescribed.
- Inspect skin for infection, striae, atrophy. If present, patient should stop the drug and notify the physician.
- Store drug in cool place, temperature less than 30°C (86°F), and protect from light and heat.
- *See hydrocortisone for nursing implications of topical medications.*
- *Note*: similar drug desoxymethasone (Stiedex).

Dexamethasone ━━━━━━━━━━━━━━━━━━━━━━━━━━

(Decadron, Decadron Shock-Pak, Oradexon)   *Corticosteroid*

ACTIONS AND USES Long-acting synthetic adrenocorticoid with intense antiinflammatory activity and minimal mineralocorticoid properties. May promote potassium and nitrogen loss, and exacerbation of glycosuria in diabetic patient. *See also hydrocortisone.*

Used as an immunosuppressant, antiinflammatory, and antiemetic agent for treatment of bronchial asthma and other bronchospastic states nonresponsive to conventional treatment and to treat life-threatening shock. Also used to treat cerebral oedema and to relieve nausea and vomiting caused by cancer chemotherapy. Used as a diagnostic test for Cushing's syndrome, to distinguish adrenal tumour from adrenal hyperplasia, and in the differential diagnosis and clinical management of depression.

DEXAMETHASONE (continued)

ROUTE AND DOSAGE   *Ophthalmic*: apply thin coating in lower conjunctival sac. **Oral: Adult**: 0.5–1.5 mg/day in divided doses up to a maximum of 15 mg/day. **IM/slow IV injection: Adult;** *initial* 0.5–20 mg, **child:** 200–500 mcg/kg/day.

ABSORPTION AND FATE   Rapid onset of action after administration. **Peak effect**: oral, 1 or 2 hours; IM, 8 hours. **Duration of effect**: oral, 2.75 days; IM, 6 days; intralesional, soft tissue, intraarticular, 1 to 3 weeks. **Half-life** (plasma): 3 to 4.5 hours; HPA axis suppression: 36 to 54 hours.

CONTRAINDICATIONS AND PRECAUTIONS   Hypersensitivity; systemic fungal infection, acute infections, active or resting tuberculosis, vaccinia, varicella, positive sputum culture of *Candida albicans*, viral diseases. Ophthalmic use: primary open-angle glaucoma, eye infections, superficial ocular herpes simplex, keratitis and tuberculosis of eye. Perforated ear drum (otic use). Safe use during pregnancy and lactation has not been established. **Cautious Use**: stromal herpes simplex, keratitis, GI ulceration, renal disease, diabetes mellitus, myasthenia gravis, congestive heart failure. *See also hydrocortisone.*

ADVERSE/SIDE EFFECTS   These include: slow healing, masked infections, perforation of small and large bowel (patients with inflammatory bowel disease); salt and water retention, GI irritation, hypertension, hypokalaemia; perianal burning and itching with rapid IV administration.
   See also hydrocortisone. **Topical use**: burning sensations, itching, irritation, dryness, folliculitis, hypertricosis, acneiform eruptions, hypopigmentation.

NURSING IMPLICATIONS
- As with other corticosteroids, dose changes up or down are made gradually.
- Diuresis may follow transfer from another steroid preparation to dexamethasone.
- Since dexamethasone has minimal sodium- and water-retaining activity, symptom development of overadministration may be quite subtle.
- Nonoperative cases of cerebral oedema may be responsive to continuous therapy with dexamethazone to remain free of symptoms of increased intracranial pressure.
- **Ophthalmic preparations**: Warn patient to consult physician promptly and to interrupt treatment with ophthalmic preparation if changes in visual acuity or diminished visual fields occur. An eye pad may be prescribed with ointment use to enhance effect of drug on corneal surface. Wash hands thoroughly before and after treatments.
- Observe eyelids and eye surfaces being treated with solution or ointment. If irritation develops, stop the treatment and consult physician.
- *See Index: Drug administration: eye drops.*
- Ophthalmic solution may also be instilled into the clean aural canal for treatment of inflammatory conditions. Consult physician regarding preparation of aural canal before instillation of medication. If gauze wick is used, it should be kept moist with medication while in place and removed after 12 to 24 hours.
- Dexamethasone is discontinued gradually to avoid consequences of hypocortisolism. Continuous supervision of patient after corticosteroid is stopped is necessary because there may be sudden reappearance of severe symptoms of the disease for which patient is being treated.

DEXAMETHASONE (continued)

- The dexamethasone dose regimen may need to be altered if patient is subjected to stress: e.g., surgery, infections, emotional stress, illness, acute bronchial attacks, trauma. It may also be indicated if there are extreme changes in patient's environment (stress on thermoregulation).
- The neonate born to a mother who has been receiving a corticosteroid during pregnancy should be monitored for symptoms of hypocortisolism.
- Caution patient on prolonged therapy not to self medicate with OTC medications unless the physician has approved.
- Inform new physician or dentist that a corticosteroid drug is being used.
- Patient should carry or wear medical identification card or jewellary with diagnosis, physician's name and telephone number, and drug being used.

Patient-teaching points
- ☐ Remind patient that corticosteroid therapy is not curative but preventive.
- ☐ The prescribed regimen should be strictly adhered to, i.e., dose intervals should not be increased, decreased, interrupted or discontinued.
- ☐ Instruct patient about symptoms of hypocortisolism and hypercortisolism.
- ☐ Urge patient to report exacerbation of symptoms and onset of side effects promptly.
- ☐ Emphasize the implications of immunosuppression with regard to prevention of exposure to infection, trauma, and to sudden changes in environmental factors.

- Do not store or expose aerosol to temperature above 120°F; do not puncture or discard into a fire or an incinerator.
- Stored at temperature between 15° and 30°C (59° and 86°F), unless otherwise directed by manufacturer.
- See hydrocortisone for additional Nursing Implications and Drug Interactions.

D

Dexamphetamine sulphate

(Dexedrine)

Central stimulant,
(sympathomimetic);
amphetamine

ACTIONS AND USES   Dextrorotatory isomer of amphetamine with which it shares actions, uses, contraindications, precautions, and adverse reactions. On a weight basis, has less pronounced action on cardiovascular and peripheral nervous systems and is a more potent appetite suppressant. CNS stimulating effect approximately twice that of racemic amphetamine.

Used in treatment of, narcolepsy, and hyperkinesia in children.

ROUTE AND DOSAGE   Oral: *Narcolepsy*: **Adults**: 10 mg daily in divided doses increasing gradually to a maximum of 60 mg/day. *Hyperkinesia*: **Child (3–5 yrs)**: 2.5 mg in the morning increased gradually to a maximum 20 mg/day; **(6–12 yrs)**: 5–10 mg in the morning increased gradually to a maximum of 40 mg/day in two 2 doses.

DEXAMPHETAMINE SULPHATE (continued)

CONTRAINDICATIONS AND PRECAUTIONS Hypersensitivity to sympathomimetic amines, glaucoma, agitated states, psychoses (especially in children), advanced arteriosclerosis, symptomatic heart disease, moderate to severe hypertension, hyperthyroidism, history of drug abuse, during or within 14 days of MAO inhibitor therapy, use as anorexiant in children under 12 years, use for hyperkinesia in children under 3 years.

ADVERSE/SIDE EFFECTS These include: rash, urticaria, nervousness, restlessness, hyperactivity, insomnia, euphoria, dizziness, headache; with prolonged use: severe depression, psychotic reactions, palpitation, tachycardia, chest pains, elevated blood pressure, dry mouth, unpleasant taste, anorexia, weight loss, diarrhoea, constipation, abdominal cramps, impotence, changes in libido, unusual fatigue; marked dystonia of head, neck, extremities; sweating. *See also amphetamine.*

NURSING IMPLICATIONS

- Inform patient that drug may impair ability to drive or perform other potentially hazardous activities.
- Because effect of prolonged use in children is not known, and because dexamphetamine may depress growth by causing loss of appetite, growth rate should be closely monitored.
- Periodic interruption of therapy or reduction in dosage is recommended to assess effectiveness of therapy in behaviour disorders.
- Tolerance to anorexiant effects may develop after a few weeks; however, tolerance does not appear to develop when used in treatment of narcolepsy.
- Discontinuation of drug following prolonged use should be accomplished gradually to avoid the extreme fatigue and mental depression that follows abrupt withdrawal.
- Amphetamines have a high abuse potential because of their excitatory and euphoric effects.
- Addiction potential is controversial. Most authorities seem to agree that long-term therapy is unlikely to produce addiction and that habituation or psychic dependence is caused by psychological factors rather than by pharmacological action. Pronounced tolerance develops with repeated use.
- Lay terms used for amphetamines include 'pep pills,' 'wake-ups,' 'bennies,' and 'speed' (when injected IV), among others. Mixture of an opioid with amphetamine is called 'speed-ball.'
- Store is well-closed containers perferably between 15° and 30°C (59° and 86°F), unless otherwise directed by manufacturer.
- *Treatment of overdosage* Gastric lavage or emesis; barbiturate for sedative effect (used with caution); acidification of urine (e.g., with ammonium chloride) to enhance amphetamine excretion; chlorpromazine to control CNS symptoms; antihypertensive for marked hypertension.
- *See amphetamine sulphate.*

Diagnostic test interferences Dexamphetamine may cause significant elevation of plasma **corticosteroids** (evening levels are highest) and increases in **urinary adrenaline** excretion (during first 3 hours after drug administration).

Dextromethorphan hydrobromide ────────────

(Cosylan)   *Antitussive*

ACTIONS AND USES   Nonnarcotic derivative of levorphanol. Chemically related to morphine, but without its hypnotic or analgesic effect, or capacity to cause tolerance or addiction. Controls cough spasms by depressing cough centre in medulla. Does not depress respiration or inhibit ciliary action. Antitussive activity comparable to that of codeine but is less likely than codeine to cause constipation, drowsiness or GI disturbances.

Used for temporary relief of cough spasms in nonproductive coughs due to colds, pertussis, and influenza. A common ingredient in many OTC cough mixtures.

ROUTE AND DOSAGE   Oral: **Adults**: (syrup contains 13.5 mg/5 ml) 5 ml 3–4 times a day. **Child (1–5 yrs)**: 25% adult dose, **(6–12 yrs)**: 50% adult dose.

ABSORPTION AND FATE   Antitussive action begins in 15 to 30 minutes and lasts 3 to 6 hours.

CONTRAINDICATIONS AND PRECAUTIONS   Sensitivity, children under 2 years of age, during or within 14 days of MAO inhibitor therapy. **Cautious Use**: productive cough, asthma.

ADVERSE/SIDE EFFECTS   Rare: dizziness, drowsiness, GI upset; CNS depression with very large doses.

NURSING IMPLICATIONS
- Although soothing local effect of the syrup may be enhanced if administered undiluted, depression of cough centre depends upon systemic absorption of drug. Increasing fluid intake may help to liquefy tenacious mucus.
- Excessive, nonproductive cough tends to be self-perpetuating because it causes irritation of pharyngeal and tracheal mucosa.
- Unnecessary cough may be lessened by voluntary restraint and by avoiding irritants such as smoking, dust, fumes, and other air pollutants. Humidification of ambient air may provide some relief.
- Treatment is directed toward decreasing the frequency and intensity of cough without completely eliminating protective cough reflex.
- Dextromethorphan may be purchased over the counter. Persons who self-medicate should be advised that symptom suppression does not mean cure of the underlying problem. Any cough persisting longer than 1 week or 10 days should be medically diagnosed.

Drug interactions   Concurrent administration of dextromethorphan and **MAO** inhibitors has resulted in nausea, coma, hypotension, hyperpyrexia, and death.

Dextromoramide————————————

(Palfium)   *Narcotic analgesic*

ACTIONS AND USES   Narcotic analgesic chemically related to methadone with similar actions and uses to morphine (q.v.) but of short duration. Is equally potent used orally as when given by injection.

Used to treat severe pain especially in terminal carcinoma.

ROUTE AND DOSAGE   Oral: Adult: 5 mg increased to 20 mg as required. **Subcutaneous or intramuscular injection**: 5 mg increased to 15 mg as required. **Rectal suppositories**: 10 mg as required.

NURSING IMPLICATIONS
- Less sedating than morphine with slow development of dependence and tolerance.
- Should not be used as an obstetric analgesic (because of the risk of neonatal respiratory depression).
- Store at room temperature.
- *See morphine*.

D

Dextropropoxyphene————————————

(Cosalgesic, Co-proxamol, Distalgesic, Doloxene,   *Narcotic analgesic*
    Doloxene Co, Paxalgesic)

ACTIONS AND USES   Centrally acting and structurally related to methadone. Analgesic potency about ½ to ⅔ that of codeine. Unlike codeine, dextropropoxyphene has little or no antitussive effect and abuse liability is somewhat lower. The hydrochloride is freely soluble in water and is more rapidly and completely absorbed than the napsylate, which is only slightly water-soluble. Lower incidence of GI side effects reported with the napsylate salt.

Used for relief of mild to moderate pain in combination products.

ROUTE AND DOSAGE   Oral: available in combination with paracetomol (Cosalgesic, Distalgesic, Paxalgesic) and aspirin (Doloxene Co).

ABSORPTION AND FATE   Absorbed chiefly in upper part of small intestines. **Peak serum levels** within 2 hours (hydrochloride) and within 3 hours (napsylate). **Onset of analgesic effects** in 15 to 30 minutes; **duration** 4 to 6 hours. **Half-life** of metabolite 30 to 36 hours; of propoxyphene; 6 to 12 hours. Degraded primarily in liver. Excreted in urine within 6 to 48 hours as metabolites and traces of unchanged drug. Crosses placenta; low levels detected in breast milk.

CONTRAINDICATIONS AND PRECAUTIONS   Hypersensitivity to drug, suicidal indi-

DEXTROPROPOXYPHENE (continued)
viduals, alcoholism, dependence on opiates. Safe use during pregnancy and in children not established. **Cautious Use:** renal or hepatic disease.

ADVERSE/SIDE EFFECTS   These include: dizziness, lightheadedness, drowsiness, sedation, unusual fatigue or weakness, restlessness, tremor, euphoria, dysphoria, headache, paradoxic excitement, nausea, vomiting, abdominal pain, constipation, minor visual disturbances, headache, skin eruptions (hypersensitivity), hypoglycaemia (patients with impaired renal function); liver dysfunction, mental confusion, toxic psychosis, coma, convulsions, respiratory depression, pulmonary oedema, acidosis, pinpoint pupils (dilate with advancing hypoxia), circulatory collapse, ECG abnormalities, nephrogenic diabetes insipidus.

NURSING IMPLICATIONS
- Capsules may be emptied and contents mixed with water or food before swallowing.
- Absorption may be somewhat delayed by presence of food in stomach.
- Evaluate patient's need for continued use of this drug. Dextropropoxyphene is commonly abused.
- Tremulousness, restlessness ('speed'), and mild euphoria (effects desired by many addicts) occur frequently.
- Dizziness, lightheadedness, drowsiness, nausea, and vomiting appear to be more prominent in the ambulatory patient. Symptoms may be relieved if patient lies down.
- Caution ambulatory patients not to drive a car and to avoid other potentially hazardous activities.
- ***Treatment of overdosage***   Fatalities occur commonly within first hour following overdosage, therefore prompt action is required: immediate emesis or gastric lavage; activated charcoal. Maintain airway (apnoea occurs quickly). Have on hand: narcotic antagonist naloxone to combat respiratory depression; assisted ventilation equipment, oxygen, anticonvulsants, IV therapy, as indicated. Analeptic drugs (e.g., amphetamines, caffeine) are not used because they tend to precipitate fatal convulsions. Cardiac function, blood gases, pH, and electrolytes should be monitored.
- Dextropropoxyphene in excessive doses, alone or in combination products, ranks second only to barbiturates as a major cause of drug-related deaths.
- Caution patient not to exceed recommended dose and to avoid alcohol and other CNS depressants.
- Tolerance and physical and psychic dependence of the morphine type can occur with excessive use.
- Store at 15° to 30°C (59° to 86°F) unless otherwise directed by manufacturer.

DRUG INTERACTIONS   *Dextropropoxyphene*

PLUS	INTERACTIONS
Alcohol and CNS depressants	Additive CNS depression: drowsiness, stupor; respiratory depression
Anticoagulants, oral	Potentiates warfarin by reducing its metabolism

DEXTROPROPOXYPHENE (continued)

PLUS (continued)	INTERACTIONS
Carbamazepine	Potentiates carbamazepine toxicity by reducing its metabolism
Orphenadrine	Increased CNS stimulation; anxiety, tremors, confusion

Diamorphine hydrochloride

(Heroin)

Narcotic analgesic; opiate agonist

ACTIONS AND USES   A semi-synthetic derivative of morphine with similar action and uses. It is more potent than morphine with a shorter duration of action, causing greater respiratory depression and less nausea than morphine. Used to treat acute and chronic pain.

ROUTE AND DOSAGE   Acute pain by SC or IM routes, average dose 5 mg repeated 4 hourly as required. **Slow IV injection**: ¼ to ½ the IM dose. *Myocardial infarction*: by slow IV injection (1mg/minute) 5 mg, then 2.5 to 5 mg if required. Reduce dose in elderly or frail patients. *Chronic pain*: oral, SC injections: 5–10 mg at regular intervals of 4 hours, increased according to need. **IM injection**: should be ½ the oral dose and ¼–⅓ the oral *morphine* dose. Continuous SC infusion is used in terminal care.

ABSORPTION AND FATE   Well absorbed from the GI tract and from subcutaneous or intramuscular injection. Converted to 6-0-monoacetyl morphine in the blood and then to morphine, excreted in the urine as morphine or morphine glucuronide. Crosses the blood–brain barrier and placenta. Infants born to addicted mothers may have withdrawal symptoms after delivery.

CONTRAINDICATIONS AND PRECAUTIONS, ADVERSE/SIDE EFFECTS   *see   morphine* (q.v.)

NURSING IMPLICATIONS
- Causes constipation; monitor bowel pattern and check for distention.
- Controlled drug, subject to the Misuse of Drugs Act 1971.
- *See morphine.*

Diazepam

(Alupram, Atensine, Diazemuls, Evacalm, Solis, Stesolid, Tensium, Valium)

Psychotropic; anxiolytic; anticonvulsant; benzodiazepine

DIAZEPAM (continued)

ACTIONS AND USES   Anxiolytic agent related to chlordiazepoxide (q.v.); reportedly superior in antianxiety and anticonvulsant activity, with somewhat shorter duration of action. Like chlordiazepoxide, appears to act at both limbic and subcortical levels of CNS. Shortens REM and stage 4 sleep, but increases total sleeptime. Causes transient analgesia after IV administration.

Used for management of anxiety disorders, for short-term relief of anxiety symptoms, to allay anxiety and tension prior to surgery, cardioversion and endoscopic procedures, as an amnesic, and treatment for restless legs. Effective when used adjunctively in status epilepticus and severe recurrent convulsive seizures.

ROUTE AND DOSAGE   Oral: Adult: 2 to 10 mg, two to four times daily. **Children (over 6 months)**: 1 to 2.5 mg, three to four times daily. **Elderly, debilitated**: 2 to 2.5 mg, one or two times daily. **Intramuscular, intravenous**: 2 to 10 mg. Repeat if necessary in 3 to 4 hours. **Elderly, debilitated**: 2 to 5 mg. *Status epilepticus*: **Slow IV injection**: 0.5% solution or emulsion, 10–20 mg at a rate of 0.5 ml (2.5 mg) in 30 seconds. Repeat as required after 30–60 min, follow if required by infusion to a maximum of 3 mg/kg in 24 hrs. **Child**: 200–300 mcg/kg. **Rectal solution: Adult or child (over 3 yrs)**: 10 mg. **Child (1–3 yrs)** and **elderly patients**: 5 mg. Repeat after 5 min if required.

NURSING IMPLICATIONS

- Tension and anxiety associated with stress of everyday life usually do not require treatment with an anxiolytic agent.
- Most adverse reactions of diazepam are dose-related. Physician will rely on accurate observations and reporting of patient's response to the drug to determine lowest effective maintenance dose.
- Maximum effect with steady state plasma levels may require 1 to 2 weeks; patient tolerance to therapeutic effects may develop after 4 weeks of treatment.
- Suicidal tendencies may be present in anxiety states accompanied by depression. Observe necessary preventive precautions.

Parenteral preparation

- Do not mix or dilute with other drugs or solutions in same syringe or infusion flask.
- Avoid IV infusion of diazepam; it may precipitate in IV fluids. Also, diazepam interacts with plastic IV administration sets and containers with significant reduction in availability of drug.
- To prevent swelling, irritation, venous thrombosis, phlebitis, inject slowly taking at least 1 minute for each 5 mg (1 ml) given to adults, and taking at least a 3-minute period to inject 0.25 mg/kg body weight of children.
- If injection cannot be made directly into vein, manufacturer suggests making injection slowly through infusion tubing as close as possible to vein insertion. Check needle site frequently to prevent extravasation.
- Avoid small veins (e.g., dorsum of hand or wrist) and intraarterial administration.
- IM administration should be made deep into large muscle mass. Aspirate for back flow. If present, remove needle, select another site. Inject slowly. Rotate injection sites.
- When given parenterally, hypotension, muscular weakness, tachycardia, and

DIAZEPAM (continued)

respiratory depression may occur, particularly if barbiturates, or narcotics are used concomitantly. Observe patient closely and monitor vital signs. Resuscitative equipment should be readily available.

- When used with a narcotic analgesic, the narcotic dose is reduced by at least ⅓ and given in small increments. In some cases, especially in the elderly, the narcotic is unnecessary.
- Diazepam is used to diminish recall of a distressing procedure such as perioral endoscopy. It does not alter the potential for symptoms related to the procedure such as increase in cough reflex, laryngospasm, and hyperventilation.
- Warn patient to avoid use of alcohol and other CNS depressants during therapy with diazepam, unless otherwise advised by physician. Concomitant use of these agents can cause severe drowsiness, respiratory depression and apnoea.
- Periodic blood cell counts and liver function tests are recommended during prolonged therapy.
- Adverse reactions such as drowsiness, ataxia, constipation and urinary retention are more likely to occur in the elderly and debilitated or in those receiving larger doses. Dosage adjustment may be necessary. Supervise ambulation.
- Monitor fluid intake and output ratio and bowel elimination.
- Because of possible sedation during early therapy, avoid activities requiring mental alertness and precision until reaction to diazepam has been evaluated.
- **Smoking-drug interaction** Smoking increases metabolism of diazepam, therefore clinical effectiveness is lowered. Heavy smokers may need a higher dose than the nonsmoker.
- Abrupt discontinuation of diazepam should generally be avoided. Doses should be tapered to termination. If patient stops drug suddenly after long-term use, withdrawal symptoms (unusual irritability, mental confusion, tremulousness, paranoia, marked photophobia, ataxia, visual hallucinations, vomiting, sweating, abdominal and muscle cramps), may occur and persist for several weeks.
- The patient should be advised that if she becomes pregnant during therapy or intends to become pregnant she should communicate with her physician regarding desirability of discontinuing drug.
- Psychological and physical dependence may occur in patients on long-term high dosage therapy, in those with histories of alcohol or drug addiction, or in those who self-medicate.
- Close supervision should be maintained over the amount of drug dispensed to the patient at one time.
- Caution patient to take drug as prescribed, and not to change dose or dose intervals; also not to offer any of it to another person, or use it to treat a self-diagnosed problem.
- Tell patient to check with physician before taking any OTC drug while on diazepam therapy.
- Preserved in tight, light-resistant containers at temperature between 15° and 30°C (59° and 86°F), unless otherwise specified by manufacturer.

Drug interactions Patients receiving diazepam and nondepolarizing neuromuscular blocking agents, e.g., **pancuronium, succinylcholine** should be closely observed for increase in intensity and duration of respiratory depression. *See also chlorodiazepoxide.*

Diazoxide━━━━━━━━━━━━━━━━━━━━━━━━━━

(Eudemine)   *Antihypertensive; vasodilator;*
                                                        hyperglycaemic; thiazide

ACTIONS AND USES   Rapid-acting benzothiadiazine (thiazide) nondiuretic hypotensive agent. In contrast to thiazide diuretics, causes sodium (Na) and water retention and decreased urinary output, probably because of increased proximal tubular reabsorption of Na and decreased glomerular filtration rate. Like thiazide diuretics, it produces hyperglycaemia by inhibiting pancreatic insulin secretion and by stimulating endogenous catecholamine release. Reduces peripheral vascular resistance and blood pressure by direct vasodilatory effect on peripheral arteriolar smooth muscles, perhaps by direct competition for calcium receptor sites. Hypotensive effect may be accompanied by marked reflex, increase in heart rate, cardiac output, and stroke volume; thus cerebral and coronary blood flow are usually maintained. Renal blood flow initially decreases then increases. Oral drug has more prominent hyperglycaemic action and less marked antihypertensive effect than parenteral drug. Diazoxide may inhibit ureteral and GI motility, and is a powerful uterine relaxant.

Used intravenously for emergency lowering of blood pressure in patients with malignant hypertension, particularly when associated with renal impairment. Not effective in pheochromocytoma. Commonly used with a diuretic to counteract diazoxide-induced Na and water retention. Used orally in treatment of various diagnosed hypoglycaemic states.

ROUTE AND DOSAGE   *Hypertension*: **Intravenous: Adults only:** 300 mg administered undiluted over 30 seconds or less. Repeated up to 3 times in 24 hours. *Hypoglycaemia*: **Oral: Adults and children:** 5 mg/kg/day divided into 2 or 3 equal doses every 8 or 12 hours.

ABSORPTION AND FATE   Rapid IV injection of 300 mg bolus dose produces fall in blood pressure in 30 to 60 seconds, with maximal effect within 5 minutes; **duration** (unpredictable) 2 to 12 hours or longer. Following oral administration, hyperglycaemic effect begins within 1 hour and may last up to 8 hours if renal function is normal. **Plasma half-life:** 20 to 36 hours in adults, 9 to 24 hours in children. More than 90% protein bound. Approximately 50% excreted by kidney unchanged. Crosses blood–brain barrier and placenta.

CONTRAINDICATIONS AND PRECAUTIONS   Hypersensitivity to diazoxide or other thiazides; eclampsia; aortic coarctation; AV shunt, significant coronary artery disease. Safe use during pregnancy, in nursing mothers, and safety of parenteral drug for children not established. Use of oral diazoxide for functional hypoglycaemia or in presence of increased bilirubin in newborns. **Cautious Use:** diabetes mellitus, impaired cerebral or cardiac circulations, impaired renal function, patients taking corticosteroids or oestrogen–progestogen combinations, hyperuricaemia, history of gout.

ADVERSE/SIDE EFFECTS   These include: tinnitus, momentary hearing loss, headache, dizziness, polyneuritis, sleepiness, euphoria, anxiety cerebral ischaemia, (confusion, unconsciousness, convulsions, paralysis), paraesthesias, extrapyramidal signs

DIAZOXIDE (continued)

(oculogyrus, rigidity, trismus, tremor), palpitations, atrial and ventricular arrhythmias, flushing, shock; orthostatic hypotension, myocardial ischaemia and infarction, angina, congestive heart failure, transient hypertension, pruritus, flushing, skin rash, monilial dermatitis, herpes, excessive hair growth (especially in children), loss of scalp hair, sweating, sensation of warmth, burning, or itching, nausea, vomiting, abdominal discomfort, diarrhoea, constipation, ileus, anorexia, transient loss of taste, parotid swelling, dry mouth, thrombocytopenia with or without purpura, transient neutropenia, eosinophilia. **Hypersensitivity**: rash, fever, leucopenia. **Ophthalmic**: blurred vision, transient cataracts, subconjunctival haemorrhage, ring scotoma, diplopia, lacrimation, papilloedema. **Renal**: decreased urinary output, nephrotic syndrome (reversible), haematuria, increased nocturia, proteinuria, azotaemia. **Other**: impaired hepatic function, chest and back pain, muscle cramps; acute pancreatitis; advance in bone age (children); sodium and water retention, oedema, hyperuricaemia, hyperglycaemia, glycosuria, diabetic ketoacidosis and nonketotic hyperosmolar coma; inhibition of labour, enlargement of breast lump, galactorrhoea; decreased immunoglobinaemia. Injection site reactions: warmth or pain along injected vein; with extravasation: severe local pain, cellulitis, phlebitis.

NURSING IMPLICATIONS

Treatment of hypertension (intravenous preparation)

- Blood glucose, serum electrolytes, and complete blood counts should be determined at start of therapy and regularly thereafter in patients receiving multiple doses.
- Patient should be recumbent while receiving IV diazoxide and should remain in bed for at least 30 minutes following administration.
- Monitor blood pressure every 5 minutes for the first 15 to 30 minutes or until stabilized, then hourly for balance of drug effect. In ambulatory patients, blood pressure measurement should be made with patient in standing position, before ending surveillance.
- If blood pressure continues to fall 30 minutes or more after drug administration, suspect cause other than drug effect. Notify physician immediately.
- A precipitous drop in blood pressure is especially dangerous for the elderly because they are less capable of adapting to the stress of compromised circulation to vital organs.
- Monitor pulse: tachycardia has occurred immediately following IV; palpitation and bradycardia have also been reported.
- Have on hand noradrenaline for treatment of severe hypotension.
- Since diazoxide causes Na and water retention, a diuretic is generally prescribed to avoid congestive heart failure and drug resistance, and to maximize hypotensive effect.
- When a diuretic (e.g. frusemide) is prescribed, it is generally given 30 to 60 minutes prior to diazoxide. Patient should remain recumbent 8 to 10 hours because of possible additive hypotensive effect.
- Fluid intake and output should be monitored. Report promptly any change in intake–output ratio, constipation, abdominal distention, or absence of bowel sounds.

DIAZOXIDE (continued)

- If feasible, daily weight provides another objective measure of fluid retention or mobilization.
- Observe patient closely for signs and symptoms of congestive heart failure (distended neck veins, rales at bases of lungs, dyspnoea, orthopnoea, cough, fatigue, weakness, dependent oedema).
- Diazoxide may cause hyperglycaemia and glycosuria in diabetic and diabetic-prone individuals. Blood and urine glucose should be closely monitored. Temporary dosage adjustment of antidiabetic drugs may be required.
- Check IV injection sites daily. Solution is strongly alkaline. Extravasation of medication into subcutaneous or intramuscular tissues can cause severe inflammatory reaction (see Index: Nursing Interventions: Extravasation). Diazoxide is administered only by peripheral vein.
- Alternate oral antihypertensive therapy should be started as soon as possible after emergency is controlled. It is rarely necessary to give IV diazoxide therapy for more than 4 or 5 days.

Treatment of hypoglycaemia (oral preparation)

- During initial therapy, patient should be closely supervised, with blood glucose, serum electrolytes, and clinical response being carefully monitored until condition stabilizes satisfactorily on minimum dosage.
- Blood glucose level should be determined periodically thereafter to evaluate need of dosage adjustment. Serum electrolyte levels should be evaluated at regular intervals particularly in patient with impaired renal function. (Hypokalaemia potentiates hyperglycaemic effect of diazoxide.)
- In contrast to IV administration of diazoxide, oral administration usually does not produce marked effects on blood pressure. However, periodic measurements of blood pressure and vital signs should be made.
- Monitor fluid intake and output ratio, and also weight. Diazoxide promotes Na and water retention, most commonly in young infants and in adults, and may precipitate congestive failure in patients with compromised cardiac reserve.
- Patient should be taught to monitor urine regularly for sugar and ketones, especially during stress conditions, and instructed to report abnormal findings and unusual symptoms to physician. Hyperglycaemia may require reduction in dosage or treatment with a hypoglycaemic agent to avoid progression to ketoacidosis.
- Ketoacidosis and hyperosmolar coma have been reported in patients treated with recommended doses, usually during an intercurrent illness. Emphasize importance of early recognition and reporting of symptoms: increased thirst, acetone (fruity) breath odour, nausea, vomiting, abdominal tenderness, confusion, air hunger. Insulin therapy and restoration of fluid and electrolyte balance are usually effective if instituted promptly.
- Prolonged surveillance is essential because of long half-life of diazoxide (for both oral and parenteral forms). In the event of overdosage, surveillance as long as 7 days may be required.
- Lanugo-type hirsutism (mainly on forehead, back, limbs) occurs frequently and is most common in children and women (reversible with discontinuation of drug).

D

DIAZOXIDE (continued)

- In some patients, higher diazoxide levels are attained with liquid that with capsule formulation. Dosage may require adjustment if patient is changed from one formulation to another.
- Diazoxide is discontinued if not effective in 2 or 3 weeks. Therapy may be continued for several years, until insulin response to presumptive tests are normal.
- Suspension formula should be shaken well before use.
- Protect diazoxide from light, heat, and freezing.
- Darkened solutions may have lost potency and therefore should not be administered.

Diagnostic test interferences   Diazoxide can cause elevations of **blood glucose, serum bilirubin, renin** and **uric acid,** and decreases in **plasma free fatty acids, creatinine,** and **PAH acid clearance, Hgb, Hct.**

DRUG INTERACTIONS   *Diazoxide* _____

PLUS	INTERACTIONS
Alpha adrenergic blocking agents (e.g., ergotamine, phentolamine)	May antagonize hyperglycaemic action of diazoxide
Anticoagulants, oral	Diazoxide enhances anticoagulant effect
Antihypertensives (e.g., hydralazine, methyldopa, reserpine)	Potentiates antihypertensive effect. Use before, during or following diazoxide may result in profound drop in BP
Corticosteroids } combinations	Potentiate hyperglycaemic effect of diazoxide
Oral antidiabetic agents	Pharmacological effects of diazoxide and these agents may be reduced. Monitor blood glucose
Phenothiazines } Thiazides and other diuretics	May intensify hyperglycaemic, hyperuricaemic, and antihypertensive effects of diazoxide. Monitor blood pressure, and blood glucose and serum uric acid levels
Phenytoin and other hydantoins	Diazoxide may enhance phenytoin metabolism with possible loss of seizure control. Monitor phenytoin plasma levels
Vasodilators (e.g., nitrates, papaverine)	Risk of severe hypotension

Dichloralphenazone ━━━━━━━━━━━━━━━━━━━━━━━━

(Welldorm)   *Sedative*

ACTIONS AND USES   A complex of chloral hydrate and phenazone, *see chloral hydrate.*

ROUTE AND DOSAGE   Oral: Adult: *Insomnia*: 1.3−1.95 mg (2−3 tabs) with water 20 min before bedtime.

Dichlorphenamide

(Daranide)

Carbonic anhydrase inhibitor; diuretic; sulphonamide derivative

ACTIONS AND USES   Nonbacteriostatic sulphonamide derivative similar to acetazolamide, except that chloride excretion is increased, and thus potential for significant metabolic acidosis is less. Contraindications, precautions, and adverse reactions are the same as for acetazolamide (q.v.).

Used in adjunctive treatment of open-angle glaucoma and preoperatively in narrow-angle glaucoma when delay of surgery is desired in order to lower intraocular pressure. Commonly used in conjunction with a miotic; an osmotic agent may also be used to enhance reduction of intraocular pressure in acute-angle closure glaucoma.

ROUTE AND DOSAGE   Oral: *Initial*: 100 to 200 mg followed by 100 mg every 12 hours until desired response is obtained. *Maintenance*: 25 to 50 mg 1 to 3 times daily.

ABSORPTION AND FATE   Onset of action within 1 hour; peaks in 2 to 4 hours and lasts 6 to 12 hours.

ADVERSE/SIDE EFFECTS   Paraesthesias, drowsiness, headache, fatigue dizziness, depression, visual disturbances, anorexia, nausea, vomiting, abdominal discomfort, rise in BUN, hyperchloraemic acidosis, hypokalaemia, asymptomatic hyperuricaemia. *See also acetazolamide.*

NURSING IMPLICATIONS
- Teach patient not to accept brand interchange as it is not recommended for carbonic anhydrase inhibitor products.
- *See acetazolamide.*

Diclofenac sodium

(Voltarol)

Antiinflamatory; NSAID (Also used in renalcolic)

ACTIONS AND USES   Used to treat pain and inflammation in rheumatic disease and arthritis.

ROUTE AND DOSAGE   Oral: 75–100 mg/day in divided doses. Deep IM injection: 75 mg 1–2 times a day. Suppositories: 100 mg usually at night.

For further information *see ibuprofen.*

Dicyclomine hydrochloride

(Kolanticon, Kolantyl, Merbentyl)

*Anticholinergic
(parasympathomimetic);
antimuscarinic;
antispasmodic*

ACTIONS AND USES   Synthetic tertiary amine with antispasmodic properties. Exhibits local anaesthetic properties. Used adjunctively in treatment of irritable bowel syndrome, neurogenic bowel disturbances, and infant colic. There are varied opinions about its value in treatment of peptic ulcer because of uncertainty as to its specific action.

ROUTE AND DOSAGE   Oral: Adults: 10 to 20 mg 3 or 4 times daily. **Children:** 10 mg 3 or 4 times daily. **Infants:** 5 mg 3 or 4 times daily.

NURSING IMPLICATIONS
- If necessary, tablet can be crushed or capsule may be emptied before administration and mixed with fluid or food of patient's choice.
- Syrup formulation may be diluted with equal volume of water.
- Advise patient to avoid hot environments. Dicyclomine may increase risk of heatstroke by decreasing sweating. This is a particular problem of the elderly because of age-related reduction in sweating response to heat.
- Infants 6 weeks and under have developed respiratory symptoms as well as seizures, fluctuations in heart rate, weakness, and coma within minutes after taking syrup formulation. Symptoms generally last 20 to 30 minutes and are believed to be due to local irritation.
- *See atropine sulphate.*

Dienoestrol

(Hormofemin, OrthoDienoestrol)

Hormone; oestrogen

ACTIONS AND USES   Synthetic nonsteroidal oestrogen structurally related to diethylstilbestrol. Shares actions of oestradiol (q.v.).

Used for treatment of atrophic vaginitis and kraurosis vulvae associated with the menopause.

ROUTE AND DOSAGE   Intravaginal: cream (0.01%): one or 2 applicatorfuls daily for 1 to 2 weeks. Dosage then reduced to half of initial dose for another 1 to 3 times weekly for 1 or 2 weeks. Vaginal suppository (0.7 mg): one or 2 daily for 1 to 2 weeks then one suppository every other day for a similar period.

ABSORPTION AND FATE, CONTRAINDICATIONS, PRECAUTIONS, ADVERSE SIDE EFFECTS   *See oestradiol.*

DIENOESTROL (continued)
NURSING IMPLICATIONS
- Administration at bedtime increases absorption and thus effectiveness.
- Intravaginal dioenestrol is readily absorbed from the vaginal mucosa and reaches blood levels approaching those of orally administered oestrogens. Systemic hyperoestrogenic effects (reportable) include uterine bleeding, oedema, reactivation of endometriosis and mastalgia and may result from overdosage of intravaginal drug or from overexposure of denuded or abraded skin surfaces of hands to oestrogen.
- Intravaginal administration of medication: have patient in recumbent position, draped, with knees flexed and legs spread apart. Put on sterile gloves before inspecting perineal area. If discharge is present gently wash area with soap (if allowed) and warm water. Spread labia and slowly insert cream applicator approximately 2 inches (5 cm) directing it slightly back toward sacrum. Patient should remain in recumbent position about 30 minutes to prevent losing the medication (no sphincter in vagina). Observe perineal area before each administration: if mucosa is red, swollen, or excoriated, or if there is a change in vaginal discharge, report to physician before giving the medication.
- If patient is to administer medication to herself, instruct her to wash her hands well before and after the procedure; also tell her not to use tampons while on vaginal therapy. She may wish to wear a sanitary towel to protect clothing.
- Ordinarily, a suppository inserter (or cream applicator) is dispensed with the medication.
- Review package insert with patient to assure understanding of oestrogen therapy.
- Protect suppositories and cream from light. Store between 8° and 15°C (46° and 59°F) in a tight container, unless otherwise directed by manufacturer.
- *See oestradiol.*

Diethylcarbamazine citrate

(Banocide)   *Anthelmintic*

ACTIONS AND USES Highly effective against microfilariae. Used to treat infections with Onchocerca volvulus and Loa loa and *Wuchereria bancroftii* in adults.

ROUTE AND DOSAGE Oral: *initial*: 1 mg/kg/day increased to 6 mg/kg/day over 3 days and continued for 21 days.

Diethylpropion hydrochloride

(Apisate, Tenvate, Dospan)   *Central stimulant; anorexigenic agent*

DIETHYLPROPION HYDROCHLORIDE (continued)

ACTIONS AND USES   Amphetamine congener with lower incidence of amphetamine-type adverse effects, but reportedly also less effective as an appetite suppressant. Anorexic action probably secondary to CNS stimulation.

Used solely in management of exogenous obesity as short-term (a few weeks) adjunct in a regimen of weight reduction based on caloric restriction.

ROUTE AND DOSAGE   Oral: 25 mg 3 times daily, 1 hour before meals. Alternatively, sustained-release preparation: 75 mg daily in midmorning. Maximum treatment period 8 weeks.

ABSORPTION AND FATE   Readily absorbed from GI tract. Effects persist about 4 hours for regular tablet, and for 10 to 14 hours for controlled-release formulations. (Bioavailability may not be uniform.) Excreted in urine.

CONTRAINDICATIONS AND PRECAUTIONS   Known hypersensitivity or idiosyncrasy to sympathomimetic amines, severe hypertension, advanced arteriosclerosis, hyperthyroidism, glaucoma, agitated states, history of drug abuse, during or within 14 days following use of MAO inhibitors, concomitant use of CNS stimulants. Safe use during pregnancy and in children under 12 years of age not established. **Cautious Use:** hypertension, arrhythmias, symptomatic cardiovascular disease, epilepsy, diabetes mellitus.

ADVERSE/SIDE EFFECTS   These include: restlessness, nervousness, dizziness, headache, insomnia, drowsiness, psychotic episodes, palpitation, tachycardia, precordial pain, elevated blood pressure, nausea, vomiting, diarrhoea, constipation, dry mouth, unpleasant taste, muscle pain, dyspnoea, hair loss, polyuria, dysuria, increased sweating, impotence, changes in libido, gynaecomastia, menstrual irregularities, bone marrow depression, increase in convulsive episodes in patients with epilepsy. *See also amphetamine.*

NURSING IMPLICATIONS

- Additional dose sometimes prescribed in midevening to control night time hunger. Rarely causes insomnia except in high doses.
- Sustained-release tablets should be swallowed whole and not chewed.
- Dosage should be carefully titrated in patients with diabetes.
- Patients with epilepsy should be observed closely for reduction in seizure control.
- Anorexigenic effect seldom lasts more than a few weeks. If tolerance develops, drug should be discontinued.
- Dry mouth may be relieved by frequent rinses with warm clear water, sugarless gum, or lemon drops, increasing noncaloric fluid intake (if allowed).
- Varying degrees of psychological and rarely physical dependence can occur. Drugs related to amphetamines are frequently misused by emotionally unstable individuals.
- Because diethylpropion may mask fatigue and may cause dizziness, caution patient to avoid operation machinery or driving a car or other hazardous activities, until reaction to drug is determined.
- *See dextramphetamine.*

Diflucortolone ━━━━━━━━━━━━━━━

(Nerisone, Nerisone Forte)   *Corticosteroid; glucocorticoid*

ACTIONS AND USES   Topical synthetic fluorinated corticosteroid with antiinflammatory, antipruritic, and vasoconstrictive activity.

Used to relieve inflammatory symptoms of a variety of skin disorders responsive to corticosteroids. *See hydrocortisone for absorption, fate, limitations, and interactions.*

ROUTE AND DOSAGE   Topical: Apply small amount cream 1 to 3 times daily.

Diflunisal ━━━━━━━━━━━━━━━━━

(Dolobid)   *Analgesic; NSAID;*
                                                             antirheumatic

D

ACTIONS AND USES   Long-acting nonsteroidal antiinflammatory drug (NSAID) with analgesic properties. Derived from salicylic acid, but is not hydrolyzed to salicylate in the body. Precise mode of action not known but appears to be related to inhibition of prostaglandin synthesis. Comparable to aspirin and paracetamol in equianalgesic doses but has longer duration of effect. However, onset of analgesic action may be delayed unless loading dose is used. Unlike aspirin, inhibition of platelet function and effect on bleeding time are dose-related and reversible, lasting only about 24 hours after drug is discontinued. Reportedly has lower incidence of gastric erosion and significant faecal blood loss than aspirin. Exerts very mild antipyretic effect; therefore is not clinically useful for this purpose. Habituation, tolerance, or addiction have not been reported.

Used for acute and long-term relief of mild to moderate pain, and for symptomatic treatment of osteoarthritis and rheumatoid arthritis.

ROUTE AND DOSAGE   Oral: Adult: 250–500 mg/twice a day.

ABSORPTION AND FATE   Onset of analgesia usually within 1 hour, peak effect within 2 to 3 hours, and duration 12 hours. **Peak plasma levels**: 2 to 3 hours. **Plasma protein binding**: 98 to 99%. **Half-life**: 10 to 12 hours (longer in patients with renal insufficiency). Steadystate plasma levels achieved in several days following multiple doses. Metabolized in liver. Excreted in urine within 72 to 96 hours, about 90% of dose as glucuronide conjugates and 3% as unchanged drug. Less than 5% eliminated in faeces. Probably crosses placenta. Excreted in breast milk (in concentrations 2 to 7% of that in plasma).

CONTRAINDICATIONS AND PRECAUTIONS   Hypersensitivity to diflunisal, patients in whom aspirin, other salicylates, or other NSAIDs precipitate an acute asthmatic attack, urticaria, angioedema, or severe rhinitis; active peptic ulcer, GI bleeding. Safe use during pregnancy, in nursing mothers, children, and infants not established. Use

DIFLUNISAL (continued)

during third trimester of pregnancy specifically contraindicated because NSAIDs are known to cause premature closure on ductus arteriosus in fetus. **Cautious Use**: history of upper GI disease, impaired renal function, compromised cardiac function and other conditions predisposing to fluid retention; hypertension, patients who may be adversely affected by prolonged bleeding time.

ADVERSE/SIDE EFFECTS   These include: drowsiness, insomnia, dizziness, headache, fatigue, nervousness, vertigo, asthenia, disorientation, stupor (overdosage). Causal relationships not established: depression paraesthesias, malaise. **Others**: rash, erythema multiforme, Stevens–Johnson syndrome, pruritus, sweating, dry mucous membranes, tinnitus, hearing loss, nausea, vomiting, dyspepsia, GI pain, diarrhoea, constipation, flatulence, GI bleeding, stomatitis, peptic, ulcer, anorexia, eructation, cholestatic jaundice, severe hepatic dysfunction, prolonged BT, anaemia, thrombocytopenia, elevation of liver function tests, blurred vision, reduced visual acuity, changes in colour vision, scotomata, corneal deposits, retinal disturbances, peripheral oedema, weight gain; causal relationships not established: dysuria, dyspnoea, palpitation, syncope, muscle cramps, fever, hypersensitivity reactions including interstitial nephritis with renal failure; anaphylactic reactions with bronchospasm.

NURSING IMPLICATIONS

- Instruct patient to swallow tablet whole. It should not be crushed or chewed.
- Caution patient to take drug as prescribed. Doubling of dosage can produce greater than doubling of drug accumulation (concentration-dependent pharmacokinetics), particularly in patients receiving repetitive doses.
- Full antiinflammatory effect for arthritis may not occur until after 8 days to several weeks of therapy in some patients.
- Since eye complications have been associated with the use of NSAIDs, advise patient to report the onset of eye problems immediately to physician. Ophthalmological studies are indicated.
- Patients with impaired renal function should be closely monitored for drug effect to avoid excessive drug accumulation and toxicity. Instruct patient to be aware of fluid intake–output ratio and pattern and to observe for peripheral oedema and unusual weight gain.
- Patients presenting signs of hepatic dysfunction (persistent abnormally high elevation of SGPT (ALT), SGOT (AST), eosinophilia, jaundice or rash) should be evaluated for hepatic reaction.
- Caution patient about the possibility of drug-induced drowsiness and dizziness with respect to driving and other potentially hazardous activities.
- Although the antipyretic effect of diflunisal is mild, be mindful of the possibility that in chronic or high doses it may mask fever in some patients.
- If used concomitantly with an anticoagulant, close monitoring of prothrombin time is advised during and for several days after concomitant use.
- Store between 15° and 30°C (59° and 86°F) in well-closed containers, unless otherwise directed by manufacturer.
- See also aspirin.

DIFLUNISAL *(continued)*

Diagnostic test interferences Diflunisal can cause lowering of **serum uric acid** concentrations by as much as 1.4 mg% and increased renal clearance of uric acid.

DRUG INTERACTIONS *Diflunisal*

PLUS	INTERACTIONS
Paracetamol	Plasma levels may increase by about 50%. Used concomitantly with caution and careful monitoring of hepatic function
Antacids	Significant reduction of diflunisal absorption, particularly if antacids are used routinely
Anticoagulants, oral	Increased anticoagulant (hypoprothrombinaemic) effect and prothrombin time
Aspirin	Small decreases in diflunisal plasma levels. Increased risk of GI irritation and bleeding
Frusemide	Decreased hyperuricaemic effects of frusemide
Hydrochlorothiazide	Significant increases in hydrochlorothiazide plasma levels, and decrease in hyperuricaemic effect
Indomethacin	Increased indomethacin plasma levels. Severe GI haemorrhage reported in some patients. Concomitant use not recommended
Lithium	Increased steady-state plasma lithium levels
Naproxen	Significant decrease in urinary excretion of naproxen
Sulindac	Lowering of active sulindac metabolite plasma levels by about ⅓

D

Digitoxin

(Digitaline Nativelle)

Antiarrhythmic; cardiac glycoside

ACTIONS AND USES Long-acting glycoside of *Digitalis purpurea* with same actions, uses, precautions, and adverse reactions as digoxin.

ROUTE AND DOSAGE Oral: Adult: 50–100 mcg/day.
For further information: *see digoxin.*

Digoxin

(Lanoxin, Lanoxin PG)

Antiarrhythmic; cardiac glycoside

DIGOXIN (continued)

ACTIONS AND USES   Widely used glycoside of *Digitalis lanata*. Share actions, uses, contraindications, and adverse reactions of digitalis and other cardiotonic glycosides. Action is more prompt and less prolonged than that of digitalis and digitoxin. Also, it is less likely to give rise to cumulative effects because it is more readily absorbed and exchanged in the body and is rather rapidly excreted in urine.

Used for rapid digitalization and for maintenance therapy in congestive heart failure, atrial fibrillation, atrial flutter, paroxysmal atrial tachycardia.

ROUTE AND DOSAGE   Dosage is highly individualized, based upon age, renal function, and lean body weights. *Rapid digitalization*: **Oral**. *Digitalizing dose*: **Adults and Children (over 10 years)**: 1–1.5 mg in divided doses over 24 hrs. *Maintenance*: 125–250 mcg once or twice a day. **IV**: only when very rapid control is needed, 0.75–1mg in 50 ml infusion over 2 or more hours.

ABSORPTION AND FATE   Absorption of oral liquid preparation is virtually complete (80 to 90%); absorption of tablets may vary (50 to 85%) depending upon brand. Onset of effects occurs in 1 to 2 hours; peak effects in 6 to 8 hours. Wide interindividual variation. After IM administration, action begins in 30 minutes and peaks in 4 to 6 hours (erratic absorption patterns). Action following IV dose begins within 5 to 30 minutes and peaks in 1½ to 2 hours; action regresses in 8 to 10 hours. Duration of action regardless of route: 3 to 4 days. **Half-life**: 34 to 44 hours. Approximately 23% protein-bound. High concentrations in myocardium, skeletal muscle, and kidney. Minimal distribution to body fat. Only 14% eliminated by hepatic metabolism; 80 to 90% of dose excreted via kidneys primarily as unchanged drug and small amounts of active metabolites. Small amounts excreted in bile via faeces. Crosses placenta and may appear in breast milk (but not in toxic amounts).

CONTRAINDICATIONS AND PRECAUTIONS   Digitalis hypersensitivity, ventricular fibrillation, ventricular tachycardia unless due to congestive heart failure. Full digitalizing dose not given if patient has received digoxin during previous week or if slowly excreted cardiotonic glycoside has been given during previous 2 weeks. **Cautious Use**: renal insufficiency, hypokalaemia, advanced heart disease, acute myocardial infarction, incomplete AV block, cor pulmonale, hypothyroidism, lung disease, pregnancy, nursing women, premature and immature infants, children, elderly, or debilitated patients.

ADVERSE/SIDE EFFECTS   These include: fatigue, muscle weakness, headache, facial neuralgia, mental depression, paraesthesias, hallucinations, confusion, drowsiness, agitation, dizziness, heart block, arrhythmias, hypotension, anorexia, nausea, vomiting, diarrhoea, visual disturbances, diaphoresis, recurrent malaise, dysphagia, gynaecomastia (uncommon).

NURSING IMPLICATIONS
- Not to be confused with digitoxin.
- Digoxin may be given without regard to food unless otherwise directed by physician. Administration of digoxin after meals or food may slightly delay rate of absorption but total amount absorbed is not affected.

DIGOXIN (continued)

- A careful medication history should be taken before initiation of therapy regarding any prior or recent use of digitalis glycosides.
- Be familiar with patient's baseline data: (e.g., quality of peripheral pulses, blood pressure, clinical symptoms, serum electrolytes, creatinine clearance) as a foundation for making sensitive assessments. Evaluations of these data guide dosage titration.
- Although a fall in ventricular rate to 60/minute in adults (70/minute in children) is used as one criterion for withholding medication and reporting to physician, actually any change in pulse rate or rhythm should be interpreted as a sign of digitalis intoxication and should be reported promptly, e.g., sudden increase or decrease in heart rate, irregular rhythm, regularization of a chronically irregular pulse.
- In children cardiac arrhythmias are usually more reliable signs of early toxicity. Early indicators of toxicity in adults (anorexia, nausea, vomiting, diarrhoea, paraesthesias, facial neuralgia, headaches, hallucinations, confusion, visual disturbances) occur rarely as initial signs in children.
- Therapeutic range of serum digoxin is 0.8 to 2 ng/ml; toxic levels: > 2 ng/ml. Blood samples for determining plasma digoxin levels should be drawn at least 5 to 6 hours after daily dose and preferably just before next scheduled daily dose.
- When patient is controlled on maintenance doses, generally radial pulse is taken for 1 full minute before drug administration. If abnormalities are detected, check apical pulse for 1 full minute and notify physician.
- When digoxin is prescribed for atrial fibrillation, patient should be advised to report to physician if pulse rate falls below 60 or rises above 110 or if he or she detects skipped beats or other changes in rhythm.
- Direct IV injection of digoxin may be administered undiluted or diluted in dextrose 5% in water or sodium chloride 0.9% (if prescribed).
- Infiltration of parenteral drug into subcutaneous tissue can cause local irritation and sloughing.
- Monitor fluid intake–output ratio during digitalization period particularly in patients with impaired renal function. Delayed or diminished renal excretion of drug can lead to toxicity. Observe for oedema daily and auscultate chest for rales. Note patient's food intake. Anorexia is an early sign of toxicity.
- Alterations of digoxin absorption may occur in patients with hypermotility secondary to laxative abuse and in patients with malabsorption syndrome.
- Diarrhoea from any cause leads to potassium loss and increased risk of digitalis toxicity. If it is a problem consult physician regarding an antidiarrhoeal medication.
- Concurrent antibiotic/digoxin therapy could precipitate toxicity because of altered intestinal flora. Monitor serum digoxin levels closely to determine reduced bioavailability.
- Creatinine clearance may be used to determine the need for dosage adjustment particularly in the elderly and other patients with impaired renal function. (Renal excretion of digoxin is reduced in proportion to creatinine clearance.)
- If quinidine is to be added to treatment regimen, digoxin dose should be reduced by 30 to 50% to prevent digoxin toxicity (see Drug Interactions). Patient should be monitored for clinical and ECG indications of toxicity, and serum digoxin levels. Because syncope is a side effect of quinidine, observe necessary safety precautions.

D

DIGOXIN (continued)

When quinidine is discontinued, serum digoxin concentrations may fall below therapeutic levels.

- Dosage should be carefully titrated and patient closely observed when being transferred from one preparation (tablet, elixir, or parenteral) to another. For example, when tablet is replaced by elixir, potential for toxicity is increased because approximately 30% more of drug is absorbed.
- Advise patient to reduce total daily salt intake by omitting obviously salty foods and table salt.
- Instruct patient to take digoxin precisely as prescribed, not to skip or double a dose or change dose intervals and to take it at the same time each day. Suggest taking drug in relation to some daily activity as a reminder and to keep a diary of drug administration such as a check-off calendar.
- Caution patient not to remove digoxin from original container and not to mix it with other tablets in a pillbox.
- When using elixir formulation, measure dose with specially calibrated dropper supplied.
- Advise patient to keep digoxin out of reach of children.
- Caution patient not to take OTC medications, especially those for coughs, colds, allergy, GI upset, or obesity without prior approval of physician.
- Do not use parenteral solution if a precipitate or discolouration is present.
- Preserved in airtight containers protected from light perferably at 15° to 30°C (59° to 86°F), unless otherwise directed by manufacturer.

Diagnostic test interferences   Significant elevations of **creatinine phosphokinase (CPK)** may follow IM administration.

DRUG INTERACTIONS   *Digoxin*

PLUS	INTERACTIONS
Antacids } Cholestyramine	May decrease absorption of digoxin
Metoclopramide	May reduce digoxin absorption by increasing GI tract motility
Neomycin	Inhibits GI absorption of digoxin; spacing will not prevent interaction; monitor serum digoxin levels
Propantheline	May increase GI absorption of digoxin (by decreasing GI motility). Reportedly digoxin elixir not affected as much as tablet form
Quinidine	Increased risk of digoxin toxicity; (reduces renal clearance of digoxin)
Spironolactone	Decreases renal tubular elimination of digoxin leading to toxicity
Sulphasalazine	May reduce bioavailability of digoxin
Thyroid preparations	Increases risk of digoxin toxicity

Dihydrocodeine ████████

(DF118, DHC continus)   *Narcotic analgesic*

ACTIONS AND USES   Semisynthetic codeine derivative more potent than codeine and less potent than morphine with similar action and uses to codeine phosphate (q.v.).
Used to treat moderate to severe pain.

ROUTE AND DOSAGE   Oral: **Adult**: 30 mg/4 to 6 hourly as required. **Child (over 4 years)**: 0.5–1 mg/kg. **Sustained release preparation**: 60 mg (1 tablet) twice a day for prolonged moderate pain. **Subcutaneous (deep)** or **intramuscular injection**: **Adult**: 50 mg/4 to 6 hourly. **Child (over 4 years)**: 0.5 to 1 mg/kg.

NURSING IMPLICATIONS
- Prolonged use may produce dependence.
- Oral preparations are not controlled drugs but injected preparations are in this category.
- A liquid preparation is available for patients unable to swallow tablets.
- Store at room temperature.
- *See codeine phosphate.*

Dihydroergotamine mesylate ████████

(Dihydergot)   *Alpha-adrenergic blocking agent; antimigraine agents; ergot alkaloid*

ACTIONS AND USES   Alpha-adrenergic blocking agent and dihydrogenated ergot alkaloid with direct constricting effect on smooth muscle of peripheral and cranial blood vessels. Has somewhat weaker vasoconstrictor action than ergotamine (q.v.), but greater adrenergic blocking activity. Toxicity potential is about one-tenth that of parent drug. Lacks uterine stimulating action in therapeutic dose. Offers no advantage if equipotent doses are compared with ergotamine.
Used to prevent or abort vascular headache (e.g., migraine or histaminic cephalalgia) when rapid control is desired or other routes are not feasible.

ROUTE AND DOSAGE   Oral: mild attacks 2–3 mg may be repeated at 30 min intervals to a total of 10 mg. *Prophylaxis*: 1–2 mg three times a day. **IM/SC**: 1–2 mg repeated after 30 min as required.

ABSORPTION AND FATE   Onset of action in 15 to 30 minutes following IM injection, less than 5 minutes following IV; duration 3 to 4 hours. Half-life: 1.3 to 3.9 hours.

DIHYDROERGOTAMINE MESYLATE (continued)

CONTRAINDICATIONS AND PRECAUTIONS   History of hypersensitivity to ergot preparations; presence of peripheral vascular disease, coronary heart disease, hypertension, peptic ulcer, impaired hepatic or renal function, sepsis. Safe use during pregnancy, in nursing women, and in children not established. *See also ergotamine.*

ADVERSE/SIDE EFFECTS   Numbness and tingling in fingers and toes, muscle pains and weakness of legs, precordial distress and pain, transient tachycardia or bradycardia, nausea, vomiting, localized oedema and itching; ergotism (excessive doses). *See ergotamine.*

NURSING IMPLICATIONS

- Drug is given at first warning of migraine headache. Optimum results are obtained by titrating the doses required to give relief for several headaches to determine the minimal effective dose. This dose is used for subsequent attacks.
- Onset of action after IM injection is delayed about 20 minutes; therefore, when more rapid relief is required, the IV route is prescribed.
- Protect ampoules from heat and light; do not freeze. Discard ampoule if solution becomes discoloured.
- Store preferably at 15° to 30°C (59° to 86°F), unless otherwise directed by manufacturer.
- *See ergotamine tartrate.*

Diloxanide furoate————————————————————————

(Entamizole Furamide)   *Amoebicide*

ACTIONS AND USES   Acetanilide with direct amoebicidal action and low degree of toxicity. Mechanism of action not established. Acts principally in bowel lumen in cyst-carrier and cyst-passing states. Reportedly not effective for use alone in patients with acute amoebic dysentery or who are passing trophozoites; also of no value in extra-intestinal amoebiasis.

Used for treatment of intestinal amoebiasis particularly in asymptomatic cyst-passers. Has been used as supplement with chloroquine, oxytetracycline, and tetracycline in treatment of acute and chronic intestinal amoebiasis.

ROUTE AND DOSAGE   Oral: Adults: 500 mg three times daily for 10 days.

ABSORPTION AND FATE   About 90% absorbed from GI tract. Blood concentrations peak within 1 hour following administration, but decline quickly over 6-hour period. Rapidly excreted in urine largely as glucuronide. Some excretion in faeces.

CONTRAINDICATIONS AND PRECAUTIONS   Safe use during pregnancy and in children under 2 years not established.

DILOXANIDE FUROATE (continued)

ADVERSE/SIDE EFFECTS   Infrequent: nausea, vomiting, oesophagitis, persistent or recurrent diarrhoea, abdominal cramps, flatulence, pruritus, urticaria, albuminuria, tingling sensations.

NURSING IMPLICATIONS

- Administer drug with meals to reduce risk of GI irritation.
- Inform patient that absence of symptoms is not an indication of cure. Amoebiasis is considered cured when no cysts or trophozoites of *Entamoeba histolytica* are found in repeated stool specimens at 6-month intervals.
- Urge patient to remain under medical supervision until discharged by physician.
- Household members and other suspected contacts should have microscopic examination of faeces.
- Review with patient and contacts preventive measures for controlling spread of amoebiasis:
  - □ Sanitary disposal of faeces.
  - □ Boil drinking water when necessary (chlorination does not generally destroy cysts; diatomaceous earth filters remove them completely, and filtration removes nearly all cysts).
  - □ Personal hygiene such as handwashing after defaecation and before preparing or eating food; risks of eating raw foods.
  - □ Fly control.
- Incubation period is commonly 3 to 4 weeks (range 5 days to several months).
- Store medication in well-covered container. Protect from light.
- *See metronidazole.*

Diltiazem

(Tildiem)   *Vasodilator; calcium channel blocking agent*

ACTIONS AND USES   Slow channel blocker with pharmacological actions similar to those of others in this class (verapamil, nifedipine). Antianginal action and increased exercise tolerance result from potent coronary dilatation effects and increased availability of oxygen for myocardial work. Inhibition of coronary artery spasm increases oxygen delivery to myocardial tissue while dilatation of systemic vasculature results in decreased total peripheral resistance, afterload, and systemic blood pressure. Slightly decreases myocardial contractility; prolongs AV nodal refractory period.

Used in management of spontaneous coronary artery spasm and chronic stable angina.

ROUTE AND DOSAGE   Oral: 60 mg three times/day; **Geriatric patient**: lower doses.

ABSORPTION AND FATE   Approximately 80% of oral dose rapidly absorbed from GI tract. Extensive first-pass metabolism in liver resulting in low bioavailability with first

DILTIAZEM (continued)

dose (40%). **Detectable plasma levels** in 30 minutes; **peak concentration** in 2 to 3 hours; 70 to 85% protein bound. **Half-life**: about 3.5 to 9 hours at steady state (may increase in the elderly, but only slight increase in renal impairment). 2 to 4% drug eliminated in urine unchanged; remainder eliminated in urine and bile as metabolites.

CONTRAINDICATIONS AND PRECAUTIONS   Known hypersensitivity to the drug; sick sinus syndrome (unless pacemaker is in place and functioning); second- or third-degree AV block; severe hypotension (systolic less than 90 mm Hg or diastolic less than 60 mm Hg). Safety and efficacy in children not established; pregnancy **Cautious Use**: congestive heart failure (especially if patient is also receiving beta-blocker), renal or hepatic impairment, the elderly, nursing mothers.

ADVERSE/SIDE EFFECTS   These include: second- and third-degree AV block, bradycardia, congestive heart failure, asymptomatic systole, flushing, hypotension, syncope, palpitation, arrhythmias, rash, photosensitivity, petechiae, urticaria, pruritus, anorexia, nausea, vomiting, diarrhoea, constipation, pyrosis, headache, fatigue, nervousness, depression, drowsiness, insomnia, confusion, oedema, acute renal failure.

NURSING IMPLICATIONS
- Administer before meals and at bedtime. Tablet may be crushed if necessary and administered with a liquid of patient's choice.
- *Therapeutic blood level*: 0.025 to 0.1 mcg/ml.
- If patient is also receiving digoxin, serum digoxin concentration should be determined and patient should be monitored for signs and symptoms of digitalis toxicity.
- Has been used concomitantly with short- or long-acting nitrates, but antianginal effectiveness needs to be studied further.
- *See verapamil*.

Dimenhydrinate————————————————————

(Dramamine)   *Antihistamine, H$_1$-receptor
antagonist; antiemetic*

ACTIONS AND USES   Ethanolamine derivative and chlorotheophylline salt of diphenhydramine (q.v.), with which it shares similar properties.

    Used chiefly in prevention and treatment of motion sickness. Also has been used in management of vertigo, nausea, and vomiting.

ROUTE AND DOSAGE   **Oral: Adults**: 50 to 100 mg 2–3 times a day. Not to exceed 400 mg/24 hours. **Oral: Children (6 to 12 years)**: 25 to 50 mg 2–3 times a day. Not to exceed 150 mg/24 hours. **Children (1 to 5 years)**: up to 25 mg in 2–3 doses.

ABSORPTION AND FATE   Duration of action approximately 3 to 6 hours. Small amounts excreted in breast milk. *See also diphenhydramine*.

DIMENHYDRINATE (continued)

CONTRAINDICATIONS AND PRECAUTIONS   History of hypersensitivity to dimenhydrate or its components; narrow-angle glaucoma, prostatic hypertrophy. Safe use during pregnancy, in nursing women, and in neonates not established. **Cautious Use**: convulsive disorders.

ADVERSE/SIDE EFFECTS   CNS: drowsiness, headache, incoordination, dizziness, nervousness, restlessness, insomnia (especially children); hypotension, palpitation, blurred vision, dry mouth, nose, throat. Less frequently: anorexia, constipation or diarrhoea, urinary frequency, dysuria. *See also diphenhydramine.*

NURSING IMPLICATIONS

- High incidence of drowsiness; this is often a desirable reaction for some patients. Bedsides and supervision of ambulation may be advisable. Caution ambulatory patient not to drive or operate dangerous machinery until drowsiness has passed.
- To prevent radiation sickness, drug is usually administered 30 to 60 minutes before treatment, then repeated 1½ hours after treatment and again in 3 hours.
- To prevent motion sickness, dimenhydrinate should be taken 30 minutes before departure and should be repeated before meals and upon retiring.
- Some claim that motion sickness can largely be prevented by (1) avoiding fatty food intake before the trip; (2) eating lightly prior to and during travel; (3) munching on crackers or other complex carbohydrate during the trip. An empty stomach may actually contribute to the feeling of nausea. Other steps that may be taken: do not drink alcohol on day of travel; travel at night so as to eliminate visual causes of motion sickness.
- Tolerance to CNS depressant effects usually occurs after a few days of drug therapy. Some decrease in antiemetic action may result with prolonged use.
- Avoid mixing parenteral preparation with other drugs. Dimenhydrinate is incompatible with many solutions.
- Store preferably between 15° and 30°C (59° and 86°F), unless otherwise directed by manufacturer. Examine parenteral preparation for particulate matter and discoloration. Do not use unless absolutely clear.

Drug interactions   Dimenhydrinate may mask ototoxic symptoms associated with **aminoglycoside antibiotics**. Enhanced CNS depression (drowsiness) may occur when antihistamines are used concurrently with **alcohol, barbiturates**, and other **CNS depressants**. *See diphenhydramine hydrochloride.*

Dimethidene maleate

(Fenostil Retard)

ACTIONS AND USES   Antihistamine, with similar action and uses to Chlorpheniramine.

DIMETHIDENE MALEATE (continued)
ROUTE AND DOSAGE   Oral: Adult: 2.5 mg twice a day.
For further information *see chlorpheniramine*

Dinoprost ▬▬▬▬▬▬▬▬▬▬▬▬▬▬▬▬▬▬▬▬▬▬▬▬▬

(Prostin F$_2$ Alpha)   *Prostaglandin*

ACTIONS AND USES   Synthetically prepared member of the prostaglandin E$_2$ series that appears to act directly on myometrium and on gastrointestinal, bronchial, and vascular smooth muscle. Stimulation of gravid uterus in early weeks of gestation more potent than that of oxytocin. Used to terminate pregnancy.

ROUTE AND DOSAGE   Oral: IV, Extra or Intraamnionic: dose depends on route.

CONTRAINDICATIONS AND PRECAUTIONS   Hypersensitivity to prostaglandins; acute pelvic inflammatory disease; history of Caesarean section, or other major uterine surgery, uterine fibroids, cervical stenosis; ruptured membranes. **Cautious Use**: history of asthma, glaucoma, hypertension, cardiovascular or renal disease, epilepsy.

ADVERSE/SIDE EFFECTS   CNS: headache, dizziness, paraesthesias, anxiety, drowsiness, seizures. **Others**: hypotension, syncope, flushing, hypertension, bradycardia and other arrhythmias, second degree heart block, vomiting, nausea, diarrhoea, epigastric pain, abdominal cramps, pain (substernal, legs, shoulder, back), urine retention, haematuria, dysuria, cervical laceration or perforation, uterine rupture, endometritis, hot flushes, breast tenderness, burning sensation, lactation: bronchoconstriction, bronchospasm (wheezing), cough, chest rales, dyspnoea, hyperventilation, sensation of chest constriction, fever, chills, diaphoresis, polydipsia, burning sensation in eyes, diplopia, hiccoughs, malaise.

NURSING IMPLICATIONS
- Drug should be used only by qualified personnel in hospital setting with facilities that are immediately available for intensive care and surgery. Patient is usually hospitalized 1 to 4 days.
- Patient should be well aware of benefits and risks of prostaglandin-induced abortion, and the nurse should be aware that the patient is in a life crisis.
- A complete medical history and physical examination should be performed before starting therapy with dinoprost.
- Instruct patient to empty her bladder before the transabdominal tap.
- Adverse effects of prostaglandin administration, such as nausea and vomiting, seldom last longer than 15 to 20 minutes because drug is rapidly metabolized.
- Monitor blood pressure, pulse, respirations, and uterine activity following drug administration. Report significant signs: pulse and blood pressure changes may signal

DINOPROST (continued)

haemorrhage; hypertonic uterine contractions can promote haemorrhage and cervical trauma. Save all clots and tissue for physician inspection and laboratory analysis.

- Promptly report vasovagal symptoms (pallor, nausea, vomiting, bradycardia, rapid fall in arterial blood pressure). Instruct patient to remain in recumbent position.
- The primipara may experience cervical laceration, particularly if oxytocin has been given before uterine response to dinoprost has ceased, and when cervix is poorly dilated.
- Since lacerations may be asymptomatic, a careful vaginal examination should be done postabortion to determine condition of the cervix. (Depending on hospital policy, may be done by the nurse if there is no bleeding.)
- Failure to pass placenta within 1 hour after foetus is delivered may require use of oxytocin or curettage. Oxytocin should not be used until cervix is dilated and uterine response to dinoprost has stopped, to avoid cervical injury and uterine rupture.
- Late postabortion haemorrhage can result from retained placental tissue, infection, or subinvolution of placental site. Note and report character and quantity of blood passed through birth canal. Emergency measures performed by the physician (including placental expression) and blood transfusions may be necessary.
- Differentiation between drug-induced pyrexia and endometritis pyrexia is difficult but essential.
- Encouraging fluids may be sufficient for drug-induced fever, if there is no clinical or bacterial evidence of intrauterine infection. Other more rigorous measures to reduce fever are not necessary because prostaglandin-induced elevated temperature is transient and self limiting.
- Lactation of several days' duration may occur following successful termination of pregnancy.
- Dinoprost does not seem to affect integrity of foetal–placental unit; thus, a live-born foetus may be delivered, particularly if abortion is accomplished at end of second trimester. If drug fails to terminate pregnancy another method is usually employed. Hypertonic saline may be utilized after cessation of uterine contractions.
- Dinoprost ampoules should be stored at 2° to 8°C (36° to 46°F) and should be discarded 24 months following date of manufacture.

D

Dinoprostone

(Prostin E$_2$)

ACTIONS AND USES   Prostaglandin with similar action and uses to Dinoprost.

ROUTE AND DOSAGE   Oral: 500 mcg *initial* then 0.5–1 mg at hourly intervals. Intravenous, extra-amniotic and vaginal routes also used.

Dioctyl sodium sulphosuccinate————————————

(Dioctyl, Fletcher's Enemette, Klyx)   *Laxative; emollient; stool*
                                                      softener, surfactant

ACTIONS AND USES   Anionic surface-active agent with emulsifying and wetting properties. Lowers surface tension, permitting water and fats to penetrate and soften stools
for easier passage.

Used in treatment of constipation associated with hard, dry stools; used for painful
anorectal conditions and in cardiac or other patients who should avoid straining during
defeacation.

ROUTE AND DOSAGE   Oral: **Adult:** up to 500 mg/day; **Child:** 60 mg/day; **Infant:**
30 mg/day all in divided doses.

CONTRAINDICATIONS AND PRECAUTIONS   Atonic constipation, nausea, vomiting,
abdominal pain, faecal impaction, intestinal obstruction or perforation; use of sodium
salts in patients on sodium restriction; use of potassium salts in patients with renal
dysfunction; concomitant use of mineral oil.

ADVERSE/SIDE EFFECTS   Rare: occasional mild abdominal cramps, bitter taste,
throat irritation (liquid preparation), nausea, rash.

NURSING IMPLICATIONS
- Advise patient to take sufficient liquid with each dose and to increase fluid intake
  during the day if allowed. Oral solution (not syrup) may be administered in one-half
  glass of milk or fruit juice to mask bitter taste.
- Dioctyl enhances systemic absorption of mineral oil and may result in tumourlike
  deposits; therefore, concomitant use is not recommended.
- Effect on stools is usually apparent 1 to 3 days after first dose.
- Dioctyl should not be administered for prolonged period in treatment of constipation
  in lieu of proper dietary management or other treatment of underlying causes. *See
  bisacodyl*. If prescribed by physician for chronic use, patient should be monitored for
  hepatotoxicity. There is a possibility that it increases intestinal absorption or hepatic
  uptake of other concomitantly administered drugs and thus may enhance their
  toxicity.
- Stored in tightly covered containers. Syrup formulations should be stored in light-
  resistant containers at 15° to 30°C (59° to 86°F), unless directed otherwise by
  manufacturer.

Diphenhydramine hydrochloride————————————

(Benadryl)   *Antihistamine; antiemetic;*
                                                      antitussive

DIPHENHYDRAMINE HYDROCHLORIDE (continued)

ACTIONS AND USES   Ethanolamine antihistamine with significant anticholinergic activity. Used for symptomatic relief of various allergic conditions.

ROUTE AND DOSAGE   Adult: Oral: 25 mg three times a day (at 4- to 6-hour intervals). Maximum daily dosage is 400 mg.

For further information: *see chlorpheniramine*.

Diphenoxylate hydrochloride with atropine sulphate ━━━━━

(Lomotil)   *Antidiarrhoeal agent*

ACTIONS AND USES   Diphenoxylate is a synthetic narcotic and phenylpiperidine analogue structurally related to pethidine. Commercially available only with atropine sulphate, added in subtherapeutic doses to discourage deliberate overdosage. Inhibits mucosal receptors responsible for peristaltic reflex thereby reducing GI motility. Has little or no analgesic activity or risk of dependence, except in high doses.

Used as adjunct in symptomatic management of diarrhoea.

ROUTE AND DOSAGE   Adult: Oral: *Initial*: 10 mg followed by 5 mg/6 hrly. Tablet contains 2.5 mg diphenoxylate hydrochloride with 0.025 mg atropine sulphate.) **Child (4–8 yrs):** 2.5 mg three times a day; **(9–12 yrs):** 2.5 mg four times a day; **(13–16 yrs):** 5 mg three times a day.

ABSORPTION AND FATE   Well-absorbed after oral administration; **onset of action** within 45 to 60 minutes, with **duration** of 3 to 4 hours. **Peak plasma levels** reached in 2 hours; **plasma half-life** 2.5 hours. Rapidly metabolized to active metabolite diphenoxylic acid (plasma half-life 4.4 hours) and inactive metabolites. Excreted slowly, primarily in faeces via bile. About 14% eliminated in urine; less than 1% as unchanged drug. Appears in breast milk.

CONTRAINDICATIONS AND PRECAUTIONS   Hypersensitivity to diphenoxylate or atropine; severe dehydration or electrolyte imbalance, advanced liver disease, obstructive jaundice, diarrhoea caused by pseudomembranous enterocolitis associated with use of broad-spectrum antibiotics; diarrhoea associated with organisms that penetrate intestinal mucosa; diarrhoea induced by poisons until toxic material is eliminated from GI tract; glaucoma; children less than 2 years of age. Safe use during pregnancy, lactation, or in women of childbearing potential not established. **Cautious Use:** advanced hepatic disease, abnormal liver function tests; renal function impairment, patients receiving addicting drugs, addiction-prone individuals or whose history suggests drug abuse; ulcerative colitis; young children (particularly patients with Down's syndrome).

ADVERSE/SIDE EFFECTS   These include: headache, sedation, drowsiness, dizziness, lethargy, numbness of extremities; restlessness, euphoria, mental depression, weakness,

DIPHENOXYLATE HYDROCHLORIDE (continued)

general malaise, flushing, palpitation, tachycardia, nausea, vomiting, anorexia, dry mouth, abdominal discomfort or distention, paralytic ileus, toxic megacolon, pruritus, angioneurotic oedema, giant urticaria, rash, nystagmus, mydriasis, blurred vision, miosis (toxicity), urinary retention, swelling of gums. **Overdosage**: hypotonia, loss of reflexes, fever, seizures, respiratory depression, coma.

NURSING IMPLICATIONS

- A careful history will usually reveal probable cause of acute diarrhoea.
- Dosage should be reduced as soon as initial control of symptoms occurs. Instruct patient to note time and number of stools as well as colour, odour, consistency, presence of blood, pus, mucus or other foreign matter. Also note colour, amount and frequency of urine (rough index of dehydration).
- Report signs of atropine poisoning (atropinism): dry mouth, flushing, hyperthermia, tachycardia, urinary retention; may occur even with recommended doses in children, particularly those with Down's syndrome.
- Drug should be withheld in presence of severe dehydration or electrolyte imbalance until appropriate corrective therapy has been initiated.
- Observe for and report abdominal distention. In ulcerative colitis, diphenoxylate-induced delay of intestinal motility may cause toxic megacolon. As a result fluid is retained in colon and thus further aggravates dehydration and electrolyte imbalance. Distention is an ominous sign in patients with ulcerative colitis.
- Magnitude of fluid and electrolyte deficits can be estimated by the following signs of dehydration: weakness, lethargy, confusion, postural hypotension, increased pulse, scanty concentrated urine, decreased sweating, increased temperature; tongue and mucosal dryness, poor skin turgor (gently pinch up skin over chest or forehead; if dehydrated, pinched appearance remains for several minutes), decreased eyeball tension (sunken eyeballs).
- Further gross calculations of fluid loss can be made by careful measurements of body weight and fluid intake and output. Note frequency, colour, odour, and consistency of stools; presence of blood, pus, mucus, or other foreign matter; note colour, amount and frequency of urine.
- Serial measurements of body weight, serum electrolytes, BUN, creatinine, haemoglobin and serum albumin are essential for determining degree of dehydration and adequacy of fluid and electrolyte balance.
- For acute diarrhoea, food is generally withheld 24 to 48 hours to reduce bowel stimulation, or patient is restricted to only clear liquids such as broth, bouillon, weak tea, ginger ale, gelatin. Ice-cold liquids, spicy foods, caffeine, beverages, milk and milk products, and concentrated sweets are usually avoided. Bland diet with frequent small meals is then added as tolerated, gradually progressing to normal diet.
- Rehydration is an important adjunct to diarrhoea treatment. Caffeine beverages and alcohol should be avoided as both increase peristalsis.
- Advise patients who are travelling to places where sanitation may be questionable to drink only boiled water or commercially bottled water, soft drinks, beer or wine. Also warn patient not to brush teeth or rinse mouth with 'raw' water and to avoid ice cubes, salads, uncooked vegetables, and unpeeled fruit.

DIPHENOXYLATE HYDROCHLORIDE (continued)

- Counsel patient to take medication only as directed by physician.
- Instruct patient to notify physician if diarrhoea persists or if fever, palpitation, or other adverse reactions occur.
- Since drug may cause dizziness and drowsiness, advise patient to use caution when driving or performing other activities requiring coordination and alertness.
- Caution patients to keep drug out of reach of children. Fatalities have been reported.
- *Overdosage treatment*   Induction of emesis or gastric lavage (effective even several hours after drug ingestion). Facilities for resuscitation and a narcotic antagonist (e.g., naloxone should be readily available. Bladder catheterization may be necessary. (Atropine causes urinary retention). Respiratory depression may occur 12 to 30 hours after overdose. Because duration of diphenoxylate action exceeds that of naloxone, extend period of observation over at least 48 hours until diphenoxylate effect on respiratory system is passed.
- Stored in tightly covered, light-resistant container, preferably between 15° and 30°C (59° and 86°F), unless otherwise directed by manufacturer.

Drug interactions   Concomitant use of **MAO inhibitors** with diphenoxylate may precipitate hypertensive crisis. Diphenoxylate may potentiate action of **alcohol, barbiturates,** and **anxiolytic agents** and other **CNS depressants**. Patient should be observed closely if these drugs are used concomitantly.

Diphenylpyraline hydrochloride ⎯⎯⎯⎯⎯⎯⎯⎯⎯⎯

(Hispril, Lergoban)   *Antihistamine*

ACTIONS AND USES   Ethanolamine derivative antihistamine with properties similar to those of other antihistamines. *See diphenhydramine.*

Used for symptomatic treatment of seasonal hay fever, perennial allergic rhinitis, vasomotor rhinitis, and various other allergic manifestations.

ROUTE AND DOSAGE   Oral: **Adult:** 5–10 mg twice a day; **Child (over 7 yrs):** 2.5 mg twice a day.

ABSORPTION AND FATE   Acts within 15 to 30 minutes. Peak effect in 1 to 2 hours; duration 3 to 6 hours for regular tablet and 8 to 12 hours for timed release form.

NURSING IMPLICATIONS
- Slow-release form should be swallowed whole and not crushed or chewed.
- Bear in mind that antihistamines may mask ototoxic and other adverse effects of drugs taken concurrently.
- Antihistamines may prevent positive reactions to skin tests for allergy if taken within 4 days of such tests.

DIPHENYLPYRALINE HYDROCHLORIDE (continued)
- Store preferably at 15° to 30°C (59° to 86°F), unless otherwise directed by manufacturer.
- *See also diphenhydramine.*

Dipipanone hydrochloride —————————————————

(Diconal)   *Narcotic; analgesic*

ACTIONS AND USES Less sedating than morphine and of shorter duration. Tablet contains dipipanone 10 mg plus cyclazine 30 mg. This combination, with an antiemetic makes the preparation unsuitable for regular treatment on terminal care. Used for moderate to severe pain.

ROUTE AND DOSAGE Oral: 1 tablet increasing to 3 tablets/6 hrly.
For further information: *see morphine*

Dipyridamole ————————————————————————

(Persantin)   *Antiplatelet agent*

ACTIONS AND USES Inhibits ADP-induced platelet aggregation. Does not affect prothrombin activity. Used to prevent thrombosis after the insertion of prosthetic values.

ROUTE AND DOSAGE Oral: 300–600 mg/day in divided doses. **IV by slow injection**: 10–20 mg 2–3 times a day.

ABSORPTION AND FATE Readily absorbed from GI tract. **Plasma levels peak** 2 to 2½ hours following administration. Concentrates in liver where it is metabolized. **Protein binding**: 91 to 97%. Mainly excreted in faeces via bile as intact drug or as glucuronide. Small amounts cross placenta.

CONTRAINDICATIONS AND PRECAUTIONS Acute myocardial infarction. Safe use in pregnancy and nursing mothers not established. **Cautious Use**: hypotension, anticoagulant therapy.

ADVERSE/SIDE EFFECTS Usually dose-related, minimal and transient: gastric distress, diarrhoea, headache, dizziness, faintness, weakness, aggravation of angina pectoris (rarely); peripheral vasodilation, flushing, hypotension (excessive dosage), skin rash.

DIPYRIDAMOLE *(continued)*
NURSING IMPLICATIONS
- Administer at least 1 hour before or 2 hours after meals, preferably with a full glass of water. Physician may prescribe it to be taken with food if gastric distress persists.
- If necessary, tablet may be crushed and mixed with liquid or soft food.
- Monitor blood pressure during period of dosage adjustment and in patients receiving high dosages.
- If postural hypotension is a problem advise patient to make all position changes slowly and in stages, especially from recumbent to upright posture.
- Store in well-closed container preferably at 15° to 30°C (59° to 86°F), unless otherwise directed by manufacturer.
- Do not confuse with disopyramide.

Drug interactions   Dipyridamole inhibits platelet aggregation and thus increases the danger of haemorrhage in patients receiving **heparin**. **Aspirin** enhances dipyridamole absorption.

D

Disodium etidronate

(Didronel)   *Chelating agent*

ACTIONS AND USES   Used to treat Paget's disease of the bone.

ROUTE AND DOSAGE   Oral: **Adult**: 5 mg/kg/day as a single dose, 2 hours before food, treatment period up to 6 months.

NURSING IMPLICATIONS
- Report any adverse effect to the Committee on Safety of Medicines.

Disopyramide

(Dirythmin SA, Rythmodan Retard)   *Antiarrhythmic*

ACTIONS AND USES   Antiarrhythmic agent with pharmacological actions similar to those of quinidine and procainamide, although chemically unrelated. Has prominent atropine like (anticholinergic) effects particularly on GI and urogenital systems.

Used to suppress and prevent recurrence of premature ventricular contractions (unifocal, multifocal, paired), and ventricular tachycardia not severe enough to require cardioversion.

ROUTE AND DOSAGE   Oral: **Adult**: 300–800 mg/day in divided doses. **IV by slow**

DISOPYRAMIDE (continued)

injection: 2 mg/kg over 5 min to a maximum of 150 mg followed immediately by 200 mg orally then 200 mg/8 hrly or 400 mcg/kg/hr by infusion. **Maximum dose**: 300 mg in the first hour and 800 mg daily.

ABSORPTION AND FATE   Approximately 70 to 90% rapidly absorbed from GI tract. **Onset of action** in 30 minutes to 3.5 hours; **duration** 1.5 to 8.5 hours. **Peak plasma concentration** in 1 to 2 hours. About 50 to 65% bound to plasma proteins. **Half-life**: 4 to 10 hours (prolonged in patients with decreased cardiac output, recent MI, ventricular arrhythmias, renal or hepatic insufficiency). Primarily metabolized by liver. Approximately 80% of dose eliminated by kidney: 40 to 60% as unchanged drug and remainder as partially active metabolites. The major metabolite has considerably more anticholinergic activity than parent drug. About 10% excreted in faeces. Crosses placenta. Appears in breast milk.

CONTRAINDICATIONS AND PRECAUTIONS   History of hypersensitivity to disopyramide; cardiogenic shock, preexisting 2nd or 3rd degree AV block (if no pacemaker is present); uncompensated or inadequately compensated congestive heart failure; hypotension (unless secondary to cardiac arrhythmia), hypokalaemia. Safe use in women of childbearing potential and during pregnancy, or in nursing women and in children not established. **Cautious Use**: sick sinus syndrome (bradycardia–tachycardia); Wolff–Parkinson–White syndrome or bundle branch block, myocarditis or other cardiomyopathy, underlying cardiac conduction abnormalities, hepatic or renal impairment, urinary tract disease (especially prostatic hypertrophy), myasthenia gravis, narrow-angle glaucoma, family history of glaucoma.

ADVERSE/SIDE EFFECTS   These include: dry mouth, urinary hesitancy, urinary retention, constipation, blurred vision, dry eyes, nose and throat, dizziness, headache, fatigue, muscle weakness, paraesthesias, peripheral neuropathy, nervousness, depression, acute psychosis, hypotension, chest pain, dyspnea, syncope, bradycardia, tachycardia, excessive widening of QRS complex or prolongation of QT interval; worsening of CHF; heart block; rarely: increased PVC's, ventricular tachycardia or fibrillation, cardiac arrest; oedema with weight gain. **Others**: cholestatic jaundice; infrequent: nausea, vomiting, anorexia, bloating, gas, diarrhoea, epigastric or abdominal pain, urinary frequency, urgency, hesitancy, impotence, pruritus, urticaria, rash, photosensitivity, precipitation of acute angle-closure glaucoma, hypoglycaemia, hypokalaemia, agranulocytosis, drying of bronchial secretions, initiation of uterine contractions (in pregnant patients), muscle aches, precipitation of myasthenia gravis.

NURSING IMPLICATIONS

■ Do not confuse with dipyridamole.

■ Check apical pulse before administering drug. Withhold drug and notify physician if pulse rate is slower than 60 beats/minute, faster than 120 beats/minute, or if there is any unusual change in rate, rhythm or quality.

■ ECG should be closely monitored, especially in patients with severe heart disease, hypotension, or hepatic or renal dysfunction. The following signs are indications for

DISOPYRAMIDE (continued)

drug withdrawal: prolongation of QT interval and worsening of arrhythmia interval, QRS widening (more than 25%).

- Monitor blood pressure during therapy in patients with myocarditis, uncompensated heart failure, and in those receiving other cardiac depressants.
- For patients who have been receiving either quinidine or procainamide, manufacturer suggests starting disopyamide 6 to 12 hours after last quinidine dose and 3 to 6 hours after last procainamide dose.
- Patients with atrial flutter or fibrillation are usually digitalized prior to initiation of therapy to ensure that disopyramide-induced improvement in AV conduction does not lead to a dangerously rapid ventricular rate.
- Monitor fluid intake and output particularly in patients with impaired renal function or prostatic hypertrophy. Persistent urinary hesitancy or retention may necessitate discontinuation of drug. Patients with renal dysfunction should be observed closely for toxic symptoms.
- Patients with history of heart disease should be checked for symptoms of congestive heart failure: orthopnoea, shortness of breath with exertion, paroxysmal nocturnal dyspnoea, pulmonary rales, weight gain, distended neck veins.
- Disopyramide should be discontinued promptly if symptoms of agranulocytosis (unusual fatigue, fever, malaise, sore mouth or throat) or jaundice appear.
- Because of the possibility of hypotension, advise patient to make position changes slowly particularly from recumbent posture, to dangle legs for a few minutes before ambulating, and not to stand still for prolonged periods. Instruct patient to lie down or sit down (in head low position) if he or she feels faint or light-headed.
- Dry mouth occurs in about 12% of patients receiving disopyramide, but frequently becomes less prominent with continued therapy. Symptom may be relieved by sugarless gum or lemon drops, frequent clear warm water rinses, increase in noncalorie fluid intake (if allowed), use of saliva substitute.
- Instruct patient that, in order to maintain regularity of heartbeat, drug must be taken precisely as prescribed. Emphasize important of not skipping, stopping medication, or changing dose without consulting physician.
- Urge patient to keep appointments for periodic clinical evaluation.
- Advise patient not to take OTC medications unless approved by physician.
- Inform patient that disopyramide may cause photosensitivity and therefore to avoid exposure to sunlight or ultraviolet light.
- Since drug may cause dizziness and blurring of vision, caution patient to avoid driving and other potentially hazardous activities until reaction to drug effects is known.
- Warn patient not to drink alcoholic beverages while taking disopyramide (*see Drug Interactions*).
- Physician may prescribe a laxative to prevent constipation and straining.

Diagnostic test interferences Blood glucose levels may be increased; **liver enzymes, triglycerides, cholesterol, BUN, creatinine** may be elevated and **haemoglobin** and **haematocrit** may be lowered.

DISOPYRAMIDE (continued)
DRUG INTERACTIONS   Disopyramide

PLUS	INTERACTIONS
Alcohol, ethyl	Additive hypoglycaemia and hypotension
Antiarrhythmic drugs (e.g., lignocaine, phenytoin, procainamide, propranolol, quinidine)	May enhance effect of disopyramide
Anticoagulants, oral	Elevation of warfarin serum levels by inhibiting warfarin metabolism
Anticholinergic drugs	Additive atropinelike effects

Disulphiram

(Antabuse)   *Enzyme inhibitor; alcohol deterrent*

ACTIONS AND USES   Aldehyde dehydrogenase inhibitor. Blocks alcohol oxidation at the acetaldehyde level. When a small amount of alcohol is introduced into the system sensitized by disulphiram action, acetaldehyde concentration of blood rises 5 to 10 times above normal. A complex of highly unpleasant symptoms is produced and is referred to as the disulphiram reaction. This reaction persists as long as alcohol is being metabolized and serves as a deterrent to further drinking. Does not produce tolerance and is not a cure for alcoholism.

Used as adjunct in treatment of the patient with chronic alcoholism who sincerely wants to maintain sobriety.

ROUTE AND DOSAGE   Oral: *initial*: 800 mg on the first day, reduced over 5 days to a *maintenance* dose of 100–200 mg/day.

ABSORPTION AND FATE   Rapidly and completely absorbed from GI tract. Full action may require 12 hours because initially drug is deposited in fat. Greater part of drug is oxidized largely by liver. 5 to 20% of dose excreted unchanged in faeces; about 20% remains in body for 1 to 2 weeks. Some may be excreted in the breath as carbon disulphide.

CONTRAINDICATIONS AND PRECAUTIONS   Hypersensitivity to disulphiram; severe myocardial disease; psychoses; pregnancy; patients receiving or patients who have recently received alcohol, metronidazole, paraldehyde, multiple drug dependence. **Cautious Use**: diabetes mellitus, epilepsy, hypothyroidism, cerebral damage, chronic and acute nephritis, hepatic cirrhosis or insufficiency.

ADVERSE/SIDE EFFECTS   Mild GI disturbances, garlic-like or metallic taste, headache, allergic or acneiform dermatitis; urticaria, fixed-drug eruption, drowsiness, fatigue, restlessness, tremor, impotence, psychoses (usually with high doses); polyneuritis, peripheral neuritis, optic neuritis; hepatotoxicity. *Disulphiram reaction*: flushing of face,

DISULPHIRAM (continued)

chest, arms, pulsating headache, nausea, violent vomiting, thirst, sweating, marked uneasiness, confusion, weakness, vertigo, blurred vision, palpitation, hyperventilation, abnormal gait, slurred speech, disorientation, confusion, personality changes, bizarre behaviour, psychoses, tachycardia, chest pain, hypotension to shock level, arrhythmias, acute congestive failure, marked respiratory depression, unconsciousness, convulsions, sudden death.

NURSING IMPLICATIONS

- Daily dose should be taken in the morning when the resolve not to drink may be strongest. Tablets may be crushed and well mixed with liquid beverage if compliance is a problem.
- To minimize sedative effect the drug may be prescribed to be taken at bedtime. Decrease in dose may also reduce sedative effect.
- Patient should be completely aware of and should consent to therapy with disulphiram. Patient and family should be fully informed of possible danger to life if alcohol is ingested during disulphiram treatment.
- Disulphiram therapy is attempted only under careful medical and nursing supervision. It is used as an adjunct to supportive and psychiatric therapy and only in patients who are motivated and fully cooperative.
- Therapy is not initiated until patient has abstained from alcohol and alcohol-containing preparations for at least 12 hours and preferably 48 hours.
- Complete physical examination, especially of circulatory and nervous systems, and careful drug history are advised prior to therapy. Baseline and follow-up transaminase tests every 10 to 40 days are suggested to detect hepatic dysfunction. In addition, complete blood count and sequential multiple analysis tests should be performed every 6 months.
- External application of solutions, creams, lotions that contain alcohol may be sufficient to produce a reaction. Teach patient to read labels and avoid use of anything that contains alcohol. Examples of unusual sources of alcohol: liniments; shaving, face, or body lotions; colognes, elixirs, fluid extracts, tinctures, vanilla, vinegars.
- Patient should be informed that prolonged administration of disulphiram does not produce tolerance; the longer one remains on therapy, the more sensitive one becomes to alcohol.
- Disulphiram reaction (*see also Adverse Reactions*): occurs within 5 to 10 minutes following ingestion of alcohol and may last 30 minutes to several hours. When blood alcohol concentration is as little as 5 to 10 mg% patient may experience a mild reaction. Symptoms are fully developed with 50 mg% concentration and unconsciousness results when level reaches 125 to 150 mg%. When symptoms subside, patient may sleep for several hours after which patient is well again.
- Intensity of reaction varies with each individual, but it is generally proportional to amount of alcohol ingested.
- Warn patient that alcohol sensitivity may last as long as 2 weeks after disulphiram has been discontinued.
- Patient may have disagreeable breath because of one of the metabolites, carbon disulphide.

D

DISULPHIRAM (continued)

- Psychotic responses (usually associated with high dosages) may unmask underlying psychosis in some patients stressed by alcohol withdrawal.
- During first 2 weeks of therapy, patient may experience side effects of disulphiram itself (*see Adverse Reactions*). These symptoms usually disappear with continued therapy or with dose reduction.
- Advise patient to carry an identification card stating that patient is on disulphiram therapy and describing the symptoms of disulphiram reaction. The names of the physician or institution to contact in an emergency should also be provided.
- During early therapy when drowsiness may be a problem, the patient should avoid driving or performing other tasks requiring alertness.
- The disulphiram test is seldom used but if given patient must be under close supervision. When employed it serves as a guide to proper dosage level, and it permits the patient to experience under controlled conditions what happens when alcohol is ingested during disulphiram treatment. It is not administered to person over 50 years of age. A clear detailed description of the reaction as an alternative to the test is felt to be sufficient in most cases.
- **Supervised disulphiram test**   After first 1 to 2 weeks of therapy with 500 mg/day, a drink of 15 ml of 100 proof whisky or equivalent is taken slowly. Test dose may be repeated only once.
- During treatment of severe disulphiram reaction, treat patient as though in shock: oxygen or carbogen (O_2, 95% and CO_2, 5%); large doses of intravenous vitamin C; ephedrine sulfate; antihistamines. Monitor potassium levels, especially if patient has diabetes mellitus.
- Maintenance therapy with disulphiram may be required for months or even years. Compliance should be determined periodically.
- Physician may prescribe pyridoxine (vitamin B_6) for patients on long-term therapy to reduce cholesterol elevating effect of disulphiram.
- Narcotic or sedative dependence may accompany or follow alcoholism. Thus, if either type of medication is indicated during time patient is on disulphiram treatment, the family as well as prescriber should be alert to signs of drug abuse.
- If a limited course of an antianxiety agent is indicated, discuss its use with patient from point of view of drug abuse. Patient should be warned not to change established dosing schedule and not to take a double dose (to make up for a missed dose).
- Behaviour modification has been achieved for many patients through *Alcoholics Anonymous*.

Patient teaching points   (Reenforcement of preliminary information given to secure consent to therapy with disulphiram.) Disulphiram reaction:
- Begins within 5 to 15 minutes after ingestion of as little as 7 ml of 100 proof whisky or equivalent.
- Persists 30 minutes to several hours.
- Can occur up to 2 weeks after discontinuation of therapy.
- Is not only unpleasant but can threaten life.
- May require medical attention.

- Protect tablets from light. Store between 15° and 30°C (59° and 86°F).

DISULPHIRAM (continued)

Diagnostic test interferences   Disulphiram reduces **uptake of I-131**; decreases **PBI** test results; decreases **urinary VMA**; increases urinary concentrations of **homovanillic acid**; increases **serum cholesterol** (occurs 3 to 6 weeks after initiation of therapy).

DRUG INTERACTIONS   *Disulphiram*

PLUS	INTERACTIONS
Alcohol	Increased toxicity of alcohol
Antidepressants, tricyclic	Enhance reaction between alcohol and disulphiram
Chlorodiazepoxide	Exaggerated clinical effects of chlorodiazepoxide
Diazepam	Exaggerated clinical effects of diazepam
Isoniazid (INH)	Unsteady gait, incoordination, or marked behavioural changes
Metronidazole	Confusional states and psychotic episodes
Oral anticoagulants	Prolonged prothrombin time
Paraldehyde	Increased toxicity of paraldehyde
Phenytoin	Phenytoin intoxication

D

Dobutamine hydrochloride

(Dobutrex)

Beta-adrenergic agonist;
sympathomimetic

ACTIONS AND USES   Direct-acting adrenergic (sympathomimetic) amine with electrophysiological effects on heart similar to those of isoprenaline and dopamine. In comparison with other catecholamines, a given increase in cardiac output is accompanied by a comparatively mild increase in heart rate and blood pressure. In patients with congestive heart failure, dobutamine increases myocardial contractility and usually stroke volume with resulting increase in cardiac output, and possibly in coronary blood flow and myocardial oxygen consumption.

Used for inotropic support in short-term treatment of adults with cardiac decompensation due to depressed myocardial contractility, as an adjunct in cardiac surgery.

ROUTE AND DOSAGE   **Intravenous infusion rate:** 2.5 to 10 mcg/kg/min. Concentration of dobutamine depends on dosage and fluid requirements of patient. Infusions have been given up to 72 hours.

ABSORPTION AND FATE   Onset of action within 1 to 10 minutes. **Peak effect** within 10 minutes. **Plasma half-life:** 2 minutes. Rapidly metabolized in liver to inactive metabolites. Excreted primarily in urine.

CONTRAINDICATIONS AND PRECAUTIONS   History of hypersensitivity to other sympathomimetic amines, ventricular tachycardia, idiopathic hypertrophic subaortic stenosis. Safe use during pregnancy, in nursing mothers and children, or following acute myocardial infarction not established. **Cautious Use:** preexisting hypertension.

DOBUTAMINE HYDROCHLORIDE (continued)

ADVERSE/SIDE EFFECTS   These include: increased heart rate and blood pressure, ventricular ectopic activity, premature ventricular beats, ventricular tachycardia (rare), palpitation, anginal pain, nausea, vomiting, nonspecific chest pain, shortness of breath, headache, paraesthesias, mild leg cramps; nervousness, fatigue (with overdosage); local pain (with infiltration).

NURSING IMPLICATIONS

- ECG and BP should be monitored continuously during administration of dobutamine.
- IV infusion rate and duration of therapy are determined by heart rate, blood pressure, ectopic activity, urine output, and whenever possible, by measurements of cardiac output and central venous or pulmonary wedge pressures.
- Since dobutamine enhances atrioventricular conduction, patients with atrial fibrillation are generally given a digitalis preparation prior to initiation of dobutamine therapy, to reduce risk of ventricular tachycardia.
- Marked increases in blood pressure (systolic pressure is the most likely to be affected) and heart rate, or the appearance of arrhythmias or other adverse cardiac effects are usually reversed promptly by reduction in dosage.
- Patients with preexisting hypertension must be closely observed for exaggerated pressor response.
- Most patients have a 10 to 20 mm Hg increase in systolic pressure (rise may be as high as 50 mm Hg in some patients), and an increase in heart rate of 5 to 15 beats/min (as high as 30 beats in some patients).
- Hypovolaemia should be corrected by administration of appropriate volume expanders prior to initiation of therapy.
- Monitor fluid intake and output. Urine output and sodium excretion generally increase because of improved cardiac output and renal perfusion.
- Dobutamine may be reconstituted by adding 10 ml sterile water for injection or 5% dextrose injection to 250 mg vial. If not completely dissolved additional 10 ml of diluent may be added.
- For IV infusion, reconstituted solution must be further diluted before administration to at least 50 ml with 5% dextrose, 0.9% sodium chloride, or sodium lactate injection. IV solutions should be used within 24 hours.
- Solutions containing dobutamine may exhibit colour changes due to slight oxidation of drug. This does not affect potency.
- Dobutamine is incompatible with sodium bicarbonate and other alkaline solutions.
- Reconstituted solution may be stored under refrigeration at 2°C to 15°C (36° to 59°F) for 48 hours or for 6 hours at room temperature.

DRUG INTERACTIONS   *Dobutamine hydrochloride*

PLUS	INTERACTIONS
Anaesthetics, general (especially cyclopropane and halothane)	May sensitize myocardium to effects of catecholamines such as dobutamine and lead to serious arrhythmias
Beta-adrenergic blocking agents: e.g., metoprolol, propranolol	May make dobutamine ineffective in increasing cardiac output, but total peripheral resistance may increase

DOBUTAMINE HYDROCHLORIDE

PLUS
(continued)

MAO inhibitors	}
Tricyclic antidepressants	
Nitroprusside, sodium	
Oxytocic drugs	

INTERACTIONS

Potentiation of pressor effects

Concomitant use produces greater increase in cardiac output and usually lower pulmonary wedge pressure

Combined use may cause severe persistent hypertension

Domperidone

(Evoxin, Motiliom)   *Antidopaminergic; antiemetic*

ACTIONS AND USES   Antiemetic with similar action and uses to metoclopramide but without such pronounced CNS side effects.

Used to treat nausea and vomiting in gastrointestinal disorders and during radiotherapy or cytotoxic chemotherapy.

ROUTE AND DOSAGE   Oral: **Adult:** 10–20 mg/4–8 hourly. **Child:** 200–400 mcg/kg for nausea and vomiting following radiotherapy or chemotherapy. **Rectal:** Adult 60 mg/4–8 hourly, **Child:** 30–120 mg/day.

NURSING IMPLICATIONS
- Monitor children for CNS side effects.
- Should be used for acute rather than long-term treatment.
- Store at room temperature.
- *See metoclopramide*

Dopamine hydrochloride

(Intropin)   *Adrenergic agonist (sympathomimetic); catecholamine*

ACTIONS AND USES   Naturally occurring neurotransmitter and immediate precursor of norepinophrine. Major cardiovascular effects produced by direct action on alpha- and beta-adrenergic receptors and on specific dopaminergic receptors in mesenteric and renal vascular beds. Positive inotropic effect on myocardium produces increased cardiac output with increase in systolic and pulse pressure and little or no effect on diastolic pressure. Improves circulation to renal vascular bed by decreasing renal vascular resistance with resulting increase in glomerular filtration rate and urinary output. Blood flow

DOPAMINE HYDROCHLORIDE (continued)

to peripheral vascular bed may decrease while mesenteric flow increases. Less prone to cause substantial decrease in systemic vascular resistance, tachyarrhythmias, or increased myocardial oxygen consumption than are other catecholamines. More effective when therapy is started shortly after signs and symptoms of shock appear and before urine flow has decreased to approximately 0.3 ml/minute.

Used to correct haemodynamic imbalance in shock syndrome due to myocardial infarction (cardiogenic shock), trauma, open heart surgery.

ROUTE AND DOSAGE   Intravenous infusion: *Initial*: 2 to 5 mcg/kg/minute.

ABSORPTION AND FATE   Onset of action within 5 minutes; **duration** less than 10 minutes. Widely distributed in body, but does not cross blood–brain barrier. About 75% of dose is inactivated, chiefly by monoamine oxidase (MAO) in liver, kidney, and plasma. Approximately 25% of dose is metabolized to norepinephrine within adrenergic nerve terminals. **Plasma half-life**: 2 minutes. Excreted in urine primarily as metabolites; small portion excreted unchanged.

CONTRAINDICATIONS AND PRECAUTIONS   Phaeochromocytoma; tachyarrhythmias or ventricular fibrillation. Safe use during pregnancy, lactation, and in paediatric patients not established. **Cautious Use**: within 14 days before or after MAO inhibitor therapy; during pregnancy; patients with history of occlusive vascular disease (e.g., Buerger's or Raynaud's disease), cold injury, diabetic endarteritis, arterial embolism.

ADVERSE/SIDE EFFECTS   Most frequent: ectopic beats, nausea, vomiting, tachycardia, anginal pain, palpitation, dyspnoea, headache, hypotension, vasoconstriction (indicated by disproportionate rise in diastolic pressure). Less frequent: piloerection, aberrant conduction, bradycardia, widening of QRS complex, azotemia, elevated blood pressure, necrosis, tissue sloughing with extravasation, gangrene.

NURSING IMPLICATIONS
- Before initiation of dopamine therapy, hypovolaemia should be corrected, if possible, with either whole blood or plasma.
- Dilution should be made just prior to administration, although reportedly the solution may remain stable for 24 hours after dilution.
- IV infusion rate and guidelines for adjusting rate of flow in relation to changes in blood pressure will be prescribed by physician. Reliable metering device should be used for accuracy of flow rate.
- Monitor blood pressure, pulse, peripheral pulses, and urinary output at intervals prescribed by physician. Precise measurements are essential for accurate titration of dosage.
- Indicators for decreasing or temporarily suspending dose (report promptly to physician): reduced urine flow rate in absence of hypotension; ascending tachycardia; dysarrhythmias; disproportionate rise in diastolic pressure (marked decrease in pulse pressure); signs of peripheral ischaemia, pallor, cyanosis, mottling; complaints of tenderness, pain, numbness, or burning sensation. (Presence of peripheral pulses is not always indicative of adequate circulation.)
- Monitor for cold extremities (fingers, toes) and report if present. Reportedly nitro-

DOPAMINE HYDROCHLORIDE (continued)

glycerin ointment (2 inch strip) applied to warmest areas of chest or abdominal wall is effective in increasing peripheral blood flow in the hypotensive patient with dopamine-induced peripheral ischaemia. (Blood pressure is not affected, however.)

- Signs and symptoms of overdosage generally respond to dosage reduction or temporary discontinuation of drug, since dopamine has short duration of action. However, if these measures fail, a short-acting alpha-adrenergic blocking agent (e.g., phentolamine) may be given to antagonize peripheral vasoconstriction.
- Infusion rate must be continuously monitored for free flow, and care must be taken to avoid extravasation, which can result in tissue sloughing and gangrene. For this reason, infusion is made preferably into a large vein of the antecubital fossa.
- Antidote for extravasation: infiltration of ischaemic area should be made as soon as possible with 10 to 15 ml of normal saline containing 5 to 10 mg phentolamine, using syringe and fine needle. *See Index: Nursing Interventions: extravasation.*
- Dopamine is a potent drug. Patient must be under constant observation.
- In addition to improvement in vital signs and urine flow, other indices of adequate dosage and perfusion of vital organs include loss of pallor, increase in toe temperature, adequacy of nail bed capillary filling, and reversal of confusion or comatose state.
- Protect dopamine from light. Discoloured solutions should not be used. Reconstituted solution is stable for 48 hours when stored at 2° to 15°C (36° to 59°F) or for 6 hours at room temperature 15° to 30°C (59° to 86°F).

Drug interactions   Administration of **MAO inhibitors** within previous 2 or 3 weeks may cause hypertensive crisis since they prolong and intensify pressor effects of dopamine. (Initial dose of dopamine should be reduced by at least one-tenth the usual dose in these patients.) A similar reaction may occur with concomitant use of **furazolidone** since it reportedly may cause dose-related inhibition of MAO. Concomitant use with **ergot alkaloids** may result in excessive vasoconstriction. Possibility of enhanced response to dopamine in patients receiving or patients who have recently received **guanethidine**. Concurrent administration of dopamine and **diuretic agents** may produce additive or potentiating effect; **phenytoin** may cause hypotension and bradycardia. **Cyclopropane** and related anaesthetics may sensitize myocardium to action of dopamine. Dopamine should be used with extreme caution in these patients.

Dothiepin ▬▬▬▬▬▬▬▬▬▬▬▬▬▬▬▬▬▬▬▬▬▬▬▬▬

(Prothiaden)   *Tricyclic; antidepressant*

ROUTE AND DOSAGE   Oral: **Adult:** *initial*, 75 mg/day gradually increased to 150 mg/day as a single dose at bedtime or in divided doses. Reduce dose to 50–75 mg in the elderly.

For further information: *see amytriptyline*

Doxapram hydrochloride ─────────────

(Dopram)   *Central stimulant (respiratory)*

ACTIONS AND USES   Short-acting analeptic capable of stimulating all levels of the cerebrospinal axis. Actions similar to those of nikethamide, but reported to have greater margin of safety because of minor effect on cortex.

Used as short-term adjunctive therapy to alleviate postanaesthesia and drug-induced respiratory depression and to hasten arousal and return of pharyngeal and laryngeal reflexes. Also used as temporary measure (approximately 2 hours) in hospitalized patients with chronic pulmonary disease associated with acute-respiratory insufficiency as an aid to prevent elevation of arterial CO_2 tension during administration of oxygen (not used in conjunction with mechanical ventilation).

ROUTE AND DOSAGE   *Respiratory stimulant*: **IV infusion**: 0.5–4 mg/min according to response. **Postoperative IV injection**: 1–1.5 mg/kg repeated after 1 hour if necessary.

ABSORPTION AND FATE   Onset of respiratory stimulation following a single IV injection occurs in 20 to 40 seconds and peaks in 1 or 2 minutes, with duration rarely more than 5 to 12 minutes. Rapidly metabolized. Believed to be excreted in urine as metabolites within 24 to 48 hours after administration.

CONTRAINDICATIONS AND PRECAUTIONS   Known hypersensitivity to doxapram; epilepsy and other convulsive disorders; incompetence of ventilatory mechanism due to muscle paresis, pulmonary fibrosis, flail chest, pneumothorax, airway obstruction, extreme dyspnoea, acute bronchial asthma; severe hypertension, coronary artery disease, uncompensated heart failure, cerebrovascular accident. Safe use during pregnancy and in children 12 years of age or younger not established. **Cautious Use**: cerebral oedema, history of bronchial asthma, chronic obstructive pulmonary disease, cardiac disease, severe tachycardia, arrhythmias, hyperthyroidism, phaeochromocytoma, hypertension, head injury, increased intracranial pressure, peptic ulcer, patients undergoing gastric surgery, acute agitation.

ADVERSE/SIDE EFFECTS   These include: dizziness, sneezing, apprehension, confusion, involuntary movements, hyperactivity, paraesthesias; feeling of warmth and burning, especially of genitalia, perineum; flushing, sweating, hyperpyrexia, headache, pilomotor erection, pruritus, muscle tremor, spasms, rigidity, convulsions (rarely), increased deep-tendon reflexes, bilateral Babinski sign, carpopedal spasm, pupillary dilation, mild delayed narcosis, mild to moderate increase in blood pressure, sinus tachycardia, bradycardia, extrasystoles, lowered T-waves, PVCs, chest pains, tightness in chest, nausea, vomiting, diarrhoea, salivation, sour taste, urinary retention, frequency, incontinence, dyspnoea, tachypnoea, cough, laryngospasm, bronchospasm, hiccoughs, rebound hypoventilation, hypocapnia with tetany, local skin irritation, thrombophlebitis with extravasation (cause-effect relationship not established): decreased haemoglobin, haematocrit, and RBC count; elevated BUN; albuminuria.

DOXAPRAM HYDROCHLORIDE (continued)
NURSING IMPLICATIONS

- Adequacy of airway and oxygenation must be assured before initiation of doxapram therapy.
- IV flow rate is prescribed by physician. Infusion rate may start at 1 mg/minute until satisfactory respiratory response is observed. It should then be maintained at 1 to 3 mg/minute and be adjusted to maintain desired respiratory response. An infusion pump is advisable for regulatory flow rate.
- Extravasation or use of same IV site for prolonged periods can cause thrombophlebitis or tissue irritation. (See Index: Nursing Interventions: Extravasation.)
- Careful monitoring and accurate observation of blood pressure, pulse, deep tendon reflexes, airway, and arterial blood gases are essential guides for determining minimum effective dosage and preventing overdosage.
- Determinations of blood gases, Po_2, Pco_2, and O_2 saturation are important for assessing effectiveness of respiratory stimulation. In patients with chronic obstructive pulmonary disease, arterial blood gases should be drawn prior to initiation of doxapram infusion and oxygen administration and then at least every ½ hour during infusion. Infusion should not be administered for longer than 2 hours.
- Doxapram should be discontinued if arterial blood gases show evidence of deterioration and mechanical ventilation is initiated.
- Postoperative patients or patients in a state of narcosis with chronic pulmonary insufficiency should receive oxygen concomitantly. Respiratory stimulation produced by doxapram increases the work of breathing and thus increases oxygen consumption and CO_2 production.
- Observe patient continuously during therapy and maintain vigilance until patient is fully alert (usually about 1 hour) and protective pharyngeal and laryngeal reflexes are completely restored.
- Notify physician immediately of any side effects. Be alert for early signs of toxicity: tachycardia, muscle tremor, spasticity, hyperactive reflexes.
- A mild to moderate increase in blood pressure commonly occurs; this is a matter of concern in patients with preexisting hypertension.
- If sudden hypotension or dysponoea develops doxapram should be discontinued.
- Doxapram generally produces increased alertness in postoperative patients and earlier perception of pain than usual. Because the action of doxapram is short, however, keep in mind that poststimulation narcosis may occur.
- Oxygen, resuscitative equipment, and IV barbiturates should be readily available in the event of excessive CNS stimulation.
- Store drug at 15° to 30°C (59° to 86°F), unless directed to do otherwise by manufacturer.

Drug interactions Synergistic pressor effects (increase in blood pressure, arrhythmias) may occur in patients receiving **sympathomimetic agents** or **MAO inhibitors**. Initiation of doxapram should be delayed for at least 10 minutes following discontinuation of anaesthetics that sensitize myocardium to catecholamines, such as **cyclopropane, enflurane,** and **halothane.**

Doxepin hydrochloride ━━━━━━━━━━━━━━━━━━━━━━

(Sinequan)   *Antidepressant; tricyclic*

ACTIONS AND USES   Dibenzoxepin tricyclic antidepressant. Actions, limitations and interactions are similar to those of imipramine (q.v.). Reportedly one of the most sedative of the tricyclic antidepressants.

Used to treat psychoneurotic anxiety and/or depressive reactions, mixed symptoms of anxiety and depression, anxiety and/or depression associated with alcoholism, organic disease, psychotic depressive disorders.

ROUTE AND DOSAGE   Oral: Adult: *Initial*: 75 mg/day as single or divided dose, increased gradually as required to 150 mg/day. Reduce dose in elderly patients.

For further information: *see imipramine.*

ABSORPTION AND FATE   Average serum half-life: 17 ± 6 hours; **effective plasma concentration**: 100 to 150 mg/ml. Hepatic metabolism; excretion largely by kidneys; crosses placenta and enters breast milk.

CONTRAINDICATIONS AND PRECAUTIONS. ADVERSE/SIDE EFFECTS   *See also imipramine.*

Doxorubicin hydrochloride ━━━━━━━━━━━━━━━━━━━━

(Adriamycin)   *Antineoplastic (antibiotic)*

ACTIONS AND USES   Cytotoxic anthracycline antibiotic isolated from *Streptomyces peucetius*, with wide spectrum of antitumour activity and strong immunosuppressive properties. Intercalates with preformed DNA residues, blocking effective DNA and RNA transcription. Highly destructive to rapidly proliferating cells and slow-developing carcinomas; selectively toxic to cardiac tissue. A potent radiosensitizer capable of enhancing radiation reactions. No clinical cross-resistance to standard antineoplastics; therefore, it may be especially effective in patients with less advanced disease. Cytotoxicity precludes its use as antiinfective agent.

Used to produce regression in neoplastic conditions, including acute lymphoblastic and myeloblastic leukaemias, Wilms' tumour neuroblastoma, soft tissue and bone sarcomas, breast and ovary carcinomas, lymphomas, bronchogenic carcinoma.

ROUTE AND DOSAGE   Intravenous: Dose regimens highly individualized.

ABSORPTION AND FATE   IV administration followed by rapid plasma clearance and significant tissue binding. **Half-life**: 0.6 hours; 3.3 hours for metabolites. Metabolized in liver and other tissues to both active and inactive metabolites. Does not cross blood–brain barrier or achieve significant level in CSF. Excreted mainly in bile; 40 to 50% of

DOXORUBICIN HYDROCHLORIDE *(continued)*

administered dose recovered in bile and faeces in 7 days. Less than 5% excreted in urine after 5 days, primarily as unchanged drug.

CONTRAINDICATIONS AND PRECAUTIONS   Myelosuppression, impaired cardiac function, obstructive jaundice, previous treatment with complete cumulative doses of doxorubicin and/or daunorubicin. Safe use in patients of childbearing potential or during pregnancy not established. **Cautious Use**: impaired hepatic or renal function, patients having had radiotherapy to areas surrounding heart, history of atopic dermatitis.

ADVERSE/SIDE EFFECTS   These include: serious, irreversible myocardial toxicity with delayed congestive heart failure, acute left ventricular failure, and hypotension, hyperpigmentation of nail beds and buccal mucosa (especially in blacks); hyperpigmentation of dermal creases (especially in children), rash, complete alopecia, recall phenomenon (skin reaction due to prior radiotherapy), stomatitis and oesophagitis (common) with ulcerations, nausea, vomiting, anorexia, inanition, diarrhoea, severe myelosuppression (60 to 85% of patients); leucopenia (principally granulocytes), thrombocytopenia, anaemia, lacrimation, drowsiness, fever, facial flush with too rapid IV infusion rate, hyperuricaemia, hypersensitivity, anaphylaxis. *With extravasation*: severe cellulitis, vesication, tissue necrosis, lymphangitis, phlebosclerosis.

NURSING IMPLICATIONS
- Not to be confused with daunorubicin.
- It is recommended that patient be hospitalized during the first phase of treatment to permit both medical and nursing surveillance, and extensive laboratory monitoring.
- Caution should be observed in preparing doxorubicin solution. Wear gloves. If powder or solution contacts skin or mucosa, wash copiously with soap and water. For more detailed information *see Index: Antineoplastics: handling vesicant drugs*.
- Administered slowly into side arm of freely running IV infusion of sodium chloride injection or 5% dextrose injection.
- Do not mix this drug with other drugs.
- Infusion rate usually permits administration of the dose in a 3- to 5-minute period. Rate will be specifically ordered. Facial flushing and local red streaking along the vein may occur if drug is administered too rapidly. Urticaria around injection site (due to histamine release) is usually self-limiting.
- If possible avoid using antecubital vein or veins on dorsum of hand or wrist where extravasation could damage underlying tendons and nerves leading to loss of mobility of entire limb. Also avoid veins in extremity with compromised venous or lymphatic drainage.
- Care should be taken to avoid extravasation. Examine the injection site frequently during infusion. Provide meticulous site care to prevent infection.
- Give prompt attention if patient complains of a stinging or burning sensation around injection site; stop infusion immediately, even though blood return can be demonstrated, and restart in another vein. Apply cold (ice) compresses.
- Perivenous extravasation can occur painlessly. If it is suspected, local infiltration with injectable corticosteroid and flooding the site with normal saline may lessen local reaction.

D

DOXORUBICIN HYDROCHLORIDE (continued)

- Monitor area of extravasation frequently. If ulceration begins (usually 1 to 4 weeks after extravasation), a plastic surgeon should be consulted. Early wide excision of the area with skin grafting may be necessary.

- Evaluation of hepatic, renal, haematopoietic, and cardiac function (ECG) should be performed prior to initiation of therapy, at regular intervals thereafter, and at end of therapy.

- Since congestive heart failure may occur several weeks to months after cessation of therapy, ECG and radionuclide scanning may be monitored at least monthly during this posttreatment period.

- Dosage may be guided by serum bilirubin level: if it is 20.5 to 51 mmol/L, one-half normal dose is prescribed; if bilirubin is more than quarter normal dose is given. (*Normal indirect serum bilirubin* [adult]: 1.7 to 6.8 mmol/L or less.)

- Therapeutic response to doxorubicin is unlikely to occur without some evidence of toxicity.

- Myocardial toxicity (irreversible) becomes more of a threat as cumulative dose approaches 550 mg/m^2 body surface and particularly if drug therapy is in conjunction with therapeutic radiation.

- Doxorubicin cardiomyopathy is associated with persistent reduction of QRS wave, prolonged systolic (time) interval, and reduced ejection fraction (by echocardiography or radionuclide angiography).

- Be alert to early signs of cardiotoxicity (dyspnoea, steady weight gain, hypotension, rapid pulse, arrhythmias) to permit immediate medical treatment. Monitor pulse and blood pressure frequently. Acute life-threatening arrhythmias may occur within a few hours of drug administration.

- Objective signs of hepatic dysfunction (jaundice, dark urine, pruritus) or kidney dysfunction (altered fluid intake–output ratio and pattern, local discomfort with voiding) demand prompt attention, since both conditions cause delayed drug elimination. Report to physician.

- Stomatitis, generally maximal in second week of therapy, frequently begins with a burning sensation accompanied by erythema of oral mucosa that may progress to ulceration and dysphagia in 2 or 3 days. Fastidious oral hygiene is required, especially before and after meals. Patient should be referred to a dentist if dental caries or periodontal disease is present. *See mustine for mouth care.*

- Immunosuppressive properties of doxorubicin require careful screening of visitors and attending personnel to shield the patient from infection, especially during leucopenic periods.

- The nadir of leucopenia (an expected 1,000/mm^3) typically occurs 10 to 14 days after single dose with recovery occurring within 21 days. RBC and platelet levels may be depressed also.

- Superinfections by microflora may result from antibiotic therapy during leukopenic period. Report black or furry tongue, diarrhoea, and foul-smelling stools, or vaginal discharge and vulvar or anal itching.

- Complete alopecia (reversible) is an expected side effect. Discuss this side effect with the patient so that wigs can be ordered if desired. An awareness of the impact of the loss of scalp and body hair on one's concept of sexuality should guide this discussion.

DOXORUBICIN HYDROCHLORIDE (continued)

■ If patient at risk of losing scalp hair intends to wear a wig, suggest an early fitting and wearing it before a large amount of hair is lost.

■ Inform patient that alopecia may also involve eyelashes and eyebrows, beard and moustache, pubic and axillary hair. Regrowth of hair usually begins 2 to 3 months after drug is discontinued.

■ Prophylactic treatment by scalp cooling may be instituted and is most effective when the patient has normal liver function. Temporary constriction of superficial scalp blood vessels by cold is thought to minimize drug contact with hair follicles. The cap or ice pack is applied 15 minutes before, during, and for 45 minutes after IV bolus administration of short-acting chemotherapeutic agent that is cleared from the blood after injection.

■ Bloody diarrhoea may result from an antiblastic effect on rapidly growing intestinal mucosal cells. The physician may prescribe an antidiarrhoeal medication. Avoid rectal medications and use of rectal thermometer in order to prevent trauma.

■ Hyperuricaemia, due to rapid lysis of neoplastic cells, may be treated by increased hydration, alkalinization of urine, and allopurinol. Urge patient to increase fluid intake to 2,500 to 3,000 ml in 24-hour period, if allowed. Monitor *blood uric acid* (normal: 178.5 to 416.4 mmol/L).

■ Symptoms of hyperuricaemia should be reported: oedema of lower legs and feet; joint, flank, or stomach pain.

■ Advise patient that the drug imparts a red colour to urine for 1 to 2 days after administration.

■ Increased lacrimation for 5 to 10 days after a single dose is a possibility. Caution patient to keep hands away from eyes to prevent conjunctivitis.

■ Consult the physician about plan for disclosure of diagnosis, expected results of therapy, and prognosis to the patient and family in order to facilitate better communication with the patient.

■ Collaborate with dietitian and patient's family to help the patient maintain optimum nutritional status. Determine dietary preferences; try to support and augment rather than reform eating patterns during period of discomfort. Space pain medication so that peak effect is at mealtime; appropriately schedule fatiguing treatments to avoid presenting food to a tired patient.

■ Reconstituted solution is stable for 24 hours at room temperature and for 48 hours under refrigeration (4° to 10°C). Protect from sunlight; discard unused solution.

Doxycycline hyclate ———————————————————————

(Doxatet, Doxylar, Nordox, Vibramycin)   *Antibiotic; tetracycline*

ACTIONS AND USES   Broad spectrum antibiotic synthetically derived from oxytetracycline. Similar to tetracycline (q.v.) in actions, uses, contraindications, precautions, and adverse reactions.

DOXYCYCLINE HYCLATE (continued)

Used to treat acute pelvic inflammatory disease, primary and secondary syphilis, uncomplicated urethral, endocervical, or rectal infections caused by *Chlamydia trachomatis*. **Investigational Use**: short-term prophylaxis of traveller's diarrhoea caused by enterotoxigenic *E. coli*; treatment of genital, inguinal, and anorectal infections caused by lymphogranuloma venereum.

ROUTE AND DOSAGE   Adult: Oral: *Initial*, 200 mg then 100 mg daily. *Acne*: 50 mg/day for 6–12 weeks or more.

ABSORPTION AND FATE   Almost completely absorbed following oral administration (in fasting adults). Absorption reduced up to 20% by food or milk, but this is usually of no clinical significance. **Serum levels peak** in 1.5 to 4 hours. Range of **plasma protein binding** 25 to 90%. **Half-life** about 15 hours after single dose and up to 22 hours after repeated doses (essentially the same for patients with normal and impaired renal function). Inactivated by intestinal chelation; excreted primarily in bile and faeces (up to 90%).

Drug interactions   Barbiturates, carbamazepine, and phenytoin may hasten metabolism of doxycycline by inducing microsomal enzyme activity thereby decreasing antibiotic activity. *See also tetracycline*.

Drostanolone propionate

(Masteril)   *Antineoplastic; androgen*

ACTIONS AND USES   Synthetic steroid hormone chemically and pharmacologically related to testosterone (q.v.). Has lower incidence of androgenic side effects than parent compound. In advanced carcinoma, promotes weight gain and feeling of well-being, even though objective remission may not be obtained.

Used palliatively in advanced inoperable metastatic carcinoma of breast in women who are 1 to 5 years postmenopause.

ROUTE AND DOSAGE   Intramuscular (in sesame oil): 300 mg weekly.

CONTRAINDICATIONS AND PRECAUTIONS   Carcinoma of male breast; premenopausal women. **Cautious Use**: during pregnancy, liver disease, cardiac decompensation, nephritis, nephrosis, carcinoma of prostate. *See testosterone*.

ADVERSE/SIDE EFFECTS   Virilism; hypercalcaemia; oedema (occasionally); severe, reversible CNS side effects (rare); local reaction at injection site (rare). *See testosterone*.

NURSING IMPLICATIONS
- At least 8 to 12 weeks of therapy may be necessary to produce satisfactory results. If disease being treated progresses significantly during first 6 to 8 weeks of treatment, another form of therapy may be indicated.

DROSTANOLONE PROPIONATE (continued)

- Treatment is generally continued as long as satisfactory results are obtained.
- Patients with oedema may require diuretic therapy before and during treatment with dromostanolone. Monitor weight and inspect dependent areas for signs of fluid retention. Report significant weight changes to physician.
- In patients with bone metastasis, serum calcium and alkaline phosphatase levels should be determined before and periodically during therapy.
- Advise patient to report symptoms of hypercalcaemia: deep bone and flank pain, thirst, polyuria, renal calculi, muscle weakness, nausea, vomiting, anorexia, constipation, lethargy, psychosis. Dromostanolone should be discontinued if severe hypercalcaemia occurs.
- Product should not be refrigerated since a precipitate may form. Store preferably at 15° to 30°C (59° to 86°F), unless otherwise directed by manufacturer.
- *See testosterone.*

Droperidol

(Droleptan Thalamonal)   *Antipsychotic (neuroleptic);*
antiemetic

ACTIONS AND USES   Butyrophenone derivative structurally and pharmacologically related to haloperidol (q.v.). Antagonises emetic effects of morphinelike analgesics and other drugs that act on the chemoreceptor trigger zone. Mild alpha-adrenergic blocking activity and direct vasodilator effect may cause hypotension. Reduces anxiety and motor activity without necessarily inducing sleep; patient remains responsive. Potentiates other CNS depressants. Reduces pressor effects of adrenaline and decreases adrenaline induced arrhythmias, but does not prevent cardiac arrhythmias. May decrease pulmonary arterial pressure. Has greater tendency to produce extrapyramidal symptoms than haloperidol.

Used to produce tranquilizing effect and to reduce nausea and vomiting during surgical and diagnostic procedures. Also used for premedication, during induction, and as adjunct in maintenance of general or regional anaesthesia. Principally used in fixed combination with a potent narcotic analgesic such as fentanyl to produce neuroleptanalgesia (quiescence, reduce motor activity, and indifference to pain and environmental stimuli) to permit carrying out a variety of diagnostic and minor surgical procedures.

ROUTE AND DOSAGE   Oral: Adult: 5–20 mg 4–8 hrly. Child: 300–600 mcg/kg. IM: Adult: up to 10 mg 4–6 hrly. Child: 200–500 mcg/kg. IV injection: 5–15 mg 4–6 hrly.

ABSORPTION AND FATE   Onset of action within 3 to 10 minutes; peaks in about 30 minutes following single IM or IV dose. Duration of sedative and tranquillizing effects (ataraxia) is generally 3 to 6 hours, but may persist 6 to 24 hours. Metabolized in liver

DROPERIDOL (continued)

and excreted primarily in urine. About 10% eliminated in urine as unchanged drug. Crosses placenta.

CONTRAINDICATIONS AND PRECAUTIONS   Known intolerance to droperidol; pregnancy, in women of childbearing potential, and children younger than 2 years of age. **Cautious Use:** elderly, debilitated, and other poor-risk patients; Parkinson's disease, hypotension; liver, kidney, cardiac disease; cardiac bradyarrhythmias.

ADVERSE/SIDE EFFECTS   Most frequent: hypotension, tachycardia, drowsiness. Chills, shivering, dizziness, restlessness, anxiety, hallucinations, mental depression, laryngospasm, bronchospasm. Extrapyramidal symptoms: dystonia, akathisia, oculogyric crisis. *See haloperidol.*

Dydrogesterone

(Duphaston)   *Hormone; progesterone*

ROUTE AND DOSAGE   Oral: depends on the patient's condition.
  For further information: *see progesterone*

E

Econazole nitrate

(Ecostatin, Pevaryl)   *Antibiotic; antifungal*

ACTIONS AND USES   Synthetic imidazole derivative with broad antifungal spectrum of activity similar to that of miconazole. Exerts fungistatic action but may be fungicidal for certain microorganisms or at high concentrations. Active against dermatophyes (including *Trichophyton mentagrophytes, T. rubrum, T. tonsurans, Epidermophyton floccosum, Microsporum audouini, M. canis*), yeasts, e.g., *Candida albicans, Pityrosporum obiculare* (tinea versicolor), and many other genera of fungi. Also appears to be active against some gram-positive bacteria (e.g., *Staphylococcus aureus, Streptococcus pyogenes*, and *Corynebacterium diphtheriae*).
  Used topically for treatment of tinea pedis (athlete's foot: ringworm of foot), tinea cruris (ringworm of the groin), tinea corporis (ringworm of body), and for treatment of tinea versicolour, and cutaneous candidiasis (moniliasis). Has been used for topical treatment of erythrasma, and with corticosteroids for fungal or bacterial dermatoses associated with inflammation.

ROUTE AND DOSAGE   Topical (1% cream in water-miscible base): *Tinea cruris, tinea corporis, tinea pedis, cutaneous candidiasis*: Apply sufficient amount and rub

ECONAZOLE NITRATE (continued)

gently into affected areas twice daily, morning and evening. **Pessaries**: 150 mg, insert one at night for three nights.

ABSORPTION AND FATE   Minimal percutaneous absorption from intact skin; absorption somewhat increased from denuded skin. Inhibitory concentrations achieved in stratum corneum, epidermis, and middle region of dermis in $\frac{1}{2}$ to 5 hours after topical application. Metabolic fate and complete excretory pattern not known. Less than 1% of applied dose eliminated in urine and faeces.

CONTRAINDICATIONS AND PRECAUTIONS   Hypersensitivity to econazole nitrate or to any ingredients in the formulation. Safe use during pregnancy, and in nursing women not established.

ADVERSE/SIDE EFFECTS   Burning, stinging sensation, pruritus, erythema.

NURSING IMPLICATIONS

- Consult physician regarding specific procedure for cleansing affected area(s) before applying medication.
- Wash hands thoroughly before and after treatments.
- Do not use occlusive dressings unless prescribed by physician.
- Instruct patient to use medication for the prescribed time even if symptoms improve, and to report to physician skin reactions suggestive of irritation or sensitization.
- Clinical improvement should occur within the first 1 or 2 weeks or therapy. Advise patient to notify physician if full course of therapy does not result in improvement. Diagnosis should be reevaluated.
- To reduce possibility of recurrence, candidal infections, tinea corporis and tinea cruris should be treated for 2 weeks and tinea pedis for 1 month. Some patients require longer periods of treatment. Patients with tinea versicolour usually improve after 2 weeks of therapy.
- Caution patient not to apply the topical cream in or near the eyes or intravaginally.
- Store at temperature less than 30°C (86°F), unless otherwise directed by manufacturer.
- *See Index: Nursing Interventions: Fungal infections.*

Edrophonium chloride

(Tensilon)

*Cholinergic
(parasympathomimetic);
cholinesterase inhibitor;
antidote; diagnostic agent*

ACTIONS AND USES   Indirect-acting cholinesterase inhibitor (quaternary ammonium compound) similar to neostigmine (q.v.) in actions, contraindications, precautions, and adverse reactions. Acts as antidote to curariform drugs by displacing them from muscle cell receptor sites, thus permitting resumption of normal transmission of neuromuscular

EDROPHONIUM CHLORIDE (continued)

impulses. However, like neostigmine, it prolongs skeletal muscle relaxant action of succinylcholine chloride and decamethonium bromide.

Used for differential diagnosis and as adjunct in evaluation of treatment requirements of myasthenia gravis, for differentiating myasthenic from cholinergic crisis, and to reverse neuromuscular block produced by overdosage of curariform drugs, e.g., tubocurarine, gallamine. Not recommended for maintenance therapy in myasthenia gravis because of its short duration of action.

ROUTE AND DOSAGE   Adults: *Edrophonium test for myasthenia gravis*: Intravenous: *Initial*: 2 mg injected within 15 to 30 seconds; needle is left *in situ*; if there is no reaction after 45 seconds, the remaining 8 mg is injected; **Intramuscular**: 10 mg; if there are no suitable veins.

ABSORPTION AND FATE   Onset of effects on skeletal muscle within 30 to 60 seconds after IV injection; **duration** 6 to 24 minutes. **Onset of effects following IM**: 2 to 10 minutes; **duration** 12 to 45 minutes. Passes blood–brain barrier only at extremely high doses.

CONTRAINDICATIONS AND PRECAUTIONS   Hypersensitivity to anticholinesterase agents; intestinal and urinary obstruction. Safe use in women of childbearing potential and during pregnancy and lactation not established. **Cautious Use**: bronchial asthma, cardiac arrhythmias, patients receiving digitalis.

ADVERSE/SIDE EFFECTS   Severe side effects uncommon with usual doses. Adverse effects include: weakness, muscle cramps, fasciculations, incoordination, respiratory paralysis, bradycardia, irregular pulse, hypotension, diarrhoea, abdominal cramps, nausea, vomiting, excessive salivation, miosis, blurred vision, lacrimation, excessive sweating, increased bronchial secretions, bronchospasm, pulmonary oedema.

NURSING IMPLICATIONS

- Edrophonium is administered by a physician. Monitor vital signs. Observe for signs of respiratory distress. Patients over 50 years of age are particularly likely to develop bradycardia, hypotension, and cardiac arrest.
- Some clinicians recommend giving a 1 to 2 mg test dose of edrophonium to elderly patients, to those with history of heart disease or who take digitalis, and possibly to all patients.
- Antidote (atropine sulphate) and facilities for endotracheal intubation, tracheostomy, suction, assisted respiration, and cardiac monitoring should be immediately available for treatment of cholinergic reaction.
- ***Edrophonium test for myasthenia gravis***   All cholinesterase inhibitors (anticholinesterases) should be discontinued for at least 8 hours before test. Estimates of muscle strength should be made before and after administration of edrophonium, e.g., width of palpebral fissure before and after 1 minute of sustained upward gaze, range of extraocular movements, grip strength, vital capacity, ability to elevate head and extremities, ability to cough, swallow, and talk.
- Positive response to edrophonium test consists of brief improvement in muscle strength unaccompanied by lingual or skeletal muscle fasciculations. In nonmyasthe-

EDROPHONIUM CHLORIDE (continued)

nic patients, edrophonium produces a cholinergic reaction (muscarinic side effects): skeletal muscle fasciculations, muscle weakness.

- **Evaluation of myasthenic treatment** *Myasthenic response*: immediate subjective improvement with increased muscle strength (improvement of ptosis, respiration, ability to speak, swallow, and talk), absence of fasciculations; generally indicates that patient requires larger dose of anticholinesterase agent or longer-acting drug. *Cholinergic response* (muscarinic side effects): lacrimation, diaphoresis, salivation, abdominal cramps, diarrhoea, nausea, vomiting; accompanied by decrease in muscle strength. Muscle weakness may appear in the following order: muscles of neck, chewing, swallowing, shoulder girdle, upper extremities, pelvic girdle, extraocular muscles, legs; fasciculations may be present or absent. Usually indicates overtreatment with cholinesterase inhibitor. *Adequate response*: no change in muscle strength; fasciculations may be present or absent; minimal cholinergic side effects (observed in patients at or near optimal dosage level).

- **Test to differentiate myasthenic crisis from cholinergic crisis** (same principle as for evaluation of myasthenic treatment)   Respiratory exchange must be adequate before test is performed. *Myasthenic crisis* may be secondary to sudden increase in severity of myasthenia gravis: edrophonium will cause improvement of respiration; indicates need for longer-acting anticholinesterase drug. *Cholinergic crisis* (caused by overstimulation by anticholinesterase drugs): edrophonium will produce increase in oropharyngeal secretions and further weakness of muscles of respiration; usually indicates need for discontinuing anticholinesterase drug.

- When used as curare antagonist, the effect of each dose of edrophonium on respiration should be carefully observed before it is repeated, and assisted ventilation should always be employed.

E

DRUG INTERACTIONS *Edrophonium*

PLUS	INTERACTIONS
Digitalis glycosides	Additive bradycardic effects
Procainamide ⎫ Quinidine ⎭	Anticholinergic properties of these drugs may antagonize cholinergic effects of edrophonium.

Enalapril Maleate

(Innovace)   *Antihypertensive*

ACTIONS AND USES   Angiotensin-converting enzyme inhibitor with similar action and uses to captopril (q.v.).

ROUTE AND DOSAGE   Oral: Adult: *hypertension*: *initial*: 5 mg/day, usual *maintenance* dose 10–20 mg/day. Maximum 40 mg/day, when used with a diuretic, in renal

ENALAPRIL MALEATE (continued)

impairment or for elderly patients the initial dose should be 2.5 mg. *Cardiac failure*: initial 2.5 mg/day under hospital supervision.

For further information: *see captopril*.

Ephedrine

*Adrenergic agonist;
bronchodilator;
decongestant*

ACTIONS AND USES   Both indirect and direct acting sympathomimetic amine. Pharmacologically similar to epinephrine (q.v.), but less potent, with slower onset and more prolonged action; effective by oral route.

Cardiovascular actions (positive inotropic and pressor effects) persist 7 to 10 times as long as those of adrenaline although bronchodilation is less prominent, it is more sustained. Like adrenaline, it contracts dilated arterioles of nasal mucosa, thus reducing engorgement and oedema and facilitating ventilation and drainage. Local application to eye produces mydriasis without loss of light reflexes or accommodation or change in intraocular pressure.

Used for temporary relief of congestion of hay fever, allergic rhinitis, and sinusitis; and in treatment and prophylaxis of mild cases of acute asthma and in patients with chronic asthma requiring continuing treatment.

ROUTE AND DOSAGE   Oral: **Adult:** 15–60 mg three times a day. **Child (up to 1 yr):** 7.5 mg; **(1–5 yrs):** 15 mg; **(6–12 yrs):** 30 mg all three times a day. **Nasal drops:** 0.5 and 1% 1–2 drops as required.

ABSORPTION AND FATE   Readily absorbed when given by oral and parenteral routes. Maximum bronchodilator effect occurs within 15 minutes to 1 hour and persists approximately 2 to 4 hours. Cardiac and pressor effects last up to 4 hours after oral administration and about 1 hour after IV. Widely distributed in body fluids; crosses blood–brain barrier. Small amounts slowly metabolized in the liver. About 60 to 75% excreted unchanged in urine within 24 hours; remainder eliminated as metabolite. Acidification of urine increases urinary excretion. Appears in breast milk. Probably crosses placenta.

CONTRAINDICATIONS AND PRECAUTIONS   History of hypersensitivity to ephedrine or other sympathomimetics; narrow-angle glaucoma; within 14 days before or after MAO inhibitor therapy; patients receiving tricyclic antidepressants, digitalis, oxytocics. Safe use during pregnancy not established. **Cautious Use:** Used with extreme caution if at all in hypertension, arteriosclerosis, angina pectoris, coronary insufficiency, chronic heart disease, diabetes mellitus, hyperthyroidism, prostatic hypertrophy.

EPHEDRINE *(continued)*

ADVERSE/SIDE EFFECTS   **Systemic** (usually with large doses): headache, insomnia, nervousness, anxiety, tremulousness, giddiness, palpitation, tachycardia, precordial pain, cardiac arrhythmias; difficult or painful urination, acute urinary retention (especially older men with prostatism, nausea, vomiting, anorexia, sweating, thirst, fixed-drug eruption. **Topical use**: burning, stinging, dryness of nasal mucosa, sneezing, rebound congestion. **Overdosage**: euphoria, confusion, delirium, convulsions, pyrexia, CNS depression (somnolence, coma), hypertension, rebound hypotension, respiratory depression, paranoid psychosis, visual and auditory hallucinations.

NURSING IMPLICATIONS

- Patients receiving ephedrine IV must be under constant supervision. Take baseline blood pressure and other vital signs. Check blood pressure repeatedly during first 5 minutes then every 3 to 5 minutes until stabilized.
- Monitor fluid intake–output ratio and pattern especially in older male patients. Encourage patient to void before taking medication (*see Adverse/Side Effects*).
- Frequent dosing in patients with hypertension can result in tachyphlaxis (diminution of response) to cardiac and pressor effects with resulting rebound hypotension. Monitoring of central venous pressure or left ventricular filling pressure is advisable in these patients.
- Ephedrine is a commonly abused drug. Patients should be advised of side effects and dangers and should be cautioned to take medication only as prescribed.
- Warn patient not to take OTC medications for coughs, colds, allergies, or asthma unless approved by physician. Ephedrine is a common ingredient in these preparations.
- Insomnia is common, particularly with continued therapy. Timing of administration and size of dosage are important considerations. If possible, administer last dose a few hours before bedtime.
- Systemic effects can occur because of excessive dosage from rapid absorption of drug solution through nasal mucosa. These are most likely to occur in the elderly.
- Instruct patient to rinse dropper or spray tip in hot water and shake dry after each use in order to prevent contamination of nasal solution.
- ***Treatment of overdosages***   Have on hand phentolamine mesylate IV or SC, or paraldehyde for hypotension; diazepam for convulsions; cool applications and dexamethasone for pyrexia.
- In general, topical treatment should not be continued for more than 3 to 5 consecutive days. Tachyphylaxis (diminution of response) with rebound congestion may occur if drug is administered in rapidly repeated doses or over prolonged period of time. Prescribed withdrawal of drug over several days frequently enables the patient to attain former responsiveness.
- Preserved in well-closed, light-resistant containers preferably between 15° and 20°C (59° and 86°F) unless otherwise directed by manufacturer. Examine liquid preparation; do not administer unless absolutely clear.

Diagnostic test interferences   Ephedrine is generally withdrawn at least 12 hours before sensitivity tests are made, in order to prevent false-positive reactions.

E

EPHEDRINE (continued)
DRUG INTERACTIONS   Ephedrine

PLUS	INTERACTIONS
Acetazolamide; sodium bicarbonate, and other urinary alkalinizers	Increase effect of ephedrine (pH dependent decrease in urinary ephedrine excretion). Monitor for ephedrine toxicity
Ammonium chloride (and other urinary acidifiers)	Increase urinary excretion of ephedrine by acidification of urine. Therefore, decrease effects of ephedrine
Anaesthetics, general (particularly Cylopropane or halogenated hydrocarbons)	Concurrent use may cause cardiac arrhythmias (these drugs sensitize heart to effects of ephedrine). Used with caution
Corticosteroids	Ephedrine may reduce response to corticosteroids
Digitalis glycosides	Risk of cardiac arrhythmias (digitalis sensitizes heart to ephedrine). Combination used with caution
Guanethidine	Ephedrine antagonizes antihypertensive action of guanethidine. Combination avoided, if possible
Methyldopa Rauwolfia alkaloids	Reduce activity of ephedrine
MAO inhibitors, including drugs with significant MAOI activity, e.g., furazolidone	Use of ephedrine within 14 days of an MAO inhibitor can result in hypertensive crisis: additive alphaadrenergic (pressor) effects. Combination generally avoided
Oxytocics	Concurrent use with ephedrine can cause severe hypertension: additive alpha-adrenergic (pressor) effects. Used concurrently with caution and only if BP does not exceed 130/80
Tricyclic antidepressants	May decrease pressor effects of ephedrine. Concurrent use generally avoided

Epirubicin hydrochloride

(Pharmorubicin)   *Cytotoxic antibiotic*

ACTIONS AND USES   A new antibiotic similar to doxorubicin used to treat a variety of solid tumours. Report side effects to the Committee on Safety of Medicines.

ROUTE AND DOSAGE   Intravenous: doses individualized.

Ergometrine Maleate

(Syntometrine)   *Alpha-adrenergic blocking agent; oxytocic; ergot alkaloid*

ERGOMETRINE MALEATE (continued)

ACTIONS AND USES   Ergot alkaloid with slow but powerful oxytocic effect; less toxic and less prone to cause gangrene than other ergot derivatives. Exerts moderate cerebral vascular constriction, but is inferior to ergotamine (q.v.) as a migraine specific. Produces prolonged nonphasic uterine contractions. Like other oxytocics, may evoke severe hypertensive episodes in hypertensive or toxaemic patients, or when regional anaesthesia (caudal or spinal) containing vasoconstrictors has been used.

Used to prevent or reduce postpartum and postabortal haemorrhage due to uterine atony.

ROUTE AND DOSAGE   Intramuscular: 200–500 mcg. *Postpartum haemorrhage*: (intravenous): 100–500 mcg. **Oral**: 0.5–1 mg.

ABSORPTION AND FATE   Rapidly and completely absorbed by all routes. Onset of uterine contractions following oral administration; 5 to 15 minutes with duration of 3 hours or longer; onset following IM in 2 to 5 minutes with duration of 3 hours. Onset is almost immediate following IV; duration is about 45 minutes. Thought to be slowly metabolized in liver. Excreted in urine.

CONTRAINDICATIONS AND PRECAUTIONS   Hypersensitivity to ergot preparations, to induce labour, use prior to delivery of placenta, threatened spontaneous abortion, prolonged use, uterine sepsis, hypertension, toxaemia.

ADVERSE/SIDE EFFECTS   Nausea, vomiting (especially with IV doses), severe hypertensive episodes, bradycardia, allergic phenomena including shock, ergotism. *See ergotamine.*

NURSING IMPLICATIONS

- Assess and record character of uterine contractions.
- IM injection produces initial, firm contraction of the postpartum uterus; a succession of minor relaxations and contractions then occur with relaxation increasing over the next period of 1.5 hours. Vigorous rhythmic contractions continue for 3 hours or more after injection.
- Desired oxytocic action may be antagonized by hypocalcaemia. Treatment: cautious IV calcium gluconate (if patient is not also taking digitalis) before ergometrine administration.
- Severe cramping following oral doses is evidence of effectiveness; however, it may also indicate need to reduce dose.
- Monitor blood pressure, pulse, and uterine response following injection until postpartum condition is stabilized (about 1 or 2 hours).
- Report sudden increase in blood pressure, pulse changes, and frequent periods of uterine relaxation. (Uterus may fail to respond in hypocalcaemic patients.)
- Patient may be more sensitive to cold. Avoid unnecessary or prolonged exposure.
- High incidence of nausea and danger of hypertensive and cerebrovascular accident have limited the use of IV route for emergency treatment.
- IV ergometrine given in second stage of labour as head is born induces contractions in 1 minute. IM injection as infant is being born produces, in 2 to 5 minutes, uterine contractions that separate placenta and prevent blood loss.

E

ERGOMETRINE MALEATE (continued)
- Oral tablets may also be administered on tongue (perlingually).
- If solution for injection is discoloured or contains particles, do not use.
- Store drug in cool place, below 8°C (46°F). However, delivery room stocks may be kept at room temperature for up to 60 days.
- *See also ergotamine tartrate.*

Ergotamine tartrate

(Cafergot, Lingrane, Migril, Medihaler, Ergotamine)   *Alpha-adrenergic blocking agent (sympatholytic); vasoconstrictor*

ACTIONS AND USES   Natural amino acid alkaloid of ergot. Alpha-adrenergic blocking agent with direct stimulating action on cranial and peripheral vascular smooth muscles and depressant effect on central vasomotor centers. In vascular headache, exerts vasoconstrictive action on previously dilated cerebral vessels, reduces amplitude of arterial pulsations, and antagonizes effects of serotonin (implicated in aetiology of vascular headaches). Does not demonstrate intrinsic sedative or analgesic actions. By unknown mechanism, ergotamine activity can lead to damage of vascular endothelium, with subsequent occlusion, thrombosis, and gangrene. Large doses may induce slight elevation of blood pressure and diminish arterial blood flow sufficiently to cause tissue ischaemia. Myometrium stimulation (oxytocic effect) becomes more prominent with dose increases and as uterine sensitivity to ergot develops during adolescence and pregnancy. Small doses given in third stage of labour promote strong uterine response without significant side effects. Stimulates chemoreceptor trigger zone and therefore may cause nausea and vomiting. May inhibit prolactin secretion.

Used as single agent or in combination with caffeine to relieve pain of migraine, cluster headache (histamine cephalalgia), and other vascular headaches. Not recommended for migraine prophylaxis because of the possibility of adverse effects.

ROUTE AND DOSAGE   Oral tablet, sublingual tablet: *Initial*: 2 mg at start of migraine followed by 1 to 2 mg at 30 to 60 minute intervals until attack has abated. Dosage should not exceed 6 mg/24-hours or 10 mg/week. **Inhalation**: each spray delivers 0.36 mg dose. Start with one inhalation; repeat, if not relieved in 5 minutes. Space additional inhalations no less than 5 minutes apart. Not to exceed 6 inhalations in 24 hours or 15 inhalations/week.

ABSORPTION AND FATE   Poorly and erratically absorbed from GI tract; response is delayed and unpredictable. **Peak plasma levels** in ½ to 3 hours. Rate and extent of absorption is enhanced by caffeine. Rapid and complete absorption following administration by inhalation. Crosses blood–brain barrier. Extensively metabolized in liver. About 90% of dose excreted as metabolites in bile via faeces. Trace amounts of unchanged drug eliminated in urine and faeces. Appears in breast milk.

ERGOTAMINE TARTRATE (continued)

CONTRAINDICATIONS AND PRECAUTIONS   Hypersensitivity, pregnancy, use in children, sepsis, obliterative vascular disease, thromboembolic disease, prolonged use of excessive dosage, hepatic and renal disease, severe pruritus, marked arteriosclerosis, coronary heart disease, hypertension, infectious states, anaemia, and malnutrition. **Cautious Use**: during lactation, elderly patients.

ADVERSE/SIDE EFFECTS   **Acute ergotism (rare)**: vomiting, diarrhoea, abdominal pain, unquenchable thirst, paraesthesias, pain (spasms) of facial muscles, tongue, limbs and lumbar region with difficulty in walking; delirium, paraesthesias, convulsive seizures, rapid or weak or irregular pulse, confusion, itching and cold skin; (occasionally): gangrene of nose, digits, ears. **Chronic ergotism**: intermittent claudication, muscle pains, weakness, numbness, coldness and cyanosis of digits (Raynaud's phenomenon). **Other**: complete absence of medium- and large-vessel pulsations in extremities; precordial distress and pain; transient bradycardia or tachycardia; elevated or lowered blood pressure; depression; drowsiness; mixed miosis (rare); kidney failure; fibrotic changes (long-term therapy), partial necrosis of tongue.

NURSING IMPLICATIONS

- Oral doses are less effective than inhalation, but they usually relieve mild or incipient attacks of migraine.
- Sublingual tablet is preferred early in the attack because of its rapid absorption and lower effective dose.
- Since degree of pain relief is proportional to rapidity of treatment, drug therapy should begin as soon after onset of attack as possible, preferably during prodrome (scintillating scotomatas, visual field defects, paraesthesias, usually on side opposite to that of the migraine, nausea).
- Metered dose nebulizers administer an exact dose and are safe if used as directed. Review instructions with patient.
- The patient's optimum dosage is determined by titrating the dose during several migraine attacks, and using the lowest effective dose for subsequent attacks.
- If migraine attacks occur more frequently or are not relieved, advise patient to report to physician. Prophylactic therapy, e.g., propranolol, or amitriptyline may be indicated.
- Advise patient to lie down in a quiet, dark room for 2 to 3 hours after drug administration. Although caffeine increases ergotamine absorption, some clinicians question its value because it may keep the patient awake and sleep contributes to the relief of migraine.
- Acute ergot poisoning is rare; but can result from overdosing or attempts at abortion.
- Instruct patient to report claudication, muscle pain or weakness of extremities, cold or numb digits, irregular heartbeat, nausea, or vomiting. Dose adjustment is indicated. With avoidance of the drug for 1 to 3 days, vasoconstriction usually subsides. Carefully protect extremities from exposure to cold temperatures; provide warmth, but not heat, to ischaemic areas. For severe peripheral vasoconstriction, IV sodium nitroprusside or intraarterial tolazoline has been used in conjunction with heparin.

ERGOTAMINE TARTRATE (continued)

Food–drug interactions   Triggers to classic migraine headache:

- □ Caffeine withdrawal (therefore, avoid caffeine beverages, e.g., tea, coffee).
- □ Tyramine-containing foods, e.g., aged cheese especially portion close to rind, Chianti, broad beans, overripe avocado (*see also Index: Food sources*).
- □ Foods containing other vasopressors, chocolate (phenylethylamine), broad beans (dopamine).
- □ Food additives, e.g., preservatives in cured meats, monosodium glutamate (MSG).

- ▪ Patients receiving high ergotamine doses for prolonged periods may experience increased frequency of headaches, fatigue, and depression. Discontinuation of the drug in these patients results in severe withdrawal headache that may last a few days.
- ▪ Patients with migraine should be helped to identify underlying emotional and physical stresses that may precipitate attacks and should be assisted in learning how to deal with them. Adequate relaxation, recreation, and sleep may help to reduce severity and frequency of attacks.
- ▪ Warn the woman of childbearing age to avoid use of ergotamine if she suspects she is pregnant, because of its oxytocic effect.
- ▪ Warn patients not to increase dosage without consulting physician; overdosage is the chief cause of untoward effects from the drug.
- ▪ Keep drug out of reach of children. Fatalities have been reported.

Patient-teaching points   Patients with migraine should be helped to identify underlying emotional, physical and environmental stresses that may trigger an attack and should be assisted in learning how to deal with them:

- □ Precipitating factors vary from person to person but commonly involve fatigue, stress, sleep deprivation, ingestion of certain foods (*see Food–drug interactions above*); hormonal changes particularly those associated with menstruation, drugs such as oral contraceptives, vasodilators; the over-achiever personality.
- □ Emphasize that adequate relaxation, recreation, and sleep may help to reduce severity and frequency of attacks.
- □ Warn patients not to increase dosage without consulting physician; overdosage is the chief cause of untoward effects from the drug.
- □ Avoid self-dosing with OTC drugs without advice of physician.

- ▪ Preserved in light-resistant container preferably between 15° and 30°C (59° and 86°F) unless otherwise directed by manufacturer.

DRUG INTERACTIONS   *Ergotamine tartrate*

PLUS	INTERACTIONS
Propranolol and possibly other beta-adrenergic blockers	Possibility of enhanced vasoconstrictor activity with high doses of ergot alkaloids. Used concomitantly with caution
Triacetyloleandomycin	Possibility of severe peripheral vasospasm and hypertension (probably interferes with ergotamine metabolism). Used concomitantly with caution

Erythromycin ———————————————————

(Arpimycin, Erycen, Erymax, Erythrocin, Erythrolar,   *Antibiotic (macrolide)*
    Erythromid, Erythroped, Ilosone, Ilotyein, Retcin)   *Erythromycin*

ACTIONS AND USES   Macrolide antibiotic produced by a strain of *Streptomyces erythreus*. Considered one of the safest antibiotics in use today. Bacteriostatic or bactericidal, depending on nature of organism and drug concentration used. Antibacterial spectrum is similar to but broader than that of penicillin; commonly used as penicillin substitute in hypersensitive patients for infections not requiring high antibiotic blood levels. More active against gram-positive than gram-negative bacteria. Effective against *Chlamydia trachomatis* is basis for its topical use in prophylaxis of neonatal inclusion conjunctivitis. Acts by inhibiting protein synthesis of sensitive microorganisms. Resistant mutants are especially frequent among staphylococci.

Used in treatment of pneumococcal and diplococcal pneumonia, *Mycoplasma pneumoniae* (primary atypical pneumonia), acute pelvic inflammatory disease caused by *Neisseria gonorrhoeae* in females sensitive to penicillin, infections caused by susceptible strains of staphylococci, streptococci, and certain strains of *Haemophilus influenzae*. Also used in intestinal amoebiasis, Legionnaires' disease, uncomplicated urethral, endocervical, and rectal infections caused by *Chlamydia trachomatis*, for prophylaxis of ophthalmia neonatorum caused by *N. gonorrhoeae, C. trachomatis*, and for chlamydial conjunctivitis in neonates. Considered an acceptable alternative to penicillin for treatment of streptococcal pharyngitis for prophylaxis of rheumatic fever and bacterial endocarditis, and for treatment of diphtheria as adjunct to antitoxin and for carrier state, and as alternate choice in treatment of primary syphilis in patients allergic to penicillins.

ROUTE AND DOSAGE   **Adults: Oral:** 250–500 mg every 6 hrs, or 0.5–1 g every 12 hrs, maximum 4 g daily. **Child (up to one year):** 12 mg/kg three times a day, **(1–7 yrs):** 125–250 mg three times a day, **(over 7 yrs):** as adult dose. **IV: infusion: Adult:** 2 g/day in divided doses (Maximum 4 g), **Child:** 20–50 mg/kg/day.

ABSORPTION AND FATE   **Peak plasma concentrations:** about 4 hours following oral administration (absorption is delayed by presence of food in stomach). Adequate blood levels maintained by administration every 6 hours. Diffuses readily into tissues and most body fluids, including pleural and peritoneal spaces and inflamed meninges. Concentrates in normal liver. **Half-life:** 0.8 to 3 hours. Excreted in active form primarily in bile and faeces. About 2 to 5% of orally administered dose excreted in urine as active drug. Crosses placenta and is excreted in breast milk.

CONTRAINDICATIONS AND PRECAUTIONS   Hypersensitivity to erythromycins. Safe use during pregnancy not established. **Cautious Use:** impaired hepatic function.

ADVERSE/SIDE EFFECTS   These include: nausea, vomiting, heartburn, anorexia, and hypersensitivity reactions: fever, eosinophilia, urticaria, skin eruptions, superinfections by nonsusceptible bacteria, yeasts, or fungi, abdominal cramping, discomfort, distention, diarrhoea.

E

ERYTHROMYCIN (continued)
NURSING IMPLICATIONS

■ Culture and sensitivity testing should be done to determine organism susceptibility.
■ Activity of erythromycin may be decreased in acid medium and by the presence of food in the stomach. Therefore it is administered preferably on an empty stomach 1 hour before or 3 hours after meals. Do not give with, or immediately before or after, fruit juices and advise patient not to crush or chew tablets.
■ Manufacturers of enteric coated tablets state that they may be given without regard to meals.
■ GI symptoms following oral administration are dose-related. Report their onset to physician. If symptoms persist following dosage reduction, physician may prescribe drug to be given with meals in spite of impaired absorption.
■ Bear in mind that pseudomembranous colitis, a potentially life-threatening condition, may occur during or after antibiotic therapy.
■ Observe for symptoms of overgrowth of nonsusceptible bacteria or fungi (fever, black furry tongue, sore mouth, enteritis, perianal irritation or itching, vaginal discharge). Emergence of resistant staphylococcal strains is highly predictable during prolonged therapy.
■ In treatment of streptococcal infections, erythromycin therapy should be continued for at least 10 days.
■ Hepatic function tests should be performed periodically during prolonged drug regimens.
■ Hepatotoxicity is believed to be a hypersensitivity reaction. Premonitory signs and symptoms may include abdominal pain, nausea, vomiting, fever, leucocytosis, and eosinophilia. Jaundice (dark urine, light-coloured stools, yellow skin, pruritus, yellow sclerae and soft palate) may or may not be present.
■ Symptoms of hepatotoxicity may appear a few days after initiation of drug but usually occur after 1 to 2 weeks of continuous therapy. Symptoms are reversible with prompt discontinuation of erythromycin.
■ Strict adherence of patient to prescribed dosage regimen should be stressed.
■ Store in tightly capped containers preferably between 15° and 30°C (59° and 86°) unless otherwise directed by manufacturer.

Diagnostic test interferences   False elevations of **urinary catecholamines, urinary steroids**, and AST (SGOT), ALT (SGPT) (by colorimetric methods).

DRUG INTERACTIONS *Erythromycins*_____

PLUS	INTERACTIONS
Anticoagulants, oral	Potentiation of anticoagulant (hypoprothrombinaemic) effect. Monitor prothrombin time
Carbamazepine Corticosteroids	Effects to these drugs may increase (erythromycin inhibits their hepatic metabolism). Reduced dosages of these drugs and close monitoring indicated
Clindamycin	Antagonistic action. Concomitant use generally avoided

ERYTHROMYCIN (continued)

PLUS (continued)	INTERACTIONS
Digoxin and other digitalis glycosides	Possibility of increased digitalis effect in some patients. Interaction may occur several months after discontinuation of erythromycin (erythromycin increases digitalis bioavailability in some patients). Reduction of digitalis dosage may be necessary
Penicillins	Erythromycin in low doses may antagonize antimicrobial action of penicillins. Combination used only when adequate amounts of each are given, administer penicillin at least a few hours before erythromycin
Theophyllines	Pharmacological effects of theophyllines may increase (erythromycin inhibits their hepatic metabolism). Theophyllines may reduce erythromycin serum concentrations. Reduced dosage of theophyllines and close monitoring indicated

Estramustine phosphate sodium ——————————

(Estracyt)   *Antineoplastic; oestrogen*

E

ACTIONS AND USES   Conjugate of oestradiol and normustine. Extent of antitumour activity contributed by each, as well as precise mechanisms of action unknown. Appears to act as a relatively weak alkylating agent and oestrogen. Major effectiveness reported to be in patients who have been refractory to oestrogen therapy alone. Contains 0.5 mEq (12.5 mg) of sodium per capsule.

Used in palliative treatment of metabolic and/or progressive carcinoma of prostate.

ROUTE AND DOSAGE   Oral: individualized.

ABSORPTION AND FATE   Well absorbed from GI tract. **Peak plasma concentration in 2 to 3 hours.** Rapidly dephosphorylated in intestines; ultimately oxidized and hydrolyzed to estramustine, oestradiol, oestrone, and nitrogen mustard. Elimination appears to be multiphasic. Half-life of terminal phase approximately 20 hours. Metabolized in liver. Most of drug excreted in bile via faeces.

CONTRAINDICATIONS AND PRECAUTIONS   Hypersensitivity to either oestradiol or nitrogen mustard; active thrombophlebitis, or thromboembolic disorders. **Cautious Use**: history of thrombophlebitis, thromboses, or thromboembolic disorders, cerebrovascular or coronary artery disease, gallstones, or peptic ulcer; impaired liver function, metabolic bone diseases associated with hypercalcaemia; diabetes mellitus, hypertension, conditions that might be aggravated by fluid retention (e.g., epilepsy, migraine, renal dysfunction); elderly patients.

ESTRAMUSTINE PHOSPHATE SODIUM (continued)

ADVERSE/SIDE EFFECTS These include: hypertension, cerebrovascular accident, myocardial infarction, thrombophlebitis, congestive heart failure, peripheral oedema, rash, pruritus, urticaria, dry skin, easy bruising, flushing, peeling skin and fingertips, thinning hair. **GI**: nausea, diarrhoea, anorexia, flatulence, vomiting, thirst, GI bleeding. **Others**: leucopenia, thrombocytopenia, hypercalcaemia, abnormalities in liver function tests, lethargy, emotional lability, insomnia, headache, anxiety, epilepsy, hoarseness, burning sensation in throat, dyspnoea, upper respiratory discharge, pulmonary emboli, tearing of eyes, gynaecomastia, breast tenderness, impotence, renal dysfunction, leg cramps, decrease in glucose tolerance, bone marrow toxicity (uncommon).

NURSING IMPLICATIONS

- Note expiry date on product label.
- Drug can be taken with meals to reduce incidence of GI side effects. Physician may prescribe an antacid or antiemetic if GI symptoms persist. Some patients require drug withdrawal.

Patient-teaching points related to drug induced nausea

- ☐ Eat small feedings at frequent intervals; eat slowly.
- ☐ Keep physically quiet when nauseated and keep upper torso elevated (for about 2 hours after eating).
- ☐ Drink liquids 1 hour before or 1 hour after rather than with meals; clear liquids may be more palatable.
- ☐ Control odours and avoid foods known to patient that precipitate or aggravate nausea.
- ☐ Avoid fried, greasy, spicy, and overly sweet foods.
- ☐ Cold foods may be less offensive than hot foods because they are generally almost odourless.
- ☐ If nausea occurs on awakening, eat dry foods such as dry toast before activity.
- ☐ Cleanse mouth after each meal; breath fresheners, or ice chips may help.
- ☐ Inspect oral cavity after vomiting for retained food/vomitus (debilitated patients or severely depressed patients may be unaware of their presence.) Cleanse mouth if necessary.
- ☐ Patient may be reassured if vomit bowl is kept handy but not visible.
- ☐ Eliminate smoking by caretaker in presence of sick person.

- Elderly patients who have nausea and vomiting should be kept turned on side with head of bed raised to prevent aspiration. Suction equipment should be readily available.
- Check blood pressure at regular intervals throughout therapy. Report significant elevations to physician.
- Keep track of weight and examine daily for peripheral oedema. Be mindful that drug can cause congestive heart failure.
- Monitor fluid intake–output ratio and pattern to prevent dehydration and electrolyte imbalance.
- Patient with diabetes should be closely observed because of possibility of estramus-

ESTRAMUSTINE PHOSPHATE SODIUM (continued)

tine-induced reduction in glucose tolerance. Baseline and periodic glucose tolerance tests are advised.

- Patient should be advised to use a barrier contraceptive. (Drug has mutagenic and teratogenic properties.) Some patients formerly impotent have regained potency while taking estramustine.
- Advise patient who experiences thinning of hair to avoid vigorous treatment of scalp and to wash and comb hair gently.
- Baseline and periodic hepatic enzymes and bilirubin tests should be performed, then repeated after drug has been discontinued for 2 months.
- Patient should receive therapy for 30 to 90 days before evaluations are made to determine adequacy of response and possible benefits of continuing treatment.
- Some patients have received therapy for more than 3 years. Therapy is usually continued as long as patient demonstrates a favorable response.
- *Treatment of overdosage*   Stomach contents evacuated by gastric lavage. Therapy is symptomatic and supportive. Haematologic and hepatic studies should be done for at least 6 weeks after drug ingestion.
- Store in refrigerator at 2° to 8°C (38° to 46°F) in tight, light-resistant containers, unless otherwise directed by manufacturer.

Ethacrynic acid ────────────────────────────

E

(Edecrin)   *Diuretic (loop)*

ACTIONS AND USES   Unsaturated ketone derivative of phenoxyacetic acid with rapid and potent diuretic action. Inhibits sodium and chloride reabsorption in proximal tubule and most segments of loop of Henle, promotes potassium and hydrogen ion excretion, and decreases urinary ammonium ion concentration and pH. Appears to have little effect on bicarbonate excretion but chloruretic effect may foster bicarbonate retention. Promotes calcium loss in hypercalcaemia and nephrogenic diabetes insipidus. Paradoxic decrease in urine volume may follow drug-induced sodium loss. Fluid-electrolyte loss may exceed that produced by thiazides, but the effect on carbohydrate metabolism and blood glucose is less. Tends to promote urate excretion at high doses and retention at low doses; does not inhibit carbonic anhydrase. Action is independent of systemic acid–base balance. Appears to have little or no direct effect on renal blood flow or glomerular filtration rate. Aldosterone secretion may be increased, thus contributing to hypokalaemia. Hypotensive effect may be due to hypovolaemia secondary to diuresis, and in part to decreased vascular resistance.

Used in treatment of severe oedema associated with congestive heart failure, hepatic cirrhosis, ascites of malignancy, renal disease, nephrotic syndrome, lymphoedema.

ROUTE AND DOSAGE   Adults: Oral: *Initial*: 50 mg (single dose); *maintenance* (following diuresis) consists of minimal effective dose (50 to 150 mg once daily after meals)

ETHACRYNIC ACID (continued)

administered on continuous or intermittent dosage schedule. Dosage adjustments are usually made in increments of 25 to 50 mg. Total daily dosage should not exceed 400 mg. **Adults only: Intravenous (ethacrynate sodium):** 50 mg administered by direct IV over at least 5 minutes, or through tubing of running infusion of compatible IV fluid. Usually one dose is sufficient. If second dose is necessary, select new injection site to avoid possibility of thrombophlebitis. Single doses should not exceed 100 mg.

ABSORPTION AND FATE   Diuretic effect occurs within 30 minutes following oral administration, peaks in 2 hours, and lasts 6 to 8 hours, possibly up to 12 hours. Following IV injection, diuresis is apparent within 5 minutes; it reaches maximum within 15 to 30 minutes and persists approximately 2 or more hours. About 95% protein bound. **Half-life:** 30 to 70 minutes. Accumulates in liver. Metabolized to active cysteine conjugate; approximately one-half to two-thirds of dose is excreted in urine; remainder is eliminated in bile. Rate of urinary excretion increases as pH increases. It is not known whether it crosses placenta or enters breast milk.

CONTRAINDICATIONS AND PRECAUTIONS   History of hypersensitivity to ethacrynic acid; anuria, hepatic coma, advanced hepatic cirrhosis, severe diarrhoea, dehydration, electrolyte imbalance, hypotension, pregnancy, lactation, women of childbearing age, infants, parenteral use in paediatric patients. **Cautious Use:** hepatic cirrhosis, elderly cardiac patients, diabetes mellitus; history of gout; pulmonary oedema associated with acute myocardial infarction, nephrotic syndrome.

ADVERSE/SIDE EFFECTS   These include: postural hypotension, thrombophlebitis, emboli, skin rash, pruritus, hyponatraemia, hypokalaemia, hypochloraemic alkalosis, hypomagnesaemia, hypocalcaemia, hypercalciuria, hypovolaemia, hyperuricaemia, anorexia, nausea, vomiting, dysphagia, abdominal discomfort or pain, malaise, diarrhoea, GI bleeding (IV use), acute pancreatitis (increased serum amylase), abnormal liver function tests, jaundice, hepatic damage, hypoproteinaemia, thrombocytopenia, agranulocytosis, severe neutropenia, Henoch's purpura (in patients with rheumatic fever), tetany, acute gout, elevated BUN, haematuria, hyperglycaemia, acute hypoglycaemia (rare), gynae comastia, headache, fever, chills, blurred vision, fatigue, weakness, apprehension, confusion, local irritation of IV site, vertigo, tinnitus, sense of fullness in ears, temporary or permanent deafness.

NURSING IMPLICATIONS

- Follow manufacturer's directions for reconstitution of sodium ethacrynate. Solution should be used within 24 hours; discard solution if it is cloudy or opalescent.
- Schedule doses to avoid nocturia and thus sleep interference.
- Explain diuretic effect (increased volume and frequency of voiding) to the patient.
- Diuretic effect tends to diminish with continuous therapy.
- Administer oral drug after a meal or food to prevent gastric irritation.
- Parenteral drug is given by direct IV injection or into tubing of a running infusion, slowly over a few minutes. Usually one dose is sufficient. If a second dose is required select another site to prevent thrombophlebitis.
- Monitor blood pressure during initial therapy. Since orthostatic hypotension some-

ETHACRYNIC ACID (continued)

times occurs, supervision of ambulation is advisable. Caution the patient to make position changes slowly, particularly from recumbent to upright position.

- Patient should be observed closely when receiving the drug by IV infusion. Rapid, copious diuresis following IV administration can produce hypotension and peripheral vascular collapse. Check infusion site frequently. Extravasation causes local pain and tissue irritation.
- Monitor fluid intake–output ratio as an important measure of drug action. Drug should be discontinued if excessive diuresis, oliguria, haematuria, or sudden profuse diarrhoea occurs. Report signs to physician.
- Establish baseline weight prior to start of therapy; weigh patient under standard conditions.
- Observe for and report warning signs and symptoms of electrolyte imbalance: anorexia, nausea, vomiting, thirst, dry mouth, polyuria, oliguria, weakness, fatigue, dizziness, headache, muscle cramps, paraesthesias, drowsiness, mental confusion.
- Fluid and electrolyte depletion is most apt to occur in patients on large doses or salt-intake restriction. Consult physician regarding allowable salt and fluid intake. Generally, salt intake is liberalized.
- Elderly and debilitated patients require close observation. Excessive diuresis promotes dehydration and hypovolaemia, both of which often precede circulatory collapse, cerebrovascular thrombosis, and pulmonary emboli, especially in these patients.
- Report immediately possible signs of thromboembolic complications: pain in chest, back, pelvis, legs.
- Monitor blood pressure and pulse of patients with impaired cardiac function. Diuretic-induced hypovolaemia may reduce cardiac output, and electrolyte loss promotes cardiotoxicity in those receiving digitalis or other cardiac glycosides.
- To reduce or prevent potassium depletion, the physician may prescribe daily ingestion of potassium-rich foods (banana, orange, peach, dried dates, milk, yogurt), potassium supplement, and intermittent dosage schedule.
- GI side effects occur most frequently after 1 to 3 months of therapy or in patients on high dosage. Loose stools or other GI symptoms at any time during therapy should be reported in order to permit dosage adjustment or discontinuation of drug if indicated.
- In patients receiving aminoglycoside antibiotics concurrently with ethacrynic acid, renal status, audiograms, and vestibular function tests are advised before initiation of therapy and regularly throughout therapy.
- Report immediately any evidence of impaired hearing. Ototoxicity has been associated with renal insufficiency, concomitant administration of aminoglycoside antibiotics, and rapid IV administration. Hearing loss may be preceded by vertigo, tinnitus, or fullness in ears; it may be transient lasting 1 to 24 hours, or it may be permanent.
- Impaired glucose tolerance with hyperglycaemia and glycosuria may occur in diabetic and diabetic-prone individuals and in patients with decompensated hepatic cirrhosis. Watch for signs of hypoglycaemia when ethacrynic acid is withdrawn.
- Acute hypoglycaemia with convulsions reportedly has been associated with use of large doses in patients with uraemia.

E

ETHACRYNIC ACID (continued)
DRUG INTERACTIONS   *Ethacrynic acid*

PLUS	INTERACTIONS
Aminoglycosides	Additive ototoxic effects. Used concomitantly with caution if at all. Monitor eighth nerve function
Anticoagulants	Potentiation of anticoagulant (hypoprothrombinaemic) effect. Increased possibility of GI bleeding. Used concomitantly with caution
Cisplatin	Additive ototoxic effects. Concurrent use generally avoided, if possible
Digitalis glycosides	Increased incidence of arrhythmias (hypokalaemia, induced by ethacrynic acid, sensitizes myocardium to effects of digitalis). Monitor serum potassium
Lithium	Increases risk of lithium toxicity (lithium excretion decreases with sodium depletion). Used concurrently with caution if at all

Ethambutol hydrochloride

(Myambutol, Mynah)   *Antitubercular*

ACTIONS AND USES   Synthetic antituberculosis agent with bacteriostatic action. Mode of action not completely understood, but it appears to inhibit RNA synthesis and thus arrests multiplication of tubercle bacilli. Not recommended for use as sole agent. The emergence of resistant strains is delayed by administering ethambutol in combination with other antituberculosis drugs.

Used in conjunction with at least one other antituberculosis agent in treatment of pulmonary tuberculosis. Also used in treatment of diseases caused by other mycobacteria.

ROUTE AND DOSAGE   Oral: **Adult**: 15 mg/kg once every 24 hours. **Child**: 25 mg/kg/day for 60 days, followed by 15 mg/kg/day.

ABSORPTION AND FATE   Approximately 70 to 80% readily absorbed from GI tract following oral administration. Absorption is not significantly affected by presence of food. **Peak serum levels** within 2 to 4 hours, 50% of peak level remains at 8 hours and 10% at 24 hours. **Plasma half-life**: 3 to 4 hours (up to 8 hours in patients with impaired renal function); 20 to 30% protein bound. Widely distributed to most body fluids and tissues. Highest concentrations in erythrocytes, kidneys, lungs, saliva. Lowest concentrations in ascitic and pleural fluid, brain, and cerebrospinal fluid. Detoxified in liver. Approximately 50% of drug is excreted unchanged in urine within 24 hours; 8 to 15% appears as inactive metabolites and 20 to 22% excreted in faeces as unchanged drug.

ETHAMBUTOL HYDROCHLORIDE (continued)

CONTRAINDICATIONS AND PRECAUTIONS   Hypersensitivity to ethambutol; patients with optic neuritis, children under 13 years of age. Safe use during pregnancy not established. **Cautious Use**: patients with renal impairment, gout, ocular defects, e.g., cataract, recurrent ocular inflammatory conditions, diabetic retinopathy.

ADVERSE/SIDE EFFECTS   These include: headache, dizziness, confusion, hallucinations, peripheral neuritis (rare), joint pains and weakness of lower extremities, anorexia, nausea, vomiting, abdominal pain, pruritus, dermatitis, anaphylaxis, fever, malaise, leucopenia (rare), bloody sputum, transient impairment of liver function, nephrotoxicity, hyperuricaemia, acute gouty arthritis, ECG abnormalities. Ocular toxicity: optic neuritis with decrease in visual acuity, temporary loss of vision, constriction of visual fields, red-green colour blindness, central and peripheral scotomata, eye pain, photophobia.

NURSING IMPLICATIONS

- Ethambutol may be taken with food if GI irritation occurs. Absorption is reportedly not significantly affected by food in stomach.
- Culture and sensitivity tests should be performed prior to initiation of therapy and repeated periodically throughout therapy.
- Ocular toxicity generally appears within 1 to 7 months after start of therapy. Symptoms usually disappear within several weeks to months after drug is discontinued, depending on degree of ocular damage.
- Advise patient to report promptly to physician the onset of blurred vision, changes in colour perception, constriction of visual fields, or any other visual symptoms. Patient should be questioned periodically about eyes.
- Ophthalmoscopic examination including tests of visual fields (finger perimetry), tests for visual acuity and tests for colour discrimination should be performed prior to start of therapy and at monthly intervals during therapy. Eyes should be tested separately as well as together.
- If detected early, visual defects generally disappear over several weeks to months. In rare instances, recovery may be delayed for a year or more or defect may be irreversible.
- Monitor fluid intake and output ratio in patients with renal impairment. Report oliguria or any significant changes in intake−output ratio or in laboratory reports of renal function. Systemic accumulation with toxicity can result from delayed drug excretion.
- In general, therapy may continue for 1 to 2 years or longer although shorter treatment regiments have been used with success.
- Hepatic and renal function tests, blood cell counts, and serum uric acid determinations should be performed at regular intervals throughout therapy.
- Emphasize importance of adhering to drug regimen and of keeping follow-up appointments.
- If patient becomes pregnant during therapy, advise her to notify physician immediately. Drug should be withdrawn.
- Protect ethambutol from light, moisture, and excessive heat.

E

ETHAMBUTOL HYDROCHLORIDE (continued)
Diagnostic test interferences Ethambutol may increase **serum uric acid** levels and may cause elevations in **liver function tests**.

Ethamivan

(Clairvan)   *Respiratory stimulant*

For further information *see nikethamide*

ROUTE AND DOSAGE   IV: 100 mg as required.

Ethamsylate

(Dicynene)   *Haemostatic*

ACTIONS AND USES   Reduces capillary bleeding in the presence of normal platelet function. Used to treat menorrhagia and haemorrhage from small blood vessels and periventricular haemorrhage in neonates.

ROUTE AND DOSAGE   Oral: 500 mg four times a day. **IV:** 1 g then 500 mg 4–6 hourly. **Neonate:** 12.5 mg/kg/6 hrly. **Child:** 250–750 mg.

Ethinyloestradiol

Hormone; oestrogen

ACTIONS AND USES   Oral oestrogen with actions similar to those of oestradiol (q.v.). *See. Ostradiol for absorption, fate, contraindications, precautions, and adverse/side effects.* Given cyclically for short-term use only.

Used in combination with progestins to control ovulation, also used to treat spontaneous or clomiphene-associated hostile cervical mucus, the excessive bleeding of endometrial hyperplasia, and to control severe vasomotor symptoms of menopause and to inhibit postmenopausal bone loss.

ROUTE AND DOSAGE   Oral: Individualized, depends on the preparation.

NURSING IMPLICATIONS
- Given cyclically, except when used for treatment of postpartum breast engorgement and palliation of carcinoma. Usual cyclic regimen: once daily for 3 weeks, followed by 1 week without the drug; then repeat this regimen.

ETHINYLOESTRADIOL (continued)

- *Food–drug interactions* High vitamin C intake (e.g., 1 g/day) may increase ethinyl oestradiol levels. Abrupt withdrawal of vitamin C may lead to breakthrough bleeding.
- Urge patient to read package insert to assure understanding about oestrogen therapy.
- Store between 15° and 30°C (59° and 86°F) in well-closed, light-resistant container.
- For further information: *see oestradiol*.

Ethoglucid

(Epodyl)

ACTIONS AND USES Alkylating antineoplastic used as a bladder instillation to treat noninvasive cancer.

ROUTE AND DOSAGE 1% solution for bladder instillation.

Ethosuximide

(Emeside, Zarontin)   *Anticonvulsant; succinimide*

ACTIONS AND USES Succinimide anticonvulsant. Reduces frequency of epileptiform attacks, apparently by depressing motor cortex and by elevating CNS threshold to stimuli. Usually ineffective in management of psychomotor or major motor seizures.

Used in management of absence (petit mal) seizures, partial seizures with complex symptomology (psychomotor seizures) and tonic–clonic (grand mal) seizures. May be administered in combination with other anticonvulsants when other forms of epilepsy coexist with petit mal.

ROUTE AND DOSAGE Highly individualized. **Oral: Adults and children (6 years and older):** 250 mg two times daily. **Children (3 to 6 years):** 250 mg/day. Dosage increases are made in small increments. A total daily dose exceeding 2 g for adults or 1 g for children up to 6 years should be administered only under strict medical supervision.

ABSORPTION AND FATE Essentially completely absorbed from GI tract. **Peak plasma concentrations** in 1 to 7 hours; however, 4 to 7 days are required for **steady-state plasma concentrations**. **Plasma half-life** 24 to 60 hours. No significant degree of plasma protein binding. Metabolized by liver. Excreted slowly in urine, about 50% as metabolites and 10 to 20% as unchanged drug. Small amounts excreted in bile and faeces.

CONTRAINDICATIONS AND PRECAUTIONS Hypersensitivity to succinimides; severe liver or renal disease; use alone in mixed types of epilepsy (may increase frequency of

ETHOSUXIMIDE (continued)

grand mal seizures). Safe use in women of childbearing potential or during pregnancy not established.

ADVERSE/SIDE EFFECTS   These include: hiccoughs, ataxia, dizziness, drowsiness, headache, euphoria, restlessness, irritability, anxiety, hyperactivity, aggressiveness, depression, inability to concentrate, lethargy, confusion, sleep disturbances, night terrors, hypochondriacal behaviour, rarely: psychosis, increased depression with overt suicidal intentions, auditory hallucinations. **Others:** Stevens-Johnson syndrome, pruritic erythematous skin eruptions, exfoliative dermatitis, systemic lupus erythematosus, nausea, vomiting, anorexia, weight loss, epigastric distress, abdominal pain, diarrhoea, constipation, frequency, haematuria, albuminuria, renal damage, eosinophilia, leucopenia, thrombocytopenia, agranulocytosis, pancytopenia, aplastic anaemia, positive direct Coombs' test, blurred vision, myopia, photophobia, periorbital oedema, increased libido, hirsutism, alopecia, vaginal bleeding, swelling of tongue, gum hypertrophy, muscle weakness.

NURSING IMPLICATIONS

- Baseline and periodic haematological studies and tests of liver and renal function should be made.
- Since ethosuximide may impair mental and physical abilities, caution the patient to avoid driving a motor vehicle and other hazardous activities.
- GI symptoms, drowsiness, ataxia, dizziness, and other neurological side effects occur frequently and indicate the need for dosage adjustment.
- Close observation is required during the period of dosage adjustment and whenever other medications are added to or eliminated from the drug regimen. Therapeutic serum levels: 40 to 100 mcg/ml.
- Behavioural changes are most likely to occur in the patient with a prior history of psychiatric disturbances. Close supervision is indicated. Drug should be withdrawn slowly if these symptoms appear.
- Abrupt withdrawal of ethosuximide (whether used alone or in combination therapy) may precipitate seizures or petit mal status.
- Since long-term drug therapy is generally required, the occurrence of adverse drug effects is a possibility. Caution the patient and responsible family members to report any unusual sign or symptom to the physician. Stress the importance of follow-up visits.
- Advise the patient to carry a wallet identification card or jewellery indicating that he or she has epilepsy, is taking medication, and the physician's name and telephone number.
- Store capsules in tight containers, and syrup in light-resistant containers at 15° to 30°C (59° to 86°F); avoid freezing.

DRUG INTERACTIONS   *Ethosuximide*

PLUS	INTERACTIONS
Antipsychotics e.g., haloperidol, pimozide	May decrease anticonvulsant effect and augment CNS depression

E

ETIDRONATE DISODIUM (continued)

Oestrogens Contraceptives, oral, (except progesterone-only agents) }	Decreased effectiveness of oestrogen and 25-fold increased risk of unplanned pregnancy in women taking oral contraceptives.
Phenothiazines (e.g., chlorpromazine)	See antipsychotics (above)
Tricyclic antidepressants (TCA), e.g., imipramine, doxepin	Mutually antagonistic; TCAs can decrease effect of an anticonvulsant; ethosuximide can decrease antidepressant effect of TCA; possible additive CNS effect on anticonvulsant activity

Note: See also phenytoin.

Etidronate disodium

(Didronel)   Regulator (calcium)

ACTIONS AND USES Diphosphate preparation with primary action on bone. Slows rate of bone turnover (bone resorption and new bone accretion) in Pagetic bone lesions and in normal remodelling process. Lowers serum alkaline phosphatase and urinary hydroxyproline levels and reduces elevated cardiac output by decreasing vascularity of bone. Induces reversible hyperphosphataemia without adverse effects.

Used to treat symptomatic polyostotic Paget's disease and heterotopic ossification due to spinal cord injury. Also used to prevent and treat heterotopic ossification following total hip replacement.

ROUTE AND DOSAGE Oral: *(Paget's disease)*: *Initial*: 5 mg/kg/day for no more than 6 months. (Doses above 10 mg/kg/day for no more than 3 months reserved for use when prompt reduction of elevated cardiac output or supression of bone turnover are required.) Retreatment after drug-free period of at least 3 months: ***heterotopic ossification due to spinal cord injury***: *Initial*: 20 mg/kg/day for 2 weeks followed by 10 mg/kg/day for 10 weeks; heterotopic ossification complicating total hip replacement: 20 mg/kg/day for 1 month preoperatively; then 20 mg/kg/day for 3 months postoperatively.

ABSORPTION AND FATE Absorption is dose-dependent. Etidronate is not metabolized and is cleared from blood in 6 hours. Within 24 hours, half of absorbed dose is excreted by kidneys; the remainder is chemically adsorbed on bone and slowly eliminated. Unabsorbed drug excreted in faeces.

CONTRAINDICATIONS AND PRECAUTIONS Enterocolitis, children, pathological fractures. **Cautious Use**: renal impairment, pregnancy, lactation, patients on restricted calcium and vitamin D intake.

ADVERSE/SIDE EFFECTS Nausea, loose bowel movements, diarrhoea; increased risk of fractures in patient with Paget's disease, increased or recurrent bone pain in Pagetic sites, onset of bone pain in previously asymptomatic sites, hypocalcaemia, suppressed mineralization of uninvolved skeleton.

NURSING IMPLICATIONS
- Take as single dose on empty stomach 2 hours before meals with full glass of water or juice to reduce gastric irritation.

ETIDRONATE DISODIUM (continued)

- Therapeutic response to this drug may be slow (1 to 3 months) and may continue for months after treatment has been discontinued.
- Maintenance of optimum nutritional status, especially adequate intake of calcium and vitamin D, is an important adjunct to effective therapy. Advise patient to include milk, dairy products, and leafy vegetables in diet.
- GI side effects may interfere with adequate nutritional status and should be treated promptly. Persistent nausea or diarrhoea should be reported.
- Monitor fluid intake–output ratio of patient with impaired renal function.
- Hypocalcaemia is a theoretical possibility. Symptoms should be reported at onset: skeletal muscle spasms, facial muscle twitching, carpopedal spasm, laryngospasm, paraesthesias, intestinal colic.
- The risk of pathological fractures increases when daily dose of 20 mg/kg is taken longer than 3 months. Instruct patient to report promptly the sudden onset of unexplained pain.
- Laboratory test values that may suggest clinical progress: e.g., decreased urinary excretion of hydroxyproline reflects decreased bone resorption; decreased serum alkaline phosphatase level indicates decreased bone formation. (*Normal urinary hydroxyproline*: 15 to 50 mg/24 hours; *serum alkaline phosphatase*: 1.4 to 4.1 Bodansky units.)
- Serum phosphate levels generally return to normal 2 to 4 weeks after medication is discontinued.
- Retreatment should not be instituted prematurely or before symptoms return. Instruct patient to report promptly if bone pain, restricted mobility, heat over involved bone site occur.
- Urge patient to keep appointments for periodic evaluation of clinical tests.

Etodolac

(Lodine, Ramodar)   *NSAID antirheumatic*

ROUTE AND DOSAGE   Oral: **Adult:** 400 mg/day as a single or divided dose. Maximum dose 600 mg/day.

See ibuprofen for nursing implications.

Etoposide

(VePesid, VP 16213)   *Antineoplastic*

ACTIONS AND USES   Semisynthetic podophyllin derivative of the mandrake. Produces cytotoxic action by unclear mechanism. Primary effect is on G_2 (resting or premitotic) phase of cell cycle; also acts on S (DNA synthesis) phase. High doses cause lysis of cells entering mitotic phase, and lower doses inhibit cells from entering prophase.

ETOPOSIDE (continued)

Used in treatment of refractory testicular neoplasms, usually in combination with other chemotherapeutic agents, in patients who have already received appropriate surgery, chemotherapy, and radiation therapy. Has also been used in treatment of choriosarcoma in women, small cell carcinoma of the lung, malignant lymphomas, Hodgkin's disease, acute myelogenous (nonlymphocytic) leukaemia.

ROUTE AND DOSAGE Intravenous or oral highly individualized according to clinical response, haematology, and tolerance.

ABSORPTION AND FATE Variable degree of penetration into CSF, generally about 1%. Distribution into other body fluids and tissues not known. Probably metabolized in liver. Extensively (94%) bound to plasma proteins. **Biphasic half-life**: initial phase about 3 hours; terminal phase, 15 hours. Approximately 44 to 60% of dose excreted in urine within 48 to 72 hours, about ⅔ as unchanged drug and remainder as metabolites. Variable amounts eliminated in faeces (2 to 16%) over 3 days.

CONTRAINDICATIONS AND PRECAUTIONS Hypersensitivity to etoposide or to formulation ingredients; severe bone marrow depression, severe hepatic or renal impairment, existing or recent viral infection, bacterial infection, intraperitoneal, intrapleural, or intrathecal administration. Safe use during pregnancy, in fertile women, nursing mothers, and in children not established. **Cautious Use**: impaired renal or hepatic function, gout.

ADVERSE/SIDE EFFECTS These include: hypotension, palpitation, tachycardia, hypertension; myocardial infarction, pulmonary oedema (causal relationship not established), reversible alopecia (can progress to total baldness); nail pigmentation, radiation recall dermatitis, severe pruritus (rare), Stevens–Johnson syndrome, nausea, vomiting, dyspepsia, anorexia, diarrhoea, constipation, stomatitis, aftertaste, severe myelosuppression: leucopenia (principally granulocytopenia), thrombocytopenia, hyperuricaemia, anaemia, pancytopenia, neutropenia, sweating, chills, fever, coryza, tachycardia, throat, back and general body pain; abdominal cramps, high-frequency deafness, pulmonary oedema, anaphylactoid reaction, peripheral neuropathy, paraesthesias, CNS toxicity: somnolence, unusual tiredness, weakness, depression, headache, ataxia (rare), transient vertigo (rare), pleural effusion, bronchospasm, necrosis, thrombophlebitis (with extravasation), pain at IV site; sepsis (immunosuppression), intermittent muscle cramps, gonadal suppression; nephrotoxicity, hepatotoxicity, and haematotoxicity with overdosage; possibility of carcinogenesis.

NURSING IMPLICATIONS

- Before treatment begins, patient and responsible family members should be informed of the possible adverse effects of etoposide, such as blood dyscrasias, alopecia, carcinogenesis.
- Etoposide concentrate must be diluted before administration with either 5% dextrose injection or 0.9% sodium chloride injection to produce final concentrations of 0.2 to 0.4 mg/ml. Higher concentrations than 0.4 mg/ml tend to crystallize. Diluted solutions with concentration of 0.2 mg/ml are stable for 96 hours, and the 0.4-mg/ml solutions are stable for 48 hours at room temperature, under normal room fluorescent light in glass or plastic (PVC) containers.

E

ETOPOSIDE (continued)

- Wear disposable surgical gloves when preparing or disposing of etoposide. Unused solution and equipment or materials used in its preparation should be properly disposed of to prevent contamination of the work environment. Follow hospital policy. *See Index*: *Antineoplastics*: *handling vesicants*.

- Etoposide is administered by slow IV infusion over 30 to 60 minutes to reduce risk of hypotension and bronchospasm. These symptoms can occur with rapid injection or following slow infusion of higher than recommended dosages.

- Be prepared to treat an anaphylactic reaction (sense of uneasiness, agitation, flushing, palpitation, coughing, difficulty in breathing, primary cardiovascular collapse); can develop in 1 to 2 minutes; can culminate in shock and death.

- Have readily available: pressor agents, e.g., adrenaline corticosteroid, and antihistamine, plasma volume expander oxygen, and equipment for maintaining airway. If the reaction occurs, infusion should be stopped immediately.

- Most patients will manifest some evidence of toxicity, therefore, constant vigilance is essential. Adverse effects are generally reversible with reduction of dosage or discontinuation of drug. Physician may reinstitute therapy following drug withdrawal, but it must be done with extreme caution.

- Check IV site during and after infusion. Extravasation can cause thrombophlebitis and necrosis.

- Monitor vital signs during and after infusion. If hypotension occurs, infusion should be stopped immediately.

- Since transient hypotension after therapy is a possible side effect, caution patient to make position changes slowly, particularly from recumbent to upright position. Be mindful of the possibility that geriatric patients are prone to manifest transient decreases or increases in blood pressure.

- Patients who develop severe toxic reactions to etoposide should be closely monitored for 3 to 4 weeks because the drug is extensively bound to plasma proteins.

- Women of childbearing potential should be advised to avoid pregnancy because of possible harm to foetus. Facilitate discussion with physician regarding appropriate contraceptive measures.

- The following laboratory tests are advised before initiating therapy, at regular intervals during therapy, and before each subsequent treatment course: CBC (including platelet count, Hgb, Hct, WBC and differential); hepatic and renal function tests: SGOT (AST), SGPT (ALT), serum bilirubin, LDH, BUN, serum creatinine.

- Bone marrow depression, notably leucopenia and thrombocytopenia, is used as an index for dosage regulation. White blood cell counts reach their lowest point (nadir) over 7 to 14 days, and platelet nadirs occur over 9 to 16 days after drug administration.

- Be alert to evidence of patient complaints that might suggest development of leucopenia (fever, chills, sore mouth or throat), infection (immunosuppression), and bleeding (thrombocytopenia).

- During period of platelet nadir particularly, protect patient from any trauma that might precipitate bleeding. If possible, invasive procedures such as rectal temperatures, enemas, catheterizations, IMs, and IVs should be withheld until platelet count has recovered sufficiently.

- Inspect patient's mouth (inside cheeks, tongue, gums, throat, lips) daily for ulcerations and bleeding. Stomatitis is especially likely to occur in patients who have had prior radiation therapy of head and neck. Patients with stomatitis should be advised to avoid obvious irritants such as extremely hot foods, spicy and rough foods, smoking, alcohol, strong commercial mouth washes, and irritating toothpastes.

■ GI side effects are generally mild and do not appear to be dose related. Some patients may require an antiemetic.

■ Before administration, inspect solution for particulate matter and discolouration. Solution should be clear and yellow in colour. If crystals are present, discard.

■ Store preferably between 15° and 30°C (59° and 86°F) unless otherwise directed by manufacturer.

Famotidine

(Pepcid PM)   *H_2 antagonist*

ACTIONS AND USES   New H_2 receptor antagonist used to treat benign gastric ulcers, treat and prevent relapse of duodenal ulcers and Zollinger–Ellison syndrome. Report side effects to the Committee on Safety of Medicines.

ROUTE AND DOSAGE   Oral: **Adult**: Treatment of ulcers 40 mg at night. ***Prophylaxis***: 20 mg at night, ***Zollinger–Ellison Syndrome***: *initial* 20 mg/6 hrly maximum 480 mg/day. For further information: *see cimetidine*.

Fenbufen

(Lederfen)   *NSAID; antirheumatic*

ROUTE AND DOSAGE   Oral: **Adult**: 300 mg in the morning, 600 mg at night. *See ibuprofen for nursing implications*.

Fenfluramine hydrochloride

(Ponderax)   *Appetite suppressant*

ACTIONS AND USES   Indirect-acting sympathomimetic amine related to amphetamine. Differs pharmacologically from amphetamine in that it generally produces CNS depression more often than stimulation. Exact mechanism of appetite-inhibiting action not clearly defined, but may be due to stimulation of hypothalamus. Believed to have intrinsic hypoglycaemic activity; appears to increase glucose uptake by skeletal muscles, thus reducing glucose available for conversion to lipid.

Used as short-term (a few weeks) adjunct in treatment of exogenous obesity.

ROUTE AND DOSAGE   Oral: 60 to 120 mg/day.

FENFLURAMINE HYDROCHLORIDE (continued)

ABSORPTION AND FATE   Readily absorbed from GI tract. **Onset of action** 1 to 2 hours; **duration of anorexigenic effect** 4 to 6 hours. Widely distributed to most body tissues. Considerable individual variation in drug metabolism and elimination. Slowly excreted in urine, primarily as metabolites; small quantities excreted as unchanged drug. Rate of urinary excretion is increased in acid urine. Excreted in saliva and sweat in small amounts.

CONTRAINDICATIONS AND PRECAUTIONS   Hypersensitivty to sympathomimetic amines; hyperthyroidism; severe hypertension; glaucoma; symptomatic cardiovascular disease including arrhythmias; history of drug abuse; agitated states; during or within 14 days following administration of MAO inhibitors; concomitant use of CNS depressants or CNS stimulants. Safe use during pregnancy, in women of childbearing age, and in children under 12 years of age not established. **Cautious Use**: mental depression, hypertension, diabetes mellitus.

ADVERSE/SIDE EFFECTS   These include: drowsiness, dizziness, confusion, incoordination, headache, elevated mood, dysphoria, mental depression, anxiety, nervousness, psychotic episodes, tremors, agitation, weakness, fatigue, dysarthria, insomnia, vivid dreams, nightmares, palpitation, tachycardia, chest pain, arrhythmias, hypotension, hypertension, fainting, skin rashes, urticaria, ecchymosis, erythema, burning sensation of skin, hair loss, dry mouth, diarrhoea, nausea, vomiting, unpleasant taste, abdominal pain, constipation, blurred vision, mydriasis, eye irritation, increased or decreased libido, impotence, menstrual irregularities, myalgia, oedema, dysuria, urinary frequency, grinding teeth during sleep (bruxism), sweating, fever, chills, myalgia, oedema, dysuria. **Overdose**: confusion, agitation, hyperventilation, exaggerated or depressed reflexes, convulsions, hyperpyrexia, dilated nonreactive pupils, rotatory nystagmus, coma, cardiac arrest.

NURSING IMPLICATIONS
- Dose increase should be made gradually to minimize possibility of side effects.
- Diarrhoea may occur during first week of therapy; report it to physician; dose reduction or termination of therapy may be required.
- Patients with diabetes maintained on insulin or other antidiabetic drugs should be observed for excessive hypoglycaemic activity when fenfluramine is added to the therapeutic regimen.
- If fenfluramine is prescribed for patients with hypertension, blood pressure should be monitored.
- Mentally depressed patients may become more depressed during therapy and/or following withdrawal of fenfluramine.
- Warn patient that fenfluramine may impair ability to perform hazardous tasks such as driving a motor vehicle.
- If tolerance to anorexigenic effect develops, drug should be discontinued.
- To achieve and maintain loss of weight, patient should be adequately instructed in dietary management.
- Following excessive use, abrupt discontinuation of fenfluramine may be associated with irritability and mental depression.
- Store in well-closed container preferably between 15° and 30°C (59° and 86°F), unless otherwise directed by manufacturer.

FENFLURAMINE HYDROCHLORIDE (continued)

Drug interactions   Use of fenfluramine during or within 14 days following administration of **MAO inhibitors** may result in hypertensive crisis. Fenfluramine reportedly may alter the effects of **hypotensive drugs**, e.g., **guanethidine, methyldopa, reserpine.** Effects of **CNS depressants** or **stimulants** may be additive (caution patient).

Fenoprofen

(Progesic, Fenopron)

Analgesic/antipyretic; NSAID; antirheumatic agent

ACTIONS AND USES   Propionic acid derivative chemically and pharmacologically similar to ibuprofen and naproxen. Claimed to be comparable to aspirin in antiinflammatory activity and to be associated with lower incidence of adverse GI symptoms. Studies suggest that fenoprofen may prolong labour by reducing uterine contractility. Cross-sensitivity to other nonsteroidal antiinflammatory drugs has been reported.

Used for antiinflammatory and analgesic effects in the symptomatic treatment of acute and chronic rheumatoid arthritis and osteoarthritis.

ROUTE AND DOSAGE   Oral: *Analgesic*: 200 mg every 4 to 6 hours, as needed. *Antirheumatic*: 300 to 600 mg four times a day. Not to exceed 3 gm daily.

ABSORPTION AND FATE   Rapidly and almost completely absorbed from upper GI tract. **Peak plasma levels** within 2 hours. **Plasma half-life**: approximately 3 hours; 99% protein bound. Metabolized in liver; appears to undergo enterohepatic recirculation. About 90% of single dose excreted in urine within 24 hours primarily as metabolites and about 3% as unchanged drug. Small amounts excreted in faeces. Does not cross placenta (preliminary studies); excreted in breast milk.

CONTRAINDICATIONS AND PRECAUTIONS   History of hypersensitivity to fenoprofen calcium; history of hypersensitivty or nephrotic syndrome associated with aspirin or other nonsteroidal antiinflammatory agents; significant renal or hepatic dysfunction. Safe use during pregnancy, in nursing mothers, and in children not established. **Cautious Use**: history of upper GI tract disorders, haemophilia or other bleeding tendencies, compromised cardiac function, hypertension impaired hearing.

ADVERSE/SIDE EFFECTS   These include: headache, drowsiness, dizziness, fatigue, lassitude, tremor, confusion, insomnia, nervousness, depression, palpitation, tachycardia, peripheral oedema. Some which may or may not be hypersensitivity reaction: pruritus, rash, purpura, increased sweating, urticaria. **Others**: tinnitus, decreased hearing, deafness, indigestion, nausea, vomiting, anorexia, constipation, diarrhoea, flatulence, abdominal pain, dry mouth; infrequent: gastritis, peptic ulcer, jaundice, cholestatic hepatitis, nephrotoxicity (rare): dysuria, cystitis, haematuria, oliguria, azotaemia, anuria, allergic nephritis, papillary necrosis, blurred vision, dyspnoea, asthenia, fatigue, malaise, anaphylaxis.

F

FENOPROFEN *(continued)*
NURSING IMPLICATIONS

- For rapid absorption, best taken on an empty stomach 30 minutes to 1 hour before or 2 hours after meals. May be administered with meals, milk, or antacid (prescribed), however, if patient experiences GI disturbances. Peak plasma levels may be delayed by food or antacids, but total amount absorbed is not affected.
- Tablet may be crushed and capsule may be emptied and contents swallowed with fluid or mixed with food.
- Important to take a detailed drug history prior to initiation of therapy. *See contraindications and precautions.*
- Therapeutic effectiveness of fenoprofen in patients with arthritis may be evidenced within a few days to peak effect in 2 to 3 weeks (relief of joint pains and stiffness, reduction in joint swelling, increase in grip strength, and improved mobility).

DRUG INTERACTIONS *Fenoprofen*

PLUS	INTERACTIONS
Anticoagulants (coumarins)	Prolongation of prothrombin time
Aspirin (in multiple doses) ⎫ Phenobarbitone ⎬	Decrease effect of fenoprofen by hepatic enzyme induction
Phenytoin and other hydantoin anticonvulsants ⎫ Sulphonamides ⎬ Sulphonylureas (oral hypoglycaemics) ⎭	Action of these drugs may be increased by being displaced from plasma protein sites
See also ibuprofen	

Fenoterol hydrobromide

(Berotec)   *Beta-2-adrenoceptor*

ACTIONS AND USES   Similar in action to salbutamol but of slightly longer action.

ROUTE AND DOSAGE   Aerosol: 180–360 mcg (1–2 puffs) 3–4 times a day. **Nebuliser solution:** 0.5–2.5 mg (maximum 5 mg) up to 4 times a day for acute symptoms.

Fentanyl citrate

(Sublimaze, Thalamonal)   *Narcotic analgesic; opiate agonist*

ACTIONS AND USES   Synthetic phenylpiperidine derivative. Pharmacological actions qualitatively similar to those of morphine but action is more prompt and less prolonged,

FENTANYL CITRATE (continued)

and fentanyl appears to have less emetic activity. On a weight basis, it is estimated to be about 80 times more potent than morphine. Histamine release occurs rarely.

Used for analgesic action of short duration preoperatively, during surgery, and in immediate postoperative period. Also used as a supplement to general or regional anaesthesis, often in combination with a neuroleptic. Commercially available combination of fentanyl with the neuroleptic drug droperidol and is used to produce tranquillization and analgesia for surgical and diagnostic procedures.

ROUTE AND DOSAGE   Highly individualized. **Adults: Intramuscular, intravenous (slow):** 50 to 200 mcg, **Children (2 to 12 years):** 3 to 5 mcg per kg, with spontaneous respiration. **Ventilated**; **Adult:** 300–500 mcg, **Child:** 15 mg/kg.

ABSORPTION AND FATE   Onset of action is almost immediate following IV administration, with peak analgesic effect in 3 to 5 minutes; duration 30 to 60 minutes. Onset of action following IM injection occurs in 7 to 15 minutes; duration 1 to 2 hours. Metabolized primarily in liver. Excreted in urine chiefly as metabolites; about 10% excreted as unchanged drug.

CONTRAINDICATIONS AND PRECAUTIONS   Patients who have received MAO inhibitors within 14 days; myasthenia gravis. Safe use in women of childbearing potential, during pregnancy, and in children younger than 2 years of age not established. **Cautious Use**: head injuries, increased intracranial pressure; elderly; debilitated, poor-risk patients; chronic obstructive pulmonary disease and other respiratory problems; liver and kidney dysfunction; bradyarrhythmias.

ADVERSE/SIDE EFFECTS   Euphoria, miosis, blurred vision, nausea, vomiting, dizziness, diaphoresis, delirium, hypotension; muscle rigidity (especially muscles of respiration) following rapid IV infusion; laryngospasm, bronchoconstriction, respiratory depression, respiratory arrest, bradycardia, circulatory depression, cardiac arrest.

NURSING IMPLICATIONS

- Monitor vital signs and observe patient for signs of skeletal and thoracic muscle (depressed respirations) rigidity and weakness.
- Instructions should be given preoperatively regarding deep breathing, turning, and moving of extremities to reduce possibility of complications.
- Duration of respiratory depressant effect may be considerably longer than analgesic effect. Have immediately available: oxygen, resuscitative equipment, endotracheal tube, suction, narcotic antagonist such as naloxone, and skeletal muscle relaxant, e.g., succinylcholine.
- Physician will rely on accurate reporting of drug effect following initial dose to estimate effects of subsequent doses if needed.
- Narcotics and other CNS depressants have additive or potentiating effects. If prescribed, initial dosage of narcotic analgesic should be reduced to one quarter or one-third of those usually employed.
- Fentanyl can produce dependence of the morphine type and therefore has abuse potential.

F

FENTANYL CITRATE (continued)
- Store at room temperature, preferably between 15° and 30°C (59° and 86°F), unless otherwise directed by manufacturer. Protect drug from light.

Ferrous fumarate

(Fersamal, Fersaday, Galfer, Meterfer)   *Antianaemic agent*

ACTIONS AND USES   Comparable to ferrous sulphate in actions, uses, contraindications, and adverse reactions. Contains 33% elemental iron.

ROUTE AND DOSAGE   Oral: Adult and Child (over 12 yrs): 300 mg twice a day. Child (up to 1 yr): 100–150 mg/day; (1–7 yrs): 200–300 mg/day; (over 7 yrs): 300–400 mg/day.
     For further information: *see ferrous sulphate*.

Ferrous gluconate

(Fergon)   *Antianaemic agent*

ACTIONS AND USES   Claimed to cause less gastric irritation and to be better tolerated than ferrous sulphate. Has same actions, uses, contraindications, and adverse reactions as ferrous sulphate. Contains 11.6% ferrous iron.

ROUTE AND DOSAGE   Oral: Adult: 900–1800 mg/day. Child (up to 1 yr): 225–450 mg/day; (1–7 yrs): 450–700 mg/day; (7–12 yrs): 750–900 mg/day in divided doses.
     For further information: *see ferrous sulphate*

Ferrous succinate

(Ferromyn)   *Antianaemic agent*

ACTIONS AND USES   Comparable to sulphate in actions and uses. Contains 35% ferrous iron.

ROUTE AND DOSAGE   Oral: Adult and child (over 12 yrs): 280–560 mg/day; (up to

FERROUS SUCCINATE (continued)
1 yr): 70–140 mg/day; (1–7 yrs): 140–210 mg/day; (7–12 yrs): 210–280 mg/day in divided doses.

For further information: *see ferrous sulphate.*

Ferrous sulphate————————————————————

(Feaspan, Ferrograd, Ironorm, Slow-Fe)   *Antianaemic agent*

ACTIONS AND USES   Standard iron preparation against which other oral preparations are usually measured. Reportedly the cheapest form of supplemental iron and as effective as other more expensive iron salts. Corrects erythropoietic abnormalities and may reverse gastric, oesophageal, and other tissue changes caused by lack of iron. Ferrous sulphate contains 20% elemental iron; ferrous sulphate exsiccated contains 29.7% iron.

Used to correct simple iron deficiency and to treat iron deficiency (microcytic, hypochromic) anaemias. Also may be used prophylactically during periods of increased iron needs, as in infancy, childhood, and pregnancy.

ROUTE AND DOSAGE   Oral: **Adult**: 300 mg to 1.2 g (the equivalent of 60 to 240 mg elemental iron) daily. Therapeutic dosages depend on severity of iron deficiency. Preferably given in divided doses rather than in *single large daily doses*. **Child**: **up to 1 year**: 36 mg, **1 to 5 years**: 72 mg, **6 to 12 years**: 120 mg daily in divided doses. Available in tablets, timed-release capsules and tablets, syrup liquid, elixir.

ABSORPTION AND FATE   Absorbed into mucosal cells of small intestines (primarily duodenum) where a small fraction is changed to ferric iron, and subsequently incorporated into ferritin; lost into faeces when mucosal cells are shed at end of 5-day life cycle. When iron presented to gut is in excess of need, mucosal cell uptake is minimal ('mucosal block'). Larger fraction enters bloodstream and bound to transferrin. Distributed to functional and storage sites in bone marrow, spleen, liver, haemoglobin, myoglobin, metalloenzymes. Plasma iron concentration and total iron-binding capacity vary with disease states and physiological conditions (higher in men than in women and higher in morning than in evening); regulated principally by haemoglobin synthesis. Major excretion route in faeces via shedding of mucosal cells; also lost in epithelial cells of skin, nails, hair, and in sweat, urine, and breast milk.

CONTRAINDICATIONS AND PRECAUTIONS   Peptic ulcer, regional enteritis, ulcerative colitis, haemolytic anaemias (in absence of iron deficiency), haemochromatosis, haemosiderosis, patients receiving repeated transfusions, pyridoxine responsive anaemia, cirrhosis of liver.

ADVERSE/SIDE EFFECTS   Generally minimal: nausea, heartburn, anorexia, constipation, diarrhoea, epigastric pain, abdominal distress, headache, yellow-brown discolouration of eyes, teeth; iron-overload haemosiderosis (rare). **Large chronic doses in infants**:

FERROUS SULPHATE (continued)

rickets (due to interference with phosphorous absorption). **Massive overdosage**: lethargy, drowsiness, nausea, vomiting, abdominal pain, diarrhoea, local corrosion of stomach and small intestines, pallor or cyanosis acidosis, shock, cardiovascular collapse, convulsions, liver necrosis, coma, death.

NURSING IMPLICATIONS

■ Oral iron preparations are best absorbed when taken on an empty stomach (i.e., between meals). However, to minimize gastric distress it may be necessary to administer the drug with or immediately after meals; or the physician may prescribe smaller doses.

■ If an antacid is prescribed it should be taken at least 1 hour before or 1 hour after the iron preparation.

Food–drug interactions

■ Tannins in tea can block absorption of inorganic (but not organic) iron. However, addition of cream or lemon binds the tannins so they cannot interact.

■ Ascorbic acid increases absorption of iron; consuming citrus fruit or tomato juice with iron preparation (except the elixir) may increase its availability.

■ In patients with uncomplicated iron deficiency, there is little therapeutic indication for concurrent administration of ascorbic acid, since these patients are able to absorb oral iron adequately. However, ascorbic acid may be prescribed in patients who have difficulty in absorbing adequate quantities or iron, such as infants and young children with severe anaemia.

■ Iron absorption may be inhibited if the iron preparation is taken with milk, eggs, or caffeine beverage (e.g., coffee, tea).

■ Since iron is potentially corrosive, tablets or capsules should not be taken within 1 hour of bedtime, and adequate liquid should accompany ingestion of medication to assure passage into stomach. Instruct patient *not* to crush tablet or empty contents of capsule prior to administration.

■ If the patient experiences difficulty in swallowing tablet or capsule, consult physician about prescribing a liquid formulation or a less corrosive form, such as ferrous gluconate. (Sustained contact of iron with oesophageal mucosa can cause ulceration.)

■ Sustained-release preparations are generally not preferred over ferrous sulphate tablets because they tend to transport iron beyond sites of optimal absorption. Also, they are more expensive.

■ In general, liquid preparations should be well diluted and administered through a straw or placed on the back of tongue with a dropper to prevent staining of teeth and to mask taste. Instruct the patient to rinse mouth with clear water immediately after ingestion.

■ Therapeutic dosages are prescribed only if indicated by appropriate diagnostic procedures. If haemoglobin and haematocrit determinations suggest anaemia, a complete blood count, reticulocyte count, and serum bilirubin determination are usually obtained; bone marrow examination may also be performed.

■ In addition to iron replacement, an important therapeutic goal is to determine underlying cause of iron loss and to remedy or alleviate causative factors.

F

FERROUS SULPHATE *(continued)*

- A complete health history should be recorded to determine, among other things, dietary iron intake, adequacy of diet, in general, and possible drug-induced causes of anaemia, such as aspirin in high dosages, sulphonamides, quinidine, antimalarial drugs, and phenylbutazone.
- Inform patient that iron preparations cause dark green or black stools. Advise patient to report constipation or diarrhoea. These symptoms may be relieved by adjustments in dosage or diet or by change to another iron preparation.
- Simple iron deficiency may be asymptomatic, but it is usually associated with ill-defined symptoms such as anorexia, easy fatigability, headache, dizziness, tinnitus, and sensitivity to cold. As iron depletion becomes more severe, signs and symptoms may include dyspnoea on exertion, palpitation, menstrual disturbances, decreased libido, waxy pallor, paraesthesias, epithelial changes including itchy skin, brittle-ness of hair and nails and ridging, flattening, or concavity of nails, and Plummer–Vinson syndrome (severe anaemia): dysphagia, stomatitis, atrophic glossitis.
- Therapeutic response may be experienced within 48 hours as a sense of well-being, increased vigour, improved appetite, and decreased irritability (in children). Reticu-locyte response may begin in 4 days; it usually peaks in 7 to 10 days (reticulocytosis) and returns to normal after 2 or 3 weeks. Haemoglobin generally increases by g/dl and haematocrit by 6% in 3 weeks.
- Haemoglobin and reticulocyte values should be monitored during therapy. In the absence of satisfactory response after 3 weeks of drug treatment, possible reasons for failure warrant investigation: e.g., noncompliance, inadequate dosage, occult blood loss, malabsorption, infection, presence of other anaemias.
- Recommended daily allowance for iron in children 4 to 6 years: 10 mg; for adult males: 10 mg; adult females; 18 mg. In pregnancy requirement cannot be met by ordinary diets, so 30 to 60 mg supplemental iron is recommended during pregnancy and for 2 or 3 months after parturition. Lactation: 18 mg.
- The average diet provides approximately 6 mg of iron per 1,000 calories. Foods high in iron content (> 5 mg/100 g): organ meats (liver, heart, kidney), brewer's yeast, wheat germ, egg yolk, dried beans, dried fruits, oysters. Other good sources (1 to 5 mg/100 g): most muscle meats, fish, fowl, most cereals and green vegetables, dark molasses.
- Facilitate development of a dietary teaching plan for patient and family.
- At present there is no convincing evidence that iron utilization is influenced by concomitant administration of copper, molybdenum, magnesium, calcium, or chlorophyll.
- As a general rule, iron should not be administered for longer than 6 months except in repeated pregnancies, persistent bleeding, or menorrhagia.
- Iron therapy is usually continued for 2 to 3 months after the haemoglobin level has returned to normal (roughly twice the period required to normalize haemoglobin concentration). Replenishment of iron stores is a slow process, because the rate of iron absorption decreases as haemoglobin approaches normal levels.
- Ingested overdoses of iron preparations in children may be fatal. Caution patients to store these drugs out of reach of children (at least one death per month is reported).
- **Treatment of overdosage** Vomiting should be induced quickly, and eggs and milk

F

FERROUS SULPHATE (continued)

should be fed to form iron complexes until gastric lavage can be done (within first hour of ingestion). Lavage solution: 1% sodium bicarbonate or 5% phosphate solution; iron chelating agent (e.g., deferoxamine mesylate) should be administered. Measures to combat shock, dehydration, blood loss, and respiratory failure may be necessary. (Gastric lavage should not be performed after the first hour because of danger of perforation due to gastric necrosis. Dimercaprol should not be used because it may form toxic complexes.)

■ Preserve in well-closed containers. Protect from moisture. Do not use discoloured tablets.

Diagnostic test interferences   Large iron doses may cause false-positive tests for **occult blood** with *o*-toluidine and **guaiac reagent**; **benzidine test** is reportedly not affected.

Drug interactions   Absorption of oral iron is inhibited by **antacids, cholestyramine, cimetidine,** and **pancreatic extracts** (space doses as far apart as possible). There may be delayed or impaired haematological response to iron therapy with **chloramphenicol** or **vitamin E** (in children). Simultaneous administration of oral iron interferes with absorption of **oral tetracycline** and vice versa; if concurrent administration is necessary, patient should receive tetracycline 3 hours after or 2 hours before iron administration. Oral iron decreases action of **doxycycline,** and **penicillamine**; separate doses by at least 2 hours. Concurrent administration of **ascorbic acid** (> 200 mg orally) increases GI absorption of elemental iron. Studies in humans do not support findings from earlier animal studies that **allopurinol** may increase hepatic iron stores.

Flavoxate hydrochloride

(Urispas)

Smooth muscle relaxant;
urinary antispasmodic

ACTIONS AND USES   Exerts spasmolytic (papaverine-like) action on smooth muscle. Reported to produce an increase in urinary bladder capacity in patients with spastic bladder, possibly by direct action on detrusor muscle.

Used for symptomatic relief of dysuria, frequency, urgency, nocturia, incontinence, and suprapubic pain associated with various urological disorders.

ROUTE AND DOSAGE   Oral: 200 mg three times a day.

ABSORPTION AND FATE   Following oral administration of a single 100-mg dose, 10 to 30% is excreted in urine within 6 hours.

CONTRAINDICATIONS AND PRECAUTIONS   Pyloric or duodenal obstruction, obstructive intestinal lesions, ileus, achalasia, GI haemorrhage, obstructive uropathies of lower

FLAVOXATE HYDROCHLORIDE (continued)

urinary tract, use in children younger than 12 years of age, use during pregnancy and in women of childbearing potential. **Cautious Use**: suspected glaucoma.

ADVERSE/SIDE EFFECTS   These include: headache, vertigo, drowsiness, mental confusion (especially in the elderly), difficulty with concentration, nervousness, palpitation, tachycardia, blurred vision, increased intraocular tension, disturbances of eye accommodation, dry mouth and throat, nausea, vomiting, abdominal pain, constipation (with high doses), dermatoses, urticaria, dysuria, hyperpyrexia, eosinophilia, leucopenia.

NURSING IMPLICATIONS

- Because of the possibility of drowsiness, mental confusion, and blurred vision, advise patients to avoid driving or performing tasks that require mental alertness and physical coordination until reaction to drug is known.
- Advise patient to report to physician adverse reactions and the lack of a favourable response.

Flecainide acetate

(Tambocor)

Antiarrhythmic;
anaesthetic (local)

ACTIONS AND USES   Local (membrane) anaesthetic and antiarrhythmic. Slows conduction velocity throughout myocardial conduction system, increases ventricular refractoriness but has little effect on repolarization. Prolongs His-ventricular and QRS intervals at therapeutic doses. Clinically, flecainide causes both hypotension and negative inotropy (in higher dose ranges) and is an effective suppressant of PVCs and a variety of atrial and ventricular arrhythmias. Generally does not alter cardiac function, but with IV administration, pulmonary capillary wedge pressure may be increased in patient with coronary disease.

Used in treatment of PVCs; atrial tachycardia and other arrhythmias unresponsive to standard agents (e.g., quinidine), Wolff–Parkinson–White syndrome, and recurrent ventricular tachycardias.

ROUTE AND DOSAGE   Oral: 100 to 200 mg every 12 hours. **Intravenous**: *Initial*: 2 mg/kg in 10–30 min to a maximum of 150 mg, then infusion of 1.5 mg/kg for 1 hr, then 250 mcg/kg/hr. Transfer to oral therapy by giving 100 mg orally and withdrawing the infusion over 4 hrs by gradual reductions.

ABSORPTION AND FATE   Absorbed promptly and almost completely with 95% bioavailability. Peak plasma concentration after oral dose reached in 1½ to 3 hours. Minimal first-pass effect. **Half-life**: 7 to 22 hours, increased in patients with congestive heart failure or renal failure. 40% protein bound. Approximately 30% drug excreted in urine unchanged.

F

FLECAINIDE ACETATE (continued)

CONTRAINDICATIONS AND PRECAUTIONS   Compromised ventricular function congestive heart failure. *See also tocainide.*

ADVERSE/SIDE EFFECTS   **After IV**: chest discomfort and tinnitus. *Also*: ataxia, leg cramps; blurred red vision, transient conjunctival infection; nasal congestion; dizziness, sense of warmth, headache; nausea, oral paraesthesia, dry mouth.

NURSING IMPLICATIONS
- Effective serum concentration: 0.4 to 1.0 mcg/ml.
- Food does not affect bioavailability.
- Monitor closely for cardiac side effects during intravenous therapy.
- *See tocainide for additional nursing implications.*

DRUG INTERACTIONS   *Flecainide*

PLUS	INTERACTIONS
Digoxin Propranolol	Increased serum levels of both drugs leading to increased toxicity potential, or more intensive drug effects

Flucloxacillin

(Floxapen, Ladropen, Stafoxil, Staphcil)   *Antiinfective; antimicrobial; penicillin*

ACTIONS AND USES   Used to treat infections due to penicillinase-producing staphlococci. May be combined with ampicillin to increase spectrum of activity (Magnapen, Flu-amp).

ROUTE AND DOSAGE   **Oral/IM: Adult:** 250 mg/6 hrly; **IV injection or slow infusion:** 0.25–1 g every 6 hrs. **Child (all routes) (2–10 yrs):** 50% adult dose, **(under 2 yrs):** 25% adult dose. Give oral doses at least 30 min before food.
   For further information: *see penicillin G.*

Fluclorolone

(Topilar)   *Corticosteroid*

ACTIONS AND USES   Topical treatment of severe skin conditions unresponsive to other steroids.
   For further information: *see hydrocortisone.*

Fludrocortisone acetate

(Florinef)   *Corticosteroid*

ACTIONS AND USES Long-acting synthetic steroid with potent mineralocorticoid and moderate glucocorticoid activity. Small doses produce marked sodium retention, increased urinary potassium excretion, and elevated blood pressure. If protein intake is inadequate, fludrocortisone induces negative nitrogen balance. Contraindications and adverse/side effects are same as for hydrocortisone (q.v.).

Used as partial replacement therapy for adrenocortical insufficiency and for treatment of salt-losing forms of congenital adrenogenital syndrome.

ROUTE AND DOSAGE Oral: 50–300 mcg/day. **Child**: 5 mcg/kg/day.

ABSORPTION AND FATE Has short duration of action. **Half-life**: 30 minutes.

NURSING IMPLICATIONS

- Concomitant oral cortisone or hydrocortisone therapy may be advisable to provide substitute therapy approximating normal adrenal activity.
- Periodic checking of serum electrolyte levels is usual during prolonged therapy. Supplemental calcium and potassium chloride, as well as restricted salt intake, may be necessary during long-term therapy.
- Monitor weight and fluid intake–output ratio to observe onset of fluid accumulation, especially if patient is on unrestricted salt intake and without potassium supplement.
- Instruct patient to report signs of potassium deficit (anorexia, paraesthesias, drowsiness, muscle weakness, nausea, polyuria, postural hypotension, mental depression).
- Patient may be advised to eat foods with high potassium content *(see Index: Food sources)*. Consult with physician and dietician. A potassium supplement may be necessary.
- Monitor and record blood pressure daily. If transient hypertension develops as a consequence of therapy, report to physician. Usually the dose will be reduced to 0.05 mg daily.
- Store in airtight containers at temperature 15° to 30°C (59° to 86°F). Protect from light.
- *See hydrocortisone for additional nursing implications and drug interactions.*

Flunisolide

(Syntaris)   *Corticosteroid; glucocorticoid*

ACTIONS AND USES Modified steroid preparation with topical antiinflammatory and vasoconstrictor activity, structurally related to hydrocortisone. Exact mechanism of action not known. Glucocorticoid activity is more potent than mineralocorticoid action. Does not suppress hypothalamus–pituitary–adrenal function except in excessive doses.

FLUNISOLIDE (continued)

Used for symptomatic relief of seasonal and perennial rhinitis in patients who have developed tolerance or poor response to conventional therapy. Also has been used for treatment of serous otitis media in children.

ROUTE AND DOSAGE   Topical (intranasal): **Adults**: Initial: 2 sprays in each nostril 2–3 times a day. **Children (6 to 14 years)**: *Initial*: 1 spray in each nostril three times daily.

For further information: *see Beclomethasone dipropionate.*

ABSORPTION AND FATE   Rapidly absorbed following nasal inhalation; about 50% reaches systemic circulation. Approximately 50% bound to plasma proteins. **Biphasic half-life**: initial: about 6 minutes; terminal: 1.8 hours. Rapidly metabolized in liver to active metabolites, 50% of which are excreted in urine and 50% in faeces. Distribution to placenta and breast milk not known.

CONTRAINDICATIONS AND PRECAUTIONS   Hypersensitivity to any ingredients in the formulation: patients receiving systemic corticosteroids; use in children under 6 years. Safe use during pregnancy and in nursing women not established. **Cautious Use**: recent nasal ulcers, nasal surgery or trauma, active or latent tuberculosis (respiratory tract); untreated fungal, bacterial, or systemic viral infection; ocular herpes.

ADVERSE/SIDE EFFECTS   These include: headache, dizziness, mild transient sensation of nasal burning or stinging (common), nasal congestion, sneezing, epistaxis or bloody nasal discharge, nasal irritation or dryness, sore throat, hoarseness, bitter taste, loss of taste or smell, nausea, vomiting, abdominal bloating, watery eyes; nasal septal perforation (rare; causal relationships not established), localized candidal infections.

F

Flunitrazepam ━━━━━━━━━━━━━━

(Rohypnol)   *Benzodiazepine; hypnotic*

ACTIONS AND USES   Benzodiazepine used as a hypnotic where daytime sedation is acceptable. Doses tend to be culminative.

ROUTE AND DOSAGE   Oral: **Adult**: 0.5–1 mg 30 minutes before retiring. **Elderly patients**: 500 mcg.

For further information: *see chlordiazepoxide.*

Fluocinolone acetonide ━━━━━━━━━━

(Synalar, Synandone)   *Corticosteroid*

FLUOCINOLONE ACETONIDE (continued)

ACTIONS AND USES Synthetic fluorinated steroid with strong antiinflammatory, antipruritic, and vasoconstrictive actions, but negligible mineralocorticoid effects. More effective than hydrocortisone (q.v.).

Used to relieve inflammatory manifestations of corticosteroid-responsive dermatoses.

ROUTE AND DOSAGE Topical: applied in thin layer over affected area two to four times daily. Supplied as cream, ointment, and gel.

CONTRAINDICATIONS AND PRECAUTIONS Infants under 2 years of age; ophthalmic use. *See also hydrocortisone.*

ADVERSE/SIDE EFFECTS *See hydrocortisone.*

NURSING IMPLICATIONS
- Protect drug from light.
- *See hydrocortisone for nursing implications related to topical application.*

Fluocinonide

(Metosyn)   Corticosteroid

ACTIONS AND USES Synthetic fluorinated glucocorticoid used only topically for antiinflammatory effects in glucocorticoid-responsive dermatoses. *See hydrocortisone for absorption, fate, limitations, interactions.*

ROUTE AND DOSAGE Topical: apply thin layer of ointment, cream, or scalp lotion (0.05%) to affected area three or four times daily, or as needed.

ADVERSE/SIDE EFFECTS Burning, itching, hypertrichosis, dermatitis. *See also hydrocortisone.*

NURSING IMPLICATIONS
- See hydrocortisone for nursing implications of topical application.
- Similar drug fluocortolone (Ultradil).

Fluorometholone

(FML)   Corticosteroid; glucocorticoid

ACTIONS AND USES Adrenal cortical steroid with actions, contraindications, and adverse/side effects similar to those of hydrocortisone (q.v.).

Used topically in management of glucocorticoid-responsive ocular inflammations.

FLUOROMETHOLONE (continued)

ROUTE AND DOSAGE   Ophthalmic: 1 to 2 drops 0.1% ophthalmic suspension three to four times daily.

ADVERSE/SIDE EFFECTS   Ophthalmic: increased intraocular pressure, especially in the elderly patient, corneal pathology; with excessive use: diminished visual field, optic nerve damage, cataracts, glaucoma exacerbation.

NURSING IMPLICATIONS

- Eye drops are not to be used for extended period of time.
- Depress lacrimal duct after instilling eye drops. *See Index: Drug administration: eye drops*.
- Caution patient to follow established dose regimen.
- If visual acuity decreases or visual field diminishes, the patient should stop the drug and notify the physician.
- *See also hydrocortisone*

Fluorouracil ———————————————————————

(Efudix, Fluorouracil)   *Antineoplastic; antimetabolite*

ACTIONS AND USES   Pyrimidine antagonist and cell cycle nonspecific. Blocks action of enzymes essential to normal DNA and RNA synthesis, and may become incorporated in RNA to form a fraudulent molecule; unbalanced growth and death of cell follow. Has higher affinity for tumour tissue than normal tissue. Highly toxic, especially to proliferative cells in neoplasms, bone marrow, and intestinal mucosa. Low therapeutic index with high potential for severe haematological toxicity. Both local and systemic administration cause increases in skin pigmentation. Is not intended as adjuvant to surgery, or for prophylaxis.

Used as single agent and in combination with other antineoplastics for palliative treatment of carefully selected patients with inoperable neoplasms of breast, colon or rectum, stomach, pancreas, urinary bladder, ovary, cervix, liver. Also used topically for solar or actinic keratoses and superficial basal cell carcinoma.

ROUTE AND DOSAGE   Highly individualized. **Intravenous**: up to 1 g/day for 5 days. **Intraarterial**: 5 – 7.5 mg/kg/day. **Oral**: 500 – 1,000 mg/m day for five days. *Superficial basal cell carcinoma*: apply two times daily for 3 to 6 weeks.

ABSORPTION AND FATE   Minimal absorption from topically applied preparation if skin is intact. Following rapid infusion, drug leaves plasma within 3 hours. Metabolized in liver; **half-life** (alpha phase): 10 to 20 minutes; (beta phase): up to 20 hours. 15% of unchanged drug is excreted in urine in 6 hours; 60 to 80% as respiratory carbon dioxide in 8 to 12 hours. Crosses blood–brain barrier. Distribution to placenta and into breast milk not known.

FLUOROURACIL (continued)

CONTRAINDICATIONS AND PRECAUTIONS   Poor nutritional status, pregnancy, myelosuppression. **Cautious Use**: major surgery during previous month, history of high-dose pelvic irradiation, metastatic cell infiltration of bone marrow, previous use of alkylating agents, men and women in childbearing ages, hepatic and renal impairment.

ADVERSE/SIDE EFFECTS   These include: anorexia, nausea, vomiting, stomatitis, oesophagopharyngitis, medicinal taste, diarrhoea, proctitis, paralytic ileus, GI haemorrhage, leucopenia, thrombocytopenia, anaemia (common), eosinophilia. **Topical use**: local pain, pruritus, hyperpigmentation, burning at site of application, dermatitis, suppuration, swelling, scarring, toxic granulation. **Other**: (may be evidenced with parenteral and topical preparations): alopecia, nail changes or loss (rare); pruritic maculopapular rash (extremities and occasionally trunk); cardiotoxicity, mild angina to crushing central chest pain with ECG changes; photosensitivity, erythema, increased pigmentation, skin dryness and fissuring, epistaxis, photophobia, lacrimation, euphoria, insomnia, acute cerebellar syndrome (dysmetria, nystagmus, ataxia), severe mental deterioration.

NURSING IMPLICATIONS

- Fluorouracil is to be administered only by or under the direct supervision of a physician experienced in cancer chemotherapy.
- Hospitalization and strict supervision during the first course of therapy with fluorouracil is necessary.
- Avoid skin exposure and inhalation of drug particles.
- Dose is determined by actual weight unless patient is obese, in which case ideal weight is used. Weigh patient under standard conditions and record weight every 3 or 4 days. Report unexplained gradual increase in weight.
- Total and differential leucocyte counts should be determined before each dose is administered. Drug should be discontinued if leucopenia occurs (WBC below 3,500/mm^3) or if patient develops thrombocytopenia (platelet count below 100,000 mm^3). Baseline and periodic checks of haematocrit and liver and kidney function test are also advised.
- A dose sufficient to create mild toxicity (anorexia, vomiting) may be necessary to produce antineoplastic effects.
- Establish a reference data base for body weight, fluid intake–output ratio and pattern, food preferences and dietary habits, bowel habits, and condition of mouth.
- This drug may be given without dilution by direct IV injection or by IV infusion with dextrose 5% in water and sodium chloride 0.9% as infusion vehicles. Rapid injections are more effective, but administration over a 2- to 8-hour period appears to reduce onset of toxicity.
- Inspect injection site frequently; avoid extravasation. If it occurs, stop infusion and restart in another vein. Ice compresses may reduce danger of local tissue damage from infiltrated solution.
- Commonly, leucopenic nadir is between 9 and 14 days after initial dose, but may be delayed as long as 20 days. Usually count is in normal range by 30th day. Monitor blood counts as indicators for design of patient care.
- During leucopenic period (WBC below 3,500/mm^3) patient should be in protective

FLUOROURACIL (continued)

isolation. Restrict visitors and personnel with colds or infections. Plan care so that patient's energy expenditure is at minimum.

- Protect patient from trauma, unnecessary injections, and use of rectal thermometer or invasive tubing.

- During thrombocytopenic period (7th to 17th day), watch for and report signs of abnormal bleeding from any source; inspect skin for ecchymotic and petechial areas.

- Antiemetics may be ordered to alleviate nausea and vomiting. Monitor patient carefully if vomiting is intractable, and report to physician.

- Indications for drug discontinuation: severe stomatitis, leucopenia (WBC below 3,500/mm³ or rapidly decreasing count), intractable vomiting, diarrhoea, thrombocytopenia (below 100,000/mm³), haemorrhage from any site.

- Inform the patient of the importance of prompt reporting of the first signs of toxicity: anorexia, vomiting, nausea, stomatitis, diarrhoea, GI bleeding.

- Poor-risk patients and occasionally patients in fairly good condition may die from the severe toxicity characteristic of this drug.

- Remissions are often short, lasting no longer than 5 to 6 months; some patients have received 9 to 45 courses of treatment over periods of time ranging from 12 to 60 months.

- The maculopapular rash usually responds to symptomatic treatment and is reversible.

- A skin lesion treated with topical fluorouracil heals without scarring in 1 to 2 months after cessation of therapy. Expected response of lesion to topical fluorouracil: erythema followed in sequence by vesiculation, erosion, ulceration, necrosis, epithelialization. Applications of drug are continued until ulcerative stage is reached (2 to 6 weeks after initial application) and then discontinued.

- Use nonmetallic applicator or gloved fingers to apply medication. If unprotected fingers are used, wash hands thoroughly.

- Even if absorption is minimal, systemic toxicity may follow use on large ulcerated area. Report symptoms promptly.

- If occlusive dressing is used there may be inflammatory reaction on adjacent normal tissue; however, use of a porous gauze dressing for cosmetic purposes does not cause inflammatory changes.

- Avoid application of cream or solution near eyes, nose, and mouth.

- If skin area treated with topical medication fails to respond to treatment, a biopsy is usually done to rule out frank neoplastic disease.

- Report disorientation or confusion observed in a patient on fluorouracil. The drug should be withdrawn immediately. Symptoms may occur earlier in each subsequent course of treatment and increase in severity.

- Help the patient to design drug regimen to fit life style, and other concurrent drug regimens. Involvement with reasonable planning supports compliance.

- Caution patient not to change dosage regimen, i.e., not to increase, decrease, or omit doses or change dosage intervals.

- Inspect pressure areas daily (coccyx region, elbows, heels). Danger of skin breakdown is greatly increased in a patient with immunosuppression, myelosuppression, and inanition.

- Caution patient to avoid exposure to sunlight or to ultraviolet lamp treatments. Protect exposed skin; if it is necessary to go outdoors, apply sun-screen lotion (SPF 12

F

FLUOROURACIL (continued)

or above) Avoid midday exposure. Photosensitivity usually subsides 2 to 3 months after last dose of the antineoplastic.

■ Photophobia and lacrimation are frequent side effects. If bothersome, report to physician. Dark glasses may be helpful.

■ If patient manifests difficulty in balance while ambulating, give assistance, and report symptom to physician promptly.

■ Facilitate discussion with patient about problem of gonadal suppression (which may be irreversible), and potential change in sexuality.

■ Contraception is advisable during fluorouracil treatment. Advise patient to report to physician if she suspects pregnancy.

■ Prepare patient for alopecia, an expected transient toxic effect. Discuss plans for cosmetic substitution if patient desires; new hair growth usually begins within 6 to 8 weeks. *See Index: Nursing Interventions: alopecia.*

■ Maintenance of adequate nutrition is imperative. Work with dietitian and family to provide adaptations in dietary habits and patterns called for by the mild but troublesome symptoms that must be tolerated (e.g., anorexia, nausea, sore mouth).

■ Stomatitis, a reliable early sign of toxicity, often precedes the leucopenic period by days. Inspect patient's mouth daily. Promptly report cracked lips, xerostomia, white patches, and erythema of buccal membranes.

■ To help patient eat with comfort, ask physician for anaesthetic solution to be swished in mouth before eating. *See mustine for nursing care of stomatitis, xerostomia.*

■ Fluorouracil solution is normally colourless to faint yellow. Slight discolouration during storage does not appear to affect potency or safety. Discard dark yellow solution. If a precipitate forms, redissolve drug by heating to 60°C (140°F) and shake vigorously. Allow to cool to body temperature before administration.

■ Store drugs at temperature between 15° and 30°C (59° and 86°F) unless otherwise directed by manufacturer. Protect from light and freezing.

Diagnostic test interferences   Fluorouracil may increase excretion of 5-hydroxyindoleacetic acid (5-HIAA) and decrease **plasma albumin** (because of drug-induced protein malabsorption).

DRUG INTERACTIONS *Fluorouracil*

PLUS	INTERACTIONS
Myelosuppressive agents, other } Radiation therapy	May enhance total effects necessitating dose adjustments

Fluphenazine

(Modecate, Moditen)   *Psychotropic; phenothiazine*

ACTIONS AND USES   Potent piperazine derivative of phenothiazine. Similar to other phenothiazines, with the following exceptions: more potent on weight basis, higher

FLUPHENAZINE (continued)

incidence of extrapyramidal complications, and lower frequency of sedative and hypotensive effects. Has weak antiemetic and anticholinergic actions. The hydrochloride has more rapid action and shorter duration of action and thus may be used initially to determine the patient's response or to establish appropriate dosage. The decanoate and enanthate forms are indicated primarily for maintenance therapy in patients who cannot be relied on to take daily oral formulations. *See chlorpromazine.*

Used for management of manifestations of psychotic disorders.

ROUTE AND DOSAGE   Adult: Oral: *Severe anxiety*; *initial* lmg twice a day increased as required to 4 mg/day. *Psychoses*: *initial* 2.5 – 10 mg/day in divided doses increased as required to 20 mg/day.

ABSORPTION AND FATE   Onset of action following subcutaneous or IM injection of fluphenazine decanoate or enanthate occurs in 24 to 72 hours; peak antipsychotic effect in 48 to 96 hours; duration of effect 4 weeks or longer for decanoate, 1 to 3 weeks for enanthate. Following oral or IM administration of the hydrochloride, onset of action occurs within 1 hour; duration of action is 6 to 8 hours. Metabolized in liver; crosses placenta; appears in breast milk.

CONTRAINDICATIONS AND PRECAUTIONS   Known hypersensitivity to fluphenazine; subcortical brain damage, comatose or severely depressed states, blood dyscrasias, or hepatic disease. Safe use in women of childbearing potential and during pregnancy or lactation not established. Parenteral form not recommended for children under 12 years of age. **Cautious Use**: hypersensitivity to other phenothiazines; use of anticholinergic agents, other CNS depressants; elderly patients, previously diagnosed breast cancer, cardiovascular diseases, phaeochromocytoma, history of convulsive disorders, patients exposed to extreme heat or phosphorous insecticides, peptic ulcer, respiratory impairment. *See also chlorpromazine.*

ADVERSE/SIDE EFFECTS   These include: tachycardia, hypotension, xerostomia, nausea, epigastric pain, constipation, faecal impaction, cholecystatic jaundice, urinary retention, polyuria, inhibition of ejaculation, transient leucopenia, agranulocytosis, drowsiness, dizziness, headache, mental depression, catatonic-like state, extrapyramidal symptoms, impaired thermoregulation, grand mal seizures, SLE-like syndrome, contact dermatitis, peripheral oedema, nasal congestion, blurred vision, increased intraocular pressure, photosensitivity, 'silent pneumonia,' hyperprolactinaemia. *See also chlorpromazine.*

NURSING IMPLICATIONS

- Persons preparing oral concentrate or liquid preparations for injection should be careful not to contact skin or clothing with drug. Warn patient to avoid spilling drug. If skin is contacted it should be rinsed promptly with warm water.
- Antacids diminish absorption, therefore, administer oral preparations at least 1 hour before or 1 hour after the antacid.
- Advise patient not to alter dosage regimen or stop it abruptly. Caution not to give the drug to any other person.

FLUPHENAZINE (continued)

- Dry syringe and needle (at least 21 gauge) should be used when administering fluphenazine enanthate (in a sesame oil vehicle). Moisture may cause solution to become cloudy.
- Mental depression and extrapyramidal symptoms *(see chlorpromazine)* occur with high frequency, particularly with long-acting forms (decanoate and enanthate). Be alert for appearance of acute dystonic reactions: abnormal posturing, torticollis, grimacing, fine tremor, oculogyric crisis.
- The physician should give approval before patient self-doses with OTC drugs. Fluphenazine enanthate formulation has a long duration of action, early detection of adverse effects is critically important. Patient should inform the physician promptly if the following symptoms appear: light-coloured stools, changes in vision, sore throat, fever, cellulitis, rash, any interference with volitional movement.
- Control environment temperature; patient may be unable to adjust to extremes. If patient complains of being cold even at average room temperature, heed complaints and furnish additional clothing or blankets if necessary. Do not apply heating pad or hot water bottles. A severe burn may result because of depressed conditioned avoidance behaviours.
- Extended exposure to high environmental temperature, to sun's rays, or to a high fever associated with serious illness places this patient at risk from heat stroke. Be alert to signs: red, dry, hot skin; full, bounding pulse, dilated pupils, dyspnoea, mental confusion, elevated blood pressure, temperature over 40.6°C (105°F). Inform physician and institute measures to reduce body temperature rapidly.
- Warn patient to avoid exposure to sun especially during hours of 10.00 hrs to 14.00 hrs also, to wear protective clothing and cover exposed skin surfaces with sun screen lotion (SPF above 12). Photosensitivity is a fairly common side effect for the person on long-term therapy.
- Renal function should be monitored in patients on long-term treatment. Blood studies, hepatic function tests, and ophthalmological examinations should also be performed periodically.
- Monitor blood pressure during early therapy. Hypotension is rarely a problem, however, fluctuations in BP have occurred in some patients. If systolic drop is more than 20 mm Hg, inform physician.
- It has been reported that although the patient is not responsive during acute catatonia (side effect) everything that happens during the episode can be recalled.
- Monitor fluid intake–output ratio and bowel elimination pattern. Check for abdominal distention and pain. Encourage adequate food and fluid intake as prophylaxis for constipation and for xerostomia. The depressed patient may not seek help for either for these conditions, or for urinary retention.
- Patients on large doses who undergo surgery, and those with cerebrovascular, cardiac, or renal insufficiency are especially prone to hypotensive effects.
- Caution patient against driving motor vehicle or other hazardous activities until reaction to the drug is known.
- Alcohol should be avoided while patient is on fluphenazine therapy.
- Inform patient that fluphenazine may discolour urine pink to red or reddish brown.

F

FLUPHENAZINE (continued)

■ All preparations of fluphenazine should be protected from light and from freezing. Solutions may safely vary in colour from almost colourless to light amber. Discard dark or otherwise discoloured solutions.

■ Store in tightly closed container at temperature between 15° and 30°C (59° and 86°F) unless otherwise specified by manufacturer.

■ *See chlorpromazine.*

■ Similar drug *flupenthixol.*

Flurandrenolone

(Haelan)   *Corticosteroid*

ACTIONS AND USES   Topical fluorinated steroid with substituted 17-hydroxyl group. Crosses skin cell membranes, complexes with nuclear DNA, and stimulates synthesis of enzymes thought to be responsible for antiinflammatory effects. Also has antipruritic and vasoconstrictive properties. Systemic absorption leads to actions, limitations, and drug interactions of hydrocortisone, prototype for corticosteroids (q.v.).

Used for relief of pruritis and inflammatory manifestations of corticosteroid-responsive dermatoses.

ROUTE AND DOSAGE   Topical cream/ointment: **Adult:** Apply sparingly 3 times a day.

ABSORPTION AND FATE   Resistant to metabolism by skin. Repeated applications lead to depot effects on skin, resulting in increased potential for systemic absorption and more severe side effects.

For further information: *see hydrocortisone.*

Flurazepam hydrochloride

(Dalmane, Paxane)   *Psychotropic; antianxiety*
hypnotic; benzodiazepine

ACTIONS AND USES   Benzodiazepine derivative, with hypnotic activity equal to or greater than that produced by barbiturates or chloral hydrate. Mode and site of action not known but appears to act at limbic and subcortical levels of CNS to produce sedation, skeletal muscle relaxation, and anticonvulsant effects. Reduces sleep induction

FLURAZEPAM HYDROCHLORIDE (continued)

time; produces slight if any suppression of REM time (dream sleep) but marked reduction of deepest sleep stage while at the same time increasing duration of total sleep time. Significance of sleep alterations not understood.

Used as hypnotic in management of all kinds of insomnia; e.g., difficulty in falling asleep, frequent nocturnal awakening, and/or early morning awakening. Used also for treatment of poor sleeping habits.

ROUTE AND DOSAGE   Oral: **Adult**: 15 to 30 mg before retiring. **Elderly; debilitated patients**: 15 mg initially; increased as necessary and tolerated.

ABSORPTION AND FATE   Rapidly absorbed from GI tract. Induces sleep within 20 to 30 minutes that lasts 7 to 8 hours. Widely distributed throughout body tissues. Elimination half-life of major metabolite 47 to 100 hours. Rapidly metabolized by liver. Excreted primarily in urine as active and inactive metabolites. Crosses placenta; appears in breast milk.

CONTRAINDICATIONS AND PRECAUTIONS   Known hypersensitivity to flurazepam; prolonged administration; intermittent porphyria, acute narrow-angle glaucoma, children under 15 years of age; pregnancy, lactation. **Cautious Use**: impaired renal or hepatic function, mental depression, psychoses, history of suicidal tendencies, addiction-prone individuals, elderly or debilitated patients, chronic obstructive pulmonary disease.

For further information: *see also chlordiazepoxide*.

NURSING IMPLICATIONS

- Hypnotic effect is apparent on second or third night of consecutive use and continues 1 or 2 nights after drug is stopped.
- Excessive drowsiness, ataxia, vertigo, and falling occur more frequently in elderly or debilitated patients. Supervise ambulation. Bed rails may be advisable.
- Store in light-resistant container with child-proof cap at temperature between 15° and 30°C (59° and 86°F) unless otherwise specified by manufacturer.

For further information: *see chlordiazepoxide*.

F

Flurbiprofen _____

(Froben)   *NSAID*

ACTIONS AND USES   Used to treat rheumatic diseases and musculo skeletal disorders.

ROUTE AND DOSAGE   **Oral or rectal**: **Adult**: 150–200 mg/day in divided doses increased in acute cases to 300 mg/day.

For further information: *see ibuprofen*.

Fluspirilene

(Redeptin)   *Neuroleptic*

ACTIONS AND USES   Maintenance in schizophrenia.

ROUTE AND DOSAGE   Depot injection: **Adult**: 2 mg/week.
For further information: *see chlorpromazine.*

Folic acid

(Lexpec)   *Vitamin*

ACTIONS AND USES   Member of vitamin B complex group essential for nucleoprotein synthesis and maintenance of normal erythropoiesis. Stimulates production of red blood cells, white blood cells, and platelets in patients with megaloblastic anaemias. In folic acid deficiency, impaired thymidylate synthesis results in the production of defective DNA that leads to megaloblast formation and arrest of bone marrow maturation.

Used in treatment of folate deficiency, macrocytic anaemia, and megaloblastic anaemias associated with malabsorption syndromes, alcoholism, primary liver disease, inadequate dietary intake, certain drugs, pregnancy, infancy, and childhood.

ROUTE AND DOSAGE   Oral: 15 mg/day for 14 days or until a response is obtained. **Child**: *initial*, **(under one year)**: 500 mcg/kg, **(1–5 yrs)**: 5 mg, **(6–12 yrs)**: 10 mg daily; then half that dose as *maintenance.*

ABSORPTION AND FATE   Readily absorbed from small intestine (primarily proximal portion). Peak folate activity in 30 to 60 minutes, following oral administration. Largely reduced and methylated in liver to metabolically active folate forms. Distributed to all body tissues, with high concentration in cerebrospinal fluid. Enters enterohepatic cycle. Extensively bound to plasma proteins in patients with folic acid deficiency. Traces of unchanged drug excreted in urine with usual therapeutic doses, but large amounts eliminated following high doses. Excreted in breast milk.

CONTRAINDICATIONS AND PRECAUTIONS   Use of folic acid alone for treatment of pernicious anaemia or other vitamin B_{12} deficiency states; use in normocytic, refractory, aplastic, or undiagnosed anaemia.

ADVERSE/SIDE EFFECTS   Reportedly nontoxic. Rarely: allergic sensitization (rash, pruritus, general malaise, bronchospasm). Slight flushing and feeling of warmth following IV administration.

NURSING IMPLICATIONS
■ A careful history of dietary intake and drug and alcohol usage should be obtained prior to start of therapy. Drugs reported to cause folate deficiency include oral

FOLIC ACID (continued)

contraceptives, alcohol, barbiturates, methotrexate, phenytoin, primidone, and tri-methoprim. Folate deficiency may also result from renal dialysis.

- Folic acid can obscure diagnosis of pernicious anaemia by alleviating haematological manifestations of vitamin B_{12} deficiency while allowing irreparable neurological damage to remain progressive.
- Treatment of anaemia with OTC vitamin preparations containing folic acid subject the patient with iron-deficiency anaemia to needless expense and may delay detection of pernicious anaemia.
- *Normal serum folate levels* have been reported to range from 6 to 15 mcg/ml.
- Folates are present in a wide variety of foods; high sources include yeast, whole grain, bran, fresh leafy vegetables, asparagus, dried beans and lentils, nuts, and fruits. Approximately 50 to 90% of folate content is destroyed by long cooking or by canning.
- The recommended daily allowances of folic acid are as follows: infants: 30 mcg; children: 100 to 300 mcg; adults: 400 mcg; during pregnancy 800 mcg; during lactation 500 mcg.
- Therapeutic effects of folic acid therapy include a sense of well-being during first 24 hours of treatment, improvement in blood picture (reticulocytosis within 2 to 5 days, reversion to normoblastic haematopoiesis and eventually normal haemoglobin), gradual reversal of symptoms of folic acid deficiency (glossitis, diarrhoea, constipation, weight loss, irritability, fatigue, restless legs, diffuse muscular pain, insomnia, forgetfulness, mental depression, pallor). Keep physician informed of patient's response.
- Emphasize the need to remain under close medical supervision while receiving folic acid therapy. Adjustment of maintenance dose should be made if there is threat of relapse.
- Folic acid injection should be protected from light.

Diagnostic test interferences   Falsely low serum erythrocyte **folate levels may occur** with **L. cassei** assay method in patients receiving antibiotics such as tetracyclines.

Drug interactions   Chloramphenicol may antagonize haematological response to folate therapy. Daily administration of 5 mg or more of folic acid may increase metabolism of **phenobarbitol** and also **phenytoin** and other **hydantoin** derivatives with resultant decrease in seizure control. Folic acid may inhibit antimicrobial effect of **pyrimethamine** and may worsen leukaemic patients taking pyrimethamine.

Frusemide

(Aluzine, Diuresal, Dryptal, Frusetic, Frusid, Lasix)   *Diuretic (loop); sulphonamide*
                                                                          derivative

ACTIONS AND USES   Rapid-acting potent sulphonamide 'loop' diuretic and

FRUSEMIDE (continued)

antihypertensive with pharmacological effects and uses almost identical to those of ethacrynic acid (q.v.). Exact mode of action not clearly defined. As with ethacrynic acid, urinary pH falls after administration, but in some patients bicarbonate excretion may temporarily increase the pH. Renal vascular resistance decreases and renal blood flow may increase during drug administration. Inhibits reabsorption of sodium and chloride primarily in loop of Henle and also in proximal and distal renal tubules. Also enhances excretion of potassium, hydrogen, calcium, magnesium, ammonium, bicarbonate, and possibly phosphate. Reportedly less ototoxic than ethacrynic acid.

Used in treatment of oedema associated with congestive heart failure, cirrhosis of liver, and renal disease, including nephrotic syndrome. May be used for management of hypertension, alone or in combination with other antihypertensive agents.

ROUTE AND DOSAGE   *Oedema*: **Adult**: **Oral**: 40 mg in the morning, *maintenance* 20 mg/day. **Intramuscular/intravenous**: 20–50 mg slowly over 1–2 min. **High dose IV infusion**: up to 1 g at a rate not exceeding 4 mg/min. **Infants and children**: 1–3 mg/kg/day. **IM/IV**: 1–1.5 mg/kg.

ABSORPTION AND FATE   Well absorbed following oral administration; diuretic effect begins in 30 to 60 minutes, peaks in 1 to 2 hours, and persists 6 to 8 hours. Following IV injection, diuretic effect starts within 5 minutes (somewhat later after IM) and peaks in 20 to 60 minutes, with duration of 2 hours. Approximately 95% bound to plasma proteins. Small amount metabolized by liver. Rapidly excreted in urine, primarily as unchanged drug; approximately 50% of oral dose and 80% of IV dose are excreted within 24 hours. Small amounts excreted in faeces. Crosses placenta; appears in breast milk.

CONTRAINDICATIONS AND PRECAUTIONS   History of hypersensitivity to frusemide or sulphonamides. Oliguria, anuria, fluid and electrolyte depletion states, hepatic coma; women of childbearing potential; pregnancy. **Cautious Use**: elderly patients, hepatic cirrhosis, nephrotic syndrome, cardiogenic shock associated with acute myocardial infarction, history of systemic lupus erythematosus, history of gout, patients receiving digitalis glycosides or potassium-depleting steroids.

ADVERSE/SIDE EFFECTS   CV: postural hypotension with excessive diuresis, acute hypotensive episodes, circulatory collapse, thromboembolic episodes. **Others**: pruritus, urticaria, exfoliative dermatitis, purpura, photosensitivity, necrotizing angiitis (vasculitis), hypovoalemia, dehydration, hyponatraemia, hypokalaemia, hypochloraemia, metabolic alkalosis, hypomagnesaemia, hypocalcaemia (tetany), hyperammonaemia, nausea, vomiting, oral and gastric burning, anorexia, diarrhoea, constipation, abdominal cramping, acute pancreatitis, jaundice, flank and loin pain, allergic interstitial nephritis, irreversible renal failure, bladder pressure or spasm, urinary frequency, anaemia, leucopenia, aplastic anaemia (rare), thrombocytopenic purpura, tinnitus, feeling of fullness in ears, hearing loss (rarely permanent), hyperglycaemia, glycosuria, elevated BUN, hyperuricaemia, increased perspiration; paraesthesias; blurred vision, muscle spasms, weakness; thrombophlebitis, pain at IM injection site.

FRUSEMIDE (continued)
NURSING IMPLICATIONS

- Schedule doses to avoid nocturia and sleep disturbance (e.g., a single dose is generally administered in the morning; twice-a-day doses may be prescribed for 08.00 hrs and 14.00 hrs.

- Intermittent dosage schedule is frequently used to allow time for natural correction of electrolyte and acid–base imbalance (e.g., drug is given for 2 to 4 consecutive days each week).

- Hospitalization is recommended when therapy is initiated in patients with hepatic cirrhosis and ascites.

- Frequent determinations should be made of blood count, serum and urine electrolytes, CO_2, BUN, blood sugar, and uric acid during first few months of therapy and periodically thereafter.

- Patients receiving the drug parenterally should be observed carefully and blood pressure and vital signs closely monitored. Sudden death from cardiac arrest has been reported. Parenteral administration should be replaced by oral administration when practical.

- Infusion rate will be prescribed by physician and should be checked frequently (generally the rate should not exceed 4 mg/minute to avoid ototoxicity).

- Close observation of the elderly patient is particularly essential during period of brisk diuresis. Sudden alteration in fluid and electrolyte balance may precipitate adverse reactions: anorexia, nausea, vomiting, thirst, dry mouth, confusion, weakness, fatigue, lightheadedness, dizziness, perspiration, muscle cramps, bladder spasm, and urinary frequency. Report onset of these symptoms to physician. *See also Index*: *Nursing Interventions*: *for symptoms of specific electrolyte depletion state.*

- Monitor fluid intake–output ratio. Report decrease in output, excessive diuresis, or diarrhoea.

- The sorbitol (flavouring agent) used in oral preparations may cause diarrhoea, especially in children receiving high doses.

- Weigh patient daily under standard conditions. Rapid and excessive weight loss (from vigorous diuresis) can induce dehydration and acute hypotensive episodes.

- Monitor blood pressure during periods of diuresis and through period of dosage adjustment.

- Excessive dehydration is most likely to occur in the elderly, in those with chronic cardiac disease on prolonged salt restriction, or in those receiving sympatholytic agents. Resultant hypovolaemia may lead to vascular thrombi and emboli (from haemoconcentration) or circulatory collapse.

- Consult physician regarding allowable salt and fluid intake. To prevent hyponatraemia and hypochloraemia, salt intake is generally liberalized in most patients. Patients with cirrhosis usually require at least moderate salt restriction.

- To reduce or prevent potassium depletion, the physician may prescribe daily ingestion of potassium-rich foods (e.g., bananas, oranges, peaches, dried dates), potassium supplement, and intermittent administration of frusemide.

- Be alert to signs of hearing loss, complaints of fullness in ears and tinnitus. Ototoxicity is usually associated with renal insufficiency, uraemia, rapid IV injection of large doses, or concomitant administration of other ototoxic drugs.

- Frusemide may cause hyperglycaemia. Diabetic and diabetic-prone individuals and

F

FRUSEMIDE *(continued)*

patients with decompensated hepatic cirrhosis require careful monitoring of urine and blood glucose.

■ Acute gout can occur in susceptible patients. Advise patient to report onset of joint redness, swelling, or pain.

■ Advise patient to avoid prolonged exposure to direct sunlight. A sunscreen agent may be advisable.

■ Slight discolouration of tablets reportedly does not alter potency; however, injection solutions having a yellow colour should be discarded.

■ Infusion solutions in which frusemide has been mixed should be used within 24 hours. Reportedly compatible with dextrose 5% in water, sodium chloride 0.9%, and Ringer's injection, lactated.

■ Store tablets and parenteral solution at controlled room temperature, preferably between 15° and 30°C (59° and 86°F) unless otherwise directed by manufacturer. Protect from light.

■ Store oral solution in refrigerator, preferably between 2° and 8°C (36° and 46°F). Protect from light and freezing.

Diagnostic test interferences Frusemide may cause elevations in **BUN, serum amylase, cholesterol, triglycerides, uric acid** and **blood glucose** levels, and may decrease **serum calcium, magnesium, potassium,** and **sodium** levels.

DRUG INTERACTIONS   *Frusemide*_____

PLUS	INTERACTIONS
Aminoglycoside antibiotics	Potentiation of ototoxicity
Antidiabetic agents	Frusemide may antagonize hypoglycaemic effect of antidiabetic agents
Antihypertensives	Additive hypotension
Cephaloridine	Enhanced nephrotoxicity
Chloral hydrate	Increased vasomotor instability with flushing, sweating, BP fluctuations
Clofibrate	In patients with nephrotic syndrome: muscular pain and marked diuresis
Corticosteroids	Excessive potassium loss
CNS depressants, e.g., alcohol, barbiturates, narcotics	Potentiate orthostatic hypotension
Digitalis glycosides	Increased risk of digitalis toxicity because of excess K, Ca, and Mg loss
Diuretics	Excessive potassium loss with other potent diuretics
Indomethacin	Response to both drugs may be impaired
Lithium	Increased risk of lithium toxicity
Adrenaline	Arterial response to noadrenaline may be somewhat diminished
Phenytoin	Reduced GI absorption of frusemide
Salicylates	Increased risk of salicylate toxicity with high doses
Skeletal muscle relaxants (surgical), e.g., Succinylcholine, Tubocurarine	Enhanced neuromuscular blockade

Gallamine triethiodide

(Flaxedil)   *Skeletal muscle relaxant*

ACTIONS AND USES   Synthetic, nondepolarizing neuromuscular blocking agent (curariform drug). Similar to tubocurarine (q.v.) in actions, uses, contraindications, precautions, and adverse reactions. About 20% as potent as tubocurarine; reported to produce less ganglionic blockade and to have no histamine-releasing properties except in very high doses. Has parasympatholytic effect on vagus, and may cause tachycardia and occasionally hypertension.

Used as preanaesthetic and intraanaesthetic medication, for treatment of GI disorders, and to reverse neuromuscular blockade.

ROUTE AND DOSAGE   **Intravenous**: 80–120 mg then 20–40 mg as required. **Child**: 1.5 mg/kg.

ABSORPTION AND FATE   Muscle relaxation peaks within 3 minutes, with duration of 15 to 20 minutes. Significantly bound to serum albumin. Excreted primarily unchanged in urine. Crosses placenta.

CONTRAINDICATIONS AND PRECAUTIONS   Hypersensitivity to gallamine or iodides, myasthenia gravis, impaired pulmonary or renal function, shock; patients weighing less than 5 kg, hyperthyroidism, hypertension, tachycardia, cardiac insufficiency, hypoalbuminaemia. *See also tubocurarine.*

NURSING IMPLICATIONS
- Tachycardia occurs almost immediately after administration, reaches maximum within 3 minutes, and declines gradually to premedication level.
- Patients with electrolyte imbalance, dehydration, or elevated temperature may be more sensitive to the effects of gallamine.
- May be stored at room temperature, protected from light and excessive heat.
- *See tubocurarine chloride.*

Gemfibrozil

G

(Lopid)   *Antilipaemic*

ACTIONS AND USES   Lipid lowering agent closely resembling clofibrate (q.v.) chemically, pharmacologically, and clinically.

Used for patients with very high serum triglyceride levels who have not responded adequately to dietary control and who are at risk of pancreatitis and abdominal pain. Also has been used for severe familial hypercholesterolaemia that developed in childhood and has not responded to dietary control or other cholesterol-lowering drugs.

ROUTE AND DOSAGE   **Oral**: 1,200 mg/day in two divided doses, 30 minutes before morning and evening meal. Usual dosage range 900 to 1,500 mg/day.

GEMFIBROZIL (continued)

ABSORPTION AND FATE   Well absorbed from GI track. **Peak plasma levels** in 1 to 2 hours. **Half-life:** 1.3 to 1.5 hours. Portion of drug undergoes enterohepatic circulation. About 75% of dose excreted in urine primarily as unchanged drug; 6% excreted in faeces.

CONTRAINDICATIONS AND PRECAUTIONS   Hypersensitivity to gemfibrozil; gallbladder disease, hepatic or severe kidney dysfunction. Safe use during pregnancy, in nursing mothers, and in children not established. **Cautious Use:** diabetes mellitus.

ADVERSE/SIDE EFFECTS   These include: headache, dizziness, blurred vision, rash, dermatitis, pruritus, urticaria, abdominal or epigastric pain, diarrhoea, nausea, vomiting, flatulence, anaemia, eosinophilia, leucopenia, hyperglycaemia, painful extremities, causal relationship not established (viral or bacterial infection, fatigue, malaise, syncope, vertigo, insomnia, paraesthesias, tinnitus, dry mouth, constipation, anorexia, gas pain, dyspepsia, cholelithiasis, cholecystitis, malignancy, postcholecystectomy complications, pancreatitis; cardiac arrhythmias, intermittent claudication), back pain, muscle cramps, myalgia, arthralgia, swollen joints; hypokalaemia, increases in liver function tests.

NURSING IMPLICATIONS
■ Store preferably between 15° and 30°C (59° and 86°F), unless otherwise directed by manufacturer.

DRUG INTERACTIONS   *Gemfibrozil*_____

PLUS	INTERACTIONS
Anticoagulants	Potentiation of anticoagulant effect Close monitoring of prothrombin time recommended

For further information: *see clofibrate*

Gentamicin sulphate _____

(Cidomycin, Genticin, Lugacin)   *Antibiotic; aminoglycoside*

ACTIONS AND USES   Broad-spectrum aminoglycoside antibiotic derived from *Micromonospora purpurea*, an actinomyces organism. By acting directly on bacterial ribosome, inhibits protein biosynthesis. Active against a wide variety of gram-negative bacteria, including *Pseudomonas aeruginosa*, *Proteus* species (including indole-positive and -negative strains), *Escherichia coli*, and *Klebsiella*, *Enterobacter*, and *Serratia* species. Also effective against certain gram-negative organisms, particularly penicillin-sensitive and some methicillin-resistant strains of *Staphylococcus aureus*. Cross-resistance and allergenicity

GENTAMICIN SULPHATE (continued)

with other members of aminoglycoside group thought to be possible. Has neuromuscular blocking action, in common with other aminoglycoside antibiotics.

Parenteral use restricted to treatment of serious infections of GI tract, respiratory tract, urinary tract, CNS, bone, skin, and soft tissue (including burns), when other less toxic antimicrobial agents are ineffective or are contraindicated. May be used in combination with other antibiotics. Also used topically for primary and secondary skin infections and for infections of external eye and its adnexa.

ROUTE AND DOSAGE   Intramuscular, intravenous: Adults: 2 to 5 mg/kg/day in three equal doses every 8 hours. (IV dosage is based on estimate of ideal body weight.) Children: 2 mg/kg every 8 hrs. *Neonates*: up to 2 weeks of age, 3 mg/kg every 12 hours. Dosages must be adjusted for patients with impaired renal function. Intrathecal: 1 mg daily, with 2–4 mg/kg/day by IM injection in divided doses (8 hrly). Topical: 0.3% cream or ointment, applied gently to lesions three times daily. Ophthalmic solution (0.3%): 1 or 2 drops in affected eye every 4 hours. Ophthalmic ointment (0.3%): applied in small amount to lower conjunctival sac two or four times daily.

ABSORPTION AND FATE   Rapidly absorbed following IM injection. Peak serum concentrations in 30 to 90 minutes; effective serum levels persist 6 to 8 hours. Administration of IV infusion over 2-hour period produces similar concentrations. Serum levels higher and more prolonged in patients with impaired renal function. Widely distributed to extracellular fluids. Poorly distributed to adipose tissue and to CSF even when meninges are inflamed. However, high CSF concentrations attained by intraventricular or intrathecal routes. Approximately 25% loosely bound to plasma proteins. Serum half-life about 1 to 2 hours. Excreted primarily in urine, largely as unchanged drug (excretion correlates with creatinine clearance). Slight absorption may occur following topical applications, especially with cream formulations. Crosses placenta.

CONTRAINDICATIONS AND PRECAUTIONS   Known hypersensitivity to gentamicin, concomitant use with other neurotoxic (ototoxic) and/or nephrotoxic drugs; myasthenia gravis. Safe use during pregnancy not established. Cautious Use: impaired renal function; topical applications to widespread areas; elderly, infants, and children.

ADVERSE/SIDE EFFECTS   These include: rash, pruritus, urticaria, eosinophilia, burning sensation of skin, fever, joint pains, laryngeal oedema, granulocytopenia, agranulocytosis, thrombocytopenic purpura, anaemia, proteinuria, cells or casts in urine, rising levels of BUN, nonprotein nitrogen, serum creatinine; oliguria, decreased creatinine clearance, renal damage, ototoxicity (vestibular disturbances, impaired hearing), optic neuritis, peripheral neuritis, numbness, tingling of skin, muscle twitching, convulsions, photosensitivity, erythema, pruritus; burning, stinging, and lacrimation with ophthalmic use, increased SGOT, SGPT, and serum bilirubin; decreased serum calcium; hypomagnesaemia, increased or decreased reticulocyte counts; transient hepatomegaly, splenomegaly; superinfections; anorexia, nausea, vomiting, weight loss, increased salivation; headache, drug fever, lethargy; loss of hair and eyebrows; pulmonary fibrosis,

GENTAMICIN SULPHATE (continued)

hypotension or hypertension; local irritation and pain following IM use; neuromuscular blockade and respiratory paralysis (with high doses).

NURSING IMPLICATIONS

- Culture and sensitivity tests should be performed initially and periodically during continued therapy. Drug is generally given for 7 to 10 days.
- Renal function and vestibular and auditory function should be determined before initiation of therapy and at regular intervals during treatment, especially in the elderly and other patients with impaired renal function and in those receiving higher doses or longer treatment. Vestibular and auditory function should also be checked 3 to 4 weeks after drug is discontinued.
- Ototoxic effect is greatest on vestibular branch of eighth cranial nerve (symptoms: headache, dizziness, nausea, and vomiting with motion, ataxia, nystagmus); however, auditory branch damage (tinnitus, roaring noises) may also occur. Hearing loss occurs particularly in high tone range and can be detected only by audiometer. Generally, conversational hearing range is not affected. Prompt reporting is critically essential to prevent permanent damage.
- Drug plasma concentrations should be determined at frequent intervals for patients with impaired renal function. When peak plasma concentrations are monitored, dosage is adjusted to prevent prolonged levels above 12 mcg/ml. When trough concentrations are monitored, dosage is usually adjusted so that levels above 2 mcg/ml are avoided.
- Fluid intake and output should be monitored. Consult physician about desirable intake; generally, patient is kept well hydrated during gentamicin therapy to prevent chemical irritation of renal tubules. Report oliguria and unusual change in intake and output ratio.
- Be alert for signs of bacterial overgrowth (superinfection) with nonsusceptible organisms (diarrhoea, anogenital itching, vaginal discharge, stomatitis, glossitis).
- In treatment of urinary tract infections, concomitant alkalinizing agent may be prescribed to raise urinary pH above 7, since gentamicin is less active in an acidic medium.
- Topically treated lesions may be covered with gauze, if necessary.
- Systemic absorption and toxicity are possible when topical applications, particularly cream preparations, are made to large denuded body surfaces.
- In treatment of impetigo contagiosa, individual crusts should first be removed (gently) to allow topical medication to contact infected site. Removal may be facilitated by soaking crusts with warm soap and water or by application of wet compresses. Consult physician regarding specific procedure.
- Caution patients using topical applications to avoid excessive exposure to sunlight because of danger of photosensitivity. Also advise patient to withhold medication and to notify physician if signs of irritation or sensitivity occur.
- Gentamicin is incompatible in a syringe or in solution with any other drug.
- Store preferably between 15° and 30°C (59° and 86°F) unless otherwise directed by manufacturer. Do not use solution if it is discoloured or contains a precipitate.

G

GENTAMICIN SULPHATE (continued)

Drug interactions Possibility of additive nephrotoxic effects with combined use of gentamicin and **cephalosporins**. **Ethacrynic acid** and **frusemide** may enhance ototoxicity of gentamicin (and other aminoglycoside antibiotics). Concurrent use is usually avoided. Combined or sequential use of **other aminoglycoside antibiotics** with gentamicin increases the probability of ototoxicity and nephrotoxicity. **Antimotion-sickness drugs** may mask symptoms of ototoxicity. There is enhanced neuromuscular blockade with neuromuscular blocking drugs (e.g., **decamethonium, ether, succinyl-choline, tubocurarine**, and related anaesthetics). Activity of gentamicin is diminished significantly by **carbenicillin**. If concurrent administration is prescribed, they should be given about 1 to 2 hours apart. **Carbenicillin** may inactivate gentamicin when mixed together for IV infusion.

Glibenclamide

(Euglucon, Daonil)   *Antidiabetic agent; sulphonylurea*

ACTIONS AND USES One of the most potent of the sulphonylurea hypoglycaemic agents. Second-generation sulphonylurea closely related in actions, uses, and limitations to glipizide (q.v.). Lowers blood sugar concentration in both diabetic and nondiabetic individuals by stimulating insulin release from functioning pancreatic beta cells. Blood glucose lowering effect persists during longterm glyburide treatment, but there is a gradual decline in meal-stimulated secretion of endogenous insulin toward pretreatment levels. Produces mild diuresis by enhanced free water clearance, perhaps by inhibiting reabsorption of Na in the proximal renal tubule or by blocking nonvasopressor-dependent reabsorption of water in the distal renal tubules.

Used as adjunct to diet to lower blood glucose in patients with non-insulin-dependent diabetes mellitus after dietary control alone has failed.

ROUTE AND DOSAGE (Dosage regimen is individualized to establish the minimum effective dose.) Recommended initial dose: **Oral**: 2.5 to 5 mg daily given with breakfast or first main meal. *Usual maintenance dose*: 1.25 to 2.0 mg daily as single or divided doses. Dose adjustment is accomplished by increments of 2.5 mg depending on blood glucose response, but no sooner than 1 or 2 weeks to allow reaching steady-state serum levels and full pharmacological effect. Maximum daily dose 15 mg.

ABSORPTION AND FATE Following oral administration drug is well absorbed within 1 hour, with peak concentration reached in 2 to 8 hours. Blood glucose lowering effect persists for 24 hours. Plasma insulin concentration begins to increase within 15 to 60 minutes after a single dose and is maximal in 1 to 2 hours; in a diabetic patient plasma insulin may persist for up to 24 hours. Distributed in highest concentrations to liver, kidneys and intestines. Metabolized in liver; more than 99% protein bound. **Half-life** of drug and its metabolites: about 10 hours (may be prolonged in patients with severe

GLIBENCLAMIDE (continued)

renal impairment). Excreted as metabolities in urine and faeces in approximately equal proportions. Appears to cross placenta but distribution into milk is not known. Minimally removed by haemodialysis.

CONTRAINDICATIONS AND PRECAUTIONS *See glipizide.*

ADVERSE/SIDE EFFECTS Hypoglycaemia (may be fatal in patient receiving as little as 2.5 to 5 mg glyburide/day); epigastric fullness, heartburn, nausea, paraesthesia, joint pain, nocturia. *See also glipizide.*

NURSING IMPLICATIONS

- Store in tightly closed, light resistant container at a temperature 15° to 30°C (59° to 86°F).
- *See glipizide for additional Nursing Implications and for Drug Interactions.*

Gliclazide ━━━━━━━━━━━━━━━━━━━━━━━━━━━━━━━━━━━

(Diamicron)   *Antidiabetic; sulphonylurea*

ACTIONS AND USES Used to treat diabetes mellitus.

ROUTE AND DOSAGE Adult: *Initial* 40–80 mg/day adjusted according to response. *See glipizide.*

Glipizide ━━━━━━━━━━━━━━━━━━━━━━━━━━━━━━━━━━━━

(Glibenese, Minodiab)   *Antidiabetic agent; sulphonylurea*

ACTIONS AND USES Second-generation sulphonylurea hypoglycaemic agent structurally similar to acetohexamide (first generation). Glipizide directly stimulates functioning pancreatic beta cells to secrete insulin, leading to an acute drop in blood glucose. Indirect action leads to altered numbers and sensitivity of peripheral insulin receptors resulting in increased insulin binding. It also causes inhibition of hepatic glucose production and reduction in serum glucagon levels. Fasting insulin levels are not increased by long-term glipizide therapy; however, a postprandial insulin response lasting through the meal challenge continues to be enhanced for at least 6 months. Glipizide has no antidiuretic activity and has no effect on plasma lipoproteins in patient being treated for non-insulin-dependent diabetes mellitus. Since loss of control when patient is being treated by diet alone may be transient, a short course of glipizide therapy may be adequate to restore control. It has not been established that this

GLIPIZIDE (continued)

drug will prevent long-term cardiovascular and neurological complications of diabetes mellitus.

Used as adjunct to diet for control of hyperglycaemia in patient with non-insulin-dependent diabetes after dietary control alone has failed; also used to treat transient loss of control in patient usually controlled well on diet.

ROUTE AND DOSAGE   (Regimen is individualized) **Oral:** recommended initial dose: 5 mg 30 minutes before breakfast (2.5 mg for elderly patient or patient with hepatic disease). Dosage is adjusted with increments of 2.5 to 5 mg dependent on blood glucose response, but no sooner than 1 or 2 weeks to allow reaching steady-state serum levels and full pharmacological effect. Maximum once-daily dose: 15 mg. Doses above 15 mg should ordinarily be divided and given before meals. Doses above 30 mg have been safely given on a twice-a-day schedule for long-term therapy. Maximum recommended total daily dose: 40 mg.

ABSORPTION AND FATE   Following oral administration drug is completely absorbed (with food, absorption is delayed by about 0.5 hours). **Peak plasma concentration** achieved in 1 to 3 hours after a single dose; **duration of action (blood glucose control)** up to 24 hours. 92 to 99% protein-bound by nonionic bonds; extensive hepatic metabolism (primary metabolites are inactive). **Half-life:** 2 to 4 hours. Excreted mainly by renal route but some excretion is via bile.

CONTRAINDICATIONS AND PRECAUTIONS   Hypersensitivity to glipizide, diabetic ketoacidosis with or without coma; pregnancy nursing mothers. Safe use in children not established. **Cautious Use:** impaired renal and hepatic function, the elderly, debilitated, malnourished patient; patient with adrenal or pituitary insufficiency.

ADVERSE/SIDE EFFECTS   These include: erythema, morbilliform or maculopapular rash, pruritus, urticaria, eczema (transient), porphyria cutanea tarda, photosensitivity reactions, nausea, diarrhoea, constipation, gastralgia, leucopenia, thrombocytopenia, haemolytic anaemia, aplastic anaemia, agranulocytosis, pancytopenia, hepatic porphyria; headache. **Overdosage:** hypoglycaemia (mild): fatigue, drowsiness, hunger, GI distress (heartburn, abdominal pain, anorexia), headache, anxiety; (severe): visual disturbances, ataxia, confusion, tachycardia, seizures, coma.

NURSING IMPLICATIONS

- Take ½ hour before a meal to give best protection against postprandial hyperglycaemia.
- Glipizide is prescribed after control of blood glucose by diet alone has failed. Inform the patient that glipizide treatment accompanies (does not substitute for) continued control of diet and (if patient is obese) a weight-loss programme.
- *Urine testing*: When diabetes is stabilized, patient is advised to test urine for glucose 2 hours after each meal.
- If urine test is positive for glucose for 2 or 3 days, then patient is usually advised to check for urine ketones and report to physician. Urine should be tested for ketones also, when patient has an illness or is subjected to stress such as surgery.

G

GLIPIZIDE (continued)

- Severe drug-induced skin rashes and pruritus may necessitate discontinuation of drug use. Symptoms usually subside rapidly when drug is withdrawn.
- Inform patient about the importance of exercise as a part of the total control programme. Plan this treatment adjunct specifically, with guidance from the physician.
- The initial dose and establishment of a maintenance regimen in the elderly or debilitated patient is approached both conservatively and gradually. Close observation for early signs of hypoglycaemia (easily overlooked – see *Adverse/Side Effects*) is paramount.
- Usually 5 to 7 days are allowed to elapse between titration steps. If response to a single dose is unsatisfactory, the dose may be divided.
- Advise patient on glipizide who wishes to become pregnant that a transfer to insulin for blood glucose control is recommended by many clinicians.
- If glipizide is used during pregnancy, it is discontinued at least 1 month before the expected delivery date to prevent prolonged severe hypoglycaemia (4 to 10 days) in the neonate.
- The potential for hypoglycaemia in nursing infants presents the necessity to decide whether to discontinue nursing or to temporarily transfer to insulin (if diet alone is inadequate for blood sugar control).
- *Transfer of a patient from insulin to glipizide*: accomplished according to the following guidelines:
  - □ If insulin daily requirement is 20 units or less: discontinue insulin and start glipizide at usual dosages with titration steps at intervals of 5 to 7 days.
  - □ If insulin daily requirement is more than 20 units; reduce insulin dose by 50% and start glipizide at usual doses. (Subsequent reduction of insulin depends on patient response.) Titration steps as above.
- During insulin withdrawal period, urine tests for sugar and ketone bodies should be checked at least three times daily. Advise patient to contact the physician if tests are abnormal.
- If the patient is being transferred from one to another sulphonylurea, no transition period is necessary. However, the patient who is transferred from one with a long half-life (e.g., chlorpropamide: half-life: 30 to 40 hours) must be observed for hypoglycaemic responses for 1 to 2 weeks because of potential overlapping of drug effect.
- When a drug that affects the hypoglycaemic action of sulphonylureas (*see Drug interactions*) is withdrawn or added to the glipizide regimen the patient should be alerted to the added danger of loss of control (hyperglycaemia). Urine and blood glucose tests and test for ketone bodies should be carefully monitored and possibly increased in frequency for several days to determine if antidiabetic drug dose adjustment is indicated.
- Keep in mind that if the patient is also receiving a beta-adrenergic blocking agent (suppresses reflex tachycardia) or is elderly the first signs of hypoglycaemia may be hard to detect.
- In the diabetic patient, hypoglycaemia is a potential effect of the following situations:

G

GLIPIZIDE (continued)

after severe or prolonged exercise, after alcohol ingestion, when caloric intake is deficient, when more than one glucose lowering drug is being used.

- Be alert to the danger of loss of control of diabetes which may result from stress such as fever, surgery, trauma, infection. Blood and urine glucose and ketone body detection may need to be checked more frequently during these stress periods, and transfer from the sulphonylurea to insulin may be necessary.

- Advise patient and/or primary care provider to observe for signs of cholestatic jaundice (yellow sclera, dark urine, pruritus). If they occur, inform the physician promptly. The drug may have to be discontinued and replaced by another anti-diabetic agent.

- ***Treatment of overdosage***   Mild hypoglycaemia (reaction without loss of consciousness of neurological symptoms) is treated with oral glucose and adjustment of dosage and meal pattern. The patient should be closely monitored for at least 5 to 7 days to assure reestablishment of safe control. Severe hypoglycaemia (reaction with coma, seizure or other neurological manifestations) requires emergency hospitalization to permit rapid IV injection of concentrated (50%) glucose solution. This will be followed by continuous infusion of 10% glucose solution at a rate adequate to maintain a blood glucose level above 100 mg/dl.

- Monitor patient for 24 to 48 hours because hypoglycaemia may recur after apparent clinical recovery.

- Store in tightly closed light resistant container at a temperature 15° to 30°C (59° to 86°F).

- *See tolbutamide for additional patient teaching points.*

DRUG INTERACTIONS   *Glipizide*

PLUS	INTERACTIONS
Anticoagulants (coumarins) Beta adrenergic blocking agents (e.g., propranolol) Chloramphenicol NSAIDs MAO inhibitors Probenecid Sulphonamides	May potentiate hypoglycaemic action of sulphonylurea agent
Adrenergics Calcium channel blocking agents (e.g., verapamil) Corticosteroids Oestrogens Isoniazid (INH) Oral contraceptives Niacin Phenothiazines Phenytoin Thiazides and other diuretics Thyroid products	May cause loss of control and produce hyperglycaemia

G

Gliquidone

(Glurenorm)   *Antidiabetic; sulphonylurea*

ACTIONS AND USES   Used to treat diabetes mellitus.

ROUTE AND DOSAGE   Oral: **Adult:** *initial* 15 mg/day before breakfast. Adjusted according to response to 45–60 mg/day in divided doses.
  For further information: *see glipizide.*

Glyceryl trinitrate

(Nitroglycerin Coro-Nitro spray, Nitrocine, Nitrocontin,   *Vasodilator (coronary)*
  Nitrate Percutol, Trasiderm-Nitro, Tridil, Nitrolingual,
  Suscard, Sustac)

ACTIONS AND USES   Organic nitrate produced from volatile liquid with explosive potential, rendered nonexplosive by addition of carbohydrates. Relaxes all smooth muscle by direct action, with most prominent effect on vascular smooth muscle. Resulting vasodilation promotes pooling of blood, produces lowered peripheral resistance, fall in blood pressure, and decreased cardiac output due to reduced venous return to heart. Precise mechanism of action in treatment of angina pectoris not established, but appears to be due to reduction in myocardial oxygen consumption. Cross tolerance with other nitrites and nitrates may occur.
  Used in prevention and treatment of acute anginal episodes. Sustained release tablets available for longer prophylaxis. Also used for treatment of ventricular failure.

ROUTE AND DOSAGE   **Sublingual:** 0.3–1 mg repeated as required. **Oral:** 2.6–6.4 mg 2–3 times a day (slow release). **Transdermal (5 and 10 mg) system:** dosage increases are made either by using larger sized system or by using a combination of systems. **Intravenous infusion:** *Initial:* 5 mcg in 5% dextrose or 0.9% sodium chloride injection, 10 to 200 mcg/minute, as necessary. **Aerosol:** 1–2 metered doses to the sublingual mucosa.

ABSORPTION AND FATE   Sublingual tablet acts in 1 to 3 minutes; duration up to 30 minutes. Transmucosal form acts in 3 minutes; duration: 10 to 30 minutes. Sustained release tablet acts in about 1 hour; action peaks in 3 to 4 hours and persists 8 to 12 hours. Transdermal system acts in 30 to 60 minutes with duration of about 24 hours. IV nitroglycerin acts immediately; duration of effects; variable. Rapidly metabolized in liver; excreted in urine mostly as inactive metabolites.

CONTRAINDICATIONS AND PRECAUTIONS   Hypersensitivity, idiosyncrasy, or tolerance to nitrites; early myocardial infarction; severe anaemia, hypotension, increased

GLYCERYL TRINITRATE (continued)

intracranial pressure, glaucoma (sustained release forms). Safe use during pregnancy and in children not established. **Cautious Use**: hepatic or renal disease, hyperthyroidism.

ADVERSE/SIDE EFFECTS   Transient headache, dizziness, flushing, postural hypotension, palpitation, increased heart rate, nausea, vomiting. **Hypersensitivity**: skin rash, exfoliative dermatitis, blurred vision, dry mouth, weakness, restlessness, pallor, perspiration, collapse. **Overdosage**: violent headache, syncope, tachycardia, paradoxical angina, circulatory collapse, convulsions, coma, respiratory failure; methaemoglobinia (toxic doses).

NURSING IMPLICATIONS

Sublingual Tablet

- Instruct patient to sit or lie down upon first indication of oncoming anginal pain, and to place tablet under tongue or in buccal pouch (hypotensive effect of drug is intensified in the upright position). Recumbent position should be avoided since venous blood return to the heart may increase. Advise patient to allow tablet to dissolve naturally and not to swallow until drug is entirely dissolved.
- As soon as pain is completely relieved, any remaining tablet may be expelled from mouth, especially if patient is experiencing unpleasant side effects such as headache.
- Advise patient to relax for 15 to 20 minutes after taking tablet to prevent dizziness or faintness.
- If pain is not relieved after one tablet, additional tablets may be taken at 5 minute intervals, but not more than 3 tablets should be taken in a 15-minute period. Taking more tablets than necessary can further decrease coronary blood flow by producing systemic hypotension.
- Pain not relieved by 3 tablets over a 15 minute period may indicate acute myocardial infarction or severe coronary insufficiency. Advise patient to contact physician immediately.
- For hospitalized patient, tablets should be kept at bedside. Allocate a specific number (usually 10 tablets) in an appropriate container, label, and make sure patient knows location and use. Request patient to report all attacks. Count tablets as (07.00 hrs and 19.00 hrs).
- Transient headache a frequent side effect, usually lasts about 5 minutes after sublingual administration and seldom longer than 20 minutes. Report to physician if persistent or severe. (Patients who do not have coronary disease may experience severe disabling headaches.)
- Sublingual tablets may be taken prophylactically 5 to 10 minutes prior to exercise or other stimulus known to trigger anginal pain (drug effect will last up to 30 minutes).
- Instruct patient to keep record for physician of number of anginal attacks, number of tablets required for relief of each attack, and possible precipitating factors.

Patient instruction for care of sublingual tablets

- Note expiration date on label.
- Once bottle is opened, remove cotton filler. Keep bottle tightly capped.

G

GLYCERYL TRINITRATE (continued)

- Store stock supply in cool, dry place or at controlled room temperature not exceeding 30°C (86°F). Inactivation of glyceryl trinitrate is increased by time, heat, air, moisture.
- Inform family members of location of stock supply. Do not handle tablets since moisture will hasten deterioration. Carry these on person at all times, away from body heat (e.g., in jacket pocket, handbag).
- References vary with respect to how long stock supply retains potency: it is generally recommended that unused tablets be discarded 8 weeks after bottle is opened. An indication of potency is suggested if drug produces a burning or stinging sensation under patient's tongue. However, many elderly patients are unable to detect this sensation; additionally, this effect may not be experienced with the newer, more stable sublingual preparations.
- *Sustained release oral tablet or capsule*:
  - ☐ Should be taken on an empty stomach (1 hour before or 2 hours after meals), with a full glass of water, and swallowed whole.
  - ☐ Sustained release form helps to prevent anginal attacks; it is not intended for immediate relief of angina.
- *Application of ointment*: Squeeze prescribed dose onto special measuring application supplied by manufacturer and use it, *not fingers* to spread ointment. Apply prescribed dose in a thin, uniform layer to premarked 6 by 6 inch square nonhairy skin surface. Areas commonly used: chest, abdomen, anterior thigh, forearm. Do not massage or rub in ointment as this increases absorption and thus interferes with drug's sustained action.
- Area may be covered with transparent kitchen wrap and secured with tape to protect clothing.
- Rotate application sites to prevent dermal inflammation and sensitization. Remove ointment from previously used sites before reapplication.
- To determine optimal dose, physician may initially prescribe ½ or 1 inch of ointment and increase dose ¼ or ½ inch at a time until headache (a definitive sign of overdosage) occurs, then gradually reduce dose to that which does not cause headache.
- If treatment is to be terminated, dosage and frequency of application must be reduced gradually over period of 4 to 6 weeks to prevent withdrawal reactions (pain, severe myocardial ischaemia).
- Keep ointment container tightly closed and store in cool place.
- *Transdermal system*:
  - ☐ A glyceryl trinitrate impregnated unit which when applied to skin releases continuous and controlled dosage over 24 hour period.
  - ☐ System is applied at the same time each day, preferably to skin site free of hair and not subject to excessive movement. Avoid abraded, irritated or scarred skin. Clip hair if necessary.
  - ☐ Change application site each time to prevent skin irritation and sensitization.
  - ☐ Contact with water, e.g., bathing, swimming does not affect the unit.
  - ☐ If faintness, dizziness or flushing occurs, advise patient to remove unit immediately from skin and notify physician. (Consult physician about this teaching point.)

G

GLYCERYL TRINITRATE (continued)

■ *Intravenous glyceryl trinitrate*:

  ☐ Must be diluted in 5% dextrose or 0.9% sodium chloride injection prior to infusion.

  ☐ Stable for at least 48 hours when stored at controlled room temperature between 15° and 30°C (59° and 86°F), and mixed and stored in a glass container.

  ☐ Nitroglycerin preparations for IV administration vary in concentration and volume. Check manufacturer's labeling information carefully for dilution and dosage particularly if change is made from one product to another.

  ☐ IV dosage titration requires careful and continuous monitoring of blood pressure, heart rate, and pulmonary capillary wedge pressure in some patients.

General points

■ Advise patient to report blurred vision or dry mouth. Both reactions warrant discontinuation of nitroglycerin.

■ Pain of angina is usually described as a squeezing, choking, tight or heavy substernal discomfort. Pain may radiate to arms, shoulders, neck and lower jaw and is of short duration, usually less than 10 minutes.

■ Dizziness, lightheadedness, and syncope (due to postural hypotension) occur most frequently in the elderly. Recovery may be hastened by head-low position, deep breathing, and movement of extremities. Advise patient to make position changes slowly and to avoid prolonged standing.

■ Inform patient that a shock-like syndrome (sharp drop in blood pressure, vertigo, flushing or pallor) may occur if alcohol is ingested too soon after taking nitroglycerin.

■ Tolerance to nitroglycerin rarely occurs with usual intermittent use, but is possible with repeated administration. It may be prevented by using smallest effective dose. Temporary withdrawal (few days) usually restores original response to drug.

■ Advise patient to report to physician any evidence of refractoriness, i.e., increase in frequency, duration or severity of attacks.

■ Each patient must learn to identify stimuli that precipitate anginal pain in him, and pace his activities accordingly. Known factors that may provoke an attack include: emotional distress, heavy meals, smoking, temperature extremes, excessive use of coffee, tea, colas; sudden burst of physical activity; climbing stairs, especially while talking or carrying heavy bundles.

■ Regular programme of graduated daily exercises is generally recommended as well as control or reduction of body weight, and low cholesterol diet.

■ Withdrawal following prolonged use must be accomplished gradually to prevent precipitating anginal attacks.

■ Advise patient to carry medical information card.

Diagnostic test interferences   Glyceryl trinitrate may cause increases in determinations of **urinary catecholamines**, and **VMA**.

Drug interactions   Combined use of glyceryl trinitrate and **alcohol** or **antihypertensive agents** may potentiate orthostatic hypotension, from additive vasodilation. Chronic administration of **pentaerythritol tetranitrate** or other long-acting nitrites may impair

GLYCERYL TRINITRATE (continued)

response to subsequently administered glyceryl trinitrate, by producing tolerance. Nitroglycerin may potentiate hypotensive effects of **tricyclic antidepressants** and may increase the pharmacological effects of **ergot alkaloids**.

Glycopyrronium

(Robinul)   *Anticholinergic*

ACTIONS AND USES   Synthetic anticholinergic (antimuscarinic) quaternary ammonium compound with pharmacological effects similar to those of atropine (q.v.).

Used in adjunctive management of peptic ulcer and other GI disorders associated with hyperacidity, hypermotility, and spasm. Also used parenterally as preanaesthetic and intraoperative medication and to reverse neuromuscular blockade.

ROUTE AND DOSAGE   Oral: **Adults:** 1–4 mg/2–3 times a day. **IM/IV:** 200–400 mcg. **Child:** 4–8 mcg/kg (maximum 200 mcg).

For further information: *see atropine sulphate.*

Gold (sodium aurothiomalate)

(Myocrisin)   *Antirheumatic*

ACTIONS AND USES   Water-soluble gold compound. Contains approximately 50% gold. Major effect is suppression of joint inflammation. Mechanism of action not clearly understood.

Used in treatment of selected patients (adults and juveniles) with acute rheumatoid arthritis.

ROUTE AND DOSAGE   Highly individualized.

ABSORPTION AND FATE   Readily absorbed following IM injection. Peak plasma concentrations reached in 4 to 6 hours. Thought to be highly concentrated in kidney, liver, spleen, and synovial fluid. Bound to plasma proteins. Half-life lengthens with successive injections. Excreted primarily in urine; appreciable amounts also eliminated in faeces. After a course of treatment, traces may be found in urine for 6 months or more.

CONTRAINDICATIONS AND PRECAUTIONS   History of severe toxicity from previous exposure to gold or other heavy metals, severe debilitation, systemic lupus erythema-

GOLD (SODIUM AUROTHIOMALATE)

tosus, Sjögren's syndrome in rheumatoid arthritis, renal disease, hepatic dysfunction, history of infectious hepatitis or haematological disorders, uncontrolled diabetes, or congestive heart failure. Safe use during pregnancy not established. **Cautious Use:** history of drug allergies or hypersensitivity, hypertension.

ADVERSE/SIDE EFFECTS Allergic (**nitritoid-type reactions**): flushing, fainting, dizziness, fall in blood pressure, sweating, nausea, vomiting, weakness. Less frequently: anaphylactic shock, bradycardia, oedema of tongue, angioneurotic oedema. **Skin and mucous membranes**: transient pruritus, erythema, dermatitis (common), fixed drug eruption, alopecia, shedding of nails, grey to blue pigmentation of skin (chrysiasis), stomatitis (common), glossitis, bronchitis, pharyngitis, pneumonitis, gastritis, colitis, vaginitis. **Other**: gold deposits in ocular tissues, photosensitivity, hepatitis with jaundice, bilirubinaemia, peripheral neuritis, encephalitis, nephrotic syndrome, glomerulitis with haematuria, proteinuria.

NURSING IMPLICATIONS

- Agitate vial before withdrawing dose to assure uniform suspension.
- Baseline haemoglobin and erythrocyte determinations, WBC count, differential count, platelet count, and urinalysis should be obtained before initiation of therapy and at regular intervals thereafter.
- Prior to each injection, urine should be analyzed for protein, blood, and sediment. Drug should be discontinued promptly if proteinuria or haematuria develops.
- Patient should be interviewed and examined before each injection to detect occurrence of transient pruritus or dermatitis (both are common early indications of toxicity), stomatitis (sore tongue, palate, or throat), metallic taste, indigestion, or other signs and symptoms of possible toxicity. Treatment should be interrupted immediately if any of these reactions occurs.
- Drug is usually administered deep into upper outer quadrant of gluteus with patient lying down. Patient should remain recumbent for at least 30 minutes after injection because of the danger of 'nitritoid reaction' (transient giddiness, vertigo, facial flushing, fainting). Observe for allergic reactions.
- Allergic reaction may occur almost immediately after injection, 10 minutes after injection, or at any time during therapy. If it is observed, treatment should be discontinued.
- Rapid improvement in joint swelling usually indicates that patient is closely approaching drug tolerance level; report to physician.
- Patients who develop gold dermatitis should be warned that exposure to sunlight may aggravate the problem.
- The appearance of purpura or ecchymoses is always an indication for doing a platelet count; report to physician.
- Patients should be informed about possible adverse reactions and warned to report any symptoms suggestive of toxicity as soon as it appears.
- Preserved in tight, light-resistant containers at room temperature preferably between 15° and 30°C (59° and 86°F). Drug should not be used if it is any darker than pale yellow.

G

Griseofulvin

(Fulcin, Grisovin)   *Antibiotic; antifungal*

ACTIONS AND USES   Fungistatic antibiotic derived from species of *Penicillium*. Deposits in keratin precursor cells and has special affinity for diseased tissue. Tightly bound to new keratin of skin, hair, and nails, which becomes highly resistant to fungal invasion. Effective against various species of *Epidermophyton*, *Microsporum*, and *Trichophyton* (has no effect on other fungi, including candida, bacteria, and yeasts).

Used in treatment of mycotic disease of skin, hair, and nails not amenable to conventional topical measures.

ROUTE AND DOSAGE   Oral: Adults: 0.5–1 g daily as divided or single dose. Child: 10 mg/kg/day as a divided or single dose.

ABSORPTION AND FATE   Absorbed primarily from duodenum (extent varies among individuals). Absorption of microsize griseofulvin is variable and unpredictable; ultramicrosize is almost completely absorbed. Concentrates in skin, hair, nails, liver, fat, and skeletal muscle. Can be detected in outer layers of stratum corneum soon after absorption. **Elimination half-life** is 9 to 24 hours. Metabolized in liver. Excreted in urine and faeces chiefly as inactive metabolites and small amounts of unchanged drug. Also excreted in perspiration.

CONTRAINDICATIONS AND PRECAUTIONS   History of sensitivity to griseofulvin, porphyria, hepatic disease, systemic lupus erythematosus. Safe use during pregnancy, for children 2 years of age and younger, or for prophylaxis against fungal infections not established. **Cautious Use**: penicillin-sensitive patients (possibility of cross-sensitivity with penicillin exists; however, reportedly penicillin-sensitive patients have been treated without difficulty).

ADVERSE/SIDE EFFECTS   Low incidence of side effects. These include: heartburn, nausea, vomiting, diarrhoea, flatulence, dry mouth, thirst, decreased taste acuity, anorexia, unpleasant taste, furred tongue, oral thrush, leucopenia, neutropenia, granulocytopenia, punctate basophilia, monocytosis, severe headache, insomnia, peripheral neuritis, paraesthesias, fatigue, mental confusion, impaired performance of routine functions, vertigo, blurred vision, proteinuria, cylinduria, hepatotoxicity, oestrogenlike effects (in children), aggravation of systemic lupus erythematosus, overgrowth of nonsusceptible organisms, candidal intertrigo, elevated porphyrins in faeces and erythrocytes.

NURSING IMPLICATIONS
- Accurate laboratory identification of infecting organism is essential prior to initiation of treatment.
- Giving the drug with or after meals may allay GI disturbances.
- Serum levels may be increased by giving the microsize formulations with a high fat content meal (increases drug absorption rate). Consult physician.
- Monitor food intake. Griseofulvin may alter taste sensations and thus may cause appetite suppression and inadequate nutrient intake.

G

GRISEOFULVIN (continued)

- Headaches often occur during early therapy but frequently disappear with continued drug administration.
- Blood studies should be performed at least once weekly during first month of therapy or longer. Periodic tests of renal and hepatic function are also advised.
- Patient may experience symptomatic relief after 48 to 96 hours of therapy. Stress the importance of continuing treatment as prescribed to prevent relapse.
- Treatment should be continued until there is clinical improvement, as well as negative potassium hydroxide amounts of lesion scrapings, or until 2 or 3 consecutive weekly cultures are negative.
- Duration of treatment depends on time required to replace infected skin, hair, or nails and thus varies with infection site. Average duration of treatment for tinea capitis (scalp ringworm) is 4 to 6 weeks; tinea corporis (body ringworm), 2 to 4 weeks; tinea pedis (athlete's foot), 4 to 8 weeks; tinea unguium (nail fungus), at least 4 months for fingernails, depending on rate of growth, and 6 months or more for toenails.
- Caution patient to avoid exposure to intense natural or artificial sunlight, because photosensitivity-type reactions may occur.
- Warn patient of possible reaction (tachycardia, flushing) on ingestion of alcohol during therapy.
- Emphasize importance of cleanliness and keeping skin dry (moist skin favours growth of fungi). For athlete's foot, advise patient to wear well-ventilated shoes without rubber soles, to alternate shoes, and to change socks daily. Physician may prescribe a drying powder as necessary. *See index: nursing interventions: fungal infection.*

Drug interactions   Griseofulvin may potentiate the effects of **alcohol**. Activity of griseofulvin may be diminished by **barbiturates** (cause reduction of griseofulvin serum levels). In some patients, griseofulvin may decrease the hypoprothrombinaemic effects of **warfarin** and possibly other **oral anticoagulants**. Close monitoring of prothrombin time is advised when griseofulvin is added to or withdrawn from anticoagulant drug regimen.

Guanethidine

(Ganda, Ismelin)   *Adrenergic blocking agent;
                                             antihypertensive*

ACTIONS AND USES   Potent, long-acting, postganglionic adrenergic blocking agent. Local instillation in eye causes miosis and reduces intraocular pressure in glaucomatous eyes.

Used to treat moderate to severe hypertension either alone or in conjunction with a thiazide diuretic and to treat glaucoma.

ROUTE AND DOSAGE   Adults: Oral: 20 mg/day increased by 10 mg each week to a maximum of 100 mg/day. *Occular*: insert drops 1–2 times a day.

GUANETHIDINE (continued)

ABSORPTION AND FATE   Irregularly absorbed from GI tract (3 to 30% variability in absorption rate, but rate remains constant for each individual).

CONTRAINDICATIONS AND PRECAUTIONS   Hypersensitivity to guanethidine; pheochromocytoma, frank congestive heart failure (not due to hypertension). Safe use during pregnancy and in women of childbearing potential not established. **Cautious Use:** diabetes mellitus, impaired renal or hepatic function, sinus bradycardia, limited cardiac reserve, coronary disease with insufficiency, recent myocardial infarction, cerebrovascular insufficiency, febrile illnesses, use in the elderly; history of peptic ulcer, colitis, or bronchial asthma.

ADVERSE/SIDE EFFECTS   These include: marked orthostatic and exertional hypotension with dizziness, light-headedness, fainting, bradycardia, angina oedema with weight gain, dyspnoea, congestive heart failure, complete heart block, skin eruptions, loss of scalp hair, blurred vision, ptosis of eyelids, parotid tenderness, nasal congestion, severe diarrhoea, nausea, vomiting, constipation, dry mouth, nocturia, urinary retention, incontinence, inhibition of ejaculation, psychological impotence.

NURSING IMPLICATIONS
- Tablet may be crushed before administration and taken with fluid of patient's choice.
- To reinforce patient compliance in taking drug regularly at the same time each day, suggest that it be taken to coincide with some routine activity such as brushing teeth in the morning. Stress importance of not stopping drug without advice of physician.
- During period of dosage adjustment, doses must be carefully titrated on the basis of orthostatic and supine blood pressures. The hypotensive effect of guanethidine is greater with patient in orthostatic position as opposed to supine position. Take readings before initiation of therapy as baseline for comparison. Blood pressure should be taken first in supine position and then again after patient has been standing for 10 minutes.
- Since hospitalized patients are given higher initial doses than ambulatory patients, standing blood pressure determinations should be made regularly during the day, if possible. The full effect of guanethidine on standing blood pressure should be carefully evaluated before patient is discharged.
- Caution patient not to get out of bed without assistance. Supervise ambulation particularly in the elderly since they are prone to develop orthostatic hypotension.
- Patients should be informed that orthostatic hypotension is most prominent shortly after arising from sleep and when too rapid changes are made to sitting or upright positions. Warn patients to move gradually to sitting position.
- Fluid intake and output should be monitored especially in the elderly and in patients with limited cardiac reserve or impaired renal function.
- Advise the patient to report character and frequency of stools. Diarrhoea due to accelerated GI motility may be manifested by increased frequency of bowel movements rather than loose stools and may be explosive and embarrassing to patient. Physician may prescribe an anticholinergic agent (e.g., atropine), or a kaolin preparation. Dosage adjustment or discontinuation of drug may be required. State of hydra-

G

GUANETHIDINE (continued)

tion and electrolyte levels should be checked in patients with severe and persistent diarrhoea.

- Patients with limited cardiac reserve are particularly susceptible to guanethidine-induced sodium and water retention, with resulting oedema, congestive failure, and drug resistance (a thiazide diuretic is generally prescribed to reduce the possibility of these effects).

- Observe for evidence of oedema, and weigh patients under standard conditions: same time (preferably in the morning before breakfast and after voiding), same weight of clothing, same scale. Sudden weight gain of 2 lb/1 kg or more should be reported to physician.

- Consult physician regarding allowable salt intake. Generally, patients are advised to omit obviously salty foods and to avoid adding salt to served foods. Physician may prescribe greater restriction of sodium-containing foods for patients with limited cardiac reserve.

- Because guanethidine has prolonged onset and duration of action and since its effects are cumulative, dosage should be increased slowly and only if there has been no reduction in standing blood pressure from previous levels. Blood pressure should be monitored during dosage adjustment period.

- A limited degree of tolerance may develop early in therapy. Dosage plateau is usually reached in 2 weeks.

- Ideal dosage is that which reduces orthostatic blood pressure to within normal range without faintness, dizziness, weakness, or fatigue.

- Dosage requirements may be reduced in presence of febrile illnesses. Advise patient to report fever to physician.

- Guanethidine may sensitize the patient to some sympathomimetic agents found in OTC cold remedies and cause hypertensive crisis. Caution patient to consult physician or pharmacist before taking any OTC drug.

- Guanethidine is reported to have antidiabetic activity (mechanism unknown). Patients on antidiabetic therapy should be observed closely for signs of hypoglycemia.

- Patient must understand that although hypertension is usually an asymptomatic disease, it can result in a variety of serious complications if untreated.

- Periodic blood counts and liver and kidney function tests are advised during prolonged therapy.

- In patients undergoing elective surgery, manufacturer recommends that if possible guanethidine be withdrawn 2 weeks prior to surgery to reduce the possibility of vascular collapse and cardiac arrest during anaesthesia. (This point is controversial. Some clinicians believe it is both unnecessary and potentially dangerous to withdraw antihypertensive before anaesthesia.) If emergency surgery is indicated, preanaesthetic and anaesthetic agents should be administered cautiously in reduced dosages.

Patient-teaching plan for patient with hypertension

- ☐ Knowledge of the medical problem.
- ☐ Drug action (reason for taking drug).
- ☐ Dosage regimen.
- ☐ Importance of keeping follow-up appointments.

GUANETHIDINE (continued)
- □ Symptoms to be reported.
- □ Diet restrictions, if prescribed (e.g., salt regulation).
- □ Weight control plans.
- □ Importance of limiting alcohol intake and avoiding tobacco, and excessive caffeine (coffee, tea, and colas), as well as emotionally charged situations.
- □ Dangers of self-medication.
- □ Importance of planned graduated exercise programme.
- □ Importance of hobbies and regular vacations.
- □ Continual reinforcement of the potential need for life-long therapy.

■ Store in well-closed container at room temperature unless otherwise directed by manufacturer.

Diagnostic test interferences Guanethidine may increase **BUN**, decrease **blood glucose** (in patients with diabetes mellitus), and may decrease **urinary noradrenaline** excretion and **urinary VMA** excretion.

DRUG INTERACTIONS *Guanethidine*

PLUS	INTERACTIONS
Alcohol, ethyl Levodopa Rauwolfia derivatives Thiazides and related diuretics	Enhance hypotensive effects of guanethidine. Used with caution
Amphetamines Antidepressants, tricyclic Cocaine Diethylpropion Doxepin Ephedrine Haloperidol MAO inhibitors Oral contraceptives Phenothiazines Dopamine	Inhibit antihypertensive effect of guanethidine
Adrenaline Metaraminol Phenylephrine	Guanethidine may augment pressor response to direct-acting alpha-adrenergic sympathomimetic amines
Anaesthetics, general	Increased risk of cardiovascular collapse and cardiac arrest
Antidiabetic agents	Enhanced hypoglycaemic effect
Digitalis glycosides	Additive bradycardic effect

Halcinonide

(Halciderm)   *Corticosteroid*

HALCINONIDE (continued)

ACTIONS AND USES   Fluorinated steroid with substituted 17-hydroxyl group. Crosses cell membranes, complexes with nuclear DNA and stimulates synthesis of enzymes thought to be responsible for antiinflammatory effects. Systemic absorption leads to actions, limitations and drug interactions observed with use of hydrocortisone (q.v.). Topical action, and limitations are similar to those of flurandrenolide (q.v.).

Used for relief of pruritic and inflammatory manifestations of corticosteroid-responsive dermatoses.

ROUTE AND DOSAGE   Topical: Cream, 0.1% applied two or three times daily.

NURSING IMPLICATIONS

- Check with physician regarding specific procedure. Generally, skin is gently washed and thoroughly dried before each application.
- Medication should be discontinued if signs of infection or irritation occur.
- Not to be applied in or around the eyes.
- Systemic corticosteroid effects may be produced when occlusive dressings are used and when topical application covers large areas of skin.
- For further information: *see hydrocortisone.*

Haloperidol ▄▄▄▄▄▄▄▄▄▄▄▄▄▄▄▄▄▄▄▄▄▄▄▄▄▄▄▄▄▄▄▄▄▄▄

(Haldol, Serenace)   *Antipsychotic; neuroleptic;*
                                                            butyrophenone

ACTIONS AND USES   Potent, long-acting butyrophenone derivative with pharmacological actions similar to those of piperazine phenothiazines but with higher incidence of extrapyramidal effects, less hypotensive, and relatively low sedative activity. Exerts strong antiemetic effect, and impairs central thermoregulation. Produces weak central anticholinergic effects and transient orthostatic hypotension. Actions thought to be due to blockade of dopamine activity.

Used for management of manifestations of psychotic disorders and in acute and chronic psychoses.

ROUTE AND DOSAGE   *Highly individualized.* Maintenance dose established at lowest effective level. **Oral: Adult:** 1.5–20 mg in divided doses increased gradually to 100 mg/day. Maximum 200 mg/day. **Child:** 25–50 mcg/kg/day increased to a maximum of 10 mg/day. **Adolescent:** up to 30 mg. **Intramuscular:** 2–10 mg increased to 30 mg in emergency, then 5 mg/hr as required.

ABSORPTION AND FATE   Well absorbed from GI tract. **Peak plasma levels:** 2 to 6 hours following oral administration and 20 minutes following IM administration. Blood levels may plateau for as long as 72 hours, with detectable levels persisting for weeks. Metabolized in liver to inactive metabolites. Serum protein binding more than 90%. **Elimination half-life:** 13 to 35 hours. Approximately 40% excreted in urine

H

HALOPERIDOL (continued)

during first 5 days; about 15% excreted in bile (then faeces). Small amounts continue to be excreted for 28 days. Crosses placenta; appears in breast milk.

CONTRAINDICATIONS AND PRECAUTIONS Hypersensitivity to haloperidol, Parkinson's disease, seizure disorders, coma, alcoholism, severe mental depression, CNS depression, thyrotoxicosis. Safe use during pregnancy and in women of childbearing potential, in nursing mothers, and in children under 3 years not established. **Cautious Use**: history of drug allergies, elderly or debilitated patients, urinary retention, glaucoma, severe cardiovascular disorders; patients receiving anticonvulsant, anticoagulant or lithium therapy.

ADVERSE/SIDE EFFECTS These include: dry mouth; hypersalivation, 'drooling,' constipation, diarrhoea, urinary retention, diaphoresis, blurred vision, extrapyramidal reactions: parkinson-like symptoms, dystonia, akathisia, tardive dyskinesia (rarely); insomnia, restlessness, anxiety, euphoria, agitation, drowsiness, mental depression, lethargy, headache, confusion, vertigo, hyperthermia, grand mal seizures, exacerbation of psychotic symptoms, tachycardia, hypotension, hypertension (with overdosage), maculopapular and acneiform rash, menstrual irregularities, galactorrhoea, lactation, gynaecomastia, impotence, increased libido, hyperglycaemia, hypoglycaemia, mild and usually transient leucopenia, leucocytosis, anaemia, tendency toward lymphomonocytosis, laryngospasm, bronchospasm, increased depth of respiration, bronchopneumonia, respiratory depression, anorexia, nausea, vomiting, jaundice (occasionally), ocular and cutaneous changes, variations in liver function tests, decreased serum cholesterol, 'therapeutic window' effect.

NURSING IMPLICATIONS

- Preliminary reports suggest that haloperidol concentrate may precipitate when mixed with coffee or with tea; avoid these beverages as diluents and administer oral forms of the drug with some other fluid.
- Because of long half-life of haloperidol, therapeutic effects are slow to develop in early therapy or when established dosing regimen is changed.
- Once the neuroleptic plan is established, monitor patient's mental status daily: appearance and general behaviour, though content, affect and mood, sensorium.
- Target symptoms expected to decrease with successful haloperidol treatment include: hallucinations, insomnia, hostility, agitation, and delusions. If no improvement in 2 to 4 weeks, medication may be increased.
- Psychotic exacerbation at the beginning of therapy has been reported. Increasing the dosage may produce improvement.
- 'Therapeutic window' effect (point at which increased dose or concentration actually decreases therapeutic response) may occur after long period of high doses. Close observation is imperative when doses are changed.
- Although orthostatic hypotension is not common, take necessary safety precautions. Have patient recumbent at time of parenteral administration and for about 1 hour following injection (levarterenol or phenylephrine is prescribed when a vasopressor is indicated; epinephrine is contraindicated).
- Extrapyramidal reactions (*see chlorpromazine*) occur frequently during first few days

H

HALOPERIDOL (continued)

of treatment. Symptoms are usually dose-related and are controlled by dosage reduction or concomitant administration of antiparkinsonian drugs. Discontinuation of therapy may be necessary. Reactions appear to be more prominent in younger patients.

- Be alert for behavioural changes in patients who are concurrently receiving antiparkinsonian drugs (e.g., benztropine, benzhexol). Such medication may have to be continued beyond termination of haloperidol therapy to prevent extrapyramidal symptoms which may appear during the period when haloperidol levels are decreasing (3 to 4 days).
- Haloperidol is administered cautiously to patients receiving anticonvulsant medication because it may lower the convulsant threshold. The established dose of the anticonvulsant is not changed.
- When haloperidol is used to control mania or cyclic disorders, the patient should be closely observed for rapid mood shift to depression. Depression may represent a drug side effect or a reversion from a manic state.
- Differential diagnosis between extrapyramidal side effects and psychotic reaction requires sensitive observation and prompt reporting.
- Fatal bronchospasm associated with use of antipsychotics has been postulated to result from drug-induced lethargy, reduced sensation of thirst, dehydration, haemoconcentration, and reduced ventilation. Adequate fluid intake and regularly scheduled breathing exercises may help to prevent its occurrence.
- Protect patient from extremes in environmental temperature.
- Alcohol should be avoided during haloperidol therapy.
- Caution against use of OTC drugs without physician's approval.
- Patient should not change dosing regimen. Tell patient not to give drug to any other person.
- Ambulatory patients and responsible family members should be completely informed about what symptoms to report and the importance of follow-up appointments.
- Advise patient not to drive a car or engage in other activities requiring mental alertness and physical coordination until drug response is known.
- Dosing regimen should be tapered when therapy is to be discontinued. Abrupt termination of treatment can initiate extrapyramidal symptoms.
- If patient suspects pregnancy or wants to be pregnant, she should discuss drug regimen with her physician. Sporadic case reports suggest that haloperidol is teratogenic during the first trimester.
- Xerostomia may promote dental problems. Deprivation of saliva fosters demineralization of normal tooth surfaces and loosening of dentures. Discuss oral hygiene with patient. (See chlorpromazine.) Encourage adequate fluid intake.
- Patient on home therapy should be told what laxative may be used if necessary.
- Periodic blood studies and liver function tests are advised in patients on prolonged therapy.
- Discard darkened solutions; slight yellowing does not affect potency, however.
- Store in light-resistant container at temperature between 15° and 30°C (59° and 86°F) unless otherwise specified by manufacturer.
- See chlorpromazine.

H

HALOPERIDOL (continued)
DRUG INTERACTIONS   *Haloperidol*

PLUS	INTERACTIONS
Alcohol	Enhanced CNS depressant effects; hypotension
Amphetamines	Haloperidol antagonizes effects of amphetamines
Anticholinergic agents	Increased intraocular pressure and may inhibit haloperidol effects
Anticonvulsants	Haloperidol lowers convulsive threshold
Anticoagulants	Interference with anticoagulant activity (based on limited data)
Antiparkinson agents	Increased intraocular pressure
CNS depressants	Additive depressant activity
Guanethidine	Reversal of hypotensive action
Lithium	Possibility of encephalopathy (extrapyramidal symptoms, fever, confusion)
Methyldopa	Possibility of dementia

See also chlorpromazine

Heparin ▬▬▬▬▬▬▬▬▬▬▬▬▬▬▬▬▬▬▬▬

(Calciparine, Monoparin, Multiparin, Pump-Hep,   *Anticoagulant*
   Unihep, Minihep, Uniparin, Hep-Flush, Hepsal)

ACTIONS AND USES   Strongly acidic, high molecular weight mucopolysaccharide with rapid anticoagulant effect, prepared from bovine lung tissue or porcine intestinal mucosa. Does not lyse already existing thrombi, but may prevent their extension and propagation. Inhibits formation of new clots. Prolongs whole blood clotting time, thrombin time, partial thromboplastin time and prothrombin time, but bleeding time (test of platelet function) is usually unaffected except with high doses. Reduces plasma triglycerides (antilipemic action), exhibits antiinflammatory and diuretic effects, and may suppress aldosterone secretion.

Used in the prophylaxis and treatment of venous thrombosis and pulmonary embolism, and to prevent thromboembolic complications arising from cardiac and vascular surgery, frostbite, and during acute stage of myocardial infarction. Also used in treatment of disseminated intravascular clotting syndrome and as anticoagulant in blood transfusions, extracorporeal circulation, dialysis procedures and to maintain the patency of catheters and cannulas.

ROUTE AND DOSAGE   IV: loading dose 5,000 units then 40,000 units by continuous infusion over 24 hours or 10,000 units every 6 hrs. **Subcutaneous:** *prophylactic*, 5,000 units pre-surgery then 12 hourly until ambulant. By continuous infusion 5,000 units over 8–12 hours. *Catheter patency*: (10 and 100 unit/ml preparation) flush as required.

H

HEPARIN (continued)

ABSORPTION AND FATE   Peak effects within minutes following direct IV injection; clotting time returns to normal within 2 to 6 hours. **Onset of action following SC** occurs within 20 to 60 minutes, (wide interpatient variation), **duration of effects**: 8 to 12 hours (dose dependent). Absorption following IM is unpredictable. **Plasma half-life**: 1½ hours (possibly shorter in patients with pulmonary embolism infections, or malignancy and longer in hepatic or renal dysfunction, and obesity). About 95% bound to plasma proteins. Some uptake and storage in mast cells. Believed to be partially metabolized by reticuloendothelial system and heparinase in liver. Excreted slowly in urine as partially degraded heparin; 20 to 50% of single dose excreted unchanged. Unlike oral anticoagulants, heparin does not cross the placenta (because of its large molecular size) and does not appear in breast milk.

CONTRAINDICATIONS AND PRECAUTIONS   Hypersensitivity to heparin, active bleeding, bleeding tendencies (haemophilia, purpura, thrombocytopenia), jaundice, ascorbic acid deficiency, inaccessible ulcerative lesions, visceral carcinoma, open wounds, extensive denudation of skin, suppurative thrombophlebitis, advanced kidney, liver or biliary disease, active tuberculosis, subacute bacterial endocarditis, continuous tube drainage of stomach or small intestines, threatened abortion, suspected intracranial haemorrhage, severe hypertension, recent surgery of eye, brain or spinal cord, spinal tap, shock. Teratogenic potential or safe use in persons of childbearing age not established. **Cautious Use**: alcoholism, history of atopy or allergy (asthma, hives, hay fever, eczema), during menstruation, during pregnancy especially the last trimester, immediate postpartum period, patients with indwelling urinary catheters, the elderly, patients in hazardous occupations.

ADVERSE/SIDE EFFECTS   Spontaneous bleeding, injection site reactions: pain, itching, ecchymoses, tissue irritation and sloughing, cyanosis and pains in arms or legs (vasospasm), diarrhoea, transient thrombocytopenia, hypofibrinogenaemia. Rarely, frequent and persistent erections (priapism), **hypersensitivity** reactions: fever, chills, urticaria, pruritus, skin rashes, itching and burning sensations of feet, numbness and tingling of hands and feet, elevated blood pressure, headache, reversible transient alopecia (usually around temporal area), nasal congestion, lacrimation, conjunctivities, chest pains, arthralgia, bronchospasm, anaphylactoid reactions. **Large doses for prolonged periods**: osteoporosis (back or rib pain, decrease in height, spontaneous fractures), hypoaldosteronism, suppressed renal function, hyperkalaemia. Rebound hyperlipaemia (following termination of heparin therapy).

NURSING IMPLICATIONS

- Read label carefully. Heparin comes in various strengths.
- Baseline blood coagulation tests, Hgb, red blood cell, and platelet counts should be performed before therapy is initiated, at regular intervals throughout therapy, and whenever patient shows signs of bleeding.
- Before administering heparin, coagulation (clotting) test results must be checked by physician; if results are not within therapeutic range, dosage adjustment is made. Because heparin has short half-life it must be given on time to maintain anticoagulant effect. Follow hospital protocol for administration of heparin.

H

HEPARIN (continued)

- *Suggested technique and general guidelines for deep SC intrafat injection:*
(1) Injections are made preferably into the fatty layer of the abdomen or just above the iliac crest. Shallow SC injection should be avoided because it is more painful and is associated with higher risk of haematoma and shorter duration of effect. (2) Use 1 ml syringe for accuracy in measuring dose, and a 25 or 26 gauge, ½ to ⅝ inch needle to make injection. (3) Discard needle use to withdraw heparin from vial. (4) Clean selected site with alcohol and allow to dry. Do not massage (rubbing can rupture small blood vessels). (5) Avoid injecting within 2 inches of umbilicus, or any scar or bruise. Gently bunch up a defined roll of tissue without pinching, and insert needle into tissue roll at a 90° angle to skin. Still maintaining hold of tissue but with slightly less pressure, and keeping needle steady, slowly inject drug. To avoid possibility of tissue injury and haematoma *do not withdraw plunger to check entry into blood vessel.* (6) Hesitate for a few seconds before withdrawing needle to prevent trailing drug through needle tract. Withdraw needle rapidly in same direction as introduced while simultaneously releasing tissue hold. (7) Apply gentle pressure to puncture site for about 1 minute, but do not massage. Application of ice following injection may help the patient who bruises easily. (8) Systematically rotate injection sites and keep record.

- When heparin is added to an infusion solution (by authorized person), manufacturer recommends inverting container at least 6 times to insure adequate mixing and to prevent pooling of heparin.

- Continuous IV infusion of heparin requires close monitoring to assure accuracy is dosage. A constant infusion pump or other approved volume control unit should be used to regulate flow rate and fluid volume. Gravity flow is not recommended because it is difficult to regulate and is subject to significant variations in flow rate when patient changes position.

- Observe all needle sites daily for haematoma and signs of inflammation (swelling, heat, redness, pain).

- Administration of heparin or any other drug IM is usually not prescribed because of risk of heaematoma. If an IM drug is ordered, its administration should be timed when patient has minimal prolongation of coagulation time. This also pertains to invasive procedures, e.g., catheterizations, enemas.

- It is critically important to make accurate observations of clinical response.

- Patients vary widely in their reaction to heparin and no test can reliably predict bleeding.

- Document coagulation times and heparin doses in nursing records. The risk of haemorrhage appears to be greatest in women, all patients 70 years of age or older, patients receiving heparin prophylactically following surgery, and patients with renal insufficiency.

- Monitor vital signs. Report pyrexia drop in blood pressure, rapid pulse, and other signs and symptoms of haemorrhage. *Inform patient without frightening him or her to avoid injury and to report*: pink, red, dark brown, or cloudy urine (haematuria); red or dark brown vomitus (haematemesis); constipation (paralytic, ileus, intestinal obstruction); red or black stools, bleeding gums or oral mucosa: petechiae of soft palate, conjunctiva, and retina (characteristic signs of thrombocytopenia); ecchymoses, haematoma, purpura, epistaxis, bloody sputum; chest pain (haemoperi-

HEPARIN (continued)

cardium), abdominal or lumbar pain or swelling (retroperitoneal bleeding); unusual increase in menstrual flow, pelvic pain (corpus luteum haemorrhage); severe or continuous headache, faintness, or dizziness (intracranial bleeding). *Antidote*: have on hand protamine sulphate (1% solution), specific heparin antagonist. Because heparin has a short half-life, mild overdosage can frequently be controlled by merely withdrawing heparin. In some cases, however, whole blood or plasma transfusion may be necessary.

- Menstruation may be somewhat increased and prolonged. Usually this is not a contraindication to continued therapy if bleeding is not excessive, and patient has no underlying pathology.
- Monitor fluid intake and output during early therapy. Inform patient that heparin may have a diuretic effect beginning 36 to 48 hours after initial dose and lasting 36 to 48 hours after termination of therapy.
- In the absence of a low platelet (thrombocyte) count, patient may carry out normal activities such as shaving with a safety razor. Usually, heparin does not affect bleeding time.
- Transient alopecia sometimes occurs several months after heparin therapy. Reassure patient that condition is reversible.
- *Smoking and alcohol consumption* may alter response to heparin and, therefore, are not advised. Also, caution patient not to take aspirin, antihistamines, or any other OTC medication without physician's approval.
- 'Heparin resistance' has occurred in conditions associated with large amounts of fibrin deposition, such as early stage of thrombophlebitis, peritonitis, fever, pleurisy, cancer, myocardial infarction, extensive surgery.
- Abrupt withdrawal of heparin may precipitate increased coagulability; generally, full dose heparin is followed by oral anticoagulant prophylactic therapy.
- Administration of an oral anticoagulant usually overlaps that of heparin for 3 to 5 days while heparin is being tapered off. To obtain valid prothrombin time, a period of at least 4 to 6 hours after last IV dose, and 12 to 24 hours after the last SC (intrafat) dose of heparin should elapse before blood is drawn. Blood samples are usually drawn at any time when heparin is administered by continuous IV infusion.
- *Heparin lock flush solution* (e.g., Hep-Flush) is a sterile heparin-saline solution for intravenous flush only. It is not *intended for therapeutic purposes*. Follow local policy regarding its use. In general, heparin lock care procedure reflects the following:
  □ A prescription is required for use of heparin lock flush solution and the order must be renewed according to a specific policy.
  □ Heparin lock flush solution is commonly used to maintain the patency of central venous catheters, femoral, and dialysis catheters. Heparinized flushing is not indicated when patency is maintained by continuous IV drip, nor is it generally used to maintain patency of short catheters as used in primary line or intermittent infusion sets.
  □ Each injection part of a multiple lumen catheter should be treated and recorded as a separate procedure.
  □ Refer to literature issued by manufacturer of the particular heparin lock set being used for detailed instructions.
  □ It is generally considered good practice to flush a heparin-lock set with 1 or 2 ml

H

HEPARIN (continued)

of normal saline before and after a medication is administered to avoid the possibility or drug interactions. If heparin lock flush solution is prescribed it is introduced following the second saline flush.

- Since heparin is strongly acidic, it is incompatible with many drugs; therefore, avoid mixing any drug with heparin unless specifically advised by physician or pharmacist.
- Heparin is stable at room temperature 15° to 30°C (59° to 86°F). Protect from freezing. Inspect all preparations for discolouration and particulate matter prior to administration.

Diagnostic test interferences   (Notify laboratory that patient is receiving heparin, if a laboratory test is to be performed.) Possibility of: false-positive rise in **BSP** test; reduction in **serum cholesterol**; significant elevations of **SGOT (AST)**, **SGPT (ALT)**; false increase in **plasma corticosteroids** (with heparin containing benzyl alcohol); reportedly may increase **blood glucose**; may decrease urinary excretion of **5-HIAA**; and may interfere with thyroid function tests (elevations of *serum free thyroxin* and **resin T$_3$ uptake**), **LE cell test**, and direct **Coombs' test** (in patients with haemolytic aneamia).

DRUG INTERACTIONS   *Heparin sodium*_____

PLUS	INTERACTIONS
Anticoagulants, oral	Heparin (especially IV bolus doses) may prolong prothrombin time used to monitor oral anticoagulant therapy
Antihistamines Aspirin other NSAIDs, and selected salicylates	May partially antagonize anticoagulant action of heparin; increased risk of haemorrhage due to inhibition of platelet adhesiveness and aggregation; potentially ulcerogenic
Contraceptives, oral	Oestrogen-containing contraceptives may reduce concentration of antithrombin III and thus paradoxically may increase thrombotic tendency
Corticotropin	Potentially ulcerogenic; increased risk of haemorrhage
Digitalis glycosides	May partially antagonize anticoagulant action of heparin
Dextran Dipyridamole Ethacrynic acid Glucocorticoids Hydrochloroquine Indomethacin Ibuprofen Mefenamic acid Oxyphenbutazone Phenylbutazone Probenecid	Increased risk of haemorrhage due to inhibition of platelet adhesiveness and aggregation; potentially ulcerogenic
Carbimazole Propylthiouracil	Enhanced anticoagulant effect because of hypoprothrombinaemic effect of thiomide antithyroid agents
Protamine	Antagonizes anticoagulant action of heparin; used as heparin antidote
Quinine	Increased risk of haemorrhage due to inhibition of platelet aggregation

H

HEPARIN (continued)

Streptokinase Tetracyclines } Urokinase	May partially antagonize anticoagulant action of heparin

Homatropine hydrobromide

(Minims)

*Anticholinergic (ophthalmic);
antimuscarinic mydriatic*

ACTIONS AND USES   Synthetic alkaloid with actions, contraindications, precautions, and adverse reactions similar to those of atropine (q.v.). Preferred to atropine for certain ophthalmological purposes because its mydriatic and cycloplegic actions occur more rapidly and are less prolonged. Cycloplegia is usually incomplete unless applications are made repeatedly.

Used as mydriatic for ocular examination and as cycloplegic to measure errors of refraction. Also used in treatment of inflammatory conditions of uveal tract, ciliary spasm and as cycloplegic and mydriatic in preoperative and postoperative conditions.

ROUTE AND DOSAGE   Topical: 1 or 2 drops of 1 to 5% solution instilled in eye up to every 3 or 4 hours. For refraction: 1 or 2 drops of 2 to 5% solution; repeat in 5 to 10 minutes if necessary.

For further information: *see atropine sulphate.*

ABSORPTION AND FATE   Following instillation, maximal paralysis of accommodation and mydriatic effects occur in 30 to 60 minutes, with recovery in 1 to 3 days.

CONTRAINDICATIONS AND PRECAUTIONS   Hypersensitivity; narrow-angle glaucoma; children under 6 years of age. **Cautious Use**: increased intraocular pressure, infants, children, the elderly, hypertension, hyperthyroidism, diabetes. *See also* atropine.

ADVERSE/SIDE EFFECTS   Increased intraocular pressure. **With prolonged use**: local irritation, congestion, oedema, eczema, follicular conjunctivitis. **Excessive dosage**: symptoms of atropine poisoning. *See atropine.*

Hyaluronidase

(Hylase)

Enzyme

H

ACTIONS AND USES   Mucolytic enzyme prepared from purified bovine testicular hyaluronidase. Hydrolyzes hyaluronic acid, which normally obstructs intercellular

HYALURONIDASE (continued)

diffusion of invasive substances. Promotes diffusion and consequently absorption of transudates, exudates, and injected fluids.

Used to enhance dispersion and absorption of other injected drugs; used for hypodermoclysis, and as adjunct in subcutaneous urography for improving resorption of radiopaque agents.

ROUTE AND DOSAGE   *For absorption and dispersion of injected drugs*: 150 units added to other drug solution. **Subcutaneous injection**: 1,500 units administered in 500–1,000 ml of injection fluid.

CONTRAINDICATIONS AND PRECAUTIONS   Injection into or around inflamed, infected, or cancerous areas; congestive heart failure; hypoproteinaemia.

ADVERSE/SIDE EFFECTS   Infrequent: sensitivity, spread of infectious processes, overhydration.

NURSING IMPLICATIONS
- Preliminary skin test for sensitivity is advised.
- Addition of hyaluronidase to hypodermoclyses may promote overhydration because it speeds water absorption. Infusion flow rate should be prescribed by physician. Patient should be closely monitored.
- When it is used to increase diffusion of a drug, bear in mind that absorption will be enhanced. Therefore, watch for adverse reactions and expect a shorter duration of drug action.
- Lyophilized form is unstable in solution and therefore is reconstituted with sodium chloride injection just before use (usually in the proportion of 1 ml per 150 units of hyaluronidase).

Hydralazine hydrochloride ────────────────

(Apresoline)   *Antihypertensive; vasodilator, peripheral*

ACTIONS AND USES   Reduces blood pressure by direct relaxation of vascular smooth muscles, with greater effect on arterioles than on veins. Diastolic response is often greater than systolic. Resulting vasodilation reduces peripheral vascular resistance and increases renal and cerebral blood flow. Has little effect on capacitance blood vessels. Antihypertensive effect may be limited by sympathetic reflexes, which cause increased heart rate, stroke volume, and cardiac output. Postural hypotensive effect is reportedly less than that produced by ganglionic blocking agents. Usually increases plasma renin activity.

Used to treat mild to moderate hypertension usually in combination with a beta-blocking drug or diuretic.

ROUTE AND DOSAGE   Adults: Oral: *Initial*: 25 mg twice a day increased to a maxi-

HYDRALAZINE HYDROCHLORIDE (continued)

mum of 50 mg twice a day. **IV**: slow injection 5–20 mg over 20 minutes (maximum 40 mg). Infusion: 20–40 mg repeated as required.

ABSORPTION AND FATE Following oral administration, onset of action in 20 to 30 minutes. Peak plasma concentration within 2 hours; duration: 2 to 4 hours. Blood pressure begins to fall within 5 to 20 minutes following IV injection; maximal effect in 10 to 80 minutes, and lasts 2 to 6 hours. Approximately 85% bound to plasma proteins. **Half-life**: 2 to 8 hours. Extensively metabolized in intestinal wall and liver primarily by acetylation (rate of which is genetically determined). Rapidly excreted in urine, primarily as metabolites. Excretion rate greatest between 2 and 10 hours. About 10% of oral dose excreted in faeces.

CONTRAINDICATIONS AND PRECAUTIONS Hypersensitivity to hydralazine, coronary artery disease, mitral valvular rheumatic heart disease, myocardial infarction, tachycardia, lupus erythematosus. Safe use during pregnancy not established. **Cautious Use**: cerebrovascular accident, advanced renal impairment, use with MAO inhibitors.

ADVERSE/SIDE EFFECTS These include: headache, dizziness, peripheral neuritis, paraesthesias, tremors, psychotic reactions (depression, anxiety, disorientation), palpitation, angina, tachycardia; less frequent: flushing, orthostatic hypotension, paradoxical pressor response, arrhythmias, profound shock (overdosage), lacrimation, conjunctivitis, nasal congestion, anorexia, nausea, vomiting, diarrhoea; less frequent: constipation, paralytic ileus, difficulty in urination, reduced haemoglobin and RBCs, leucopenia, agranulocytosis, purpura, rash, urticaria, pruritus, fever, chills, arthralgia, eosinophilia, obstructive jaundice, muscle cramps, lymphadenopathy, splenomegaly; sweating (common), rheumatoid or SLE-like syndrome, fixed drug eruption, sodium retention and oedema (long-term therapy).

NURSING IMPLICATIONS
- Reportedly two or three times as much hydralazine enters the general circulation when it is taken with food (food reduces first-pass metabolism of drug in the intestinal wall). It is advisable to be consistent in taking drug either with meals or on an empty stomach to minimize fluctuations in blood levels.
- Observe mental status; note anxiety, depression, obtundation (signs of cerebral ischaemia from too rapid reduction in blood pressure).
- Blood pressure should be closely monitored in patients receiving parenteral hydralazine. Check every 5 minutes until stabilized at desired level, then every 15 minutes thereafter throughout hypertensive crisis.
- A marked fall in blood pressure may further compromise renal blood flow in patients with renal damage and result in reduced urinary output.
- Fluid intake and output should be monitored when drug is given parenterally and in those with renal dysfunction. Output may be increased in some patients because of improved renal blood flow.
- Instruct patient to monitor weight and to check for oedema. Advise patient to report sudden gain or apparent slow increase in weight, and the onset of oedema. Sodium retention has occurred with long-term use.
- Refer to a dietician for dietary management: allowable salt intake; weight control.

H

HYDRALAZINE HYDROCHLORIDE (continued)

- Most patients receiving parenteral hydralazine are transferred to oral form within 24 to 48 hours.
- Some patients experience headache and palpitation within 2 to 4 hours after first oral dose. Symptoms usually subside spontaneously. Advise patients to inform physician of adverse reactions; most can be controlled by dose reduction.
- Physician may prescribe pyridoxine (vitamin B_6) prophylactically or when patient develops symptoms of peripheral neuritis (paraesthesias, numbness). This complication is believed to result from antipyridoxine effect of hydralazine.
- Because of the possibility of postural hypotension, caution patients to make position changes slowly, particularly from lying to sitting position and from sitting to standing, and to avoid standing still, taking hot baths and showers, strenuous exercise, and excessive alcohol intake.
- Caution patient to lie down or sit down (in head-low position) if feeling faint or dizzy. Patients who engage in potentially hazardous activities such as driving or operating machinery should be advised of the possibility of these symptoms.
- Withdrawal of hydralazine should be accomplished gradually to avoid sudden rise in pressure and heart failure. Patients should be informed of the dangers of sudden withdrawal.
- An LE cell preparation is indicated if patient manifests arthralgia, fever, chest pain, malaise, or other unexplained signs and symptoms.
- Stress the importance of follow-up care. Some patients develop tolerance during chronic drug administration requiring higher dosages or a change in drug regimen.
- Store preferably at 15° to 30°C (59° to 86°F) in tight, light-resistant containers, unless otherwise directed by manufacturer. Avoid freezing.
- *See guanethidine for summary of teaching points for patients with hypertension.*

Diagnostic test interferences   Positive **direct Coombs' tests** in patients with hydralazine-induced SLE. Hydralazine interferes with urinary **17-OHCS** determinations (modified Glenn–Nelson technique).

DRUG INTERACTIONS   *Hydralazine*_____

PLUS	INTERACTIONS
Diazoxide and other potent antihypertensives	Severe additive hypotensive effect
Diuretics } MAO inhibitors }	Potentiation of antihypertensive action

Hydrochlorothiazide▬▬▬▬▬▬▬▬▬▬▬▬▬▬▬

(Esidrex, Hydrosaluric)   *Diuretic; antihypertensive; thiazide*

ACTIONS AND USES   Benzothiadiazine (thiazide) derivative. Similar to chlorothi-

HYDORCHLOROTHIAZIDE (continued)

azide (q.v.) in actions, uses, contraindications, precautions, adverse reactions, and interactions.

Used as adjunct in treatment of oedema associated with congestive heart failure, hepatic cirrhosis, renal failure, and in the management of hypertension.

ROUTE AND DOSAGE Oral: Adults: *Oedema*: *Initial*: 50–100 mg once or twice a day, *maintenance*: 25–50 mg daily or on alternate days. *Hypertension* 25–100 mg daily as a single or divided dose.

ABSORPTION AND FATE Diuretic effect begins in 2 hours, peaks in 4 hours, and lasts 6 to 12 hours. **Half-life**: normal kidneys, 2 hours; anuria, 15 hours. Excreted unchanged by kidneys within 24 hours. Crosses placenta; found in breast milk.

CONTRAINDICATIONS AND PRECAUTIONS Hypersensitivity to thiazides or other sulphonamides; anuria, pregnancy, lactation. **Cautious Use**: bronchial asthma, allergy, hepatic cirrhosis, renal dysfunction; history of gout. *See also chlorothiazide.*

ADVERSE/SIDE EFFECTS Nausea, vomiting, orthostatic hypotension, unusual fatigue, photosensitivity, exacerbation of gout, lupus erythematosus, hyperglycaemia, agranulocytosis, hypokalaemia. *See also chlorothiazide.*

Hydrocortisone ━━━━━━━━━━━━━━━━━━━━━━━━

(Efcortelan soluble, Efcortesol, Solucortef)   *Corticosteroid*

ACTIONS AND USES Short-acting synthetic steroid with strong glucocorticoid actions and, in high doses, mineralocorticoid properties. *Action mechanism*: corticosteroids cross cell membranes to complex with specific cytoplasmic receptors. The resulting complexes enter the nucleus, bind to DNA thereby initiating cytoplasmic synthesis of enzymes responsible for systemic effects of adrenocorticoids. *Metabolic effects*: promotes hepatic gluconeogenesis but decreases peripheral utilization of glucose thus predisposing patient on high doses to diabetes mellitus. Promotes protein catabolism, lipolysis, and, with high doses, redistribution of body fat. Interrupts normal linear growth in children. Displays antivitamin D activity leading to interference with calcium (Ca) absorption from GI tract; promotes gastroduodenal ulceration, and enhances peripheral vascular responsiveness to catecholamines. *Antiinflammatory effects* (*glucocorticoid*): prevents or suppresses clinical phenomena of inflammation including inhibition of phagocytosis, histamine activity and release of kinins; decreased complement components, reduced proliferation of fibroblasts and collagen deposition resulting in suppressed healing and scar tissue formation. *Immunosuppressive effects*: modified immune response to various stimuli with consequent decreased number of circulating eosinophils and lymphocytes decreased passage of immune complexes through basement membranes, reduction in antibody titres and suppressed cell-mediated hypersensitivity reactions. *Mineralocorticoid*

H

HYDROCORTISONE (continued)

effects: sodium (Na) retention and potassium (K) excretion, preservation of normal water and increased glomerular filtration rate. High doses may lead to depression, disorientation, euphoria. Prolonged hypothalamic–pituitary–adrenal axis suppression, promotes adrenal cortex atrophy with development of Cushingoid (hypercorticism) features; response to stress as in primary adrenocortical insufficiency (hypocorticism), depending on dosage and duration.

Used as replacement therapy in hypocorticism (adrenocortical insufficiency); to suppress undesirable inflammatory or immune responses, to produce temporary remission in nonadrenal disease, and to block ACTH production in diagnostic tests. Specific indications include: rheumatic disorders and collagen diseases; dermatological diseases, alopecia areata, shock unresponsive to conventional therapy; oral, otic, and ocular inflammatory conditions; neoplastic disease of lymphatic system, severe allergic states, chronic ulcerative colitis, respiratory diseases, haematological disorders, cerebral oedema, nephrotic syndrome, acute exacerbation of multiple sclerosis, thyroiditis, tuberculosis, meningitis, acute status asthmaticus; to decrease bleeding tendencies and normalize blood counts; aplastic anaemia.

ROUTE AND DOSAGE   Adults: all doses vary according to condition being treated; Paediatric: doses, if available, usually governed more by severity of condition and clinical response of patient.

ABSORPTION AND FATE   Rapid absorption from GI tract, 90 to 95% protein bound. **Onset of action**: oral: 1 to 2 hours; parenteral, rapid; rectal, 3 to 5 days. **Peak effect**: oral, 1 hours; IM, 4 to 8 hours. **Duration of action**: oral, IM: 1 to 1½ days; intraarticular, intralesional, soft tissue injection: 3 days to 4 weeks. **Half-life**: plasma: 1.5 to 2 hours; HPA suppression: 8 to 12 hours. Metabolized in liver. Excreted in urine principally as 17-hydroxysteroids (17-OHCS) and 17-ketosteroids (17-KS). Crosses placenta.

CONTRAINDICATIONS AND PRECAUTIONS   Hypersensitivity to glucocorticoids, idiopathic thrombocytopenic purpura, psychoses, acute glomerulonephritis, viral or bacterial diseases of skin, infections not controlled by antibiotics, active or latent amoebiasis, hypercorticism (Cushing's syndrome), small pox vaccination or other immunological procedures. (Topical steroids contraindicated in presence of varicella, vaccinia, on surfaces with compromised circulation, and in children less than 2 years old.) Safe use in women of childbearing potential, nursing mothers, during pregnancy not established. **Cautious Use**: children, diabetes mellitus; chronic active hepatitis positive for hepatitis B surface antigen, hyperlipidaemia, cirrhosis, stromal herpes simplex, glaucoma, tuberculosis of eye, osteoporosis, convulsive disorders, hypothyroidism, diverticulitis, nonspecific ulcerative colitis, fresh intestinal anastomoses, active or latent peptic ulcer, gastritis, oesophagitis, thromboembolic disorders, congestive heart failure, metastatic carcinoma, hypertension, renal insufficiency, history of allergies, active or arrested tuberculosis, systemic fungal infection, myasthenia gravis.

ADVERSE/SIDE EFFECTS   (Dose- and treatment-duration dependent). These include:

HYDROCORTISONE *(continued)*

syncopal episodes, thrombophlebitis, thromboembolism or fat embolism, palpitation, tachycardia, necrotizing angiitis, skin thinning and atrophy, acne, impaired wound healing, petechiae, ecchymosis, easy bruisings, suppression of skin test reaction; hypo- or hyperpigmentation, hirsutism, acneiform eruptions, subcutaneous fat atrophy; allergic dermatitis, urticaria, angioneurotic oedema, increased sweating, suppressed linear growth in children, decreased glucose tolerance; hyperglycaemia, manifestations of latent diabetes mellitus, secondary pituitary and adrenocortical unresponsiveness especially in stress; amenorrhoea and other menstrual difficulties, hypocalcaemia, Na and fluid retention, hypokalaemia and hypokalaemic alkalosis; congestive heart failure, hypertension, nausea, increased appetite, ulcerative oesophagitis, pancreatitis, abdominal distention, peptic ulcer with perforation and haemorrhage, melaena, thrombocytopenia, osteoporosis, compression fractures, muscle wasting and weakness, tendon rupture, aseptic necrosis of femoral and humeral heads, vertigo, headache, nystagmus, ataxia (rare), increased intracranial pressure with papilloedema (usually after discontinuation of medication), mental disturbances, aggravation of preexisting psychiatric conditions, insomnia, posterior subcapsular cataracts (especially in children), glaucoma, exophthalmus, increased intraocular pressure with optic nerve damage, perforation of the globe, fungal infection of the cornea, decreased or blurred vision. IV site: pain, irritation, necrosis, atrophy, sterile abscess; Charcot-like arthropathy; following intraarticular use, burning and tingling in perineal area (after IV injection), negative nitrogen balance, anaphylactoid or hypersensitivity reactions; aggravation or masking of infections; malaise, hiccoughs, hoarseness, dry mouth, sore throat (with inhalation therapy), weight gain, obesity; increased or decreased motility and number of spermatozoa, decreased serum concentration of vitamins A and C; urinary frequency and urgency, enuresis, **Overdosage (hypercorticism)**: anxiety, mental confusion, depression, hyperglycaemia, hypokalaemia, hypernatraemia, polycythaemia, hypertension, oedema, GI cramping or bleeding, ecchymoses, 'moon' face.

NURSING IMPLICATIONS
- Carefully check manufacturer's label for recommended route of administration.
- Before systemic corticosteroid therapy is started, a skin test for tuberculosis may be done.
- The initial suppressive dosing regimen should be brief, especially if alternate-day therapy is anticipated. Usually 4 to 10 days is sufficient for satisfactory clinical response in many allergic and collagen diseases.
- Inject *IM preparation* deeply into upper outer quadrant of buttock to avoid local atrophy. Avoid using deltoid muscle. Rotate injection site.
- Avoid *SC injection*; may produce sterile abscess or pseudoatrophy with persistent depression of overlying dermis lasting several weeks or months.
- Take oral drug at mealtimes or with a (low-salt) snack to reduce gastric irritation.
- Counsel patient to take drug as prescribed and not to alter dosing regimen or stop medication without consulting physician. Additionally, patient should not give any of the drug to another person.
- Establish baseline and continuing data regarding blood pressure, fluid intake and output ratio and pattern, weight, and sleep pattern, documentation in care plan.

H

HYDROCORTISONE (continued)

- Check and record blood pressure during dose stabilization period at least two times daily. Report an ascending pattern.
- 24-hour urine specimens may be required to rule out Cushing's syndrome (hypercorticism).
- Two-hour postprandial blood glucose, serum K, chest radiograph, and routine laboratory studies are performed at regular intervals during long-term steroid therapy.
- The elderly patient and the patient with low serum albumen are especially susceptible to adverse/side effects because of excess circulating free glucocorticoids.
- If patient has a history of diabetes mellitus, urine should be tested for glycosuria daily. Report positive findings; dietary and antidiabetic medication dose adjustments may be indicated.
- Be alert to signs of hypocalcaemia: muscle twitching, cramps, carpopedal spasm, positive Trousseau's and Chvostek's signs; and of hypokalaemia: muscle twitching, flaccid paralysis, postural hypotension, tetany, polydipsia, polyurea, cardiac dysrhythmias. Patients with hypocalcaemia have increased requirements for pyridoxine (vitamin B_6), vitamins C and D, and folates.
- Ophthalmoscopic examinations including tonometry are recommended every 2 to 3 months, especially if patient is receiving ophthalmic steroid therapy.
- Monitor patient's weight under standard conditions. Inform patient that a slight weight gain with improved appetite is expected, but after dosage stabilization has been achieved, a sudden slow but steady weight increase (5 lb/2−2.5 kg week) should be reported.
- A salt-restricted diet (unless otherwise contraindicated) and one rich in vitamin D and K and protein, is usually prescribed.
- Facilitate collaboration with dietitian and patient to plan diet. Teach food sources of K (leafy vegetables, potato, avocado, wheat, citrus fruit, melon, bananas, whole grains) as well as foods to avoid in order to decrease Na intake (snack foods, prepared luncheon meats, bouillon, sauces, processed cheese).
- Because of immunosuppression and the possibility of masked infection, warn patient to report incidence of slow healing or persistent inflammation in an abrasion, wound, or joint or any vague feeling of being sick without clear aetiological definition, or return of pretreatment symptoms.
- The immunocompromised patient should be fastidious about personal hygiene, give special attention to foot care, and be particularly cautious about bruising or abrading the skin.
- To continue beneficial effect of *intraarticular injection*, teach the patient proper joint alignment, appropriate posttreatment exercise, when to begin the exercises, and how long to avoid weight-bearing activities.
- Exaggerated sense of well-being and analgesic effects (painless joints) may encourage patient to increase physical activity even if acute disease process still exists. Discuss with physician and work with patient/family to plan reasonable and safe range of activities of daily living.
- Intraarticular injections can lead to systemic effects.

H

HYDROCORTISONE (continued)

- Compression and spontaneous fractures of long bones and vertebrae present hazards particularly in long-term corticosteroid treatment of rheumatoid arthritis or diabetes, in immobilized patients, and the elderly. Supervise getting out of bed or chair. Report persistent backache or chest pain (possible symptoms of vertebral or rib fracture). Patient's mattress should be firm.
- Be aware of previous history of psychotic tendencies. Watch for changes in mood and behaviour, emotional stability, sleep pattern, or psychomotor activity especially with long-term therapy, that may signal onset of recurrence. Report symptoms to physician.
- Dose adjustment may be required if patient is subjected to severe stress (serious infection, surgery, or injury) or if a remission or disease exacerbation occurs.
- Dyspepsia with hyperacidity should not be ignored. Encourage patient to report symptoms to physician and not to self-medicate in order to find relief.
- If a patient is receiving aspirin concomitantly with a corticosteroid, salicylism may be induced when the corticosteroid dosage is decreased or discontinued.
- Warn patient not to use aspirin or other OTC drugs unless prescribed specifically by the physician.
- Steroid ulcers with long-term therapy are frequently treated with an antacid. Encourage patient to avoid alcohol and caffeine.
- When corticosteroid is given for rheumatoid arthritis, complete relief is not sought because of the hazards of continuous treatment. A regimen of rest, physical therapy, and salicylates continues during steroid therapy.
- Observe newborn infant born of mother on substantial doses of corticosteroid during pregnancy for signs of hypoadrenalism.

Topical applications: (hydrocortisone and its esters)

- Warn patient not to use OTC topical preparations of a corticosteroid more than 7 days. They should not be used for children less than 2 years old. If symptoms do not abate, consult physician.
- Wash hands before and after application of medication.
- Usually topical preparations are applied to hydrated skin, i.e., after a shower or bath when skin is damp or wet.
- Cleansing and application of prescribed preparation should be done with extreme gentleness because of easy bruisability and poor healing. Do not apply thick layers of medication or an occlusive dressing unless specifically prescribed.
- A light film of the topical preparation should be massaged into affected area gently and thoroughly until it disappears. If an *occlusive dressing* is to be used, apply medication sparingly, rub until it disappears, and then reapply, leaving a thin coat over lesion. Completely cover area with transparent plastic or other occlusive device or vehicle.
- Occlusive vehicles or transparent plastic enhance absorption. Greasy ointments are more occlusive than gels and seem to be the preferred preparation for dry scaly skin.
- If lesion is essentially dry, make dressing as airtight and water tight as possible. Prevent evaporation by sealing dressing to adjacent skin. Discuss with physician.

H

HYDROCORTISONE (continued)

- Avoid covering a weeping or exudative lesion.
- If treated area is large, a sequential approach may be used with treatment of only a portion of the total area at a time.
- An occulsive dressing over a large area should be removed if a patient has a pyrexia to avoid interference with thermostatic defence mechanisms.
- An occlusive dressing increases percutaneous penetration as much as 10%. Discomfort and warmth may be troublesome. Inspect skin carefully between applications for ecchymotic, petechial and purpuric signs, maceration, secondary infection, skin atrophy, striae or miliaria; if present, stop medication and notify physician. Antifungal or antimicrobial treatment may be instituted.
- Rates of penetration of topical corticosteroid differ in various anatomic sites: thus comparatively small doses are used on face, scalp, scrotum, axilla, and groin. Usually occlusive dressings are not applied to these areas.
- Advise patient to avoid exposure of treated skin to temperature extremes.
- Caution should be used when a plastic film dressing is used on children to avoid possibility of accidental suffocation. Also warn patient to exercise great precaution when smoking while plastic is in use.
- Instruct patient to report promptly if initial therapeutic response is followed by relapse. Contact sensitivity or sensitivity to corticosteroid impurities may be presenting. The medication will be changed in kind or in dose.
- Although adrenal suppression from topical therapy infrequently occurs, whole-body applications of potent corticosteroid, occlusion, and stress may present a hazard. Replacement therapy before surgery may be given to prevent adrenal crisis.
- Urge patient on long-term therapy with topical corticosterone to check shelf-life date. (Full potency is supposed to be maintained to end of shelf-life.) Application of an old preparation with loss of potency may simulate sudden withdrawal of medication.
- Determine need for continued therapy with topical preparation. Since absorption of corticosteroid through abraded skin is greater than through normal skin, a healed area can simulate sudden withdrawal of medication by causing withdrawal symptoms with continued application.
- Abrupt discontinuation of corticosteroids after long-term therapy may result in *withdrawal syndrome* (myalgia, fever, arthralgia, malaise) and hypocorticism (anorexia, vomiting, nausea, fatigue, dizziness, hypotension, hypoglycaemia, myalgia, arthralgia).
- Single doses of corticosteroids or use for a short period (less than 1 week) do not produce withdrawal symptoms when discontinued, even with moderately large doses precautions should be taken when a patient is transferred from systemic to oral or nasal inhalation therapy (e.g., beclomethasone, flunisolide) as well as at time of discontinuing long-term therapy.
- To prevent withdrawal symptoms and permit adrenals to recover from drug-induced partial atrophy, doses are gradually reduced by scheduled decrements (various regimens).
- If during withdrawal, the disease flares up, a dosage increase followed by a more gradual withdrawal may be necessary.

H

HYDROCORTISONE (continued)

■ Patient is supervised about 1 year after withdrawal from systemic corticosteroids.

■ Patient/family should be advised to tell a dentist or new physician about recently prolonged corticosteroid treatment.

■ Ordinarily long-term corticosteroid therapy is not interrupted when patient undergoes major surgery, but dosage may be increased.

■ Advise patient receiving corticosteroid to carry a medical identification card or jewellery with recorded diagnosis, drug therapy, and name of physician.

■ Urge patient to adhere to scheduled appointments for regimen reevaluation.

■ Store medication between 15° and 30°C (59° and 86°F); unless otherwise directed by manufacturer. Protect drug from light and freezing.

Diagnostic test interferences   Hydrocortisone (corticosteroids) may increase **serum cholesterol, blood glucose, serum Na, uric acid** (in acute leukaemia) and **Ca** (in bone metastasis). It may decrease serum **Ca, K, PBI, thyroxin (T_4), triiodothyronine (T_3)** and reduce **thyroid I-131** uptake. It increases **urine glucose** level and **calcium** excretion; decreases **urine 17-OHCS** and **17-KS** levels. May produce false-negative results with nitroblue tetrazolium test for systemic bacterial infection, and suppress reactions to skin tests.

DRUG INTERACTIONS   *Hydrocortisone (corticosteroids)*

PLUS	INTERACTIONS
Alcohol and ulcerogenic drugs (e.g., aspirin, indomethacin, salicylates, corticosteroids)	Increased risk of GI ulceration
Amphotericin B, K-depleting diuretics (e.g., thiazides, frusemide, ethacrynic acid)	Increased hypokalaemic effect of hydrocortisone
Anion exchange resins, e.g., cholestyramine, colestipol	Decreased pharmacological effects of corticosteroids (interference with absorption)
Anticoagulants, oral, e.g., coumarins	May decrease anticoagulant effect of coumarins
Anticonvulsants, e.g., phenytoin	Corticosteroids lower seizure threshold requiring close monitoring of anticonvulsant activity
Antidiabetic agents (oral and insulin)	Decreased hypoglycaemic effect of antidiabetic agents
Barbiturates, ephedrine, phenytoin, rifampicin	Decreased glucocorticoid response
Cholinesterase inhibitors, e.g., ambenonium neostigmine	Decreased effect of cholinesterase
Digitalis glycosides	Increased risk of digitalis toxicity and arrhythmias due to hypokalaemic effect of corticosteroids
Oestrogens, indomethacin, nicotine, salicylates, pyrazolones	Increased antiinflammatory activity of corticosteroids
Isoniazid (INH)	Antitubercular effectiveness may be decreased
Salicylates	Decreased serum levels of salicylates (decreased pharmacological effects)
Oral contraceptives, erythromycins	Increased or prolonged corticosteroid activity
Theophyllines	Decreased glucocorticosteroid response
Vaccines, toxoids	Diminished response to toxoids, live and inactivated vaccines

Hydroflumethiazide _____

(Hydrenox)   *Diuretic; antihypertensive;*
thiazide

ACTIONS AND USES   Benzothiadiazine (thiazide) derivative. Similar to chlorothiazide (q.v.) in actions, uses, contraindications, precautions, adverse reactions, and interactions.

ROUTE AND DOSAGE   Oral: Adult: *Oedema*: *Initial* 50 to 200 mg daily. *Maintenance*: 25 to 150 mg on alternate days. *Hypertension*: 25 to 50 mg daily.

ABSORPTION AND FATE   Diuretic effect begins in 1 to 2 hours, peaks in 3 to 4 hours and lasts 18 to 24 hours. Presumed to be distributed and excreted similarly to other thiazides. *See chlorothiazide.*

CONTRAINDICATIONS AND PRECAUTIONS   Hypersensitivity to other thiazides or sulphonamide derivatives; anuria; pregnancy, lactation, hypokalaemia. *See chlorothiazide.*

ADVERSE/SIDE EFFECTS   Postural hypotension, photosensitivity hypokalaemia, hyperglycaemia, hyponatraemia, asymptomatic hyperuricaemia, agranulocytosis. *See also chlorothiazide.*

For further information: *see chlorothiazide.*

Hydroxocobalamin _____

(Cobalin-H, Neo-Cytamen))   *Vitamin*

ACTIONS AND USES   Cobalamin derivative similar to cyanocobalamin (vitamin B_{12}). Essential for normal growth, cell reproduction, maturation of RBC's, nucleoprotein synthesis, maintenance of nervous system (myelin synthesis), and believed to be involved in protein and carbohydrate metabolism. Also acts as coenzyme in various biological reactions. Stimulates reticulocytes and together with folic acid is involved in formation of oxyribonucleotides from ribonucleotides. Vitamin B_{12} deficiency results in megaloblastic anaemia, dysfunction of spinal cord with paralysis, GI lesions.

Used in treatment of vitamin B_{12} deficiency due to malabsorption syndrome as pernicious (Addison's) anaemia, and nitrous oxide–induced megaloblastosis.

ROUTE AND DOSAGE   Intramuscular (only): **Adults and child**: *Initial*: 1 mg repeated 5 times at 2–3 day intervals, *maintenance*: 1 mg three monthly.

NURSING IMPLICATIONS
- Some patients experience mild pain at injection site following administration.
- A careful history of previous sensitivities should be obtained. An intradermal test dose is recommended in patients suspected of being sensitive to cyanocobalamin. Reportedly sensitization to cyanocobalamin can take as long as 8 years to develop.
- Potassium levels should be monitored during the first 48 hours particularly in

H

HYDROXOCOBALAMIN *(continued)*

patients with Addisonian pernicious anaemia or megaloblastic anaemia, with supplementation if necessary. Conversion to normal erythropoiesis increases erythrocyte potassium requirement and can result in fatal hypokalaemia in these patients.

- Monitor vital signs in patients with cardiac disease and in those receiving parenteral cyanocobalamin, and be alert to symptoms to pulmonary oedema, which generally occur early in therapy.
- Dietary deficiency of vitamin B_{12} alone is rare; however, it has been observed in vegetarians and their breast-fed infants. Rich food sources: organ meats, clams, oysters; good sources: egg yolk, crabs/salmon, sardines, muscle meat, milk and dairy products.
- Perserved in light-resistant containers at room temperature preferably between 15° and 30°C (59° and 85°F) unless otherwise directed by manufacturer.

Smoking–drug infection Smokers appear to have increased requirements for vitamin B_{12}.

DRUG INTERACTIONS *Hydroxocobalamin*

PLUS	INTERACTIONS
Chloramphenicol	Interferes with erythrocyte maturation and thus may cause poor therapeutic response to vitamin B_{12}
Prednisone	May increase absorption of vitamin B_{12}

Hydroxychloroquine sulphate

(Plaquenil)

Antimalarial; suppressant
(lupus erythematosus)

ACTIONS AND USES 4-Aminoquinoline derivative closely related to chloroquine and with similar actions, uses, contraindications, precautions, adverse reactions, and interactions.

Used for suppressive prophylaxis and for treatment of acute malarial attacks due to all forms of susceptible malaria. Used adjunctively with primaquine for eradication of *P. vivax* and *P. malariae*.

ROUTE AND DOSAGE Oral: *Acute malaria*: **Adults**: *Initial*: 800 mg, followed by 400 mg after 6 to 8 hours, then 400 mg on each of next 2 days to total of 2 g. *Malaria suppression*: **Adults**: 400 mg once weekly on same day of each week. If possible, suppressive therapy should begin 2 weeks prior to exposure and continued for 8 weeks after leaving endemic area; failing this, an initial double (loading) dose of 800 mg in adults. **Child**: 6 mg/kg once weekly.

CONTRAINDICATIONS AND PRECAUTIONS Known hypersensitivity to 4-aminoquinoline compounds; psoriasis, porphyria, long-term therapy in children, pregnancy.

H

HYDROXYCHLOROQUINE SULPHATE (continued)

Cautious Use: hepatic disease, alcoholism, with hepatotoxic drugs, impaired renal function, metabolic acidosis, patients with tendency toward dermatitis. *See also chloroquine.*

ADVERSE/SIDE EFFECTS   GI distress, visual disturbances, retinopathy, muscle weakness, vertigo, tinnitus, nerve deafness, dermatological and haematological reactions. **With overdosage**: respiratory depression, cardiovascular collapse, shock. *See also chloroquine.*

NURSING IMPLICATIONS

- Administration of drug immediately before or after meals may reduce incidence of GI distress.
- All patients on long-term therapy should have baseline and periodic (every 3 months) ophthalmoscopic examinations (including visual acuity, slit lamp, fundoscopy, and visual fields), and blood cell counts.
- Hydroxychloroquine has cumulative actions. In patients requiring long-term therapy, therapeutic effect may not appear for several weeks, and maximal benefit may not occur for 6 months.
- Patients receiving prolonged therapy should be informed about adverse symptoms and advised to report their onset immediately. Patients should be questioned about possible symptoms and examined periodically (include tests for muscle weakness, knee and ankle reflexes, and opthalmoscopic examinations). Drug should be discontinued if weakness, visual symptoms, or skin eruptions occur.
- Counsel patient to follow drug regimen as prescribed by the physician.
- Caution patients to keep drug out of reach of children. Children are especially sensitive to 4-aminoquinoline compounds (chloroquine, hydroxychloroquine). A number of fatalities have been reported.
- Store preferably between 15° and 30°C (59° and 86°F) unless otherwise directed by manufacturer.
- *See chloroquine.*

Hydroxyprogesterone hexanoate ━━━━━━━

(Proluton depot)

ACTIONS AND USES   Used to treat threatened and habitual abortion.
For further information: *see progesterone.*

H

Hydroxyurea ━━━━━━━━━━━━━━━

(Hydrea)   *Antineoplastic*

HYDROXYUREA (continued)

ACTIONS AND USES   Synthetic analogue of urea with antimetabolite activity. Blocks incorporation of thymidine into DNA and may damage already formed DNA molecules; does not affect synthesis of RNA or protein. Cytotoxic effect limited to tissues with high rates of cell proliferation. May reduce iron utilization by erythrocytes; has no effect on erythrocyte survival time. No cross resistance with other antineoplastics has been demonstrated.

Used in palliative treatment of metastatic melanoma, chronic myelocytic leukaemia; recurrent metastatic, or inoperable ovarian cancer. Also used as adjunct to radiographic therapy for treatment of advanced primary squamous cell (epidermoid) carcinoma of head (excluding lip), neck, lungs.

ROUTE AND DOSAGE   Oral (individualized on basis of patient's actual or ideal weight, whichever is less): *Intermittent therapy*: 80 mg/kg body weight as single dose every third day. *Continuous therapy*: 20 to 30 mg/kg body weight as single daily dose.

ABSORPTION AND FATE   Readily absorbed from GI tract; peak serum concentrations in 2 hours. Undetectable in blood after 24 hours. Degraded in liver. Over 80% recovered as respiratory CO_2 and as urea in urine, within 12 hours; remainder excreted unchanged. No cumulative effect. Passes blood–brain barrier.

CONTRAINDICATIONS AND PRECAUTIONS   Pregnancy, patients of childbearing age, children, myelosuppression. **Cautious Use**: following recent use of other cytotoxic drugs or irradiation; renal dysfunction, elderly patients, history of gout.

ADVERSE/SIDE EFFECTS   These include: maculopapular rash, facial erythema, postirradiation erythema, alopecia (rare), (occasional): stomatitis, anorexia, nausea, vomiting, diarrhoea, constipation, leucopenia, thrombocytopenia, megaloblastic erythropoiesis, anaemia, renal tubular dysfunction, dysuria (rare), elevated BUN, serum uric acid, creatinine levels; hyperuricaemia.

NURSING IMPLICATIONS
- If patient cannot swallow capsule, contents may be emptied into glass of water and taken immediately. Small amounts of inert material used as drug vehicle may not dissolve, but can be ingested.
- Toxicity incidence with use of hydroxyurea is as high as 66% with doses of 40 mg/kg body weight. Inform patient of potential side effects and of importance of reporting symptoms promptly.

Hydroxyzine hydrochloride ▬▬▬▬▬▬▬▬▬▬

(Atarax)   *Anxiolytic; antihistamine*

H

ACTIONS AND USES   Piperazine derivative of diphenylmethane, structurally and pharmacologically related to other cyclizines (e.g., buclizine, chlorcyclizine). In

HYDROXYZINE HYDROCHLORIDE (continued)

common with such agents, it causes CNS depression and has anticholinergic, antiemetic, bronchodilator and antihistaminic activity. It ataractic effect is produced primarily by depression of hypothalamus and brain-stem reticular formation, rather than cortical areas. Also has skeletal muscle relaxant effect and mild antisecretory and analgesic activity. The hydrochloride is available in both intramuscular and oral preparations.

Used for treatment of emotional or psychoneurotical states characterized by anxiety, tension, or psychomotor agitation; to relieve anxiety, control nausea and emesis. Also used in management of pruritus due to allergic conditions, e.g., chronic urticaria, atopic and contact dermatoses.

ROUTE AND DOSAGE   Oral (hydrochloride or pamoate): **Anxiety Adults:** 50 mg to 100 mg four times daily. **Children (under 6 years):** 50 mg daily in divided doses; **(over 6 years):** 50 to 100 mg daily in divided doses. **Urticaria: Adult:** 25 mg three times a day.

ABSORPTION AND FATE   Rapidly absorbed from GI tract. **Onset of effects** within 15 to 30 minutes following oral administration; **duration of action** 4 to 6 hours. Metabolic fate not known.

CONTRAINDICATIONS AND PRECAUTIONS   Known hypersensitivity to hydroxyzine; use as sole treatment in psychoses or depression. Safe use during early pregnancy or in nursing mothers not established; lactation.

ADVERSE/SIDE EFFECTS   Drowsiness, sedation, dizziness, injection site reactions, dry mouth, headache. Rarely: involuntary motor activity, tremor, convulsions. **Hypersensitivy reactions:** urticaria, erythematous macular eruptions, erythema multiforme.

NURSING IMPLICATIONS

- Drowsiness may occur, but it usually disappears with continued therapy or following reduction of dosage.
- Forewarn the patient about the possibility of drowsiness and dizziness, and caution against driving a car or performing hazardous tasks requiring mental alertness and physical coordination while taking hydroxyzine.
- Alcohol and hydroxyzine should not be taken at the same time. Concomitant use enhances the effects of both agents. When CNS depressants are prescribed concomitantly, dosage of the depressant is reduced up to 50%.
- Patient should be advised that if she becomes pregnant during therapy or intends to become pregnant she should communicate with her physician about the desirability of discontinuing the drug.
- Xerostomia is uncomfortable and sets the stage for potential loss of taste and other serious clinical problems. If patient is on high dosage of hydroxyzine, monitor condition of oral membranes daily.
- Dry mouth may be relieved by frequent warm water rinses, increasing fluid intake and by use of saliva substitute if necessary. Avoid frequent use of commercial mouth rinses. They may change normal flora of the mouth and permit onset of a superinfection.
- Urge patient to give scrupulous care to teeth: use unwaxed dental floss and floss teeth

H

HYDROXYZINE HYDROCHLORIDE (continued)

daily, brush gently with a soft small tooth brush after meals, and use a fluoride toothpaste at least once a day. Avoid irritation or abrasion of tissues.

- Effectiveness of use longer than 4 months should be reassessed on basis of individual's response to the drug.
- Advise patient to consult physician before self-dosing with OTC medications.
- Protect hydroxyzine from light. Store at temperature between 15° and 30°C (59° and 86°F) unless otherwise specified by the manufacturer.

Diagnostic test interferences   Possibility of false-positive urinary 17-hydroxycorti-costeroid determinations (modified Glenn–Nelson technique).

DRUG INTERACTIONS *Hydroxyzine*

PLUS	INTERACTIONS
Alcohol Analgesics, nonnarcotic Antipsychotics, other Barbiturates and other sedatives Narcotics	Mutual potentiation of CNS depressant effects

Hyocine hydrobromide

Anticholinergic; antispasmodic

ACTIONS AND USES   Extremely potent, belladonna alkaloid with anticholinergic and antispasmodic activity.

Used to treat GI tract disorders caused by spasm and hypermotility, as conjunct therapy with diet and antacids for peptic ulcer management, and as an aid in the control of gastric hypersecretion and intestinal hypermotility. Also in symptomatic relief of biliary and renal colic. Premedication.

ROUTE AND DOSAGE   Oral or subcutaneous: 300–600 mcg four times a day. Child: 3–5 yrs 75–100 mcg; (6–12 yrs): 100–300 mcg.

ABSORPTION AND FATE   Duration of effect, 4 to 6 hours. Metabolized by the liver: half-life 13 to 38 hours; protein binding 50%. Excreted in urine.

CONTRAINDICATIONS AND PRECAUTIONS   Hypersensitivity to belladonna alkaloids. Narrow-angle glaucoma, prostatic hypertrophy. **Cautious Use**: diabetes mellitus, cardiac disease. *See also atropine.*

ADVERSE/SIDE EFFECTS   Confusion, excitement in elderly patients; palpitations, blurred vision, xerostomia, constipation, paralytic ileus, urinary retention, anhidrosis. *See also atropine.*

H

HYOCINE HYDROBROMIDE (continued)
NURSING IMPLICATIONS
- Administer oral preparation about one hour before meals and at bedtime (at least 2 hours after last meal).
- Advise patient to avoid excessive exposure to a high temperature in environment; drug-induced heat stroke can develop.
- Monitor urinary output. If changes in intake—output ratio and/or voiding pattern occur, notify physician.
- Dose for the elderly patient should be less than the standard adult dose. Observe patient carefully for signs of paradoxical reactions.
- This drug may cause drowsiness. Advise patient to be cautious while driving a car until response to drug is known.
- If patient complains about blurred vision, suggest use of dark glasses; but if this side effect persists, advise patient to report to physician for dose adjustment or possible change of drug.
- *See atropine sulphate.*

Ibuprofen

(Apsifen, Brufen, Ebufac, Fenbid, Ibular, Ibumetin, Motrin, Paxofen)   *NSAID*

ACTIONS AND USES   Propionic acid derivative with nonsteroid antiinflammatory activity and significant antipyretic and analgesic properties. Comparable to aspirin in analgesic action, but higher doses are required for antiinflammatory effect; also reported to cause fewer GI symptoms than aspirin in equieffective doses. Antiinflammatory action postulated to be due to inhibition of prostaglandin synthesis and/or release. Antipyretic effect is thought to result from action on hypothalamus; heat dissipation accompanies vasodilation and peripheral blood flow. Inhibits platelet aggregation and prolongs bleeding time, but does not affect prothrombin or whole blood clotting times. Cross-sensitivity with aspirin and other nonsteroidal antiinflammatory drugs has been reported.

Used in chronic, symptomatic treatment of active rheumatoid arthritis and osteoarthritis; and as analgesic for dysmenorrhoea, postextraction dental pain, postoperative pain, musculoskeletal pain, gout, juvenile rheumatoid arthritis.

ROUTE AND DOSAGE   Oral: 0.6–1.2 g daily in divided doses, Max 2.4 g. **Child:** 20 mg/kg/day if under 30 kg, maximum of 500 mg in 24 hrs.

ABSORPTION AND FATE   Rapidly absorbed. Peak plasma levels occur in 1 to 2 hours and decline to about one-half peak level in 4 hours. Approximately 90 to 99% **bound to plasma proteins**; plasma **half-life**: 2 to 4 hours. Metabolized by oxidation to inactive metabolites. Excretion almost complete within 24 hours after last dose. About 50

IBUPROFEN (continued)

to 60% excreted in urine as inactive metabolites and less than 10% as unchanged drug. Some biliary excretion occurs.

CONTRAINDICATIONS AND PRECAUTIONS   History of hypersensitivity to ibuprofen; patients with syndrome of nasal polyps, rhinitis, and asthma associated with aspirin (aspirin triad) or other nonsteroidal antiinflammatory drugs; active peptic ulcer; children 14 years of age or younger; pregnancy, nursing mothers. **Cautious Use**: history of GI ulceration, impaired hepatic or renal function, cardiac decompensation, patients with SLE.

ADVERSE/SIDE EFFECTS   These include: headache, dizziness, nystagmus, lightheadedness, tinnitus, fatigue, malaise, drowsiness, anxiety, confusion, depression, maculopapular and vesicobullous skin eruptions, erythema multiforme, pruritus, rectal itching, acne, dyspepsia, heartburn, nausea, vomiting, anorexia, diarrhoea, constipation, bloating, flatulence, stomatitis, epigastric or abdominal pain, GI ulceration, bleeding, leucopenia; decreased haemoglobin and haematocrit; transitory rise in SGOT, SGPT, serum alkaline phosphatase; rise in bleeding time, blurred vision, visual-field defects, sore throat, epistaxis, flushing, fluid retention with oedema, Stevens-Johnson syndrome, toxic hepatitis, nephrotoxicity, aseptic meningitis.

NURSING IMPLICATIONS

- Absorption rate is slower and drug plasma level is reduced when ibuprofen is administered with food; therefore it is usually given on an empty stomach, e.g., 1 hour before or 2 hours after meals.
- If GI intolerance occurs, physician may prescribe administration of drug with food or milk or may decrease dosage.
- It is important to take a detailed drug history prior to initiation of therapy. *See contraindications and precautions*.
- Patients with history of cardiac decompensation should be observed closely for evidence of fluid retention and oedema.
- Side effects appear to be dose-related. Physician will rely on accurate observation and reporting to estimate lowest effective dosage level.
- Inform patients about possible CNS effects (lightheadedness, dizziness, drowsiness), and caution them to avoid dangerous activities until their reactions to the drug have been determined.
- Patients should be advised to report immediately to physician the onset of GI disturbances, skin rash, blurred vision or other eye symptoms.
- Patients who experience any visual disturbances should have ophthalmic evaluation, including examination of visual fields.
- Optimum therapeutic response generally occurs within 2 weeks (e.g., relief of pain, stiffness, or swelling or improved joint flexion and strength). When satisfactory response occurs, dosage should be reviewed by physician and adjusted as required.
- If patient is self-medicating with ibuprofen, advise discontinuing drug and consulting physician if pain persists beyond 10 days or fever persists more than 3 days, or if joint swelling develops or if pain and fever worsen.

IBUPROFEN (continued)

- Advise patient not to self-medicate with ibuprofen if taking prescribed drugs, without physician approval.
- Inform patient that alcohol and aspirin may increase risk of GI ulceration and bleeding tendencies and therefore should be avoided, unless otherwise advised by physician.
- Since ibuprofen may prolong bleeding time, advise patient to inform dentist or surgeon that he or she is taking drug.
- Store preferably between 15° and 30°C (59° and 86°F) in well-closed, light-resistant container unless otherwise directed by manufacturer.

Drug interactions   Ulcerogenic effect may be potentiated by concomitant administration of ibuprofen and **indomethacin, phenylbutazone,** or **salicylates.** There is also the possibility (based on animal studies) that **aspirin** may cause lower blood levels and decrease the antiinflammatory activity of ibuprofen. Although ibuprofen has not been shown to enhance the hypoprothrombinaemic effects of **oral anticoagulants,** cautious use is advised if they are given concurrently, since ibuprofen inhibits platelet aggregation.

Idoxuridine

(Herpid, Iduridin, Idoxene, Kerecid)   *Antiviral*

ACTIONS AND USES   Topical antiviral agent. Pyrimidine nucleoside structurally related to thymidine, a metabolite essential for synthesis of DNA. Antiviral activity is primarily due to a substitution process. Not effective against RNA viruses. Idoxuridine has no effect on accumulated scarring, vascularization, or consequent progressive loss of vision. Some resistant strains of herpes simplex have been reported. Potentially carcinogenic. Squamous cell carcinoma at site of topical treatment has been reported.

Used in treatment of herpes simplex keratitis as single agent or conjunctively with a corticosteroid.

ROUTE AND DOSAGE   Topical: Ophthalmic solution 0.1%: *Initial*: 1 drop instilled in conjunctival sac of each infected eye every hour during the day and every 2 hours at night until improvement occurs. Dosage may then be reduced to 1 drop every 2 hours during the day and every 4 hours at night. Ophthalmic ointment 0.5%: 5 instillations daily into conjunctival sac in infected eye; given approximately every 4 hours, with last dose at bedtime. Skin paint: 5% use sparingly on the lesion and surrounding area four times a day. For up to 4 days: 0.1% for oral lesions, hold about 2 ml in contact with the lesion for 2–3 minutes 3 or more times a day.

ABSORPTION AND FATE   Poorly absorbed following instillation into eyes. Tissue uptake of drug (a function of cellular metabolism) is reportedly less with increasing drug concentrations, higher concentrations. Slowly degraded when instilled in eye permitting long enough contact with eye surface for antiviral action.

IDOXURIDINE (continued)

CONTRAINDICATIONS AND PRECAUTIONS Hypersensitivity to idoxuridine, iodine or iodine containing preparations, or to any components in the formulation. **Cautious Use:** women of childbearing potential, during pregnancy and lactation; corticosteroids.

ADVERSE/SIDE EFFECTS These include: (occasionally) local irritation, pain, burning, lacrimation, pruritus, inflammation, or oedema of eyes, lids, and surrounding face; follicular conjunctivitis, photophobia; corneal clouding, stippling, and small punctate defects; corneal ulceration and swelling; delayed healing.

Overdosage (local): small defects in corneal epithelium.

NURSING IMPLICATIONS

- Boric acid should not be used during therapy with idoxuridine, since irritation may occur.
- To prevent the possibility of systemic absorption, apply light finger pressure to head of lacrimal duct for 1 minute when eyedrop is instilled. *See index: Drug administration: eye drops.*
- If photosensitivity is troublesome, advise patient to wear sunglasses.
- Idoxuridine should not be mixed with other medications.
- The recommended frequency and duration of therapy must not be exceeded.
- To prevent recurrence, instillations are usually continued for at least 3 to 5 days after corneal healing appears complete, as demonstrated by loss of staining with fluorescein.
- Epithelial infections usually improve within 7 or 8 days. If patient continues to improve, therapy is generally continued up to 21 days. If no improvement is noted after 7 or 8 days, physician may institute another form of therapy. In some cases, physician may continue therapy using fresh solution.
- Topical corticosteroids may be used with idoxuridine for herpes simplex with stromal lesions, corneal oedema or iritis. Idoxuridine therapy should continue a few days after the steroid is discontinued.
- Do not mix idoxuridine with any other drug. Antibiotics and atropine may be given concurrently if necessary.
- Follow manufacturers directions regarding storage. Decomposed idoxuridine not only has reduced antiviral activity but also may be toxic.
- Store at controlled room temperature.
- Do not confuse dermatological (5%) paint with 0.1% oral solution.

Ifosfamide ━━━━━━━━━━━━━━━━━━━━━━━━━━━━━━━━━

(Mitoxana)   *Antineoplastic; alkylating agent*

ACTIONS AND USES Ifosfamide is a cell-cycle nonspecific alkylating agent structurally related to cyclophosphamide (q.v.). Following intravenous administration, it

IFSOSFAMIDE (continued)
is metabolized to an active form by the liver. Used to treat chronic lymphocytic leukaemia, lymphomas and solid tumours.

ROUTE AND DOSAGE   By intravenous injection or infusion in highly individualized doses.

NURSING IMPLICATIONS
■ Given with mesna to protect the patient from haemorrhagic cystitis.
   For further information: *see cyclophosphamide*.

Imipramine hydrochloride ———————————————

(Praminil, Tofranil)   *Antidepressant; tricyclic*

ACTIONS AND USES   Dibenzazepine derivative and tertiary amine. Tricyclic antidepressant, structurally related to the phenothiazines. In contrast to phenothiazines which act on dopamine receptors, TCAs block reuptake of serotonin and noradrenaline by presynaptic neurones in CNS. Resulting increase in concentration in synaptic cleft enhances activity at receptor site, thought to be the basis for antidepressant effects. Imipramine appears to be a more active inhibitor of noradrenaline than serotonin reuptake. Exhibits anticholinergic, antihistaminic, hypotensive, sedative and mild peripheral vasodilator effects. Decreases number of awakenings from sleep, markedly reduces time in REM sleep. Prolongs myocardial repolarization time and may produce quinidinelike conduction abnormalities (arrhythmias, heart block, bundle branch block). Relief of nocturnal enuresis perhaps due to nervous system stimulation resulting in earlier arousal to sensation of full bladder.

   Used in endogenous depression; occasionally used for reactive depression. Less effective in presence of organic brain damage or schizophrenia. Also used for temporary adjuvant treatment of enuresis in children over 6 years old.

ROUTE AND DOSAGE   Oral: **Adult**: *Initial*: 75 mg/day in divided doses, increased to 200 mg with up to 150 mg given as a single dose at bedtime. **Elderly patients**: 10–25 mg 1–3 times a day. *Enuresis*: **Child (7 yrs)**: 25 mg, **(8–11 yrs)**: 25–50 mg, **(over 11 yrs)**: 50–75 mg at bedtime for a maximum of 3 months.

ABSORPTION AND FATE   Well absorbed from GI tract and highly bound to plasma proteins; wide distribution, including CNS. Hepatic metabolism with possible enterohepatic cycling. Principle active metabolite: desipramine. **Plasma half-life**: 6 to 20 hours; wide interpatient plasma level variation due to differences in first-pass (hepatic) metabolism, perhaps a genetic effect. (In general, the elderly metabolize TCAs more slowly than young adults.) Excreted primarily as inactive metabolite in urine; small amount in faeces. Crosses placental barrier and may be secreted in breast milk.

CONTRAINDICATIONS AND PRECAUTIONS   Sensitivity to other dibenzazepines; acute

IMIPRAMINE HYDROCHLORIDE (continued)

recovery period following myocardial infarction; severe renal or hepatic impairment; use of hydrochloride in children under 12 except to treat enuresis; concomitant use of MAO inhibitors; pregnancy, lactation (may be teratogenic). **Cautious Use**: children, adolescents; elderly especially with cardiac disorder; respiratory difficulties, cardiovascular, hepatic or GI diseases; increased intraocular pressure, narrow angle glaucoma, schizophrenia, hypomania or manic episodes, patient with suicide tendency, seizure disorders; prostatic hypertrophy, urinary retention, alcoholism, hyperthyroidism, concomitant use of thyroid medication, electroshock therapy.

ADVERSE/SIDE EFFECTS   These include: xerostomia, blurred vision, disturbance of accommodation, mydriasis, constipation, paralytic ileus, urinary retention, delayed micturition, orthostatic hypotension, hypertension or hypotension, palpitation, myocardial infarction, congestive heart failure, arrhythmias, heart block, cardiotoxicity, ECG changes, stroke, shock, testicular swelling, gynaecomastia (males), galactorrhoea and breast enlargement (females), increased or decreased libido, ejaculatory and erectile disturbances, delayed orgasm (male and female); elevation or depression of blood glucose levels, nausea, vomiting, diarrhoea, slowed gastric emptying time, flatulence, abdominal cramps, oesophageal reflux, anorexia, stomatitis, increased salivation, black tongue, peculiar taste, bone marrow depression: agranulocytosis, eosinophilia, purpura, thrombocytopenia, orthostatic hypotension, tachycardia, arrhythmias, blurred vision, constipation, xerostomia, impaired micturition, dizziness, tinnitus; numbness, tingling and paraesthesias of extremities; incoordination, ataxia, tremors, peripheral neuropathy, extrapyramidal symptoms, lowered seizure threshold, altered EEG patterns, delirium, disturbed concentration, confusion, hallucinations, anxiety, restlessness, agitation, insomnia, nightmares; shift to hypomania, mania; exacerbation of psychoses, cholestatic jaundice, precipitated acute intermittent porphyria, nasal congestion, excessive perspiration, flushing, paradoxic urinary frequency, nocturia, drowsiness, fatigue, weakness, headache, proneness to falling, alopecia, excessive appetite, changes in heat and cold tolerance.

NURSING IMPLICATIONS

- Administer drug with or immediately after food to reduce gastric irritation.
- Administer single daily dose at bedtime if dizziness and drowsiness are bothersome and dangerous during the day. If insomnia and stimulation are problems, administer drug in the AM.
- Dose sensitivity and side effects are most likely to occur in adolescents and the elderly. A lower initial dose should be used for these patients.
- Supervise drug ingestion. When patient is discharged from hospital instruct patient and family members not to double or skip doses, change dose interval, or combine dose with another nonprescribed drug.
- Risk of suicide is particularly great when patient nears the end of a depressive cycle. Be alert to sudden improvement in mood and behaviour, which may signify patient has finally come to an 'acceptable' solution: to commit suicide.
- Accurate early reporting to physician about patient's response to drug therapy is essential to prevent serious adverse effects, and to the design of an individualized therapeutic regimen.

IMIPRAMINE HYDROCHLORIDE (continued)

- *Signs of therapeutic effectiveness of tricyclic antidepressants (TCAs):* renewed interest in surroundings and personal appearance, mood elevation, increased physical activity and energy, improved appetite and sleep patterns, reduction in morbid pre-occupations.
- A trial of therapy with adequate dose is not judged a failure for at least a month: with no improvement, drug is discontinued. With apparent improvement, maintenance dosage can be instituted. Therapeutic plasma level: 150 to 300 mg/ml.
- Some patients on TCA therapy experience complete recovery within 4 to 6 weeks; others may require drug therapy for several years, or for life.
- Because of long serum half-life, dose adjustments are not made more frequently than every 4 days.
- Advise patient not to use OTC drugs while on a TCA, without physician's approval. Many preparations contain sympathomimetic amines and concomitant administration with imipramine could precipitate hypertensive crisis.
- The actions of both alcohol and imipramine are potentiated when used together during therapy and for up to 2 weeks after TCA is discontinued. Consult physician about safe amount of alcohol, if any, that can be taken.
- If a patient uses excessive amounts of alcohol it should be borne in mind that the potentiation of TCA effects may increase the danger of overdosage or suicide attempt.
- **Smoking–drug interaction**   Imipramine metabolism may be increased by smoking, thus changing dose requirements.
- Elderly patients are apt to develop 'confusional reaction' (restlessness, disturbed sleep, forgetfulness) during first 2 weeks of therapy. Symptoms last 3 to 20 days. Report to physician.
- Warn patient to avoid hazardous tasks such as driving a motor vehicle or operating machinery until drug response is known.
- Exposure to strong sunlight should be avoided because of potential photosensitivity. Advise use of sun screen lotion (SPF 12 to 15), if allowed. Remind patient that ultraviolet radiation is present even on dark days and that danger from sun is less when it is closest to horizon (before 10.00 hrs and after 13.00 hrs).
- Report promptly early signs of agranulocytosis (pyrexia, malaise, sore throat). Need to stop drug and appropriate treatment will depend upon evaluation of WBC and differential.
- Report signs of cholestatic jaundice: flu-like symptoms (general malaise, nausea, vomiting, fever, upper abdominal pain), yellow skin or sclerae, dark urine, light-coloured stools, pruritus.
- Observe patient with history of glaucoma. The onset of a severe headache, halos of light, dilated pupils, eye pain, nausea, vomiting, may signal acute attack. Notify physician.
- TCAs may caused grand mal seizures in susceptible patients e.g., those with seizure disorders, organic brain disease, alcoholism, barbiturate withdrawal, and those receiving high doses of TCA.
- Monitor blood pressure, and pulse rate for tachycardia and other arrhythmias. Withhold drug if systolic BP falls more than 20 mm Hg or if there is a sudden increase in pulse rate, and notify physician.

IMIPRAMINE HYDROCHLORIDE (continued)

- If patient has cardiovascular disease or its history, cardiac surveillance by ECG is necessary during period of dose adjustment and periodically during maintenance treatment.

- Orthostatic hypotension tends to be mild in normotensive individuals, but may be marked in pretreatment hypertensive or cardiac patients.

- Instruct patient to change position slowly and in stages especially from recumbency to upright posture; dangle legs over bed for a few minutes before ambulation. Caution against standing still for prolonged periods, taking hot showers or baths, or exposure for prolonged periods to the sun.

- Sitting with legs elevated and wearing support stockings or socks may prevent orthostatic hypotension. Consult physician.

- Extrapyramidal symptoms (tremors, twitching, ataxia, incoordination, hyperreflexia, drooling) may occur in patients receiving large doses and especially in the elderly. Fine tremors may be alleviated by small doses of propranolol. The physician may change dosage, or drug.

- Promptly report appearance of psychogenic reactions: transition from depression to hypomania or mania, hallucinations, delusion (especially apt to occur in patients with organic brain damage or history of psychosis). TCA therapy will be discontinued.

- Monitor fluid intake–output ratio and bowel elimination, at least until maintenance dosage is stabilized, to detect urinary retention or frequency, constipation or paralytic ileus. Palpate for bladder distention and auscultate for peristalsis as indicated. Notify physician if patient is unable to void. A cholinergic drug may be ordered.

- Note depressed patient's interest in food and fluids. Some patients may require increases in bulk foods (such as whole grain cereals) or fluids and a laxative to overcome drug-induced constipation.

- Drug-induced *xerostomia* is frequently an anticholinergic overlay of a chronically dry mouth in the depressed person.

- Xerostomic condition is characterized by sore mouth, crusting of oral mucosa, repeated clicking of tongue as patient attempts to lubricate the mouth, pebbly tongue surface (leads to decreased taste perception). Alert physician.

- Frequently inspect oral mucosa, especially gingival surfaces under dentures. Dry mouth promotes tissue erosion and shrinkage, leading to poor adhesion of dentures to bony ridges.

- Discomfort from oral dryness interferes with speech, mastication, and swallowing and is a potential dental hazard: deprivation of normal saliva favors demineralization of tooth surfaces.

- Relief of xerostomia may result from (1) frequent warm clear water rinses, (2) use of a saliva substitute which when sprayed onto oral surfaces provides lubrication effect for 1 to 3 hours; (3) avoidance of hard, rough food, (4) increased noncaloric fluid intake.

- If salivary flow responds to stimulation, relief may be provided by chewing sugarless gum. Dip gum in a droplet of cooking oil to reduce force of mastication and to make gum very slippery.

- Urge patient to floss teeth daily with waxed floss and to brush gently with a small soft tooth brush after eating. A fluoride toothpaste helps to restore mineralization of tooth surface.

I

IMIPRAMINE HYDROCHLORIDE (continued)

- Persistence of xerostomia may cause reduction in food and liquid intake and is a known factor in noncompliance. It should be brought under control before patient is discharged. A consultation with a dentist may be indicated.
- Weigh patients under standard conditions. A gain of 0.5–1 kg within 2 to 3 days and frank oedema should be reported.
- Hyperglycaemia or hypoglycaemia may occur in some patients. Diabetic patients should be monitored, particularly during early therapy.
- TCA may cause a change in tolerance to heat and cold. Regulate environmental temperature, personal clothing, and bed-covers accordingly. Protect patient from inadvertent contact with uncontrolled hot objects (e.g., radiators, heating pads).
- The severely depressed patient may need assistance with personal hygiene because of excessive sweating produced by the drug.
- *Overdosage* onset may be sudden and is manifested by anticholinergic, extrapyramidal, and cardiac symptoms. Physostigmine salicylate by slow IV reverses TCA effects. (There is no specific antidote.) Additionally, aggressive supportive therapy includes: gastric lavage, active charcoal slurry, anticonvulsant, cardiac monitor, resuscitation equipment. Keep patient in quiet darkened environment. Observe closely for at least 72 hours and monitor by ECG for at least 5 days. Relapse may occur after apparent recovery.
- Coma in the patient with an overdose of TCA has accompanying symptoms of warm skin, dilated pupils, and tachycardia ('atropine syndrome'). Hypertension and hyperreflexia may also be present.
- Drug withdrawal should be gradual. Abrupt termination of therapy, especially in patients receiving high doses for 2 months or more may result in nausea, headache, vertigo, malaise, insomnia, nightmares.
- Education of patient/family in collaboration with physician from start of therapy may help to promote patient compliance.

Enuresis patient-teaching point

- ☐ Early evening bedwetters are usually given 25 mg in midafternoon and a repeat dose at bedtime.
- ☐ With adequate dosage, positive results generally occur in 1 to 2 weeks. Maintenance dosage is continued until the child is dry every night for 3 months.
- ☐ A drug-free period following adequate response to drug therapy is sometimes instituted. When imipramine is to be withdrawn dosage is tapered to reduce possibility of relapse.
- ☐ Children who relapse when drug is withheld do not always respond to restart of therapy. In some patients, effectiveness decreases with continued drug administration. Counsel parent to inform physician if this occurs.
- ☐ Most frequent side effects in children: fatigue, nervousness, sleep disorders, mild GI symptoms. Others include: constipation, convulsions, emotional instability, syncope, collapse. Parent should report these symptoms; termination of therapy may be indicated.
- ☐ Enuresis is generally associated with an emotional component, such as guilt

IMIPRAMINE HYDROCHLORIDE (continued)

feelings and anxiety, even when it is not primarily psychogenic in origin; ample time should be given to parent and child to discuss problems of management.

Summary of patient-teaching

- ☐ Stress biochemical theory of endogenous depression.
- ☐ Permanent remission occurs in most cases (75 to 80%).
- ☐ Symptom relief may require as long as 21 days.
- ☐ Side effects may occur that have to be 'lived with'; tolerance develops however to most of them, or there are medications that help to reduce discomfort. Keep physician informed.
- ☐ Maintain dosage until advised otherwise by physician.
- ☐ Keep follow-up appointments throughout maintenance therapy.
- ☐ Advise significant others to encourage physical and diversional activities. Do not let patient 'vegetate.'

- ■ Counsel parent regarding the proper use and physical security of imipramine. Poisoning in children is an emerging public health problem. A dose as low as 15 mg/kg can be lethal.
- ■ Store oral and parenteral solution at temperature between 15° and 30°C (59° and 86°F) unless advised differently by manufacturer.

Diagnostic test interferences Imipramine elevates **serum bilirubin, alkaline phosphatase** and may elevate **blood glucose**. It decreases **urinary 5-HIAA** and **VMA** excretion and may falsely increase excretion of **urinary catecholamines**.

DRUG INTERACTIONS   *Imipramine: tricyclic antidepressants (TCAs)*_____

PLUS	INTERACTIONS
Acetazolamide	Increased TCA effects
Adrenaline	Increased pressor response
Alcohol	Mutual potentiation of effects
Ammonium chloride	Decreased TCA effects
Amphetamines	Enhanced amphetamine effects
Anticholinergics	Mutual potentiation of atropine-like effects
Anticoagulant, oral	Increased hypoprothrombinaemia
Anticonvulsants	Anticonvulsant effect may be reduced by TCA
Antihistamines	Additive anticholinergic effects of TCA
Ascorbic acid	Decreased TCA effects
Barbiturates	Potentiated adverse effects of toxic dose of TCA; decreased TCA serum levels and thus TCA effectiveness. Potentiated action of barbiturates
Beta-adrenergic blockers	Actions antagonized by TCA
Chlordiazepoxide	Additive sedative effect of TCA
Clonidine	Decreased antihypertensive effect of clonidine
Diazepam	Additive atropinelike and sedative effects of TCA

IMIPRAMINE HYDROCHLORIDE (continued)

PLUS (continued)	INTERACTIONS
Fenfluramine	Potentiates sedative action of TCA
Glutethimide	Additive anticholinergic effects of TCA
Guanethidine	Decreased antihypertensive effect of guanethidine
MAO inhibitors	Hyperpyretic crises, convulsions, hypertensive episodes, death
Methyldopa	Blocked hypotensive effect of methyldopa
Narcotic analgesics	Increased narcotic-induced respiratory depression
Noradrenaline	Increased pressor response to levarterenol
Oral contraceptives	May inhibit TCA effects
Oxazepam	Additive sedation and atropinelike side effects
Phenothiazines	Additive effects of TCA
Phenylbutazone	Desipramine inhibits GI absorption of phenylbutazone
Phenylephrine	Increased pressor response to phenylephrine
Phenytoin Procainamide	Possibility of decreased phenytoin seizure control
Quinidine	Potentiated cardiovascular effects of TCA
Reserpine	Decreases hypotensive action of reserpine; reserpine may exert stimulating effect in depressed patient
Sodium bicarbonate	Increased TCA effects
Sympathomimetics	Increased hypertensive and cardiac arrhythmic effects of sympathomimetics
Thyroid preparations	Mutually potentiating effects
Vasodilators	Additive hypotensive effect of TCA

Indapamide ▬▬▬▬▬▬▬▬▬▬▬▬▬▬▬▬▬▬▬▬▬▬▬

(Natrilix)   *Antihypertensive; diuretic*

ACTIONS AND USES   First member of new class of antihypertensive/diuretic agents, the indolines. Has both diuretic and direct vascular effects; action mechanism is similar to that of the thiazide diuretics. Principal site of action is on the proximal portion of the distal renal tubules. Enhances excretion of Na, K and water by interfering with Na transfer across renal epithelium. Like the thiazides, indapamide increases Ca reabsorption without causing important changes in serum Ca concentration. Free water clearance during hydration is decreased. Hypotensive activity in the hypertensive patient appears to result from a decrease in plasma and extracellular fluid volume, decreased peripheral vascular resistance, direct arteriolar dilation, and calcium channel blockade. Has little effect on cardiac output, rate, or rhythm, and, unlike the thiazides, does not increase serum cholesterol. Augments the action of other hypotensive agents.

INDAPAMIDE (continued)

Used alone or with other antihypertensives in the management of hypertension in patients who have failed to respond to diet, exercise, or weight reduction.

ROUTE AND DOSAGE   Oral: 2.5 mg as a single daily dose.

ABSORPTION AND FATE   Rapidly and completely absorbed from GI tract. Peak blood concentration of 230 to 260 ng/ml achieved 2 to 2½ hours after single 5-mg dose; 71 to 79% protein bound. **Half-life**: 14 to 18 hours; not prolonged by impaired renal function. Extensive hepatic metabolism with production of glucuronide and sulphate conjugates. About 60% of dose excreted in urine in 48 hours; only 7% of dose excreted unchanged. 16 to 23% excreted in faeces via bile.

CONTRAINDICATIONS AND PRECAUTIONS   Hypersensitivity to indapamide or other sulphonamide derivatives, anuria. Safe use during pregnancy, lactation, and in children not established. **Cautious Use**: electrolyte imbalance, severe renal disease, impaired hepatic function or progressive liver disease, hypokalaemia, prediabetic and type II diabetic patient, hyperparathyroidism, thyroid disorders, SLE, sympathectomized patient, history of gout.

ADVERSE/SIDE EFFECTS   These include: orthostatic hypotension, PVCs, dysrhythmias, palpitation, headache, dizziness, fatigue, weakness, loss of energy, muscle cramps or spasm, paraesthesia, tension, anxiety, agitation, vertigo, insomnia, depression, blurred vision, rash, hives, pruritus, vasculitis, dry mouth, anorexia, nausea, vomiting, diarrhoea, constipation, abdominal cramps or pain, urinary frequency, nocturia, polyuria, impotence or reduced libido, rhinorrhoea, flushing, dilutional hyponatraemia, hyperuricaemia, hyperglycaemia, hypochloraemia, increased BUN or creatinine, glycosuria, weight loss, tingling of extremities. **Overdosage**: nausea, vomiting, weakness, electrolyte balance disturbance, hypotension, depressed respirations.

NURSING IMPLICATIONS
- Administer in morning to prevent nocturia. Urge patient to take a glass of fluid (if allowed) with the medication.
- Laboratory tests to monitor serum electrolytes should be evaluated periodically.
- Fluid and salt intake are generally not altered during treatment with indapamide. However, the elderly patient is especially vulnerable to fluid volume changes. If diuresis has been brisk (characteristic of the response in an older person), be alert to sudden appearance of symptoms of hypovolaemia (profound weakness, dizziness, perspiration, vomiting) and hypokalaemia (dry mouth, nausea, vomiting, thirst, muscle cramps, confusion, paraesthesias, abdominal distention, tachycardia, hypoactive reflexes).
- Report promptly when signs of electrolyte imbalance are observed. K supplements or K-rich foods may be prescribed (*See Index: Food sources*).
- An elderly patient may have a severe potassium deficit before it is diagnosed if the early symptoms of weakness, confusion, easy fatiguability are attributed to old age alone. Correlation of serum K levels with alerted observation is especially important in prevention of diuretic-induced hypokalaemia in this age group.

INDAPAMIDE (continued)

- Moderate hyperuricaemia with exacerbation of gout symptoms
- Instruct patient to report promptly to the physician symptoms of developing renal impairment (urinary frequency, altered fluid input−output ratio and pattern, painful urination, weight change, oedema). Withholding or discontinuation of diuretic may be considered. Periodic renal function tests are indicated throughout therapy with indapamide.
- Advise patient to report unexplained, progressive weight gain (e.g., 2 to 3 pounds/ 1−1.5 kg in 2 to 3 days). Discuss salt and fluid intake parameters with physician and be certain these guidelines are fully understood by the patient.
- Keep in mind that if the patient is receiving a cardiac glycoside, hypokalaemia increases the risk of digitalis intoxication (cardiac arrhythmia).
- If patient has hepatic dysfunction, even minor changes in fluid−electrolyte balance can precipitate hepatic coma. Instruct patient to report promptly the onset of symptoms suggestive of decreasing hepatic function (jaundice, dyspepsia, darkened urine, pruritus).
- Routine examination for blood glucose level changes or for glycosuria should continue throughout indapamide treatment period. The drug may alter insulin requirements and cause borderline diabetes to manifest.
- Since indapamide may cause hypercalcaemia (and hypophosphataemia), it is withheld before tests for parathyroid function are performed.
- Monitor elimination pattern since constipation may be a side effect. Advise patient to consult physician for a laxative if needed and not to self-dose with an OTC product. Discuss prevention of constipation with patient, e.g., adding more bulk to diet, increased exercise and fluid intake (if allowed).
- A diuretic regimen may be sufficient therapy for reducing mild hypertension. Urge patient to keep scheduled appointments so that hypotensive response can be monitored. Lack of optimum clinical response may indicate changing the stepped-care regimen to step 2 (i.e., addition of an adrenergic drug).
- Store drug in tightly closed, light-resistant container at controlled room temperature less than 40°C, preferably 15° to 30°C (59° to 86°F) unless otherwise directed by manufacturer.

DRUG INTERACTIONS   Indapamide

PLUS	INTERACTIONS
Antihypertensives, other	Potentiated hypotensive action
Alcohol, barbiturates, narcotic analgesics	Increased risk of orthostatic hypotension
Cardiac glycosides (e.g., digoxin)	Increased risk of digitalis toxicity (because of hypokalaemic effect of indapamide)
Corticosteroids, corticotropin, amphotericin B	Enhanced hypokalaemic effect of indapamide
Insulins, oral hypoglycaemics (e.g., tolbutamide)	Increased hypoglycaemic effect of antidiabetic agents
Lithium	Decreased renal clearance of lithium; increased risk of lithium toxicity. Concomitant use should be avoided

INDAPAMIDE (continued)

PLUS	INTERACTIONS
(continued)	
Tubocurarine, other nondepolarizing skeletal muscle relaxants	Increased skeletal muscle relaxation
Vasopressors	Decreased responsiveness to vasopressor activity. Use of indapamide only with extreme caution

Indomethacin

(Artracin, Imbrilon, Indocid, Indoflex, Indolar, Indomod,   *NSAID*
    Mobilan, Rheumacin, Slo-Indo)

ACTIONS AND USES Potent nonsteroid compound with antiinflammatory, analgesic, and antipyretic effects similar to those of aspirin. Antipyretic and antiiflammatory actions may be related to ability to inhibit prostaglandin biosynthesis. Uncouples oxidative phosphorylation in cartilaginous and hepatic mitochondria. Appears to reduce motility of polymorphonuclear leucocytes, development of cellular exudates, and vascular permeability in injured tissue. Apparently has no uricosuric action. Inhibits platelet aggregation but effect is of shorter duration than that of aspirin (effect usually disappears within 24 hours after drug is discontinued). Enhances effect of ADH and therefore promotes sodium and water retention.

Used for palliative treatment in active stages of moderate to severe rheumatoid arthritis, ankylosing rheumatoid spondylitis, acute gouty arthritis, and osteoarthritis of hip in patients intolerant to or unresponsive to adequate trials with salicylates and other therapy. Also used to close patent ductus arteriosus in premature infants.

ROUTE AND DOSAGE Oral: 50–200 mg/day with food. **Rectal suppositories**: 100 mg night and morning as required.

ABSORPTION AND FATE Promptly and almost completely absorbed from GI tract. **Onset of action** in 1 to 2 hours. **Peak plasma levels** within 3 hours following single oral dose; **duration of action** 4 to 6 hours. Approximately 90% bound to plasma protein, and also extensively bound in tissues; low concentrations in cerebrospinal fluid. **Half-life**: about 4½ hours. Largely metabolized in liver and kidneys. Excreted primarily in urine, mainly as glucuronide and about 10 to 20% as unchanged drug. Some elimination in bile and faeces. Crosses placenta; appears in breast milk.

CONTRAINDICATIONS AND PRECAUTIONS Allergy to indomethacin, aspirin, or other nonsteroidal antiinflammatory agents; nasal polyps associated with angioedema, history of GI lesions; pregnancy, nursing mothers, children (14 years of age or younger). **Cautious Use**: history of psychiatric illness, epilepsy, parkinsonism; impaired renal or hepatic function, controlled infections, coagulation defects, congestive heart failure, elderly patients, persons in hazardous occupations.

INDOMETHACIN (continued)

ADVERSE/SIDE EFFECTS   Altered laboratory findings: Increased SGOT, SGPT, bilirubin, BUN; positive direct Coombs' test. Side effects include: elevated BP, palpitation, chest pains, tachycardia, headache (common), dizziness, vertigo, lightheadedness, syncope, fatigue, muscle weakness, ataxia, insomnia, nightmares, drowsiness, narcolepsy, confusion, coma, convulsions, peripheral neuropathy, psychic disturbances (hallucinations, depersonalization, depression), aggravation of epilepsy, parkinsonism, blurred vision, lacrimation, eye pain, visual field changes, corneal deposits, retinal disturbances including macula, tinnitus, hearing disturbances, nausea, vomiting, diarrhoea, anorexia, bloating, abdominal distention, ulcerative stomatitis, proctitis, rectal bleeding, GI ulceration, haemorrhage, perforation, haemolytic anaemia, aplastic anaemia (sometimes fatal), agranulocytosis, leucopenia, thrombocytopenic purpura, haematuria, urinary frequency, renal failure (causal relationships not established), epistaxis, hair loss, exfoliative dermatitis, erythema nodosum, vaginal bleeding, breast changes, hyperglycaemia and glycosuria (rare), toxic hepatitis, oedema, weight gain, flushing, sweating.

NURSING IMPLICATIONS

- Indomethacin is contraindicated in patients allergic to aspirin. Question patient carefully regarding aspirin sensitivity prior to initiation of therapy.
- Administer immediately after meals, or with food, milk, or antacid (if prescribed) to minimize, GI side effects. Food or antacid may cause somewhat delayed and reduced absorption, but advantage of safety outweighs risk of impaired absorption.
- Incidence of adverse reactions is high (especially in elderly patients) and is dose-related in most patients. Physician will rely on accurate and prompt reporting of patient's response and tolerance to establish lowest possible effective dosage.
- Indomethacin can cause severe GI complications (reported to be among the most common side effects). Be alert to suspicious signs and symptoms and report immediately.
- Patient should be carefully observed and should be instructed to report adverse reactions in order to prevent serious and sometimes irreversible or fatal effects.
- In patients with underlying cardiovascular disease, the potential for sodium and water retention should be anticipated. Monitor weight and observe dependent areas for signs of oedema.
- Frontal headache is the most frequent CNS side effect; it should be reported. If it persists, dosage reduction or cessation of drug may be indicated. Usually it is more severe in the morning, but it may occur within 1 hour after drug ingestion. A dose scheduled at bedtime, with milk, may reduce the incidence of morning headache.
- Complete blood counts, renal and hepatic function tests, ophthalmoscopic examinations, and hearing tests should be performed periodically during prolonged therapy.
- Following control of acute flairs of chronic rheumatoid arthritis, physician may make repeated attempts to reduce daily doses until drug is finally discontinued.
- Expected therapeutic effects in rheumatoid arthritis are reduced fever, increased strength, reduced stiffness, and relief of pain, swelling, and tenderness. If improvement is not noted in 2 to 3 weeks, alternate therapy is generally prescribed.
- Therapeutic effect in acute gouty attack (relief of joint tenderness and pain) is usually

INDOMETHACIN (continued)

apparent in 24 to 36 hours; swelling generally disappears in 3 to 5 days. Keep physician informed; dosage should be reduced once pain is tolerable.

- Bear in mind that indomethacin may mask signs and symptoms of latent infections.
- Because of the possibility of dizziness and lightheadedness, caution the patient to avoid activities requiring mental alertness and motor coordination.
- Advise the patient not to take aspirin, because it may potentiate the ulcerogenic effects of indomethacin. *See also Drug Interactions.*
- Green colouration of urine has been reported in patients who develop indomethacin-induced hepatitis.
- Preserved in tight, light-resistant containers.

Drug interactions Ulcerogenic effects of indomethacin may be potentiated by concomitant administration of **corticosteroids, phenylbutazone,** or **salicylates;** concurrently administered **aspirin** may delay or decrease indomethacin absorption and thus may interfere with its therapeutic effectiveness. Recent reports indicate that indomethacin does not enhance the hypoprothrombinaemic effects of **oral anticoagulants;** however, since indomethacin inhibits platelet aggregation and may cause GI ulceration and bleeding, cautious use is advised. Concomitant use with **frusemide:** response to both drugs may be inhibited. Indomethacin may cause slight increase in **penicillin G** half-life. **Probenecid** may increase indomethacin serum levels. Possibility of impaired antihypertensive response to **propranolol** and other **beta-adrenergic blockers.**

Indoramin

(Baratol)   *Antihypertensive; alpha-adrenergic blocking agent*

ACTIONS AND USES   Used to treat hypertension usually with a beta-blocking drug orithiazide diuretic.

ROUTE AND DOSAGE   Oral: **Adult:** *initial* 25 mg twice a day increased by 25–50 mg/day at two weekly intervals to a maximum of 200 mg/day.
For further information: *see phenoxybenzamine.*

Inosine pranobex

(Imunovir)   *Antiviral*

ACTIONS AND USES   Newly introduced antiviral drug used to treat herpes simplex infection and as a adjunct to the treatment of genital warts.

INOSINE PRANOBEX (continued)
ROUTE AND DOSAGE   Oral: Adult: *Herpes simplex*: 1 g four times a day for 7–14 days. *Genital warts*: 1 g three times a day. Report adverse effects to the Committee on Safety of Medicines.

Inositol nicotinate

(Hexopal)

ACTIONS AND USES   Peripheral vasodilator with similar action and uses to nicotinic acid (q.v.).

ROUTE AND DOSAGE   Oral: Adult: 500 mg to 1 g three times a day.

Insulin injection (neutral)

(Neutral insulin injection, Hypurin Neutral, Neusulin,
   Quick sol ⟨bovine⟩, Velosulin ⟨porcine⟩, Human
   Actrapid, Human Velosulin, Humulin-S ⟨human⟩)

Antidiabetic; hypoglycaemic

ACTIONS AND USES   Short-acting, clear, colourless solution of exogenous unmodified insulin extracted from beta cells in beef and/or pork pancreas (as labelled). Biosynthetic human insulin is derived not from human pancreas but from cultures of genetically modified *Escherichia coli* by recombinant DNA technology. Enhances transmembrane passage of glucose into most body cells and by unknown mechanism may itself enter the cell to activate selected intermediary metabolic processes. Promotes conversion of glucose to glycogen, inhibits fatty acid mobilization from fat depots, promotes triglyceride synthesis, stimulates protein production, and promotes intracellular shift of K and Mg (magnesium). In the diabetic, insulin temporarily restores proper utilization of glucose and fat thereby preventing glycosuria, diabetic ketoacidosis, and coma. Neutral insulin supersedes insulin injection which is now renamed Acid insulin injection.

Used in the emergency treatment of diabetic ketoacidosis or coma, to initiate therapy in patient with insulin-dependent diabetes mellitus and in combination with intermediate-acting or long-acting insulin to provide better control of blood glucose concentrations in the diabetic patient. Used IV to stimulate growth hormone secretion (by producing hypoglycaemia) to evaluate pituitary growth hormone reserve in patient with known or suspected growth hormone deficiency. Other uses include: promotion of intracellular shift of K in treatment of hyperkalaemia (IV); to induce hypoglycaemic shock as therapy in psychiatry.

INSULIN INJECTION (NEUTRAL) (continued)

ROUTE AND DOSAGE   Subcutaneous, IM, IV: Dosage highly individualized according to blood and urine glucose concentrations.

ABSORPTION AND FATE   Following administration, absorbed directly into blood, circulated widely in extracellular fluid as free hormone. After SC injection, **action begins** in ½ to 1 hour. **Duration of effect**: 6 to 8 hours. Following IV injection, **action begins** in 10 to 30 minutes, **peaks** in ½ to 1 hour and **lasts** 1 to 2 hours. Plasma half-life following IV injection, 3 to 5 minutes. Half-life after SC injection, 4 hours and after IM, 2 hours. Metabolized primarily in liver and to lesser extent in kidney and muscle. Less than 2% of dose eliminated in urine.

CONTRAINDICATIONS AND PRECAUTIONS   Hypersensitivity to insulin animal protein.

ADVERSE/SIDE EFFECTS   Hypersensitivity (usually occurs when insulin is at peak action point): localized allergic reactions at injection site; generalized urticaria or bullae, lymphadenopathy, anaphylaxis (rare). **Hypoglycaemia (hyperinsulinism)**: profuse sweating, hunger, headache, nausea, tremulousness, tremors, palpitation, tachycardia, weakness, fatigue, nystagmus, circumoral pallor; numb mouth, tongue, and other paraesthesias; visual disturbances (diplopia, blurred vision, mydriasis), staring expression, confusion, personality changes, ataxia, incoherent speech, apprehension, irritability, inability to concentrate, personality changes, uncontrolled yawning, loss of consciousness, delirium, hypothermia, convulsions, Babinski reflex coma. (Urine glucose tests will be negative.) **Other**: posthypoglycaemic or rebound hyperglycaemia (Somogyi effect), lipoatrophy and lipohypertrophy of injection sites; insulin resistance. **Overdosage**: psychic disturbances, i.e., aphasia, personality changes, maniacal behaviour.

NURSING IMPLICATIONS

- All insulin in the UK is now supplied in 100 unit/ml concentration.
- Insulin is often mixed with intermediate acting insulins to attain good control.
- When neutral insulin is used alone, multiple injections are required. Insulin may be absorbed to the container or tubing when added to an IV infusion solution. Amount lost is variable and depends on concentration of insulin, infusion system, contact duration, and flow rate. The less the concentration of insulin in the solution and the slower the rate of flow, the greater the percentage absorbed.
- To reduce the potential for loss of insulin, normal serum albumin can be added to the insulin solution, or insulin may be added from a syringe directly into vein or IV tubing.
- During early period of dosage regulation, some patients experience visual difficulties. Advise patient to delay changing prescription lenses until vision stabilizes (usually 3 to 6 weeks).
- In the event of unavoidable insulin shortage, advise patient to reduce dosage temporarily, decrease food intake by one-third of usual quantity, and drink generous

INSULIN INJECTION (NEUTRAL) (continued)

amounts of liquids with little or no caloric value (water, coffee, tea, clear soup, broth).

- The amount and distribution of food throughout the day is determined by the physician and should not be changed unless prescribed.

Storage, preparation, and administration

- Advise patient to keep an extra vial of insulin, syringe, and needle on hand.
- Insulin in use is stable at room temperature up to 1 month. Avoid exposure to temperature extremes or to direct sunlight. Refrigerate stock supply.
- Avoid injection of cold insulin; it can lead to lipodystrophy, reduced rate of absorption, and local reactions.
- Examine vial before preparing dose. Do not use if solution is discoloured, cloudy, or contains a precipitate.
- Check expiry date on label. Discard outdated vials and partially used vials that have not been in use for several weeks.
- Insulins should not be mixed unless prescribed by physician. In general clear insulin is drawn up into syringe first to avoid contaminating it with the second insulin (cloudy).
- Insulin is generally administered 15 to 30 minutes before a meal so that peak action will coincide with postprandial hyperglycaemia.
- Eliminate air bubble within syringe and hub of needle (dead space) for accurate dosage. In syringes with detachable needles, dead space may be equivalent to 0.1 ml. Some disposable syringes with permanently attached needles have no dead space and thus provide more accurate measurement. Inject insulin into area that has a substantial layer of fat and is free of large blood vessels and nerves.
- Commonly used injection sites: upper arms, thighs, abdomen (avoid area over urinary bladder and 2 inches around navel), buttocks, and upper back (if fat is loose enough to pick up).
- Superficial subcutaneous injection may cause local allergic reaction or irritation and therefore should be avoided.
- For self-injection of an arm, instruct patient to press back of upper arm against a chair back so that tissue is 'bunched up,' making needle insertion easier.
- If patient is engaged in active sports it has been suggested that injection of insulin be made into the abdomen rather than into a muscle that will be heavily taxed, since this may speed up insulin absorption.
- Available injection sites are lost when lipodystrophy (dimpling or atrophy of adipose tissue seen predominantly in women and children) and hypertrophy or thickening develops. Lipodystrophy has been associated with inadequate rotation of injection sites, use of cold insulin, and intrafat insulin injections. (Reportedly, injection of purified insulins directly into lesions may correct lipodystrophy.)
- Allow approximately 1 inch between injection sites and avoid reuse of a site for 6 to 8 weeks, if possible.
- Maintain an injection record or chart to assure systematic site rotation.
- Special equipment is available for patients who are visually impaired or who have other handicaps.

INSULIN INJECTION (NEUTRAL) (continued)
Special points on adverse reactions

- Local reactions at injection site sometimes develop 1 to 3 weeks after therapy starts appearing 1 to 12 hours after an injection. Symptoms may last several hours to days, but usually disappear with continued use. Advise patient to report symptoms; physician may prescribe an antihistamine. Zinc sensitivity has been implicated. Injection technique should be checked.

- Generalized allergic reaction (sensitivity to species source of insulin) may be reversed by substituting insulin from another source.

- Patients highly sensitive to insulin who cannot be maintained on oral hypoglycaemics may be rapidly desensitized with subcutaneous administration of small and frequent doses of insulin. Observe patient closely for anaphylaxis and onset of hypoglycaemia during desensitization period.

- *Hypoglycaemic reaction* (insulin shock) may occur from excess insulin, insufficient food intake, e.g., skipped or delayed meals, vomiting, diarrhoea, unaccustomed exercise (burns up sugar and thus adds to insulin effect of lowering blood sugar), infection or illness or nervous or emotional tension, overindulgence in alcohol.

- Symptomatic hypoglycaemia occurs when blood sugar fall is sudden and rapid. Onset generally corresponds to peak action of insulin.

- Somogyi effect develops when patient chronically receives unnecessarily large doses of insulin with resulting unrecognized or uncorrected hypoglycaemia. The body attempts to compensate by accelerating release of hormones concerned with plasma glucose regulation (e.g., glucagon, catecholamines, somatropin, adrenal corticosteroids) with resulting rebound hyperglycaemia. Suspect Somogyi effect if evening blood or urine glucose levels are low followed by morning hyperglycaemia, or if patient appears to require increasingly more insulin.

- Restlessness and diaphoresis occurring during sleep are suggestive of hypoglycaemia in the diabetic patient.

- Instruct patient and responsible family members to respond promptly to beginning symptoms of hypoglycaemia (often vague): profuse sweating, hunger, fatigue, inability to concentrate, lassitude, depression, early morning headache, drowsiness, anxiety (*see Adverse/Side Effects*).

- Hypoglycaemic reaction occurs suddenly (in minutes to hours) and is an emergency situation, since prolonged hypoglycaemia can cause irreversible brain damage. Advise patient to take 120 mls of orange juice (45 ml–90 mls for child) followed by a meal of 1 glass milk with crackers or a sandwich (or other longer-acting carbohydrate or protein food). Other emergency sources of fast-acting carbohydrate include 4 ounces of a sugar sweetened soft drink, 2 sugar cubes, 2½ teaspoons of sugar, 2 teaspoons of honey or golden syrup. Failure to show signs of recovery within 30 minutes indicates necessity for emergency treatment.

- Patients with severe hypoglycaemia may receive glucagon, epinephrine, or IV glucose 10 to 50%. As soon as patient is fully conscious, oral carbohydrate may be given e.g., orange juice with sugar.

- Advise patient to carry some form of rapid-acting carbohydrate (e.g., lump sugar) at all times to treat hypoglycaemia.

- *Diabetic ketoacidosis* as a sequel to insulin deficiency or resistance is a medical

INSULIN INJECTION (NEUTRAL) (continued)

emergency that appears over a period of weeks in controlled diabetics or in a few hours in noncontrolled patients. Blood sugar levels may rise as high as 15.5–42 mmol/h or higher. Precipitating factors: omission of insulin, improperly balanced diet, over-eating, failure to increase insulin dosage during times of increased need, such as rapid growth in juveniles, fever, infection, or other illness, emotional stress, surgery, trauma, pregnancy. Patient/family education is critically important.

- *Symptoms of diabetic ketoacidosis*: drowsiness, nausea, diarrhoea, abdominal pain, intense thirst (polydipsia); polyuria, dry mouth, dry flushed skin, poor skin turgor, soft eyeballs, low BP, weak rapid pulse, fruity (acetone) breath, Kussmaul's respirations (air hunger), inattention, weakness, drowsiness, coma. Elevated laboratory values: urine glucose, urine ketones, blood glucose, serum ketoacids; decreased blood pH, and sodium bicarbonate.
- Severe ketoacidosis is treated with insulin injection IV, large amounts of IV fluids. Blood sugar is monitored hourly at bedside until values improve, then every 2 to 4 hours, as prescribed.
- During treatment for ketoacidosis with IV insulin, check blood pressure, fluid intake and output ratio, and blood glucose every hour.
- Observe level of consciousness; be alert for signs of hypoglycaemia (patient may pass from hyperglycaemia into insulin coma without regaining consciousness). Also observe for signs of hyperkalaemia (*see Index: Clinical signs and symptoms*).
- The juvenile diabetic generally is more prone to hypoglycaemia and ketoacidosis than the mature diabetic. Both child and parent must know signs of impending complications (*see Adverse Effects*). Short-term weight loss provides an accurate assessment of dehydration.
- Loss of diabetes control (hyperglycaemia or hypoglycaemia) occurs commonly at the beginning of a menstrual period. Advise patient to test urine/blood regularly during this time and to adjust insulin dosage accordingly, as prescribed by physician.
- Activity and insulin requirement vary inversely; this insulin requirements of the normally active diabetic child tend to decrease in the summer (when activity increases) and increase in the autumn. The abnormally active child with diabetes requires added food before and during anticipated activity.
- In the event of an illness, advise patient to continue taking insulin, go to bed, and drink liberally (every hour if possible) of noncaloric liquids. Do not force liquids if nauseated or vomiting. If unable to eat prescribed diet, replace with liquid or semiliquid carbohydrate according to food exchange list. Test urine or blood for sugar and acetone four times a day, before meals and at bedtime. Consult physician for insulin regulation if unable to eat prescribed diet, or if 4 meals of liquid or semiliquid carbohydrates have been taken or if urine/blood tests are unusual (e.g., high sugar, sugar with acetone).
- Hyperosmolar nonketotic diabetic coma most frequently occurs in diabetic patients who receive insufficient insulin to prevent advancing hyperglycaemia.

Glucose urine testing, glucose blood testing
- For reliability of results, advise patient to use only the prescribed type of urine test. Review the instructions on the package insert with the patient.

INSULIN INJECTION (NEUTRAL) (continued)

- Test of first voiding reflects a summation of blood sugars; test of second voiding (preferred and usually prescribed) reflects an instantaneous measurement of sugar in the blood. In the labile diabetic, urine may be tested four times daily, before meals and at bedtime to determine the pattern of urine sugars. Occasionally, tests are done at times of peak and minimum insulin effects.
- In general, glycosuria indicates unsuitable insulin dosage or dietary imbalance or indiscretion.
- Usually urine test for ketones is not done routinely in stabilized diabetics. It is checked routinely in new, unstable, and juvenile diabetes and if patient has lost weight, exercises vigorously, has an illness, and whenever urine contains glucose.
- Presence of acetone without sugar usually signifies insufficient carbohydrate intake. Acetone with sugar may indicate onset of ketoacidosis. Notify physician promptly.
- Since women in third trimester of pregnancy and nursing mothers may have lactose in urine, cupric sulphate reagents such as Benedict's test or Clinitest should not be used. Glucose oxidase reagents, e.g., Clinistix, Diastix, may be used.
- Caution patients to avoid OTC medications (which may have high sugar content) unless approved by physician. Aspirin or ascorbic acid in large doses may cause positive urine glucose test.
- Blood (capillary) glucose test kits, including lancet for finger or ear lobe prick, are now available for home use, e.g., Autolet self-monitoring kits (e.g., Dextrostix) require a special instrument for accurate interpretation of test readings.
- Physician may have patient supplement urine testing with blood glucose tests to improve diabetic control. The patient may be instructed to do the test before a meal or 2 hours after a meal (or more frequently, if indicated), during infection, unusual stress, any illness, pregnancy, when urine tests for ketones are positive and urine glucose shows 5% for 3 or 4 tests; before and immediately following a new exercise programme. During pregnancy, tests are done more routinely (at least 4 or 5 times a week).

Smoking–drug interaction

- Insulin absorption is decreased during the first 30 minutes after smoking. This interaction combined with a known increase in catecholamine release during smoking may have significant clinical effects. A heavy smoker may require up to 30% more insulin than the non-smoker.

Other

- Emphasize need for maintaining optimum skin care and foot care to prevent vascularrelated complications and infection.
- Hypoglycaemic reaction is sometimes the first indication of pregnancy in the diabetic woman. Patient should report promptly to physician.
- Insulin requirements during first trimester of pregnancy frequently decrease by one-third (utilization of glucose by foetus). During second and third trimesters, hormonal changes induced by pregnancy and action of placental insulinase may necessitate increased dosage (decreased insulin requirement during this period suggests a failing

I

INSULIN INJECTION (NEUTRAL) (continued)

placenta). On day of delivery, physician may omit insulin dose and administer IV glucose.

- After delivery, maternal insulin requirements usually are less than prepregnant dosage. Observe patient closely for hypoglycaemia. Insulin requirement gradually returns to prepregnancy level within 1 to 6 weeks.

- During lactation, frequent blood glucose determinations are advised. Both Benedict's test and Clinitest give positive readings for lactose; therefore, they should not be used during this period. Greater reliance will be placed on blood glucose analyses.

- When the patient plans to travel, advise patient to carry ample insulin (in event of delay in flight), at least 2 or 3 syringes and needles, and an adequate supply of emergency carbohydrate in hand luggage or handbag travel kits are available).

- Insulin dosage adjustment when travelling requires preplanning with physician, particularly when changes in time zones are involved.

- If foreign languages are spoken in countries to be visited, advise the patient to learn emergency vocabulary: 'Sugar.' 'May I have orange juice?' 'I am a diabetic.' 'I need a doctor.'

- For information about diabetic care here and in foreign countries, patients can write to International Diabetes Federation, 10, Queen Anne St., London WI, England.

- Advise patient to wear medical identification bracelet, necklace, or card with patient's and physician's names addresses, and telephone numbers, as well as diagnosis, dosage, and type of antidiabetic agent being taken.

- A high fibre diet may help to lower plasma glucose in some patients. Remind patient that dietary changes must be prescribed by physician.

- Advise patient to avoid alcohol, since it may reduce gluconeogenesis and thus precipitate hypoglycaemic crisis.

- Suicidal overdosing with SC injection has been successfully managed by excision of injection site.

- Be familiar with the information on insulin package insert, which is also available to the patient, and consult with physician for directions the patient is to follow. Prepare a teaching plan in collaboration with physician, dietitian, patient, and responsible family members.

Summary of patient/family teaching plan

- ☐ Nature of diabetes mellitus.
- ☐ Review patient instruction sheet (package insert).
- ☐ Insulin: action, administration, storage, syringe–insulin coordination.
- ☐ What to do in the event of unavoidable insulin shortage.
- ☐ Adjustments of insulin dosage (as prescribed) in relation to urine tests, illness, changes in activity, diet, travel; pregnancy.
- ☐ Urine and blood testing and recording, how and when to test.
- ☐ Cause, symptoms, prevention, and treatment of hypoglycaemia and ketoacidosis.
- ☐ Importance of adhering to prescribed diet and maintaining optimal body weight.
- ☐ Planned, graded exercise schedule (approved by physician). Personal hygiene: foot care, skin and dental care, prevention of infection.
- ☐ OTC medications and alcohol.

INSULIN INJECTION (NEUTRAL) (continued)

☐ Importance of regular follow-up visits for check of blood sugar and adjustment of insulin dosage and diet, if necessary.

☐ Educational resources: British Diabetic Association, 10, Queen Anne St, London WI.

Diagnostic test interferences   Large doses of insulin may increase urinary excretion of VMA. Insulin may cause alterations in **thyroid function tests**, and **liver function tests**, and may decrease **serum potassium**, and **serum calcium**.

DRUG INTERACTIONS *Insulin*

PLUS	INTERACTIONS
Alcohol, ethyl	Excessive alcohol intake can precipitate hypoglycaemic crisis
Anabolic steroids	Additive hypoglycaemic effects
Chlorthalidone	Antagonizes hypoglycaemic effects of insulin
Clonidine	Inhibits normal catecholamine response to insulin-induced hypoglycaemia, also suppresses signs and symptoms of hypoglycaemia
Contraceptives, oral Corticosteroids Thyroxine Diazoxide Andrenaline Oestrogens Ethacrynic acid	Hyperglycaemic action of these drugs may increase insulin requirements
Fenfluramin	Additive hypoglycaemic effects
Frusemide	Hyperglycaemic action may increase insulin requiremnts
Glucagon	Antagonizes hypoglycaemic effects of insulin
Guanethidine Hypoglycaemics, oral	Additive hypoglycaemic effects
Lithium •	Hyperglycaemic action may increase insulin requirements
MAO inhibitors	May enhance hypoglycaemic action of insulin
Marijuana	Hyperglycaemic action may impair glucose tolerance
Oxytetracycline	Possibility of additive hypoglycaemic effects
Phenothiazines Phenytoin	Hyperglycaemic action may increase insulin requirements
Propranolol	Interferes with carbohydrate metabolism with risk of prolonged hypoglycaemia; also may blunt warning signs of hypoglycaemia, e.g., palpitation, tachycardia
Salicylates (large doses) Sulphinpyrazone	Possibility of additive hypoglycaemic effects
Tiazide diuretics Thyroid preparations Triamterene	Hyperglycaemic action may increase insulin requirements

Insulin zinc suspension

(Insulin zinc suspension lente, Hypurin lente, Lentard MC, Neulente, Tempulin ⟨bovine⟩) (Human monotard)

Antidiabetic; hypoglycaemic

Insulin zinc suspension (amorphous)

(Semitard MC ⟨bovine⟩)

Insulin zinc suspension (chrystalline)

(Human Ultratard, Human Zn)

Insulin injection (biphasic)

(Rapitard MC)

ACTIONS AND USES   Intermediate-acting insulin. May be used in combination with neutral insulin twice daily or once a day for elderly patients. Administered by the subcutaneous route only.

ABSORPTION AND FATE   Action onset: 1 to 2 hours; **peak effect**: 4 to 12 hours; **Duration of action**: 16–35 hours.

NURSING IMPLICATIONS
- Usually administered 30 to 60 minutes before breakfast. Some patients require another injection 30 minutes before suppertime or at bedtime.
- Should not be administered IV. This preparation is not suitable for emergency treatment.
- For further information: *see neutral insulin.*

Insulin, isophane

(Isophane Insulin Injection, Hypurin Isophane, Monophane, Neuphane ⟨bovine⟩) (Insulatard ⟨porcine⟩) (Human Insulatard, Human Protaphane, Humulin I ⟨human⟩)

Antidiabetic; hypoglycaemic

ACTIONS AND USES   Intermediate-acting cloudy suspension of zinc insulin crystals and modified by protamine, in a neutral buffer. Combines some of the advantages and eliminates some of the disadvantages of both very short-acting and very long-acting

INSULIN, ISOPHANE (continued)

preparations. Therapeutic effect is prompt enough to control postprandial hypergly-caemia, which formerly called for supplemental doses of insulin injection. Generally, considered drug of choice to control hyperglycaemia in the diabetic patient.

ROUTE AND DOSAGE   Subcutaneous: (individualized).

ABSORPTION AND FATE   Action onset: 2 to 3 hours, **peak effect**: 4 to 12 hours; duration of action: about 24 hours.

NURSING IMPLICATIONS

- This preparation should never be administered IV; it is not suitable for emergency use.
- Usually given 30 to 60 minutes before first meal of the day. If necessary a second smaller dose may be prescribed 30 minutes before supper or at bedtime.
- If insulin was given before breakfast, a hypoglycaemic episode is most likely to occur between midafternoon and dinnertime, when insulin effect is peaking. Patient should be told to eat a snack in midafternoon and to carry sugar to treat a reaction. A snack at bedtime will prevent insulin reaction during the night.
- Insulin isophane/neutral mixtures: (initard 50/50, Mixtard 30/70 〈porcine〉) (Human Actraphane 70/30, Human initard 50/50, Human Mixtard 30/70, Humulin 90/10, Humulin 80/20 〈human〉)
  For further information: *see neutral insulin.*

Insulin, protamine zinc

(Hypurin Protamine Zinc 〈bovine〉)   *Antidiabetic; hypoglycaemic*

ACTIONS AND USES   Long-acting, cloudy suspension of insulin modified by addition of zinc chloride and protamine sulphate which has poor solubility and thus delays absorption.

Used to treat diabetes mellitus in patients who are not adequately controlled by unmodified insulin.

ABSORPTION AND FATE   Action onset: effects in 4 to 8 hours; **peak effect**: 14 to 24 hours; **duration of action** in excess of 36 hours. *See insulin injection.*

NURSING IMPLICATIONS

- Should not be administered IV. Not suitable for emergency use.
- Usually administered 30 to 60 minutes before breakfast.
- Active principal is in the milky white precipitate. To assure complete dispersion, mix thoroughly by gently rotating vial between palms and inverting it end to end several times. Do not shake; frothing will interfere with accurate measurement. If suspension or vial walls display granules or clumps after mixing, or if solution is clear and remains clear after mixing, discard vial.

Ipratropium bromide

(Atrovent)

*Anticholinergic;
bronchodilator*

ACTIONS AND USES   Acts directly on the airways causing dilation. Effective in the relief of bronchial constriction association with chronic bronchitis unresponsive to selective beta-2 adrenoceptor stimulants.

ROUTE AND DOSAGE   Aerosol inhalation: **Adult**: 18–36 mcg (1–2 puffs) maximum 72 mcg (4 puffs) 3–4 times a day. **Child (under 6 yrs)**: 18 mcg (1 puff); **(6–12 yrs)**: 18–36 mcg (1–2 puffs) three times a day. **Nebuliser: Adult**: 100–500 mcg four times a day. **Child (3–14 yrs)**: 100–500 mcg three times a day.

ABSORPTION AND FATE   Slow onset of action following aerosol inhalation. Maximum effect after 30–60 minutes.

CONTRAINDICATIONS AND PRECAUTIONS   Glaucoma and prostate hypertrophy.

ADVERSE/SIDE EFFECTS   Constipation, dry mouth, (rarely) urinary retention.

NURSING IMPLICATIONS
- Advise patient not to exceed the prescribed dose.
- Teach the technique of inhalation and explain manufacturer's instructions.
- Pressurised containers should not be punctured.
- Store at room temperature.

Iprindole

(Prondol)

Antidepressant; tricyclic

ACTIONS AND USES   Similar action and use to imipramine.

ROUTE AND DOSAGE   Oral: **Adult**: 15–30 mg three times a day, maximum 180 mg/day.
For further information: *see imipramine.*

Iproniazid

(Marsilid)

MAOI antidepressant; hydrazine

ACTIONS AND USES   Similar action and use to phenelzine.

IPRONIAZID (continued)
ROUTE AND DOSAGE   25–150 mg/day as a single dose.
  For further information: *see phenelzine.*

Iron dextran ━━━━━━━━━━━━━━━━━━━━━━━━━━━━━━━━━━━━

(Imferon)   *Antianaemic*

ACTIONS AND USES   A dark-brown slightly viscous liquid complex of ferric hydroxide
with dextran in 0.9% sodium chloride solution for injection. Reticuloendothelial cells
of liver, spleen, and bone marrow dissociate iron from iron dextran complex; the released
ferric ion combines with transferrin, and is transported to bone marrow, where it is
incorporated into haemoglobin.

  Used only in patients with clearly established iron deficiency anaemia when oral
administration of iron is unsatisfactory or impossible. Each millilitre of iron dextran
contains 50 mg elemental iron.

ROUTE AND DOSAGE   **IM (deep) or IV injection**: dose calculated according to body
weight and haemoglobin level.

ABSORPTION AND FATE   Following IM administration, most of drug is absorbed
from injection site through lymphatic system. The remainder (10 to 50%) becomes
fixed locally and is gradually absorbed over several months or longer. Slowly cleared
from plasma by reticuloendothelial system. Small amounts of iron dextran cross the
placenta. Traces are excreted in breast milk, urine, bile, and faeces.

CONTRAINDICATION AND PRECAUTIONS   Hypersensitivity to the product; all anaemias except iron-deficiency anaemia. Safe use during pregnancy and childbearing
period not established. **Cautious Use**: rheumatoid arthritis, ankylosing spondylitis,
impaired hepatic function, history of allergies and/or asthma.

ADVERSE/SIDE EFFECTS   These include: headache, shivering, transient paraesthesias,
syncope, dizziness, peripheral vascular flushing (rapid IV), hypotension, precordial
pain or pressure sensation, tachycardia, fatal cardiac arrhythmias, circulatory collapse,
nausea, vomiting, metallic taste, abdominal pain, sterile abscess and brown skin
discolouration (IM site), local phlebitis (IV site), lymphadenopathy, haemosiderosis,
risk of carcinogenesis at injection site associated with IM administration, reactivation of
quiescent rheumatoid arthritis, exogenous haemosiderosis.

NURSING IMPLICATIONS
- Oral iron should be discontinued prior to iron dextran administration.
- Diagnosis of iron-deficiency anaemia should be corroborated by appropriate labora-
  tory investigations, with the cause being determined and if possible corrected, before
  therapy is initiated.
- Anticipated response to parenteral iron therapy is an average weekly haemoglobin rise

IRON DEXTRAN (continued)

of about 1 g/dl. As with oral therapy, peak levels are generally reached in about 4 to 8 weeks.

- Regardless of route used, a test dose of 0.5 ml is given over a 5 minute period to the first IM or IV therapeutic dose to observe patient's response to the drug. If no reaction to the IM test dose occurs, after at least 1 hour, the remaining portion of initial dose is administered. If no reaction occurs after the IV test dose, the therapeutic regimen is started in 2 to 3 days. Fatal anaphylactic reactions have occurred. Adrenaline (0.5 ml of a 1:1,000 solution) should be immediately available for hypersensitivity emergency.
- Although anaphylactic reactions usually occur within a few minutes after injection, it is recommended that 1 hour or more elapse before giving remainder of initial dose following test dose.
- IM injections should be given only into the muscle mass in upper outer quadrant of buttock (never in the upper arm or other exposed area). Use a 2- or 3-inch, 19- or 20-gauge needle. The Z-tract technique is recommended to prevent drug leakage along the needle track and brown staining of subcutaneous tissue. Staining of skin may also be minimized by using one needle to withdraw drug from container and another needle for injection. Brown staining of skin may persist 1 to 2 years, since drug is absorbed slowly from subcutaneous tissue.
- **Z-track technique** Firmly displace skin laterally prior to injection. After needle is inserted, withdraw plunger carefully to check that there is no entry into a blood vessel. Inject slowly. Rotate injection sites. No more than 5 ml should be injected into a single IM site.
- If patient is receiving IM in standing position, patient should be bearing weight on the leg opposite the injection site; if in bed, patient should be in the lateral position with injection site uppermost.
- Mixing any other drug in syringe or solution with iron dextran is not advised.
- The IV route is preferred and recommended for patients with insufficient muscle mass, those with impaired absorption (as in oedema), when uncontrolled bleeding is a possibility, or when massive and prolonged parenteral therapy is indicated.
- If the IV injection does not exceed 100 mg, it is administered undiluted at a prescribed rate (usually no more than 50 mg or less per minute).
- The diluent for IV infusion is 0.9% NaCl injection. (5% dextrose solution is associated with a higher incidence of phlebitis and local pain.) Increased frequency of adverse effects may be expected with large IV doses, particularly delayed reactions (arthralgia, myalgia, pyrexia).
- Following IV administration, the patient should remain in bed for at least 30 minutes to prevent orthostatic hypotension. Monitor blood pressure and pulse.
- IV administration may exacerbate acute joint pain in patients with rheumatoid arthritis or ankylosing spondylitis. For this reason, the IM route is generally preferred in these patients.
- Systemic reactions may occur over a 24-hour period after parenteral iron has been administered. Instruct patient to report any unusual symptoms.
- Clinical response to iron dextran may be delayed if patient is also receiving chloramphenicol.

IRON DEXTRAN (continued)

- Periodic determinations of haemoglobin, haematocrit, and reticulocyte count should be made as a guide to therapy. Oral iron therapy should replace parenteral therapy as soon as feasible.
- Blood grouping and cross matching are reportedly not affected by iron dextran.
- Similar drug iron sorbitol (Jectofer).

Diagnostic test interferences   Falsely elevated **serum bilirubin** and falsely decreased **serum calcium** values may occur. Large doses of iron dextran may impart a brown color to serum drawn 4 hours after iron administration. **Bone scans** involving Tc-99m diphosphonate have shown dense areas of activity along contour of iliac crest 1 to 6 days after IM injections of iron dextran.

Isocarboxazid

(Marplan)   *Antidepressant; MAO inhibitor;*
                                                                         hydrazine

ACTIONS AND USES   MAO inhibitor of the hydrazine group. Similar in actions, uses, contraindications, precautions, and adverse reactions to phenelzine (q.v.). Recommended only for treatment of depressed patients refractory to or intolerant of tricyclic antidepressants or to electroconvulsive therapy.

ROUTE AND DOSAGE   Oral: *Initial*: 30 mg daily in single or divided doses.

CONTRAINDICATIONS AND PRECAUTIONS   Children (under 16); elderly (over 60 years of age). **Cautious Use**: hypertension, hyperthyroidism, parkinsonism, renal impairment, cardiac arrhythmias. *See also phenelzine.*

NURSING IMPLICATIONS

- A complete review of prior drug therapy is advised before initiation of isocarboxazid.
- Store in a well closed, light-resistant container at temperature between 15° and 30°C (59° and 86°F).
- See also phenelzine sulphate.

Isoetharine hydrochloride

(Numotac)   *Beta-adrenergic agonist;*
                                                                         bronchodilator

ACTIONS AND USES   Used to treat reversible airways obstruction.

ISOETHARINE HYDROCHLORIDE (continued)

ROUTE AND DOSAGE   Oral: 10–20 mg 3–4 times a day.

For further information: *see salbutamol.*

Isoniazid

(Rimifon)   *Antitubercular agent*

ACTIONS AND USES   Hydrazide of isonicotinic acid with highly specific action against *Mycobacterium tuberculosis*. Exerts bacteriostatic action against actively growing tubercle bacilli; may be bactericidal in higher concentrations.

Used in treatment of all forms of active tuberculosis caused by susceptible organisms and as preventive in high-risk persons (e.g., household members, persons with positive tuberculin skin test reactions). Used in combination with other tuberculostatic agents.

ROUTE AND DOSAGE   Oral: intramuscular: (dosages are identical). Administered in single or divided doses. **Adults:** 300 mg/day. **Child:** 6 mg/kg/day. *Meningitis:* 10 mg/kg/day.

ABSORPTION AND FATE   Peak blood levels in 1 to 2 hours following oral administration and sooner following IM injection. Levels decline to 50% or less within 6 hours. Diffuses readily into body tissues, organs and fluids, notably saliva, bronchial secretions, and pleural, ascitic, and cerebrospinal fluids. Metabolized in liver primarily by acetylation and dehydrazination (rate of acetylation is genetically determined). **Half-life** 2 to 5 hours in hepatic insufficiency and in 'slow' inactivators, and 0.5 to 1.6 hours in fast inactivators. About 75 to 95% of dose is excreted in urine within 24 hours as metabolites; small amounts executed in saliva and faeces. Crosses placenta and passes into breast milk.

CONTRAINDICATIONS AND PRECAUTIONS   History of isoniazid-associated hypersensitivity reactions, including hepatic injury; acute liver damage of any aetiology; pregnancy (unless risk is warranted). **Cautious Use:** chronic liver disease, renal dysfunction, history of convulsive disorder.

ADVERSE/SIDE EFFECTS   Usually dose-related. These include: nausea, vomiting, epigastric distress, constipation, agranulocytosis, haemolytic or aplastic anaemia, thrombocytopenia, eosinophilia, methaemoglobinaemia, elevated SGOT and SGPT, bilirubinaemia, jaundice, fatal hepatitis, decreased vitamin B_{12} absorption, pyridoxine (vitamin B_6) deficiency, pellagra, gynaecomastia, hyperglycaemia, glycosuria, hyperkalaemia, acetonuria, metabolic acidosis, proteinuria, paraesthesias, peripheral neuropathy, visual disturbances, optic neuritis and atrophy, tinnitus, vertigo, ataxia, somnolence, excessive dreaming, insomnia, amnesia, euphoria, toxic psychosis, changes in affect and behaviour, depression impaired memory, hyperreflexia, muscle twitching, convulsions, headache, tachycardia, dyspnoea, dry mouth, urinary retention (males),

ISONIAZID (continued)

postural hypotension, rheumatic and lupus-erythematosus-like syndromes, irritation at injection site. **Overdosage**: dizziness, nausea, vomiting, slurred speech, visual hallucinations, blurred vision, respiratory distress, CNS depression, convulsions, stupor.

NURSING IMPLICATIONS

- Oral isoniazid is best taken on an empty stomach since food interferes with its absorption. However, if GI irritation occurs, drug may be taken with meals.
- Isoniazid in solution tends to crystallize at low temperatures; if this occurs, solution should be allowed to warm to room temperature to redissolve crystals prior to use.
- Local transient pain may follow IM injections. Massage injection site following drug administration. Rotate injection sites.
- Appropriate mycobacteriological studies and susceptibility tests should be performed before initiation of therapy and periodically thereafter to detect possible bacterial resistance.
- Vision testing and ophthalmoscopic examinations are recommended initially, periodically during drug therapy, and whenever visual symptoms appear. Early cessation of therapy usually results in resolution of ocular reactions.
- Adverse reactions occur most frequently in malnourished patients, the elderly, and in 'slow' isoniazid inactivators (acetylators). Rate of acetylation (a metabolic process) is genetically determined and affects plasma drug concentration. Slow acetylation leads to high plasma drug levels and thus to increased risk of toxicity. Approximately 50% of blacks and Caucasians are 'slow' inactivators; the majority of American Indians, Eskimos, and Orientals are 'rapid' inactivators.

Food–drug interactions

- Warn patient that concurrent ingestion of tyramine-containing foods (e.g., aged cheeses, smoked fish) may cause palpitation, flushing, and blood pressure elevation (possibly by isoniazid-induced MAO inhibition).
- Warn patient that histamine-containing foods (e.g., skipjack, tuna, sauerkraut juice, yeast extracts) may cause exaggerated drug response (headache, hypotension, palpitation, sweating, itching, flushing, diarrhoea) possibly by isoniazid inhibition of diamine oxidase.
- Isoniazid-induced pyridoxine (vitamin B_6) depletion causes neurotoxic effects. B_6 supplementation usually accompanies isoniazid use.
- Niacin (vitamin B_3) and folate stores are also decreased during isoniazid therapy.
- Peripheral neuritis, the most common vitamin B_{12} deficiency symptom, is usually preceded by paraesthesias of feet and hands (numbness, tingling, burning). Patients particularly susceptible include malnourished patients, diabetics, adolescents, and 'slow acetylators.'
- Diabetic patients should be observed for loss of diabetes control. Both true glycosuria and false-positive Benedict's tests have been reported. *See Diagnostic Test Interferences.*
- Isoniazid hepatitis (sometimes fatal) usually develops during the first 4 to 6 months of treatment, but it may occur at any time during drug therapy; it is most common in patients 50 years of age and older in those who ingest alcohol daily, and possibly in rapid acetylators.

ISONIAZID (continued)

- Continuation of isoniazid therapy after the onset of hepatic dysfunction increases risk of severe liver damage.
- Patients should be carefully interviewed and examined at monthly intervals for early detection of signs and symptoms of hepatotoxicity (loss of appetite, fatigue, malaise, nausea, vomiting, abdominal discomfort, dark urine, jaundice or scleral icterus). Instruct patient to withhold medication and report promptly to physician if any of these effects occur. Some physicians order monthly liver function tests throughout therapy.
- Advise patient to reduce alcohol intake while on isoniazid therapy because of increased risk of hepatotoxicity (see Drug Interactions).
- Hypersensitivity reactions should be reported immediately and all drugs withheld. Generally, they occur within 3 to 7 weeks following initiation of therapy.
- Therapeutic effects of isoniazid usually become evident within the first 2 to 3 weeks of therapy and may include reduction of fever and night sweats, diminished cough and sputum, increased appetite and weight gain, reduction of fatigue, and sense of well-being. Over 90% of patients receiving optimal therapy have negative sputum by the sixth month.
- Check weight at least twice weekly under standard conditions.
- Isoniazid may produce a sense of euphoria, which tempts the patient to do more than he or she should. Stress the importance of planned rest periods.
- Antitubercular agents permit therapy to continue on an outpatient basis after initial hospitalization. Patients and responsible family members must understand the importance of continuous medical supervision to follow course of disease, and uninterrupted drug therapy to prevent relapse and spread of infection to others.
- In general, isoniazid therapy is continued for a minimum of 18 months to 2 years for original treatment of active tuberculosis. When used for preventive therapy, isoniazid is usually continued for 12 months. Duration of treatment is shorter (minimum of 9 months) when both isoniazid and rifampicin are used.
- Pyridoxine (IV) is a specific antidote for isoniazid overdosage.
- Preserved in tightly closed, light-resistant containers at 15° to 30°C (59° to 86°F) unless otherwise directed by manufacturer.

Diagnostic test interferences   Isoniazid may produce false-positive results using **Benedict's solution**, but usually not with glucose oxidase methods (e.g., Clinistix, Dextrostix). Urinary excretion of **5-HIAA** may be decreased in patients with carcinoid syndrome.

Drug interactions   Daily ingestion of **alcohol** may increase risk of isoniazid-induced hepatotoxicity. Simultaneous administration of large doses of **aluminium hydroxide** and other aluminium-containing antacids may delay or decrease absorption of isoniazid; to minimize risk of interaction, schedule isoniazid at least 1 hour prior to antacid and administration. PAS reduces rate of isoniazid acetylation and thus may result in higher blood levels. **Cycloserine** and **ethionamide** increase risk of CNS toxicity (dizziness, drowsiness). **Disulphiram**: concurrent use with isoniazid may result in changes in coordination, affect, and behaviour. **Rifampicin** increases risk of hepatotoxicity. Con-

ISONIAZID (continued)

current administration of isoniazid and **phenytoin** (and possibly other hydantoin derivatives) may result in a significant rise in serum phenytoin levels and toxicity (ataxia, drowsiness, nystagmus); reduced phenytoin dosage is recommended in 'slow acetylators' particularly, with isoniazid is added to the therapeutic regimen.

Isoprenaline hydrochloride

(Isuprel, Saventrine)

*Adrenergic agonist (beta);
sympathamimetic;
bronchodilator*

Isoprenaline sulphate

(Iso-Autohaler, Medihaler-Iso)

ACTIONS AND USES   Synthetic direct-acting sympathomimetic amine chemically and pharmacologically similar to adrenaline but acts almost exclusively on beta-adrenergic receptors. Primary therapeutic effects include cardiac stimulation (positive inotropic and chronotropic actions), relaxation of bronchial tree, and peripheral vasodilation. Decreases both diastolic and mean pressures, but maintains or slightly increases systolic pressure, especially when patient is in shock. Large doses cause substantial drop in blood pressure, and repeated large doses may result in cardiac enlargement and focal myocarditis. Relaxes GI and uterine smooth muscles; inhibits histamine release. Increases hepatic glycogenolysis; but, unlike adrenaline, stimulates insulin secretion and thus rarely produces hyperglycaemia. Can also cause central excitation.

Used as bronchodilator in acute and chronic asthma and other respiratory disorders and in bronchospasm induced by anaesthesia. Effective as cardiac stimulant in cardiac arrest, carotid sinus hypersensitivity, cardiogenic and bacteraemic shock, Stokes-Adams syndrome, or ventricular arrhythmias due to A-V block. Also may be used in treatment of shock which persists after adequate fluid replacement.

ROUTE AND DOSAGE   *Isoprenaline hydrochloride*: **Oral: Adult**: 30 mg 8 hourly then increased, maximum of 840 mg/day. I.V. 0.5–10 mcg/min. *Isoprenaline sulphate*: **Sublingual**: 10–20 mg 1–3 times a day. **Child**: 5–10 mg 1–3 times a day. **Aerosol inhalation: Adult and child**: 80–240 mcg (1–3 puffs). Dose should not be repeated within 30 minutes and not more than 8 times in 24 hours. **Inhalation from nebulizer**: 1% solution 1 ml as required.

ABSORPTION AND FATE   Readily absorbed following parenteral injection and oral inhalation. Absorption following oral, sublingual, and rectal routes reportedly not as predictable. Bronchodilation occurs promptly and persists 1 to 2 hours following inhalation and sublingual tablet (variable), up to 2 hours following subcutaneous

ISOPRENALINE SULPHATE (continued)

injection, and 2 to 4 hours following rectal administration. Pharmacological action appears to terminate primarily by tissue uptake. Metabolized by conjugation in GI tract, liver, lungs, and other tissues. Metabolism in children may be more rapid and extensive. Secreted in urine within 24 to 48 hours. Small quantities of inactive metabolites excreted in faeces.

CONTRAINDICATIONS AND PRECAUTIONS Preexisting cardiac arrhythmias associated with tachycardia; central hyperexcitability, simultaneous use with adrenaline. Safe use in women of childbearing potential and during pregnancy and lactation not established. **Cautious Use**: sensitivity to sympathomimetic amines, elderly and debilitated patients, hypertension, coronary insufficiency and other cardiovascular disease, renal dysfunction, hyperthyroidism, diabetes, prostatic hypertrophy, glaucoma, tuberculosis.

ADVERSE/SIDE EFFECTS These include: headache, mild tremors, nervousness, anxiety, lightheadedness, vertigo, insomnia, excitement, weakness, fatigue, flushing, palpitation, tachycardia, paradoxic Stokes-Adams seizure (rare), precordial pain or distress, nausea, vomiting, swelling of parotids (prolonged use), bad taste, buccal ulcerations (sublingual administration), severe prolonged asthma attack, sweating, bronchial irritation and oedema (particularly with inhalations of powder). **Overdosage**: cardiac excitability, extrasystoles, arrhythmias, elevation followed by fall in blood pressure, severe bronchoconstriction, cardiac arrest, sudden death (especially following excessive use of aerosols).

NURSING IMPLICATIONS

IV administration is regulated by continuous ECG monitoring

- Patient must be observed constantly, and response to therapy must be carefully monitored by frequent determinations of heart rate, ECG pattern, blood pressure, and central venous pressure, as well as (for patients with shock) urine volume, blood pH, and PCO_2 levels.
- IV infusion rate should be prescribed by physician, with specific guidelines for regulating flow or terminating infusion in relation to heart rate, premature beats, ECG changes, precordial distress, BP, and urine flow. Rate of infusion is generally decreased or infusion may be temporarily discontinued if heart rate exceeds 110 beats/minute because of the danger of precipitating arrhythmias.
- Constant-infusion pump apparatus is recommended to prevent sudden influx of large amounts of drug.
- Facilities for administration of oxygen mixtures and respiratory assistance should be immediately available.
- High frequency of arrhythmias reported, particularly when administered IV to patients with cardiogenic shock or ischaemic heart disease, digitalized patients, and those with electrolyte imbalance.
- Intracardiac injection for cardiac standstill must be accompanied by cardiac massage to perfuse drug to myocardium.
- Solutions intended for oral inhalation must not be injected.

ISOPRENALINE SULPHATE (continued)

- **Sublingual tablet** Patient should be forewarned of potential transient facial flushing, palpitation, and precordial discomfort. (Systemic effects reported to occur more frequently by this route than by inhalation.)
- **Sublingual tablet administration** Instruct patient to allow tablet to dissolve under tongue, without sucking, and not to swallow saliva (may cause epigastric pain) until drug has been completely absorbed.
- Sublingual tablet may be administered rectally, if prescribed.
- Prolonged use of sublingual tablets reportedly can damage teeth, possibly because of drug acidity. Patient should be advised to rinse mouth with water after medication has completely absorbed and between doses.
- Tolerance to bronchodilating effect and cardiac stimulant effect may develop with prolonged or too frequent use, and rebound bronchospasm may occur when effects of drug end.
- Caution patient to take medication as prescribed, and advise patient to report to physician if usual dosage does not produce expected relief. Once tolerance has developed, continued use can result in serious adverse effects.
- Parotid swelling following prolonged use has been reported. Drug should be discontinued if this occurs.
- Inform patient taking repeated doses (as well as responsible family members) about adverse reactions, and advise them to report onset of such reactions to physician.
- Some isoprenaline products contain bisulphites or metabisulphites. These products should not be used by the patient with known allergy to sulphites. Check label.
- Preserved in tight, light-resistant containers preferably between 15° and 30°C (59° and 86°F) unless otherwise directed by manufacturer. Isoprenaline solutions lose potency with standing, and solutions gradually become pink to brownish pink from exposure to air, light, or heat or contact with metal or alkali. Do not use if precipitate or discolouration is present.

Drug interactions Effects of isoprenaline are antagonized by **propranolol** and other beta-adrenergic blocking agents. Possibility of additive effects and increased cardiotoxicity when administered concomitantly with *adrenaline* and most other sympathomimetic bronchodilators (may be prevented if given at least 4 hours apart). Administration of isoprenaline in patients receiving **tricyclic antidepressants** may increase the possibility of arrhythmias.

Isosorbide dinitrate

(Cedocar, Isoket, Isordil, Sorbichew, Sorbitrate, Seni-Slow, Sorbid, Vascardin)   *Vasodilator*

ACTIONS AND USES Vasodilator more stable than and with similar actions to glyceryl trinitrate (q.v.). Used in the prophylaxis and treatment of angina and in acute left ventricular failure.

ISOSORBIDE DINITRATE (continued)
ROUTE AND DOSAGE   Adult: sublingual 5–10 mg as required. Oral: *angina*: 30–120 mg a day in divided doses; *ventricular failure*: 40–160 mg a day maximum dose 240 mg/day. **Infusion**: 2–10 mg/hour.

For further information: *see glyceryl trinitrate*.

Isosorbide mononitrate

(Elanton, Ismo, Monit, Mono-Cedocard)   *Vasodilator*

ACTIONS AND USES   Vasodilator with similar action to glyceryl trinitrate. Used in angina prophylaxis.

ROUTE AND DOSAGE   Oral: **Adult**: 20 mg 2–3 times a day (10 mg if the patient has not received nitrates before) doses may be increased to 120 mg/day in divided doses if required.

For further information: *see glyceryl trinitrate*.

Isoxsuprine hydrochloride

(Defencin CP, Dovadilan)   *Adrenergic agonist (beta); vasodilator*

ACTIONS AND USES   Sympathomimetic agent with beta-adrenergic stimulant activity and with slight effect on alpha-receptors. Action is not blocked by propranolol (a beta-adrenergic blocker) suggesting that isoxuprine acts directly on vascular smooth muscle. Vasodilating action on arteries within skeletal muscles is greater than on cutaneous vessels. Also causes cardiac stimulation (increases cardiac contractility, rate, and output) and may produce bronchodilatation, mild inhibition of GI motility, and uterine relaxation by direct action on smooth muscles. At high doses inhibits platelet aggregation and lowers blood viscosity.

Used as adjunctive therapy in treatment of cerebral vascular insufficiency and peripheral vascular disease, such as arteriosclerosis obliterans, thromboangiitis obliterans (Buerger's disease), and Raynaud's disease.

ROUTE AND DOSAGE   Oral: 20 mg 4 times a day or 40 mg every 24 hrs. **IM**: 5–10 mg up to 4 times a day. **IV**: *initial* 100 mcg/min increased to 500 mcg/min.

ABSORPTION AND FATE   Well absorbed from GI tract. Therapeutic blood levels are achieved within 1 hour and persist for almost 3 hours. **Mean plasma half-life**: 1.25 hours. Partly conjugated in blood; excreted primarily in urine. Crosses placenta.

ISOXSUPRINE HYDROCHLORIDE (continued)

CONTRAINDICATIONS AND PRECAUTIONS Immediately postpartum; in presence of arterial bleeding; parenteral use in presence of hypotension, tachycardia. Safe use in pregnancy not established. **Cautious Use**: bleeding disorders, severe cerebrovascular disease, severe obliterative coronary artery disease, recent myocardial infarction.

ADVERSE/SIDE EFFECTS These include: flushing, orthostatic hypotension with lightheadedness, faintness; palpitation, tachycardia, dizziness, nervousness, trembling, weakness, nausea, vomiting, abdominal distress, abdominal distention, severe rash.

NURSING IMPLICATIONS

- Advise patient to report adverse reactions (skin rash, palpitation, flushing) promptly, symptoms are usually effectively controlled by dosage reduction or discontinuation of drug.
- Parenteral administration may cause hypotension and tachycardia. Monitor blood pressure and pulse. Supervise ambulation.
- To prevent orthostatic hypotension, instruct patient to make position changes slowly and in stages particularly from recumbent to upright posture and to avoid standing still.
- Therapeutic response to isoxsuprine in treatment of peripheral vascular disorders may take several weeks. Evaluate clinical manifestations of arterial insufficiency: pain with walking (intermittent claudication), rest pain, sensations of numbness, coldness, burning; weak or absent peripheral pulses, rapid blanching when legs are elevated; rubor (cyanosis or dusky skin colour) in dependent position, keep physician informed.
- Patients should be completely informed about skin care of legs and feet and care of toenails. Properly fitted shoes and stockings and the importance of avoiding mechanical, chemical, and thermal trauma should be emphasized. Cessation of smoking and control of weight are crucial adjuncts to pharmacotherapeutic regimen.
- If isoxsuprine has been used to delay premature labor, hypotension, irregular and rapid heart beat may be observed in both mother and baby.
- Hypocalcaemia, hypoglycaemia, and ileus have been observed in babies born of mothers taking isoxsuprine.

Kanamycin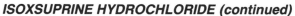

(Kannasyn)   *Antibiotic; aminoglycoside*

ACTIONS AND USES Aminoglycoside antibiotic derived from *Streptomyces kanamyceticus* and similar to neomycin in chemical structure and antibacterial properties. Active against many gram-negative microorganisms, especially *Klebisella pneumoniae. Enterobacter aerogenes, Proteus* species, *E. coli, Serratia marcescens*, and *Acinetobacter*. Also effective against many strains of *Staphylococcus aureus*, but it is not the drug of choice. Cross-resistance between kanamycin and neomycin is complete. As with other aminogly-

KANAMYCIN (continued)

cosides, exerts curarelike effect on neuromuscular junction. Oral kanamycin reportedly decreases serum cholesterol.

Used orally to reduce ammonia-producing bacteria in intestinal tract as adjunctive treatment of hepatic coma; also used for preoperative bowel antisepsis and for treatment of intestinal infections. Parenteral drug is used in short-term treatment of serious infections.

ROUTE AND DOSAGE   **IM**: 250 mg 6 hourly or 500 mg 12 hourly. **IV**: slow injection, 15–30 mg/kg/day in divided doses.

ABSORPTION AND FATE   Poorly absorbed from GI tract. Excreted in faeces as unchanged drug; absorbed portion, if any, excreted unchanged in urine. Completely absorbed following IM injection in about 1.5 hours. Peak serum concentrations reached in about 1 hour, declining to very low levels by 12 hours. **Serum half-life**: 2 to 4 hours. Diffuses to most body fluids, including cerebrospinal fluid, but only if meninges are inflamed. Also readily absorbed from peritoneal cavity. Excreted by kidneys (mostly by glomerular filtration); 81% excreted in urine as unchanged drug. Approximately one-half of IM dose eliminated in 4 hours; excretion complete within 24 to 48 hours (prolonged in patients with renal impairment). Crosses placenta and appears in breast milk.

NURSING IMPLICATIONS

- Kanamycin should not be mixed in the same syringe with other drugs. Discard partially used vials within 48 hours.
- Advise home patients to discard remaining drug after therapy is completed.
- Kanamycin is stable for 24 hours at 15° to 30°C (59° to 86°F) in most IV solutions. Consult manufacturer's literature for storage information.

  For further information: *see gentamicin.*

Drug interactions   It is possible for additive nephrotoxic effects to occur with **cephalosporins**. Combined or sequential use of kanamycin with other **aminoglycoside antibiotics** increases the possibility of nephrotoxicity and ototoxicity. Concurrent use with potent diuretics, e.g., **bumetanide** (Bumex) **ethacrynic acid** frusemide potentiates ototoxicity. Enhanced neuromuscular blockade and respiratory depression may occur with **ether** and related **inhalation anaesthetic agents**, and **skeletal muscle relaxants** e.g., **succinylcholine, tubocurarine**. *See gentamicin for other possible interactions.*

Kaolin

ACTIONS AND USES   Highly absorbent powder, absorbs toxins and adds bulk to faeces. Used in antidiarrhoeal mixtures or as a suspension.

KAOLIN (continued)
ROUTE AND DOSAGE   Oral: Adult: 5–25 g as required. Child: 1–5 g as required. Kaolin and morphine mixture (contains 916 mcg morphine hydrochloride in 10 ml) 10–20 ml/4 hourly.

K

Ketazolam

(Anxon)   *Psychotrophic; anxiolytic; diazepine*

ACTIONS AND USES   Similar actions and uses to chlordiazepoxide.

ROUTE AND DOSAGE   Oral: Adult: 15–60 mg.
For further information: *see chlordiazepoxide.*

Ketoconazole

(Nizoral)   *Antibiotic; antifungal*

ACTIONS AND USES   Broad-spectrum antifungal agent active against clinical infections with *Coccidioides immitis, Histoplasma capsulatum, Paracoccidioides brasiliensis, Phialophora,* and *Candida* species. *In vitro* studies suggest mode of action involves interference with synthesis of ergosterol, an essential component of fungal cell membranes.

Used for treatment of many oral and systemic fungal infections including candidiasis (chronic mucocutaneous candidiasis, oral thrush, candiduria) coccidioidomycosis, histoplasmosis, paracoccidioidomycosis, chromomycosis, and dermatophytoses.

ROUTE AND DOSAGE   Oral: Adults: *Initial*: 200 mg once daily. May be increased to 400 mg once daily for serious infection or to improve clinical response. **Children: older than 2 years**: 3.0 mg/kg/daily as single doses.

ABSORPTION AND FATE   Following oral administration of single dose mean peak plasma levels (3.5 mcg/ml) reached within 1 to 2 hours. Plasma elimination is biphasic: **half-life** of 2 hours within first 10 hours and 8 hours thereafter. Poor penetration into CSF. Metabolized in liver; plasma protein binding about 99%. About 13% excreted in urine (2 to 4% unchanged drug); major excretory route through bile into intestinal tract.

CONTRAINDICATIONS AND PRECAUTIONS   Hypersensitivity to ketoconazole; use during pregnancy not advised (teratogenic and embryotoxic effects reported in animal studies); lactation, children under age 2, fungal meningitis. **Cautious Use**: drug-induced achlorhydria, hepatic impairment.

K

KETOCONAZOLE (continued)

ADVERSE/SIDE EFFECTS   Usually well tolerated. Side effects include: nausea, vomiting, abdominal pain, diarrhoea pruritus, headache, dizziness, somnolence, fever, chills, photophobia, transient increases in serum liver enzymes.

NURSING IMPLICATIONS

- The infective organism should be identified but treatment may be started before obtaining lab results.
- Ketoconazole requires an acid medium for dissolution; therefore administer it at least 2 hours before an antacid, anticholinergic, cimetidine, or ranitidine (agents that may elevate GI pH) is given.
- Give drug with water, fruit juice, coffee, or tea.
- Advise patient to refrain from driving a car or using hazardous equipment until response to the drug is known. Drowsiness and dizziness are early and time-limited side effects.
- Treatment is continued until all clinical and lab tests indicate that fungal infection has subsided.
- Minimal treatment period for candidiasis to 1 to 2 weeks. Chronic mucocutaneous candidiasis may require maintenance therapy. Minimal treatment for systemic fungal infection is 6 months.
- Instruct patient to avoid OTC drugs for gastric distress, such as, Alka-Seltzer. Consult physician before taking any nonprescribed medicines.
- Caution patient not to alter the dose or dose interval and not to stop taking keto-conazole before consulting the physician. Poor response and recurrence of clinical symptoms are often related to an erratic dose regimen.
- Store in tightly-covered container, preferably between 15° and 30°C (59° and 86°F) unless otherwise directed by manufacturer.

Drug interactions   Antacids, anticholinergics, antihistamines (H_2-receptor antagonists) decrease absorption of ketoconazole leading to inadequate plasma level. Antifungal action of ketoconazole may be reduced by concurrent administration of **Isoniazid** and **rifampicin** (effect of rifampicin may also be reduced). Pharmacological effects of **cyclosporine** may be increased; monitor cyclosporine serum levels and serum creatinine.

Ketoprofen ─────────────────

(Alrheumat, Orudis, Oruvail)   *NSAID*

ACTIONS AND USES   Similar action and uses to indomethicin.

ROUTE AND DOSAGE   Oral: **Adult**: 100–200 mg/day in 2–4 divided doses, **Rectal**: 100 mg at bedtime. Combined rectal and oral treatment dose should not exceed 200 mg/day.

For further information: *see indomethicin.*

Ketotifen

(Zaditen)

ACTIONS AND USES   Used as prophylaxis in asthma.

ROUTE AND DOSAGE   Oral: **Adult**: 1–2 mg/day. **Child (over 2 yrs)**: 1mg twice a day.

For further information: *see sodium chromoglycate.*

L

Labetalol hydrochloride

(Labrocol, Trandate)   *Adrenergic blocking agent*
                                                   (alpha/beta);
                                                   antihypertensive

ACTIONS AND USES   Adrenergic receptor blocking agent that combines selective alpha activity and nonselective beta-adrenergic blocking actions. Both activities contribute to blood pressure reduction. Alpha blockade results in vasodilation, decreased peripheral resistance, and orthostatic hypotension, and only slightly affects cardiac output and coronary artery blood flow. Beta-blocking effects on sinus node, AV node, and ventricular muscle lead to bradycardia, delay in AV conduction, and depression of cardiac contractility. Similar to propranolol and other nonselective beta-blockers in ability to decrease resting and exercise-induced heart rate. Depresses plasma renin activity both at rest and during exercise. Also has weak membrane stabilizing properties at recommended doses. Does not abolish digitalis-induced inotropic action on heart muscle.

Used for treatment of mild, moderate, and severe hypertension. May be used alone or in combination with other antihypertensive agents.

ROUTE AND DOSAGE   Oral: *initially,* 100 mg twice daily. **Intravenous**: 50 mg slowly over 1 minute repeat after 5 minutes if required. Maximum 200 mg. *Continuous infusion*: 2 mg/minute to a maximum of 200 mg.

ABSORPTION AND FATE   Rapidly and completely absorbed following oral administration. **Onset of hypotensive action** usually within 1 to 2 hours; **peak plasma levels** in 2 to 4 hours. **Duration of action**: 8 to 12 hours (dose-dependent). *Onset of action* following IV administration: within 5 minutes; **plasma levels peak** in 20 to 40 minutes. Approximately 50% protein bound. **Plasma half-life** 3 to 8 hours. Steady-state plasma response in 24 to 72 hours. Undergoes extensive first-pass metabolism in liver. About 60% of dose excreted by kidneys as inactive metabolites and unchanged drug (5%); 40% of dose eliminated in faeces via bile. Crosses placenta. Small amounts appear in breast milk.

CONTRAINDICATIONS AND PRECAUTIONS   Bronchial asthma, uncontrolled cardiac failure, heart block (greater than first degree), cardiogenic shock, severe bradycardia.

LABETALOL HYDROCHLORIDE (continued)

Safe use during pregnancy, in nursing women, and in children not established. **Cautious Use**: nonallergic bronchospastic disease, chronic obstructive airways disease, well compensated patients with history of heart failure, phaeochromocytoma, impaired hepatic function, jaundice, diabetes mellitus.

ADVERSE/SIDE EFFECTS These include: postural hypotension, light-headedness, angina pectoris, palpitation, bradycardia, syncope, pedal or peripheral oedema, pulmonary oedema, congestive heart failure, flushing, cold extremities, Raynaud's phenomenon, arrhythmias (following IV), paradoxical hypertension (patients with phaeochromocytoma), rashes of various types, reversible alopecia, increased sweating, pruritus, nausea/vomiting, dyspepsia, constipation, diarrhoea, taste disturbances, cholestasis with or without jaundice, increases in serum transaminases, dry mouth, dizziness, fatigue/malaise (asthenia), headache, tremors, paraesthesias (especially scalp tingling), hypoaesthesia (numbness) following IV, mental depression, sleep disturbances, nightmares, dry eyes, activity disturbances, acute urinary retention, difficult micturition, transient rises in BUN and serum creatinine, impotence, ejaculation failure, loss of libido, Peyronie's disease, dyspnoea, bronchospasm, nasal stuffiness, myalgia, muscle cramps, toxic myopathy, antimitochondrial antibodies, positive antinuclear factor (ANF), SLE syndrome, pain at IV injection site. For potential adverse effects listed for other beta blockers *see propranolol*.

NURSING IMPLICATIONS

- Administered oral preparation preferably with or immediately after food. Food increases drug bioavailability. Advise consistency.
- Monitor blood pressure and pulse during dosage adjustment period. Standing blood pressure is used as indicator for making dosage adjustments.
- Patients should be supine when receiving labetalol IV. Take blood pressure immediately before drug is administered, then 5 minutes and 10 minutes after injection.
- Supine position should be maintained for at least 3 hours after IV administration. At the end of this time, determine patient's ability to tolerate elevated and upright positions before allowing ambulation.
- Controller device is recommended for maintaining accurate flow rate during IV infusion.
- Caution patient that postural hypotension is most likely to occur during peak plasma levels, i.e., 2 to 4 hours after drug administration.
- Instruct patient to adopt the habit of making position changes slowly and in stages, particularly from recumbent to upright position. Elderly patients are particularly sensitive to hypotensive effects.
- Diabetic patients should be closely monitored. Inform patient that labetalol may mask usual cardiovascular response to acute hypoglycaemia, e.g., tachycardia. Advise patient to be alert to possible signs of hypoglycaemia, e.g., weakness, clammy skin, headache, confusion, visual disturbances.
- Reassure patient that most adverse effects are transient and dose-related and occur early in therapy. Encourage patient to telephone any unusual symptoms or problems to clinician or responsible care provider.

LABETALOL HYDROCHLORIDE (continued)

■ Periodic ophthalmoscopic examinations are advised during prolonged therapy. Reportedly, labetalol may accumulate in tissues with high melanin content such as the choroid. This eye problem has not been reported in humans, but has occurred in laboratory animals.

■ Stress importance of keeping follow-up appointments. Tests of liver and renal function should be performed periodically during therapy.

■ Warn patient not to interrupt or discontinue drug therapy without consulting the physician.

■ Discontinuation of labetalol following chronic administration should be done by gradual reduction of dosage over a 1- to 2-week period. Patient should be closely monitored.

■ Since labetalol can cause dizziness and light-headedness, advise patient to avoid driving and other potentially hazardous activities until reaction to drug is known.

■ Withdrawal of antihypertensive therapy before surgery remains controversial. Anaesthetist should be informed of physician's decision.

■ *Treatment of overdosage* Induce emesis (ipecuanha syrup) or gastric lavage. Keep patient supine with legs elevated if necessary. Have on hand atropine (3 mg) for excessive bradycardia, isoprenaline digitalis glycoside, diuretic, noradrenaline; theophylline or a beta-2-stimulating agent for bronchospasm.

■ Store preferably between 2° to 30°C (36° to 86°F), unless otherwise advised by physician. Do not freeze. Protect tablets from excess moisture.

■ *See propranolol for patient teaching points regarding hypertensive therapy.*

Diagnostic test interferences False increases in **urinary catecholamines** when measured by nonspecific trihydroxyindole (THI) reaction (due to labetalol metabolites), but not with specific radioenzymatic or high performance liquid chromatography assay techniques.

DRUG INTERACTIONS *Labetalol*_____

PLUS	INTERACTIONS
Beta-adrenergic agonist bronchodilators, e.g., ephedrine Orciprenaline, terbutaline	Labetalol may blunt bronchodilator effect requiring higher doses of these drugs
Cimetidine	Increases bioavailability of labetalol (by increasing its absorption or decreasing hepatic metabolism). May require lower doses
Halothane	Additive hypotensive effects, especially with high concentrations (3% or above) of halothane
Insulins	Pharmacological effects of insulins may be increased and symptoms of hypoglycaemia may be obscured by labetalol
Glyceryl trinitrate	Possibility of additive hypotensive effects. Labetalol blunts reflex tachycardia induced by nitroglycerin
Tricyclic antidepressants	Possibility of increased incidence of tremor

See also propranolol for other possible drug interactions.

Lactulose

(Duphalac)   *Laxative*

ACTIONS AND USES   An ammonia detoxicant that reduces blood ammonia levels by as much as 25 to 50%. Action relies on environmental changes in the colon produced by bacterial degradation of lactulose. Resulting acidification of colon and osmotic fermentative diarrhoea prevents absorption of ammonium ion (NH_4^+) while promoting migration of blood ammonia (NH_3) into the intestinal tract. Once in the acid colon, NH_3 is converted to the nonabsorbable NH_4^+ ion and lost to systemic circulation. Other lactulose metabolites with laxative properties, plus the osmotically increased water, stimulate expulsion of the trapped ammonia. Lactulose therapy is reported to improve protein tolerance.

Used to treat chronic constipation and hepatic encephalopathy.

ROUTE AND DOSAGE   Oral: Adult: Constipation: 15 ml twice a day, reduced according to need. **Child (up to 1 yr)**: 2.5 ml; **(1−5 yrs)**: 5 ml; **(6−12 yrs)**: 10 ml twice a day. *Portal-system encephalopathy*: 30−50 ml 3 times a day.

ABSORPTION AND FATE   Poorly absorbed. 97% reaches intestinal tract relatively unchanged where it is metabolized by resident bacteria to organic acids. Excretion (3% or less) in urine completed within 24 hours.

CONTRAINDICATIONS AND PRECAUTIONS   Low galactose diet; safe use in pregnancy and during lactation not determined. **Cautious Use**: diabetes mellitus, concomitant use with electrocautery procedures (proctoscopy, colonoscopy), elderly and debilitated patients, children.

ADVERSE/SIDE EFFECTS   *Initial dose*: flatulence, belching, intestinal cramps, abdominal pain, diarrhoea (excessive dose), nausea, vomiting, colon accumulation of H_2 gas, hypernatraemia.

NURSING IMPLICATIONS
- Administer with fruit juice or other nonfat drink to increase palatability; avoid meal time.
- Laxative action is not instituted until drug reaches the colon; therefore transit time before reaching the colon and during passage through colon affects response time. 24 to 48 hours (normally required for a bowel movement) is also required for drug-induced laxation.
- Any factor that slows gastric or small intestine transit time may extend initial response time to oral lactulose therapy (e.g., food, constipation, hypercatabolic states, as with infection).
- Therapeutic response (decreased blood ammonia) in patient with hepatic encephalopathy is marked by clearing of confusion, apathy, and irritation, and by improved mental state and EEG patterns.
- Warn patient who may be discouraged by slow onset of drug action not to self-medicate with another laxative.

LACTULOSE (continued)

- Abuse of lactulose therapy for constipation should be prevented because of danger of electrolyte imbalance. Periodic lab evaluations of K, chlorides, CO_2 are indicated during chronic lactulose use.
- Changes in ageing retard and reduce capacity of the elderly to adjust to electrolyte imbalance.
- Lactulose-induced osmotic changes in the bowel support intestinal water loss and potential hypernatraemia. Fluid intake (often self-limited by the elderly) should be actively promoted (up to 1,500 to 2,000 ml/day) during drug therapy for constipation.
- Avoid exposing lactulose solution to light. Normal darkening does not affect action. Discard solution that is very dark or cloudy.
- If solution is refrigerated, it will be too viscous to pour. Store at room temperature (below 30°C, or 86°F), which will reduce viscosity; do not freeze.
- *See bisocodyl for patient teaching regarding management of chronic constipation.*

DRUG INTERACTIONS   *Lactulose*

PLUS	INTERACTIONS
Laxatives	Laxation may incorrectly suggest therapeutic action of lactulose
Neomycin and possibly other oral antiinfectives	May inhibit lactulose action by reduction or removal of resident colon bacteria

Latamoxef

(Moxalactam)

Antibiotic (beta-lactam); cephalosporin

ACTIONS AND USES   Synthetic, broad spectrum beta-lactam antibiotic with prolonged action; usually classified as third generation cephalosporin. In general, spectrum of activity resembles that of other third generation members, particularly cefotaxime.

Used for treatment of serious infections of lower respiratory and urinary tracts, skin and skin structure, bone and joint, and for intraabdominal infections, septicaemia, and meningitis. Used alone or with an aminoglycoside.

ROUTE AND DOSAGE   **IM or IV: Adult**: 0.25–3 g every 12 hours, 4 g 8 hrly is severe infections. **Neonate**: 25 mg/kg every 8–12 hrs. **Child**: 50 mg/kg every 12 hrs.

ABSORPTION AND FATE   Well-absorbed following IM or IV administration and widely distributed to most body tissues and fluids. **Serum levels peak** in ½ to 2 hours following IM injection, and at the end of IV infusion. **Half-life**: 2 to 2½ hours (longer in patients with renal dysfunction). Crosses blood–brain barrier; drug concentrations in CSF: 10 to 30% of those in serum (higher when meninges are inflamed), and half-life is

LATAMOXEF (continued)

twice as long. Does not appear to be metabolized. Approximately 80% excreted in urine within 24 hours as unchanged drug; small amounts appear in stool via bile. Crosses placenta. Distribution to breast milk not known.

NURSING IMPLICATIONS

- For IM administration, moxalactam should be diluted with either sterile or bacteriostatic water, sterile or bacteriostatic 0.9% sodium chloride for injection, or 0.5 or 1.0% lignocaine hydrochloride injection (by prescription).
- For direct intermittent IV administration, injections should be made slowly over 3 to 5 minutes, directly into vein or through tubing of a free-flowing compatible IV infusion solution.
- For further information: *see cefotaxime.*

Levodopa ———————————————————————

(Brocardopa, Larodopa)   *Antiparkinsonian*

ACTIONS AND USES   Metabolic precursor of dopamine, a catecholamine neurotransmitter. Unlike dopamine, levodopa readily crosses the blood–brain barrier. Precise mechanism of action unknown. It is hypothesized that levodopa is rapidly decarboxylated to dopamine and thus restores dopamine levels in extrapyramidal centers (believed to be depleted in parkinsonism). Cardiac stimulation may be produced by action of dopamine on β-adrenergic receptors. Also may augment secretion of growth hormone, which in turn is postulated to affect glucose utilization.

Used in treatment of idiopathic Parkinson's disease, postencephalitic and arteriosclerotic parkinsonism, and parkinsonian symptoms associated with manganese and carbon monoxide poisoning. Also commercially available in combination with carbidopa (as Sinemet), and with benserazide (as Madopar) that are decarboxylase inhibitors which permit lower dosage range of levodopa and thus reduce incidence of adverse reactions.

ROUTE AND DOSAGE   Oral: *Initial*: 125 to 500 mg daily divided into two or more equal doses; *Sinemet*: 100 to 125 mg three to four times a day. *Madopar*: twice daily 50 to 100 mg doses given as levodopa content.

ABSORPTION AND FATE   Rapidly and completely absorbed from GI tract. **Peak plasma concentrations** within 1 to 3 hours. Converted to dopamine by decarboxylation in GI tract and liver; small amount of levodopa reaches CNS, where it is metabolized to dopamine by dopa decarboxylase. Major metabolite is homovanillic acid; minute amounts of dopamine are converted to noradrenaline. About 80% of dose is excreted in urine within 24 hours; negligible amounts are eliminated in faeces.

CONTRAINDICATIONS AND PRECAUTIONS   Known hypersensitivity to levodopa, narrow-angle glaucoma patients with suspicious pigmented lesion or history of melano-

LEVODOPA (continued)

ma, acute psychoses, severe psychoneurosis, within 2 weeks of MAO inhibitors. Safe use in women of childbearing potential, during pregnancy and lactation, and in children under 12 years of age not established. **Cautious Use**: cardiovascular, renal, hepatic, or endocrine disease, history of myocardial infarction with residual arrhythmias, peptic ulcer, convulsions, psychiatric disorders, dial infarction with residual arrhythmias, peptic ulcer, convulsions, psychiatric disorders, chronic wide-angle glaucoma, diabetes, pulmonary diseases, bronchial asthma, patients receiving antihypertensive drugs.

ADVERSE/SIDE EFFECTS These include: arthostatic hypotension; (less frequent): palpitation, tachycardia, hypertension, phlebitis, anorexia, nausea, vomiting, abdominal distress, flatulence, dry mouth, dysphagia, sialorrhoea; (less frequent): burning sensation of tongue, bitter taste, diarrhoea or constipation; (rarely): duodenal ulcer, GI bleeding, haemolytic anaemia, agranulocytosis, reduced haemoglobin and haematocrit, leucopenia, choreiform and involuntary movements, increased hand tremor, bradykinetic episodes (on−off phenomena), trismus, grinding of teeth (bruxism), ataxia, muscle twitching, numbness, weakness, fatigue, headache, opisthotonos, confusion, agitation, anxiety, euphoria, insomnia, nightmares; (less frequent): psychotic episodes with paranoid delusions or hallucinations, severe depression, hypomania; (rare): convulsions, blepharospasm, diplopia, blurred vision, dilated pupils, widening of palpebral fissures, oculorhinorrhoea, flushing, skin rashes, increased sweating, bizarre breathing patterns, urinary retention or incontinence, increased sexual drive, priapism, weight gain or loss, oedema; (rarely): hiccoughs, loss of hair, and malignant melanoma.

NURSING IMPLICATIONS

- **Food−drug interaction** Ingestion of l-dopa with meals, especially if high in protein, appears to interfere with plasma-to-CNS transport of the drug. Administration of drug between meals and with low protein snack (if desired) may decrease fluctuations in clinical response.
- If patient is unable to swallow capsule or tablet form, consult pharmacist about preparing a liquid formulation.
- Rate of dosage increase is determined primarily by patient's tolerance and response to levodopa. Make accurate observations and report promptly adverse reactions (generally dose-related and reversible) and therapeutic effects.
- Monitor vital signs, particularly during period of dosage adjustment. Report alterations in blood pressure, pulse, and respiratory rate and rhythm.
- Orthostatic hypotension is usually asymptomatic, but some patients experience dizziness and syncope. Caution patient to make positional changes slowly, particularly from recumbent to upright position, and to dangle legs a few minutes before standing. Supervision of ambulation is indicated. Tolerance to this effect usually develops within a few months of therapy. Elastic stockings may help some patients; consult physician.
- Muscle twitching and spasmodic winking (blepharospasm) are *early signs of overdosage*; report them promptly.
- All patients should be closely monitored for behaviour changes. Patients in depression should be closely observed for suicidal tendencies.

LEVODOPA (continued)

- Therapeutic effects: significant improvement usually appears during second or third week of therapy, but it may not occur for 6 months or more in some patients. Therapeutic effect on Parkinson's disease appears to decline after 6 to 8 years of therapy.
- Elevation of mood and sense of well-being may precede objective improvement. Stress the importance of resuming activities gradually and observing safety precautions in order to avoid injury. The patient with a history of cardiac problems should be cautioned against overactivity.
- Patients with chronic wide-angle glaucoma should be monitored during therapy for changes in intraocular pressure.
- Patients with diabetes should be observed carefully for alterations in diabetes control. Frequent monitoring of blood sugar is advised.
- All patients on extended therapy should be checked periodically for symptoms of diabetes and acromegaly and for functioning of haematopoietic, hepatic, and renal systems.
- About 80% of patients on full therapeutic doses for 1 year or longer develop abnormal involuntary movements such as facial grimacing, exaggerated chewing, protrusion of tongue, rhythmic opening and closing of mouth, bobbing of head, jerky arm and leg movements, and exaggerated respiration. Symptoms tend to increase if dosage is not reduced.
- Chronic management may be accompanied by the on–off phenomenon: rapid unpredictable swings in intensity of motor symptoms of parkinsonism evidenced by increase in bradykinesia (attacks of 'leg freezing' or slow body movement). The patient is unable to perform activities, such as walking, during the 'off' periods as opposed to independent ability during normal 'on' periods. Attacks develop within minutes, last 1 to 3 hours, usually appear at same time of day, and are due to excessive drug levels. The phenomenon may be precipitated by emotional stress.
- Solicit help of family members to establish a baseline profile of the patient's disabilities. This information is essential for accurate differentiation between desired response to therapy and drug-induced neuropsychiatric adverse reactions.
- Urge patient to maintain prescribed drug regimen. Sudden withdrawal of medication can lead to parkinsonian crisis with return of marked rigidity, akinesia, tremor, hyperpyrexia.
- Inform patients with a metabolite of levodopa may cause urine to darken on standing and may also cause sweat to be dark-coloured.
- Caution patients not to take over-the-counter preparations or fortified cereals unless approved by physician. Multivitamins, antinauseants, and fortified cereals usually contain pyridoxine (vitamin B_6); 5 mg or more of pyridoxine daily may reverse the effects of levodopa.
- In the event a patient requires general anaesthesia, levodopa therapy is continued as long as patient is able to take fluids and medication by mouth (generally discontinued 6 to 24 hours prior to anaesthesia). Therapy usually is resumed as soon as patient is able to take oral medication.
- Patient and responsible family members require guidance and supervision of drug regimen.
- Physical therapy is an important adjunct to drug therapy.

LEVODOPA (continued)

■ Stored in tight, light-resistant containers preferably between 15° and 30°C (59° and 86°F) unless otherwise directed by manufacturer.

Diagnostic test interferences   False-negative **urine glucose** tests may result with use of glucose oxidase methods (e.g., Clinistix) and false-positive results with the copper reduction method (e.g., Clinitest), especially in patients receiving large doses. There is also possibility of false-positive tests for **urinary ketones** by dip-stick tests, (Labstix) false elevations of **serum** and **urinary uric acid** levels by colorimetric methods, but not with uricase; false increases in **urinary protein** by Lowry method; false decreases in **urinary VMA** by Pisano method, and false increases in urinary catecholamine levels by Hingerty method.

Drug interactions   Drugs that may inhibit or decrease therapeutic effects of levodopa include **anticholinergics, diazepam** and possibly other **phenothiazines** (mutually antagonistic), **phenylbutazone phenytoin** and other hydantoins, **pyridoxine,** (vitamin B$_6$) in doses of 5 mg or more, and **reserpine**. Levodopa may enhance the hypotensive effects of **guanethidine** and **methyldopa**. Methyldopa may enhance antiparkinsonian effects of levodopa (used therapeutically). Concomitant use of **MAO inhibitors** and drugs with MAO activity may produce hypertension (levodopa contraindicated with MAOIs, but may be used concurrently in carbidopa-levodopa combination product). **Propranolol** may enhance the therapeutic effect of levodopa and may also enhance levodopa-induced stimulation of growth hormone secretion.

Levorphanol tartrate

(Dromoran)   *Narcotic analgesic*

ACTIONS AND USES   Synthetic morphinan derivative with agonist activity only. Actions, uses, contraindications, precautions, and adverse reactions similar to those of morphine (q.v.). More potent as an analgesic and has somewhat longer duration of action than morphine. Reported to cause less nausea, vomiting, and constipation than equivalent doses of morphine, but may produce more sedation, smooth-muscle stimulation, and respiratory depression. Unlike morphine, can be given by mouth.

Used to relieve moderate to severe pain. Used also preoperatively to allay apprehension.

ROUTE AND DOSAGE   **Oral:** 1.5−4.5 mg once or twice a day. **Subcutaneous/intramuscular:** 2−4 mg as required. **Slow IV injection:** 1−2 mg repeated as required.

ABSORPTION AND FATE   **Peak analgesia** within 60 to 90 minutes following subcutaneous injection, and within 20 minutes following IV injection. **Duration of action** 4 to 5 hours. **Half-life:** 1.2 hours; 50% protein bound. Metabolized primarily in liver. Excreted in urine mainly as glucuronide conjugate.

LEVORPHANOL TARTRATE (continued)
NURSING IMPLICATIONS

- Not to be confused with levallorphan tartrate, a narcotic antagonist, and sometimes used as an antidote for levorphanol.
- See morphine sulphate.

Lignocaine hydrochloride ━━━━━━━━━━━━━━━━━━━━

(Xylocard, Xylocaine, Xylodase, Instillagel)   *Antiarrhythmic, anaesthetic*
                                                      (local)

ACTIONS AND USES   Aminoacyl amide with anaesthetic, and antiarrhythmic properties. Cardiac actions similar to those of procainamide and quinidine, but has little effect on myocardial contractility, A-V and intraventricular conduction, cardiac output, and systolic arterial pressure in equivalent doses. Exerts antiarrhythmic action by suppressing automaticity in His-Purkinje system and by elevating electrical stimulation threshold of ventricle during diastole. Progressive depression of CNS occurs with increasing blood concentrations; produces anticonvulsant, sedative, and analgesic effects. Action as local anaesthetic is more prompt, more intense, and longer lasting than that of procaine. Suppresses cough and gag reflexes.

Used for rapid control of ventricular arrhythmias occurring during acute myocardial infarction, cardiac surgery, and cardiac catheterization and those caused by digitalis intoxication. Preparations also available for surface and infiltration anaesthesia and for nerve block, including caudal and spinal block anaesthesia. Topical preparations are used to relieve local discomfort of skin and mucous membranes.

ROUTE AND DOSAGE   **Intravenous bolus:** 100 mg, administered over 5 min; followed by infusion 4 mg/min for 30 min, 2 mg/min for 2 hrs then 1 mg/min. **Infiltration analgesia:** 0.25−0.5% nerve block 1−2% (maximum volume: 50 ml of 1% or 25 ml of 1%) epidural or caudal block 1% all with adrenaline 1 in 200,000. **Surface analgesia:** 2−4% for oral upper GI and urethra. **Spray:** 10%.

ABSORPTION AND FATE   Following IV bolus dose, action begins within 10 to 90 seconds and lasts up to 20 minutes. Following IM injection, effective antiarrhythmic blood levels occur within 5 to 15 minutes and persist 60 to 90 minutes. Duration of action: lumbar epidural block 100 minutes; spinal anaesthesia: motor 100 minutes, sensory 140 minutes; caudal block: 75 to 135 minutes. Peak effect after local application to mucous membranes: 2 to 5 minutes; duration: 30 to 60 minutes. Rapidly distributed to most body tissues. **Biphasic half-life:** initial: 7 to 8 minutes; terminal 1 to 2 hours (longer in patients with renal or hepatic disease). About 50 to 75% bound to plasma proteins. Approximately 90% metabolized by liver and excreted in urine as metabolites; less than 3% excreted unchanged. Average duration of anaesthetic action is 90 to 120 minutes. Crosses placenta.

CONTRAINDICATIONS AND PRECAUTIONS   History of hypersensitivity to amide-

LIGNOCAINE HYDROCHLORIDE (continued)

type local anaesthetics; application or injection of lignocaine anaesthetic in presence of severe trauma or sepsis, blood dyscrasias, supraventricular arrhythmias, Stokes–Adams syndrome, untreated sinus bradycardia, severe degrees of sinoatrial, atrioventricular, and intraventricular heart block. Safe use during pregnancy and in children not established. **Cautious Use**: liver or renal disease, congestive heart failure, marked hypoxia, respiratory depression, hypovolaemia, shock, myasthenia gravis, debilitated patients, the elderly, family history of malignant hyperthermia (fulminant hypermetabolism).

ADVERSE/SIDE EFFECTS   These include: drowsiness, dizziness, lightheadedness, restlessness, confusion, disorientation, irritability, apprehension, euphoria, wild excitement, tinnitus, decreased hearing, blurred or double vision, impaired colour perception, numbness of lips or tongue and other paraesthesias including sensations of heat and cold, chest heaviness, difficulty in speaking, difficulty in breathing or swallowing, muscular twitching, tremors, psychosis. With high doses: convulsions, respiratory depression and arrest, hypotension, bradycardia, conduction disorders including heart block, cardiovascular collapse, cardiac arrest, anorexia, nausea, vomiting, excessive perspiration, soreness at IM site, local thrombophlebitis (with prolonged IV infusion), hypersensitivity reactions (urticaria, rash, oedema, anaphylactoid reactions).

NURSING IMPLICATIONS

- Only lignocaine hydrochloride injection without preservatives or adrenaline that is specifically labelled for IV use should be used for IV injection or infusion. Lignocaine should not be added to transfusion assemblies.
- Constant ECG monitoring and frequent determinations of blood pressure are essential to avoid potential overdosage and toxicity.
- In patients with sinus bradycardia or incomplete heart block, administration of IV lignocaine to eliminate ventricular ectopic beats is usually preceded by prior acceleration of heart (e.g., by atropine, isoprenaline or electric pacing) to avoid provoking more frequent and serious ventricular arrhythmias or complete heart block.
- Watch for neurotoxic effects, particularly in patients receiving IV infusions of lignocaine or those with high lignocaine blood levels (drowsiness, dizziness, confusion, paraesthesias, visual disturbances, excitement, behavioural changes).
- IV infusion should be terminated as soon as patient's basic cardiac rhythm stabilizes or at earliest signs and symptoms of toxicity (infusions are rarely continued beyond 24 hours). An oral antiarrhythmic is used for maintenance therapy.
- If ECG signs of excessive cardiac depression such as prolongation of PR interval or QRS complex and the appearance or aggravation of arrhythmias occur, infusion should be stopped immediately.
- Reports of convulsions are common. Resuscitative equipment, oxygen, and emergency drugs including diazepam, ultrashort-acting barbiturate, vasopressors (adrenaline or metaraminol) should be immediately available for management of convulsions and respiratory depression.
- Lignocaine blood levels of approximately 1.5 to 6 mcg/ml are reported to provide 'usually effective' antiarrhythmic activity. Blood levels greater than 7 mcg/ml are potentially toxic.

LIGNOCAINE HYDROCHLORIDE (continued)

Anaesthetic use   Lignocaine solutions containing preservatives should not be used for spinal or epidural (including caudal) block.

- Instruct patient using lignocaine for relief of oral discomfort to swish solution around in mouth. It can be swallowed, but patient should know that oral topical anaesthetic (xylocaine viscous) may interfere with swallowing reflex. Food should not be ingested within 60 minutes following drug application, especially in paediatric, elderly, or debilitated patients. Also, warn against chewing gum while buccal and throat membranes are anaesthetized to prevent biting trauma.
- Partially used solutions of lignocaine without preservatives should be discarded after initial use.
- Inspect solutions for particulate matter and discolouration prior to administration and discard if either is present.
- Lignocaine injection and commercially prepared solutions containing the drug in 5% dextrose are stored preferably at 15 to 30°C (59 to 86°F) unless otherwise directed by manufacturer.

Diagnostic test interferences   Increases in **creatine phosphokinase** level may occur for 48 hours following IM dose and may interfere with test for presence in myocardial infarction.

DRUG INTERACTIONS   *Lignocaine*

PLUS	INTERACTIONS
Barbiturates	Decrease lignocaine action through enzyme induction
Cimetidine	Increases pharmacological effects of lignocaine. Monitor for lignocaine toxicity
Phenytoin	Increases cardiac depressant effect of lignocaine
Procainamide	Additive neurological effects
Propranolol, quinidine	Increase cardiac depressant effect of lignocaine. Monitor for toxicity
Succinylcholine, and other neuromuscular blocking agents	Enhance muscle relaxant effects. Monitor for respiratory depression

Lincomycin

(Lincocin)   *Antibiotic (macrolide)*

ACTIONS AND USES   Derived from *Streptomyces lincolnensis*. Bacteriostatic or bactericidal depending on concentration used and sensitivity of organism. Acts by binding selectivity to 50S subunits of bacterial ribosomes, thus suppressing protein synthesis. Similar to erythromycin in antibacterial activity, and demonstrates some cross-resistance with it. Effective against most of the common gram-positive pathogens, particularly streptococci, pneumococci, and staphylococci. Also effective against *Bacteroides* and

LINCOMYCIN (continued)

other anaerobes; however, little activity against most gram-negative organisms, and ineffective against viruses, yeasts, or fungi. Resistance by *Staphylococcus* is acquired in stepwise manner. Lincomycin is reported to have neuromuscular blocking properties.

Used reserved for treatment of serious infections caused by susceptible bacteria in penicillin-allergic patients or patients for whom penicillin is inappropriate.

ROUTE AND DOSAGE   Oral: Adults: 500 mg every 6 to 8 hours. **Intramuscular: Adults**: 600 mg every 12 to 24 hours. **Paediatric (over 1 month of age)**: 10 mg/kg every 12 to 24 hours. **Intravenous: Adults**: 600 mg every 8 to 12 hours.

ABSORPTION AND FATE   Rapidly but only partially (20 to 35%) absorbed from GI tract. Peak plasma concentrations in 2 to 4 hours after oral dose; levels maintained above minimal inhibitory concentration for 6 to 8 hours. IM injection produces maximal plasma concentrations within 30 minutes; effective levels persist 12 to 14 hours. IV infusion of 600 mg over a 2-hour period produces therapeutic levels that persist for 14 hours. Following subconjunctival injection, ocular fluid drug levels last 5 hours. Distributed to most body tissues and fluids. Significant concentrations in bone, aqueous humour, bile, peritoneal, pleural, and synovial fluids. Low concentrations have been attained in cerebrospinal fluid when meninges are inflamed. **Half-life** about 5 hours; 57 to 72% protein bound depending on plasma concentration. Partially metabolized in liver. Excreted in urine, bile, and faeces mostly as unchanged drug and bioactive metabolite. Not cleared from blood by haemodialysis or peritoneal dialysis. Crosses placenta and may appear in breast milk.

CONTRAINDICATIONS AND PRECAUTIONS   Previous hypersensitivity to lincomycin and clindamycin; impaired hepatic function, known monilial infections (unless treated concurrently); use in newborns. Safe use in pregnancy and nursing mothers not established. **Cautious Use**: impaired renal function; history of GI disease, particularly colitis; history of liver, endocrine, or metabolic diseases; history of asthma, hayfever, eczema, drug or other allergies; elderly patients. *See also Drug Interactions*.

ADVERSE/SIDE EFFECTS   These include: hypotension, syncope, cardiopulmonary arrest (particularly after rapid IV), glossitis, stomatitis, nausea, vomiting, anorexia, decreased taste acuity, unpleasant or altered taste, abdominal cramps, diarrhoea, acute enterocolitis, pseudomembranous colitis (potentially fatal), neutropenia, leucopenia, agranulocytosis, thrombocytopenic purpura, and aplastic anaemia and pancytopenia (rare), pruritus, urticaria, skin rashes, exfoliative and vesiculobullous dermatitis, angioedema, photosensitivity, anaphylactoid reaction, serum sickness, superinfections (proctitis, pruritus ani, vaginitis), tinnitus, vertigo, dizziness, headache, generalized myalgia, thrombophlebitis following IV use (infrequent); pain at IM injection site (infrequent); jaundice and abnormal liver function tests (direct relationship to lincomycin not established).

NURSING IMPLICATIONS
- A careful history should be taken of previous sensitivities to drugs or other allergens.
- Culture and sensitivity tests should be performed initially and during therapy to determine continued microbial susceptibility.

LINCOMYCIN (continued)

- Absorption is reduced and delayed by presence of food in stomach. Administer oral drug with a full glass (200 mls) of water at least 1 to 2 hours before meals or 2 to 3 hours after meals.
- Administer IM injection deep into large muscle mass; inject slowly to minimize pain. Rotate injection sites.
- Monitor blood pressure and pulse in patients receiving parenteral drug. Have patient remain recumbent following drug administration until blood pressure stability is assured.
- Relatively high incidence of diarrhoea (20%) is associated with use of lincomycin. Monitor patients closely and report changes in bowel frequency. If significant diarrhoea occurs, drug should be discontinued.
- Antiperistaltic agents such as opiates or diphenoxylate with atropine may prolong and worsen diarrhoea by delaying removal of toxins from colon. Advise patient not to self-medicate. Medical management consists of fluid, electrolyte, and protein supplements, as indicated, and possibly corticosteroids. Oral vancomycin or cholestyramine has been prescribed for pseudomembranous colitis caused by *C. difficile*.
- Diarrhoea, acute colitis, or pseudomembranous colitis (suspect this if patient develops high temperature, diarrhoea, or ileus) may occur up to several weeks following cessation of therapy. Advise patients to report promptly the onset of perianal irritation, diarrhoea, or blood and mucus in stools.
- Advise patients to report immediately symptoms of hypersensitivity. Drug should be discontinued.
- Periodic hepatic and renal function studies and complete blood cell counts are indicated during prolonged drug therapy.
- Superinfections by nonsusceptible organisms are most likely to occur when duration of therapy exceeds 10 days.
- Instruct patient to take drug for full course of therapy as prescribed. Drug therapy should continue at least 10 days in patients with group A β-haemolytic streptococcal infections to reduce the possibility of rheumatic fever or glomerulonephritis.
- Follow manufacturer's directions for reconstitution, storage time, compatible IV fluids, and IV administration rates.
- Store unopened vials and oral drug preferably between 15° and 30°C (59° and 86°F) unless otherwise directed by manufacturer.

Diagnostic test interferences Lincomycin may cause increase in **serum alkaline phosphatase bilirubin, CPK, SGOT**, and **SGPT**, and possibly **serum triglycerides**.

DRUG INTERACTIONS *Lincomycin*

PLUS	INTERACTIONS
Chloramphenicol Erythromycin	Possibility of mutual antagonism
Kaolin antidiarrhoeal compounds	Reduce intestinal absorption of lincomycin by about 90%. If used, administer kaolin at least 12 hours before or 3 to 4 hours after lincomycin
Skeletal muscle relaxants (e.g., ether, tubocurarine, pancuronium)	Enhanced neuromuscular blocking action

Liothyronine sodium ▬▬▬▬▬▬▬▬▬▬▬▬▬

(Tertroxin, T$_3$, Tri-iodothyronine) *Hormone*

ACTIONS AND USES Synthetic form of natural thyroid hormone. Shares actions and uses of thyroxine, but has more rapid action and more rapid disappearance of effect, permitting quick dosage adjustment if necessary; 20 mcg are equivalent to approximately 100 mcg of thyroxine.

ROUTE AND DOSAGE Adult: *inital*: 10–20 mcg/day increased gradually to 20 mcg three times a day. **Elderly patients** should have a reduced dose. **Child**: according to size. **IV**: in hypothyroid coma 5–20 mcg repeated after 12 hrs.

NURSING IMPLICATIONS
- Metabolic effects persist a few days after drug withdrawal.
- Infants with thyroid dysfunction (mother provides little or no thyroid hormone to foetus) are started on replacement therapy as soon as possible to prevent permanent mental and physical changes.
- Residual actions of other thyroid preparations may persist for weeks; therefore, during early period of liothyronine substitution for another preparation, watch for possible additive effects, particularly if the ʼpatient is elderly, has cardiovascular disease, or is a child.
- With onset of overdosage symptoms (hyperthyroidism), drug is withheld for 1 or 2 days; usually therapy can be resumed with lower dosage.
- Advise patient not to take OTC medications unless approved by physician.
- *See also thyroxine.*

Lithium carbonate ▬▬▬▬▬▬▬▬▬▬▬▬▬

(Camcolit, Liskonum, Phasal, Priadel) *Antimanic agent*

Lithium citrate

(Litarex)

ACTIONS AND USES Alkali metal salt which behaves in body much like sodium ion. Accumulates within neurons since Na pump is less efficient in transporting it out than Na, and thus alters electrophysiological characteristics of neurons. Enhances reuptake (thus inactivation) of biogenic amines, 5-HT and noradrenaline at nerve terminals, but apparently does not affect dopaminergic systems in brain. Specific relationship of these actions in treatment of mania not known. May induce several endocrinological effects. Decreases amount of circulating thyroid hormones, but normal functioning usually returns through pituitary feedback.

LITHIUM CITRATE (continued)

Used for control and prophylaxis of manic episodes in manic-depressive psychosis. May be given simultaneously with an antipsychotic agent during acute manic episode.

ROUTE AND DOSAGE   Individualized according to both serum lithium level and clinical condition (*see Nursing Implications*). **Oral: Adults:** *Initial*, 0.25−2 g daily adjusted to produce a therapeutic plasma concentration.

ABSORPTION AND FATE   Absorbed well from GI tract; **peak serum levels** reached ½ to 4 hours after a dose. **Half-life** adult: 24 hours; adolescent: 18 hours; elderly: 36 hours or more. No evidence of protein binding. Crosses blood−brain barrier slowly with appreciable amounts in cerebrospinal fluid, once steady state established. Approximately 50 to 75% of single dose excreted in urine within 24 hours followed by slower excretion over several days. Alkalinization of urine increases excretion. Less than 1% eliminated in faeces and 4 to 5% in sweat. Crosses placenta; enters breast milk.

CONTRAINDICATIONS AND PRECAUTIONS   Significant cardiovascular or renal disease, brain damage, schizophrenia, organic brain syndrome, severe debilitation, dehydration or Na depletion; patients on low salt diet or receiving diuretics; pregnancy, (especially first trimester), nursing mothers, children under age 12. **Cautious Use:** elderly patients, thyroid disease, epilepsy, concomitant use with haloperidol and other antipsychotics, parkinsonism, diabetes mellitus, severe infections, urinary retention.

ADVERSE/SIDE EFFECTS   These include: dizziness, headache, lethargy, drowsiness, fatigue, slurred speech, psychomotor retardation, giddiness, tinnitus, impaired vision, incontinence, restlessness, seizures, confusion, blackout spells, disorientation, recent memory loss, stupor, coma, EEG changes, arrhythmias, hypotension, vasculitis, peripheral circulatory collapse, ECG changes, skin problems (thought to be toxicity rather than allergy): pruritus, maculopapular rash, hyperkeratosis, chronic folliculitis, transient acneiform, papules (face, neck, intertriginous areas), anaesthesia of skin, cutaneous ulcers, drying and thinning of hair, allergic vasculitis, impaired vision, transient scotomata, tinnitus, nausea, vomiting, anorexia, abdominal pain, diarrhoea, incontinence, dry mouth, metallic taste, diffuse thyroid enlargement, hypothyroidism, nephrogenic diabetes insipidus, transient hyperglycaemia, glycosuria, hyponatraemia, fine hand tremors (common), coarse tremors, choreoathetotic movements; fasciculations, clonic movements, incoordination including ataxia, muscle weakness, hyperreflexia, encephalopathic syndrome (weakness, lethargy, fever, tremors, confusion, extrapyramidal symptoms), reversible leucocytosis, albuminuria, oliguria, urinary incontinence, polyuria, polydipsia, increased uric acid excretion, oedema, weight gain (common) or loss, exacerbation of psoriasis, flulike symptoms.

NURSING IMPLICATIONS

- GI symptoms may be minimized by taking drug with meals. Transient nausea and general discomfort appear to coincide with peak rise in serum levels. Report persistent symptoms. Dosage may be adjusted to provide levels without high peaks.
- Hospitalization is usually a necessity during initial treatment stage of daily serum lithium determinations until therapeutic dose is established.

LITHIUM CITRATE *(continued)*

- Onset of therapeutic effects usually is preceded by a lag of 1 to 2 weeks. If drug control is not apparent within 1 to 3 weeks, drug is usually withdrawn.
- Therapeutic response to therapy is evidenced by changed facial affect, improved posture, assumption of self-care, improved ability to concentrate, improved sleep pattern. Keep physician informed of patient's progress.
- Urge patient to drink plenty of liquids (2 to 3 L/day) during stabilization period and at least 1 to 1½ L/day during remainder of therapy.
- Instruct patient to be alert to increased output of dilute urine and persistent thirst. Chronic lithium therapy may be associated with diminished renal concentrating ability occasionally presenting as nephrogenic diabetes insipidus (with polydypsia and polyuria). Dose reduction may be indicated.
- Reduced intake of fluid and sodium (Na) can accelerate lithium retention with subsequent toxicity. Conversely, marked increase in Na intake can increase excretion and reduce drug effect.
- **Food–drug interactions**   6 to 10 g salt intake (average intake) is required to keep serum lithium in the therapeutic range.
- Normal dietary salt intake can be inadvertently compromised by lack of understanding. Caution patient to avoid self-prescribed low salt regimen, self-dosing with sodium antacids, high sodium foods, e.g., prepared meats, and drinks such as diet soda. Also warn against 'crash' diets or diet pills that reduce appetite and food, salt and fluid intake.
- Diffuse thyroid enlargement, generally without change in thyroid function, may occur in some patients (mostly women) after 5 months to 2 years of therapy. Lab studies of thyroid hormone and periodic palpation of the thyroid gland should be a part of preventive therapy. Be alert to and report symptoms of *hypothyroidism*: hoarseness, lethargy, fatigue, myxoedema, headache, puffed face, weight gain, cold intolerance. Symptoms are reversible.
- Contraceptive measures should be used during therapy but if the patient becomes pregnant she should be apprised of the potential risk to the foetus. If therapy is continued, serum lithium levels must be closely monitored to prevent toxicity. Renal clearance increases during pregnancy but reverts to lower rate immediately after delivery; dose, therefore, will be reduced to prevent toxicity.
- Neonates born of mothers who took lithium during pregnancy may have high serum lithium level manifested by flaccidity, poor reflexes, cardiac dysrhythmia, and chronic twitching may impair both physical and mental ability. Caution against any activity demanding alertness (e.g., driving a car) until clinical response to drug has been established.
- The elderly require special monitoring to prevent toxicity which may occur at serum levels ordinarily tolerated by other patients. Ability to excrete lithium decreases with aging, thus a smaller dose than usual may give desired control. Urinary creatinine clearance may be used as an index of patient's excretory function. Lithium clearance may be only one-fifth that of creatinine.
- Polydipsia and polyuria, apparently not dose-related, are common early side effects particularly in the elderly. Symptoms may lessen but then reappear after several months or even years of maintenance therapy.

LITHIUM CITRATE (continued)

- The encephalopathic syndrome may be induced when lithium is given concomitantly with haloperidol or with other antipsychotic medication, particularly in the elderly. Promptly report to the physician early signs of extrapyramidal reactions (*see Index: Clinical signs and symptoms*).
- The fine tremor of hand or jaw, polyurea, mild thirst, transient mild nausea, and general discomfort that may occur in early treatment of mania sometimes persist throughout therapy. Usually, however, symptoms subside with temporary reduction of dose. If symptoms persist, drug is withdrawn.
- *Early signs of Lithium intoxication* may occur several days after starting therapy: vomiting, diarrhoea, lack of coordination, drowsiness, muscular weakness, slurred speech. With high serum concentrations, ataxia, blurred vision, giddiness, tinnitus, muscle twitching or coarse tremors, and a large output of dilute urine occur.
- Warn patient not to switch brands of lithium; because of varying fillers, a different brand may introduce a change in dose.
- Urge patient to adhere to established dosage regimen, i.e., not to change or omit doses and not to change dose intervals.
- Clinical follow-up and regular checks on serum lithium levels are essential if treatment is to be safe and effective. Emphasize importance to family and patient of keeping all scheduled appointments for clinic visits.
- **Treatment of overdosage** . Induced vomiting, or gastric lavage if patient is conscious. Have available supportive measures for maintenance of airway and respiratory function and correction of fluid and electrolyte inbalance. Dialysis may be required for severe intoxication. Supportive therapy should continue for several days because of prolonged half-life of lithium.
- Store drug at temperature between 15° and 30°C (59° and 86°F) unless manufacturer directs otherwise. Protect from light and moisture.

Diagnostic test interferences   Lithium carbonate may cause **hypokalaemia, glycosuria**, transient **hyperglycaemia, proteinuria**, increased **VMA** excretion, increased serum **enzymes, BUN, FBS,** and **magnesium** levels; lowered **serum T$_3$, T$_4$,** and **PBI** levels, elevated **I-131** uptake, leucocytosis, increased **uric acid** excretion.

DRUG INTERACTIONS   Lithium (Li)

PLUS	INTERACTIONS
Acetazolamide, aminophylline, caffeine, mannitol, sodium chloride (excess), urinary alkalinizers (e.g., sodium bicarbonate), theophylline, urea	Increase Li excretion; lower serum Li and thus decrease therapeutic effects of Li
Amphetamines	Inhibit amphetamine activity
Antipsychotic agents, e.g., haloperidol	Augment potential Li toxicity: e.g., encephalopathic syndrome and brain damage
Carbamazepine	
Chlorpromazine and other phenothiazines	Increase Li excretion; enhanced potential hyperglycaemic effect of Li; reduced chlorpromazine serum and brain levels
Diazepam	Monitor for hypothermia

LITHIUM CITRATE (continued)

PLUS	INTERACTIONS
(continued)	
Ethacrynic acid, frusemide, sodium chloride loss	Decrease Li excretion; increase serum Li level and thus enhance Li effects
Indomethacin, methyldopa, piroxicam spironolactone, tetracyclines	Increase risk of Li toxicity
Noradrenaline	Decrease pressor effects of noradrenaline
Potassium iodide and other iodides; tricyclic antidepressants	Enhance hypothyroid effects of Lithium
Skeletal muscle relaxants	Increase neuromuscular blocking activity
Thiazide diuretics	Potentiate neurotoxic and cardiotoxic effects of Li

Lomustine

(CCNU)   *Antineoplastic; alkylating agent*

ACTIONS AND USES   Lipid-soluble alkylating nitrosurea with actions like those of carmustine (q.v.).

Used in Hodgkin's disease and other malignancies (melanoma, brain tumours).

ROUTE AND DOSAGE   Oral: **Adults and children**: individualized.

ABSORPTION AND FATE   Rapidly absorbed from GI tract. **Serum half-life of drug and/or metabolites**: 16 to 48 hours. About 50% protein bound. 50% of dose excreted in urine within 24 hours; 75% within 4 days. Because of high lipid solubility and relatively no ionization at physiologic pH, crosses blood–brain barrier readily. CSF levels are 50% greater than concurrent plasma levels. Rapidly and completely metabolized in liver. Excreted in urine as metabolites. Appears in breast milk.

CONTRAINDICATIONS AND PRECAUTIONS   History of hypersensitivity to lomustine. Safe use in pregnancy and in nursing mothers not established. Reported to be carcinogenic in laboratory animals. **Cautious Use**: patients with decreased circulating platelets, leucocytes, or erythrocytes, renal or hepatic function impairment, infection, previous cytotoxic or radiation therapy.

ADVERSE/SIDE EFFECTS   Delayed (cumulative) myelosuppression, stomatitis, alopecia (reversible), anaemia, hepatotoxicity, nausea, vomiting; neurological reactions (relationship to drug unclear): lethargy, ataxia, dysarthria.

NURSING IMPLICATIONS
- Blood counts should be monitored weekly for at least 6 weeks after last dose. Liver and kidney function tests should be performed periodically.
- Since haematological toxicity is delayed and cumulative, a repeat course is not given before 6 weeks.

LOMUSTINE (continued)

- Nausea and vomiting may occur 3 to 4 hours after drug administration, usually lasting less than 24 hours. Symptoms may be controlled by administering drug to fasting patient, or physician may prescribe an antiemetic prior to dosage.
- Anorexia may persist for 2 or 3 days after a dose.
- Thrombocytopenia occurs about 4 weeks and leucopenia about 6 weeks after a dose, persisting 1 to 2 weeks.
- Inspect oral cavity daily for symptoms of superinfections and for signs of stomatitis or xerostomia.
- Contraceptive measures are recommended during therapy.
- Pharmacist will prepare prescribed dose by combining various capsule strengths. Explain to patient that a given dose may include capsules of different colours.
- Store capsules away from excessive heat (over 40°C).
- For further information: *see mustine.*

Loperamide

(Imodium)   *Antidiarrhoeal*

ACTIONS AND USES   Synthetic piperidine derivative chemically related to diphenoxylate and to meperidine. Reportedly as effective an antidiarrhoeal as diphenoxylate with longer duration of action. Inhibits GI peristaltic activity by direct action on circular and longitudinal intestinal muscles. Prolongs transit time of intestinal contents, increases consistency of stools, and reduces fluid and electrolyte loss.

Used to treat acute nonspecific diarrhoea, chronic diarrhoea associated with inflammatory bowel disease.

ROUTE AND DOSAGE   Oral: *Aute diarrhoea*: *Initial*: 4 mg followed by 2 mg after each unformed stool. Once diarrhoea is controlled, dosage is reduced to maintenance level. Usual maintenance dose: 4 to 8 mg daily. Maximum dose 16 mg.

ABSORPTION AND FATE   Poorly absorbed from GI tract. **Onset of action** in 30 to 60 minutes; **duration**: 4 to 5 hours. Approximately 97% protein bound. **Half-life**: 7 to 14 hours. Metabolized in liver. Less than 2% of dose excreted in urine; about 30% eliminated in faeces as unchanged drug.

CONTRAINDICATIONS AND PRECAUTIONS   Hypersensitivity to loperamide, severe colitis, acute diarrhoea caused by broad spectrum antibiotics (pseudomembranous colitis), or associated with microorganisms that penetrate intestinal mucosa, e.g., toxigenic *E. coli*, salmonella, or shigella. Safe use during pregnancy, in nursing mothers, and in children not established. **Cautious Use**: dehydration, diarrhoea caused by invasive bacteria, impaired hepatic function.

ADVERSE/SIDE EFFECTS   These include: drowsiness, dizziness, CNS depression (overdosage), abdominal discomfort or pain, abdominal distention, bloating, consti-

LOPERAMIDE (continued)

pation, nausea, vomiting, anorexia, dry mouth, fatigure, fever, toxic megacolon (patients with ulcerative colitis).

NURSING IMPLICATIONS

- Since loperamide may cause drowsiness and dizziness, caution patient to avoid driving and other potentially hazardous activities until drug response is known.
- In acute diarrhoea, loperamide should be discontinued if there is no improvement after 48 hours of therapy. Advise patient to notify physician if diarrhoea persists or if fever develops.
- Patients with chronic diarrhoea usually respond to loperamide therapy within 10 days. Loperamide may be continued if diarrhoea cannot be controlled by diet or specific treatment, e.g., antibiotics.
- Instruct patient to record number and consistency of stools. Fluids and electrolytes should be monitored especially in young children.
- If the patient with ulcerative colitis develops abdominal distention or other GI symptoms, notify physician promptly (possible signs of toxic megacolon).
- Inform patient that alcohol and other CNS depressants may enhance drowsiness and therefore should not be taken concomitantly unless otherwise advised by physician.
- **_Treatment of overdosage_**   Slurry of activated charcoal; if vomiting does not occur, gastric lavage followed by activated charcoal slurry. Monitor patient for signs of CNS depression for at least 24 hours. Have naxolone on hand.
- Dry mouth may be reduced by frequent rinsing with clear warm water and by increasing fluid intake. If these measures fail to provide relief a saliva substitute.
- Excessive sedation may occur in young children or patients with chronic liver disease.
- Store at room temperature preferably between 15° and 30°C (59° and 86°F) unless otherwise specified by manufacturer.

Lorprazolam —————————————————

(Dormonoct)   Sedative; hypnotic;
                                                         benzodiazepine

ROUTE AND DOSAGE   Oral: **Adults**: 1 mg at bedtime. Maximum dose 2 mg. **Elderly patients**: no more than 1 mg.

For further information: *see temazepam.*

Lorazepam —————————————————————

(Ativan)   Anxiolytic; benzodiazepine

LORAZEPAM (continued)

ACTIONS AND USES   Most potent of the available benzodiazepines with actions, uses, limitations, and interactions similar to those of chlordiazepoxide (q.v.).

Used for management of anxiety disorders, and for short-term relief of symptoms of anxiety. Also used for preanaesthetic medication to produce sedation, and to reduce anxiety and recall of events related to day of surgery.

ROUTE AND DOSAGE   *Highly individualized.* **Oral**: usual range: 2 to 6 mg/day in divided doses with largest dose at bedtime. *Anxiety*: 1 to 4 mg/day two or three times daily. *Insomnia*: single daily dose: 1 to 4 mg at bedtime. **Elderly, debilitated**: Half adult dose. *Acute panic attack*; **IM/IV** (slow injection): 25 to 30 mcg/kg/6 hourly as required.

ABSORPTION AND FATE   Readily absorbed from GI tract and following IM administration. **Peak concentrations in plasma** in 2 hours after oral administration, and 60 to 90 minutes after IM injection. Approximately 85% bound to plasma proteins. **Elimination half-life** of oral drug: 10 to 15 hours; of **parenteral drug**: about 16 hours. Metabolized in liver and excreted in urine with no residual accumulation. Crosses placenta and enters breast milk.

CONTRAINDICATIONS AND PRECAUTIONS   Known sensitivity to benzodiazepines; acute narrow-angle glaucoma, primary depressive disorders or psychosis, children under 12 years of age (oral preparation) patients under 18 years of age (parenteral preparation); coma, shock, acute alcohol intoxication, pregnancy, lactation. **Cautious Use**: renal or hepatic impairment, narrow-angle glaucoma, suicidal tendency, GI disorders, elderly and debilitated patients; limited pulmonary reserve. *See also chlordiazepoxide.*

ADVERSE/SIDE EFFECTS   (Usually disappear with continued medication or with reduced dosage): sedation, dizziness, weakness, unsteadiness, disorientation, depression, sleep disturbance, restlessness, confusion, hallucinations, hypertension or hypotension (occasionally) nausea, anorexia, blurred vision, diplopia, depressed hearing. *See also chlodiazepoxide.*

NURSING IMPLICATIONS

- The tension and anxiety associated with stresses of everyday living usually do not require treatment with an anxiolytic agent.
- When high dosage is required, the evening dose should be increased before the daytime doses.
- IM lorazepam is injected undiluted, deep into a large muscle mass.
- Prepare lorazepam for IV administration immediately before use. Dilute with an equal volume of compatible solution. Do not use a solution that is discoloured or that has a precipitate.
- Diluted drug is injected directly into vein or into IV infusion tubing at rate not to exceed 2 mg/minute, and with repeated aspiration to confirm intravenous entry. Extreme precautions should be taken to prevent intraarterial injection and perivascular extravasation.
- Inadvertent intraarterial injection may produce arteriospasm resulting in gangrene which may require amputation. (*See Index: Nursing Interventions: extravasation.*)

LORAZEPAM (continued)

- Patients over 50 years of age may have more profound and prolonged sedation with IV lorazepam. Usually an initial dose of 2 mg should not be exceeded.
- IM or IV lorazepam injection of 2 to 4 mg is usually followed by a depth of drowsiness or sleepiness that permits patient to respond to simple instructions whether patient appears to be asleep or awake.
- The elderly patient should be aware that he or she will be sleepy for a period longer than 6 to 8 hours after surgery. Supervise ambulation of patient for at least 8 hours after lorazepam injection to prevent falling and injury.
- Equipment for maintaining patient airway should be immediately available before IV administration. Partial airway obstruction has occurred in the lorazepam medicated patient undergoing regional anaesthesia.
- Advise patient to refrain from any hazardous activity including dangerous sports and driving a car, for at least 24 to 48 hours after receiving IM injection of lorazepam. If patient is on oral drug therapy, patient should not drive until the sedative action of lorazepam has diminished. In time, patient may know how many hours he or she should wait before it is safe to drive.
- When alcohol or a CNS depressant is combined with lorazepam the depressant effects of each agent are potentiated. **Alcoholic beverages** should not be consumed for at least 24 to 48 hours after receiving an injection and should be avoided when patient is on an oral regimen.
- *Food–drug interactions*   Advise patient to avoid large volume intake of coffee. Anxiolytic effects of lorazepam can significantly be altered by 500 mg caffeine. (1 cup of coffee contains 125 to 250 mg caffeine.)
- Tell the patient that if she becomes pregnant or wishes to become pregnant, she should communicate with her physician about the desirability of continuing the drug.
- Periodic blood counts and liver function tests are recommended for the patient on long-term therapy.
- Keep parenteral preparation in refrigerator; do not freeze. Store tablets at temperature between 15° and 30°C (59° and 86°F) unless manufacturer specifies otherwise.
- *See chlordiozepoxide.*

Diagnostic test interferences   Lorazepam may increase **serum lactic dehydrogenase (LDH)**. *See also chlordiazepoxide.*

Lormetazepam

(Noctamid)

ACTIONS AND USES   Benzodiazepine with similar action and uses to temazepam.

ROUTE AND DOSAGE   Oral: Adult: 1 mg at bedtime, elderly patients 500 mg.

Lypressin

(Synto pressin)   *Hormone; antidiuretic*

ACTIONS AND USES   Lysine vasopressin; synthetic polypeptide with pharmacological action similar to that of vasopressin (q.v.). Possesses antidiuretic activity, with very little oxytocic and minimal cardiovascular pressor activity in therapeutic doses.

Used to control or prevent complications of diabetes insipidus due to deficiency of endogenous posterior pituitary antidiuretic hormone. Particularly useful in patients who are nonresponsive to other forms of therapy and who experience allergic or other undesirable effects from vasopressin of animal origin.

ROUTE AND DOSAGE   Topical (intranasal): 2.5 to 10 units, 3 to 7 times a day.

NURSING IMPLICATIONS
- Warn patient not to inhale the spray.
- Instruct patient to clear nasal passages well before administering the spray.
- For further information: *see also vasopressin.*

Magnesium hydroxide

Magnesium carbonate   *Antacid; laxative (saline)*

Magnesium trisilicate

ACTIONS AND USES   Acts as antacid in low doses and as mild saline laxative at higher doses.

Used for short-term treatment of occasional constipation, for relief of GI symptoms associated with hyperacidity, and as adjunct in treatment of peptic ulcer.

ROUTE AND DOSAGE   Oral: **Adults:** Depends on preparation.

ABSORPTION AND FATE   Absorbed magnesium ions are usually excreted rapidly by kidney. Laxative action occurs in about 4 to 8 hours, depending on dosage. Crosses placenta. Excreted in breast milk.

CONTRAINDICATIONS AND PRECAUTIONS   Abdominal pain, nausea, vomiting, diarrhoea, severe renal dysfunction, faecal impaction, intestinal obstruction or perforation, rectal bleeding, colostomy, ileostomy. Safe use during pregnancy and in children under 2 years of age not established.

ADVERSE/SIDE EFFECTS   **Excessive dosage:** nausea, vomiting, abdominal cramps, diarrhoea, alkalinization of urine, dehydration. *Hypermagnesaemia*: weakness, nausea, vomiting, lethargy, mental depression, hyporeflexia, hypotension, bradycardia, com-

MAGNESIUM TRISILICATE (continued)
plete heart block and other ECG abnormalities, respiratory depression, coma. **Prolonged Use**: rectal concretions (rare), electrolyte imbalance.

NURSING IMPLICATIONS
- For antacid action, usually given 20 minutes to 1 hour before meals and at bedtime. Mix suspension with water or follow with sufficient water to assure that it reaches the stomach.
- For laxative effect, follow the drug with at least a full glass of water to enhance drug action. Administer in the morning or at bedtime. Most effective when taken on an empty stomach.
- Evaluate the patient's continued need for drug. Prolonged and frequent use of laxative doses may lead to dependence and tends to reinforce neurotic preoccupation with bowels. Additionally, even therapeutic doses can raise urinary pH and thereby predispose susceptible patients to urinary infection and urolithiasis, or elevate serum magnesium concentrations and cause bradycardia and other symptoms of hypermagnesaemia.
- Inform patient that the cause of persistent or recurrent constipation should be investigated by physician.

Teaching outline for laxative users   Correct patient's misconceptions about constipation. Inform patient that constipation is defined as infrequent or difficult passage of stools. The omission of one day's evacuation is not constipation and will not cause accumulation of poisons in the body. Functional constipation can be corrected by:
- □ Regularity of meals.
- □ Addition of bulk and fibre to diet (if allowed) such as raw and cooked vegetables and fruits, whole grain cereals, and bread (some physicians recommend 4 to 6 tablespoonfuls of whole bran daily).
- □ Adequate daily fluid intake (at least 6 to 8 full glasses of liquid). Drinking a large glass of warm water flavoured with lemon or orange juice, immediately on arising is helpful.
- □ Planned exercise programme.
- □ Unhurried defecation time at approximately the same time each day – defecation reflexes are most active following a meal, especially breakfast.

- Stored at room temperature in tightly covered container. Slowly absorbs carbon dioxide on exposure to air. Avoid freezing.

Diagnostic test interferences   Magnesium antacids cause significant elevations in **urinary pH** that may persist for 1 or more days after drug is withdrawn. Decreased **serum potassium** levels and elevated **blood glucose** with prolonged use of high doses.

DRUG INTERACTIONS   *Magnesium salts*

PLUS	INTERACTIONS
Chlordiazepoxide	Antacids reduce absorption and therefore decrease chlordiazepoxide effect
Chlorpromazine and other phenothiazines	Lower phenothiazine serum levels by decreasing GI absorption

M

MAGNESIUM TRISILICATE (continued)

PLUS	INTERACTIONS
(continued)	
Dicumarol	Milk of magnesia may increase serum dicumarol levels by enhancing its absorption if given concurrently
Digoxin ⎱ Iron salts ⎬ Isoniazid ⎰	Antacids reduce effects of these drugs by reducing absorption
Nitrofurantoin ⎱ Pencillamine ⎬ Salicylates ⎰	Magnesium-containing drugs may enhance muscular relaxation effect (theoretical possibility)
Neuromuscular blocking agents ⎱ Gallamine Succinylcholine Tubocurarine and others ⎰	Coadministration may cause metabolic alkalosis in patients with renal dysfunction
Tetracylines (oral)	Concurrent use of antacid results in formation of insoluble complex

In common with other antacids, magnesium hydroxide may cause premature dissolution and absorption of enteric-coated tablets and may interfere with the absorption of other oral medications. In general it is advisable not to take other oral drugs within 1 or 2 hours of an antacid.

Mannitol ——————————————————————————

(Osmitrol)   *Diuretic; osmotic*

ACTIONS AND USES   Hexahydric alcohol prepared commercially by reduction of dextrose. Induces diuresis by raising osmotic pressure of glomerular filtrate, thereby inhibiting tubular, reabsorption of water and solutes. In large doses, may increase rate of electrolyte excretion, particularly sodium, chloride, and potassium. Reduces elevated intraocular and cerebrospinal pressures by increasing plasma osmolality, thus inducing diffusion of water from these fluids back into plasma and extravascular space. Rebound increase in intracranial pressure sometimes occurs about 12 hours following drug administration.

Used to promote diuresis in drug overdose. Also used to reduce elevated intraocular and intracranial pressures, and for forced diuresis with some cytotoxic drug regimens.

ROUTE AND DOSAGE   Intravenous infusion: 50 to 200 g over 24 hrs.

ABSORPTION AND FATE   Diuresis occurs within 1 to 3 hours. Elevated intraocular pressure is lowered within 30 to 60 minutes for period of 4 to 6 hours; elevated cerebrospinal fluid pressure may be reduced within 15 minutes, with effect lasting 3 to 8 hours. Confined to extracellular space; does not cross blood–brain barrier, except with very high plasma concentrations or in the presence of acidosis. **Half-life**: about 100 minutes. Small quantity metabolized to glycogen in liver. Rapidly excreted by kidney. Approximately 80% of 100 g dose eliminated unchanged in urine within 3 hours.

CONTRAINDICATIONS AND PRECAUTIONS   Anuria, marked pulmonary oedema or

MANNITOL (continued)

congestive heart failure, metabolic oedema, organic CNS disease, intracranial bleeding, shock, severe dehydration, history of allergy. Safe use during pregnancy and in women of childbearing potential and children under 12 years of age not established.

ADVERSE/SIDE EFFECTS Dry mouth, thirst, blurred vision, marked diuresis, urinary retention, oedema, headache, circulatory overload with pulmonary congestion, congestive heart failure, fluid and electrolyte imbalance, dehydration, acidosis, nausea, vomiting, rhinitis, arm pain, angina-like pains, tachycardia, backache, transient muscle rigidity, tremors, convulsions, chills, fever, dizziness, hypotension, hypertension, allergic reactions, nephrosis, uricosuria, thrombophlebitis; with extravasation: local oedema, skin necrosis.

NURSING IMPLICATIONS

- IV infusion flow rate (prescribed by physician) is generally adjusted to maintain urine flow of at least 30 to 50 ml/hour.
- A test dose of 200 mg/kg should be given by slow IV infusion.
- Serum and urine electrolytes (particularly sodium, potassium, and chloride), central venous pressure, and renal function should be closely monitored during therapy.
- Fluid intake and output must be accurately measured and recorded to achieve proper fluid balance. Check output on the half-hour or hourly. Increasing oliguria is an indication to terminate therapy; report immediately. (If urinary output is not adequate, mannitol may accumulate and cause circulatory overload, with resulting pulmonary oedema, water intoxication, and congestive heart failure.)
- Consult physician regarding allowable oral fluid intake volume. In general, volume of total fluid intake (all sources) should be no more than 1 L in excess of urinary output.
- Monitor vital signs, and be alert for indications of fluid and electrolyte imbalance (e.g., thirst, muscle cramps or weakness, paraesthesias, and signs of congestive heart failure: distended neck veins, dyspnoea, chest rales, tachycardia, blood pressure changes).
- Accurate daily weight under standard conditions provides another reliable index of fluid balance.
- Care should be taken to avoid extravasation. Observe injection site for signs of inflammation or oedema.
- Parenteral mannitol may crystallize when exposed to low temperatures. If crystallization occurs, place bottle in hot water bath (approximately 50°C) and periodically shake vigorously. Cool to body temperature before administration. Do not use solution if crystals cannot be completely dissolved.
- Concentrations higher than 15% have a greater tendency to crystallize. Administration set with an in-line IV filter should be used when infusing concentrations of 15% or above.
- Mannitol should not be added to whole blood transfusion. However, if blood must be given simultaneously, at least 20 mEq of sodium chloride should be added to each litre of mannitol solution to avoid pseudoagglutination.
- Patients receiving urological irrigations of mannitol should be observed closely for systemic reactions.
- Store preferably between 15° and 30°C (59° and 86°F) unless otherwise directed by manufacturer. Avoid freezing.

MANNITOL (continued)
Diagnostic test interferences Mannitol may interfere with blood inorganic phosphorus and ethylene glycol determinations.

Drug interactions Mannitol increases lithium excretion.

Maprotiline hydrochloride

(Ludiomil) *Antidepressant; tetracyclic*

ACTIONS AND USES Tetracyclic antidepressant pharmacologically and therapeutically similar to the tricyclic antidepressants.

Used for treatment of depressive neurosis. *see imipramine.*

ROUTE AND DOSAGE Oral: **Adult**: 25–75 mg/day in divided doses or single dose at bedtime. **Elderly patients**: 30 mg/day.

ABSORPTION AND FATE Slow, complete absorption from GI tract; peak blood concentrations in 12 hours. **Half-life**: 51 hours; about 88% bound to plasma proteins. Hepatic metabolism. Excreted primarily in urine (70% of dose) also in faeces (30%) as metabolites, within 21 days.

CONTRAINDICATIONS AND PRECAUTIONS Patients under 18 years of age. *See imipramine.*

ADVERSE/SIDE EFFECTS Sedation, seizures. **Anticholinergic**: xerostomia, constipation, urinary retention, blurred vision. *See also imipramine.*

NURSING IMPLICATIONS
- Drug may be given as single dose or in divided doses. Risk of seizures is reduced by initiating therapy with low dosages.
- Therapeutic effects are sometimes seen in 3 to 7 days; 2 to 3 weeks are usually necessary.
- Store drug at temperature between 15° and 30°C (59° and 86°F) unless otherwise specified by the manufacturer.
- *See imipramine.*

Mazindol

(Teronac) *Appetite suppressant*

ACTIONS AND USES Imidazoisoindole derivative with pharmacological properties

MAZINDOL (continued)

similar to those of amphetamines. Produces CNS and cardiac stimulation in addition to amphetaminelike effects. Appears to exert primary effects on limbic system; also appears to alter noradrenaline metabolism by inhibiting normal neuronal uptake mechanism.

Used in short-term management of exogenous obesity.

ROUTE AND DOSAGE   Oral: 2 mg once daily for up to 12 weeks.

ABSORPTION AND FATE   Readily absorbed from GI tract. **Onset of action** in 30 to 60 minutes; **duration** 8 to 15 hours. Excreted primarily in urine as unchanged drug and conjugated metabolites.

CONTRAINDICATIONS AND PRECAUTIONS   Glaucoma; hypersensitivity to the drug; severe hypertension; symptomatic cardiovascular disease, including arrhythmias; agitated states; history of drug abuse; during or within 14 days following administration of MAO inhibitors; children under age 12. Safe use in women of childbearing potential or during pregnancy not established. **Cautious Use**: hyperexcitability states.

ADVERSE/SIDE EFFECTS   These include: restlessness, dizziness, insomnia, dysphoria, depression, tremor, headache, drowsiness, weakness, palpitation, tachycardia, rash, excessive sweating, clamminess, impotence, changes in libido (rare), dry mouth, unpleasant taste, diarrhoea, constipation, nausea, vomiting.

NURSING IMPLICATIONS

- Drug may be taken with meals if GI discomfort occurs.
- Possibility of abuse potential should be kept in mind.
- Rate of weight loss is greatest during first few weeks of therapy and tends to decrease thereafter.
- Tolerance may develop within a few weeks. When it occurs, drug should be discontinued.
- Insulin requirements of patients with diabetes may be decreased in association with use of mazindol and concomitant caloric restriction and weight loss.
- Caution patients that mazindol may impair ability to perform hazardous activities such as driving a car or operating machinery.

Drug interactions   Mazindol may decrease the hypotensive effects of **guanethidine** and potentiate pressor amines, e.g., **noradrenaline, isoprenaline** (patient should be closely monitored if given concomitantly). Administration of mazindol with or within 14 days of **MAO inhibitors** can produce hypertensive crisis.

Mebendazole ———————————————

(Vermox)   *Anthelmintic*

ACTIONS AND USES   Carbamate with unusually broad spectrum of anthelmintic

MEBENDAZOLE (continued)

activity. Mechanism of action not known. Inhibits formation of worm's microtubules and inhibits glucose and other nutrient uptake by susceptible helminths.

Used in treatment of hookworm, roundworm and threadworm.

ROUTE AND DOSAGE   Oral: Adults and children (over 2 years): *Hook- and roundworm* 5 ml or 1 tab twice a day for 3 days. *Threadworm*: single dose of 5 ml or 1 tab.

ABSORPTION AND FATE   Only a small portion (5 to 10%) is absorbed from GI tract. Peak plasma levels in 2 to 4 hours. Most of dose excreted in faeces; 5 to 10% of dose excreted in urine within 3 days, mainly as inactive metabolites.

CONTRAINDICATIONS AND PRECAUTIONS   Hypersensitivity to mebendazole. Safe use during pregnancy, in nursing women, and in children under 2 years of age not established.

ADVERSE/SIDE EFFECTS   Transient abdominal pain, diarrhoea, dizziness, fever (possibly due to tissue necrosis in cysts).

NURSING IMPLICATIONS

- May be given without regard to food. Food in GI tract reportedly does not affect drug action.
- Commercial chewable tablet may be chewed, crushed, mixed with food, or swallowed whole.
- If cure does not occur within 3 weeks after initiation of therapy, second course of treatment is advised.
- Fasting and purging are not required.
- Because worms are readily transmitted from person to person all family members should be examined and treated simultaneously.

Patient teaching during period of drug therapy for parasite infestation

- ☐ Emphasize importance of washing hands thoroughly after toilet and before eating.
- ☐ Keep hands away from mouth; keep fingernails short.
- ☐ Avoid walking barefoot (hookworm).
- ☐ Handle bedding carefully without shaking it to avoid dispersing ova into the air.
- ☐ Advise patient to change underclothing, bedclothes, towels and facecloths daily and to bathe frequently, preferably by showering.
- ☐ Disinfect toilet facilities daily.
- ☐ Infected person should sleep alone.
- ☐ House should be vacuum cleaned and damp mopped daily to reduce number of ova.

- Stools will be examined for ova and parasites to establish diagnosis and cure. Collect specimen in clean, dry container, e.g., bedpan. Then transfer to properly labelled container to be sent to laboratory. Parasites may be destroyed by water from toilet bowl, urine, or certain medications e.g., antibiotics, castor oil, mineral oil, anti-diarrhoeal formulations.

Mebeverine

(Cologac, Colven)   *Antispasmodic*

ACTIONS AND USES   Acts directly on the smooth muscle of the colon to relieve cramps pain and flatulence associated with irritable bowel syndrome. Not recommended for children under 10 yrs. Contraindicated in paralytic ileus.

ROUTE AND DOSAGE   Oral: **Adult:** *Tablets (135 mg)*: 1 three times a day; *liquid (50 mg/5 ml)*: 15 ml three timea a day; *granules (135 mg/sachet)*: 1 sachet in water twice daily.

Mebhydrolin

(Fabahistin)   *Antihistamine*

ACTIONS AND USES   Symptomatic relief of allergies.

ROUTE AND DOSAGE   50–100 mg three times a day. **Child (under 2 years):** 50–100 mg; **(2–5 years):** 50–150 mg; **(6–12 years):** 100–200 mg daily in divided dose.
   For further information: *see chlorpheniramine*.

Mecillinam

(Selexidin)   *Antibiotic; penicillin*

ACTIONS AND USES   Active against gram-negative bacteria including salmonellae, used to treat sensitive infections.

ROUTE AND DOSAGE   IM and slow IV injection or infusion: 5–15 mg/kg every 6–8 hours.
   For further information: *see penicillin G*.

Meclozine hydrochloride

(Ancoloxin)   *Antiemetic; antihistamine*

ACTIONS AND USES   Long-acting piperazine derivative of diphenylmethane,

MECLOZINE HYDROCHLORIDE (continued)

structurally and pharmacologically related to cyclizine compounds. Has marked effect in blocking histamine-induced vasopressive response, but only slight anticholinergic action. In common with similar agents, also exhibits CNS depression, antispasmodic, antiemetic, and local anaesthetic activity. Has marked depressant action on labyrinthine excitability and on conduction in vestibularcerebellar pathways.

Used in management of nausea,

ROUTE AND DOSAGE Oral: 1–2 tabs, 2–3 times a day. Tablet contains meclozine 25 mg plus pyridoxine 50 mg.

ABSORPTION AND FATE Slow onset of action; **duration of action** 8 to 24 hours. **Plasma half-life**: 6 hours. Metabolic fate unknown.

CONTRAINDICATIONS AND PRECAUTIONS Hypersensitivity to meclozine; use during pregnancy and in women of childbearing potential; use in paediatric age group. **Cautious Use**: angle-closure glaucoma, prostatic hypertrophy. *See diphenhydramine.*

ADVERSE/SIDE EFFECTS Drowsiness, dry mouth, blurred vision, fatigue.

NURSING IMPLICATIONS
- Forewarn patients about side effects such as drowsiness, and advise patients not to drive a car or engage in other hazardous activities until their reactions to the drug are known.
- Caution patients that the sedative action may be additive to that of alcohol, barbiturates, narcotic analgesics, or other CNS depressants.
- *See also diphenhydramine.*

Medazepam

(Nobrium)   *Benzodiazepine*

ROUTE AND DOSAGE Oral: Adult: 15–30 mg/day.
For further information: *see diazepam.*

Medroxyprogesterone acetate

(Depo-Provera, Provera, Farlutal)   *Progesterone; antineoplastic*

ACTIONS AND USES Synthetic derivative of progesterone with prolonged, variable duration of action. Lacks oestrogenic and androgenic properties and has no deleterious

MEDROXYPROGESTERONE ACETATE (continued)

effects on lipid metabolism. Effective on oestrogen-primed endometrium. Actions, uses, absorption, fate and limitations similar to those of progesterone (q.v.). Used to treat abnormal bleeding, amenorrhoea, cancer and as a contraceptive.

ROUTE AND DOSAGE   Oral: *Secondary amenorrhoea*: 2.5 to 10 mg daily for 5 to 10 days beginning on the 16th to 21st day of the cycle for 4 cycles. *Abnormal bleeding due to hormonal imbalance*: 5 to 10 mg daily for 5 to 10 days beginning on the 16th and 21st day of menstrual cycle. If bleeding is controlled, administer 2 subsequent cycles. *Endometrial, prostatic breast and renal cancer*: individualized doses. **IM** (deep injection): *Contraceptive*: 150 mg in the first 3 to 5 days of the cycle or first 6 weeks postpartum, duration 3 months.

ADVERSE/SIDE EFFECTS   (Rare): hyperpyrexia, headache. *See also progesterone.*

NURSING IMPLICATIONS

- IM injection may be painful. Monitor sites for evidence of sterile abscess. A residual lump and discolouration of tissue may develop.
- Following repeated IM injections, infertility and amenorrhoea may persist for as long as 18 months.
- Planned menstrual cycling with medroxyprogesterone may benefit the patient with a history of recurrent episodes of abnormal uterine bleeding.
- Teach patient self-breast examination (SBE).
- Discuss package insert with patient to assure complete understanding of progesterone therapy.
- Store drug at temperature between 15° and 30°C (59° and 86°F); protect from freezing.
- *See progesterone.*

M

Mefenamic acid ▃▃▃▃▃▃▃▃▃▃▃▃▃▃▃▃▃▃▃▃▃▃▃▃

(Ponstan)   *NSAID*

ACTIONS AND USES   Anthranilic acid derivative with analgesic, anti-inflammatory, and antipyretic actions similar to those of aspirin. Like aspirin, inhibits prostaglandin synthesis, and affects platelet function. No evidence that it is superior to aspirin. Associated with a number of serious adverse reactions, particularly when used for prolonged periods at high doses.

Used for short-term relief of mild to moderate pain including arthritis and primary dysmenorrhoea.

ROUTE AND DOSAGE   Oral: **Adult:** 500 mg three times a day. **Child (over 6 mths):** 25 mg/kg/day in divided doses for up to 7 days; longer in chronic juvenile arthritis.

MEFENAMIC ACID (continued)

ABSORPTION AND FATE   Absorbed slowly from GI tract. **Peak analgesic effect** in 2 to 4 hours may persist up to 6 hours. Firmly bound to plasma proteins. Partly detoxified in liver. Excreted in urine and faeces as free drug and conjugated metabolites. Approximately 50% of dose is excreted in urine within 48 hours.

CONTRAINDICATIONS AND PRECAUTIONS   Hypersensitivity to drug, GI inflammation, or ulceration. Safe use in women of childbearing potential, children under age 14, and during pregnancy or lactation not established. **Cautious Use**: history of renal or hepatic disease, blood dyscrasias, asthma, diabetes mellitus, hypersensitivity to aspirin. *See also drug interactions.*

ADVERSE/SIDE EFFECTS   These include: drowsiness, insomnia, dizziness, vertigo, unsteady gait, nervousness, confusion, headache; status epilepticus with overdose, urticaria, rash, facial oedema, severe diarrhoea (common), GI inflammation, ulceration, and bleeding; nausea, vomiting, abdominal cramps, flatus, constipation, prolonged prothrombin time, severe autoimmune haemolytic anaemia (long-term use), leucopenia, eosinophilia, agranulocytosis, thrombocytopenic purpura, megaloblastic anaemia, pancytopenia, bone marrow hypoplasia, nephrotoxicity, dysuria, albuminuria, haematuria, elevation of BUN, eye irritation, loss of colour vision (reversible), blurred vision, ear pain, perspiration, increased need for insulin in diabetic patients, hepatic toxicity, palpitation, dyspnoea; acute exacerbation of asthma; bronchoconstriction (in patients sensitive to aspirin).

NURSING IMPLICATIONS

- Administer with meals, food, or milk to minimize GI adverse effects.
- Use of drug for a period exceeding 1 week is not recommended (manufacturer's warning).
- Mefenamic acid should be discontinued promptly if diarrhoea, dark stools, haematemesis, ecchymoses, epistaxis, or rash occur, and not used thereafter. Advise patients to report these signs to the physician.
- Also advise patient to notify physician if persistent GI discomfort, sore throat, fever, or malaise occurs.
- Since the drug may cause dizziness and drowsiness, caution patients to avoid driving a car and other potentially hazardous activities until response to drug is known.
- Diabetic patients may show increased need for insulin.

Diagnostic test interferences   False-positive reactions for **urinary bilirubin** (using diazo tablet test).

DRUG INTERACTIONS   *Mefenamic acid*_____

PLUS	INTERACTIONS
Oral anticoagulants	Increased hypoprothrombinaemia; displaces anticoagulants from protein binding sites. Concomitant use generally avoided

MEFENAMIC ACID (continued)

PLUS	INTERACTIONS
(continued)	
Corticosteroids ⎱ Indomethacin ⎰ Phenylbutazone ⎰ Salicylates ⎰	Ulcerogenic effects potentiated

Mefruside

(Baycaron)   *Thiazide; diuretic*

ACTIONS AND USES   Thiazide diuretic used to treat oedema and hypertension.

ROUTE AND DOSAGE   Oral: Adult: *initial* 25–50 mg in the morning increased to 75–100 mg for oedema. *Maintenance* 25 mg/day.
For further information: *see bendrofluazide.*

Megestrol acetate

(Megace)   *Progesterone; antineoplastic*

ACTIONS AND USES   Progestational hormone with antineoplastic properties.
    Used as palliative agent for treatment of advanced carcinoma of breast or endometrium.

ROUTE AND DOSAGE   Oral: *Breast cancer*: 160 mg daily. *Endometrial cancer*: 40 to 320 mg daily in divided doses.

CONTRAINDICATIONS AND PRECAUTIONS   Diagnostic test for pregnancy; use in neoplastic diseases other than cancer of endometrium and breast; first 4 months of pregnancy. *See also progesterone.*

ADVERSE/SIDE EFFECTS   Carpal tunnel syndrome, alopecia, deep vein thrombophlebitis, breast tenderness, abdominal pain, nausea, vomiting, headache, allergic-type reactions (including bronchial asthma). *See also progesterone.*

NURSING IMPLICATIONS
- Contraception measures are recommended during therapy for carcinoma with megestrol.
- Monitor for breathing distress characteristic of asthma; rash, urticaria, anaphylaxis, tachypnoea, anxiety. Stop medication if they appear and notify physician.

MEGESTROL ACETATE (continued)

- Teach patient self-breast examination.
- Discuss package insert with patient to assure understanding of megestrol therapy.
- Store tablets in a well-closed container at temperatures between 15° and 30°C (59° and 86°F) unless otherwise specified by manufacturer.
- *See progesterone.*

Melphalan

(Alkeran)   *Antineoplastic; alkylating*
                                                                   agent; nitrogen mustard

ACTIONS AND USES   Nitrogen mustard chemically and pharmacologically related to mechlorethamine (q.v.). Has strong immunosuppressive and myelosuppressive effects, but unlike mechlorethamine, lacks vesicant properties. Carcinogenic potential suspected.

Used chiefly for palliative treatment of multiple myeloma. Also used in treatment of many other neoplasms, including Hodgkin's disease and carcinomas of breast, and ovary. Regional perfusion alone or with other antineoplastics is investigational.

ROUTE AND DOSAGE   Oral and IV: *Multiple myeloma*: Individualized.

ABSORPTION AND FATE   Well absorbed from GI tract. **Plasma half-life**: about 90 minutes. Widely distributed to all tissues; metabolism and excretion not fully known. Approximately 10 to 15% excreted unchanged in urine.

CONTRAINDICATIONS AND PRECAUTIONS   Hypersensitivity to melphalan; use during pregnancy or in men and women of childbearing age not established. **Cautious Use**: recent treatment with other chemotherapeutic agent; concurrent administration with radiation therapy; severe anaemia, neutrophilia, or thrombocytopenia, impaired renal function.

ADVERSE/SIDE EFFECTS   These include: leucopenia, agranulocytosis, thrombocytopenia, anaemia, acute nonlymphatic leukaemia, mild thrombophlebitis at site of infusion, uraemia, angioneurotic peripheral oedema, minor neurological toxicity (rare), nausea, vomiting (with high doses); occasional stomatitis, diarrhoea hypersensitivity reactions, temporary alopecia, skin rash, bronchopulmonary dysplasia (rare), pulmonary fibrosis, menstrual irregularities, hyperuricaemia. *See mustine.*

NURSING IMPLICATIONS

- Administer parenteral drug immediately after preparation of solution.
- Administer oral drug with meals to reduce nausea and vomiting. An antiemetic may be ordered if dose is high and side effects are increased.
- Monitor laboratory reports to anticipate leucopenic and thrombocytopenic periods in order to adapt nursing care accordingly.

MELPHALAN (continued)

- Stored in light-resistant airtight containers at room temperature, preferably between 15 and 30°C (59 and 86°F) unless otherwise directed by manufacturer.
- *See mustine.*

Menadiol sodium phosphate

(Synkayvite)   *Vitamin*

ACTIONS AND USES   Synthetic, fat-soluble vitamin K analogue. Similar in activity to naturally occurring vitamin K, which is essential in hepatic biosynthesis of blood clotting factors II, VII, IX, X. Mechanism of action unknown.

Used in treatment of vitamin K defiency in malabsorption syndromes.

ROUTE AND DOSAGE   Oral, subcutaneous, intramuscular, intravenous: 5 to 15 mg once or twice daily.

ABSORPTION AND FATE   Absorbed directly into bloodstream after oral administration, even in the absence of bile salts. Converted to menadione in body. Following SC or IM administration, bleeding may be controlled within 1 to 2 hours; prothrombin time usually returns to normal in 8 to 24 hours. Response after IV administration is more prompt, but action is less sustained.

ADVERSE/SIDE EFFECTS   Nausea, vomiting, allergic reaction; pruritus, urticaria, rash.

NURSING IMPLICATIONS

- Dosage and duration of treatment are determined by prothrombin times and clinical response.
- Concomitant administration of bile salts is not required for intestinal absorption since menadiol sodium phosphate is water-soluble.
- Solutions of menadiol sodium phosphate may be irritating to skin.
- Parenteral drug is incompatible with protein hydrolysate.
- Stored in tight, light-resistant containers at room temperature, preferably between 15 and 30°C (59 and 86°F) unless otherwise directed by manufacturer.
- *Similar drug phytomenadione.*

Meprobamate

(Equanil, Meprate)   *Psychotropic; anxiolytic;*
                                                     carbamate

MEPROBAMATE (continued)

ACTIONS AND USES   Propanediol carbamate derivative structurally and pharmacologically related to carisoprodol. CNS depressant actions similar to those of barbiturates. Acts on multiple sites in CNS and appears to block cortical-thalamic impulses. Has no effect on medulla, reticular activating system, or autonomic nervous system. Skeletal muscle relaxant effect is probably related to sedative rather than to direct action. Hypnotic doses suppress REM sleep.

Used to relieve anxiety and tension of pyschoneurotic states and as adjunct in disease states associated with anxiety and tension. Also used to promote sleep in anxious, tense patients. Available in fixed combination with ethoheptazine citrate and aspirin (Equagesic).

ROUTE AND DOSAGE   Adults: **Oral**: 400 mg three or four times daily, or 600 mg two times daily. Doses greater than 2.4 g/day not recommended.

ABSORPTION AND FATE   **Onset of sedative action** within 1 hour following oral administration. **Plasma half-life**: 6 to 16 hours. Uniformly distributed throughout body; rapidly metabolized in liver. About 8 to 19% of dose is excreted in urine unchanged, and 10% in faeces as inactive metabolites, within 24 hours. Induces hepatic microsomal enzymes. Crosses placenta and enters breast milk.

CONTRAINDICATIONS AND PRECAUTIONS   History of hypersensitivity to meprobamate or related carbamates such as carisoprodol and tybamate; history of acute intermittent prophyria; pregnancy, lactation; children under 6 years of age. **Cautious Use**: impaired renal or hepatic function, convulsive disorders, history of alcoholism or drug abuse, patients with suicidal tendencies.

ADVERSE/SIDE EFFECTS   *Allergy or idiosyncrasy*: itchy, urticarial, or erythematous maculopapular rash; exfoliative dermatitis, petechiae, purpura, ecchymoses, eosinophilia, peripheral oedema, angioneurotic oedema, adenopathy, fever, chills, proctitis, bronchospasm, oliguria, anuria, Stevens–Johnson syndrome; anaphylaxis. **Others**: drowsiness and ataxia (most frequent), dizziness, vertigo, slurred speech, headache, weakness, paraesthesias, impaired visual accommodation, paradoxic, euphoria and rage reactions, seizures in epileptics, panic reaction, rapid EEG activity, hypotensive crisis, syncope, palpitation, tachycardia, arrhythmais, transient ECG changes, anorexia, stomatitis, nausea, vomiting, diarrhoea, exacerbation of acute intermittent porphyria, grand mal attack, respiratory depression and circulatory collapse (toxic doses).

NURSING IMPLICATIONS
- May be administered with food to minimize gastric distress.
- The elderly, and debilitated patients are prone to oversedation and to the hypotensive effects of meprobamate, especially during early therapy. Generally, lower doses are prescribed and dose increases are made gradually.
- Caution patient to make position changes slowly, especially from recumbent to upright, and to dangle legs for a few minutes before standing. Supervise ambulation, if necessary.

MEPROBAMATE (continued)

- Hypnotic doses may cause increased motor activity during sleep. Bed rails are advisable.
- Warn patient that tolerance to alcohol will be lowered. When meprobamate and alcohol (or another CNS depressant) are taken concomitantly, the CNS depressant actions of each agent are intensified.
- Caution patient not to self-dose with OTC drugs without consulting the physician.
- Since meprobamate may impair mental and physical abilities, caution patient to avoid driving a car or engaging in other hazardous activities until drug response has been determined.
- If daytime psychomotor function is impaired consult physician. A change in regimen or drug may be indicated.
- Patients should be instructed to report immediately: onset of skin rash, sore throat, fever, bruising, unexplained bleeding. All are indicators of possible allergic or idiosyncratic reactions or blood dyscrasias.
- Patient should be advised that if she becomes pregnant during therapy or intends to become pregnant she should communicate with her physician about the desirability of discontinuing the drug.
- Instruct patient to take drug as prescribed; patient should not change dose or dose intervals. Warn patient not to give any of it to another person, and not to use it for a self-diagnosed problem.
- Psychological or physical dependence may occur with long-term use of high doses.

Meptazinol

(Meptid)   *Narcotic analgesic*

ACTIONS AND USES   Used for pain in obstetrics and renal colic.

ROUTE AND DOSAGE   Oral: 200 mg 3–6 hrly. **IM**: 75–100 mg and **IV**: 50–100 mg 2–4 hrly.
 For further information: *see buprenorphine*.

Mequitazine

(Primalan)

ACTIONS AND USES   Antihistamine used for symptomatic relief of allergy.

ROUTE AND DOSAGE   Oral: **Adult**: 5 mg twice a day.
 For further information: *see diphenhydramine*.

Mercaptopurine ━━━━━━━━━━━━━━━━━━━━━━━━

(Puri-Nethol)   *Antineoplastic; antimetabolite*

ACTIONS AND USES   Antimetabolite and purine antagonist. Inhibits purine metabolism by unclear mechanism. Blocks conversion of inosinic acid to adenine and xanthine ribotides within sensitive tumour cells. Also inhibits adenine-containing coenzymes, suggesting an influence over multiple cellular reactions. Has delayed immunosuppressive properties and carcinogenic potential.

Used primarily for treatment of acute lymphocytic and myelogenous leukaemia. Response in adults is less than in children, but mercaptopurine is initial drug of choice. In chronic granulocytic leukaemia, produces temporary remission.

ROUTE AND DOSAGE   Highly individualized.

ABSORPTION AND FATE   Oral preparations are erratically and incompletely absorbed without damage to intestinal mucosa. **Half-life**: 21 minutes in children, 47 minutes in adults. Rapid distribution to sensitive tumour cells; crosses blood–brain barrier. Partial degradation in liver with rapid excretion in urine as metabolites, including 6-thiouric acid and inorganic sulphates. Small proportion excreted for as long as 17 days. Drug is dialyzable.

CONTRAINDICATIONS AND PRECAUTIONS   Prior resistance to mercaptopurine; first trimester of pregnancy, infections. **Cautious Use**: impaired renal or hepatic function, concomitant use with allopurinol.

ADVERSE/SIDE EFFECTS   These include: stomatitis, oesophagitis, anorexia, nausea, vomiting, diarrhoea, intestinal ulcerations, leucopenia, anaemia, eosinophilia, pancytopenia, thrombocytopenia, abnormal bleeding, bone marrow hypoplasia, impaired liver function, hyperuricaemia, skin rash, oliguria, renal impairment, drug fever.

NURSING IMPLICATIONS
- Keep a fluid balance chart. Weigh the patient before treatment commences.
- Monitor daily laboratory reports for suggested adaptations in nursing management. Blood picture may change dramatically in a short period, and counts may continue to decrease several days after drug is withdrawn.
- During periods of leucopenia, protect patient from exposure to trauma, infections, or other stresses (restrict visitors and personnel who have colds).
- Check vital signs daily.
- Oral ulcerations are rare; those that occur resemble lesions of thrush (creamy white exudative patches on inflamed painful mucosa). Inspect buccal membranes if patient complains of discomfort. Amphotericin B or nystatin may be ordered for relief. *See Index: Nursing Interventions: stomatitis.*
- Nausea, vomiting, and diarrhoea are uncommon during drug administration, but they may signal excessive dosage, especially in adults.
- In acute leukaemia, mercaptopurine may be continued in spite of thrombocytopenia and bleeding. Often, bleeding stops and platelet count rises during treatment.

MERCAPTOPURINE (continued)

- If thrombocytopenia develops, watch for signs of abnormal bleeding (ecchymoses, petechiae, melaena, bleeding gums); report them immediately.
- Jaundice signals onset of hepatic toxicity and may necessitate terminating use. Report other signs such as clay-coloured stools or frothy dark urine. In some instances, jaundice appears and subsequently disappears during mercaptopurine therapy; it may persist days after drug is discontinued.
- Weigh patient under standard conditions once weekly and record weight.

Treatment of hyperuricaemia includes

- Allopurinol (reduces or prevents hyperuricaemia due to increased nucleoprotein breakdown). (Mercaptopurine dosage will be decreased by one-third or one-fourth of usual dosage.)
- Increased hydration (10 to 12 glasses of fluid daily). Consult physician about desirable volume, particularly if patient is receiving IV infusions.
- Urine alkanization, e.g., with acetazolamide change in fluid intake–output ratio that could suggest renal insufficiency.
- Store tablets in light- and air-resistant container.

Drug interactions Allopurinol retards metabolism of mercaptopurine and therefore enhances antineoplastic activity and toxicity. Hypoprothrombinaemic effect of **oral anticoagulants** may be reduced; monitor patient more closely when mercaptopurine is introduced or stopped. Mercaptopurine may reverse neuromuscular blocking effects of nondepolarizing muscle relaxants e.g., *tubocurarine*.

Mersalyl

Mercurial diuretic

ACTIONS AND USES Diuretic effect in oedema unresponsive to other diuretics. Rarely used because of nephrotoxicity. Given by IM injection only.

ROUTE AND DOSAGE IM (deep injection): 0.5–2 ml.

Mesalazine

(Asacol)   *Salicylate*

ACTIONS AND USES Mesalazine and sulphapyridine are the two components of sulphasalazine (q.v.). Mesalazine is known to be the component active against ulcerative colitis. Used to maintain remission in ulceratative colitis in patients who cannot tolerate sulphasalazine.

MESALAZINE (continued)
ROUTE AND DOSAGE   Oral: Adult: 400–800 mg three times a day.

ABSORPTION AND FATE   This preparation (Asacol) contains 400 mg mesalozine (5-amino-salicylic acid) and is coated with an acrylic based resin designed to disintegrate at pH 7 or above in the terminal ileum or large bowel. This 400 mg tablet is equivalent to the mesalazine theoretically available from 1 g sulphasalazine.

CONTRAINDICATIONS AND PRECAUTIONS   Sensitivity to salicylates. Not recommended for children under 2 years. Renal impairment and headache. Exacerbation of colitis symptoms (rate).

NURSING IMPLICATIONS
- Do not administer mesalazine with lactulose or similar preparations which alter pH in the bowel.
- *See sulphasalazine.*

Mesna

(Uromitexan)   *Cytotoxic antagonist*

ACTIONS AND USES   Mesna reacts specifically with acrolein, a metabolite of ifosfamide and cyclophosphamide, in the urinary tract to prevent toxicity, thus preventing haemorrhagic cystitis.

ROUTE AND DOSAGE   Intravenous injection of infusion dose highly individualized.

Metaraminol bitartrate

(Aramine)   *Adrenergic agonist;*
                                                                      (sympathomimetic)

ACTIONS AND USES   Potent synthetic sympathomimetic amine. Overall effects similar to those of noradrenaline.

Used for prevention and treatment of acute hypotensive states occurring with spinal anaesthesia, and as adjunct in treatment of hypotension due to haemorrhage, reaction to medication.

ROUTE AND DOSAGE   Adults: **Subcutaneous, intramuscular:** 2 to 10 mg. At least 10 minutes should elapse before additional dose is given, to prevent cumulative effect. **Intravenous infusion:** 15 to 100 mg in 500 ml of 5% dextrose injection or sodium chloride injection. **Children: Subcutaneous, intramuscular:** 0.1 mg/kg. **Intravenous (direct):** 0.01 mg/kg.

METARAMINOL BITARTRATE (continued)

ABSORPTION AND FATE   Onset of pressor effect occurs within 1 to 2 minutes after start of IV infusion, within 10 minutes after IM injection, and in 5 to 20 minutes after administration. Effects last 20 to 90 minutes, depending on route of administration. Drug effects appear to be terminated primarily by uptake into tissues and urinary excretion.

CONTRAINDICATIONS AND PRECAUTIONS   Use with cyclopropane, halothane, within 14 days of MAO inhibitor therapy; peripheral or mesenteric thrombosis; pulmonary oedema, cardiac arrest; untreated hypoxia, hypercapnia, and acidosis; as sole therapy in hypovolaemia. Safe use during pregnancy not established. **Cautious Use**: digitalized patients, hypertension, thyroid disease, diabetes mellitus, cirrhosis of liver, history of malaria (may produce relapse).

ADVERSE/SIDE EFFECTS   Apprehension, restlessness, headache, tremor, nausea, vomiting, weakness, flushing, pallor, sweating, precordial pain, palpitation, tachycardia, bradycardia, decreased urinary output, metabolic acidosis (hypovolaemic patients), hyperglycaemia. **Excessive dosage**: severe hypertension, headache, convulsions acute pulmonary oedema, arrhythmias, cardiac arrest. Injection site reactions (especially following SC): abscess formation, tissue necrosis, sloughing. **Prolonged use**: plasma volume depletion with recurrence of shock state.

NURSING IMPLICATIONS

- Except in emergency situations, blood volume should be corrected as fully as possible before therapy is initiated.
- Avoid exposure of drug to excessive heat, and protect it from light.
- For further information: *see noradrenaline.*

Drug Interactions   There may be an enhanced pressor response to metaraminol in patients receiving (parenteral) **ergot alkaloids, guanethidine, MAO inhibitors,** or **tricyclic antidepressants.** Concurrent use of these drugs generally avoided. **Digitalis glycosides** may sensitize myocardium to the effects of metaraminol. Response to metaraminol may be altered by **reserpine** (based on limited studies). IV administration of metaraminol during use of **cyclopropane** or **halothane** or related general anaesthetics may lead to serious ventricular arrhythmias.

Metformin

(Glucophage, Orabet)   *Biguanide; antidiabetic*

ROUTE AND DOSAGE   Oral: **Adult**: 500 mg/8 hrly or 850 mg every 12 hours. Maximum 3 g/day in divided doses.
   See glipizide for nursing implications.

Methadone hydrochloride ———————————————

(Physeptone)   *Narcotic analgesic*

ACTIONS AND USES   Synthetic diphenylheptane derivative with pharmacological properties qualitatively similar to those of morphine (q.v.), but is orally effective and has
longer duration of action. A single oral dose produces less sedation and euphoria than
does morphine, but repeated doses produce marked sedation (cumulative action). Causes
less constipation than morphine, but respiratory depressant effect (principal danger
of overdosage) and antitussive actions are comparable. Highly addictive, with abuse
potential that matches that of morphine; abstinence syndrome develops more slowly;
withdrawal symptoms are less intense, but more prolonged.

Used to relieve severe pain; and for detoxification in dependence.

ROUTE AND DOSAGE   Oral, subcutaneous, intramuscular: Adults: 5–10 mg
every 6–8 hours.

ABSORPTION AND FATE   Well absorbed from GI tract. Following single oral dose,
onset of action in 30 to 60 minutes, with duration of 6 to 8 hours; following parenteral
administration: onset of action in 10 to 20 minutes, and peak effects in 1 to 2 hours.
Duration of action (cumulative effect): 22 to 48 hours. Widely distributed to tissues;
about 85% firmly bound to plasma proteins. **Half-life:** 15 to 25 hours. Metabolized
chiefly in liver. Metabolities excreted primarily in urine; less than 10% excreted
unchanged in urine. Crosses placenta and enters breast milk.

CONTRAINDICATIONS AND PRECAUTIONS   Obstetric analgesia. Safe use during pregnancy, in nursing mothers, and for treatment of narcotic addiction in patients under 18
years not established. **Cautious Use:** hepatic, renal, or cardiac dysfunction. *See also
morphine.*

ADVERSE/SIDE EFFECTS   Drowsiness, nausea, vomiting, dry mouth, constipation,
lightheadedness, dizziness, transient fall in blood pressure, bone and muscle pain,
hallucinations, impotence. *See also morphine.*

NURSING IMPLICATIONS
- IM route is preferred when repeated parenteral administration is required (SC
  injections may cause local irritation and induration). Aspirate carefully before
  injecting drug to avoid inadvertent IV administration. Rotate injection sites.
- Orthostatic hypotension, sweating, constipation, drowsiness, GI symptoms, and
  other transient side effects of therapeutic doses appear to be more prominent in
  ambulatory patients. Most side effects disappear over a period of several weeks.
- Instruct patients to make position changes slowly, particularly from recumbent to
  upright position, and to sit or lie down if they feel dizzy or faint.
- Patients should be informed that methadone may impair mental and physical abilities
  required for performance of potentially hazardous activities, such as driving a car or
  operating machinery.
- Principal danger of overdosage, as with morphine, is extreme respiratory depression.

METHADONE HYDROCHLORIDE (continued)

- Due to the cumulative effects of methadone, **abstinence symptoms** may not appear for 36 to 72 hours after last dose and may last 10 to 14 days. Symptoms are usually of mild intensity (anorexia, insomnia, anxiety, abdominal discomfort, weakness, headache, sweating, hot and cold flushes). Purposive behaviour is prominent by the sixth day.
- Narcotic antagonists such as naloxone and levallorphan terminate methadone intoxication by competing for narcotic binding sites. Since antagonist action is shorter (1 to 3 hours) than that of methadone (36 to 48 hours or more), repeated doses for 8 to 24 hours may be required. Patient should be watched closely for recurrence of respiratory depression.
- Preserved in tight, light-resistant containers at room temperature (between 59° and 86°F) unless otherwise directed by manufacturer.
- *See morphine sulphate.*

Drug interactions   Methadone is used with caution and in reduced dosage in patients concurrently receiving other **CNS depressants** (including **alcohol**), and cimetidine. Patients addicted to heroin or those who are on methadone maintenance may experience withdrawal symptoms when given barbiturates, **pentazocine**, phenytoin and other hydantoins, **rifampicin** urinary acidifiers e.g., ammonium chloride.

M

Methicillin sodium

(Celbenin) *Antibiotic (beta lactam); penicillin*

ACTIONS AND USES   Semisynthetic salt of penicillin with antimicrobial spectrum similar to that of penicillin G (q.v.); differs from the latter in its high resistance to penicillinase-producing strains of staphylococci.

Used primarily in infections caused by penicillinase-producing staphylococci. May be used to initiate therapy in suspected staphylococcal infections pending results of culture and sensitivity tests.

ROUTE AND DOSAGE   Intramuscular: Intravenous: **Adults**: 1 g every 4 to 6 hours.

ABSORPTION AND FATE   Peak plasma concentrations within 30 minutes to 1 hour following IM injection and within 15 minutes after IV injection; serum levels decline within 4 hours after IM and within 2 hours after IV administration. Well distributed in various body tissues and fluids. Little diffusion to cerebrospinal fluid unless meninges are inflamed. About 40% bound to plasma proteins. Approximately two-thirds of 1 g dose is eliminated unchanged in urine in 4 hours; 20% or more excreted in faeces via bile (rate of elimination is extremely slow in infants). Crosses placenta.

NURSING IMPLICATIONS
- *See also penicillin G.*

Methohexitone sodium —————————————————

(Brietal Sodium)   *Anaesthetic (general);*
                                                          barbiturate

ACTIONS AND USES   Rapid, ultra-short-acting barbiturate anaesthetic agent. More potent than thiopentone (q.v.), but has less cumulative effect and shorter duration of action, and recovery is more rapid. Abnormal muscle movements, coughing, sneezing, and laryngospasm reportedly occur more frequently than with thiopentone. *See thiopentone for absorption and fate, contraindications and precautions, adverse/side effects.*

Used for induction of anaesthesia, as supplement for other anaesthetics, and as general anesthetic for brief operative procedures.

ROUTE AND DOSAGE   **Intravenous:** 1 or 2% solution, by slow injection 50–120 mg over 25–60 seconds on 1–1.5 mg/kg according to response. **Child:** 1–2 mg/kg. **Continuous infusion:** 0.1–0.2% solution according to response.

NURSING IMPLICATIONS

- Methohexitone solution is incompatible with acid solutions, e.g., atropine and with silicone. Do not allow contact with rubber stoppers or parts of syringes treated with silicone.
- See thiopentone.

Methotrexate —————————————————————

(Emtexate, Maxtrex)   *Antineoplastic; antimetabolic;*
                                                  folic acid antagonist

ACTIONS AND USES   Antimetabolite and folic acid antagonist. Blocks folinic acid (active principle of folic acid) participation in nucleic acid synthesis, thereby interfering with mitotic process. Rapidly proliferating tissues (malignant cells, bone marrow) are sensitive to this effect. In psoriasis, reproductive rate of epithelial cells is higher than in normal cells. Methotrexate controls the psoriatic process by its effect on mitosis. Some evidence of toxicity usually accompanies therapeutic response. Induces remission slowly; use often preceded by other antineoplastic therapies.

Used principally in combination regimens to maintain induced remissions in neoplastic diseases. Effective in treatment of gestational choriocarcinoma and hydatidiform mole and as immunosuppressant in kidney transplantation, for acute and subacute leukaemias and leukaemic meningitis, especially in children. Used in lymphosarcoma, in certain inoperable tumours of head, neck, and pelvis, and in mycosis fungoides. Also used to treat severe psoriasis nonresponsive to other forms of therapy.

ROUTE AND DOSAGE   **Oral, intramuscular, intravenous, intraarterial, intrathecal:** dosage individualized according to disease being treated, concurrent drug therapy, response, and tolerance of patient. *Severe psoriasis:* **Oral:** usual dose 15–25 mg/week.

METHOTREXATE *(continued)*

ABSORPTION AND FATE   Rapidly absorbed from GI tract; peak serum levels 1 to 2 hours after oral administration and 30 to 60 minutes after parenteral administration. **Serum half-life** 2 to 4 hours after IM and oral administration; approximately one-half of drug is bound to serum proteins. Wide distribution, with highest concentrations in kidneys, gall-bladder, spleen, liver, skin. Unchanged drug is retained several weeks in impaired kidneys, several months in the liver, and about 6 days in cerebrospinal fluid following intrathecal injection. Up to 90% of drug is cleared by kidneys; small amounts also excreted in stools through enterohepatic route. Crosses placenta; minimal passage across blood−brain barrier.

CONTRAINDICATIONS AND PRECAUTIONS   Pregnancy, hepatic and renal insufficiency, men and women of childbearing age, concomitant administration of hepatotoxic drugs and haematopoietic depressants, alcohol, ultraviolet exposure to psoriatic lesions, preexisting blood dyscrasias. **Cautious Use**: infections, peptic ulcer, ulcerative colitis, very young or old patients, cancer patients with preexisting bone marrow impairment, poor nutritional status.

ADVERSE/SIDE EFFECTS   Dose-related and reversible. These include: erythematous rashes, pruritis, uticaria, folliculitis, vasculitis, photosensitivity, depigmentation, hyperpigmentation, alopecia, hepatotoxicity, GI ulcerations and haemorrhage, ulcerative stomatitis, glossitis, gingivitis, pharyngitis, nausea, vomiting, diarrhoea, hepatic cirrhosis, marked myelosuppression, aplastic bone marrow, telangiectasis, thrombophlebitis at intraarterial catheter site, hypogammaglobulinaemia, hyperuricaemia, headache, drowsiness, blurred vision, dizziness, aphasia, hemiparesis, convulsions (after intrathecal administration), mental confusion, tremors, ataxia, coma, defective oogenesis or spermatogenesis, nephropathy, haematuria, menstrual dysfunction, infertility, abortion, foetal defects, malaise, undue fatigue, systemic toxicity (after intrathecal and intraarterial administration), chills, fever, decreased resistance to infection, septicaemia, osteoporosis, metabolic changes precipitating diabetes and sudden death, pneumonitis.

NURSING IMPLICATIONS

- A test dose (5 to 10 mg parentally) one week before therapy, precedes treatment of psoriasis.
- Avoid skin exposure and inhalation of drug particles.
- Oral preparations should be given 1 to 2 hours before or 2 to 3 hours after meals.
- Preserve drug in tight, light-resistant container.
- Hepatic and renal function tests, blood tests (including blood type and group, bleeding time, coagulation time) and chest radiographs should be part of the health data base in case of emergency surgery or need for transfusion during therapy. Tests are repeated at weekly intervals during methotrexate therapy.
- Hepatic function tests may be abnormal 1 to 3 days after methotrexate administration, and GI symptoms may be absent.
- Monitor all laboratory reports daily as indicators for adaptations in nursing and drug regimens.

METHOTREXATE (continued)

- Patient should be fully informed of dangers of this drug and warned to report promptly any abnormal symptoms.
- Alcohol ingestion increases the incidence and severity of methotrexate hepatotoxicity.
- Leucovorin calcium (citrovorin factor) given within 12 hours after methotrexate protects normal tissues from lethal effects of the drug (leucovorin 'rescue').
- If an overdosage of methotrexate is given, leucovorin may be employed as antidote (must be given within the first hour of overdosage).
- Prolonged treatment with small frequent doses may lead to hepatotoxicity, which is best diagnosed by liver biopsy.
- Ulcerative stomatitis with glossitis and gingivitis, often the first signs of toxicity, necessitate interruption of therapy or dosage adjustment. Inspect mouth daily; report patchy necrotic areas, bleeding and discomfort, or overgrowth (black, furry tongue).
- Fastidious mouth care prevents infection, provides comfort, and is essential to maintenance of adequate nutritional status. *See Index: Nursing interventions: stomatitis.*
- In presence of hyperuricaemia, patient may be kept well hydrated (about 2,000 ml/24 hours) to dilute hyperuric fluids and given allopurinol to prevent urate deposition.
- Monitor fluid intake–output ratio and pattern. Severe nephrotoxicity (haematuria, dysuria, azotemia, oliguria) fosters drug accumulation and renal damage and requires dosage adjustment or discontinuation.
- During leucopenic periods, prevent patient exposure to personnel and visitors with infections or colds. Be alert to onset of agranulocytosis (cough, extreme fatigue, sore throat, chills, fever), and report symptoms promptly. Methotrexate therapy will be interrupted and appropriate antibiotic drugs prescribed.
- Watch for and report symptoms of thrombocytopenia: ecchymoses, petechiae, epistaxis, melena, haematuria, vaginal bleeding, slow and protracted oozing following trauma.
- Contraceptive measures should be used both during and for at least 8 weeks following therapy.
- Alopecia is reversible; hair regrowth begins after drug discontinuation, but it may require several months. *See Index: Nursing intervention: alopecia.*
- Methotrexate may precipitate gouty arthritis. Instruct the patient to report joint pains to physician.
- Bloody diarrhoea necessitates interruption of therapy to prevent perforation or haemorrhagic enteritis. Report to physician.
- Warn patient not to self-medicate with vitamins. Some OTC compounds may include folic acid (or its derivatives), which alters methotrexate response.
- Diabetes may be precipitated; therefore, tests for glucosuria should be performed periodically, and significant symptoms such as polydipsia and polyuria should be reported.
- Instruct patient to notify physician if psoriasis worsens.
- Burning and erythema may occur in psoriatic areas after each dose of methotrexate.
- Concomitant exposure to ultraviolet light and to sunlight may aggravate psoriatic lesions in patients on methotrexate therapy.

METHOTREXATE (continued)

- Advise patient to adhere to dosage regimen i.e., not to omit, increase, or decrease dose or change dose intervals.
- Deaths have been reported with use of this agent in the treatment of psoriasis.
- Consult physician about plans for disclosure of diagnosis, prognosis, and treatment so that discussions with patient and family will be supportive and nonconflicting.

Diagnostic test interferences Severe reactions may occur when live vaccines are administered because of immunosuppressive activity of methotrexate.

Drug interactions Salicylates, sulphonamides, phenylbutazone, phenytoin, tetracycline, chloramphenicol, and **PABA** displace methotrexate from plasma protein binding, causing increased toxicity. Studies suggest that large doses of **penicillin** and **probenecid** increase methotrexate plasma levels, with resultant increase in its toxicity. **Vitamin preparations** containing **folic acid** and derivatives may alter response to methotrexate. Hepatotoxicity caused by methotrexate is increased by concomitant administration of **alcohol**. Hypoprothrombinaemia produced by **anticoagulants** is enhanced by methotrexate. Oral aminoglycoside antibiotics may reduce absorption of oral methotrexate.

M

Methotrimeprazine

(Nozinan, Veractil)   *Phenothiazine derivative*

ACTIONS AND USES Aliphatic (propylamino) derivative of phenothiazine with CNS actions similar to those of chlorpromazine (q.v.).

Used to treat schizophrenia and other psychoses.

ROUTE AND DOSAGE IM/IV: *sedation*: 2.5–25 mg every 6–8 hrs as required. Oral: 25–50 mg/day in divided doses, increased if necessary, maximum 1 g/day.

ABSORPTION AND FATE Enters cerebrospinal fluid. Probably metabolized in liver. Metabolites exhibit some activity, but less than parent drug. Excreted slowly in urine and faeces, primarily as metabolites and about 1% as unchanged drug. Elimination in urine may continue 1 week after a single dose. Crosses placenta; small amounts may enter breast milk.

NURSING IMPLICATIONS

- Administer IM injection deep into large muscle mass (subcutaneous injection causes severe local irritation). Carefully withdraw plunger to prevent inadvertent injection into blood vessel.
- Pain at injection site and local inflammatory reaction commonly occur. Rotate injection sites and observe daily.
- Protect drug from light.

METHOTRIMEPRAZINE (continued)
DRUG INTERACTIONS   *Methotrimeprazine*_____

PLUS	INTERACTIONS
Anticholinergic agents (e.g., atropine, scopolamine, and others)	Aggravation of extrapyramidal symptoms, CNS stimulation, delirium
Skeletal muscle relaxants, surgical (e.g., succinylcholine, tubocurarine)	Prolonged muscle relaxation

For further information: *see chlorpromazine*

Methyclothiazide ━━━━━━━━━━━━━━━━━━━━━━━━━━━━━━━

(Enduron)   *Diuretic; antihypertensive;*
                                                                             thiazide

M

ACTIONS AND USES   Benzothiadiazine (thiazide) derivative. Similar to chlorothiazide (q.v.) in actions, uses, contraindications, adverse reactions and interactions.

Used in antihypertensive treatment, and adjunctively in the management of oedema associated with congestive heart failure, renal pathology and hepatic cirrhosis.

ROUTE AND DOSAGE   Oral: Adults: *Diuretic*: 2.5 to 5 mg once daily or once daily 3 to 5 times a week. *Antihypertensive*: 2.5 to 10 mg once daily.

ABSORPTION AND FATE   Diuretic effect begins within 2 hours, peaks in 6 hours and lasts more than 24 hours. Excreted unchanged by kidneys. Passes placenta; appears in breast milk.

CONTRAINDICATIONS AND PRECAUTIONS   Hypersensitivity to thiazides, sulphonamide derivatives; anuria, hypokalaemia, pregnancy, lactation. **Cautious Use**: impaired renal or hepatic function, gout, SLE, hypercalcaemia, diabetes mellitus. *See also chlorothiazide.*

ADVERSE/SIDE EFFECTS   Postural hypotension, sialadenitis, unusual fatigue, dizziness, paraesthesias, yellow vision, hypokalaemia, agranulocytosis. *See also chlorothiazide.*

NURSING IMPLICATIONS
- The elderly are more responsive to excessive diuresis than young people because of changes in the cardiovascular and renal systems with ageing. Orthostatic hypotension may be a problem.
- Advise patient to avoid driving a vehicle or working with dangerous equipment until adjustment to the hypotensive effects of this drug has been made.
- Store drug at temperature between 15° and 30°C (59° and 86°F) unless otherwise instructed by manufacturer.
- *See chlorothiazide.*

Methylcellulose

(Cologel, Celevac, Cellucon)   *Laxative; bulk forming*

ACTIONS AND USES   Hydrophilic semisynthetic cellulose derivative. Oral preparation swells on contact with water to form a demulcent nonabsorbable gel that facilitates passage of stool and reflexly stimulates peristalsis.

Used orally as adjunct in treatment of chronic constipation.

ROUTE AND DOSAGE   Oral: Adults: depends on the preparation.

CONTRAINDICATIONS AND PRECAUTIONS   Nausea, vomiting, abdominal pain, intestinal obstruction, ulceration or stenosis, diarrhoea.

ADVERSE/SIDE EFFECTS   Oral form: diarrhoea, nausea, vomiting, faecal impaction, oesophageal obstruction.

NURSING IMPLICATIONS
- Each oral dose should be taken with 1 or more glasses of water; additional fluids should be taken during the day. Faecal impaction can occur if fluid intake by mouth is insufficient.
- Caution the patient not to chew the tablet form because it may start to swell in the oesophagus and cause obstruction.
- Laxation generally occurs in 12 to 24 hours; however, some patients may require 2 or 3 days of medication.
- Review proper bowel hygiene: adequacy of fluid and dietary intake, exercise, habit time.

M

Methyldopa

(Aldomet, Dopamet, Medomet)   *Antihypertensive (centrally acting)*

Methyldopate hydrochloride

ACTIONS AND USES   Structurally related to catecholamines and their precursors. Exact mechanism of action unknown; metabolic product of the drug appears to act on both CNS and peripheral vasculature by displacing noradrenaline from its storage sites. Lowers standing and supine blood pressures, and unlike adrenergic blockers, it is not so prone to produce orthostatic hypotension, diurnal blood pressure variations, or exercise hypertension. Reduces renal vascular resistance; maintains cardiac output without acceleration, but may slow heart rate; tends to support sodium and water retention. Although it has sedative effect, it also increases REM sleep.

Used in treatment of sustained moderate to severe hypertension, particularly in

METHYLDOPATE HYDROCHLORIDE (continued)

patients with renal dysfunction. Parenteral form has been used for treatment of hypertensive crises but is not preferred because of its slow onset of action. Methyldopa is commercially available in combination with hydrochlorothiazide (Hydromet).

ROUTE AND DOSAGE   Adults: Oral: 250 mg two or three times a day for first 48 hours; daily dosage may then be increased or decreased, preferably at intervals of not less than 2 days, until adequate response is achieved. *Maintenance*: 500 mg to 2 g in 2 to 4 divided doses daily. Maximum recommended daily dosage 3 g. **Intravenous (methyldopate hydrochloride):** 250 to 500 mg at 6-hour intervals, as required. Maximum recommended dose 1 g every 6 hours.

ABSORPTION AND FATE   About 50% of oral dose is absorbed from GI tract. Maximal antihypertensive effect in 4 to 6 hours; action may persist 24 hours after single oral dose. Following IV injection, major decline in blood pressure occurs within 4 to 6 hours; duration 10 to 16 hours. Weakly bound to plasma proteins. Metabolized in GI tract and liver. About 85% excreted in urine within 24 hours; some unabsorbed oral drug excreted in faeces. Crosses placenta; appears in breast milk.

CONTRAINDICATIONS AND PRECAUTIONS   Hypersensitivity to methyldopa, active hepatic disease, phaeochromocytoma, blood dyscrasias, mild or labile hypertension amenable to treatment with mild sedation or thiazide diuretics. Safe use in women of childbearing potential and during pregnancy not established. **Cautious Use:** history of impaired liver or renal function or disease; angina pectoris, history of mental depression, young or elderly patients.

ADVERSE/SIDE EFFECTS   These include: orthostatic hypotension, syncope (carotid sinus hypersensitivity), aggravation of angina pectoris, bradycardia, myocarditis, oedema, weight gain (sodium and water retention), paradoxic hypertensive reaction (especially with IV administration), diarrhoea, constipation, abdominal distention, malabsorption syndrome, nausea, vomiting, dry mouth, sore or black tongue, sialadenitis, positive direct Coombs' test (common especially in black patients), haemolytic anaemia (rare), granulocytopenia, agranulocytosis, abnormal liver function tests, jaundice, hepatitis, sedation, drowsiness, sluggishness, headache, weakness, fatigue, dizziness, vertigo, paresthesias, Bell's palsy, decrease in mental acuity, inability to concentrate, amnesia-like syndrome, involuntary choreoathetotic movements, parkinsonism, mild psychoses, depression, nightmares, nasal stuffiness (common), gynaecomastia, lactation, decreased libido, impotence, hypothermia (large doses), positive tests for lupus and rheumatoid factors, granulomatous skin lesions, pancreatitis.

NURSING IMPLICATIONS
- During period of dosage adjustment, physician may request blood pressures to be taken at regular intervals in lying, sitting, and standing positions.
- During IV infusion of methyldopate, check blood pressure and pulse at least every 30 minutes until stabilized, and observe for adequacy of urinary output.
- Transient sedation and drowsiness, sometimes associated with mental depression, weakness, and headache, commonly occur during first 24 to 72 hours of therapy or

METHYLDOPATE HYDROCHLORIDE (continued)

whenever dosage is increased. Symptoms tend to disappear with continuation of therapy or with dosage reduction.

- To minimize daytime sedation, physician may prescribe dosage increases to be made in the evening. Some patients maintain adequate blood pressure control with a single evening dose.
- Orthostatic hypotension with dizziness and lightheadedness may occur during period of dosage adjustment; this indicates need for dosage reduction. Elderly patients and patients with impaired renal function are particularly likely to manifest this drug effect. Supervison of ambulation may be advisable.
- Caution patient that hot baths and showers, prolonged standing in one position, and strenuous exercise may enhance orthostatic hypotension. Instruct patient to make position changes slowly, particularly from recumbent to upright posture and to dangle legs a few minutes before standing.
- Monitor fluid intake and output. Report oliguria and changes in intake–output ratio.
- Weigh patient under standard conditions, and check for oedema. Concomitant administration of a diuretic is usually prescribed because methyldopa favours sodium and water retention.
- Methyldopa hepatoxicity (reversible) resembles viral hepatitis and commonly develops in 2 to 4 weeks, but it may occur from 1 week to 1 year after start of therapy. It is manifested by flu-like symptoms: chills, fever, headache, pruritus, dark urine, fatigue, GI upset and anorexia and is sometimes associated with rash, arthralgia, enlarged liver, and positive Coombs' test. (Occurs commonly in postmenopausal women.) Report to physician; drug should be discontinued.
- Baseline and regularly scheduled blood counts and liver function tests are advised during first 6 to 12 weeks of therapy or if patient develops unexplained fever.
- Be alert to symptoms of mental depression and report their appearance to physician: anorexia, insomnia, inattention to personal hygiene, withdrawal. Drug-induced depression may persist even after drug is withdrawn.
- Positive Coombs' test may or may not indicate haemolytic anaemia; it usually develops between 6 to 12 months of therapy and may remain positive for several months after drug is discontinued. If for any reason the need for transfusion arises, both direct and indirect Coombs' tests should be performed. Positive tests may interfere with accurate cross-matching of blood.
- Tolerance to drug effect may occur during the second or third week of therapy (manifested by rising blood pressure). Report to physician. Effectiveness may be restored by adding a diuretic or increasing dosage of methyldopa.
- Caution patient that methyldopa may affect ability to perform activities requiring concentrated mental effort, especially during first few days of therapy or whenever dosage is increased; patient should avoid potentially hazardous tasks such as driving a car or operating machinery, until reaction to drug is known.
- Inform the patient that urine may darken on standing (thought to be due to breakdown product of drug or its metabolite) and that urine contaminated with a hypochlorite toilet bleaching agent may first turn red, then brown and black. Both are possible simple tests for checking patient compliance.

M

METHYLDOPATE HYDROCHLORIDE (continued)

■ Compliance tends to be poor in patients receiving antihypertensive agents, for a variety of reasons. Urge the patient to keep follow-up visits. Some patients acquire tolerance about the second or third month of therapy, necessitating dosage increases, and rebound hypertension has been reported as a result of acute methyldopa withdrawal.

■ Advise patient not to take OTC medications for coughs, colds, or allergy unless approved by physician (many contain sympathomimetic agents that may increase blood pressure).

Diagnostic test interferences Methyldopa may interfere with **serum creatinine** measurements using alkaline picrate method, **SGOT** by colorimetric methods, and **uric acid** measurements by phosphotungstate method (in patients with high methyldopa blood levels); it may produce false elevations of **urinary catecholamines**, and increase in **serum amylase** in patients with methyldopa-induced sialadenitis.

DRUG INTERACTIONS *Methyldopa*_____

PLUS	INTERACTIONS
Amphetamines } Antidepressants, tricyclics }	Reduce antihypertensive effect of methyldopa
Ephedrine	Methyldopa may inhibit effectiveness of ephedrine
Haloperidol	Adverse psychiatric symptoms may result
Levodopa	Methyldopa may inhibit therapeutic response to levodopa
Lithium	Increased risk of lithium toxicity
Methotrimeprazine	Additive hypotensive effect
MAO inhibitors	Hallucinations (based on limited clinical evidence)
Noradrenaline	Slight increase in pressor response to noradrenaline
Phenothiazines } Propranolol and possibly other beta-adrenergic blockers }	Paradoxic hypertensive response may occur
Phenoxybenzamine	Methyldopa augments sympatholytic activity of phenoxybenzamine to cause urinary incontinence
Tolbutamide, and possibly other sulphonylureas	Hypoglycaemic effects may be increased by methyldopa

Methylphenobarbitone ▬▬▬▬▬▬▬▬▬▬▬▬▬▬▬▬

(Prominal)   *Barbiturate; anticonvulsant*

ROUTE AND DOSAGE   Adults: **Oral:** 100–600 mg/day.
    For further information: *see phenobarbitone.*

Methylprednisolone

(Medrone)   *Corticosteroid; glucocorticoid*

Methylprednisolone acetate

(Depo-Medrone, Neo-Medrone)

Methylprednisolone sodium succinate

(Solu-Medrone)

ACTIONS AND USES   Intermediate acting synthetic adrenal steroid with similar glucocorticoid activity but considerably less sodium and water retention effects than those of hydrocortisone (q.v.). On weight basis, 4 mg methylprednisolone is equivalent to 20 mg hydrocortisone. Acetate has longer duration of action and more rapid onset of activity than parent compound. Sodium succinate is characterized by rapid onset of action and is used for emergency therapy of short duration. *See hydrocortisone.*

Used as an antiinflammatory agent in the management of acute and chronic inflammatory diseases, for palliative management of neoplastic diseases, for control of severe acute and chronic allergic processes, and for cerebraloedema and shock.

ROUTE AND DOSAGE   All dosages are individualized according to severity of disease and response of patient. **Paediatric:** less than adult dosage and governed by severity of the condition rather than by a specific dose according to weight and age. **Oral:** 4 to 48 mg/day in single or divided doses. **Topical cream:** 0.25 applied one to three times daily. *Sodium Succinate*: **Intramuscular, intravenous (direct or infusion):** up to 120 mg/day for up to 3 days, shock: **IV:** 30 mg/kg.

ABSORPTION AND FATE   **Peak effect:** oral, 1 or 2 hours; IM, 4 to 8 days; intraarticular, intralesional, 7 days. **Duration of effect:** oral, 1.25 to 1.5 days; IM, 1 to 4 weeks, intraarticular, intralesional, 1 to 5 weeks. **Plasma half-life:** more than 3.5 hours. **HPA (hypothalamic−pituitary−adrenal) axis suppression:** 18 to 36 hours.

CONTRAINDICATIONS AND PRECAUTIONS   Systemic fungal infections. Safe use by children, during pregnancy and lactation not established. **Cautious Use:** Cushing's syndrome, GI ulceration, hypertension, varicella, vaccinia, diabetes mellitus, emotional instability or psychotic tendencies. *See also hydrocortisone.*

ADVERSE/SIDE EFFECTS   Severe hypokalaemia, congestive heart failure, euphoria, insomnia, delayed wound healing. *See also hydrocortisone.*

NURSING IMPLICATIONS
- Tablet may be crushed before administration and taken with fluid of patient's choice.
- The oral preparation will be less irritating if given with food.

METHYLPREDNISOLONE SODIUM SUCCINATE (continued)

- Direct intravenous injection should be administered over one to several minutes.
- Methylprednisolone sodium succinate solution should be used within 48 hours after preparation.
- Avoid contacting eyes with the ointment. *See hydrocortisone for nursing implications regarding use of topical formulation.*
- Instruct patient not to alter established dosage regimen, i.e., not to increase, decrease or omit doses or change dose intervals. Withdrawal symptoms (rebound inflammation, fever) can be induced with sudden discontinuation of therapy.
- Monitor urine for glucosuria. The diabetic may require increased doses of insulin or sulphonylurea agent.
- Instruct patient to report immediately onset of signs of hypocorticism adrenal insufficiency: fatigue, nausea, anorexia, joint pain, muscular weakness, dizziness, fever.
- Store at temperature 15° to 30°C (59° or 86°F). Prevent freezing.
- *See also hydrocortisone for additional nursing implications and drug interactions.*

M

Methyltestosterone

(Virormone—oral)   *Hormone*

ACTIONS AND USES   Orally effective, short-acting steroid with androgen/anabolic activity ratio (1:1) similar to that of testosterone (q.v.), but less effective than its esters. Fails to produce full sexual maturation when administered to preadolescent male with complete testicular failure unless preceded by testosterone therapy.

Used as treatment for hypogonadism that starts in adult life after puberty; also used alone or combined with oestrogen to treat menopausal symptoms and functional menstrual disorders. *See testosterone.*

ROUTE AND DOSAGE   Oral: 30–50 mg/day in divided doses.

ABSORPTION AND FATE   Absorbed from oral mucosa and GI tract. All metabolites excreted in urine.

CONTRAINDICATIONS AND PRECAUTIONS   Hepatic dysfunction. *See also testosterone.*

ADVERSE/SIDE EFFECTS   Cholestatic hepatitis with jaundice. *See also testosterone.*

NURSING IMPLICATIONS
- Creatinuria is a frequent finding with use of this drug, but its significance is unclear. (Normal *urinary creatinine*: 15 to 25 mg/kg/24 hours.)
- *See also testosterone.*

Methyprylon

(Noludar)   *Hypnotic; piperidine*

ACTIONS AND USES   Piperidine derivative structurally related to glutethimide. Produces CNS depressant effects similar to those of short-acting barbiturates. Hypnotic doses suppress REM sleep.

Used as hypnotic for relief of severe intractable insomnia.

ROUTE AND DOSAGE   Oral: **Adults**: 200 to 400 mg before retiring; total daily dose should not exceed 400 mg.

ABSORPTION AND FATE   Hypnotic dose induces sleep within 45 minutes; **duration** 5 to 8 hours. **Plasma half-life** 3 to 6 hours. Conjugated in liver; metabolites are secreted in bile and reabsorbed. Most of dose is excreted in urine as metabolites and their glucuronide conjugates; approximately 3% excreted unchanged.

CONTRAINDICATIONS AND PRECAUTIONS   Porphyria, known hypersensitivity to methyprylon, patient who is hallucinating or who is pyschotic. Safe use during pregnancy and in women of childbearing potential, nursing mothers, and children under 12 years of age not established. **Cautious Use**: hepatic or renal impairment, addiction-prone individuals, mental depression, history of suicidal tendencies.

ADVERSE/SIDE EFFECTS   Infrequent: morning drowsiness, dizziness, nausea, vomiting, diarrhoea, oesophagitis, headache, paradoxic excitation, skin rash, exacerbation of intermittent porphyria. Reported, but causal relationship not established: neutropenia, thrombocytopenia. **Acute toxicity**: somnolence, confusion, constricted pupils, hyperpyrexia, hypothermia, shock, pulmonary oedema, respiratory depression; occasionally during recovery: excitation, convulsions, delirium, hallucinations.

NURSING IMPLICATIONS
- Hypnotic dose is administered 15 minutes before retiring. Prepare patient for sleep before administering drug.
- Tolerance may develop to hypnotic and sedative effects, but not to toxic effects.
- Psychological and physical dependence may occur, especially after prolonged use of large doses. Patient's continued need for methyprylon should be evaluated regularly.
- Warn patients about possible additive effects with alcohol and other CNS depressants.
- Caution patient to avoid driving a car or engaging in other activities requiring mental alertness, until response to drug is known.
- Gradual drug withdrawal is advised after prolonged use. Sudden discontinuation of drug may result in *withdrawal symptoms* similar to those following barbiturate dependence: confusion, marked nervousness, insomnia, sweating polyuria, hyperreflexia, delirium, miosis, hallucinations, convulsion, death.
- ***Treatment of overdosage***   Gastric lavage, general supportive measures (airway maintenance, assisted respiration, oxygen, IV fluids), pressor agent (noradrenaline,

M

METHYPRYLON (continued)

metaraminol), short-acting barbiturate for convulsions and excitation, close monitoring of vital signs and urinary output.

■ Preserved in tightly closed, light-resistant containers.

Diagnostic test interferences Methyprylon may interfere with urinary steriod determinations.

Methysergide

(Deseril)   *Antimigraine; ergot alkaloid*

M

ACTIONS AND USES Ergot derivative and congener of LSD. Unlike ergotamine (q.v.), has weak vasoconstrictor and oxytoxic actions. Action mechanism in migraine prevention unclear. Serotonin (a strong vasoconstrictor) levels are reduced during an attack. Methysergide replaces serotonin on cranial artery receptor sites during an attack, thereby preserving vasoconstriction afforded by serotonin. Ineffective treatment of acute attacks. Prolonged use has been known to promote fibrotic processes.

Used in prophylactic management of severe recurrent migraine, cluster, and other vascular headaches unresponsive to other antimigraine drugs.

ROUTE AND DOSAGE Oral: 4 to 6 mg daily in divided doses.

ABSORPTION AND FATE Metabolic fate unknown, but thought to be well absorbed. Widely distributed to all tissues, and metabolized in liver.

CONTRAINDICATIONS AND PRECAUTIONS Fibrotic processes, pulmonary or collagen diseases, oedema, serious infections, debilitated states. *See also ergotamine tartrate.*

ADVERSE/SIDE EFFECTS These include: insomnia, drowsiness, vertigo, mild euphoria, confusion, excitement, feelings of unreality or depersonalization, distortions of body image, depression, anxiety, hallucinations, nightmares, ataxia, hyperaesthesia, paraesthesia, peripheral oedema, thrombophlebitis, claudication, impaired circulation, angina of effort, ECG changes, postural hypotension, tachycardia, facial flushing, telangiectasia, rash, excessive hair loss. **Fibrotic complications**: *retroperitoneal fibrosis* (fatigue, malaise, fever, urinary obstruction with girdle or flank pain, dysuria, oliguria, polyuria, increased BUN and sedimentation rate), *pleuropulmonary fibrosis* (dyspnoea, chest pain and tightness, pleural friction rubs and effusion) and *cardiac fibrosis* (fibrotic thickening of cardiac valves with murmurs), nausea, vomiting, heartburn, hyperchlorhydria, abdominal pain, diarrhoea, constipation, neutropenia, eosinophilia, weakness, arthralgia, myalgia, weight gain, scotomata, nasal stuffiness, positive direct Coombs' test.

NURSING IMPLICATIONS

■ GI side effects can frequently be prevented by gradual introduction of medication and by administering drug with meals.

METHYSERGIDE (continued)

- One or two days of drug therapy are required before protective drug action is realized; at end of therapy, protection continues two days beyond last dose.
- Therapeutic trial period of 3 weeks is advised to determine patient's response to methysergide. If no response occurs in this time, it is unlikely that longer administration will be of benefit.
- Pretreatment and periodic assessments of cardiac status, renal function, blood count, and sedimentation rate are advised.
- Since incidence of side effects is relatively high (usually reversible with discontinuation of drug), patient should be examined regularly for development of fibrotic and vascular complications: auscultate heart and lungs; check peripheral pulses, and auscultate major vessels for bruits; observe for signs of phlebitis or venous obstruction. Also, observe and question patient concerning presence of CNS symptoms and other possible adverse effects (see Adverse/Side Effects).
- Instruct patient to report the following immediately: onset of abdominal, back or chest pain; dyspnoea; leg pains while walking; cold, numb, or painful extremities; fever; dysuria or other urinary problems; oedema; weight gain; other unusual signs and symptoms.
- Counsel patient to weigh self daily, and teach patient how to check extremities for oedema.
- Caloric restriction and reduction of salt intake may be prescribed.
- Since postural hypotension is a possible side effect, advise patient to make position changes slowly, particularly from recumbent to upright posture, and to dangle legs a few minutes before standing. Also instruct patient to lie down if faintness occurs.
- Continuous administration of methysergide should not exceed 6 months without a medication-free interval of 3 to 4 weeks. Drug may be readministered after drug-free interval, if necessary.
- To avoid 'headache rebound,' drug should be withdrawn gradually over 2- or 3-week period preceding discontinuation. Caution patient not to stop medication abruptly because of this possibility.
- Preserved in tight, light-resistant containers preferably at 15° to 30°C (59° to 86°F) unless otherwise directed by manufacturer.

Metoclopramide hydrochloride ———————————————

(Maxeran, Reglan, Maxolon, Metox, Metramid, Mygdalon, Paramid, Primperan)

Cholinergic;
(parasympathomimetic);
antiemetic

ACTIONS AND USES   Potent central dopamine receptor antagonist. Structurally related to procainamide but has little antiarrhythmic or anaesthetic activity. Exact mechanism of action not clear, but appears to sensitize GI smooth muscle to effects of acetylcholine by direct action. Increases resting tone of oesophageal sphincter (thereby

METOCLOPRAMIDE HYDROCHLORIDE *(continued)*

increasing lower oesophageal sphincter pressure), and increases tone and amplitude of upper GI contractions. As a result, gastric emptying and intestinal transit are accelerated with little effect, if any, on gastric, biliary or pancreatic secretions. Antiemetic action results from drug-induced elevation of chemoreceptor trigger-zone threshold and enhanced gastric emptying (which blocks the gastric stasis that precedes vomiting). Has no apparent effect on seizure threshold. Inhibits central and peripheral effects of apomorphine and indirectly stimulates release of prolactin. Directly stimulates secretion of aldosterone, but has no effect on plasma renin activity, plasma K or cortisol concentrations. High doses produce neuroleptic actions similar to those of antipsychotic agents (e.g., phenothiazines). Metoclopramide actions can be reduced or abolished by anticholinergics. Mutagenicity and carcinogenicity potential not known.

Used for management of nausea and vomiting including that caused by anti-cancer chemotherapy and radiotherapy and to facilitate intubation of small bowel.

ROUTE AND DOSAGE   *Small bowel intubation*; *radiological examination*: **Intravenous**: **Adult**: 10 mg (2 ml) as single dose over 1 to 2 minutes; 5–10 minutes before examination. *Nausea and vomiting*: **oral, IM or IV**: 10 mg three times a day. **Child (up to 1 yr)**: 1 mg twice a day; **(1–2 yrs)**: 1 mg 2–3 times a day; **(3–5 yrs)**: 2 mg 2–3 times a day; **(6–9 yrs)**: 2.5 mg 3 times a day; **(10–14 yrs)**; 5 mg three times a day.

ABSORPTION AND FATE   Rapidly absorbed after oral administration (except in presence of gastric paresis). **Onset of action** in 30 to 60 minutes following oral, 10 to 15 minutes following IM, and 1 to 3 minutes following IV dose. **Duration of effects** 1 to 2 hours. Subject to first-pass metabolism following oral administration; **bioavailability** 30 to 100%; **protein-binding**: 13 to 22%. **Half-life**: 4 hours. Distributed to most body tissues and fluids including milk. Crosses blood–brain and placenta barriers. Minimally metabolized by liver; excreted in urine and faeces (via bile); minimally removed by haemodialysis or peritoneal dialysis.

CONTRAINDICATIONS AND PRECAUTIONS   Sensitivity or intolerance to metoclopramide; history of seizure disorders, concurrent use of drugs that can cause extrapyramidal symptoms; phaeochromocytoma, presence of mechanical GI obstruction or perforation, patient with history of breast cancer. Safe use during pregnancy; in fertile women, and in nursing mothers not established. **Cautious Use**: congestive heart failure, hypokalaemia, renal dysfunction, GI haemorrhage, history of intermittent porphyria.

ADVERSE/SIDE EFFECTS   These include: mild sedation (50% patients), fatigue, restlessness, agitation, headache, insomnia, disorientation, extrapyramidal symptoms (acute dystonic type). **CV**: hypotension, supraventricular tachycardia. **Others**: nausea, constipation, diarrhoea, dry mouth, urticarial or maculopapular rash, glossal or periorbital oedema, methaemoglobinaemia, galactorrhoea, gynaecomastia, amenorrhoea, impotence.

NURSING IMPLICATIONS
- Oral form is usually taken 30 minutes before meals and at bedtime.
- The compatibility of metoclopropamide with other admixtures depends upon multiple factors including temperature, drug concentration, and pH. Consult pharmacist for needed information.

METOCLOPRAMIDE HYDROCHLORIDE (continued)

- Discard open ampoules; do not store for future use.
- Extrapyramidal symptoms *(see Index)* are most likely to occur in children, young adults and with high dose treatment of vomiting associated with cancer chemotherapy. Report immediately the onset of restlessness, involuntary movements, facial grimacing, rigitity, or tremors. Usual treatment: 50 mg diphenhydramine IM.
- Therapeutic effectiveness in patient with diabetic gastroparesis is indicated by relief of anorexia, nausea, vomiting, persistent fullness after meals.
- During early treatment period, serum aldosterone may be elevated; however, after prolonged administration periods, it returns to pretreatment level.
- Monitor for possible Na retention and hypokalaemia especially if patient has congestive heart failure or cirrhosis.
- Adverse reactions associated with increased serum prolactin concentration (galactorrhoea, menstrual disorders, gynaecomastia) usually disappear within a few weeks or months after drug treatment is stopped.
- Caution patients to avoid driving and other potentially hazardous activities for a few hours after drug administration.
- Therapy beyond 12 weeks has not been evaluated sufficiently to recommended prolonged use.
- Store in light-resistant bottle at 15° to 30°C (59° to 86°F). Tablets are stable for 3 years; solutions and injections, for 5 years.

Diagnostic test interferences   Metoclopramide increases **serum prolactin** levels, and may increase **aldosterone** (during early treatment period) and **thyrotropin** levels.

DRUG INTERACTIONS *Metoclopramide*

PLUS	INTERACTIONS
Paracetamol, alcohol, levodopa, Tetracyclines	Accelerated intestinal absorption: unpredictable onset of action
Alcohol and other CNS depressants (including antianxiety agents)	Additive sedation
Anticholinergics (e.g., atropine): opiate analgesics	Antagonize metoclopromide's effect on GI motility
Psychotropics (e.g., phenothiazines)	Promotion of extrapyramidal symptoms

Metolazone

(Metenix)

Diuretic; antihypertensive; sulphonamide derivative

ACTIONS AND USES   Quinazoline derivative diuretic, structurally and pharmacologically similar to chlorothiazide (q.v.). Appears to be more effective as a diuretic than thiazides in patients with severe renal failure.

Used in management of hypertension as sole agent or to enhance effectiveness of other

METOLAZONE (continued)
antihypertensive in severe form of hypertension; also used in treatment of oedema associated with congestive heart failure and renal disease.

ROUTE AND DOSAGE   Oral: Adult: *oedema of cardiac failure*: *Initial*: 5 to 10 mg once daily; *oedema of renal failure*: 5 to 20 mg once daily. *Maintenance*: dose lowered to minimum effective level. *Hypertension*: *Initial*: 5 mg daily in morning. *Maintenance*: dose determined by patient's blood pressure response. *Highly individualized*.

ABSORPTION AND FATE   Incompletely absorbed (65% in normal subjects, 40% of patients with cardiac disease). Diuresis begins in 1 hour, peaks in 2 hours and lasts for 12 to 24 hours. **Half-life** (normal kidneys) 5.3 hours. Enterohepatic cycling and high degree of protein binding prolongs duration of action. 79 to 95% drug excreted in urine. Crosses placenta and enters breast milk.

CONTRAINDICATIONS AND PRECAUTIONS   Anuria, hypokalaemia, hepatic coma or precoma; hypersensitivity to metolazone and sulphonamides; pregnancy, lactation. **Cautious Use**: history of gout, allergies, concomitant use of digitalis glycosides, renal and hepatic dysfunction. *See also chlorothiazide*.

ADVERSE/SIDE EFFECTS   Cholestatic jaundice, vertigo, orthostatic hypotension, venous thrombosis, leucopenia, dehydration, hypokalaemia, hyperuricaemia, hyperglycaemia. *See also chlorothiazide*.

NURSING IMPLICATIONS
- Schedule doses to avoid nocturia and interrupted sleep. Administer oral drug early in AM after eating to prevent gastric irritation; (if given in two doses, schedule second dose no later than 15.00 hrs).
- Elderly patients may be more sensitive to effects of usual adult dose; thus overdosage and adverse reactions should be anticipated.
- When adverse reactions are moderate to severe, metolazone therapy should be terminated.
- Antihypertensive effects may be observed 3 or 4 days, but 3 to 4 weeks are required for maximum effect.
- Warn patient not to drink alcohol while taking metolazone since it potentiates orthostatic hypotension.
- Store tablets in tightly closed container at 15° to 30°C (59° to 86°F) unless otherwise specified by manufacturer.
- *See chlorothiazide*.

Metoprolol tartrate

(Betaloc, Lopresor)

Antihypertensive; beta-adrenergic blocking agent

METOPROLOL TARTRATE (continued)

ACTIONS AND USES   Relatively selective beta$_1$-adrenergic blocking agent. Like propranolol, comparatively inhibits access of catecholamines to beta$_1$-adrenergic receptors, especially within myocardium (cardioselective action).

Used in management of mild to severe hypertension alone or concomitantly with diuretic therapy (usually a thiazide) and/or a vasodilator (e.g., hydralazine or prazosin). Also used for prophylactic management of stable angina pectoris. Reportedly as effective as propranolol in reducing both standing and supine blood pressures. In contrast to propranolol, has little or no membrane-stabilizing quinidine-like effect on heart and also does not block beta$_2$-adrenergic receptors located chiefly in vascular and bronchial smooth muscle except at higher doses. Also unlike propranolol, causes less inhibition of glycogenolysis in skeletal and cardiac muscles, less blocking of insulin release, and does not significantly inhibit isoprenaline induced bronchodilation. Therefore, generally preferred for use in patients prone to bronchospasm (together with a beta$_2$ agonist such as terbutaline), Raynaud's disease, and diabetes mellitus. Metoprolol decreases plasma renin levels. Used for treatment of hypertension and arrhythmias migraine and thyrotoxicosis.

ROUTE AND DOSAGE   Oral: *hypertension*: *Initial*: 50 mg twice daily. May be increased at weekly (or longer) intervals until optimum blood pressure reduction obtained. *Maintenance*: 100 mg–400 mg. **Angina**: 50–100 mg, 2–3 times a day; *Migraine*: 100–200 mg/day. *Thyrotoxicosis*: 50 mg 4 times a day. IV: up to 5 mg at the rate of 1–2 mg/min. Repeat after 5 min if required, total dose 10–15 mg.

ABSORPTION AND FATE   Rapidly and almost completely absorbed from GI tract. Undergoes about 50% first-pass metabolism. **Peak effects** in 1½ to 4 hours. **Duration of action** (dose related): 13 to 19 hours; with chronic therapy, antihypertensive effect may persist up to 4 weeks. Widely distributed to body tissues. Highest concentrations in heart, liver, lungs, and saliva. Crosses blood–brain barrier. About 11 to 12% protein bound. **Half-life**: 3 to 4 hours. Extensively metabolized in liver. Eliminated by kidney primarily as minimally active metabolites and about 3 to 10% unchanged drug. Approximately 95% of single dose excreted within 72 hours. Crosses placenta. Enters breast milk.

CONTRAINDICATIONS AND PRECAUTIONS   Cardiogenic shock, sinus bradycardia, heart block greater than first degree, overt cardiac failure, right ventricular failure secondary to pulmonary hypertension. Safe use during pregnancy, in women of child-bearing potential, in nursing mothers, and in children not established. **Cautious Use**: impaired hepatic or renal function, cardiomegaly, congestive heart failure controlled by digitalis and diuretics; A-V conduction defects, bronchial asthma and other bronchospastic diseases, history of allergy, thyrotoxicosis, diabetes mellitus, peripheral vascular disease.

ADVERSE/SIDE EFFECTS   These include: dizziness, fatigue, headache, insomnia, nightmares, increased dreaming, hallucinations, mental depression, bradycardia, palpitation, cold extremities, Raynaud's phenomenon, intermittent claudication, angina pectoris, congestive heart failure, intensification of AV block, AV dissociation,

METOPROLOL TARTRATE (continued)

complete heart block, cardiac arrest, dry skin, pruritus, alopecia (reversible), skin eruptions, visual disturbances, inflamed conjunctiva and eyelids, punctate keratitis, keratoconjunctivitis, corneal ulcerations, dry eyes (decreased tear production), tinnitus, nausea, heartburn, gastric pain, diarrhoea or constipation, flatulence, eosinophilia, agranulocytosis, thrombocytopenic and nonthrombocytopenic purpura, dry mouth and mucous membranes, sweating, restless legs; hypoglycaemia, bronchospasm (with high doses), Peyronie's disease (rare). *See also propranolol.*

NURSING IMPLICATIONS

- Reportedly, ingestion with food slightly enhances absorption of metoprolol. However, administration with food is not essential, but it is important that drug be given with or without food consistently to minimize possible variations in bioavailability.
- Inform patient that most adverse effects tend to be mild and transient and that they generally disappear with continued therapy.
- Instruct patient to report immediately to physician the onset of ocular symptoms.
- If mouth dryness is bothersome, advise patient that the following measures may provide relief: rinse mouth frequently with clear warm water; increase noncalorie liquid intake if it has been inadequate; sugarless gum or lemon drops. If these measures fail, consult physician about use of artificial saliva substitutes.
- Stored in tight, light-resistant container.
- *See propranolol.*

Metronidazole

(Elyzol, Flagyl, Metrolyl, Nidazol, Vaginyl, Zadstat)   *Antiprotozoal*

ACTIONS AND USES   Synthetic compound with direct trichomonicidal and amoebecidal activity against *Trichomonas vaginalis* (causes a venereal disease), *Entamoeba histolytica*, and *Giardia lamblia*. Also exhibits antibacterial activity against obligate anaerobic bacteria, gram-negative anaerobic bacilli and *Clostridia*. Microaerophilic streptococci and most aerobic bacteria are resistant. Metronidazole enters bacterial cells more readily under aerobic conditions; after reduction in the cell, it binds to and degrades DNA. Frequency of postoperative infection and nonspore forming anaerobic infections reported to be decreased with prophylactic use of the drug before and up to 7 days after surgery.

Used in treatment of asymptomatic and symptomatic trichomoniasis in both females and males: acute intestinal amoebiasis and amoebic liver abscess, and anaerobic infections.

ROUTE AND DOSAGE   Oral: *Trichomoniasis*: 200 mg three times daily for 7 days. *Amoebiasis*: Adults: 800 mg every 8 hours for 5 days. *Anaerobic infections*: 400 mg/8 hourly. **Rectal**: 1 g /8 hrly for 3 days then 1 g 12 hrly for 3 days **IV**: 500 mg/8 hrly for 7 days. **Child**: any route 7.5 mg/kg/8 hrly.

METRONIDAZOLE (continued)

ABSORPTION AND FATE   Well absorbed after oral administration. Peak serum concentration usually in 1 to 2 hours. Distributed widely to all tissues including brain; therapeutic levels achieved in abscesses, bile, cerebrospinal fluid, empyema fluid, breast milk, and saliva. Only slightly bound (1 to 8%) to human plasma protein. **Elimination half-life** range: 6.2 to 11.5 hours. Accumulates in presence of impaired renal function; major route of elimination in urine. Rapidly crosses placenta and is secreted in breast milk. Concentration in saliva and breast milk during treatment approximates that in serum.

CONTRAINDICATIONS AND PRECAUTIONS   History of hypersensitivity to metronidazole, blood dyscrasias, active CNS disease, first trimester of pregnancy, nursing mothers. **Cautious Use:** coexistent candidiasis, second and third trimesters of pregnancy.

ADVERSE/SIDE EFFECTS   These include: vertigo, headache, ataxia, confusion, irritability, depression, restlessness, weakness, fatigue, drowsiness, insomnia, sensory neuropathy, paraesthesias, polyuria, dysuria, pyuria, incontinence, cystitis, decreased libido, dyspareunia, dryness of vagina and vulva, sense of pelvic pressure, nausea, vomiting, anorexia, epigastric distress, abdominal cramps, diarrhoea, constipation, dry mouth, metallic or bitter taste, moderate neutropenia, leucopenia; nasal congestion, fever, fleeting joint pains, ECG changes (flattening of T wave); fungal overgrowth of *Candida*; proctitis.

NURSING IMPLICATIONS
- Tablets may be crushed before ingestion if patient cannot swallow them whole.
- Administer oral preparation immediately before, with, or immediately after meals or with food or milk to reduce GI distress.
- Dosage regimens are individualized sometimes on the basis of anticipated compliance. Some patients cannot be relied upon to take eight tablets in 1 day. Caution the patient to adhere closely to the established regimen without schedule interruption or changing the dose.
- Presence of trichomonads should be confirmed by wet smear and/or by cultures prior to start of therapy for trichomoniasis and prior to a course of retreatment.
- Total and differential leucocyte counts are recommended before, during and after therapy, especially if a second course is necessary.
- During therapy for trichomoniasis it is recommended that the patient refrain from intercourse unless the male partner wears a condom to prevent reinfection.
- Sexual partners should receive concurrent treatment. Asymptomatic trichomoniasis in the male is a frequent source of reinfection of the female; therefore, it is recommended that treatment be given even if the male partner has a negative culture.
- Therapy should be discontinued immediately if symptoms of CNS toxicity develop, e.g., ataxia, tremor, incoordination, paraesthesias, numbness, impairment of pain or touch sensation.
- Warn patient that ingestion of alcohol during metronidazole therapy may induce a disulphiram reaction (sweating, flushing, vomiting, headache, abdominal cramps).
- Inform patient that urine may appear dark or reddish brown (especially with higher

METRONIDAZOLE (continued)

than recommended doses). This is thought to be caused by a metabolite and appears to have no clinical significance.

- Women with trichomoniasis should be advised not to wear tights or tight underwear and to avoid bubble baths. Also review perineal hygiene technique.
- Advise patient to report symptoms of candidal overgrowth: furry tongue, colour changes of tongue, glossitis, stomatitis; vaginitis, curdlike, milky vaginal discharge; proctitis. Treatment with a candicidal agent may be indicated.
- 4 to 6 weeks are allowed to elapse before the decision is made to repeat treatment.
- Repeated faeces examinations, usually up to 3 months, are necessary to assure that amoebae have been eliminated.
- ***Diagnostic test intereferences***   Metronidazole may interfere with certain chemical analyses for SGOT, resulting in decreased values.
- Store drug in tightly closed, light-resistant containers preferably at 15° to 30°C (59° and 86°F) unless otherwise directed by manufacturer. Do no freeze.

DRUG INTERACTIONS   *Metronidazole*

PLUS	INTERACTIONS
Alchol	Disulphram reaction
Disulphiram	Acute psychotic reaction due to combined toxicity
Warfarin	Potentiation of hypoprothrombinaemic effect of warfarin

Mexiletine

(Mexitil)   *Antiarrhythmic*

ACTIONS AND USES   Analogue of lignocaine with potent anaesthetic action. Used to treat acute and chronic ventricular arrhythmias.

ROUTE AND DOSAGE   Oral: *initial* dose 400 mg then after 2 hours, 200–250 mg 3–4 times a day **intravenous**: Loading dose: 150 to 250 mg at rate of 25 mg/min, followed by IV infusion of 0.1% solution/250 mg over 1st hour, then 125 mg over 2 hrs, then 500 mcg/min.

ABSORPTION AND FATE   Rapidly absorbed from GI tract with about 88% bioavailability after oral dose. Metabolized in liver; half-life: about 12 hours (lengthened in acute MI). Less than 10% unchanged drug eliminated in urine; renal elimination increases with urine acidification. Excreted in breast milk.

CONTRAINDICATIONS AND PRECAUTIONS   Severe left ventricular failure, cardiogenic shock, severe bradyarrhythmias. *See also tocainide.*

MEXILETINE (continued)

ADVERSE/SIDE EFFECTS   Dose related, and readily reversible after drug is discontinued: tremor, blurred vision, atoxia. *See also tocainide.*

NURSING IMPLICATIONS

- Effective serum concentration: 0.5 to 2 mcg/ml.
- Administered with food or milk to reduce gastric distress.
- During IV administration, connect patient to cardiac monitor, monitor ECG waveforms and be alert for dysrhythmias. Have resuscitative equipment ready.
- Check pulse and blood pressure before administration of mexiletine, until both are stabilized. Patient should understand that changes in pulse rate and regularity may signal decreasing clinical effectiveness of drug.
- *Instruct patient about pulse parameters to be reported*: i.e., changes in rhythm, and rate (bradycardia = pulse below 60); symptomatic bradycardia (lightheadedness, syncope, dizziness), and postural hypotension.
- Adverse reactions are more common with IV administration than with oral doses, especially if the loading dose was administered too rapidly.
- CNS adverse reactions predominate (intention tremors, nystagmus, blurred vision, dizziness, ataxia, confusion, nausea). Supervise ambulation in the weak, debilitated patient or the elderly during drug stabilization period.
- Drug compliance with mexiletine is affected particularly by the distressing side effects of tremor, ataxia, and eye symptoms.
- Check with patient about adherence to drug regimen frequently. If side effects are increasing, consult physician. Dose adjustment or discontinuation may be needed.
- *See tocainide for additional nursing implications and drug interactions.*

M

Mezlocillin sodium —————————————————————

(Baypen)   *Antibiotic (beta lactam);*
                                                      penicillin

ACTIONS AND USES   Semisynthetic acylureidopenicillin with extended spectrum. Structurally resembles ampicillin (q.v.), and has similar but wider antibacterial spectrum. Broadened spectrum of activity includes strains of pathogenic aerobic gram-negative bacteria, e.g., *Bacteroides*, *Enterobacter*, *Escherichia*, *Haemophilus*, *Klebsiella*, *Pseudomonas*, *Proteus*, and *Serratia*, and gram-positive organisms such as *Streptococcus faecalis* (enterococcus). Inactive against penicillinase-producing strains of *Staphylococcus aureus*. Contains 1.85 m.mol (42.6 mg) of sodium per gram.

Used primarily for serious infections caused by *Pseudomonas aeruginosa*. Also used to treat other infections caused by susceptible strains.

ROUTE AND DOSAGE   Adults: **Intravenous or intramuscular**: 0.5 to 2 g every 6 hours *Severe infections*: 5 g every 6 hours IV.

ABSORPTION AND FATE   Rapidly absorbed following IM or IV administration. Serum

MEZLOCILLIN SODIUM (continued)

levels peak in about 45 minutes after IM and within 5 minutes following IV injection. Well-distributed into most body tissues and fluids; highest concentrations in urine and bile. Adequate CSF penetration if meninges are inflamed. Approximately 16 to 42% bound to plasma proteins. **Half-life**: 50 to 55 minutes (longer in patients with renal impairment). Only slightly metabolized in liver. Excreted primarily by kidney; 55 to 65% of dose eliminated as unchanged drug within 6 hours, and less than 10% as inactive metabolite. Up to 25% of dose excreted in bile. Crosses placenta. Small amounts excreted in breast milk.

NURSING IMPLICATIONS

- IM injections should be made into a relatively large muscle such as the gluteus maximus (upper outer quadrant). Aspirate carefully before injecting drug to avoid inadvertent entry into blood vessel. Discomfort associated with IM administration may be lessened by making injection slowly (over 12 to 15 seconds). Do not exceed 2 g per IM injection.
- Intravenous administration may be made by IV bolus (direct injection of reconstituted solution into vein or IV tubing, over 3 to 5 minutes), or by intermittent infusion over 30 minutes. Primary infusion should be temporarily withheld during infusion of mezlocillin. Observe IV sites for evidence of inflammation.
- See manufacturer's directions for reconstitution, compatible solutions, and stability information.
- Be alert to signs of superinfections: white patches in mouth or black hairy tongue, foul-smelling stools or vaginal discharge, diarrhoea, vaginitis, anogenital itching.
- Therapy generally continues for at least 2 days after signs and symptoms of infection have subsided. Usual duration of therapy for serious infections is 7 to 10 days, but it may be longer in complicated infections.
- Antibiotic therapy for group A beta-haemolytic streptococcal infections should continue for at least 10 days, to reduce risk of rheumatic fever or glomerulonephritis.
- Store unopened vials and infusion bottles at or below 30°C (86°F), unless otherwise directed by manufacturer. Powder and reconstituted solutions may darken slightly, but this does not indicate loss of potency. Solutions should be clear. If a precipitate should form under refrigeration, warm to 37°C (98.6°F) in a water bath and shake well.

Diagnostic test interferences   Possibility of false-positive **urine protein** determinations (when mezlocillin concentration in urine is high) using sulphosalicylic acid and boiling test, acetic acid test, biuret reaction, nitric acid test; bromophenol blue reagent test (Multi-stix) is not affected.

DRUG INTERACTION   *Mezlocillin*

PLUS	INTERACTIONS
Anticoagulants (oral and parenteral)	Possibility of additive anticoagulant effects. Monitor closely

See penicillin G

Mianserin

(Bolvidon)   *Tetracyclic; antidepressant*

ROUTE AND DOSAGE   Oral: **Adult:** *Initial* 30–40 mg divided or single dose, increased to a maximum of 200 mg/day in divided doses. See amitriptyline for actions, uses, contraindications and side effects, (additional side effects, leucopenia, agranulocytosis, and aplastic anaemia, jaundice, arthritis and arthralgia. Blood counts should be done every 4 weeks during the first three months of treatment.)

Miconazole

(Daktarin, Dermonistat)   *Antibiotic; antifungal*

M

ACTIONS AND USES   Broad-spectrum agent with fungicidal activity against *Candida albicans* and other species of this genus. Mode of action unclear, but appears to inhibit uptake of components essential for cell reproduction and growth and to alter cell wall structure, thus promoting cell death.

Used for treatment of vulvovaginal candidiasis, tinea pedis (athlete's foot), tinea cruris, tinea corporis, and tinea versicolour caused by dermatophytes. Also useful (parenteral) for treatment of severe systemic fungal infections including coccidioidomycosis, candidiasis, cryptococcosis, paracoccidioidomycosis, and for treatment of chronic mucocutaneous candidiasis. IV infusion is inadequate therapy for urinary bladder infections or for fungal meningitis; these conditions require supplements of miconazole by intrathecal administration and bladder irrigation.

ROUTE AND DOSAGE   **Intravaginal:** 1 applicator of cream or 2 pessaries into vagina daily at bedtime for 7 days; may be repeated if necessary. **Topical:** cover affected area generously, morning and evening, and once daily in patients with tinea versicolor. **Intravenous: Adult:** 1,800 to 3,600 mg day (usually divided into 3 infusions). **Children:** 20 to 40 mg/kg/day in divided doses. Maximum dose: 15 mg/kg/infusion. **Bladder instillation:** 100 mg twice a day as undiluted solution or by continuous irrigation over 12 hours in 500 ml sterile saline solution, **Oral:** 250 mg/6 hrly.

ABSORPTION AND FATE   Following absorption, rapid hepatic metabolism. About 90% protein bound; **phasic half-lives:** 0.4, 2.1, 24.1 hours. Metabolized in liver. Excreted in urine and faeces principally as inactive metabolites.

CONTRAINDICATIONS AND PRECAUTIONS   Known sensitivity to miconazole. Safe use in children under 1 year of age, during pregnancy after first trimester, and in nursing women not established. **Cautious Use:** hepatic or renal impairment.

MICONAZOLE (continued)

ADVERSE/SIDE EFFECTS   Tachycardia, cardiac arrhythmias (with rapid IV injection); vulvovaginal burning, itching or irritation, pelvic cramps, hives, skin rash, and head-ache. (With parenteral use): phlebitis, pruritus, rash, nausea, vomiting, diarrhoea, febrile reaction, drowsiness, flushing, hyponatraemia (transient), decreased haematocrit; thrombocytopenia, hyperlipaemia, arrhythmias, anaphylaxis.

NURSING IMPLICATIONS

- If nausea is a problem, the patient may be premedicated with an antiemetic or antihistamine.
- Ask physician about how to cleanse affected area prior to application of cream or lotion.
- Massage affected area gently until cream disappears.
- Persistent vulvovaginitis should be reevaluated if 3 to 4 weeks does not bring relief. Advise patient to report to physician for urine and blood glucose studies, since vaginitis may be a symptom of unrecognized diabetes mellitus.
- Infections caused by dermatophytes require about 1 week of treatment with miconazole.
- The full course of treatment should be completed in order to assure recovery.
- Clinical improvement from topical application should be expected in 1 or 2 weeks. If no improvement in 4 weeks, the diagnosis is reevaluated. Tinea pedis infection should be treated for 1 month to assure permanent recovery.
- Avoid contact of drug with eyes.
- Pathogens causing vaginitis should be identified before treatment since miconazole is effective only against candidal vulvovaginitis.
- Instruct patient to insert applicator of drug high into the vagina and to use a sanitary towel to prevent staining.
- Advise patient to avoid sexual intercourse during treatment period to prevent reinfection.
- Hypersensitivity test should be performed prior to IV administration. An initial test dose of 200 mg is administered by physician. Monitor patient for hypersensitivity reactions. Have immediately available emergency drugs and resuscitation equipment.
- IV administration should be slow (over a period of 30 to 60 minutes) to prevent nausea and risk of arrhythmias or tachycardia. Physician must prescribe flow rate.
- Drug is diluted for IV injection in at least 200 ml Isotonic Saline or 5% Dextrose solution. A 20-ml ampoule contains 10 mg/ml drug. Following dilution, solution is stable at room temperature for 48 hours. If solution darkens in colour, discard it. This is a sign of deterioration.
- Miconazole is stored preferably at 15° to 30°C (59° to 86°F) unless otherwise directed by manufacturer.

Drug interactions   Miconazole may enhance **oral anticoagulant** effects. When combined with **amphotericin B**, antifungal activity of the combination is less than that of either drug used alone.

Minocycline hydrochloride

(Minocin)   *Antiinfective; tetracycline*

ACTIONS AND USES Semisynthetic tetracycline derivative with actions, uses, contra-indications, precautions, and adverse reactions as for tetracycline (q.v.). Appears to be active against strains of staphylococci resistant to other tetracyclines, and photosensitivity occurs only rarely. Reported to be more completely absorbed than other tetracyclines because it is more lipid-soluble.

ROUTE AND DOSAGE **Adults: Oral:** 200 mg followed by 100 mg every 12 hours.

ABSORPTION AND FATE Well absorbed by oral route. About 70 to 75% bound to plasma proteins. Serum half-life following single 200-mg dose approximately 11 to 17 hours. Slow renal clearance. About 12% of dose excreted in urine; remainder persists in body in fatty tissues. Crosses placenta, and appears in breast milk.

For further information: *see tetracycline.*

NURSING IMPLICATIONS
- Check expiration date. Outdated tetracyclines can cause severe adverse side effects.
- Studies to date indicate that minocycline is not significantly influenced by food and dairy products, in contrast to other tetracyclines.
- Since lightheadedness, dizziness, or vertigo occur frequently, caution patient to avoid driving vehicles and other hazardous activities while on minocycline. (Lightheadedness is usually transient and often disappears during therapy.)
- *See tetracycline hydrochloride.*

Minoxidil

(Loniten)   *Antihypertensive; vasodilator*
                                                                  (peripheral)

ACTIONS AND USES Direct-acting vasodilator similar to other drugs of this class, e.g., hydralazine, diazoxide, prazosin, but hypotensive effect is more pronounced. Appears to act by blocking calcium uptake into cell membrane. Reduces systolic and diastolic blood pressures in supine and standing positions, and decreases peripheral vascular resistance by direct vasodilating action on arterior vessels. Does not affect vasomotor reflexes and therefore does not produce orthostatic hypotension. Has a greater lowering effect on elevated blood pressures than on blood pressures approaching the normal range.

Used with a diuretic to prevent fluid retention and with a beta-adrenergic blocking agent (e.g., propranolol) to treat severe hypertension.

MINOXIDIL (continued)

ROUTE AND DOSAGE   Oral: Adults and children (over 12 years): *Initial*: 5 mg once daily. If necessary, increased gradually after at least 3-day interval to 10, 20, and then 40 mg/day in single or divided doses. (When rapid management of blood pressure is indicated adjustments may be made every 6 hours if patient is closely monitored.) Maximal recommended dosage 50 mg daily.

ABSORPTION AND FATE   Rapidly and well absorbed from GI tract. Onset of anti-hypertensive effect in 30 minutes; **peak action** in 2 to 3 hours, with duration of 10 to 12 hours in most patients and up to 75 hours in some (significant interindividual variability reported). Widely distributed throughout body; not bound to plasma proteins. **Plasma half-life**: approximately 4.2 hours (but drug effects persist significantly longer). About 90% of drug metabolized to minimally active metabolites. Approximately 97% excreted in urine and faeces; less than 10% excreted as unchanged drug.

CONTRAINDICATIONS AND PRECAUTIONS   Phaeochromocytoma. Safe use during pregnancy or in women of childbearing potential, or in nursing mothers or children not established. **Cautious Use**: severe renal impairment, recent myocardial infarction (within preceding month), coronary artery disease, chronic congestive heart failure.

ADVERSE/SIDE EFFECTS   These include: tachycardia, angina pectoris, ECG changes (especially in direction and magnitude of T-waves), pericardial effusion and tamponade, rebound hypertension (following drug withdrawal), pulmonary hypertension (causal relationship not established), intermittent claudication; oedema, including pulmonary oedema; congestive heart failure (salt and water retention), hypertrichosis, darkening of skin, transient pruritus, Stevens–Johnson syndrome, hypersensitivity rash, nausea, headache, fatigue, breast tenderness, gynaecomastia, polymenorrhoea, thrombocytopenia.

NURSING IMPLICATIONS

- Minoxidil may be taken without regard to meals or food.
- Take blood pressure and apical pulse before administering medication and report significant changes. Consult physician for parameters.
- Monitor blood pressure and pulse at regular intervals during therapy. Abrupt reduction in blood pressure can result in cerebrovascular accident and myocardial infarction. Keep physician informed.
- Since experience with children taking minoxidil is limited, dosage must be very carefully titrated.
- Patients on home care should be told usual pulse rate and instructed to count radial pulse for one full minute before taking drug. Advise patient to report an increase of 20 or more beats/minute.
- Fluid and electrolyte balance should be closely followed throughout therapy. Sodium and water retention commonly occurs in patients receiving minoxidil. Consult physician regarding sodium restriction. If patient is on diuretic therapy, potassium intake and serum potassium levels will require monitoring.

M

MINOXIDIL (continued)

- Monitor fluid intake and output and daily weight. Report unusual changes in intake–output ratio or daily weight gain of 1.5 or more kg.
- For patients who develop refractory fluid retention, some clinicians withdraw drug for 1 or 2 days and then resume therapy aimed at more vigorous diuresis.
- Observe patient daily for oedema and auscultate lungs for rales. Be alert for signs and symptoms of congestive heart failure: night cough, dyspnoea on exertion, orthopnoea, distended neck veins.
- Also observe patient for symptoms of pericardial effusion or tamponade. Symptoms are similar to those of congestive failure but additionally patient may have paradoxical pulse (normal inspiratory reduction in systolic blood pressure may fall as much as 10 to 20 mm Hg). Diagnosis is confirmed by echocardiographic studies.
- Note possible adverse reactions of drugs that are given in conjunction with minoxidil.
- Patient should be thoroughly informed of possibility of *hypertrichosis* (elongation, thickening, and increased pigmentation of fine body hair, especially of face, arms, and back). It develops 3 to 9 weeks after start of therapy and occurs in approximately 80% of patients. It is reportedly not an endocrine disorder and is reversible within 1 to 6 months following discontinuation of minoxidil. In addition to shaving, depilatory creams containing calcium thioglycolate are effective in removing unwanted hair. Vitamin E therapy has been used to reduce severity of this side effect.
- Instruct patient to notify physician promptly if the following signs or symptoms appear: increase of 20 or more beats per minute in resting pulse; breathing difficulty; dizziness; lightheadedness; fainting; oedema (tight shoes or rings, puffiness, pitting); weight gain, chest pain, arm or shoulder pain; easy bruising or bleeding.
- Review package insert with patient (dispensed with product). Emphasize importance of taking, drug as prescribed and caution patient not to skip or alter dosage and not to discontinue medication without consulting physician.
- Rebound hypertension has followed minoxidil withdrawal. Conversion to conventional therapy must be accomplished gradually and with close observation of patient.
- **Treatment of toxicity** Have on hand phenylephrine, dopamine, and vasopressin to reverse hypotension.
- Stored in tightly covered container preferably at 15° to 30°C (59° to 86°F) unless otherwise directed by manufacturer.

Diagnostic test interferences Haematocrit, haemoglobin, and erythrocyte count usually decrease (about 7%) during early therapy; serum alkaline phosphatase, BUN, and creatinine may increase during early therapy.

DRUG INTERACTIONS *Minoxidil*

PLUS	INTERACTIONS
Noradrenaline, adrenaline	Excessive cardiac stimulant action
Guanethidine	Profound orthostatic hypotension; if possible guanethidine should be withdrawn gradually 1 to 3 weeks before minoxidil therapy

M

Mitomycin

(Mitomycin-C, Kyowa)   *Antineoplastic; antibiotic*

ACTIONS AND USES   Potent antibiotic antineoplastic compound produced by *Streptomyces caespitosus* with wide range of antibacterial activity. Described extensively in the literature as Mitomycin-C. Effective in certain tumours nonresponsive to surgery, radiation or other chemotherapeutic agents. Action mechanism not clear but reportedly combines with DNA (attachment site unknown), thereby interfering with cellular and enzymatic RNA and protein synthesis. Mitomycin has been shown to be carcinogenic in mice and rats; thus selected patients must be aware of the inherent risk in spite of possible therapeutic benefits.

Used in combination with other chemotherapeutic agents in palliative, adjunctive treatment of disseminated adenocarcinoma of breast, pancreas, or stomach, squamous cell carcinoma of head, neck, lung, and cervix. Not recommended to replace surgery and/or radiotherapy, nor as a single primary therapeutic agent.

ROUTE AND DOSAGE   **Intravenous**: highly individualized.

ABSORPTION AND FATE   Following IV injection. Mitomycin is cleared rapidly from blood by hepatic metabolism. **Half-life**: 17 minutes. Approximately 10% dose secreted unchanged in urine.

CONTRAINDICATIONS AND PRECAUTIONS   Hypersensitivity or idiosyncrasy reaction; thrombocytopenia, coagulation disorders or bleeding tendencies; pregnancy. **Cautious Use**: renal impairment, myelosuppression.

ADVERSE/SIDE EFFECTS   Bone marrow toxicity (thrombocytopenia, leucopenia occurring 4 to 8 weeks after treatment onset); fever, anorexia, stomatitis, nausea, vomiting alopecia; desquamation, induration, pruritus, pain, bleeding, paraesthesias, necrosis, cellulitis at injection site; haemoptysis, dyspnoea, nonproductive cough, pneumonia, elevated BUN. Following symptoms may or may not be drug induced: headache, blurred vision, drowsiness, fatigue, oedema, syncope, confusion, thrombophlebitis, anaemia, haematemesis, diarrhoea, pain.

NURSING IMPLICATIONS
- Patient receiving mitomycin should be hospitalized so that emergency treatment and laboratory facilities will be available.
- Avoid extravasation when drug in administered, to prevent extreme tissue reaction (cellulitis) to the toxic drug. *See Index: Nursing Interventions: extravasation.*
- Because of cumulative myelosuppression, laboratory studies of platelet counts, prothrombin and bleeding times, differential and haemoglobin studies, serum creatinine are performed frequently during treatment and for at least 7 weeks after treatment is terminated.
- Usually drug is not administered if serum creatinine is greater than 1.7 mg%.
- If platelet count falls below 75,000 and WBC down to 3,000 or prothrombin or bleeding times are prolonged, treatment is suspended or modified.
- Monitor fluid intake–output ratio and pattern. Any sign of impaired kidney function

MITOMYCIN (continued)

should be reported: change in ratio, dysuria, haematuria, oliguria, frequency, urgency. Keep patient hydrated (at least 2,000 to 2,500 ml orally daily if tolerated). Drug is nephrotoxic.
- Observe closely for signs of infection. Monitor body temperature frequently. Instruct patient to report immediately if signs of common cold present.
- *See mustine for nursing implications related to stomatitis.*

Mitozantrone

(Novantrone)   *Antineoplastic; anthraquinone*

ACTIONS AND USES   Structurally related to doxorubicin. Used to treat breast cancer.

ROUTE AND DOSAGE   Highly individualized by intravenous infusion or injection. For further information: *see doxorubicin.*

M

Morphine sulphate

(Duromorph, MST Continus)   *Narcotic analgesic; opiate agonist*

Morphine tartrate

(Cyclimorph)

ACTIONS AND USES   Suggested mechanisms of analgesic action include elevation of pain threshold, interference with pain conduction or CNS response to pain, or altered pain perception. Relieves pain without obtunding other sensory modalites, and may produce euphoria; drowsiness occurs commonly, and higher doses promote deep sleep. Also depresses respiratory centre and cough reflex and may induce nausea and vomiting by increasing vestibular sensitivity. Initial doses stimulate and subsequent doses depress vomiting centre. Causes constriction of pupils, even in total darkness, and greatly enhances pupillary response to light (tolerance to miotic effect is rare). Generally, has no major effect on blood, pressure, heart rate or rhythm when patient is supine; however, orthostatic hypotension may occur in head-up position, possibly by dilatation of peripheral vessels (histamine release) or by depression of medullary vasomotor centre. Delays digestion by decreasing stomach motility and hydrochloric acid, biliary and pancreatic secretions. Decreases intensity and frequency of propulsive peristalsis, and enhances amplitude of nonpropulsive contractions, thus causing desiccation of faeces and resultant constipation. Increases tone of smooth muscles and sphincters in GI, biliary, and

MORPHINE TARTRATE (continued)

genitourinary systems. Reduction of urinary outflow may be mediated by antidiuretic hormone release or by decreased renal blood flow. Release of ACTH, FSH, LH, and TSH may be suppressed.

Used for symptomatic relief of severe pain after nonnarcotic analgesics have failed and as preanaesthetic medication; also used to relieve dyspnoea of acute left ventricular failure and pulmonary oedema and pain of myocardial infarction. Treatment of acute and chronic pain by intrathecal, epidural, and continuous IV routes. Used in combination with kaolin as an antidiarrhoeal and with cyclizine (cyclimorph).

ROUTE AND DOSAGE   Oral: *initial* 10 to 20 mg every 4 hours (MST is given twice daily). **Subcutaneous, intramuscular: Adults:** 5 to 20 mg every 4 hours, if necessary. **Children (up to 1 mth):** 150 mcg/kg; **(1−12 mth):** 200 mcg/kg; **(1−5 yrs):** 2.5−5 mg; **(6−12 yrs):** 5−10 mg. **Intravenous:** ¼−½ the IM dose. **Rectal:** 10 to 20 mg every 4 hours or as directed.

ABSORPTION AND FATE   Absorption from GI tract is complete, but variable in rate. Well absorbed following parenteral injection. **Peak analgesia** within 50 to 90 minutes following subcutaneous administration and 20 minutes after IV injection. Analgesia may be maintained up to 7 hours. Wide distribution, with concentration mainly in kidney, liver, lung, spleen; lower concentrations in brain and muscle. **Plasma half-life:** 2.5 to 3 hours. Metabolized chiefly in liver. About 90% of dose is excreted in urine within 24 hours, largely in conjugated form, with small amounts as unchanged drug; 7 to 10% excreted via bile through faeces. Crosses placenta: small amounts appear in breast milk.

CONTRAINDICATIONS AND PRECAUTIONS   Hypersensitivity to opiates, increased intracranial pressure, convulsive disorders, acute alcoholism, acute bronchial asthma, chronic pulmonary diseases, severe respiratory depression, chemical-irritant-induced pulmonary oedema, prostatic hypertrophy, undiagnosed acute abdominal conditions, pancreatitis, acute ulcerative colitis, severe liver or renal insufficiency, Addison's disease, hypothyroidism. Safe use during pregnancy not established. **Cautious Use:** toxic psychosis, cardiac arrhythmias, cardiovascular disease, emphysema, kyphoscoliosis, cor pulmonale, severe obesity, reduced blood volume; very old, very young, or debilitated patients; use during labour.

ADVERSE/SIDE EFFECTS   Acute intoxication: deep sleep, coma, marked miosis, severe respiratory depression (as low as 2 to 4/minute) or arrest, pulmonary oedema, hypothermia, skeletal muscle flaccidity, oliguria, hypotension, bradycardia, convulsions (infants, and children), cardiac arrest. **Others:** respiratory depression, decreased cough reflex, euphoria, dysphoria, paradoxic CNS stimulation (restlessness, tremor, delirium, insomnia), drowsiness, dizziness, weakness, headache, miosis, hypothermia, bradycardia, orthostatic hypotension, syncope, flushing of face, neck, and upper thorax, nausea, vomiting, anorexia, constipation, dry mouth, biliary colic, urinary retention or urgency, dysuria, reduced libido and/or potency (prolonged use), sweating, prolonged labour and respiratory depression of newborn, decreased urinary VMA excretion, elevated transaminase levels, precipitation of porphyria.

MORPHINE TARTRATE *(continued)*
NURSING IMPLICATIONS

- Fullest analgesic effect is achieved if drug is administered before the patient experiences intense pain (morphine relieves continuous dull pain more effectively than sharp intermittent pain, which generally requires higher doses).
- Note that the patient's cultural background may influence response to pain. Some patients tend to be stoic, but others may overtly show that they feel pain.
- Elevated pulse or respiratory rate, restlessness, anorexia, or drawn facial expression may indicate need for analgesia.
- Differentiate among restlessness as a sign of pain and the need for medication, restlessness associated with hypoxia, and restlessness caused by morphine-induced CNS stimulation (a paradoxic reaction that is particularly common in women and elderly patients).
- Provide maximum comfort measures, and reduce environmental stimuli before preparing medication.
- Before administering the drug, note respiratory rate, depth, and rhythm and size of pupils. Respirations of 12/minute or below and miosis are signs of toxicity (miosis is replaced by pupillary dilatation in asphyxia). Withhold drug and report these signs to physician.
- Pupillary size is best judged in good room light (with patient facing away from window light) rather than by flashlight, which causes immediate miosis.
- Caution patients not to smoke or ambulate without assistance after receiving the drug. Bedsides may be advisable.
- When given parenterally in repeated doses, the intramuscular route is recommended. Repeated subcutaneous injections can cause local tissue irritation.
- Slow release preparation (MST) should be swallowed whole.
- Monitor vital signs at regular intervals. Morphine-induced respiratory depression may occur even with small doses, and it increases progressively with higher doses (generally reaching maximum within 90 minutes following SC, 30 minutes after IM, and 7 minutes after IV administration). However, respiratory minute volume may remain below normal 4 to 5 hours following therapeutic doses.
- Narcotic analgesics also depress cough and sigh reflexes and thus may induce atelectasis, especially in postoperative patients. Purposefully encourage changes in position, deep breathing, and coughing (unless contraindicated) at regularly scheduled intervals.
- Narcotic antagonists (e.g., naloxone) and facilities for oxygen and support of respiration should be available.
- Nausea and orthostatic hypotension (with lightheadedness and dizziness) most often occur in ambulatory patients or when a supine patient assumes the head-up position or in patients not experiencing severe pain. (Morphine decreases the ability of the cardiovascular system to respond to gravitational shifts.)
- Transient fall in blood pressure (even in the supine position) is apt to occur in patients with acute myocardial infarction.
- Monitor fluid intake—output ratio and pattern. Report oliguria or urinary retention. Morphine may dull perception of bladder stimuli; therefore, encourage the patient to void at least every 4 hours. Palpate lower abdomen to detect bladder distention.

M

MORPHINE TARTRATE (continued)

■ Monitor bowel pattern. Inattention to the defaecation reflex and desiccation of faeces contribute to the constipating effects of morphine. Check for abdominal distention and intestinal peristaltic sounds during postoperative period. Record relief of pain and duration of analgesia.

■ Tolerance as well as physiological and psychological dependence may develop with repeated use. There is high abuse liability.

■ Be alert to purposive behaviour (manipulations) to get more drug; this usually begins shortly before next scheduled dose. Such behaviour may signal the onset of tolerance and addiction.

■ Abrupt cessation of drug use in the presence of physiological dependence initiates the *abstinence syndrome*, usually within 24 to 48 hours after last dose. Without treatment, withdrawal symptoms ('cold turkey') develop, with increasing intensity and a common sequence: drug craving and anxiety (within 6 hours of last dose); irritability, perspiration, yawning, rhinorrhoea, itchy nose, sneezing, lacrimation (within 14 hours); pupil dilation, piloerection ('gooseflesh'), tremulousness, muscle jerks, bone and muscle aches, nausea, hot and cold flashes, tossing, restless sleep ('yen'), elevated systolic blood pressure, dilated pupils, elevated temperature, pulse, and respiration rates (within 24 to 36 hours); curled-up position, vomiting, diarrhoea, weight loss, haemoconcentration, increased blood sugar, spontaneous ejaculation or orgasm (within 36 to 48 hours).

■ Severity and character of withdrawal symptoms depend on the interval between doses, duration of drug use, total daily dose, and health and personality of the addicted individual.

■ Morphine is reported to be physically and chemically incompatible with many solutions. Do not mix with other drugs without the advice of a pharmacist.

■ Preserved in tight, light-resistant containers.

■ A controlled drug.

Diagnostic test interferences   False-positive **urine glucose** determinations may occur using Benedict's solution. **Plasma amylase** and lipase determinations may be falsely positive for 24 hours after use of morphine.

Drug interactions   CNS depressant effects of morphine and other narcotic analgesics may be exaggerated and prolonged by concurrent administration of **alcohol**, general **anaesthetics**, **antianxiety drugs**, **phenothiazines**, **tricyclic antidepressants**, **barbiturates**, other **sedatives**, **hypnotics**, and **MAO inhibitors**. Narcotic analgesics may enhance the neuromuscular blocking action of **skeletal muscle relaxants**.

Mustine ▬▬▬▬▬▬▬▬▬▬▬▬▬▬▬▬▬▬▬▬▬▬▬▬▬▬▬▬▬▬▬▬▬

(Nitrogen mustard)   *Antineoplastic; alkylating*
agent; nitrogen mustard

MUSTINE (continued)

ACTIONS AND USES   Analogue of mustard gas and standard of reference for nitrogen mustards. Forms highly reactive carbonium ion, which causes cross-linking and abnormal base-pairing in DNA thereby interfering with DNA replication and RNA and protein synthesis. Cell cycle nonspecific, i.e., highly toxic to rapidly proliferating cells at any time during cell cycle. Actions simulate those of radiographic therapy, but nitrogen mustards produce more acute tissue damage and more rapid recovery. Has strong myelosuppressive and weak immunosuppressive activity and is a powerful vesicant. Therapy may be associated with incidence of a second malignant tumour particularly if combined with radiation therapy or with other antineoplastics.

Use generally confined to nonterminal stages of neoplastic disease. Employed as single agent or in combination with other agents in treatment of Hodgkin's disease.

ROUTE AND DOSAGE   **Intravenous:** as a single agent or in combination with other cytotoxic drugs. Highly individualized.

ABSORPTION AND FATE   Rapid transformation to metabolites; less than 0.01% of unchanged drug excreted in urine. Interruption of blood supply to given tissue a few minutes during and immediately after drug injection protects area from drug cytotoxic effects.

CONTRAINDICATIONS AND PRECAUTIONS   Pregnancy at least until third trimester, lactation, myelosuppression, infectious granuloma, known infectious diseases, acute herpes zoster, intracavitary use with other systemic bone marrow suppressants. **Cautious Use:** bone marrow infiltration with malignant cells, chronic lymphocytic leukaemia, men or women of childbearing age, use with radiographic treatment or other chemotherapy in alternating courses.

ADVERSE/SIDE EFFECTS   These include: vertigo, tinnitus, diminished hearing, headache, drowsiness, peripheral neuropathy, lightheadedness, paraesthesias, cerebral deterioration, coma, pruritus, hyperpigmentation, maculopapular skin eruptions (rare), herpes zoster, alopecia, stomatitis, xerostomia, anorexia, nausea, vomiting, diarrhoea, peptic ulcer, jaundice, leucopenia, thrombocytopenia, lymphocytopenia, agranulocytosis, anaemia, hyperheparinaemia, delayed catamaenia, oligomenorrhea, amenorrhoea, azoospermia, impaired spermatogenesis, total germinal aplasia, chromosomal abnormalities, hyperuricaemia, metallic taste immediately after dose, weakness, fever, hypersensitivity reactions. With extravasation: painful inflammatory reaction, tissue sloughing, thrombosis, thrombophlebitis.

NURSING IMPLICATIONS

- Solution should be prepared and administered while wearing surgical gloves for protection of skin. Avoid inhalation of vapours and dust and contact of drug with eyes and skin.
- If drug contacts the skin, flush contaminated area immediately with copious amounts of water for at least 15 minutes, followed by 2% sodium thiosulphate solution. Irritation may appear after a latent period.
- If eye contact occurs, irrigate immediately with copious amounts of 0.9% sodium chloride, followed by ophthalmological examination as soon as possible.

MUSTINE *(continued)*

- Prepare solution immediately before administration.
- Do not use discoloured solution or contents of vial in which there are drops of moisture.
- If drug extravasates, prompt application of ice compresses, continued intermittently for a 6- to 12-hour period, may reduce local tissue damage and discomfort. Tissue induration and tenderness may persist 4 to 6 weeks, and tissue may slough.
- Begin flow chart with established baseline data relative to body weight, intake—output ratio and pattern, and blood picture as reference for design for drug and nursing care regimens.
- Laboratory studies of peripheral blood are essential guides for determining when to give another course of therapy. Urge patient to keep appointments for clinical evaluation.
- Give drug preferably late in the day to prevent interference with sleep by side effects.
- Intracavitary administration is preceded by removal of most of the fluid in the cavity to be treated.
- Intrapleural or intrapericardial injection of nitrogen mustard is given directly through the thoracentesis needle.
- Intraperitoneal injection is given through a rubber catheter inserted into the paracentesis trocar or through a No. 18 gauge needle inserted in another site.
- Immediately after intracavitary administration, change the patient's position (prone, supine, right side, left side, knee-chest) every 5 to 10 minutes for an hour, to assure full contact of drug with all parts of the cavity. Paracentesis may be done 24 to 36 hours later to remove any remaining fluid.
- Reaccumulation of fluid in the treated cavity is a possibility and requires careful monitoring by radiography and clinical evaluation. Watch for signs of compromised vital functions because of fluid pressure.
- Pain is rare with intrapleural injection but transient cardiac irregularities may occur. Monitor cardiac function during and after treatment until cardiac status is stable.
- Pain is common with intraperitoneal injection and usually is associated with nausea, vomiting, and diarrhoea of 2 to 3 days' duration.
- Nausea and vomiting may occur 1 to 3 hours after drug injection; vomiting usually subsides within 8 hours, but nausea may persist. Schedule treatments, other drugs, and meals so as to avoid peak times of nausea.
- Prolonged vomiting and diarrhoea can produce blood volume depletion: signs: decreased skin turgor, shrunken and dry tongue, postural hypotension, weakness, confusion. Carefully monitor and record patient's fluid losses. Discuss with physician the supportive measures that will restore and maintain fluid balance.
- Work with dietitian and patient's family to help patient maintain optimum nutritional status. Anorexia should not be ignored. Determine dietary preferences; support and augment (rather than attempt to reform) eating patterns during periods of discomfort and leucopenia.
- Myelosuppressive symptoms appear by the fourth day after treatment begins and are maximal by tenth day. Generally, lymphocytopenia begins within 24 hours and is maximum in 6 to 8 days. Significant granulocytopenia usually occurs within 6 to 8

MUSTINE (continued)

days, is maximum between 14 to 25 days with recovery complete within 2 weeks of its nadir.

- Thrombocytopenia usually manifests 6 to 8 days after a treatment. Explain its significance to patient. Petechiae, ecchymoses, or abnormal bleeding from intestinal and buccal membranes should be reported immediately. Warn patient to prevent bruising or falls. During period of thrombocytopenia, injections and use of rectal thermometer or rectal tube, and other invasive procedures should be kept at a minimum.

- Report symptoms of unexplained fever, chills, sore throat, tachycardia, and mucosal ulceration since they may signal onset of agranulocytosis (relatively infrequent incidence).

- Symptoms of depression of leucopenic system may be evident up to 50 days or more from the start of therapy.

- Profound immunosuppression places patient at risk for infections, poor healing and lowered defense mechanisms for combating stress. Prevent exposure of patient to persons with infection especially upper respiratory tract infections, and plan nursing interventions to keep patient's expenditure of energy at a minimum.

- Rapid neoplastic cell and leucocyte destruction leads to elevated serum uric acid (hyperuricaemia) and potential renal urate calculi.

- Preventive measures against incidence of hyperuricaemia include increased fluid intake, alkalinizing of urine, and administration of allopurinol.

- Encourage patient to increase fluid intake up to 3,000 ml/day if allowed. Urge prompt reporting of symptoms including: flank or joint pain, swelling of lower legs and feet, changes in voiding pattern.

- Azoospermia and amenorrhoea after a course of therapy may be irreversible. Occasionally spermatogenesis may return in patients in remission several years after intensive chemotherapy. This should be discussed with patient before therapy is started.

- High doses and regional infusion of mechlorethamine increase incidence of tinnitus and deafness. Alert patient to report symptoms promptly.

- Herpes zoster may be precipitated by mustine treatment and usually necessitates withdrawal of the drug. It occurs commonly in patients with lymphoma. Maculopapular skin eruptions usually do not necessitate stopping drug.

- Discuss the problem of alopecia (reversible) with the patient. If desired, a wig should be ordered. Keep in mind the psychological importance of hair to one's self-image and concept of sexuality. *(See Index: Nursing interventions: alopecia.)*

- *Mouth care* Cytoxic effects of antineoplastic therapy are reflected in oral membranes and structures and in salivary glands. Establish baselines for oral care by inspecting oral cavity before chemotherapy begins. Note and record state of hydration of oral mucosa, condition of gingiva, teeth, tongue, mucosa, and lips. If prosthetic devices do not fit properly, record. If patient has correctable oral problems, they should be treated before therapy with antineoplastics. Institute corrective measures to minimize possibility of irritation or infection after immunosuppression and myelosuppression has been established. Facilitate consultation with a dentist if necessary.

MUSTINE (continued)

Stomatitis Continuous meticulous measures are important to prevent oral infection from superinfection or trauma, and to relieve discomfort, and to prevent demineralization of tooth surfaces because of saliva deprivation.

- Keep oral membranes well hydrated by frequent rinses with warm water or, if patient cannot do this, irrigate cavity with warm water at least every 2 hours.
- Brush teeth using soft-bristled toothbrush (softened with warm water); if gums are painful, use moistened cotton covered finger or rubber tip on toothbrush. Use fluoride toothpaste or medication at least once daily.
- Cleansing before and after meals is important. Encourage patient to floss teeth gently with waxed floss at least once daily. Do it for patient if necessary.
- Apply thin film of petroleum jelly to cracked, dry lips. Avoid use of lemon and glycerin swabs, which irritate membranes, change consistency of saliva, and may promote decalcification of teeth.
- In presence of ulcerations or dysphagia, avoid hot or cold foods and drinks; avoid spicy, sour, dry, rough or chunky foods as well as smoking and alcoholic beverages.
- Xerostomia may be relieved by use of a saliva substitute
- Dietary supplements may be indicated during period of oral complications. Facilitate patient-dietitian conferences.

Diagnostic test interferences Mustine may increase **serum** and **urine uric acid** and decrease **serum cholinesterase**.

Drug interactions Mustine (nitrogen mustards) may reduce effectiveness of **antigout agents** necessitating dose adjustment. Other **myelosuppressants** augment action of mechlorethamine necessitating dose adjustment.

Nabilone ▬▬▬▬▬▬▬▬▬▬▬▬▬▬▬▬▬▬▬▬▬▬▬▬

(Cesamet)   *Cannabinoid; antiemetic*

ACTIONS AND USES A systemic cannabinoid chemically related to, but with less central effects than, cannabis. Used to combat nausea and vomiting induced by cytotoxic chemotherapy.

ROUTE AND DOSAGE Oral: Adult: 1–2 mg twice a day commencing the night prior to chemotherapy and continuing, if required, for 24 hours after chemotherapy is completed. Maximum daily dose 6 mg.

ABSORPTION AND FATE Absorbed from gastrointestinal tract and excreted principally in the bile.

CONTRAINDICATIONS AND PRECAUTIONS Known allergy to cannabinoids. **Cautious use** in pregnancy, children, hepatic disease and for patients receiving central nervous system depressants.

NABILONE (continued)

ADVERSE/SIDE EFFECTS These include: drowsiness, confusion, disorientation, euphoria, depression, hallucinations, psychosis, blurred vision, tremors, postural hypotension.

NURSING IMPLICATIONS

- Alertness may be affected so the patient should be advised not to drive or use machinery.
- Nabilone may be abused; ensure that tablets are not hoarded.
- Sedative effect increased when used with other CNS depressants (particularly alcohol). Advise patient to avoid alcoholic drinks.
- Warn the patient to rise slowly from sitting or lying positions, this will help to prevent dizziness due to postural hypotension.
- Keep in a tightly closed container at room temperature.

Nadolol

(Corgard)

Beta-adrenergic blocking agent; antihypertensive

N

ACTIONS AND USES Nonselective beta-adrenergic blocking agent pharmacologically and chemically similar to propranolol (q.v.). Unlike propranolol, has no membrane-stabilizing activity and little direct myocardial depressant effect. Suppression of beta$_2$-adrenergic receptors in bronchial and vascular smooth muscle can cause bronchospasm and a Raynaud's-like phenomenon. Decreases standing and supine blood pressures by an unknown mechanism. Reduces plasma renin activity.

Used in treatment of hypertension either alone or in combination with a diuretic. Also used for long-term prophylactic management of angina pectoris, migraine and thyrotoxicosis.

ROUTE AND DOSAGE Oral: *Angina pectoris*: Usual dose 80–160 mg/day.

ABSORPTION AND FATE About 30 to 40% absorbed from GI tract. **Peak plasma levels** in 2 to 4 hours; **duration** 17 to 24 hours. Widely distributed in body tissues. **Half-life** 10 to 24 hours. Approximately 30% protein bound. Not metabolized. About 70% eliminated unchanged via kidneys. Also excreted unchanged in bile and breast milk.

CONTRAINDICATIONS AND PRECAUTIONS Bronchial asthma, severe chronic obstructive pulmonary disease, inadequate myocardial function, sinus bradycardia, greater than first-degree conduction block, over cardiac failure, cardiogenic shock. Safe use during pregnancy, in nursing mothers, and in children under 18 years of age not established. **Cautious Use**: congestive heart failure, diabetes mellitus, hyperthyroidism, renal impairment.

NADOLOL (continued)
ADVERSE/SIDE EFFECTS   These include: dizziness, fatigue, sedation, headache, paraesthesias, behavioural changes; rare: mental depression, hallucinations, disorientation. **Others**: bradycardia, peripheral vascular insufficiency (Raynaud's type), palpitation, postural hypotension, conduction or rhythm disturbances, congestive heart failure, blurred vision, nasal stuffiness, tinnitus, vertigo, dry mouth, dry eyes, nausea, vomiting, anorexia, diarrhoea, constipation, abdominal cramps, bloating, flatulence, dry mouth, agranulocytosis, thrombocytopenia, weight gain, sleep disturbances, dry skin, impotence.

NURSING IMPLICATIONS
- May be administered without regard to food. Presence of food in GI tract does not affect rate or extent of absorption.
- Usually administered no more than once daily because it has a long half-life.
- Blood pressure determinations and apical pulse rate should be used as guides to dosage.
- Therapeutic effectiveness for patients with angina is evaluated by reduction in frequency of anginal attacks and improved exercise tolerance. Improvement should coincide with steady state serum concentration which is generally reached within 6 to 9 days. Keep physician informed of drug effect.
- Protect drug from light. Store at room temperature.
- *See also propranolol.*

Naftidrofuryl

(Praxilene)   *Vasodilator*

ACTIONS AND USES   Cerebral vasodilator used in cerebral and periferal vascular disease.

ROUTE AND DOSAGE   *Peripheral vascular disease*: 100–200 mg three times each day. *Cerebrovascular disease*: 100 mg three times each day.
   For further information: *see cyclandelate.*

Nalbuphine hydrochloride

(Nubain)   *Analgesic*

ACTIONS AND USES   Synthetic narcotic analgesic with agonist and weak antagonist properties. Structurally similar to naloxone and oxymorphone, but pharmacological effects are like those of pentazocine. Analgesic potency in about 3 ot 4 times greater

NALBUPHINE HYDROCHLORIDE (continued)

than that of pentazocine and approximately equal to that produced by equivalent doses of morphine. On a weight basis, produces respiratory depression about equal to that of morphine; however, in contrast to morphine, doses higher than 30 mg produce no further respiratory depression. Antagonistic potency is approximately one-fourth that of naloxone and about 10 times greater than that of pentazocine.

Used for symptomatic relief of moderate to severe pain. Also used to provide pre-operative sedation analgesia, and as a supplement to surgical anaesthesia.

ROUTE AND DOSAGE Subcutaneous, intramuscular, intravenous: 10 to 20 mg every 3 to 6 hours, as necessary. Not to exceed 160 mg/day.

ABSORPTION AND FATE Duration of analgesia approximately 3 to 6 hours. **Half-life**: about 5 hours. Metabolized in liver.

CONTRAINDICATIONS AND PRECAUTIONS History of hypersensitivity to drug. Safe use during pregnancy and in patients under age 18 years not established. **Cautious Use**: history of emotional instability or drug abuse; head injury, increased intracranial pressure; impaired respirations, impaired renal or hepatic function, myocardial infarction, biliary tract surgery.

ADVERSE/SIDE EFFECTS Most common: sedation; sweaty, clammy skin; nausea, vomiting, dizziness, vertigo. Other side effects include: nervousness, depression, restlessness, crying, euphoria, dysphoria, distortion of body image, unusual dreams, confusion, hallucinations; numbness and tingling sensations, hypertension, hypotension, bradycardia, tachycardia, flushing, abdominal cramps, bitter taste, dyspnoea, asthma, respiratory depression, speech difficulty, urinary urgency, blurred vision.

NURSING IMPLICATIONS

- Caution patient to avoid driving and other potentially hazardous activities until reaction to drug is determined.
- Inform patient that concurrent use of alcohol and other CNS depressants may result in additive effects.
- Use of drug during labour and delivery may cause respiratory depression of newborn.
- Abrupt termination of nalbuphine following prolonged use may result in symptoms similar to narcotic withdrawal: nausea, vomiting, abdominal cramps, lacrimation, nasal congestion, piloerection, fever, restlessness, anxiety.
- **Management of overdosage** IV administration of naloxone hydrochloride, supportive measures: oxygen, IV fluids, vasopressors.
- Protect nalbuphine from excessive light and store between 15° and 30°C (59° and 86°F) unless otherwise directed by manufacturer.

Nalidixic acid

(NegGram)   *Antiinfective*

NALIDIXIC ACID (continued)

ACTIONS AND USES   Synthetic naphthyridine derivative with marked bactericidal activity against gram-negative organisms, including majority of *Proteus* strains, *Klebsiella*, Enterobacter (*Aerobacter*), and *Escherichia coli*. Ineffective against *Pseudomonas* species. Gram-positive bacteria are relatively resistant. Appears to act by inhibiting DNA and RNA synthesis. Bacterial resistance has occurred.

Used in treatment of urinary tract infections caused by susceptible gram-negative organisms.

ROUTE AND DOSAGE   Oral: Adults: *Initial*: 1 g four times a day for 1 or 2 weeks; reduced to 500 mg four times a day for prolonged therapy. **Children (over 3 months to age 12)**: *Initial*: 50 mg/kg/day in four equally divided doses; for prolonged therapy, may be reduced to 30 mg/kg/day.

ABSORPTION AND FATE   Rapidly and almost completely absorbed from GI tract. Peak serum levels may occur in 1 to 2 hours, but unpredictably because of high plasma protein binding (93 to 97%). Mostly metabolized in liver. Approximately 80% of single dose is excreted in urine within 24 hours as intact drug and conjugates. Small amounts are excreted in faeces. Crosses placenta; negligible excretion in breast milk.

CONTRAINDICATIONS AND PRECAUTIONS   Known hypersensitivity to nalidixic acid, history of convulsive disorders, first trimester of pregnancy, infants younger than 3 months of age. **Cautious Use**: second and third trimesters of pregnancy, renal or hepatic disease, epilepsy, severe cerebral arteriosclerosis.

ADVERSE/SIDE EFFECTS   These include: drowsiness, dizziness, vertigo, muscle weakness, myalgia, visual disturbances; (with overdosage): headache, intracranial hypertension, convulsions, toxic psychosis (rare), sixth cranial nerve palsy (lateral rectus muscle of eye). Common side effects: nausea, vomiting, abdominal pain, diarrhoea; Occasional side effect: bleeding. Others: cholestasis; metabolic acidosis (with overdosage); paraesthesias; thrombocytopenia, leucopenia, haemolytic anaemia (especially in glucose-6-phosphate dehydrogenase deficiency); increased BUN and SGOT; glycosuria and hyperglycaemia (overdosage).

NURSING IMPLICATIONS

- Culture and sensitivity tests are advised prior to initiation of treatment and periodically during therapy. Bacterial resistance sometimes develops within 48 hours after start of therapy. Follow-up cultures are also advised to determine if infection is eliminated.
- Reportedly, blood levels are higher when drug is administered on empty stomach than when taken with food, but how this affects outcome of urinary level is unknown (because of high plasma protein binding). May be administered with food or milk if patient complains of GI distress.
- CNS reactions tend to occur 30 minutes after initiation of treatment or after second or third dose. Infants, children, and geriatric patients are especially susceptible. Observe for and report immediately the onset of marked irritability, vomiting, bulging of anterior fontanelle (infants), headache, excitement or drowsiness, papilloedema. vertigo.

NALIDIXIC ACID (continued)

- Subjective visual disturbances may occur during first few days of therapy. Report to physician. Symptoms usually disappear promptly with reduction of dosage or discontinuation of therapy.
- Blood counts and renal and hepatic function tests are recommended if therapy is continued longer than 2 weeks.
- Caution patient to avoid exposure to direct sunlight or ultraviolet light while receiving drug. Therapy should be discontinued if photosensitivity occurs (erythema or bullae on exposed skin surfaces). Susceptible patients may continue to be photosensitive up to 3 months after termination of drug.
- See Index: Nursing Interventions: urinary tract infection.

Diagnostic test interferences   False-positive urine tests for **glucose** with copper reduction methods (e.g., Benedict's, Fehling's), but not with glucose oxidase methods (e.g., Clinistix). May cause elevation of **urinary 17-ketosteroids** (Zimmerman method).

Drug interactions   Absorption of nalidixic acid may be decreased by antacids; however, **sodium bicarbonate** may increase absorption (clinical significance not determined). **Nitrofurantoin** may antagonize effect of nalidixic acid. Nalidixic acid may enhance effects of **oral anticoagulants** (by displacing them from protein binding sites).

Naloxone hydrochloride ━━━━━━━━━━━━━━━━━━━━━━━

(Narcan)   *Narcotic antagonist*

ACTIONS AND USES   N-allyl analogue of oxymorphone. A 'pure' narcotic antagonist, essentially free of agonistic (morphine–like) properties. Thus, unlike the narcotic antagonist levallorphan, produces no significant analgesia, respiratory depression, psychotomimetic effects, or miosis when administered in the absence of narcotics, and possesses more potent narcotic antagonist action. Not effective against non-opioid-induced respiratory depression. Tolerance and psychic or physical dependence not reported.

Used in treatment of narcotic overdosage and to reverse respiratory depression induced by natural and synthetic narcotics, and by pentazocine, and propoxyphene. Drug of choice when nature of depressant drug is not known, and for diagnosis of suspected acute opioid overdosage.

ROUTE AND DOSAGE   Subcutaneous, intramuscular, intravenous: **Adults**: 0.8–2 mg; may be repeated IV at two- to three-minute intervals, if necessary, maximum 10 mg. **Paediatric**: 0.01 mg/kg; may be repeated as for adult administration.

ABSORPTION AND FATE   Onset of action following IV injection occurs within 2 minutes and within 2 to 5 minutes after subcutaneous or IM administration. **Duration**

NALOXONE HYDROCHLORIDE (continued)

of action 3 to 5 hours, depending on dosage and route. **Plasma half-life** 60 to 90 minutes. Rapidly metabolized in liver, primarily by conjugation with glucuronic acid. Based on limited studies, 25 to 40% of IV dose is excreted in urine as metabolites in 6 hours and 60 to 70% in 72 hours. Readily crosses placenta.

CONTRAINDICATIONS AND PRECAUTIONS   Known hypersensitivity to naloxone; respiratory depression due to non-opioid drugs. Safe use during pregnancy (other than labour) not established. **Cautious Use**: in neonates and children; known or suspected narcotic dependence; cardiac irritability.

ADVERSE/SIDE EFFECTS   *Excessive dosage in narcotic depression*: reversal of analgesia, increased blood pressure, tremors, hyperventilation, slight drowsiness, elevated partial thromboplastin time. *Too rapid reversal*: nausea, vomiting, sweating, tachycardia.

NURSING IMPLICATIONS
- Resuscitative measures such as maintaining airway, artificial ventilation, cardiac massage, and vasopressor agents may be required.
- Monitor respirations and other vital signs. In some patients, respirations may 'overshoot' to higher level than that prior to respiratory depression.
- Duration of action of some narcotics may exceed that of naloxone; therefore, patient must be closely observed. Keep physician informed; repeat naloxone dose may be necessary.
- Narcotic abstinence symptoms induced by naloxone generally start to diminish 20 to 40 minutes after administration and usually disappear within 90 minutes.
- Do not mix naloxone with preparations containing a metabisulphite or bisulphite, long chain or high molecular weight anions (e.g., dextran) or solutions with alkaline pH. Compatible admixtures should be used within 24 hours.
- Surgical and obstetric patients should be closely monitored for bleeding. Naloxone has been associated with abnormal coagulation test results. Also observe for reversal of analgesia, which may be manifested by nausea, vomiting, sweating, tachycardia.
- Protect drug from excessive light.

Nandrolone decanoate ————————————————

(Deca-Durabolin)   *Anabolic steroid*

Nandrolone phenylpropionate

(Durabolin)

ACTIONS AND USES   Synthetic steroid with high ratio of anabolic activity to androgenic activity. Both esters have same actions and uses, but differ in action duration:

NANDROLONE PHENYLPROPIONATE (continued)

decanoate actions last 3 to 4 weeks; phenpropionate ester continues to exert anabolic effect for 1 to 3 weeks.

Used to stimulate protein synthesis after major surgery or chronic debilitating disease.

ROUTE AND DOSAGE   Intramuscular: Adults: 25–50 mg *decanoate* every 3 weeks; *phenpropionate* 25–50 mg/week.

NURSING IMPLICATIONS

- Inject drug deep IM, preferably into gluteal muscle in adult; follow hospital policy regarding IM site in small child.
- Intermittent therapy is usually recommended (4-month course of treatment followed by 6 to 8 weeks rest period).

Naproxen ▬▬▬▬▬▬▬▬▬▬▬▬▬▬▬▬▬▬▬▬▬▬▬▬

(Naprosyn, Laraflex)
Antiinflammatory (nonsteroidal); analagesic; antipyretic

ACTIONS AND USES   Nonsteroidal antiinflammatory drug with analgesic and antipyretic properties similar to other arylacetic acid derivatives, e.g., fenoprofen (q.v.).

Used for antiinflammatory and analgesic effects in symptomatic treatment of acute and chronic rheumatoid arthritis, and in management of ankylosing spondylitis, osteoarthritis and gout.

ROUTE AND DOSAGE   Oral: *musculoskeletal pain*: 250 mg 6–8 hrly. *Acute gout*: *Initial*: 750 mg naproxen followed by 250 mg every 8 hours until attack subsides. *Juvenile arthritis*: 10 mg/kg/day in two divided doses. *Rheumatoid arthritis*: 0.5–1 g daily in two doses.

NURSING IMPLICATIONS

- Patients with arthritis may experience symptomatic relief (reduction in joint pain, swelling, stiffness) within 24 to 48 hours with sodium naproxen therapy and in 2 to 4 weeks with naproxen.
- Since naproxen may cause dizziness and drowsiness, advise patient to exercise caution when driving or performing other potentially hazardous activities.
- *See fenoprofen drug interactions; see aspirin.*

Diagnostic test interferences   Transient elevations in **BUN** and serum **alkaline phosphatase** may occur. Naproxen may interfere with some urinary assays of **5-HIAA** and may cause falsely **high urinary 17-KGS** levels (using n-dinitrobenzene reagent). Suggested that naproxen be withdrawn 72 hours before adrenal function tests.

Natamycin

(Pimafucin)

*Antiinfective; antibiotic
(macrolide); antifungal*

ACTIONS AND USES   Tetraene polyene compound derived from *Streptomyces natalensis*. Effective against many yeasts and filamentous fungi including *Candida, Aspergillus, Cephalosporium, Fusarium*, and *Penicillium*. Action mechanism simulates that of amphotericin B and nystatin: by binding to sterols in the cell membrane, structure and integrity is changed leading to loss of intracellular K and other essential constituents, and destruction of the organism. Has some activity *in vivo* against *Trichomonas vaginalis*; is not active against gram-positive or gram-negative bacteria or viruses. Has low order of toxicity.

Used to treat candidiasis and susceptible fungi including those infecting the lungs.

ROUTE AND DOSAGE   **Topical** (2% cream): applied 2−3 times a day. **Oral suspension**: 10 mg/ml, 10 drops retained near the lesion after food. **Pessary**: 25 mg, one at night for 20 nights or twice a day. **Inhalation**: 2.5 mg/8 hourly.

ABSORPTION AND FATE   Does not appear to be absorbed significantly from intact or debrided mucous membrane or from GI tract.

CONTRAINDICATIONS AND PRECAUTIONS   Hypersensitivity to any component of the formulation; concomitant administration of a corticosteroid. Safe use during pregnancy not established.

ADVERSE/SIDE EFFECTS   Reports scanty. Blurred vision, photophobia, eye pain. Uneven adherence of suspension to epithelial ulcerations or in fornices.

NURSING IMPLICATIONS
- Initial diagnosis and sustained treatment should be based on clinical laboratory diagnosis by an ophthalmologist.
- Thorough handwashing before and after treatment is imperative. Infection is easily transferred to other individuals.
- Face-cloths and hand towels should be used only by the patient to prevent transmission of the fungal infection.
- Encourage patient to keep hands away from treated areas, even if discomfort tempts the patient to scratch, rub, etc.
- Store at room temperature.

Nedocromil

(Tilade)

Antiasthmatic

ACTIONS AND USES   Recently introduced drug with similar action and use to sodium cromoglycate.

NEDOCROMIL (continued)
ROUTE AND DOSAGE   Aerosol: 4 mg (2 puffs) twice a day. Not suitable for children under 12 yrs.

For further informaton: *see sodium cromoglycate.*

Nefopam

(Acupan)   *Analgesic*

ACTIONS AND USES   Rapid action centrally acting analgesic, does not cause respiratory depression. Used to relieve acute and chronic pain.

ROUTE AND DOSAGE   Oral: Adult: 30–90 mg three times a day. IM: 20 mg four times a day. Reduce dose in the elderly.

ABSORPTION AND FATE   Rapidly absorbed in the GI tract. Onset of action: 15–20 min after IM injection peak activity after 1.5 hrs.

CONTRAINDICATIONS AND PRECAUTIONS   Not to be used for patients receiving MAOI drugs or with a history of convulsions. **Cautious use** in liver or renal disease. Not recommended for children.

ADVERSE/SIDE EFFECTS   Nausea, vomiting, blurred vision, dry mouth, drowsiness, sweating.

NURSING IMPLICATIONS
- Patient should be in a recumbent position for IM injection and instructed to wait for 20 minutes before rising.
- Store in a cool dry place.

Neomycin sulphate

(Mycifradin, Nivemycin)   *Antibiotic; aminoglycoside*

ACTIONS AND USES   Aminoglycoside antibiotic obtained from *Streptomyces fradiae*; reported to be the most potent in neuromuscular blocking action and the most toxic of this group. Broad spectrum of antibacterial activity, and actions similar to those of gentamicin (q.v.).

Used for preoperative intestinal antisepsis; used to inhibit nitrogen-forming bacteria of GI tract in patients with cirrhosis or hepatic coma and for treatment of urinary tract infections. Also used topically for short-term treatment of eye, ear, and skin infections. Available in a variety of creams, ointments, and sprays in combination with other antibiotics and corticosteroids.

NEOMYCIN SULPHATE (continued)
ROUTE AND DOSAGE   Adults: Oral: 1 g every 4 hours.

ABSORPTION AND FATE   About 3% absorbed from GI tract following oral administration (neonates and prematures may absorb up to 10%). **Peak plasma levels** in
1 to 4 hours; still present in low levels at 8 hours. **Half-life**: about 3 hours (longer in
patients with renal impairment and premature infants). About 90% bound to serum
proteins. May be absorbed through ear, eye, denuded or inflamed skin, and body
cavities following topical applications.

CONTRAINDICATIONS AND PRECAUTIONS   History of sensitivity to topical or systemic neomycin or to any ingredient in formulations; use of oral drug in patients with
intestinal obstruction; ulcerative bowel lesions; topical applications over large skin
areas; parenteral use in patients with renal disease or impaired hearing; myasthenia
gravis. Safe use during pregnancy not established. **Cautious Use**: topical otic applications in patients with perforated eardrum. *See also gentamicin.*

ADVERSE/SIDE EFFECTS   Oral: mild laxative effect, diarrhoea, nausea, vomiting;
prolonged therapy: malabsorption-like syndrome including cyanocobalamin (vitamin
B_{12}) deficiency, low serum cholesterol. **Systemic absorption**: nephrotoxicity, ototoxicity, neuromuscular blockade with muscular and respiratory paralysis, hypersensitivity
reactions. *See kanamycin.* **Topical use**: redness, scaling, pruritus, dermatitis.

NURSING IMPLICATIONS
- Neomycin can cause irreversible damage to auditory branch of eighth cranial nerve
  (occurs more frequently than vestibular damage). At first, loss of hearing most
  often involves high-frequency sounds, then may progress to include normal hearing
  frequencies. In general, severity and persistence of ototoxic symptoms depend on
  dosage and duration of drug therapy; these have occurred in patients on prolonged
  therapy even when serum drug levels have been low. Early reporting is essential.
- Advise patient to report any unusual symptom related to ears or hearing: e.g.,
  tinnitus, roaring sounds, loss of hearing acuity, dizziness.
- *Preoperative bowel preparation*   Low-residue diet should be prescribed. Saline
  laxative is generally given immediately before neomycin therapy is initiated. Daily
  enemas may also be ordered.
- *Topical use*   The possibility of systemic absorption and sensitization should be
  considered. High incidence of allergic dermatitis is associated with topical neomycin. Sensitivity may be manifested as persistent dermatitis. Caution patient to
  stop treatment and report to physician if irritation occurs.
- Patients who develop sensitivity should be informed that they will probably continue
  to be sensitive to neomycin and to other aminoglycoside antibiotics (gentamicin,
  kanamycin, neomycin, streptomycin).
- For applications to skin. Consult physician about what to use for cleansing the part
  to be treated before each neomycin application.
- Topical therapy of external ear is most effective if canal is clean and dry prior to
  instillation of neomycin. Consult physician. Duration of treatment should be limited
  to 7 to 10 days.

NEOMYCIN SULPHATE (continued)

- Caution patient not to exceed prescribed dosage or duration of therapy.
- Parenteral solutions should be stored in refrigerator (2° to 15°C) to minimize possibility of contamination and discolouration and should be used as soon as possible, preferably within 1 week after reconstitution.

Drug interactions   Neomycin may reduce **cyanocobalamin** (vitamin B_{12}) absorption. *See also gentamicin*.

Neostigmine

(Prostigmin)

*Parasympathomimetic;
cholinesterase inhibitor;
antidote*

N

ACTIONS AND USES   Synthetic quaternary ammonium analogue of physostigmine, but less likely to cause disturbing side effects. Produces reversible cholinesterase inhibition or inactivation, and thus allows intensified and prolonged effect of acetylcholine at cholinergic synapses (basis for use in myasthenia gravis). Also produces generalized cholinergic response, including miosis, increased tonus of intestinal and skeletal muscles, constriction of bronchi and ureters, slower pulse rate, and stimulation of salivary and sweat glands. Has direct stimulant action on voluntary muscle fibres and possibly on autonomic ganglia and CNS neurons. Use in amenorrhoea or as pregnancy test is based on premise that delayed menstruation may be due to diminished vascular responsiveness to acetylcholine.

Used to prevent and treat postoperative abdominal distention and urinary retention; for symptomatic control of and sometimes for differential diagnosis of myasthenia gravis; and to reverse the effects of nondepolarizing muscle relaxants, e.g., tubocurarine.

ROUTE AND DOSAGE   Neostigmine bromide: **Oral:** *Myasthenia gravis*: *Initial*: 15 to 30 mg three or four times daily, increased gradually until maximum benefit obtained. Maintenance dose range: 15 to 375 mg daily, depending on patient's needs and tolerance. Neostigmine methylsulphate: **Subcutaneous, intramuscular:** 1–2.5 mg at suitable intervals throughout the day (total daily dose 5–20 mg).

ABSORPTION AND FATE   Poorly and irregularly absorbed from GI tract. Onset of action in 2 to 4 hours following oral administration and in 10 to 30 minutes following parenteral injection; **duration of effect** is 2.5 to 4 hours. Does not cross blood–brain barrier, except at extremely high doses. Metabolized in liver by microsomal enzymes. Excreted in urine.

CONTRAINDICATIONS AND PRECAUTIONS   Known hypersensitivity to neostigmine or bromide (oral formulation); mechanical, intestinal, or urinary obstruction; megacolon; peritonitis; acute peptic ulcer, urinary tract infection; hyperthyroidism. Safe use during pregnancy not established. **Cautious Use:** bronchial asthma, bradycardia,

NEOSTIGMINE (continued)

cardiac arrhythmias, hypotension, recent coronary occlusion, epilepsy, vagotonia, patients receiving other anticholinergic drugs.

ADVERSE/SIDE EFFECTS   Cholinergic crisis (overdosage): any or all of the above (see Actions); with extremely high doses, also CNS stimulation, fear, agitation, restlessness. **Muscarinic effects**: nausea, vomiting, eructation, epigastric discomfort, abdominal cramps, diarrhoea, involuntary or difficult defecation or micturition, increased salivation (common) and bronchial secretions, tightness in chest, sneezing, cough, dyspnoea, diaphoresis, lacrimation, miosis, blurred vision, bradycardia, hypotension. **Nicotinic effects**: muscle cramps, fasciculations (common), twitching, pallor, elevated blood pressure, fatigability, generalized weakness, respiratory depression and paralysis.

NURSING IMPLICATIONS

- Note that size of oral dose is considerably larger than that of parenteral dose because drug is poorly absorbed when taken orally (15 mg of oral drug is approximately equivalent to 0.5 mg of parenteral form).
- Check pulse before giving drug to patients with bradycardia. If below 80/minute, consult physician. Atropine will be ordered to restore heart rate.
- For treatment of myasthenia gravis: monitor pulse, respiration, and blood pressure during period of dosage adjustment.
- If patient has difficulty chewing, physician may prescribe oral neostigmine 30 to 45 minutes before meals. If patient has difficulty swallowing, the parenteral form may be necessary.
- GI (muscarinic) side effects occur especially during early therapy and may be reduced by taking drug with milk or food. Physician may prescribe atropine or other anticholinergic agent with each dose or every other dose to suppress side effects (*note*: these drugs may mask toxic symptoms of neostigmine).
- Regulation of dosage interval is extremely difficult; dosage must be adjusted for each patient to deal with unpredictable exacerbations and remissions.
- Report promptly and record accurately the onset of myasthenic symptoms and drug side effects in relation to last dose in order to assist physician in determining lowest effective dosage schedule.
- Encourage patient to keep a diary of 'peaks and troughs' of muscle strength.
- Frequently, drug therapy is required both day and night, with larger portions of total dose being given at times of greater fatigue, as in the late afternoon and at mealtimes.
- All activities should be appropriately spaced to avoid undue fatigue.
- Deep breathing, coughing, and range-of-motion exercises should be encouraged.
- Respiratory depression may appear abruptly in myasthenic patients. Report unusual apprehension (a frequent manifestation of inadequate ventilation), and be alert for tachypnoea, tachycardia, restlessness, rising blood pressure.
- Have the following immediately available: atropine, facilities for endotracheal intubation, tracheostomy, suction, oxygen, assisted respiration.
- In myasthenic patients, the time that muscular weakness appears may indicate whether patient is in cholinergic or myasthenic crisis. Weakness that appears ap-

NEOSTIGMINE (continued)

proximately 1 hour after drug administration suggests *cholinergic crisis (overdosage)* and is treated by prompt withdrawal of neostigmine and immediate administration of atropine. Weakness that occurs 3 hours or more after drug administration is more likely to be due to *myasthenic crisis (underdosage or drug resistance)* and is treated by more intensive anticholinesterase therapy.

- Manifestations of neostigmine overdosage often appear first in muscles of neck and those involved in chewing and swallowing, with muscles of shoulder girdle and upper extremities affected next.
- Signs and symptoms of myasthenia gravis that may be relieved by neostigmine: lid ptosis; diplopia; drooping facies; difficulty in chewing, swallowing, breathing, or coughing; weakness to neck, limbs, and trunk muscles. Record drug effect and duration of action.
- Lid ptosis, especially in the elderly, may continue despite drug therapy. Often, patients are helped by means of an adhesive lid crutch attached to rim of eyeglasses.
- Some patients become refractory to neostigmine after prolonged use and require change in dosage or medication.
- Drug therapy for myasthenia gravis is lifesaving and must be continued throughout patient's life. Patient may require help to overcome psychological problems associated with prolonged disability.
- Patient and responsible family members should be taught to keep an accurate record for physician of patient's response to drug, as well as how to recognize side effects, how to modify dosage regimen according to patient's changing needs, or how to administer atropine if necessary. They should be aware that certain factors may require an increase in size or frequency of dose (e.g., physical or emotional stress, infection, menstruation, surgery), whereas remission requires a decrease in dosage.
- Advise patient to wear identification bracelet indicating the presence of myasthenia gravis. Also inform patient and family of educational resources.
- **Neostigmine test for myasthenia gravis** The neostigmine test has been largely replaced by the edrophonium (Tensilon) test. All anticholinesterase medications should be discontinued at least 8 hours before test. Accurate recordings are made of grip strength, vital capacity, range of extraocular movements, ptosis, etc, before test (usually, atropine sulphate 0.6 mg IM is given prior to or concomitantly with neostigmine methylsulphate to prevent muscarinic effects). After neostigmine is given, muscle strength is retested at 15-minute intervals for 1 hour. Objective and subjective improvement in strength and movement indicates positive test. Nonmyasthenic patient may experience weakness, abdominal cramps, diarrhoea, diaphoresis, dysuria.
- When neostigmine is used as antidote for tubocurarine or other nondepolarizing neuromuscular blocking agents (usually preceded by atropine), monitor respiration, maintain airway or assisted ventilation, and give oxygen as indicated. Respiratory assistance is continued until recovery of respiration and neuromuscular transmission is assured.
- *For relief of postoperative abdominal distention*: Rectal tube is inserted following drug administration to facilitate expulsion of gas. Lubricated tube is inserted just past rectal sphincter and kept in place for about 1 hour. In some cases, a small low enema

NEOSTIGMINE (continued)

may be prescribed. Record results: passage of flatus, decrease in abdominal distention, pain, rigidity.

Drug interactions   Parenteral neostigmine antagonizes the effects of **nondepolarizing neuromuscular blocking agents**, e.g., **gallamine, metocurine, pancuronium, tubocurarine** (interaction used therapeutically). Upward adjustment of neostigmine dosage may be required in myasthenic patients receiving drugs that interfere with neuromuscular transmission, e.g., **aminoglycoside antibiotics (gentamicin, kanamycin, neomycin, streptomycin)**, **local anaesthetics** and some **general anaesthetics**, and **antiarrhythmic agents**, e.g., **procainamide, quinidine** (all used with extreme caution, if at all). Neostigmine may prolong the action of depolarizing muscle relaxants, e.g., **decamethonium, succinylcholine**. Muscarinic effects of neostigmine are antagonized by **atropine** (interaction used therapeutically).

Netilmicin sulphate ———————————————————————————

(Netillin)   *Antibiotic; aminoglycoside*

ACTIONS AND USES   Rapid acting, broad spectrum, semisynthetic aminoglycoside derivative of sisomicin. In common with other aminoglycosides, appears to act by interfering with protein synthesis of bacterial cell wall. Spectrum of activity comparable to that of gentamicin, but netilmicin is also effective against gentamicin-resistant bacteria. Not inactivated by most strains of bacteria resistant to other aminoglycosides. Bactericidal action primarily against gram-negative organisms including *Citrobacter, Enterobacter, Escherichia coli, Klebsiella, Proteus mirabilis, Pseudomonas aeruginosa, Salmonella, Serratia*, and certain gram-positive bacteria such as *Staphylococcus pyogenes* and *Streptococcus faecalis*. Like other aminoglycosides, not effective against most anaerobic bacteria (*Bacteroides* and *Clostridium* species), viruses, or fungi. Reportedly less ototoxic and nephrotoxic than other aminoglycosides, but has high potential for neuromuscular blocking action.

Used for short-term treatment of serious or life-threatening infections resistant to gentamicin.

ROUTE AND DOSAGE   Intramuscular, Intravenous injection or infusion: **Adults:** 4–6 mg/kg/day in divided doses. **Child:** 2–2.5 mg/kg/every 8 hrs. **Neonate:** 3 mg/kg every 8 hours.

ABSORPTION AND FATE   Rapidly and completely absorbed following IM or IV administration. **Serum levels peak** within 30 to 60 minutes (still measurable for 12 hours) following IM, and at the end of 1 hour after IV infusion. Promptly distributed into tissues, normal body fluids, (including urine, sputum, bile, pericardial, peritoneal, pleural, synovial), and abscess and blister fluid. Poor distribution to adipose tissue and to CSF, unless meninges are inflamed. **Protein binding**: 0 to 30%. **Half-life**: 2 to 3.4

NETILMICIN SULPHATE (continued)

hours (prolonged to about 30 or more hours in impaired renal function); in children: inversely related to weight and age. About 75 to 90% of dose excreted unchanged in urine within 24 hours; minimal amounts eliminated in bile. Crosses placenta. Small quantities distributed into breast milk.

CONTRAINDICATIONS AND PRECAUTIONS   History of hypersensitivity or toxic reaction to netilmicin, or other aminoglycosides, or to bisulphites or any other ingredient in the formulation, pregnancy, nursing infants, use for minor infections. **Cautious Use**: impaired renal function, prematures, neonates, the elderly, patients with ascites, oedema, dehydration, severe burns, cystic fibrosis, fever, anaemia, myasthenia gravis, parkinsonism, history of ear disease; infant botulism.

ADVERSE/SIDE EFFECTS   (Low incidence in patients with normal renal function.) These include: headache, lethargy, drowsiness, paraesthesias, tremors, muscle twitching, peripheral neuritis, disorientation, seizures, neuromuscular blockade; musculoskeletal weakness or paralysis, respiratory depression or paralysis, palpitation, hypotension, ototoxicity (usually irreversible: eighth cranial nerve auditory branch: tinnitus, hearing loss, ringing, buzzing or fullness in ears: vestibular branch: vertigo, nystagmus, ataxia, nausea and vomiting, diarrhoea, stomatitis, proctitis, enterocolitis (possibly super-infections), increases in: SGPT (ALT), SGOT (AST), alkalinephosphatase, bilirubin; anaemia, eosinophilia, neutropenia, thrombocytopenia, thrombocytosis, prolonged PT, agranulocytosis, leucopenia, leucemoid reaction, hyperkalaemia, blurred vision, increase in serum creatinine and BUN; decrease in creatinine clearance; haematuria, proteinuria, urinary frequency, oliguria, polyuria, fever, oedema, arthralgia; pain, induration and haematoma at injection site.

NURSING IMPLICATIONS

- Culture and sensitivity tests should be done prior to initiation of therapy. Therapy may begin before test results are available.
- Renal function should be evaluated before and periodically during therapy: serum creatinine, creatinine clearance rate, BUN, urinalysis including specific gravity. Close attention to these values is particularly important for high risk patients, i.e., renal function impairment, the elderly, dehydrated patients, burn patients, and patients receiving high doses or prolonged therapy.
- Monitor fluid intake–output ratio and pattern and report significant changes. Keep patient well hydrated throughout therapy to minimize possibility of chemical irritation of renal tubules, and to reduce risk of toxicity.
- Dosage adjustments for patients with impaired renal function are based on creatinine clearance rates, serum creatinine, or on peak and trough serum drug levels. (These patients tend to accumulate toxic concentrations of netilmicin.) Creatinine clearance is either measured or estimated from published nonograms or equations. See manufacturer's package insert.
- Close monitoring or serum drug concentrations is especially important for patients with fever, oedema, severe burns, and anaemia. Peak serum drug levels tend to be significantly reduced in these patients, possibly due to alterations in extracellular fluid volume.

NETILMICIN SULPHATE *(continued)*

- Urinalysis may be done daily in high risk patients to determine presence of albumin, casts, white or red blood cells, and lowering of specific gravity. All represent signs of renal irritation and the need for increased hydration.
- Patients should be evaluated before and during therapy for hearing acuity and vestibular status. Loss of higher frequency sounds, an early sign of cochlear damage, can be detected only by audiometric testing. Notify physician promptly if patient complains of any hearing loss, tinnitus, vertigo, or ataxia.
- Serial audiometric tests may be done for patients at high risk for ototoxicity: patients with impaired renal function, history of hearing, or vestibular problems, concomitant therapy with other potentially ototoxic drugs, patients in high dose or prolonged netilmicin therapy.
- If therapeutic effectiveness is not evident within 3 to 5 days, bacterial sensitivity tests should be repeated.
- For most patients, therapy may last 7 to 14 days. However, carefully selected patients with complicated infections may require longer therapy.
- Have ready calcium salts and equipment for mechanical respiratory assistance, to reverse neuromuscular blockade.
- Watch for signs of superinfection especially of upper respiratory tract. Also suspect overgrowth of opportunistic organisms if patient develops sore rectum, diarrhoea, vaginal discharge, sore mouth, fever.
- *See manufacturer's package insert for list of compatible diluents and stability of prepared solutions.* Solutions retain potency for up to 72 hours when stored in glass containers either at room temperature or refrigerated. Do not use solutions that are discoloured or that contain particulate matter.
- Avoid mixing netilmicin with other drugs without first consulting pharmacist or specialized references for compatibility.
- Store between 2° and 30°C (36° to 86°F) unless otherwise directed by manufacturer. Avoid freezing.

Diagnostic test interferences   Concomitant netilmicin–cephalosporin therapy may cause false elevations of **creatinine** determinations. Concomitant use of beta-lactam antibiotics (cephalosporins, penicillins) may result in falsely low **aminoglycoside levels** (mutual inactivation may continue in body fluid specimen unless promptly assayed, or frozen, or treated with beta-lactamase).

DRUG INTERACTIONS   *Netilmicin*

PLUS	INTERACTIONS
Aminoglycosides	Increased potential for nephrotoxicity, ototoxicity, and neuromuscular blockade. Concurrent or sequential use generally avoided
Amphotericin B	Synergistic nephrotoxic effects; used concomitantly, e.g., with caution
Antibiotics (polypeptides) e.g., bacitracin (parenteral), capreomycin, colistin, polymyxin B	Possibility of additive neuromuscular blocking action. Used with extreme caution

NETILMICIN SULPHATE (continued)

PLUS (continued)	INTERACTIONS
Cephalosporins	Additive nephrotoxic effects. Used concomitantly, e.g., only with caution
Cisplatin	Additive nephrotoxicity and ototoxicity. Concurrent or sequential use generally avoided
Citrate-anticoagulated blood	Enhancement of neuromuscular blocking action. Concurrent use generally avoided
Dimenhydrinate	May mask symptoms of ototoxicity. Used with caution
Diuretics (loop) e.g., bumetanide, frusemide, ethacrynic acid	Increased risk of ototoxicity, particularly with parenteral diuretics. Concurrent use generally avoided
Penicillins	Synergistic effects, however, physiochemical inactivation can occur depending on contact time. Scheduling 1 hour apart may help
Succinylcholine (depolarizing muscle relaxant) tubocurarine and other nondepolarizing muscle relaxants	Possibility of additive neuromuscular blocking action. Used with extreme caution
Vancomycin	Additive neurotoxicity and nephrotoxicity. Concurrent or sequential use requires careful monitoring

Nicardipidine

(Cardene)   *Calcium channel blocker*

ACTIONS AND USES   Used for prophylaxis and treatment of angina. Vasodilator (peripheral and coronary)

ROUTE AND DOSAGE   Oral: **Adult:** *Initial* 20 mg three times a day increased to 30 mg three times a day.
   For further information: *see verapamil*.

Nicotinic acid, Nicotinic acid Derivatives

(Hexopal, Pernivit, Ronicol)   *Vitamin; vasodilator*

Nicofuranose

(Bradilan)

NICOFURANOSE (continued)

ACTIONS AND USES   Large doses effectively reduce elevated serum cholesterol and total lipid levels in hypercholesterolaemia and hyperlipidaemic states. Unclear whether drug-induced reduction of cholesterol and lipids has a beneficial effect on morbidity or mortality caused by atherosclerosis or coronary heart disease.

Used in treatment of hyperlipidaemia (elevated cholesterol and/or triglycerides) in patient who does not respond adequately to diet or weight loss.

ROUTE AND DOSAGE   Oral: Adults: *Hyperlipidaemia*: *Nicotinic acid*: 100–200 mg three times a day increased to 1–2 g three times a day over 2–4 weeks. *Nicofuranose*: 0.5–1 g three times a day. *Vasodilation* (Nicotinic acid derivatives) depends on product.

ABSORPTION AND FATE   Rapid absorption from GI tract. **Peak serum level**: 20 to 70 minutes. Therapeutic plasma concentration of 0.5 to 1.0 mcg/ml required for active antilipidaemic action. **Plasma half-life**: about 45 minutes. Major metabolites from hepatic degradation: nicotinuric acid, N-methylnicotinamide and 2-pyridone. About ⅓ oral dose excreted in urine unchanged.

CONTRAINDICATIONS AND PRECAUTIONS   Hypersensitivity to niotin, hepatic impairment, severe hypotension, haemorrhage or arterial bleeding, active peptic ulcer. Used during pregnancy and lactation only if benefits outweigh risks to foetus or nursing infant. **Cautious Use**: history of gall bladder disease, liver disease, and peptic ulcer; glaucoma, angina, coronary artery disease, diabetes mellitus, predisposition to gout, allergy.

ADVERSE/SIDE EFFECTS   These include: transient headache, tingling of extremities, syncope; (with chronic use): nervousness, panic, toxic amblyopia, proptosis, blurred vision, loss of central vision. **Others**: generalized flushing with sensation of warmth, postural hypotension, vasovagal attacks, increased sebaceous gland activity, dry skin, skin rash, pruritus, keratitis nigricans, abnormalities of hepatic function tests; jaundice, bloating, flatulence, hunger pains, nausea, vomiting, GI disorders, activation of peptic ulcer, xerostomia, hyperuricaemia, allergy, hyperglycaemia, glycosuria, hypoprothrombinaemia, hypoalbuminaemia.

NURSING IMPLICATIONS
- Take oral drug with meals to decrease GI distress.
- Take with cold water (not hot beverage) if necessary to facilitate swallowing.
- After oral dose, plasma free fatty acic concentration is lowered within 30 minutes, plasma triglyceride levels within hours; however, cholesterol levels do not decline for several days.
- Therapeutic response usually begins within 24 hours. Note and record effect of therapy on clinical manifestations of deficiency (fiery red tongue, sialorrhoea and infection of oral membranes, nausea, vomiting, diarrhoea, confusion).
- In treatment of hyperlipidaemia, dosage is individualized according to effect on serum lipid levels.

NICOFURANOSE (continued)

- Diabetics, potential diabetics, and patients on high doses will require close monitoring. Hyperglycaemia, glycosuria, ketonuria, and increased insulin requirements have been reported.
- Baseline and periodic tests of blood glucose and liver function should be performed in patients receiving prolonged high dose therapy.
- Inform patient that cutaneous warmth and flushing in face, neck, and ears may occur within first 2 hours after oral ingestion (and immediately after parenteral administration) and may last several hours. Effects are usually transient and subside as therapy continues.
- Caution patient to sit or lie down and to avoid sudden posture changes if weakness or dizziness is experienced. These symptoms and persistent flushing shoud be reported to the physician. Relief may be obtained by reduction of dosage, increasing subsequent doses in small increments, or by changing to sustained-action formulation.
- Alcohol and large doses of niotin cause increased flushing and sensation of warmth. Alcohol should be limited if patient is being treated for hypertriglyceridaemia.
- Observe patient closely for evidence of hepatic dysfunction (jaundice, dark urine, light-coloured stools, pruritus) and hyperuricaemia in patient predisposed to gout (flank, joint, or stomach pain; altered urine excretion pattern).
- Caution patient with skin manifestations to avoid exposure to direct sunlight until lesions have entirely cleared.
- Patient may be restricted in intake of saturated fats, sugars and/or cholesterol.
- Store drug at temperature between 15° and 30°C (59° and 86°F) in light- and moisture-proof container.

Diagnostic test interferences   Causes elevated **serum bilirubin, uric acid, alkaline phosphatase, SGOT, SGPT, LDH** levels, and may cause **glucose intolerance**. Decreases **serum cholesterol** 15 to 30%, and may cause false elevations with certain fluorometric methods of determining **urinary catecholamines**. May cause false-positive **urine glucose** tests using copper sulphate reagents, e.g., Benedict's solution.

Drug interactions   Potentiates hypotensive effects of **antihypertensives** (ganglionic blocking type). **Clonidine** may inhibit **nicotin**-induced skin flushing.

Niclosamide

(Yomesan)   *Antiinfective; anthelmintic*

ACTIONS AND USES   Salicylanilide derivative reportedly effective against most tapeworms that infect man. Acts by inhibiting oxidative phosphorylation in mitochondria of cestodes. On contact, kills scolex and proximal segments of tapeworm, which may then be partially or fully digested in intestines. Lacks ovicidal action and is not effective in larval or tissue encystment stage of tapeworm infections, e.g., cysticercosis.

NICLOSAMIDE (continued)
Used in treatment of intestinal tapeworm (cestode) infections.

ROUTE AND DOSAGE   Oral: Adults: 2 g in single dose. **Children (under 2 years):** 500 mg, 2–6 years 1 g.

ABSORPTION AND FATE   Pharmacokinetic information scanty. Minimally absorbed from GI tract. Excreted in faeces.

CONTRAINDICATIONS AND PRECAUTIONS   Hypersensitivity to niclosamide or to any ingredients in the formulation. Safe use during pregnancy, in nursing women, and in children under 2 years not established.

ADVERSE/SIDE EFFECTS   These include: drowsiness, dizziness, headache, irritability, skin rash, pruritus ani, alopecia, sweating, nausea, vomiting, abdominal discomfort, anorexia, diarrhoea, constipation, oral irritation, bad taste, rectal bleeding, fever, weakness, oedema of an arm, backache, palpitation. Rare: Transient rise in SGOT (AST).

NURSING IMPLICATIONS
- Administered after a light meal, e.g., after breakfast. Instruct patient to chew tablet thoroughly, then swallow with a little water.
- For young children, tablet may be crushed to a fine powder and mixed with sufficient water to form a paste for ease of ingestion.
- Dietary restrictions and purgation before or after drug therapy, and hospitalization during treatment are not usually necessary. Some patients may require a laxative if constipation is a problem, or for recovery of scolex to determine cure.
- Stool examinations for presence of scolex, proglottids (tapeworm segments), and ova may be required at 1 and 3 months following therapy to determine cure. No patient is considered cured unless stools have been negative for ova and proglottids for at least 3 months.
- *Treatment of niclosamide toxicity*   Fast-acting laxative, enema. Do *not* induce emesis.
- Store preferably at temperature below 30°C (86°F), protected from light, unless otherwise directed by manufacturer.

Nicoumalone ——————————————————

(Sinthrome)   *Anticoagulant; coumarin*

ROUTE AND DOSAGE   8–12 mg on the first day, 4–8 mg on the second, maintainance 1–8 mg/day.
For further information: *see warfarin*.

Nifedipine ━━━━━━━━━━━━━━━━━━━━━━━━━━━━━━━━━━

(Adalat)   *Vasodilator (coronary);*
calcium channel blocking
agent

ACTIONS AND USES   Calcium channel blocking agent similar to verapamil (q.v.) in actions, uses, and limitations. Selectively blocks calcium ion influx across cell membranes of cardiac muscle and vascular smooth muscle without changing serum calcium concentrations. Reduces myocardial oxygen utilization and supply and relaxes and prevents coronary artery spasm. In contrast to verapamil and diltiazem, has little or no effect on SA and AV nodal conduction with therapeutic dosing. Decreases peripheral vascular resistance and increases cardiac output.

Used in management of angina and mild to moderate hypertension and Raynaud's phenomenon.

ROUTE AND DOSAGE   (Dosage established by titration, usually over a 7 to 14 day period.) **Oral**: *Adult: Initial*: 10 mg three times daily, increased to 20 mg three times a day. Range 60–80 mg/day. *Slow release preparations*: 20 mg twice a day increased as required to 40 mg twice a day. Reduce dose in the elderly.

ABSORPTION AND FATE   Rapidly and fully absorbed (about 9%) after oral administration. **Onset of action** within 10 minutes; **peak levels** in 30 minutes. Metabolized in liver. Highly bound (92 to 98%) to plasma protein; **half-life**: 2 to 5 hours. Effects of renal or hepatic impairment on metabolism and excretion of nifedipine not known. 1 to 2% dose excreted unchanged in urine.

CONTRAINDICATIONS AND PRECAUTIONS   Known hypersensitivity to nifedipine. Safe use during pregnancy and in children not established. **Cautious Use**: concomitant use with hypotensives; congestive heart failure, lactating, women.

ADVERSE/SIDE EFFECTS   These include: dizziness, nervousness, mood changes, jitteriness, sleep disturbances, blurred vision, retinal ischaemia, difficulty in balance, headache, hypotension (may be excessive), facial flushing, heat sensation, palpitation, nausea, heartburn, diarrhoea, constipation, cramps, flatulence, inflammation, joint stiffness, muscle cramps, hyperglycaemia, hypokalaemia, sore throat, weakness, dermatitus, pruritus, urticaria, gingival hyperplasia, fever, sweating, chills, febrile reaction, sexual difficulties, peripheral, oedema. **Overdose**: prolonged systemic hypotension.

NURSING IMPLICATIONS
- May be co-administered with sublingual glyceryl trinitrate and with long-acting nitrates.
- Occasionally a patient has developed increased frequency, duration and severity of angina on starting treatment with this drug or when dosage is increased. Counsel patient to keep a record of glyceryl trinitrate use and to report promptly if changes in previous pattern occur.
- Careful monitoring of blood pressure during titration period is indicated. Severe

NIFEDIPINE (continued)

hypotension may be produced, especially if patient is also taking other drugs known to lower blood pressure.

- Warn patient not to change nifedipine dosage regimen without consulting physician; i.e., patient should not omit, increase, decrease dose, or change the dose interval. Withdrawal symptoms may occur with abrupt discontinuation of the drug (chest pain, increase in anginal episodes, myocardial infarction, dysrhythmias).
- Monitor the blood sugar in patient who is diabetic. Nifedipine has diabetogenic properties.
- **Smoking–drug interaction** It has been shown that smoking decreases the efficacy of nifedipine and that it has direct and adverse effects on the heart in the patient on nifedipine treatment.
- Treatment of overdosage calls for active cardiovascular support, monitoring of cardiac and respiratory function and intake and output ratio and pattern; elevation of extremities; administration of a vasoconstrictor such as noradrenaline.
- Discontinuation of drug should be gradual with close medical supervision to prevent severe hypotensive and other side effects.
- Protect capsules from light and moisture; store at temperature between 15° and 25°C (59° and 77°F).
- *See also verapamil.*

Diagnostic test interferences Nifedipine may cause mild to moderate increases of alkaline phosphatase, CK, LDH, SGOT (AST), SGPT (ALT).

Drug interactions Nifedipine and hypotensive may increase likelihood of congestive heart failure, severe hypotension, exacerbation of angina. *See also verapamil.*

Nikethamide ————————————————————————

Central stimulant (respiratory); analeptic

ACTIONS AND USES Diethyl derivative of nicotinamide, the pellagra-preventive vitamin. Similar to doxapram in actions and toxic effects (q.v.), but generally regarded to be less effective and to have less margin of safety.

Used to overcome CNS depression, respiratory depression, and circulatory failure, particularly when due to CNS depressant drugs. May be combined with electroshock therapy to restore respiration more quickly and to reduce number of required treatments.

ROUTE AND DOSAGE Adults: Intravenous, intramuscular: 0.5–1 g repeated at 15–30 min intervals as necessary.

ABSORPTION AND FATE Readily absorbed following oral or IM administration; maximum effect in 20 to 30 minutes; duration about 1 hour. Duration of action fol-

NIKE:THAMIDE (continued)

lowing IV is 5 to 10 minutes, but may increase with succeeding doses. Converted in part to nicotinamide in body. Metabolic excreted in urine.

ADVERSE/SIDE EFFECTS   Burning or itching, especially at back of nose, is the most common side effect. *See also doxapram.*

NURSING IMPLICATIONS
- Difference between clinically effective dose and that producing side effects is often small. Therefore, any side effects should be construed to be the result of overdosage.
- Widespread CNS stimulation may occur with repeated doses. Observe for and report increases in vital signs, coughing, sneezing, flushing, itching, nausea, vomiting, tremors, muscle rigidity.
- *See doxapram hydrochloride.*
- Similar drug ethamivan (Clairvan).

Nitrazepam

(Mogadon, Nitrados, Noctesed, Remnos, Somnite, Surem, Unisomnia)

Hypnotic; benzodiazepine

ACTIONS AND USES   Used in imsomnia. Has culminative effects which cause daytime sedation. *See chlordiazepoxide.*

ROUTE AND DOSAGE   Oral: **Adult**: 5–10 mg at bedtime, reduce dose in the elderly to 2.5–5 mg.

NURSING IMPLICATIONS
- Prolonged use may lead to dependence.
- Long half–life contributes to hangover effect of daytime sedation.
- Caution patient not to drive or operate machinery.
- *See chlordiazepoxide.*

Nitrofurantoin

(Furadantin, Macrodantin, Urantoin)

Antibacterial (urinary); nitrofuran

ACTIONS AND USES   Synthetic nitrofuran derivative related to nitrofurazone. Active against wide variety of gram-negative and gram-positive microorganisms, including strains of *Escherichia coli, Staphylococcus aureus, Streptococcus faecalis*, enterococci, and *Klebsiella-Aerobacter. Pseudomonas aeruginosa* and many strains of *Proteus* are resistant.

NITROFURANTOIN (continued)

Presumed to act by interfering with several bacterial enzyme systems. Highly soluble in urine and reportedly most active in acid urine. Antimicrobial concentrations in urine exceed those in blood.

Used in treatment of pyelonephritis, pyelitis, and cystitis caused by susceptible organisms.

ROUTE AND DOSAGE   Oral: **Adults**: 100 mg four times daily.

ABSORPTION AND FATE   Rapidly and almost completely absorbed from GI tract (macrocrystalline form appears to be absorbed more slowly than conventional tablets, but urinary concentrations are not significantly reduced). *Half-life*: 18 minutes to 1 hour. Crosses blood–brain barrier. Degraded by all body tissues (except blood) to inactive metabolites. Excreted rapidly in urine, about 40% of dose as unchanged drug; small amounts may be eliminated in faeces. Crosses placenta; enters breast milk.

CONTRAINDICATIONS AND PRECAUTIONS   Known hypersensitivity to nitrofuran derivatives, anuria, oliguria, significant impairment of renal function (creatinine clearance under 40 ml/minute), patients with G6PD deficiency, infants under 3 months of age, parenteral use in children under 12 years of age. Safe use in women of child-bearing potential, during pregnancy, pregnancy at term, and in nursing mothers not established. **Cautious Use**: history of asthma, anaemia, diabetes, vitamin B deficiency, electrolyte imbalance, debilitating disease.

ADVERSE/SIDE EFFECTS   These include: anorexia, nausea, vomiting, abdominal pain, diarrhoea, peripheral neuropathy, headache, nystagmus, drowsiness, vertigo, transient alopecia, genitourinary superinfections (especially with *Pseudomonas*), tooth staining from direct contact with oral suspension and crushed tablets (infants), crystalluria (elderly patients); pulmonary sensitivity reactions (interstitial pneumonitis and/or fibrosis).

NURSING IMPLICATIONS

- Drug must be given at equally spaced intervals around the clock to maintain therapeutic urinary drug levels.
- Administer oral drug with meals or milk to minimize gastric irritation.
- Nausea occurs fairly frequently and may be relieved by using macrocrystalline preparation or by reduction in dosage. Consult physician.
- Because of the possibility of tooth staining associated with direct contact of drug with teeth advise patient to avoid crushing tablets to dilute oral suspension in milk, infant feeds water, or fruit juice, and to rinse mouth thoroughly after taking drug.
- Inform patient that nitrofurantoin may impart a harmless brown colour to urine (due to drug metabolite).
- Monitor fluid intake and output. Report oliguria and any change in intake–output ratio. Drug should be discontinued if oliguria or anuria develops or *creatinine clearance* falls below 40 ml/minute. (Normal: 115 ± 20 ml/minute.)
- Consult physician regarding fluid intake. Generally, fluids are not forced, since drug is highly soluble; however, intake should be adequate.

NITROFURANTOIN (continued)

- Culture and sensitivity tests are performed prior to therapy and are recommended in patients with recurrent infections.
- Be alert to signs of urinary tract superinfections: milky urine, foul-smelling urine, perineal irritation, dysuria.
- Acute pulmonary sensitivity reaction usually occurs within first week of therapy and appears to be more common in the elderly. May be manifested by mild to severe flu-like syndrome: fever, dyspnoea, cough, chest pains, chills, decreased breath sounds, rhonchi and crepitant rates on auscultation. Eosinophilia generally develops in a few days. Recovery usually occurs rapidly after drug is discontinued.
- Subacute or chronic pulmonary sensitivity reaction is associated with prolonged therapy. Commonly manifested by insidious onset of malaise, cough, dyspnoea on exertion, altered pulmonary function (radiographic findings: interstitial pneumonitis and/or fibrosis).
- Peripheral neuropathy can be severe and irreversible. Be alert for and advise the patient to report onset of muscle weakness, tingling, numbness, or other sensations. Reportedly, these are most likely to occur in patients with renal impairment, anaemia, diabetes, electrolyte imbalance, vitamin B deficiency, or debilitating disease. Drug should be discontinued immediately.
- Treatment is continued for at least 3 days after sterile urines are obtained. Course of treatment for acute infections rarely exceeds 14 days.
- Dispensed in amber-coloured containers; strong light darkens drug. Nitrofurantoin decomposes on contact with metals other than stainless steel or aluminium.

Diagnostic test interferences Nitrofurantoin metabolite may produce false-positive **urine glucose** test results wth Benedict's reagent.

Drug interactions Drugs that tend to alkalinize urine (e.g., **acetazolamide, thiazides**) may decrease the effect of nitrofurantoin. There is the possibility that **antacids** may delay absorption of nitrofurantoin. Nitrofurantoin may antagonize the effects of **nalidixic acid.** Concomitant administration with **probenecid** (particularly in high doses) and possibly **sulphinpyrazone** may increase nitrofurantoin in serum to toxic levels by decreasing renal clearance (also decreasing effectiveness in urinary tract infections). Antimicrobial effectiveness of nitrofurantoin may be reduced by **magnesium** containing drugs.

N

Nizatidine

(Axid)

ACTIONS AND USES New H_2 blocker used to treat benign gastric and duodenal ulcers.

ROUTE AND DOSAGE Oral: Adult: 300 mg at night for 4–8 weeks. *Prophylaxis*: 150 mg at night for up to 1 year.
For further information: *see cimetidine*.

NIZATIDINE (continued)
ADVERSE/SIDE EFFECTS   Report adverse reactions to the Committee On Safety of Medicines.

Noradrenaline

(Levophed)

Alpha-adrenergic agonist
(direct-acting);
catecholamine

ACTIONS AND USES   Direct-acting sympathomimetic amine identical to body catecholamine noradrenaline. Acts directly and predominantly on alpha-adrenergic receptors; little action on beta-receptors except in heart (beta$_1$ receptors). Main therapeutic effects are vasoconstriction and cardiac stimulation. Has powerful constrictor action on resistance and capacitance blood vessels. Reduces blood flow to kidney, other vital organs, skin, and skeletal muscle. Peripheral vasoconstriction (alpha-adrenergic action) and moderate inotropic stimulation of heart (beta-adrenergic action) result in increased systolic and diastolic blood pressure, myocardial oxygenation, coronary artery blood flow, and work of heart. Cardiac output varies reflexly with systemic blood pressure. Reflex increase of vagal activity in response to pronounced effect on arterial blood pressure may cause bradycardia.

Used to restore blood pressure in certain acute hypotensive states such as sympathectomy, phenochromocytomectomy, spinal anaesthesia, poliomyelitis, myocardial infarction, septicaemia, blood transfusion, and drug reactions. Also used as adjunct in treatment of cardiac arrest.

ROUTE AND DOSAGE   Highly individualized according to response of patient. **Intravenous infusion:** give 8 mcg/ml solution of noradrenaline acid tartrate (equivalent to 4 mcg/ml noradrenaline base) at rate of 2–3 ml/min initially then adjusted to response.

ABSORPTION AND FATE   Pressor activity occurs rapidly and lasts 1 to 2 minutes following termination of IV infusion. Pronounced localization in sympathetic nerve endings. Inactivated in liver and other tissues, primarily by catechol-*o*-methyl transferase and to smaller extent by monamine oxidase. Excreted in urine mainly as inactive metabolites; 4 to 16% of dose is excreted unchanged. Crosses placenta.

CONTRAINDICATIONS AND PRECAUTIONS   Use as sole therapy in hypovolaemic states, except as temporary emergency measure; mesenteric or peripheral vascular thrombosis; profound hypoxia or hypercarbia; pregnancy; use during cyclopropane or halothane anaesthesia. **Cautious Use:** hypertension, hyperthyroidism, severe heart disease, elderly patients, within 14 days of MAOI therapy, patients receiving tricyclic antidepressants.

NORADRENALINE (continued)

ADVERSE/SIDE EFFECTS   Headache, palpitation, hypertension, reflex bradycardia, fatal arrhythmias (large doses), respiratory difficulty, restlessness, anxiety, tremors, dizziness, weakness, insomnia, pallor, tissue necrosis at injection site (with extravasation), swelling of thyroid gland (rare). **With prolonged administration**: plasma volume depletion, oedema, haemorrhage, intestinal, hepatic, and renal necrosis. **Overdosage or individual sensitivity**: blurred vision, photophobia, hyperglycaemia, retrosternal and pharyngeal pain, profuse sweating, vomiting, severe hypertension, violent headache, cerebral haemorrhage, convulsions.

NURSING IMPLICATIONS

- IV infusion of noradrenaline in saline alone is not recommended. Dextrose (in distilled water or saline solution) is used to prevent oxidation and thus loss of potency.
- An infusion pump or apparatus to control noradrenaline flow rate is generally used. Regulation of flow rate is determined by blood pressure response. Consult physician for specific guidelines.
- Blood volume depletion must be continuously corrected by appropriate fluid and electrolyte replacement therapy to maintain tissue perfusion and to avoid recurrence of hypotension when norepinephrine is stopped.
- Whole blood or plasma is incompatible with noradrenaline and therefore should be administered separately.
- Patient should be attended constantly while receiving noradrenaline. Take baseline blood pressure and pulse before start of therapy, then every 2 minutes from initiation of drug until stabilization occurs at desired level, then every 5 minutes during drug administration.
- In normotensive patients it is recommended that flow rate be adjusted to maintain blood pressure at low normal (usually 80 to 100 mm Hg systolic). In previously hypertensive patients, systolic is generally maintained no higher than 40 mm Hg *below* preexisting systolic level.
- In addition to vital signs, carefully observe and record mentation (index of cerebral circulation), skin temperature of extremities, and colour (especially of earlobes, lips, nail beds).
- Flow rate must be constantly monitored. Check infusion site frequently for free flow (adhesive tape should not obscure injection site). Report immediately any evidence of extravasation: blanching along course of infused vein (may occur without obvious extravasation), cold, hard swelling around injection site.
- Monitor fluid intake and output. Urinary retention and renal shutdown are possibilities, especially in hypovolaemic patients. Urinary output is a sensitive indicator of the degree of renal perfusion. Report decrease in urinary output or change in intake–output ratio.
- Be alert to patient's complaints of headache, vomiting, palpitation, arrhythmias, chest pain, photophobia, and blurred vision as possible symptoms of overdosage. Reflex bradycardia may occur as a result of rise in blood pressure.
- Emergency drugs should be immediately available in the event of cardiac irregularities. Atropine is an antidote for bradycardia; cardiac arrhythmias may be treated with propranolol.

N

NORADRENALINE (continued)

■ If therapy is to be prolonged, it is advisable to change infusion sites at intervals to allow effect of local vasoconstriction to subside.

■ When therapy is to be discontinued, infusion rate is slowed gradually. Abrupt withdrawal should be avoided. Continue to monitor vital signs and observe patient closely after cessation of therapy for clinical sign of circulatory inadequacy.

■ Do not use solution if discolouration or precipitate is present. Protect from light.

Drug interactions   Noradrenaline should be used cautiously and in small doses in patients receiving drugs that may potentiate its pressor effects: some **antihistamines** (especially **dexchlorpheniramine, diphenhydramine, tripelennamine**), **parenteral ergot alkaloids, guanethidine, methyldopa**, and **tricyclic antidepressants**. Noradrenaline should be administered with, extreme caution in patients receiving **MAO inhibitors** (possibility of severe and prolonged hypertension in some patients). Concurrent administration of noradrenaline with **cyclopropane** or **halothane** and related general anaesthetics may lead to ventricular arrhythmias. Administration of noradrenaline to patients already receiving **propranolol** may result in high elevations of blood pressure.

Nortriptyline

N

(Allergron, Aventyl)   *Antidepressant; tricyclic*

ACTIONS AND USES   Dibenzocycloheptane derivative of amitriptyline. Tricyclic antidepressant (TCA) with less sedative and anticholinergic effects than imipramine (q.v.). Action mechanism unclear; mood elevation may be due to its inhibition of reuptake of norepinephrine at the presynaptic membrane.

Used to treat endogenous depression. Similar in actions, uses, limitations, and interactions to imipramine.

ROUTE AND DOSAGE   Oral: Adult: *Initial*, 20–40 mg/day increased to a maximum of 100 mg/day in divided doses. *Maintenance* 30–75 mg/day. **Enuresis**: **Child (7 yrs)**: 10 mg; **(8–11 yrs)**: 10–20 mg; **(over 11 yrs)**: 25–35 mg at night, for a maximum period of 3 months.

ABSORPTION AND FATE   Hepatic metabolism; 95% protein binding. **Serum half-life**: 31 ± 13 hours. Effective plasma levels: 50 to 150 ng/ml. Excreted primarily in urine. Crosses placenta; excreted in breast milk.

CONTRAINDICATIONS AND PRECAUTIONS   Children under 12 years of age; pregnancy, lactation, during or within 14 days of MAO inhibitors therapy; acute recovery period after myocardial infarction. **Cautious Use**: narrow-angle glaucoma, hyperthyroidism, concurrent administration of thyroid medications, concurrent use with electroshock therapy. *See also imipramine.*

NORTRIPTYLINE (continued)

ADVERSE/SIDE EFFECTS   Urinary retention, paralytic ileus, orthostatic hypotension, drowsiness, confusional state (especially in the elderly and with high dosage), agranulocytosis, tremors, hyperhydrosis, dry mouth, blurred vision, photosensitivity reaction. *See also imipramine.*

NURSING IMPLICATIONS

- Nortriptyline has a narrow therapeutic plasma level range, a characteristic called 'therapeutic window.' Note that drug levels either above or below the therapeutic window of this drug are associated with decreased rate of response.
- Therapeutic response may not occur for 2 weeks or more.
- If psychotic signs increase, notify physician. Because of the therapeutic window effect of nortriptyline, a substitute TCA may be prescribed rather than an increase in dosage.
- Store drug in tightly closed container preferably between 15° and 30°C (59° and 86°F) unless otherwise specified by manufacturer.
- *See imipramine.*

Nystatin

(Nystan, Nystatin-Dome, Nystaform, Tinaderm-M)   *Antifungal; antiinfective*

ACTIONS AND USES   Antifungal antibiotic produced by *Streptomyces noursei*. Has fungistatic and fungicidal activity against a variety of yeasts and fungi; not appreciably active against bacteria, viruses, or protozoa. Thought to act by binding to sterols in fungal cell membrane, thereby changing membrane potential and allowing leakage of intracellular components. Reportedly nontoxic, topical preparations are nonstaining even with prolonged administration.

Used to treat infections of skin and mucous membranes caused by *Candida* species.

ROUTE AND DOSAGE   Oral tablet: **Adults:** *intestinal candidiasis*: 500,000 units/6 hourly. **Child:** 100,000 units 4 times a day. Used as a mouthwash for oral conditions and as cream for skin conditions. **Pessary:** 100,000 units 1 or 2 inserted high in the vagina for 14 consecutive nights. **Pastilles:** 100,000 units one sucked slowly 4 times a day after food.

ABSORPTION AND FATE   Poorly absorbed following oral administration; no detectable blood levels at recommended doses. Excreted in stool as unchanged drug. Not absorbed from intact skin or mucous membrane.

CONTRAINDICATIONS AND PRECAUTIONS   Hypersensitivity to nystatin or to any components in formulation.

ADVERSE/SIDE EFFECTS   Usually mild: nausea, vomiting, epigastric distress, diarrhoea, (especially with high oral doses), hypersensitivity reactions (rare).

NYSTATIN (continued)
NURSING IMPLICATIONS

- Management of factors predisposing to candidiasis is equally as important as treatment in preventing reinfection and eliminating deep-seated infections.
- Avoid contact of drug with hands. Hypersensitivity reactions occur rarely with nystatin alone; reportedly, preservatives used in some formulations are associated with a high incidence of contact dermatitis.
- Advise patient to report onset of redness, swelling, or irritation. Drug should be discontinued if these symptoms occur.
- *Oral candidiasis* (*thrush*): Divide prescribed dose of oral suspension so that one-half is placed in each side of mouth. Mouth should be clear of food debris before drug administration. Instruct patient to keep medication in contact with oral mucosa for at least several minutes, if possible before swallowing. For infants, medication may be applied by means of swab.
- Advise patient to brush teeth, or at least or rinse mouth thoroughly after each meal and to floss teeth daily. (Patients with dentures should remove and clean them also after each meal.) Overuse of commercial mouth washes tends to change oral flora and therefore should be avoided.
- In elderly patients, oral candidiasis has been associated with poorly fitting dentures. If this is a problem, advise patient to contact dentist.
- Treatment of oral candidiasis should be continued for at least 48 hours after symptoms have subsided and mouth cultures are normal. Pending laboratory confirmation, articles contaminated by mouth contact should be kept isolated for the patient's use or concurrently disinfected.
- *Candidiasis of feet, skin, and nails*: For candidal infection of feet, instruct patient to dust shoes and stockings, as well as feet, with nystatin dusting powder.
- Proper hygiene and skin care to prevent spread of infection and reinfection are essential aspects of therapy. Advise patient to change stockings and underclothing daily and to use own linen and towels.
- Occlusive dressings (including tight-fitting underclothing) or applications of ointment preparation to moist, dark areas of body favour growth of yeast and therefore should be avoided.
- Cream formulation is preferred to the ointment for intertriginous areas. For very moist lesions, powder formulation is usually prescribed. Consult physician.
- Infected areas should be cleaned gently before each application. Use of harsh soaps and vigorous scrubbing are contraindicated. Some physicians prescribe moist compresses with cool water for 15 minutes prior to application of medication (for soothing and drying action). Consult physician for specific guidelines.
- Treatment of cutaneous candidal infections is usually continued for at least 2 weeks; discontinued only after two negative tests for *Candida*.
- *Paronychia*: Advise patient to keep hands out of water as much as possible. Medication should be applied to nails and paronychial folds. Chronic paronychia may require several months of therapy to achieve clinical and mycologic cure. Relapses may be due to reinfection from Candida in intestinal tract.
- *Intestinal candidiasis*: To prevent relapse, therapy is continued for at least 48 hours after symptoms have disappeared (vomiting, diarrhoea, abdominal cramps, oesophagitis).

NYSTATIN (continued)

- *Vulvovaginal candidiasis*: Inform patient that medication should be continued during menstruation. In most cases 2 weeks of therapy are sufficient; however, some patients may require longer treatment.
- In pregnant patients, vaginal tablets may be continued for 3 to 6 weeks before term in order to prevent thrush in newborns.
- Possible predisposing factors should be considered, e.g., diabetes, pregnancy, infection by sexual partner, use of birth control pills, history of antibiotic therapy (candidal infections have occurred 6 to 8 weeks after therapy), corticosteroid therapy, use of close-fitting nylon tights.
- Nystatin is preserved in tightly covered, light-resistant containers, away from heat. Expiration dates vary with manufacturer.

Oestradiol

(Benztrone, Hormonin, Progynova)   *Hormone; oestrogen*

ACTIONS AND USES   Natural or synthetic steroid hormone produced by ovaries. Essential for normal maturation of the female and for maintenance of normal menstrual cycles during reproductive years. Promotes endometrial lining development and increases volume, acidity, and glycogen content of vaginal secretions. Weakly anabolic; large doses induce sodium and fluid retention. Decreases, intestinal motility but stimulates uterine motility. By unclear mechanism, contributes to moulding of body contours, shaping the skeleton and acceleration of epiphyseal closure of long bones. Decreases bone resorption rate which is accelerated at time of menopause. Oestrogen therapy increases risk of thrombosis in women receiving hormone for postpartum breast engorgement and in men receiving oestrogens for prostatic cancer; also increases risk of endometrial carcinoma and gall-bladder disease in postmenopausal women. May mask onset of climacteric. Men receiving large doses of oestrogens are more prone than nonusers to nonfatal myocardial infarction, pulmonary embolism, and thrombophlebitis. There is no evidence that oestrogen therapy for postmenopausal women increases risk of breast cancer. Furthermore, recent studies support the position that the healthy postmenopausal woman need not fear thrombosis or hypercoagulation from combination oestrogen/progesterone therapy.

Used to treat natural or surgical menopausal symptoms (except nervous symptoms or depression), kraurosis vulvae, atrophic vaginitis, primary ovarian failure and female hypogonadism. Also used to prevent and treat postmenopausal osteoporosis and as palliative for advanced prostatic carcinoma and inoperable breast cancer in women at least 5 years postmenopause. Combined with progestins in many oral contraceptive formulations.

ROUTE AND DOSAGE   Generally, lowest effective dosage for shortest possible time to decrease adverse effects; highly individualized depending on the preparation.

OESTRADIOL (continued)

ABSORPTION AND FATE   Readily absorbed from GI tract. **Half-life**: 50 minutes. 50 to 80% binding with plasma proteins. Enters cells of oestrogen responsive tissues (female genital organs, breasts, pituitary and hypothalamus) and by unknown mechanism is transported to the nucleus where it stimulates DNA, RNA and protein synthesis. (The palliative response to oestrogen treatment in women with metastasic cancer of breast results from the presence of these receptor proteins.) Large amounts of free oestrogen excreted into bile, reabsorbed from GI tract and recirculated through liver, principle site of degradation. Excretion primarily in urine as sulphates and glucuronides; small amounts present in faeces. Crosses placenta and appears in breast milk.

CONTRAINDICATIONS AND PRECAUTIONS   Oestrogen hypersensitivity, known or suspected pregnancy, oestrogenic-dependent neoplasms, breast cancer (except in selected patients being treated for metastatic disease). History of active thromboembolic disorders, arterial thrombosis, or thrombophlebitis; undiagnosed abnormal genital bleeding; history of cholestatic disease; thyroid dysfunction, blood dyscrasias. **Cautious Use**: Adolescents with incomplete bone growth; endometriosis, lactation, hypertension, cardiac insufficiency, diseases of calcium and phosphate metabolism, cerebrovascular disease, mental depression, benign breast disease, family history of breast or genital tract neoplasm; diabetes mellitus, gall-bladder disease, preexisting leiomyoma, abnormal mammogram, history of idiopathic jaundice of pregnancy; varicosities, asthma, epilepsy, migraine headaches, hepatic or renal dysfunction; jaundice, acute intermittent porphyria, pyridoxine deficiency.

ADVERSE/SIDE EFFECTS   These include: skin rash, photosensitivity, pruritus, acne, chloasma, melasma, loss of scalp hair, hirsutism, chorea, scotomata, steepening of corneal curvature, intolerance to contact lenses, nausea, vomiting, anorexia, diarrhoea, abdominal cramps, bloating, cholestatic jaundice, thirst, benign hepatoadenoma, mastodynia, breast secretion, changes in vaginal bleeding pattern, spotting, changes in menstrual flow, vaginal candidiasis, reactivation of endometriosis, increased size of preexisting fibromyomata. Thromboembolic disorders, reduced carbohydrate tolerance, hypercalcaemia, hypertension, leg cramps, oedema, weight gain or loss, aggravation of porphyria, abdominal pain, changes in libido, fatigue, backache, cystitis like syndrome. **In males**: gynaecomastia, testicular atrophy, feminization, impotence (reversible).

NURSING IMPLICATIONS

- Take oral medication with or immediately after solid food to reduce nausea.
- Nausea, frequently at breakfast time, seldom interferes with eating or causes weight loss and usually disappears after 1 or 2 weeks of drug use.
- In some cases, a progestational agent is added to the last 5 days of each cycle of oestrogen therapy to produce more regularity.
- A complete history (including menstrual pattern) and physical examination with particular reference to blood pressure, eyes, breasts, abdomen and pelvic organs, and including Pap smear should precede initiation of oestrogen therapy and be repeated every 6 to 12 months during treatment.
- Withdrawal bleeding may occur even after oophorectomy and after menopause.

OESTRADIOL (continued)

Inform postmenopausal women that such bleeding is pseudomenstruation and does not indicate return of fertility.

- If a patient has intermittent bleeding or begins to bleed without having previously done so, she should promptly report to her physician for an evaluation. Breakthrough bleeding may be stopped by increasing oestrogen dose; however if bleeding persists, the physician may recommend curettage.
- Advise patient to report abdominal pain and tenderness or abdominal mass, possible symptoms of hepatic adenoma and/or hepatic haemorrhage.
- If user suspects she is pregnant, she should stop taking the oestrogen immediately and inform the physician. She should be told about the potential risk of masculinization of female foetus.
- Cyclic fluid retention should be reported. A low-salt diet and diuretic may be prescribed.
- During intensive therapy with oestrogens, monitor vital signs and chart for comparison purposes. A gradual increase in blood pressure and pulse readings over time is reportable.
- Be alert to the possibility of behaviour changes or increasing mental depression, symptoms that may suggest recurrence of pretreatment psychic disorders. Report to physician; drug will usually be discontinued.
- Instruct patient to report the following symptoms of thromboembolic disorders immediately: tenderness, swelling, and redness in extremity; sudden, severe headache or chest pain; sudden slurring of speech; sudden change in vision; tenderness, pain, sudden shortness of breath. If physician is not available, patient should go to the nearest hospital emergency room.
- *Teach patient how to elicit Homan's sign*: pain in calf and popliteal region with forced dorsiflexion of foot (early sign of thrombosis).
- Symptoms of vaginal candidiasis (thick, white, curdlike secretions and inflamed congested introitus) should be reported to permit appropriate treatment.
- Reassure male patients that oestrogen-induced feminization and impotence are reversible with termination of therapy.
- Since oestradiol decreases free thyroxine, patient on therapy for a nonfunctioning thyroid may need an increase in thyroid replacement agent while also receiving an oestrogen.
- History of jaundice in pregnancy increases the possibility of oestrogen-induced jaundice. Instruct patient to report yellow skin and sclera, pruritus, dark urine, and light-coloured stools oestrogen therapy is usually interrupted pending clinical investigation.
- Advise patient to determine weight under standard conditions 1 or 2 times/week and to report sudden weight gain or other signs of fluid retention.
- Menopausal symptoms in well-controlled patients on oestrogens begin to return in full intensity by end of rest period without oestrogen.
- Advise diabetic users to report positive urine tests promptly. Dosage adjustment of antidiabetic drug may be indicated. Stress necessity of periodic clinical evaluation for the potential diabetic (family history).
- **Smoking–drug interaction**   Recent studies suggest that smoking increases serum

O

OESTRADIOL (continued)

oestradiol and oestrone concentrations. Since incidence of heart attack in men treated with oestrogen is known to increase, smoking behaviour should be discussed with patient on oestrogen therapy.

Food–drug interactions

- Oestrogenic depression of caffeine metabolism may cause caffeinism. Urge patient to decrease caffeine intake from sources such as tea, coffee, cola.
- Pyridoxine (Vitamin B_6) levels are lowered by oestrogens. A supplement may be ordered for the patient on long-term therapy, especially if undernourished.

- Emphasize need for compliance with established dosage schedule which should not be altered unless physician prescribes a change.
- If patient forgets a dose, she should take it as soon as remembered, unless it is near the time for the next dose. In that case, she should take it on time and without doubling the amount.
- Teach self-examination of breasts, emphasizing a monthly schedule.
- Long-term or high-dosage therapy with oestrogens is reduced or terminated gradually.
- When hypercalcaemia (*normal serum calcium*: 8.5 to 10.5 mg/dl) occurs in patient with breast cancer, it usually indicates progression of bone metastasis; oestrogen treatment is usually terminated.
- Severe hypercalcaemia may be caused by oestradiol therapy in patients with breast cancer and bone metastasis. Monitor carefully in order to identify symptoms promptly: hypotonicity of muscles, deep bone and flank pain, polyuria, extreme thirst, GI symptoms, mental confusion, lethargy, cardiac arrhythmia. Discontinuation of oestrogen is indicated with institution of measures to encourage calcium excretion.
- Caution patient to be careful about exposure to sun lamps and to sun. Oestrogen users sometimes sunburn more easily and develop brown, blotchy spots on exposed skin (reversible with termination of therapy).
- Acute overdosage of an oestrogen does not have serious effects even in small children. Nausea may occur and withdrawal bleeding may result. Notify physician.
- *Cosmetic use*: Systemic effects have followed excessive use of oestrogen creams in cosmetic preparations (oedema, vaginal bleeding, nausea, vomiting).
- Dermal thickness may be slightly increased by oestrogen cosmetic cream, but usually without altering facial appearance.
- There is no scientific evidence that oestrogen creams as cosmetics are more effective than simple emolients in relieving dry skin.
- The pathologist should be advised of oestrogen therapy when relevant specimens are submitted; the dentist should know if extraction or periodontal surgery is anticipated and in an emergency, the attending physician should be informed.
- Oestrogen treatment is usually interrupted at least 4 weeks before surgery that may be associated with a prolonged period of immobilization or with vascular complications.
- If liver or endocrine function tests are abnormal, they should be repeated after oestrogen has been withdrawn for two cycles.
- Protect tablets from light and moisture in well-closed container. Store between 15°

OESTRADIOL (continued)

and 30°C (59° and 86°F) and protect from freezing, unless otherwise directed by manufacturer.

Diagnostic test interferences   Oestradiol reduces response of **metyrapone** test and excretion of **pregnanediol**. *Increases*: **BSP** retention, noradrenaline-induced **platelet aggregability**, hydrocortisone, **PBI**, T_4, sodium, thyroxine-binding globulin (TBG), prothrombin and factors **VII, VIII, IX and X**; triglyceride and lipoprotein (especially HDL) concentrations, **renin** substrate. *Decreases*: **antithrombin III**, pyridoxine and **serum folate** concentrations, **serum cholesterol**, values for the T_3 **resin uptake** test, **glucose tolerance**. May cause false-positive test for **LE cells** and/or antinuclear antibodies (**ANA**).

DRUG INTERACTIONS   *Oestradiol (oestrogens)*

PLUS	INTERACTIONS
Anticoagulants, oral	Oestradiol decreases anticoagulant activity by increasing action of selected clothing factors
Antidiabetic agents	Decreases glucose tolerance
Anticonvulsants Barbiturates Carbamazepine Phenylbutazone Primidone Rifampicin	Decrease oestrogen effect by increasing rate of hepatic breakdown of oestrogen
Corticosteroids	Potentiates antiinflammatory and glycosuric effects of hydrocortisone
Pethidine	Increases narcotic effect by depressing hepatic breakdown
Tricyclic antidepressants	Increases toxicity of antidepressants

O

Oestradiol valerate

(Progynova)   *Hormone; oestrogen*

ACTIONS AND USES   Provides 2 to 3 weeks of oestrogen effects from single IM injection. *See oestradiol*.

Oestrogens, conjugated

(Premarin)   *Oestrogen; postcoital contraceptive (emergency); systemic haemostatic*

OESTROGENS, CONJUGATED (continued)

ACTIONS AND USES   Short-acting oestrogen preparation. Contains mixture of conjugated oestrogens, including sodium oestrone sulphate (50 to 65%) and sodium equilin sulphate (20 to 35%).

Used for atrophic vaginitis and kraurosis vulvae and to arrest abnormal uterine bleeding due to hormonal imbalance; also used to treat hypogonadism, primary ovarian failure, moderate to severe vasomotor symptoms associated with menopause; to prevent postpartum breast engorgement, to retard progression of osteoporosis, and as palliative therapy of mammary and prostatic carcinomas. *See oestradiol*.

Orciprenaline

(Alupent)   *Adrenoceptor stimulant*

ACTIONS AND USES   Partially selective adrenoceptor stimulant used in reversible airway obstruction.

ROUTE AND DOSAGE   Oral: **Adult**: 20 mg 4 times a day. **Child (up to 1 yr)**: 5–10 mg 3 times a day, **(1–3 yrs)**: 5–10 mg 4 times a day; **(3–12 yrs)**: 40–60 mg/day in divided doses. **IM (deep injection)**: **Adult**: 500 mcg repeated after 30 min if required. **Child (up to 6 yrs)**: 250 mcg, over 6 yrs 500 mcg. **Aerosol**: **Adult**: 670–1340 mcg (1–2 puffs) maximum 12 puffs a day. **Child (up to 6 yrs)**: 670 mcg (1 puff) 6 times a day. **Child (over 6 years)** as for adult.

O

Orphenadrine citrate

(Norflex)   *Anticholinergic;*
                                                                             antiparkinsonian agent;
                                                                             skeletal muscle relaxant

Orphenadrine hydrochloride

(Disipal)

ACTIONS AND USES   Tertiary amine anticholinergic agent and centrally acting skeletal muscle relaxant. Structurally similar to diphenhydramine (q.v.), and also closely related to chlorphenoxamine. Relaxes tense skeletal muscles indirectly, possibly by analgesic action or by atropine-like central action. Has some local anaesthetic and antihistaminic activity, but less than that of diphenhydramine. Also produces slight euphoria.

ORPHENADRINE HYDROCHLORIDE (continued)

Used as the citrate to relieve muscle spasm discomfort associated with acute musculo-skeletal conditions. The hydrochloride is used as an adjunct in the treatment of all forms of parkinsonism (arteriosclerotic, idiopathic, postencephalitic).

ROUTE AND DOSAGE   *Orphenadrine citrate*: **Oral**: 100–300 mg/day in divided doses. **IM**: 20–40 mg as required. **Intravenous**: 60 mg; may be repeated every 12 hours, if necessary. *Orphenadrine hydrochloride*: **Oral**: 50 mg three times daily. Doses up to 400 mg daily if necessary and tolerated.

ABSORPTION AND FATE   Readily absorbed following oral administration. **Peak effect** in about 2 hours; **duration**: approximately 4 to 6 hours. Rapidly distributed in tissues. **Plasma half-life**: 14 hours. Extensively metabolized; 60% excreted in urine within 3 days, 8% as unchanged drug.

CONTRAINDICATIONS AND PRECAUTIONS   Narrow-angle glaucoma, pyloric or duodenal obstruction, stenosing peptic ulcers, prostatic hypertrophy or bladder neck obstruction, myasthenia, gravis, cardiospasm (megaloesophagus). Safe use during pregnancy, in women of childbearing potential, and in the paediatric age group not established. **Cautious Use**: history of tachycardia, cardiac decompensation, arrhythmias, coronary insufficiency.

ADVERSE/SIDE EFFECTS   These include: drowsiness, weakness, headache, dizziness; mild CNS stimulation (high doses): restlessness, anxiety, tremors, confusion, hallucinations, agitation, tachycardia, palpitation, syncope, dry mouth, nausea, vomiting, abdominal cramps, constipation, urinary hesitancy or retention, increased ocular tension, dilated pupils, blurred vision.

NURSING IMPLICATIONS
- Note that orphenadrine citrate and orphenadrine hydrochloride are not interchangeable. *See Route and Dosage.*
- Periodic studies of blood, urine, and liver function are recommended with prolonged therapy.
- Complaints of mouth dryness, urinary hesitancy or retention, headache, tremors, GI problems, palpitation, or rapid pulse should be communicated to physician. Dosage reduction or drug withdrawal is indicated.
- Mouth dryness may be relieved by frequent rinsing with clear tepid water, increasing noncaloric fluid intake, sugarless gum or lemon drops.
- Keep physician informed of therapeutic drug effect. In the patient with parkinsonism, orphenadrine reduces muscular rigidity, but has little effect on tremors. Some reduction in excessive salivation and perspiration may occur and patient may appear mildly euphoric.
- Caution patient to avoid driving and other potentially hazardous activities until reaction to drug is known.
- Warn patient that concomitant use of alcohol and other CNS depressants may result in potentiation of depressant effects.
- The elderly patient is particularly sensitive to anticholinergic effects (urinary

O

ORPHENADRINE HYDROCHLORIDE (continued)

hesitancy, constipation) and therefore should be closely observed. Have patient void before taking drug.

- Protect orphenadrine from light.

Drug interactions   Based on limited clinical studies, concomitant use with **phenothiazines** may result in reduced phenothiazine levels or hypoglycaemia, and patients receiving propoxyphene and orphenadrine concomitantly may manifest confusion, anxiety, tremors.

Oxaminiquine

(Mansil, Vansil)   *Anthelmintic*

ACTIONS AND USES   Tetrahydroquinone derivative prepared in the presence of *Aspergillus sclerotiorum*.

Used to treat all stages of *Schistosoma mansoni* infection, including acute and chronic phases with hepatosplenic involvement.

Oxazepam

(Oxanid)   *Anxiolytic; benzodiazepine*

ACTIONS AND USES   Benzodiazepine derivative related to chlordiazepoxide with which it shares actions, uses, limitations and interactions. Has shorter duration of action, and causes fewer adverse/side effects than chlordiazepoxide (q.v.).

Used in management of anxiety and tension, associated with a wide range of emotional disturbances. Also used to control acute withdrawal symptoms in chronic alcoholism.

ROUTE AND DOSAGE   Oral: Anxiety: 10 to 30 mg, three or four times per day. **Elderly, debilitated**: 10 mg three times per day.

ABSORPTION AND FATE   Following absorption from GI tract, peak plasma concentrations occur in 2 to 4 hours. About 90% protein bound. Metabolized in liver. **Plasma half-life**: 3 to 21 hours. Excreted slowly in urine, primarily as glucuronide, and in faeces as unchanged drug. Most of a given dose is excreted within 2 days.

CONTRAINDICATIONS AND PRECAUTIONS   Hypersensitivity to oxazepam and other benzodiazepines; psychoses, pregnancy, lactation, children under age 12, acute-angle glaucoma, acute alcohol intoxication. **Cautious Use**: elderly and debilitated patients;

OXAZEPAM (continued)

impaired renal and hepatic function, addiction-prone patients, mental depression, and chronic obstructive airways disease.

ADVERSE/SIDE EFFECTS   These include: drowsiness, dizziness, mental confusion, vertigo, ataxia, headache, lethargy, syncope, tremor, slurred speech, paradoxic reaction (euphoria, excitement), nausea, xerostomia, jaundice, skin rash, oedema, hypotension, leucopenia, altered libido oedema.

NURSING IMPLICATIONS

- Continued effectiveness of response to oxazepam should be reassessed at end of 4 months. Urge patient to keep appointments with physician.
- Elderly patients should be observed closely for signs of overdosage. Report to physician if daytime psychomotor function is depressed.
- Mild paradoxic stimulation of affect and excitement with sleep disturbances may occur within the first 2 weeks of therapy. Report promptly. Dosage reduction is indicated.
- Liver function tests and blood counts should be performed on a regular planned basis.
- Instruct patients not to change dose or dose schedule. Furthermore, they should not give any of the drug to another person and should refrain from using it to treat a self-diagnosed condition.
- Advise patient to consult physician before self-medicating with OTC drugs.
- Caution patient against driving a car or operating dangerous machinery until response to drug has been evaluated.
- Warn patient not to drink alcoholic beverages while being treated with oxazepam. The CNS depressant effects of each agent may be intensified.
- Patient should be advised that if she becomes pregnant during therapy or intends to become pregnant she should communicate with her physician about the desirability of discontinuing the drug.
- Excessive and prolonged use may cause physical dependence.
- Following prolonged therapy, drug should be withdrawn slowly to avoid precipitating withdrawal symptoms (seizures, mental confusion, nausea, vomiting, muscle and abdominal cramps, tremulousness, sleep disturbances, unusual irritability, hyperhydrosis).
- Store in well-closed container at temperature between 15° and 30°C (59° and 86°F) unless otherwise specified by manufacturer.
- *See also chlordiazepoxide.*

O

Oxpentifylline

(Trental)

ACTIONS AND USES   Vasodilator used in peripheral vascular disease.

ROUTE AND DOSAGE   Oral: 400 mg 2–3 times a day. See nicotinic acid.

Oxprenolol

(Apsolox, Laracor, Slow-pren, Slow-Trasicor, Trasicor)

Antihypertensive; beta-adrenocepror blocking agent; antianginal; antiarrythmic

ACTIONS AND USES   Used in the treatment of hypertension, angina, cardiac arrythmias and thyrotoxicosis. For further information: *see pindolol.*

ROUTE AND DOSAGE   Oral: Adult: *hypertension*: 80 mg twice a day initially, increased as required at weekly intervals. *Angina*: 40–160 mg three times a day. *Thyrotoxicosis*: 40–120 mg/day in divided doses. Maximum dose 480 mg/day. **IV**: slow injection 2 mg repeated after 5 min as required, maximum 16 mg. *Arrhythmias*: *initial* 20–40 mg three times a day. *See propranolol.*

Oxymetazoline hydrochloride

(Afrazine, Iliadin)

Alpha-adrenergic agonist; decongestant

ACTIONS AND USES   Imidazoline-derivative sympathomimetic agent structurally and pharmacologically related to naphazoline. Direct action on alpha receptors of sympathetic nervous system produces constriction of smaller arterioles in nasal passages and prolonged decongestant effect. Has no effect on beta receptors.

Used for relief of nasal congestion in a variety of allergic and infectious disorders of the upper respiratory tract.

ROUTE AND DOSAGE   Topical: depends on the preparation. Usually twice a day.

CONTRAINDICATIONS AND PRECAUTIONS   Hypersensitivity to drug components; use in children under 6 years of age. Safe use in women of childbearing potential and during pregnancy not established. **Cautious Use**: within 14 days of MAO inhibitors, coronary artery disease, hypertension, hyperthyroidism, diabetes mellitus.

ADVERSE/SIDE EFFECTS   Burning, stinging, dryness of nasal mucosa, sneezing. With excessive use: headache, lightheadedness, drowsiness, insomnia, palpitation, rebound congestion.

NURSING IMPLICATIONS
- Usually administered in the morning and at bedtime. Effects appear within 30 minutes and last about 6 to 7 hours.
- If necessary, patient should blow nose gently with both nostrils open to clear nasal passages before administration of medication.
- Nasal spray is delivered with patient in upright position. Place spray nozzle in nostril

OXYMETAZOLINE HYDROCHLORIDE (continued)

without occluding it, and have patient bend head slightly forward and sniff briskly during administration.

- Lateral, head-low position is recommended for instillation of nose drops.
- Rinse dropper or spray tip in hot water after each use to prevent contamination of solution by nasal secretions.
- Caution patient not to exceed prescribed or recommended dosage. Rebound congestion (chemical rhinitis) may occur with prolonged or excessive use.
- Systemic effects can result from swallowing excessive medication.
- Advise patient to keep drug out of reach of children and not to permit use of the medication by anyone.

Oxymetholone

(Anapolon)   *Androgen; anabolic*

ACTIONS AND USES   Potent steroid with androgenic: anabolic activity ratio approximately 1:3. Used to treat aplastic anaemia.

ROUTE AND DOSAGE   *Aplastic anaemia*: **Adults and children**: 1 to 5 mg/kg body weight per day. Highly individualized.

NURSING IMPLICATIONS

- Periodic liver function tests are especially important for the elderly patient. Drug should be stopped with first sign of liver toxicity (jaundice).
- Oxymetholone does not replace supportive measures for treatment of anaemia (such as transfusions and correction of iron, folic acid, vitamin B_{12}, or pyridoxine deficiency).
- A course of therapy for treatment of osteoporosis is 7 to 21 days.
- For treatment of anaemias, a minimum trial period of 3 to 6 months is recommended, since response tends to be slow.
- Optimal effects in treatment of osteoporosis are usually experienced in 4 to 6 weeks.
- *See ethinyloestradiol.*

O

Oxytetracycline

(Berkmycin, Oxymycin, Terramycin, Unimycin,   *Antiinfective; antibacterial;*
  Imperacin)   *tetracycline*

ACTIONS AND USES   Broad-spectrum antibiotic with actions, uses, contraindications, precautions, and adverse reactions similar to those of tetracycline (q.v.).

OXYTETRACYCLINE (continued)
ROUTE AND DOSAGE   Adults: Oral: 250 to 500 mg every 6 hours.

ABSORPTION AND FATE   Adequately but incompletely absorbed from GI tract; **peak plasma concentrations** in 2 to 4 hours. Appears to concentrate in hepatic system. **Half-life**: 6 to 9 hours. Excreted in bile, faeces, and urine in active form. Crosses placenta.

CONTRAINDICATIONS AND PRECAUTIONS   Hypersensitivity to tetracyclines; during tooth development (last half of pregnancy, infancy, childhood to age 8). **Cautious Use**: impaired renal function. *See tetracycline.*

ADVERSE/SIDE EFFECTS   Nausea, vomiting, diarrhoea, stomatitis, skin rash, super-infections, renal toxicity. *See tetracycline.*

NURSING IMPLICATIONS
- Check expiration date. Degradation products of outdated tetracyclines can be highly nephrotoxic. Instruct patient to discard unused drug when course of therapy has ended.
- Food may interfere with rate and extent of absorption of oral drug. Administer at least 1 hour before or 2 hours following meals. Do not give with antacids, milk, milk products, or other calcium-containing foods.
- Caution patient to avoid excessive exposure to sunlight.
- Dosage will require readjustment in the presence of renal dysfunction.
- *See tetracycline.*

Oxytocin injection

(Syntocinon)   *Hormone; oxytocic*

ACTIONS AND USES   Synthetic, water-soluble polypeptide consisting of 8 amino acids, identical pharmacologically to the oxytocic principle of posterior pituitary. By direct action on myofibrils, produces phasic contractions characteristic of normal delivery. Promotes milk ejection (letdown) reflex in nursing mother, thereby increasing flow (not volume) of milk; also facilitates flow of milk during period of breast engorgement. Uterine sensitivity to oxytocin increases during gestation period and peaks sharply before parturition.

Used to initiate or improve uterine contraction at term only in carefully selected patients and only after cervix is dilated and presentation of foetus has occurred; used to stimulate letdown reflex in nursing mother and to relieve pain from breast.

ROUTE AND DOSAGE   *Stimulation or induction of labour*: Intravenous infusion (drip method): 1 to 3 mU/minute adjusted to response. *Control of postpartum uterine bleeding*: Intravenous infusion (drip method): 5 to 10 U added to 500 ml at

OXYTOCIN INJECTION (continued)

15 drops/min according to response. *Milk letdown*: **Nasal spray (40 units/ml)**: one spray into one or both nostrils 2 to 3 minutes before nursing or pumping of breasts.

ABSORPTION AND FATE   Uterine response following IM injection is evidenced in 3 to 7 minutes, with duration of 30 to 60 minutes; after IV injection, response occurs within 1 minute, with shorter duration; following nasal spray, in 5 to 10 minutes. Plasma half-life is 1 minute to several minutes (shorter during late pregnancy and lactation). Rapidly removed from plasma by mammary gland, kidney, and liver and inactivated, perhaps by oxytocinase, an enzyme produced in placenta and uterine tissue during pregnancy. Small portion of dose is excreted in active form by kidney.

CONTRAINDICATIONS AND PRECAUTIONS   Hypersensitivity to oxytocin, significant cephalopelvic disproportion, unfavourable foetal position or presentations which are undeliverable without conversion before delivery, obstetric emergencies where benefit-to-risk ratio for mother or foetus favours surgical intervention, foetal distress where delivery is not imminent, prematurity, placenta praevia, prolonged use in severe toxaemia or uterine inertia, hypertonic uterine patterns, previous surgery of uterus or cervix including Caesarean section, conditions predisposing to thromboplastin or amniotic fluid embolism (dead foetus, abruptio placentae), grand multiparity, invasive cervical carcinoma, primipara over 35 years of age, past history of uterine sepsis or of traumatic delivery, intranasal route during labour, simultaneous administration of drug by two routes. **Cautious Use**: concomitant use with cyclopropane anaesthesia or vasoconstrictive drugs.

ADVERSE/SIDE EFFECTS   Foetus: bradycardia and other arrhythmias, hypoxia, intracranial haemorrhage, trauma from too rapid propulsion through pelvis, neonatal jaundice, death. Mother: hypersensitivity leading to uterine hypertonicity, tetanic contractions, uterine rupture, anaphylactic reactions, postpartum haemorrhage, cardiac arrhythmias, pelvic haematoma, nausea, vomiting, hypertensive episodes, subarachnoid haemorrhage, increased blood flow, fatal afibrinogenaemia, ADH effects leading to severe water intoxication and hyponatraemia, hypotension, ECG changes, PVCs anxiety, dyspnoea, precordial pain, oedema, cyanosis or redness of skin, cardiovascular spasm and collapse. *Citrate*: parabuccal irritation.

NURSING IMPLICATIONS

- When diluting oxytocin for IV infusion, rotate bottle gently to distribute medicine throughout solution.
- Before instituting treatment, start charts to record maternal blood pressure and other vital signs fluid intake–output ratio, weight, strength, duration, and frequency of contractions, as well as foetal heart tone and rate.
- Oxytocin administration should be supervised by persons having thorough knowledge of the drug and the skill to identify complications.
- Use of a Y connection to infusion tubing is advised to allow oxytocin solution to be discontinued if necessary while vein is kept open.
- Oxytocin is incompatible with infusions of fibrinolysin, noradrenaline bitartrate, prochlorperazine edisylate, protein hydrolysate and warfarin sodium.

OXYTOCIN INJECTION (continued)

■ During infusion period, monitor foetal heart rate and maternal blood pressure and pulse at least every 15 minutes; evaluate tonus of myometrium during and between contractions and record on flow chart. Report change in rate and rhythm immediately.

■ If contractions are prolonged (occurring at less than 2-minute intervals) and if monitor records concentrations about 50 mm Hg, or if contractions last 90 seconds or longer, stop infusion to prevent foetal anoxia, turn patient on her side, and notify physician. Stimulation will wane rapidly within 2 to 3 minutes. Oxygen administration may be necessary.

■ The fundus should be checked frequently during the first few postpartum hours and several times daily thereafter.

■ Knowledge of time factors related to onset and duration of effects (*see Absorption and Fate*) is essential for prevention of foetal and maternal crises.

■ Oxytocin should never be administered by more than one route at a time.

■ *Nasal spray*: Instruct patient to clear nasal passages well before administration. Hold squeeze bottle upright, and spray solution into nostril with patient's head in a vertical position.

■ When oxytocin is given to stimulate the letdown of milk, provide measures that support a beneficial response: quiet nonstressful environment, maternal confidence through knowledge and freedom from worry and pain.

■ If local or regional (caudal, spinal) anaesthesia is being given to the patient receiving oxytocin, be alert to the possibility of hypertensive crisis: sudden intense occipital headache, palpitation, marked hypertension, stiff neck, nausea, vomiting, sweating, fever, photophobia, dilated pupils, bradycardia or tachycardia, constricting chest pain.

■ Monitor fluid intake and output during labour. If patient is receiving drug by prolonged IV infusion, watch for symptoms of water intoxication (drowsiness, listlessness, headache, confusion, anuria, weight gain). Report changes in alertness and orientation and changes in intake–output ratio, i.e., marked decrease in output with excessive intake.

■ Unless otherwise directed by manufacturer, store oxytocin solution in refrigerator but do not freeze.

Drug interactions Ephedrine, methoxamine, and other **vasopressors** can cause severe hypertension when administered at same time as oxytocin.

Pancreatin ⎯⎯⎯⎯⎯⎯⎯⎯⎯⎯⎯⎯⎯⎯⎯⎯⎯⎯⎯⎯⎯

(Cotazym, Creon, Nutrizym, Pancrease Pancrex)   *Enzyme*

ACTIONS AND USES Pancreatic enzyme concentrate of bovine or porcine origin containing principally lipase, protease, and amylase in standardized amounts. Assists in digestion of starch, protein, and fats; decreases nitrogen and fat content of stool.

PANCREATIN (continued)

Used as digestive aid in conditions associated with exocrine pancreatic deficiency such as chronic pancreatitis, pancreatectomy or gastrectomy, and cystic fibrosis.

ROUTE AND DOSAGE   Oral: **Adults and children**: with each meal. Dose depends on the preparation.

CONTRAINDICATIONS AND PRECAUTIONS   Cautious Use: history of hypersensitivity reactions to beef or pork products. Safe use during pregnancy not established.

ADVERSE/SIDE EFFECTS   With large doses: anorexia, nausea, vomiting, diarrhoea, buccal and anal soreness (particularly in infants), hyperuricosuria, hypersensitivity reactions (sneezing, lacrimation, skin rashes).

NURSING IMPLICATIONS
- Since pancreatin is inactivated by gastric pepsin and acid pH, it may be prescribed to be taken with or after an antacid or cimetidine.
- Monitor patient for symptoms of diabetes mellitus (polyuria, thirst, hunger, pruritus). Insulin-dependent diabetes frequently occurs in these patients.
- Avoid inhalation of powder formulation.
- Enteric-coated tablets are to be swallowed whole, not crushed or chewed.
- Monitor fluid intake and output and weight. Note appetite, quality of stools, weight loss, abdominal bloating (pancreatic insufficiency may present as diabetes mellitus, steatorrhoea, bulky stools).
- For pancreatic insufficiency, a special diet high in protein and carbohydrates and low in fat (50 g/day) is generally recommened to avoid indigestion. Multivitamin supplements may also be prescribed.
- Periodic measurement of faecal fat and nitrogen, serum carotene and calcium, and prothrombin activity may be made to evaluate response to drug therapy.
- Stored in tight containers at room temperature not exceeding 30°C (86°F).

Drug interactions   Pancreatin may inhibit absorption of oral iron; cimetidine may enhance enzyme effects.

Papaveretum

(Omnopon)   *Analgesic; narcotic*

ACTIONS AND USES   Opiate analgesic used for preoperative sedation and postoperative pain relief.

ROUTE AND DOSAGE   SC/IM: 20 mg/4 hrly. **Slow IV injection**: 25–50% of the SC IM dose. *Preoperative sedation*: **IM/SC**: 10–20 mg, 45–60 minutes preanaesthesia. **Child (up to 1 month)**: 150 mcg/kg; **(1–2 months)**: 200 mcg/kg; **(1–2yrs)**: 200–300 mcg/kg.

For further information: *see morphine.*

P

Paracetamol

(Calpol, Disprol, Paldesic, Panadol, Salzone)   *Analgesic; antipyretic*

ACTIONS AND USES   Principal active metabolite of acetanilid and phenacetin. Analgesic and antipyretic actions, approximately equivalent to those of aspirin, appear to be related to inhibition of prostaglandin synthesis. Unlike aspirin, paracetamol lacks antiplatelet action, generally produces no gastric bleeding and has weak antiinflammatory, uricosuric, and antirheumatic properties. Produces analgesia by unknown mechanism, perhaps by action on peripheral nervous system. Reduces fever by direct action on hypothalamus heat-regulating centre with consequent peripheral vasodilation, sweating, and dissipation of heat. Reportedly has antidiuretic activity. Paracetamol is available OTC.

Used for temporary relief of mild to moderate pain, such as simple headache, minor joint and muscle pains, neuralgia, and dysmenorrhoea, and for control of fever. Generally used as substitute for aspirin when the latter is not tolerated, or is contraindicated (as in anticoagulated patients).

ROUTE AND DOSAGE   **Adults, children (over 11 years): Oral:** 0.5–1 g 4–6 hrly. Maximum 4 g/day. **Child (up to 1 yr):** 60–120 mg; **(1–5 yrs):** 120–250 mg; **(6–12 yrs):** 250–500 mg repeated 4–6 hrly, maximum four doses in 24 hrs.

ABSORPTION AND FATE   Rapidly and almost completely absorbed from GI tract and well distributed in body fluids. Peak blood levels in ½ to 2 hours; duration of action 3 to 4 hours. Variable bioavailability with rectal suppository. About 25% protein bound. **Half-life:** 1 to 3.5 hours. Metabolized in liver. 85% excreted in urine as conjugated paracetamol and other (active and inactive) metabolites; 2 to 4% excreted unchanged. Crosses placenta. Excreted in breast milk.

CONTRAINDICATIONS AND PRECAUTIONS   Hypersensitivity to paracetamol, children under 3 years of age unless directed by a physician; repeated administration to patients with anaemia, or hepatic, renal, cardiac, or pulmonary disease; G6PD deficiency. **Cautious Use:** arthritic or rheumatoid conditions affecting children under 12 years of age; alcoholism, malnutrition, thrombocytopenia.

ADVERSE/SIDE EFFECTS   Negligible with recommended dosage. **Acute poisoning:** *2 to 24 hours postingestion:* anorexia, nausea, vomiting, dizziness, lethargy, generalized weakness, diaphoresis, chills, epigastric or abdominal pain, diarrhoea; *24 to 48 hours postingestion* (often asymptomatic): onset of hepatotoxicity: elevation of serum transaminases (ALT, AST) and bilirubin; 3 to 5 days postingestion: vomiting, jaundice, RUQ tenderness, hepatic necrosis, abnormal liver function tests, hypoglycaemia, metabolic acidosis, hypoprothrombinaemia, hepatic coma, acute renal failure, CNS stimulation or depression, hypothermia, circulatory and acute renal failure. **Chronic ingestion:** haemoglobinaemia, neutropenia, pancytopenia, leucopenia, haemolytic anaemia (rare), thrombocytopenic purpura, agranulocytosis; rarely: methemoglobinaemia (cyanosis of skin, nails, mucous membranes, CNS stimulation, then sulphhaemo-globinaemia de-

P

PARACETAMOL *(continued)*

pression); hypoglycaemia or hyperglycaemia, splenomegaly, acute pancreatitis, psychological changes, hepatic and renal damage. **Hypersensitivity (rare)**: erythematous or urticarial skin rash, drug fever, mucosal lesions, laryngeal oedema.

NURSING IMPLICATIONS

- Tablet may be crushed before administration and taken with fluid of patient's choice.
- Coadministration with a high carbohydrate meal may significantly retard absorption rate.
- Caution patient not to exceed recommended dosage. Overdosing and chronic use can cause liver damage and other toxic effects.
- Patients on prescribed high doses or long-term therapy are advised to have periodic tests of hepatic, renal, and haematopoietic function.
- Individuals with poor nutrition or who have ingested alcohol over prolonged periods are prone to hepatotoxicity even from moderate doses.
- Remind patients who self-medicate that reduction of fever by paracetamol may mask serious illness.
- Paracetamol should not be used by adults and children for self-medication of pain beyond 3 to 5 days without consulting a physician. Additionally, it should not be used for fever persisting longer than 3 days, and never for fever over 39.5°C (103°F), or for recurrent fever without medical direction.
- There is no basis for the claim that paracetamol is safer than aspirin and there is little evidence that combination analgesic formulations have any therapeutic advantage over single component products.
- High abuse potential; psychological dependence can occur.
- Most poisonings result from suicide attempts or accidental ingestion by children. Caution patient to keep paracetamol out of the reach of children.
- ***Treatment of acute poisoning***   Contact regional poison centre for directions in use of acetylcysteine (antidote). Acetylcysteine may prevent hepatic necrosis if administered within 16 hours of overdose. Stomach contents are evacuated by emesis induced with ipecacuanha syrup or gastric lavage. (Administration of activated charcoal is not recommended because it may interfere with absorption of acetylcysteine; however, if it has been used it should be thoroughly removed by lavage.) Obtain serum paracetamol concentration no sooner than 4 hours postingestion. Liver function tests: SGOT (AST), SGPT (ALT), bilirubin, prothrombin time should be obtained initially and every 24 hours for 96 hours. Patient who has ingested a toxic dose should be hospitalized because the onset of hepatic damage is usually insidious and may not be apparent for several days after overdosage.
- Preserved in tightly covered, light-resistant containers, at room temperature preferably between 15° and 30°C (59° and 86°F), unless otherwise directed by manufacturer.

Diagnostic test interferences   Paracetamol may cause (1) false increases in **urinary 5-HIAA** (5-hydroxyindoleacetic acid) by-product of serotonin, (2) false decreases in **blood glucose** (by glucose oxidase-peroxidase procedure), and (3) false increases in **serum uric acid** (with phosphotungstate method).

P

PARACETAMOL (continued)
DRUG INTERACTIONS   *Paracetamol*

PLUS	INTERACTIONS
Alcohol (chronic or excessive ingestion)	Increased risk of hepatotoxicity
Anticoagulants, oral	Possibility of increased anticoagulant (hypoprothrombinaemic) effect
Chloramphenicol	Increased risk of chloramphenicol toxicity (by decreased drug metabolism). Monitor chloramphenicol serum levels
Contraceptives, oral	Decreased analgesic effect (drug metabolism increased)
Diazepam	Increased diazepam effects (decreased diazepam renal excretion)
Phenothiazines	Possibility of severe hypokalaemia

Paraldehyde

Sedative, hypnotic

ACTIONS AND USES   Cyclic ether formed by polymerization of acetaldehyde. Potent CNS depressant with sedative and hypnotic actions similar to those of alcohol, barbiturates, and chloral hydrate.

Used to control convulsions arising from status epilepticus. Now, rarely used.

ROUTE AND DOSAGE   Each 1 ml contains approximately 1 g paraldehyde. **Adults: Intramuscular**: 5 to 10 ml. **Child (0–3 mths):** 0.5 ml; **(3–6 mth):** 1 ml; **(6–12 mth):** 1.5 ml; **(1–2 yrs):** 2ml; **(3–5 yrs):** 3–4 ml; **(6–12 yrs):** 5–6 ml. **Rectal: Adult:** 4–5 ml as 10% solution in saline. **Child:** as for IM dose. **IV route**: may be used in specialist centers.

ABSORPTION AND FATE   Absorbed well from all routes. Hypnotic action within 10 to 15 minutes; effects last 6 to 8 hours or more. **Average half-life**: 7.5 hours. Approximately 70 to 80% of dose is metabolized by liver. Significant amounts (11 to 28%) excreted unchanged through lungs; traces eliminated unchanged in urine. Readily crosses placenta.

CONTRAINDICATIONS AND PRECAUTIONS   Severe hepatic insufficiency, respiratory disease, GI inflammation or ulceration, disulphiram therapy.

ADVERSE/SIDE EFFECTS   Irritation of mucous membrane (oral and rectal routes), nausea, vomiting, unpleasant taste and odour, hangover, dizziness, ataxia, erythematous skin rash; occasionally confusion and paradoxical excitement. IM injection: pain, sterile abscess, necrosis, muscle irritation; thrombophlebitis following IV administration. **Prolonged Use**: toxic hepatitis, nephrosis, metabolic acidosis. **Overdosage:**

PARALDEHYDE (continued)

rapid laboured breathing, respiratory depression, pulmonary haemorrhage and oedema, hypotension, bleeding gastritis, renal and liver damage, acidosis, dilation and failure of right heart, cardiovascular collapse.

NURSING IMPLICATIONS

- Paraldehyde is a colourless clear liquid with a strong characteristic odour and a burning, disagreeable taste.
- On exposure to light, air, and heat, drug liberates acetaldehyde, which oxidizes to acetic acid. Do not use solution if it is coloured in any way or smells of acetic acid (vinegar odour).
- Decomposed paraldehyde is extremely corrosive to tissues and can cause fatal poisoning. Discard unused contents of any container that has been opened for more than 24 hours.
- Do not use plastics for measuring or administering paraldehyde. Contact with plastic syringes, catheters, measuring or drinking cups, or other plastic materials can result in decomposition of paraldehyde to toxic compounds. Parenteral preparation should be drawn into a glass syringe: use rubber catheter for rectal administration.
- When given rectally, drug should be dissolved in 200 ml of 0.9% sodium chloride solution, olive or arachis oil to prevent rectal irritation.
- IM injection should be made deep into upper outer quadrant of buttock well away from nerve trunks. Paraldehyde can cause nerve injury and paralysis. Aspirate carefully before injecting drug, and massage injection site well. Rotate injection sites. Not to exceed 5 ml per injection site.
- When given by IV route (infrequently used), CNS depression may be preceded by a brief period of excitement and coughing. The coughing that sometimes occurs when paraldehyde is given IV may be due to untoward effects on pulmonary capillaries. Monitor patient closely for hypotension and respiratory depression.
- Paraldehyde is not analgesic; therefore, it should not be given to relieve pain. The drug may produce excitement or delirium in the presence of pain.
- Bronchial secretions may be increased. Keep the patient turned on side to prevent aspiration. Suction may be necessary.
- Advise bed rest and no smoking. Bedsides are indicated.
- Keep patient's room well ventilated to control the strong, pungent odour of exhaled drug. The odour may attract flies in the summer. Patient's breath will have a characteristic odour for several hours.
- Tolerance and physical and/or psychological dependence can occur with prolonged use. Paraldehyde addiction resembles alcoholism.
- Rapid withdrawal after prolonged use may produce delirium tremens and hallucinations.
- ***Treatment of overdosage*** Gastric lavage for oral ingestion (if endotracheal tube with cuff is in place to prevent aspiration of vomitus) or rectal lavage for rectal overdosage, followed by demulcent such as mineral oil (orally or by nasogastric tube).
- Preserved in tight, light-resistant containers in amounts not exceeding 30 ml and at temperatures not over 25°C (77°F). Keep away from heat, open flames, and sparks.

P

PARALDEHYDE (continued)

Diagnostic test interferences   Chronic use of alcohol (ethanol) and paraldehyde may cause false-positive **serum ketones** (nitroprusside tube dilution method) and **urine ketones** (Acetest) and may interfere with **urinary steroid (17-OHCS)** determinations by modification of Reddy, Jenkins, Thorn procedure.

Drug interactions   Theoretically, disulphiram may increase blood levels of paraldehyde by inhibiting its metabolism. Paraldehyde may increase blood levels of paraldehyde by inhibiting its metabolism. Paraldehyde may increase the possibility of **sulphonamide** crystalluria (with the less soluble drugs such as sulphadiazine, sulphapyridine, sulphamerazine). Additive effects may result when administered concomitantly with other **CNS depressant drugs**, such as **alcohol, general anaesthetics.**

Penicillamine

(Distamine, Pendramine)   *Chelating agent*

ACTIONS AND USES   Thiol compound prepared by hydrolysis of penicillin but lacking antibacterial activity. Forms stable soluble chelate with copper, zinc, iron, lead, mercury, and possibly other heavy metals and promotes their excretion in urine. Also combines chemically with cystine to form a soluble disulphide complex which prevents stone formation and may even dissolve existing cystitic stones. Mechanism of action in rheumatoid arthritis not known, but appears to be related to inhibition of collagen formation. Cross-sensitivity between penicillin and penicillamine can occur.

Used to promote renal excretion of excess copper in Wilson's disease (hepatolenticular degeneration). Also used in patients with active rheumatoid arthritis who have failed to respond to conventional therapy, and in treatment of moderate asymptomatic lead poisoning.

ROUTE AND DOSAGE   Oral: **Adults: Wilson's** disease: 250 mg four times daily. **Children**: 20 mg/kg/day divided into 4 doses. *Rheumatoid arthritis*: *Initial*: 125 or 250 mg daily. Dosage increase of 125 or 250 mg/day at 1- to 3-month intervals, if necessary. Maximum daily dosage up to 1 to 1.5 g daily.

ABSORPTION AND FATE   Well absorbed from GI tract. **Peak blood levels** in 1 hour. Probably metabolized in liver. Readily excreted in urine and faeces primarily as inactive disulphides. Crosses placenta.

CONTRAINDICATIONS AND PRECAUTIONS   Hypersensitivity to penicillamine or any penicillin; history of penicillamine-related aplastic anaemia or agranulocytosis, patients with rheumatoid arthritis who have renal insufficiency or who are pregnant, during pregnancy in patients with cystinuria, concomitant administration with drugs that can cause severe haematological or renal reactions, e.g., antimalarials, gold salts, immunosuppressants, oxyphenbutazone, phenylbutazone. **Cautious Use**: allergy-prone individuals.

PENICILLAMINE (continued)

ADVERSE/SIDE EFFECTS   These include: anorexia, nausea, vomiting, epigastric pain, diarrhoea, oral lesions, reduction or loss of taste perception (particularly salt and sweet), metallic taste, activation of peptic ulcer, thrombocytopenia, leucopenia, agranulocytosis, thrombotic thrombocytopenic purpura, haemolytic anaemia, aplastic anaemia, cholestatic jaundice, membranous glomerulopathy, Goodpasture's syndrome, proteinuria, haematuria, tinnitus, optic neuritis, thrombophlebitis, hyperpyrexia, alopecia, myasthenia gravis syndrome, mammary hyperplasia, alveolitis, skin friability, excessive skin wrinkling, pancreatitis, pyridoxine deficiency, tingling of feet, ptosis, weakness.

NURSING IMPLICATIONS

- Not to be confused with penicillin.
- Administered on an empty stomach (30 to 60 minutes before or 2 hours after meals) to avoid absorption of metals in foods by penicillamine.
- If patient cannot swallow capsules or tablets, contents may be administered in 15 to 30 ml of chilled fruit juice.
- All patients should be closely monitored throughout therapy. Penicillamine can produce severe toxic reactions involving skin, blood, kidneys, and liver. Most reactions respond favourably if drug is discontinued.
- Allergic reactions occur in about one-third of patients receiving penicillamine. Temporary interruptions of therapy increase possibility of sensitivity reactions.
- Temperature should be taken nightly during first few months of therapy. Fever is a possible early sign of allergy.
- White and differential blood cell counts, direct platelet counts, haemoglobin, and urinalyses should be done prior to initiation of therapy and every 3 days during the first month of therapy then every 2 weeks thereafter. Liver function tests and eye examinations should be performed before start of therapy and at least twice yearly thereafter.
- Instruct patient to observe skin over pressure areas: knees, elbows, shoulder blades, toes, buttocks. Penicillamine increases skin friability. Report unusual bruising or bleeding, sore mouth or throat, fever, skin rash, or any other unusual symptoms.
- For patients undergoing elective surgery, physician may reduce dosage because penicillamine tends to retard tissue healing by inhibiting collagen and elastin formation.
- Physician may prescribe prophylactic doses of pyridoxine (vitamine B_6) because penicillamine interferes with the metabolism of this vitamin.
- Clinical evidence of therapeutic effectiveness may not be apparent until 1 to 3 months of drug therapy.
- *Wilson's disease*: Physician may prescribe sulphurated potash before each meal to minimize absorption of copper.
- Patients with Wilson's disease will require a low copper diet (less than 2 mg copper daily). Foods high in copper that should be avoided include: alcoholic beverages, chocolate, tea, all offal, all shellfish, duck, goose, meat, gelatin, molasses, mushrooms, nuts, dried beans, dried lentils, bran products.
- Drinking water should be analyzed for copper content. Demineralized water should be used if copper content is more than 0.1 mg/L.
- Therapeutic effectiveness in Wilson's disease is indicated by improvement in

P

PENICILLAMINE (continued)

psychiatric and neurological symptoms, visual symptoms, and hepatic function. In some patients, neurological symptoms become more prominent during initial therapy and then subside.

- Optimal dose for patients with Wilson's disease is determined by quantitative anlaysis of urinary copper. Urine must be collected in copper-free container.
- *Rheumatoid arthritis*: Record evidence of drug effectiveness such as improvement in grip strength, decrease in stiffness following immobility, reduction of pain, decrease in sedimentation rate and rheumatoid factor.
- Dosage should be reduced or drug discontinued if the patient with rheumatoid arthritis develops proteinuria or if platelet count drops, or neutropenia occurs.

Drug interactions Potentiation of haematological and renal adverse effects may occur with **antimalarials, cytotoxics, gold therapy, oxyphenbutazone,** and **phenyl-butazone.** Oral iron may inhibit absorption of penicillamine. (Space as far apart as possible.)

Penicillin G ————————————————————————

(Benzyl, Crystapen)   *Antibiotic; penicillin*

ACTIONS AND USES Acid-labile, penicillinase-sensitive, natural penicillin derived from cultures of *Penicillium notatum* or related moulds. Antimicrobial spectrum is relatively narrow compared to that of the semisynthetic penicillins. Bactericidal at therapeutic serum levels; bacteriostatic at lower concentrations. Acts by interfering with synthesis of mucopeptides essential to formation and integrity of bacterial cell wall. Effective primarily on immature cell walls of rapidly growing and dividing cells; minimally or ineffective on dormant or mature organisms. Action is inhibited by penicillinase; therefore penicillin G is ineffective against many strains of *Staphylococcus aureus*. Highly active against gram-positive cocci (e.g., nonpenicillinase-producing *Staphylococcus*, Streptococcus groups A,C,G,H,L,M, and *S. pneumoniae*); and gram-negative cocci (*Neisseria gonorrhoeae, N. meningitidis*). Also effective against gram-positive bacilli (*Bacillus anthracis, Clostridium* species including gas gangrene and tetanus, and certain species of *Corynebacterium, Erysipelothrix,* and *Listeria*); gram negative bacilli (Fusobacterium, Pasteurella, Streptobacillus, and *Bacteroides* species. Parenteral penicillin G is effective against most strains of *Escherichia coli*, all strains of *Proteus mirabilis, Salmonella,* and *Shigella*, and some strains of *Enterobacter aerogenes,* and *Alcaligenes faecalis*); Spirochetes (*Treponema pallidum, T. pertenue, Leptospira*); Actinomycetes (*A. bovis, A. israelii*). The penicillins are not active against fungi, plasmodia, amoebae, rickettsiae, and viruses. In large doses, penicillin G is capable of inhibiting platelet aggregation and may also act as a CNS irritant.

Used in treatment of infections caused by penicillin-sensitive microorganisms: actinomycosis, anthrax, diphtheria (carrier state), empyema, erysipelas, gas gangrene, gonorrheal infections, leptospirosis, mastoiditis, meningitis, acute osteomyelitis, otitis

PENICILLIN G (continued)

media, pinta, pneumonia, rat-bite fever, sinus infections; certain staphylococcal infections; streptococcal infections, including scarlet fever; syphilis (all stages), tetanus, urinary tract infections. Also used as prophylaxis in patients with rheumatic or congenital heart disease.

ROUTE AND DOSAGE   Oral: Adults and Children (over 12 years): IV or IM: 300–600 mg 2–4 times a day. Child (up to 12 yrs): 10–20 mg/kg/day. Neonate: 30 mg/kg/day. IV infusion: up to 24 g/day. Intrathecal: 6–12 mg/day.

ABSORPTION AND FATE   Absorption following oral administration is irregular and incomplete and occurs chiefly in the duodenum. Readily absorbed following IM administration; serum levels peak in 15 to 30 minutes and persist 3 to 5 hours. Diffuses rapidly into most body fluids and tissues including kidneys, liver, skin, bile, lymph; peritoneal, pleural, pericardial, and joint spaces; small amounts of saliva, and prostatic secretion. Adequate absorption into cerebrospinal fluid and eye occurs when inflammation is present. About 45 to 65% bound to plasma proteins. **Half-life:** 30 to 60 minutes. Excreted in urine mostly as unchanged drug (approximately 60 to 90% of IM dose eliminated within 5 hours). Excretion delayed in neonates, young infants, the elderly, and patients with impaired renal function. Small amount excreted in faeces. Crosses placenta. Appears in breast milk.

CONTRAINDICATIONS AND PRECAUTIONS   Hypersensitivity to any of the penicillins or cephalosporins; administration of oral drug to patients with severe infections, nausea, vomiting, hypermotility, gastric dilatation, cardiospasm. **Cautious Use:** history of or suspected atopy or allergy, (asthma, eczema, hay fever, hives); renal or hepatic dysfunction, myasthenia gravis, epilepsy, neonates, young infants. Use in nursing mothers may lead to sensitization of infants.

ADVERSE/SIDE EFFECTS   Electrolyte imbalance: hyperkalamia (penicillin G potassium); hypokalaemia, alkalosis, hypernatraemia, congestive heart failure (penicillin G sodium). **Hypersensitivity reactions.** (1) **immediate** (usually occurs within 2 to 30 minutes after drug administration); *localized anaphylaxis*: itchy palms or axilla or generalized pruritus or urticaria, flushed skin, coughing, sneezing, feeling of uneasiness; *systemic anaphylaxis*: fever, vomiting, diarrhoea, severe abdominal cramps, widespread increase in capillary permeability and vasodilation with resulting oedema (mouth, tongue, pharynx, larynx), laryngospasm, bronchospasm, hypotension, circulatory collapse (anaphylactic shock), cardiac arrhythmias, cardiac arrest. (2) **Accelerated** (occurs in 1 to 72 hours): malaise, fever, urticaria, erythema or other skin reactions and (less commonly) angioneurotic and laryngeal oedema, asthma. (3) **Delayed or late** (develops after 72 hours): *serum sickness* (fever, malaise, pruritus, urticaria, lymphadenopathy, arthralgia, angioedema of face and extremities, neuritis prostration, eosinophilia). Skin rashes ranging from urticaria to exfoliative dermatitis, Stevens-Johnson syndrome, fixed-drug eruptions, contact dermatitis; haemolytic anaemia, granulocytopenia, neutropenia, leucopenia, thrombocytopenia, SLE-like syndrome, interstitial nephritis, Loeffler's syndrome, vasculitis. **Injection site reactions:** pain, inflammation, abscess, phlebitis, thrombophlebiti. **Superinfections:** especially with candida and gram-negative bacteria (e.g., *Proteus, Pseudomonas*). **Toxicity:** bone marrow depression,

P

PENICILLIN G *(continued)*

granulocytopenia, hepatitis (infrequent), neuromuscular irritability: twitching, lethargy, confusion, stupor, hyperreflexia, multifocal myoclonus, localized or generalized seizures, coma.

NURSING IMPLICATIONS

- Before treatment with penicillin is initiated, an exact history should be obtained of patient's previous exposure and sensitivity to penicillins and cephalosporins, and other allergic reactions of any kind.
- Check expiry date on penicillin container or package label.
- *Parenteral administration*: See manufacturer's labelling for directions on preparation of initial dilution. Loosen powder by tapping vial against palm of hand. Holding vial horizontally, rotate it while directing stream of diluent against wall of vial. Shake vial vigorously until powder is completely dissolved. (For IV administration, the initial dilution should be further diluted with 0.9% sodium chloride or 5% dextrose for IV use.)
- Carefully select IM site. Accidental injection into or near a nerve can cause irritation with severe pain and dysfunction. IM injection is made deep into a large muscle mass. Before injecting drug, check for blood back-flow to avoid entering a blood vessel. Inject slowly. Rotate injection sites.
- In high doses, IV penicillin G should be administered slowly to avoid electrolyte imbalance from potassium or sodium content. Physician will prescribe specific flow rate.
- Penicillin is a highly sensitizing substance. Contact dermatitis can occur in certain susceptible individuals who are frequently in contact with the drug. Babies whose mothers are receiving penicillin therapy can be sensitized through breast milk.
- The incidence of hypersensitivity to penicillin among adults is estimated to be between 1% and 5% (reports vary).
- Allergy to penicillin is unpredictable. It has occurred in patients with a negative history of penicillin allergy and also in patients with no known prior contact with penicillin (sensitization may have occurred from penicillin used commercially in foods and beverages, e.g., Roquefort or blue cheese, fowl, beer). Paradoxically, some patients with mild sensitivity have tolerated penicillin at a later date.
- Hypersensitivity reactions are more likely to occur with parenteral penicillin but may also occur with the oral drug. Skin rash is the most common type allergic reaction and should be reported promptly to physician.
- Reactions to penicillin may be rapid in onset or may not appear for days or weeks *(see Adverse/Side Effects)*. Symptoms usually disappear fairly quickly once drug is stopped, but in some patients may persist for 5 days or more and require hospitalization for treatment.
- Observe all patients closely for at least one-half hour following administration of parenteral penicillin. The rapid appearance of a red flare or wheal at the IM or IV injection site is a possible sign of sensitivity. Report to physician. Also suspect an allergic reaction if patient becomes irritable, has nausea and vomiting, breathing difficulty, or sudden fever.
- Have ready a tourniquet adrenaline, an antihistamine, e.g., diphenhydramine and

PENICILLIN G (continued)

aminophylline, hydrocortisone, suction, and equipment for endotracheal intubation and tracheostomy.

- If patient is found to be allergic to penicillin, note this in prominent place on chart, Kardex, and at the bedside. Advise patient to carry this information and to be sure to communicate it to the attending physician at any future time.
- Neuromuscular irritability occurs most commonly in patients receiving parenteral penicillin in excess of 20 million units/day who have renal insufficiency, hyponatraemia, or underlying CNS disease, notably myasthenia gravis or epilepsy. Seizure precautions are indicated. Symptoms usually begin with twitching, especially of face and extremities (see also Adverse/Side Effects).
- Some patients receiving penicillin for treatment of syphilis develop Jarisch–Herxheimer reaction. This reaction resembles penicillin allergy, but is thought to be due to the toxic products released from spirochetes killed by penicillin. It occurs 8 to 24 hours following treatment with penicillin and is characterized by headache, chills, fever, myalgia, arthralgia, malaise, and worsening of syphilitic skin lesions. Advise patient to notify physician if these symptoms appear. The reaction is usually self-limiting.
- Monitor fluid intake and output particularly in patients receiving high parenteral doses. Report oliguria, haematuria, and changes in intake–output ratio. Consult physician regarding optimum fluid intake. Dehydration increases the concentration of drug in kidneys and can cause renal irritation and damage.
- Neonates, young infants, the elderly, and patients with impaired renal function receiving high-dose penicillin therapy should be closely observed for signs of toxicity (see Adverse/Side Effects). Urinary excretion of penicillin is significantly delayed in these patients.
- Patients with diabetes who are receiving massive doses of penicillin should be advised of the possibility of obtaining false-positive urine glucose test results (see Diagnostic Test Interferences).
- It is reported that therapeutic failure has occurred in some adult diabetic patients receiving IM penicillin G. Close monitoring is indicated.
- Patients on high-dose therapy should be closely observed for evidence of bleeding, and bleeding time should be monitored. (In high doses penicillin interferes with platelet aggregation.)
- Patients receiving prolonged treatment should have evaluations of renal, hepatic, and haematological systems at regular intervals. Additionally, electrolyte balance and cardiovascular status should be checked periodically in patients receiving high parenteral doses. The dry powder (for parenteral use) may be stored at room temperature. After reconstitution (initial dilution), solutions may be stored for 1 week under refrigeration. Intravenous infusion solutions containing penicillin G are stable at room temperature for at least 24 hours.

Diagnostic test interferences   Blood grouping and compatibility tests: Possible interference associated with penicillin doses greater than 20 million units daily. **Urine glucose**: Massive doses of penicillin may cause false-positive test results possibly Clinitest, but not with glucose oxidase methods, e.g., Clinistix, **Urine protein**:

PENICILLIN G (continued)

Massive doses of penicillin can produce false-positive results when turbidity measures are used (e.g., acetic acid and heat, sulphosalicylic acid); Ames reagent reportedly not affected. **Urinary PSP excretion tests**: False decrease in urinary excretion of PSP. **Urinary steroids**: Large IV doses of penicillin may interfere with accurate measurement of urinary 17-OHCS (Glenn–Nelson technique not affected).

DRUG INTERACTIONS   *Penicillin G*

PLUS	INTERACTIONS
Alcohol, ethyl	Reportedly enhances degradation of the penicillins
Antacids	Tend to delay absorption of oral penicillins; however, they also may protect penicillins from destruction by gastric acids
Antibiotics: Chloramphenicol Erythromycins Tetracyclines	Bacteriostatic antibiotics antagonize bactericidal actions of the penicillins by slowing rate of bacterial growth (*see Actions and Uses*)
Anticoagulants	Penicillins may enhance bleeding tendency by inhibiting platelet aggregation
Aspirin (salicylates) Indomethacin	Increase serum levels of penicillins by displacing them from plasma protein binding sites
Neomycin	Oral neomycin may decrease absorption of oral penicillins presumably by producing a malabsorption syndrome
Phenylbutazone	Increases serum levels of penicillins by displacing them from plasma protein binding sites
Probenecid Sulphinpyrazone	Decrease renal excretion of penicillins with resulting higher and more prolonged penicillin blood levels

Benzathine Penicillin (Similar drug)

(Penidural)

ROUTE AND DOSAGE   Oral: (suspension 229 mg/5 ml): **Adult**: 10 ml, 3–4 times a day. **Child**: 5 ml, 2–4 times a day. (Paediatric suspension 115 mg/5 ml.)

Penicillin G procaine suspension

(Bicillin, Depocillin)   *Antibiotic Penicillin*

ACTIONS AND USES   Repository (long-acting) form of penicillin G. The procaine salt has low solubility and thus creates a tissue depot from which penicillin is slowly

PENICILLIN G PROCAINE SUSPENSION (continued)

absorbed. Accordingly, the number of injections required to maintain effective blood levels is reduced. Also, procaine exerts a local anaesthetic effect. Same actions and antibacterial activity as for Penicillin G and is similarly inactivated by penicillinase and gastric acids. Onset of action is slower and produces lower serum concentrations than equivalent doses of penicillin G, but has longer duration of action.

Used in moderately severe infections due to penicillin G-sensitive microorganisms (*see Penicillin G*) that are susceptible to low but prolonged serum penicillin concentrations. Commonly used for treatment of uncomplicated gonorrhoeal infections.

ROUTE AND DOSAGE   Intramuscular (only): **Adults**: 300 mg, 1–2 times a day. *Gonorrhoea*: men, 2.4 g, women, 4.8 g as a single dose.

ABSORPTION AND FATE   Slowly released from IM injection site. Hydrolyzed to penicillin G in body. Blood levels peak in 1 to 3 hours, plateau in almost 4 hours and decrease slowly over the next 15 to 20 hours. Widely distributed in body with highest concentrations in kidneys and lesser amounts in liver, skin, intestines, and cerebrospinal fluid. Approximately 60% bound to plasma proteins. Excreted rapidly via kidneys; 60 to 90% of dose (aqueous suspension) eliminated within 24 to 36 hours. Excretion may be delayed in neonates, young infants, the elderly, and in other patients with impaired renal function.

CONTRAINDICATIONS AND PRECAUTIONS   History of hypersensitivity to any of the penicillins, cephalosporins, or to procaine or any other 'caine-type' local anaesthetics; neonates. **Cautious Use**: history of or suspected atopy or allergy. *See penicillin G*.

ADVERSE/SIDE EFFECTS   Hypersensitivity reactions. *Procaine toxicity*: mental disturbances (anxiety, confusion, depression, combativeness, hallucinations), expressed fear of impending death, weakness, dizziness, headache, tinnitus, unusual tastes, palpitation, changes in pulse rate and blood pressure, seizures. *See also penicillin G*.

NURSING IMPLICATIONS

- Before treatment is initiated, an exact history should be obtained of patient's previous exposure and sensitivity to penicillins, cephalosporins, and to procaine, and other allergic reactions of any kind.
- If sensitivity to procaine is suspected, physician may test patient by injecting 0.1 ml of 1 to 2% procaine hydrochloride, intradermally. The appearance of a wheal, flare, or eruption indicates procaine sensitivity.
- Note expiry date. Multiple-dose vial should be shaken thoroughly before withdrawing medication, to ensure uniform suspension of drug.
- Administer IM deeply into upper outer quadrant of gluteus muscle; in infants and small children midlateral aspect of thigh is generally preferred. Injections are almost painless because of local anaesthetic action of procaine. Select IM site carefully. Accidental injection into or near major peripheral nerves and blood vessels can cause neurovascular damage. Subcutaneous or intraarterial injection is contraindicated.
- Aspirate carefully before injecting drug, to avoid entry into a blood vessel. Inadvertent IV administration reportedly has resulted in pulmonary infarcts and death.

P

PENICILLIN G PROCAINE SUSPENSION (continued)

Inject drug at a slow, but steady rate to prevent needle blockage. Rotate injection sites.

- Report the following to the physician: onset of rash, pruritus, fever, chills or other symptoms of an allergic reaction (*see penicillin G*). Reactions may be difficult to treat because drug action is relatively prolonged.
- Note manufacturer's directions for storage. Generally, penicillin G procaine aqueous suspension is stored in refrigerator. Avoid freezing.
- *See penicillia G potassium.*

Penicillin V (phenoxymethyl)───────────

(Apsin VK, Crystapen V, Distaquine V-K, Econocil VK,   *Antibiotic (Beta-lactam);*
    Stabilin VK, V-Cil-K)   *penicillin*

ACTIONS AND USES   Acid-stable phenoxymethyl analogue of penicillin G (q.v.) with which it shares actions; is bactericidal, and is inactivated by penicillinase. Less active than penicillin G against gonococci and other gram-negative microorganisms.

Used for mild to moderate infections caused by susceptible streptococci, pneumococci, and staphylococci. Also used in treatment of Vincent's disease and as prophylaxis in rheumatic fever.

ROUTE AND DOSAGE   Oral: **Adults and Children (over 12 years)**: 250 to 500 mg every 6 to 8 hours. **Child (up to 1 yr)**: 62.5 mg, **(1–5 yrs)**: 125 mg, **(6–12 yrs)**: 250 mg every 6 hrs.

ABSORPTION AND FATE   Rapidly absorbed from GI tract. Serum concentrations peak in 30 to 60 minutes and are maintained for 6 or more hours. Highest levels in kidneys. Approximately 50 to 80% bound to plasma proteins. **Half-life**: 30 minutes. Excreted in urine as rapidly as absorbed; excretion is delayed in neonates, young infants, and patients with impaired renal function. Appears in breast milk.

CONTRAINDICATIONS AND PRECAUTIONS   Hypersensitivity to any penicillin or cephalosporin. History of or suspected atopy or allergy (hay fever, asthma, hives, eczema). *See also penicillin G.*

ADVERSE/SIDE EFFECTS   Nausea, vomiting diarrhoea, epigastric distress; hypersensitivity reactions: flushing, pruritus, urticaria or other skin eruptions, eosinophilia, anaphylaxis; haemolytic anaemia, leucopenia, thrombocytopenia, neuropathy, superinfections.

NURSING IMPLICATIONS
- It is reported that drug may be better absorbed and result in higher blood levels when taken after a meal than on an empty stomach.

PENICILLIN V (PHENOXYMETHYL) (continued)

- Following reconstitution (by pharmacist), oral solution is stable for 14 days under refrigeration. Date and time of reconstitution and expiry date should appear on container. Shake well before pouring.
- If oral liquid preparation is not dispensed with a specially marked measuring device, question pharmacist. The average household measure is not accurate enough for this formulation.
- Inform patient that in order to maintain a constant blood level, penicillin V should be given around the clock at specific intervals. If it is not prescribed in this way the physician should be asked to clarify the order.
- Instruct patient not to miss any doses and to continue taking medication until it is all gone, unless otherwise directed by the physician.
- Patients receiving prolonged therapy should have evaluations of renal, hepatic, and haematological systems at regular intervals.
- As with other penicillin preparations, advise patient to withhold medication and to report promptly to physician the onset of hypersensitivity reactions and super-infections.
- *See Penicillin G.*

Pentaerythritol tetranitrate ━━━━━━━━━━━━━━━━━━━━

(Cardiacap, Peritrate, Mycardol)   *Vasodilator (coronary);*
                                                                    antianginal; nitrate

ACTIONS AND USES Nitric acid ester of a tetrahydric alcohol. Actions, contraindications, precautions, and adverse/side effects as for glyceryl trinitrate (q.v.). Slower acting than glyceryl trinitrate but duration of action is longer. Not effective for control of acute attacks. Tolerance can occur, and cross tolerance with other nitrites and nitrates is possible.

Used prophylactically for long-term management of angina pectoris.

ROUTE AND DOSAGE (Dose titrate to individual's response.) **Oral: Adult:** 20–60 mg, 3–4 times a day.

ABSORPTION AND FATE Onset of haemodynamic effects in 20 to 60 minutes; duration 4 to 5 hours. Action of sustained release forms may persist up to 12 hours. Largely metabolized in liver prior to entering general circulation. **Half-life:** about 10 minutes. Excreted in urine; small amounts in faeces.

NURSING IMPLICATIONS
- Not to be used to relieve an acute episode of anginal pain.
- Administered at least 30 minutes before or 1 hour after meals and at bedtime. Sustained release forms also administered on an empty stomach (one dose on arising and second dose 12 hours later).

P

PENTAERYTHRITOL TETRANITRATE (continued)

- Advise patient to report onset of skin rash or persistent headaches to physician. Discontinuation of therapy may be required.
- Inform patient that alcohol may enhance drug hypotensive effect.
- Orthostatic hypotension can be particularly dangerous for the elderly. Evaluate incidence; if troublesome, notify physician.
- Advise patient to report signs of decreasing therapeutic effect.
- Avoid sudden discontinuation of pentaerythritol therapy; coronary vasospasm may be induced.
- Protect drug from exposure to heat and moisture to prevent loss of potency.
- Store at temperature between 15° and 30°C (59° and 86°F).
- *See glyceryl trinitrate.*
- In presence of high environmental temperature, heat prostration can occur with use of this drug, especially in the elderly.
- Caution patient not to engage in activities requiring mental alertness and skill until drug response has stabilized.
- Have on hand the antidote neostigmine in the event of severe toxic reactions.
- *See atropine.*

Pentazocine

(Fortral)   *Narcotic analgesic*

ACTIONS AND USES   Synthetic benzomorphan analgesic structurally related to phenazocine. On a weight basis, analgesic potency approximately one-third that of morphine, and somewhat greater than that of codeine. In general, adverse reactions are qualitatively similar to those of morphine (q.v.). Unlike morphine, large doses may cause increase in blood pressure and heart rate. Also, acts as weak narcotic antagonist of pethidine and morphine, and has sedative properties.

Used for relief of moderate to severe pain.

ROUTE AND DOSAGE   **Oral: Adult:** 50 mg 3–4 hourly. **Child (6–12 yrs):** 25 mg. **SC/IM/IV injection:** 30–60 mg, 3–4 hourly, **Child (over 1 yr):** by **SC or IM route**, 500 mg/kg. **Rectal suppositories:** 50 mg up to 4 times a day.

NURSING IMPLICATIONS
- Pentazocine may produce acute withdrawal symptoms in some patients who have been receiving opioids on a regular basis.
- Caution ambulatory patients to avoid potentially hazardous activities such as driving a car or operating machinery until response to drug is known.
- Tolerance to analgesic effect sometimes occurs. Psychological and physical dependence have been reported in patients with history of drug abuse.
- Abrupt discontinuation of drug following extended use may result in chills, ab-

PENTAZOCINE (continued)

dominal and muscle cramps, yawning, rhinorrhoea, lacrimation, itching, restlessness, anxiety, drug-seeking behaviour.

- Overdosage is treated by supportive measures such as oxygen, IV fluids, vasopressors, assisted or controlled ventilation as necessary, and narcotic antagonist naloxone (levallorphan is not effective for respiratory depression).
- Do not mix pentazocine in some syringe with soluble barbiturates, because precipitation will occur.
- Preserved in tight, light-resistant containers.

Perphenazine

(Fentazin)

Antipsychotic; antiemetic; phenothiazine

ACTIONS AND USES   Piperazine phenothiazine similar to chlorpromazine in actions, absorption and fate, contraindications, precautions, adverse reactions and interactions. Effects all parts of CNS, particularly the hypothalamus. Produces less sedation and hypotension, greater antiemetic effects, higher incidence of extrapyramidal effects and lower levels of anticholinergic side effects than chlorpromazine (q.v.).

Used in management of the manifestations of psychotic disorders and for intractable hiccoughs, and severe anxiety.

ROUTE AND DOSAGE   Oral: **Adult and Children (over 12 years of age):** *Initial* 4 mg, three times a day according to response. Maximum 24 mg/day. Reduce dose in the elderly. **IM:** 5–10 mg then 5 mg 6 hrly as required.

CONTRAINDICATIONS AND PRECAUTIONS   Hypersensitivity to perphenazine and other phenothiazines; preexisting liver damage, suspected or established subcortical brain damage, comatose states, blood dyscrasias, bone marrow depression, pregnancy nursing mothers, women who may become pregnant, children under 12 years of age. **Cautious Use:** previously diagnosed breast cancer; renal dysfunction, alcohol withdrawal, epilepsy, psychological depression, patients with suicidal tendency, and those who will be exposed to extreme heat in work, or exposed to phosphorous insecticides. *See also chlorpromazine.*

ADVERSE/SIDE EFFECTS   Extrapyramidal effects, convulsions, constipation, xerostomia, nasal congestion, decreased sweating, tachycardia, bradycardia, adynamic ileus, hypotension, photosensitivity. *See also chlorpromazine.*

NURSING IMPLICATIONS

- If the patient is also receiving antacid or antidiarrhoeal medication, schedule the phenothiazine to be taken at least 1 hour before or 1 hour after the other medication.
- Administer intramuscular injection deep into upper outer quadrant of the buttock with patient in recumbent position. Advise patient to continue lying down for at

P

PERPHENAZINE (continued)

least 1 hour after injection. Monitor blood pressure and pulse. Usually patient can be transferred to the oral formulation (equal or higher doses) within 24 to 48 hours.

- The elderly and paediatric patients should be observed very carefully during parenteral therapy for hypotensive and extrapyramidal reactions.
- The patient on long-term therapy (especially the elderly female patient) is at high risk for tardive dyskinesia. Watch for early signs: fine vermicular movement or rapid protrusions of the tongue. Report immediately when noticed. Discontinue medication.
- Warn patient not to spill oral concentrate on skin or clothing. Wash well with soap and water if it occurs. Contact dermatitis has been reported.
- If jaundice appears in the second to fourth week, suspect hypersensitivity; withhold drug and report to physician.
- Monitor fluid intake–output ratio and bowel elimination pattern. The depressed patient is apt to drink too little fluid and may not seek help for constipation.
- Perphenazine may discolour urine reddish brown.
- Protect solutions from light. Do not used precipitated or darkened parenteral solution; however, slight discolouration does not alter potency or therapeutic effects.
- Store drug at temperature between 15° and 30°C (59° and 86°F) unless otherwise specified by manufacturer. Protect from freezing.
- *See chlorpromazine.*

Pethidine

(Pamergan)   *Narcotic analgesic*

ACTIONS AND USES Synthetic morphine-like compound (phenylpiperidine derivative). Chemically dissimilar to morphine, but in equianalgesic doses it is qualitatively comparable with regard to analgesic effects, sedation, euphoria, pupillary constriction, and respiratory depression. Reported to differ from morphine in having a somewhat more rapid onset and shorter duration of action and in producing less depression of cough reflex, constipation, urinary retention, and smooth muscle spasm. Usual doses produce either no pupillary change or slight miosis, but overdosage results in marked miosis or mydriasis. Also, unlike morphine, has little or no antidiarrhoeic or antitussive action and produces CNS stimulation in toxic doses. In common with morphine, it causes sensitization of labyrinthine apparatus, stimulation of chemoreceptor trigger zone, and depression of medullary vasomotor centre it also has vagolytic and anticholinergic actions and may inhibit release of ACTH and gonadotropic hormones. Promotes release of histamine and antidiuretic hormone, and elevation of blood sugar.

Used for relief of moderate to severe pain, for preoperative medication, for support of anaesthesia and for obstetric analgesia.

ROUTE AND DOSAGE (Controlled Drug.) **Oral:** 50–150 mg/4 hrly. **Child:** 0.5–2

PETHIDINE (continued)

mg/kg. **SC/IM: Adult:** 25–100 mg/4 hrly. **IM: Child:** 0.5–2 mg/kg. **IV: slow injection:** 25–50 mg/4 hrly.

ABSORPTION AND FATE   Well absorbed from GI tract; analgesic effect following oral administration begins in 15 minutes, peaks in about 1 hour, and subsides over 2 to 4 hours. Onset of action following SC or IM administration occurs within 10 minutes; action peaks within 60 minutes, duration of action for both routes 2 to 4 hours. Onset of action following IV administration in about 5 minutes; duration approximately 2 hours. **Half-life:** 2.4 to 4 hours; 65 to 75% bound to plasma proteins. Metabolized chiefly in liver to active and inactive metabolites. Excreted in urine, mostly as metabolites and about 5% unchanged drug (excretion enhanced by acidification of urine). Crosses placenta and appears in breast milk.

CONTRAINDICATIONS AND PRECAUTIONS   Hypersensitivity to pethidine, convulsive disorders, acute abdominal conditions prior to diagnosis, pregnancy (prior to labour), nursing mothers. **Cautious Use:** head injuries, increased intracranial pressure, asthma and other respiratory conditions, supraventricular tachycardias, prostatic hypertrophy, urethral stricture, glaucoma, elderly or debilitated patients, impaired renal or hepatic function, hypothyroidism, Addison's disease.

ADVERSE/SIDE EFFECTS   These include: dizziness, weakness, euphoria, dysphoria, sedation, headache, uncoordinated muscle movements, disorientation, decreased cough reflex, miosis, corneal anaesthesia, respiratory depression. Toxic doses: muscle twitching, tremors, hyperactive reflexes, excitement, hypersensitivity to external stimuli, agitation, confusion, hallucinations, dilated pupils, convulsions, facial flushing, lightheadedness, hypotension, syncope, palpitation, bradycardia, tachycardia, cardiovascular collapse, cardiac arrest (toxic doses), dry mouth, nausea, vomiting, constipation, biliary tract spasm, oliguria, urinary retention, profuse perspiration, respiratory depression in newborn, bronchoconstriction (large doses), phlebitis (following IV use), pain, tissue irritation and induration, particularly following subcutaneous injection; increased levels of serum amylase, BSP retention, bilirubin, SGOT, SGPT.

NURSING IMPLICATIONS

- In patients receiving repeated doses, note respiration rate, depth and rhythm, and size of pupils. If respirations are 12 per minute or below and pupils are constricted or dilated (*see Actions and Uses*) or breathing is shallow, or if signs of CNS hyperactivity are present consult physician before administering drug.
- Carefully aspirate before giving IM injection in order to avoid inadvertent IV administration. IV injection of undiluted drug can cause a marked increase in heart rate and syncope.
- A high incidence of severe untoward effects is associated with IV use. Facilities for administration of oxygen and control of respiration should be immediately available, as well as a narcotic antagonist (e.g., naloxone.)
- Vital signs should be monitored closely. Heart rate may increase markedly, and hypotension may occur.
- Before administering pethidine provide maximum comfort measures and reduce

P

PETHIDINE (continued)

environmental stimuli. Caution patient not to smoke and not to ambulate without assistance after receiving the drug. Bedsides are advisable.

■ Use of comfort measures, as well as displays of thoughtfulness and interest by those attending the patient, are as important as medication in control of pain.

■ Monitor vital signs, particularly in patients receiving repeated doses. Pethidine may cause severe hypotension in postoperative patients and those with depleted blood volume.

■ Deep breathing, coughing (unless contraindicated), and changes in position at scheduled intervals may help to overcome the respiratory depression.

■ Ambulatory patients are more likely than supine patients to manifest nausea, vomiting, dizziness, and faintness associated with fall in blood pressure (these symptoms may also occur in patients without pain). Symptoms are lessened by the recumbent position and aggravated by the head-up position. Report to physician; dosage reduction or drug discontinuation may be indicated.

■ Caution ambulatory patients to avoid driving a car or engaging in other hazardous activities until any drowsiness and dizziness have passed.

■ Record the patient's response to pethidine and evaluate continued need for the drug.

■ Repeated used of pethidine can lead to tolerance and psychological and physical dependence of the morphine type. High abuse potential has been reported among nurses and physicians.

■ Abrupt discontinuation of pethidine following repeated use results in *morphinelike withdrawal symptoms*. Symptoms develop more rapidly (within 3 hours, peaking in 8 to 12 hours) and are of shorter duration than with morphine. Nausea, vomiting, diarrhoea, and pupillary dilatation are less prominent, but muscle twitching, restlessness, and nervousness are greater than produced by morphine.

■ Preserved in tightly closed, light-resistant containers preferably between 15 to 30°C (59 to 86°F) unless otherwise directed by manufacturer.

Drug interactions   CNS stimulation or depression induced by pethidine and its congeners may be potentiated by **amphetamines, barbiturates, cimetidine, MAO inhibitors** including drugs with significant **MAOI** activity e.g., **isoniazid** (INH) (concurrent use avoided); **phenothiazines** (concurrent use avoided); **phenytoin** and other hydantoins; **tricyclic antidepressants, other CNS depressants**, including **alcohol**.

Phenelzine sulphate ——————————————————————

(Nardil)   *Antidepressant; MAO inhibitor;*
                                                             hydrazine

ACTIONS AND USES   Potent hydrazine MAO inhibitor with amphetamine-like pharmacological properties. Precise mode of action not known. Antidepressant and diverse effects believed to be due to irreversible inhibition of MAO (mitochondrial enzyme involved in degradation and excretion of sympathomimetic amines), thereby permitting

PHENELZINE SULPHATE (continued)

increased concentrations of endogenous adrenaline, noradrenaline serotonin, and dopamine within presynaptic neurons and at receptor sites. Also thought to inhibit hepatic microsomal drug-metabolizing enzymes; thus may intensify and prolong the effects of many drugs. Termination of drug action depends on regeneration of MAO, which occurs 2 to 3 weeks after discontinuation of therapy. Exerts paradoxic hypotensive effect (apparently by ganglionic blocking action), suppresses REM sleep, and reportedly may decrease serum cholinesterase. MAO inhibitor has unpredictable effect on convulsive threshold in epilepsy.

Used in management of endogenous depression, depressive phase of manic-depressive psychosis, and severe exogenous (reactive) depression not responsive to more commonly used therapy.

ROUTE AND DOSAGE   Oral: *Initial*: 15 mg three times a day. Increased gradually until maximum benefit is achieved, dosage reduced slowly over several weeks to maintenance level: 15 mg daily or every other day, as long as required. Maximum recommended daily dose: 75 mg.

ABSORPTION AND FATE   Readily absorbed from GI tract and rapidly metabolized. Excreted in urine as metabolites and unchanged drug.

CONTRAINDICATIONS AND PRECAUTIONS   Hypersensitivity to MAO inhibitors, phaeochromocytoma, hyperthyroidism, congestive heart failure, cardiovascular or cerebrovascular disease, impaired renal function, hypernatraemia, atonic colitis, glaucoma, history of frequent or severe headaches, history of liver disease, abnormal liver function tests, elderly or debilitated patients, paranoid schizophrenia. Safe use during pregnancy and lactation and in women of childbearing potential and children under 16 years of age not established. **Cautious Use**: epilepsy, pyloric stenosis, diabetes, depression accompanying alcoholism or drug addiction, manic-depressive states, agitated patients, suicidal tendencies, chronic brain syndromes, history of angina pectoris.

ADVERSE/SIDE EFFECTS   Constipation, dry mouth, dizziness or vertigo, headache, orthostatic hypotension, drowsiness or insomnia, weakness, fatigue, nausea, vomiting, anorexia, weight gain, oedema, tremors, twitching, hyperreflexia, mania, hypomania, confusion, memory impairment, blurred vision, hyperhidrosis, skin rash. **Hypertensive crisis**: intense occipital headache, palpitation, marked hypertension, stiff neck, nausea, vomiting, sweating, fever, photophobia, dilated pupils, bradycardia or tachycardia, constricting chest pain, intracranial bleeding. **Less common**: glaucoma, nystagmus, incontinence, dysuria, urinary frequency or retention, transient impotence, galactorrhoea, gynaecomastia, black tongue, hypernatraemia, transient respiratory and cardiovascular depression, jaundice, delirium, hallucinations, euphoria, acute anxiety reaction, akathisia, ataxia, toxic precipitation of schizophrenia, convulsions, possibility of optic damage, peripheral neuropathy, spider telangiectasis, photosensitivity, hypoglycaemia, decreased 5-HIAA and VMA, normocytic and normochromic anaemia, leucopenia. **Severe overdosage**: faintness, hypotension or hypertension, hyperactivity, marked agitation, anxiety, seizures, trismus, opisthotonos, respiratory depression, coma, circulatory collapse.

P

PHENELZINE SULPHATE (continued)
NURSING IMPLICATIONS

- Before initiation of phenelzine treatment, it is advisable to evaluate patient's blood pressure in standing and recumbent positions. Baseline blood cell counts and liver function tests should also be performed.
- Many adverse reactions associated with MAO inhibitors are dose-related. Physician will rely on accurate observations and prompt reporting of patient's response to therapy to determine spacing and lowest effective dosage.
- In titrating initial dosages, blood pressure and pulse should be monitored between doses, and patient should be closely observed for evidence of adverse drug effects. Thereafter, monitor at regular intervals throughout therapy.
- Elastic stockings and elevation of legs when sitting may minimize hypotensive effects of drug (discuss with physician).
- Instruct patient to make position changes slowly, especially from recumbent to upright posture, and to dangle legs over bed a few minutes before ambulating. Also caution against standing still for prolonged periods. Patient should avoid hot showers and baths (resulting vasodilatation may potentiate hypotension) and should lie down immediately if feeling lightheaded or faint. Supervise ambulation.
- Headache and palpitation, prodromal symptoms of hypertensive crisis, indicate need to discontinue drug therapy. Instruct patient to report immediately the onset of these symptoms or any other unusual effects.
- Ingestion of foods and beverages containing tyramine or tryptophan (form pressor amines in body) or drugs containing pressor agents can result in severe hyptertensive reactions. Provide patient and responsible family members with a list of foods and beverages that may cause reactions (see below). These substances should be avoided during drug therapy and for at least 2 to 3 weeks after therapy has been discontinued.
- **Food and beverages to avoid**   Avocado, bananas, canned figs, raisins, liquorice, chocolate, cheeses (particularly cheddar and other strong and aged varieties), yogurt, cream, sour cream, broad bean pods, liver (especially chicken liver), aged meats, pickled or kippered herring, yeast and meat extracts, soy sauce, meat tenderizers, game. Alcoholic beverages in general should be avoided (since tyramine content is difficult to determine), especially Chianti, other wines, and beer. Also advise against excessive amounts of caffeine beverages (e.g., coffee, tea, cocoa, or cola) and cyclamates (believed to be converted in body in part to a pressor amine).
- **Treatment and hypertensive crisis**   Have ready short-acting α-adrenergic blocking agent (e.g., phentolamine) to lower blood pressure; external cooling for hyperpyrexia.
- **Treatment of overdosage**   Gastric lavage if performed early; maintain airway, hydration, and electrolyte balance. Have ready phenothiazine tranquilizer (for agitation). Toxic effects may be delayed and prolonged; therefore, patient must be closely observed for at least 1 week after overdosage.
- Advise patient to avoid self-medication. OTC preparations containing dextromethorphan, sympathomimetic agents, or antihistamines (e.g., cough, cold, and hay fever remedies, appetite suppressants) can precipitate severe hypertensive reactions if taken during therapy or within 2 or 3 weeks after discontinuation of an MAO inhibitor.

PHENELZINE SULPHATE (continued)

- Monitor fluid intake–output ratio and pattern until dosage is stabilized to identify indirect indices of oedema and urinary dysfunction. Report changes and abnormalities; impaired renal function increases the possibility of toxicity from cumulative effects.
- Instruct patient to check weight two or three times weekly and report unusual gain.
- Dry mouth may be relieved by sugarless candy or gum or by rinsing mouth with clear water.
- Attempt at suicide by the depressed person is particularly possible when the response to drug therapy begins (i.e., near end of depressive cycle). Careful observation of patient should be maintained until depression is controlled. Watch to ensure that drug is swallowed.
- In manic-depressive states, observe closely for rapid swing to manic phase. Patients with schizophrenia may present with excessive stimulation.
- Hypomania (exaggeration of motility, feelings, and ideas) may occur as depression improves, particularly in patients with hyperkinetic symptoms obscured by a depressive effect. This reaction may also appear at higher than recommended doses or with long-term therapy. Report immediately.
- Observe for and report therapeutic effectiveness of drug: improvement in sleep pattern, appetite, physical activity, interest in self and surroundings, as well as lessening of anxiety and bodily complaints.
- If no therapeutic response occurs after 3 or 4 weeks, drug is usually discontinued. Maximum antidepressant effects generally appear in 2 to 6 weeks and persist several weeks after drug withdrawal.
- Patient with diabetes should be closely observed for signs of hypoglycaemia. Reduced dosage of insulin or oral antidiabetic drug may be necessary (*see Drug Interactions*).
- MAO inhibitors should be discontinued at least 10 days before elective surgery to allow time for recovery of MAO before anaesthetics are given.
- Patients on prolonged therapy should be checked periodically for altered colour perception, visual fields, and fundi. Changes in red-green vision may be the first indication of eye damage.
- Instruct patient to report jaundice. Hepatotoxicity is believed to be a hypersensitivity reaction unrelated to dosage or duration of therapy.
- Periodic haematological studies and liver function tests are recommended during prolonged therapy and high dosage.
- MAO inhibitors may suppress anginal pain that would otherwise serve as a warning sign of myocardial ischaemia. Caution patient to avoid overexertion while receiving drug therapy.
- Rapid withdrawal of MAO inhibitors should be avoided, particularly after high dosage, since a rebound effect may occur (headache, excitability, hallucinations, and possibly depression).
- Preserved in tightly covered containers away from heat and light.

Diagnostic test interferences   Phenelzine may cause a slight false increase in **serum bilirubin**.

PHENELZINE SULPHATE (continued)

Drug interactions   Hypertensive reaction and related symptoms may result from use (concurrently or within 2 weeks) of MAO inhibitors with amines having indirect sympathomimetic action: **amphetamines, cyclopentamine, ephedrine, metaraminol, methylphenidate, phenylephrine, phenylpropanolamine, pseudoephedrine.** Similar interactions are reportedly possible with **cyclamates, dextromethorphan, levodopa, methyldopa, methotrimeprazine, reserpine, tricyclic antidepressants, tryptamine,** and **tyramine**-rich foods and beverages.

With the exception of dopamine (contraindicated), direct-acting sympathomimetic amines **adrenaline, isoprenaline, noradrenaline methoxamine)** are not significantly affected by MAO inhibitors; however, cautious administration is advised.

MAO inhibitors may potentiate the effects of **barbiturates**; potentiate adverse cardiovascular effects of **doxapram** (theoretical possibility); antagonize antihypertensive effects of **guanethidine** (concurrent use avoided); enhance or prolong hypoglycaemic action of **insulin** and **oral antidiabetic agents**; cause severe CNS excitation and depression leading to coma and death with **pethidine**—thus concurrent use is to be avoided (other **narcotic analgesics** used only with extreme caution and in small doses); increase extrapyramidal reactions of **phenothiazines**; enhance the effect of **succinylcholine** by reducing its breakdown by plasma pseudocholinesterase; produce hypotension when used with **thiazide diuretics**.

Phenethicillin━━━━━━━━━━━━━━━━━━━━━━━━━━━━━

(Brokil)

ACTIONS AND USES   Penicillin with similar action and use to penicillin G (q.v.). *See penicillin G.*

ROUTE AND DOSAGE   **Oral: Adult:** 250 mg/6 hrly. **Child (under 2 yrs):** ¼ adult-dose; **(2–10 yrs):** ½ adult dose.

Phenindamine━━━━━━━━━━━━━━━━━━━━━━━━━━━━━

(Thephorin)

ACTIONS AND USES   Antihistamine used for symptomatic relief in allergy.

ROUTE AND DOSAGE   **Oral: Adult:** 25–50 mg 4 times a day. **Child (over 10 yrs):** 25 mg 1–3 times a day. *See chlorpheniramine.*

Phenindione

(Dindevan)

ACTIONS AND USES   Anticoagulant with similar action and use to warfarin (q.v.).

ROUTE AND DOSAGE   Oral: **Adult**: 200 mg first day, 100 mg second day, maintenance 50–150 mg/day.

Phenobarbitone

(Gardenal, Luminal)

CNS depressant; sedative, hypnotic; anticonvulsant; barbiturate

ACTIONS AND USES   Long-acting barbiturate. Sedative and hypnotic effects of barbiturates appear to be due primarily to interference with impulse transmission of cerebral cortex by inhibition of reticular activating system (concerned with both sleep and arousal mechanisms). Initially, barbiturates suppress REM sleep, but with chronic therapy REM sleep returns to normal. Has no analgesic properties, and small doses may increase reaction to painful stimuli. CNS depression may range from mild sedation to coma, depending on dosage, route of administration, degree of nervous system excitability, and drug tolerance. Phenobarbitone limits spread of seizure activity by increasing threshold for motor cortex stimuli. Anticonvulsant action of phenobarbitone is shared by mephobarbitone but not other barbiturates, and is reportedly unrelated to sedative effect. Phenobarbitone has a bilirubin lowering effect, by inducing production of glucuronyl transferase; also increases excretion and flow of bile salts.

Used in long term management of tonic–clonic (grand mal) seizures and partial seizures; status epilepticus, eclampsia, febrile convulsions in young children.

ROUTE AND DOSAGE   **Adults**: **Oral**: 60–180 mg at night. **IM/IV**: 50–200 mg/6 hrly as required. Maximum 600 mg/day. **Child**: **Oral**: 5–8 mg/kg/day.

ABSORPTION AND FATE   Absorbed slowly following all routes of administration. Peak serum concentrations reached in 8 to 12 hours; peak brain concentration in 10 to 15 hours. Widely distributed in tissues and body fluids. Hypnotic doses produce sleep within 20 to 60 minutes; duration varies from 6 to 10 hours. About 40 to 60% bound to plasma proteins and also to tissues, including brain. **Half-life** 53 to 118 hours (somewhat shorter and more variable in children). Small amount metabolized in liver; excreted in urine largely as unchanged drug. Alkalinization of urine and hydration enhance renal excretion. Readily crosses placenta; enters breast milk.

CONTRAINDICATIONS AND PRECAUTIONS   Sensitivity to barbiturates, manifest hepatic, or familial history of porphyria, severe respiratory or renal disease, history of

P

PHENOBARBITONE (continued)

previous addiction to sedative hypnotics, uncontrolled pain, women of childbearing potential, pregnancy (particularly early pregnancy), nursing mothers, timed release formulation for children under 12 years of age. **Cautious Use**: impaired hepatic, renal, cardiac, or respiratory function, history of allergies, elderly or debilitated patients, patients with fever, hyperthyroidism, diabetes mellitus, or severe anaemia, during labour and delivery, lactation, patient with borderline hypoadrenal function.

ADVERSE/SIDE EFFECTS   These include: somnolence, nightmares, insomnia, 'hang-over' headache, anxiety, thinking abnormalities, dizziness, nystagmus, irritability, paradoxic excitement and exacerbation of hyperkinetic behaviour (in children); confusion or depression or marked excitement (elderly or debilitated patients); ataxia, bradycardia, syncope, hypotension, mild maculopapular, morbilliform rash; (rare) exfoliative dermatitis, erythema multiforme, Stevens-Johnson syndrome, nausea, vomiting, constipation, diarrhoea, epigastic pain. **Hypersensitivity**: rash, angioneurotic oedema, fever, serum sickness, urticaria; hypoventilation, apnoea, laryngospasm, bronchospasm, circulatory collapse. **Injection site (extravasation)**: thrombosis, gangrene transient pain, tenderness, redness. **Intravenous**: coughing, hiccoughing, laryngospasm. **Overdosage (acute intoxication)**: *see Nursing Implications*.

NURSING IMPLICATIONS

- Phenobarbitone and other long acting barbiturates may be cumulative in action. Doses in excess of 400 mg/day for more than 90 days are likely to cause some degree of physical dependence.
- Therapeutic serum concentrations of 10 to 20 mcg/ml produce anticonvulsant activity in most patients. These values are usually attained after 2 or 3 weeks of therapy with a dose of 100 to 200 mg/day.
- Serum concentrations greater than 50 mcg/ml may cause coma; concentrations in excess of 80 mcg/ml are potentially lethal.
- Because of the long half-life, steady-state plasma level may not be reached until after 3 or 4 weeks of therapy with phenobarbitone.
- Administer IM deep into large muscle mass; volume should not exceed 5 ml at any one site. Patients receiving large doses should be closely observed for at least 30 minutes to assure that narcosis is not excessive.
- Keep patient under constant observation when drug is administered IV, and record vital signs at least every hour or more often if indicated. Administration rate: no greater than 60 mg/minute. Resuscitation equipment and drugs should be immediately available.
- Extravasation of IV phenobarbitone may cause necrotic tissue changes that may necessitate skin grafting. (Addicts who use IV phenobarbitone for a 'high' have been known to lose a finger from the damage of intraarterial injections.) Frequently check the injection site. (*See Nursing Interventions: extravasation.*)
- When administering oral barbiturates, observe that patient actually swallows the pill.
- If patient cannot swallow pill, it may be crushed before administration, then mixed with a fluid or with food. (Do not permit patient to swallow dry crushed drug.)

PHENOBARBITONE (continued)

- Barbiturates do not have analgesic action, and they may be expected to produce restlessness when given to patients in pain.
- Patients receiving anticonvulsant therapy may experience drowsiness during first few weeks of treatment, but this usually diminishes with continued use of the barbiturate.
- The elderly or debilitated patient and children sometimes have parodoxical response to barbiturate therapy: i.e., irritability, marked excitement (inappropriate tearfulness and aggression in children), depression and confusion. Be alert to unexpected responses and report promptly. Protect the elderly patient from falling, irrational behaviour and effects of depression (anorexia, social withdrawal).
- The elderly patient receiving a barbiturate is predisposed to bedsore development (decreased body movement in sleep). Multidrug therapy, if necessary, is difficult to control because of altered hepatic microsomal enzyme function with aging.
- Caution patient to avoid potentially hazardous activities requiring mental alertness such as driving a car or operating machinery, until response to drug is known.
- Alcohol in any amount given with a barbiturate may severely impair judgment and abilities; it should not be consumed by a patient on barbiturate therapy.

Food–drug interaction

- Phenobarbitone increases vitamin D metabolism leading to subtherapeutic levels and possible onset of osteomalacia, or rickets (long-term therapy). Advise patient to increase vitamin D fortified foods (e.g., milk products). A vitamin D supplement may be prescribed.
- Long-term therapy may result in nutritional folate deficiency (barbiturates inhibit intestinal tract deconjugase enzymes that prepare dietary folic acid for absorption). Laboratory confirmation is the basis for urging patient to maintain adequate dietary folate intake: fresh vegetables (especially green leafy), fresh fruits, whole grains, liver. A supplement of folic acid may be prescribed.

- Caution patient to adhere to drug regimen: i.e., intervals between doses should not be changed and doses should not be increased or decreased without advice.
- Warn patient not to stop taking drug abruptly because of danger of withdrawal symptoms which can be fatal: (8 to 12 hours after last dose): apprehension, hand and finger tremors, weakness, dizziness, disturbed vision, nausea, vomiting, sweating, orthostatic hypotension, insomnia. More severe symptoms may develop 2 to 8 days after withdrawal: delirium, convulsion, status epilepticus (patient with epilepsy). Withdrawal symptoms may occur after a course of therapy with 600 to 800 mg daily for 35 days and may last up to 15 days after abrupt cessation of drug therapy.
- Be alert to adverse reactions in the patient who apparently has tolerated phenobarbitone in the past.
- It is important that pregnancy be avoided in patients receiving barbiturates (reportedly teratogenic). Patients on prolonged therapy should consider alternative methods of contraception in addition to or instead of oral contraceptives to prevent unplanned pregnancy *(see Drug Interactions)*. The neonate born of mother who received barbiturate therapy throughout the last trimester may show withdrawal symptoms for 1 to 14

PHENOBARBITONE (continued)

days after birth. Symptoms resemble congenital opiate withdrawal symptoms: hyperactivity, restlessness, tremor, hyperreflexia, disturbed sleep.

- Hepatic function and haematology tests and determinations of serum folate and vitamin D levels are advised during prolonged therapy.
- Instruct patients on prolonged therapy to report to physician the onset of fever, sore throat or mouth, malaise, easy bruising or bleeding, petechiae, jaundice, rash.
- Advise patients taking barbiturates at home not to keep drug on bedside table or in a readily accessible place. Patients have been known to forgot having taken the drug, and in half-wakened conditions have accidentally overdosed themselves.
- Slang names for barbiturates include 'barbs', 'sleepers', 'downs', 'phennies', 'peanuts', among many others. Addicts frequently use barbiturates to boost the effects of weak heroin.
- Barbiturates increase the metabolism of many drugs leading to decreased pharmacological effects of those drugs. Whenever a barbiturate is added to an established regimen of another drug close observation for changes in effectiveness of the first drug is essential, at least during early phase of barbiturate use.
- Barbiturates decrease or reduce pharmacological effects of the following drugs (groups); anticoagulants (coumarins), carbamazepine, corticosteroids, digitoxin, doxycycline, oestradiol, griseofulvin, oral contraceptives, quinidine, phenothiazines, tricyclic antidepressants. Clinical significance is not always delineated (e.g., griseofulvin). *See specific drug interactant for more information.*
- Store at 15° to 30°C (59° to 86°F) unless otherwise directed by manufacturer.

Diagnostic test interferences   Barbiturates may affect **bromsulphalein** retention tests (by enhancing hepatic uptake and excretion of dye) and increase **serum phosphatase.**

DRUG INTERACTIONS   *Phenobarbitone*

PLUS	INTERACTIONS
Alcohol and other CNS depressants	Additive depressant effects
Anaesthetics	
Chloramphenicol	
Valproic acid	Prolonged barbiturate action
Disulphiram	
Nondepolarizing skeletal muscle relaxants (e.g., tubocurarine)	Additive respiratory depression
Frusemide	May aggravate or produce orthostatic hypotension
Phenytoin	Increased/decreased effects of either drug
Sulphonamides	May increase effects of barbiturates

Phenoxybenzamine hydrochloride ━━━━━━━━━━

*Antihypertensive, alpha-
adrenergic blocking agent*

PHENOXYBENZAMINE HYDROCHLORIDE (continued)

ACTIONS AND USES   Long-acting alpha-adrenergic blocking agent. Apparently produces noncompetitive blockade ('chemical sympathectomy') of alpha-adrenergic receptor sites at postganglionic synapse. Causes orthostatic hypotension in both normotensive and hypertensive patients, and also blocks pupillary dilation and retraction of eyelids.

Used in management of phaeochromocytoma.

ROUTE AND DOSAGE   Oral: **Adult:** *Initial:* 10 mg daily in a single dose; dosage may be increased by increments of 10 mg daily. *Maintenance:* 20 to 60 mg daily in single or divided doses.

ABSORPTION AND FATE   About 30% of oral dose is absorbed. **Onset of action** in 2 hours; **peak effects** within 4 to 6 hours. Alpha-adrenergic blockade persists for 3 or 4 days. **Half-life** approximately 24 hours. About 80% excreted in urine and bile in 24 hours.

CONTRAINDICATIONS AND PRECAUTIONS   When fall in blood pressure would be dangerous; compensated congestive failure. **Cautious Use:** marked cerebral or coronary arteriosclerosis, renal insufficiency, respiratory infections. Safe use during pregnancy not established.

ADVERSE/SIDE EFFECTS   Nasal congestion, dry mouth, miosis, drooping of eyelids, postural hypotension, tachycardia, palpitation, dizziness, fainting, inhibition of ejaculation, drowsiness, sedation, tiredness, weakness, lethargy, confusion, headache, GI irritation, vomiting, shock, CNS stimulation (large doses), allergic contact dermatitis.

NURSING IMPLICATIONS
- Giving the drug with milk or in divided doses may reduce gastric irritation.
- During period of dosage adjustment, monitor blood pressure and note pulse quality, rate, and rhythm in recumbent and standing positions. (Hypotension and tachycardia are most likely to occur in standing position). Patient should be closely observed for at least 4 days from one dosage increment to the next.
- Instruct patient to make position changes slowly, particularly from recumbent to upright posture, and to dangle legs and exercise ankles and feet for a few minutes before standing.
- Advise patient to lie down or sit down in head-low position immediately at the onset of faintness or weakness. Physician may prescribe support stockings and abdominal support to help prevent orthostatic hypotension. Miosis, nasal stuffiness, and inhibition of ejaculation generally decrease with continued therapy.
- Inform patient that postural hypotension and palpitation usually disappear with continued therapy, but they may reappear under conditions that promote vasodilation, such as strenuous exercise or ingestion of a large meal or alcohol.
- Since phenoxybenzamine has cumulative action, onset of therapeutic effects may not occur until after 2 weeks of therapy, and full therapeutic effects may not be apparent for several more weeks. (Drug action lasts several days after discontinuation of therapy.)
- Therapeutic effectiveness in patients with phaeochromocytoma is indicated by decreases in blood pressure, pulse, and sweating. In patients with peripheral vascular

P

PHENOXYBENZAMINE HYDROCHLORIDE (continued)

problems, observe for improvement in skin colour, temperature, and quality of peripheral pulses, as well as less sensitivity to cold.

- Advise patient not to take OTC medications for coughs, colds, or allergy without approval of physician. (Many contain sympathomimetic agents that cause blood pressure elevation.)
- Preserved in airtight containers, protected from light.

Phentermine hydrochloride

(Duromine, Lonamin)   *Sympathomimetic*

ACTIONS AND USES   Sympathomimetic amine related chemically and pharmacological to amphetamine (q.v.). Cardiovascular actions and CNS stimulant effects are less prominent than those of amphetamine.

Used as short-term (a few weeks) adjunct in management of exogenous obesity.

ROUTE AND DOSAGE   Oral: **Adult**: Extended release capsule, 15 to 30 mg once a day before breakfast.

CONTRAINDICATIONS AND PRECAUTIONS   History of hypersensitivity to sympathomimetic amines; during or within 14 days of MAO inhibitor use; glaucoma, angina, children 12 years or less. Safe use during pregnancy not established. **Cautious Use**: advance arteriosclerosis, symptomatic cardiovascular disease, moderate to severe hypertension, hyperthyroidism, glaucoma, agitated states, history of drug abuse.

ADVERSE/SIDE EFFECTS   Nervousness, dizziness, insomnia, dry mouth, nausea, constipation, hypertension, palpitation, tachycardia, decreased sexual desire, impotence; severe dermatoses, marked insomnia, irritability, hyperactivity, psychoses. Abrupt cessation following prolonged high dosage: extreme fatigue, depression, changes in sleep EEG patterns.

NURSING IMPLICATIONS
- Caution patient not to change established dose regimen, i.e., not to increase, decrease or omit doses. Warn against use of the drug for any purposes other than the one for which it is prescribed.
- To prevent insomnia, late evening medication should be avoided.
- Avoid caffeine drinks which increase amphetaminelike and related amine effects.
- Tolerance to anorexigenic effect usually occurs within a few weeks. Drug should be discontinued when this occurs.
- Caution patient to avoid potentially hazardous activities such as driving a car or operating machinery until his or her response to the drug is known.
- Instruct patient to notify physician if palpitation, nervousness or dizziness occur.
- Severe psychological dependence has occurred in patients who have exceeded recommended dosage.
- See *also amphetamine.*

PHENTERMINE HYDROCHLORIDE (continued)
DRUG INTERACTIONS   *Phentermine hydrochloride*_____

PLUS	INTERACTIONS
Acetozolamide, sodium bicarbonate	Increased renal reabsorption of phentermine
Ammonium chloride, ascorbic acid	Decreased phentermine effects
MAO inhibitors	Severe hypertension
Phenothiazines, haloperidol	Decreased effect of psychotropics

Phentolamine hydrochloride ━━━━━━━━━━━━━━

(Rogitine)   *Alpha-adrenergic blocking*
                                                                      agent

ACTIONS AND USES   Imidazoline alpha-adrenergic blocking agent structurally related to tolazoline, but has more potent blocking effects. Competetively blocks alpha-adrenergic receptors, but action is transient and incomplete. Prevents hypertension resulting from elevated levels of circulating adrenaline and/or noradrenaline. Causes vasodilation, and decreases general vascular resistance and pulmonary arterial pressure, primarily by direct action on vascular smooth muscle. Through stimulation of beta-adrenergic receptors, produces positive inotropic and chronotropic cardiac effects, and increases cardiac output. Also has histamine-like action that stimulates gastric secretions.

Used in diagnosis of phaeochromocytoma and to prevent or control hypertensive episodes prior to or during phaeochromocytomectomy.

ROUTE AND DOSAGE   **IV injection:** 5–10 mg repeated as required; **infusion:** 5–6 mg over 10–30 min at a rate of 0.1–2 mg/min.

ABSORPTION AND FATE   Maximum effect on blood pressure following IV administration in 2 minutes (persists 10 to 15 minutes), and in 15 to 20 minutes after IM (blood pressure returns to preinjection level in 3 to 4 hours).

CONTRAINDICATIONS AND PRECAUTIONS   Hypersensitivity to phentolamine or related drugs; myocardial infarction (previous or present). Safe use during pregnancy and lactation not established. **Cautious Use:** gastritis, peptic ulcer, coronary artery disease.

ADVERSE/SIDE EFFECTS   Weakness, dizziness, flushing, orthostatic hypotension, nasal stuffiness, conjunctival infection, abdominal pain, nausea, vomiting, diarrhoea, exacerbation of peptic ulcer. With parenteral administration especially: acute and prolonged hypotension, tachycardia, anginal pain, cardiac arrhythmias, myocardial infarction, cerebrovascular spasm, shocklike state.

NURSING IMPLICATIONS
- Patient should be in supine position when receiving drug parenterally. Monitor blood pressure and pulse every 2 minutes until stabilized.

PHENTOLAMINE HYDROCHLORIDE (continued)

- Instruct patient to lie down or sit down in head-low position immediately if feels lightheaded or dizzy.
- **Treatment of overdosage** (evidenced by precipitous drop in blood pressure)   Keep patient recumbent with head lowered; supportive measures; IV fluids; IV infusion of noradrenaline, carefully titrated. **Adrenaline as contraindicated**, since paradoxic fall in blood pressure may result.
- Phentolamine hydrochloride is preserved in well-closed, light-resistant containers.

Phenylbutazone

(Butacote, Butazolidin, Butazone)   *NSAID, pyrazolone*

ACTIONS AND USES   Pyrazolone derivative with antiinflammatory, antipyretic, analgesic, and mild uricosuric properties. Specific antiinflammatory action mechanism unknown but appears to be associated with prostaglandin synthesis, leucocyte migration, and release or activity of lysosomal enzymes. Inhibits platelet aggregation. Does not cure inflammatory condition but produces effective short-term symptomatic relief of pain and disability. Should not be used as a general analgesic or antipyretic.

Used in treatment of ankylosing spondylitis in hospitals only.

ROUTE AND DOSAGE   Oral: 200 mg 2–3 times a day, reduce to the minimum effective dose.

ABSORPTION AND FATE   Readily absorbed from GI tract with onset of action in 30 to 60 minutes. **Peak plasma levels** in 2 hours; **duration of action** 3 to 5 days. Repeated daily doses produce plateau in plasma levels in 3 to 5 days. Metabolized in liver to several active metabolites including oxyphenbutazone and hydroxyphenylbutazone. 98% protein-bound; **half-life**: 50 to 100 hours (increased to 149 hours with hepatic dysfunction). Distributed to most body tissues. Excreted slowly in urine as unchanged drug (1%) and metabolites. Crosses placenta; enters breast milk, and synovial spaces (with concentration equal to about 50% that in plasma). Has potential cumulative toxicity.

CONTRAINDICATIONS AND PRECAUTIONS   Phenylbutazone or oxyphenbutazone sensitivity and idiosyncrasy, history of peptic ulcer, GI inflammatory disease, pancreatitis, stomatitis, aspirin hypersensitivity, drug allergy, blood dyscrasias, renal disease, hepatic dysfunction, left ventricular failure, borderline cardiac failure, severe hypertension, oedema, polymyalgia rheumatica, temporal arteritis, concomitant use with other drugs such as chemotherapeutic agents, use with long-term anticoagulants (oral) therapy, children under age 14, senile patient. Safe use during pregnancy especially during third trimester not established. **Cautious Use**: glaucoma, patients over age 40, asthma.

PHENYLBUTAZONE *(continued)*

ADVERSE/SIDE EFFECTS   These include: hypertension, palpitation, pericarditis, cardiac decompensation, fixed drug eruptions, erythema nodosum and multiforme, nonthrombocytopenic purpura, optic neuritis, retinal haemorrhage and detachment, oculomotor palsy, toxic amblyopia, blurred vision, conjunctivitis, scotomata; hearing loss, tinnitus, hyperglycaemia, thyroid hyperplasia, toxic goitre, myxoedema; sodium, chloride and fluid retention; rapid plasma volume expansion with plasma dilution, metabolic acidosis, respiratory alkalosis, recurring dyspepsia (including heartburn and indigestion), nausea, vomiting, constipation, diarrhoea, xerostomia, ulcerative stomatitis and oesophagitis, salivary gland enlargement, epigastric pain, constipation, abdominal distention with flatulence, ulceration of bowel, reactivation of peptic ulcer, hepatitis (fatal and nonfatal), pancreatitis, bone marrow depression, pancytopenia, thrombocytopenia, agranulocytosis, aplastic anaemia (sometimes fatal), leucopenia, leukaemia, haematuria, proteinuria, glomerulonephritis, renal failure, nephrotic syndrome, renal calculi, azotemia, trembling, nervousness, taste disturbances.

NURSING IMPLICATIONS

- Steady state therapeutic serum levels: reached in 3 to 4 days.
- Possible GI irritation can be minimized by administering drug with meals or with full glass of milk.
- Tablet may crushed and capsule may be emptied if patient cannot swallow them whole. Mix crushed powder or capsule contents with fluid of patient's choice or mix with food. Should not be swallowed dry.
- Careful, detailed history and complete physical and laboratory examinations (including GI diagnostic tests in patient with persistent or severe dyspepsia) are advised prior to initiating therapy.
- Frequent regular blood studies are advisable when drug is given beyond 1 week, the usual treatment period.
- Any significant change in haematology: i.e., total white count depression, relative decrease in granulocytes, appearance of blast forms, fall in haematocrit, signals the necessity to stop treatment pending complete haematology studies.
- Although phenylbutazone increases action of oral anticoagulants when given concomitantly, it does not affect prothrombin activity when administered alone; however, the combination of antiplatelet and ulcerogenic action of phenylbutazone contributes to the hazard of of serious haemorrhage during drug therapy.
- Keep physician informed of patient's response to medication. If favourable response is not noted in 1 week drug is discontinued. When improvement occurs (usually begins in 3 to 4 days), dosage is reduced and discontinued as soon as symptomatic relief dictates.
- Adverse reactions are both age- and dose-related. If the patient is over age 60, longer than a 1-week treatment period is not recommended because of high risk of severe, fatal, toxic reactions in this age group.
- Check with physician about alcohol ingestion. Alcohol impairs motor coordination in the patient receiving phenylbutazone (probably in additive effect). This action should be pointed out to the patient especially with respect to driving.
- Warn patient to discontinue drug therapy immediately and report to physician:

P

PHENYLBUTAZONE (continued)

fever, stomatitis, oral ulcerations, salivary gland enlargement, severe sore throat, epigastric pain, dyspepsia, unusual unexplained bleeding and bruising, tarry stools, skin rashes, oedema, pruritus, jaundice.

- Any eye symptoms should be investigated. Be sure patient understands this, because (especially with the elderly person) adaptation to blurring may be subconscious at first. Drug should be discontinued and a complete ophthalmic examination carried out.
- Keep in mind that the presenting symptom of leukaemia (an adverse effect of phenylbutazone) can be arthritic-like pain; therefore reappearance of acute joint pain after satisfactory response to treatment, should be differentially evaluated.
- Monitor patient with asthma especially if patient is also sensitive to aspirin. This drug like others with prostaglandin synthetase inhibition activity may precipitate an acute asthma attack.
- Urge patient not to self-dose with OTC drugs unless advised to do so by physician. Many pain relief OTC preparations contain aspirin.
- Phenylbutazone may cause drowsiness; therefore, advise patient to observe caution while driving or performing tasks requiring alertness until response to drug is known.
- Warn patient to adhere to dosage regimen, i.e., not to double, reduce, or omit doses nor to change dose intervals without the physician's approval.

Food (nutrient)–drug interaction Phenylbutazone interferes with absorption of folates, tryptophane and other amino acids.
- **Smoking–drug interaction** Smoking shortens half-life and increases clearance rate of phenylbutazone. It is possible that the heavy smoker may require an adjusted dosage regimen.
- Instruct patient to keep a record of daily weight and to check for lower leg, ankle, or facial oedema. Advise patient to report sudden weight gain (i.e., gain of 1–1.5 kg within 2 to 3 days). Oedema may signify hepatic or renal dysfunction or electrolyte imbalance and may indicate necessity of stopping therapy. In the elderly, a reduction of dose may suffice to reduce oedema of ankles and face.
- Store drug at temperature between 15° and 30°C (59° and 86°F) in light and moisture-resistant container.

Diagnostic test interferences Phenylbutazone reduces **iodine uptake** by thyroid gland.

DRUG INTERACTIONS *Phenylbutazone*_____

PLUS	INTERACTIONS
Alcohol	Increased phenylbutazone-induced ulcerogenic effects
Antiinflammatory agents (other NSAIDs)	Displaced from protein-binding sites with resulting increase in pharmacological and toxic effects of displaced drug; the reverse is also true: i.e., phenylbutazone may be displaced, increasing its serum concentration and potential toxicity

PHENYLBUTAZONE (continued)

PLUS (continued)	INTERACTIONS
Anticoagulants, coumarins	Increased anticoagulant effect; increased risk of serious haemorrhage. Concomitant use should be avoided
Aspirin	Increases ulcerogenic effects of phenylbutazone
Beta-blocking agents	May reduce antihypertensive effects of the beta-blocker
Desipramine	Decreases phenylbutazone serum level, thereby reducing clinical effects
Digitalis glycosides	Enhances metabolism of digitalis leading to underdigitalization
Hydantoins (e.g., phenytoin)	Increased risk of phenytoin toxicity
Hypoglycaemics, sulphonylureas	Increased hypoglycaemic effects
Insulin	Potentiation of hypoglycaemic action of insulin
Methotrexate	Increased response to methotrexate possibly leading to toxicity. Concomitant use should be avoided
Salicylates	Antagonizes uricosuric activity
Sulphonamides	See antiinflammatory agents
Thyroid hormone	See antiinflammatory agents

Phenylephrine hydrochloride ▬▬▬▬▬▬▬▬▬▬▬▬

(Neophryn)
Adrenergic (vasoconstrictor)
Alpha-adrenergic

ACTIONS AND USES   Potent, noncatecholamine, direct-acting sympathomimetic with strong alpha-adrenergic and weak beta-adrenergic cardiac stimulant actions. Produces little or no CNS stimulation. Elevates systolic and diastolic pressures through arteriolar constriction; also constricts capacitance vessels and increases venous return to heart. Rise in blood pressure causes reflex bradycardia. Topical applications to eye produce vasconstriction and prompt mydriasis of short duration, usually without causing cycloplegia. Reduces intraocular pressure by increasing outflow and decreasing rate of aqueous and humour secretion. Nasal decongestant action qualitatively similar to that of adrenaline but more potent and has longer duration of action.

Used parenterally to maintain blood pressure during anaesthesia, to treat vascular failure in shock, and to overcome paroxysmal supraventricular tachycardia. Used topically for rhinitis of common cold, allergic rhinitis, and sinusitis; in selected patients with wide-angle glaucoma; as mydriatic for opthalmoscopic examination or surgery, and for relief of uveitis.

ROUTE AND DOSAGE   Parenteral: *Hypotension*: **Intramuscular, subcutaneous:** 2 to 5 mg (range 1 to 10 mg) initial dose not to exceed 5 mg every 10 to 15 minutes as

PHENYLEPHRINE HYDROCHLORIDE (continued)

needed. **Intravenous infusion**: 5–20 mg/500 ml Dextrose Injection or NaCI Injection): adjusted according to response. **Intravenous injection**: 0.1 to 0.5 mg; subsequent doses no more often than 10 to 15 minutes at increments of up to 0.2 mg. **Eye drops**: 2.5 and 10%. **Nasal drops**: 0.25% spray, 0.5% as required.

ABSORPTION AND FATE   IV: immediate effects lasting 20 to 30 minutes. SC: IM: effects last 45 to 60 minutes. Maximum mydriasis achieved within 60 minutes; recovery usually occurs approximately 6 hours later. Decongestant effect (direct vasoconstriction) with use of nasal preparations: prompt and lasts for several hours.

CONTRAINDICATIONS AND PRECAUTIONS   Severe coronary disease, severe hypertension, ventricular tachycardia; narrow-angle glaucoma (ophthalmic preparations). **Cautious Use**: hyperthyroidism, diabetes mellitus, myocardial disease, cerebral arteriosclerosis, bradycardia, elderly patients; 21 days before or following termination of MAO inhibitor therapy. *10% ophthalmic solution*: elderly patients with preexisting cardiovascular disease, or patients with diabetes mellitus, hypertension or hyperthyroidism; patients with aneurysms, infants.

ADVERSE/SIDE EFFECTS   **Intranasal**: rebound congestion (hyperaemia and oedema of mucosa), burning, stinging, dryness, sneezing. **Ophthalmic**: transient stinging, lacrimation, browache, headache, blurred vision, conjunctival allergy (pigmentary deposits on lids, conjunctiva, and cornea with prolonged use), increased sensitivity to light. **Systemic effects**: palpitation, tachycardia, bradycardia (overdosage), extrasystoles, hypertension, trembling, sweating, pallor, sense of fullness in head, tingling of extremities, sleeplessness, dizziness, lightheadedness, weakness.

NURSING IMPLICATIONS

- During IV administration, monitor pulse, blood pressure and central venous pressure (every 2 to 5 minutes). Control flow rate and dosage to prevent excessive increases.
- IV overdoses can induce ventricular dysrhythmias.
- Have ready phentolamine to treat hypertensive emergency with IV administration; levodopa to reduce excess mydriatic effect of ophthalmic preparation.
- Caution patient not to exceed recommended dosage regardless of formulation; i.e., patient should not double, decrease or omit doses nor should patient change dose intervals unless told to do so by the physician.
- If no relief is experienced from preparation in 5 days, patient should inform the physician.
- Systemic absorption from nasal and conjunctival membranes can occur, though infrequently (*See Adverse/Side Effects*). Stop the drug and report to the physician.

Nasal preparations   Instruct patient to blow nose gently (with both nostrils open) to clear nasal passages well, before administration of medication.

- *Instillation* (*Drops*): tilt head back while sitting or standing up, or lie on bed and hang head over side. Stay in position a few minutes to permit medication to spread through nose.
- (*Spray*): with head upright, squeeze bottle quickly and firmly to produce 1 or 2 sprays into each nostril; wait 3 to 5 minutes, blow nose and repeat dose.

P

PHENYLEPHRINE HYDROCHLORIDE (continued)

Ophthalmic preparations   (*See Index for administration instructions*):

- To avoid excessive systemic absorption, tell patient to apply pressure to lacrimal sac during and for 1 to 2 minutes after instillation of drops.
- Inform patient that after instillation of ophthalmic preparation, pupils of eyes will be very large and eyes may be more sensitive to light than usual. Advise patient to use sunglasses in bright light and to stop medication and notify physician if this sensitivity persists beyond 12 hours after drug has been discontinued.
- Instillation of 2.5 to 10% strength solution frequently can cause burning and stinging.
- Observe for congestion or rebound miosis after topical administration to eye.
- A local anaesthetic may be instilled before the phenylephrine to reduce discomfort of stinging and burning.
- Caution patient that some ophthalmic solutions may stain contact lenses.

- Avoid swallowing solutions or jelly; systemic effects may be induced.
- Cleanse tips and droppers of nasal solution dispensers with hot water after use to prevent contamination of solution. Droppers of ophthalmic solution bottles should not touch any surface including the eye.
- Do not allow anyone other than the patient to use the prescribed supply of phenylephrine.
- Phenylephrine is incompatable with butacaine, oxidizing agents, ferric salts, metals, and alkalies.
- Solutions and jelly change colour to brown, form a precipitate and lose potency with exposure to air, strong light or heat. Do not transfer solutions from original container to another.
- Store in original container at temperature between 15° and 30°C (59° and 86°F) protected from freezing, strong light and exposure to air.

DRUG INTERACTIONS *Phenylephrine hydrochloride*_____

PLUS	INTERACTIONS
Ergot alkaloids, guanethidine, reserpine, tricyclic antidepressants	Increase pressor effects of phenylephrine
Halothane, digitalis, mercurial diuretics	Cardiac arrhythmias
MAO inhibitors	Hypertensive crisis
Oxytoxics	Persistence hypertension

Phenylpropanolamine hydrochloride ━━━━━━━━━━━━━

ACTIONS AND USES   Sympathomimetic drug used in combination products (Eskornade, Dimotane) to treat sinusitis and catarrh.

Phenytoin ▬▬▬▬▬▬▬▬▬▬▬▬▬▬▬▬▬▬▬▬▬▬▬▬▬▬▬▬▬▬▬▬▬▬▬▬▬▬▬

(Epanutin, Infatabs)   *Anticonvulsant; antiarrhythmic;*
hydantoin

ACTIONS AND USES   Hydantoin derivative chemically related to phenobarbitone. Precise mechanism of anticonvulsant action not known but drug use is accompanied by reduced voltage, frequency, and spread of electrical discharges within the motor cortex, resulting in prevention or reduction in severity and frequency of epileptiform attacks. Unlike phenobarbitone has little hypnotic action, is ineffective for control of drug-induced seizures, and has limited ability to modify threshold in electroconvulsive seizures. Has antiarrhythmic properties similar to those of lignocaine and tocainamide. Induces hepatic microsomal enzymes and therefore affects the metabolism of many other drugs. Like other hydantoin derivatives, increases metabolic inactivation of vitamin D and has antifolate properties.

Used to control grand mal, psychomotor and nonepileptic seizures treatment of paradoxical atrial tachycardia, ventricular arrhythmias, particularly those associated with digitalis toxicity, and symptomatic treatment of rheumatoid arthritis.

ROUTE AND DOSAGE   **Oral: Adults:** usual range: 150–300 mg daily. Dose limit up to 600 mg/day. Doses may be given once a day or in 3 divided doses after maintenance dose is established. **Paediatric:** usual range 5–8 mg/kg/day, in 1 or 2 divided doses. **Intravenous: Arrhythmias:** 3.5–5 mg/kg at a rate of 50 mg/min or less. Repeat after 10 min if required. **Status epilepticus:** 13–15 mg/kg at a rate of 50 mg/min or less as a loading dose. **Maintenance** doses of 100 mg are then given at 6 hourly intervals.

ABSORPTION AND FATE   Slowly absorbed following oral administration (rate of absorption may vary widely among products by different manufacturers). **Peak plasma concentrations** (oral): 3 to 12 hours; phenytoin sodium: 2 to 3 hours. **Onset of action:** 3 to 5 minutes following IV injection. Drug precipitates at IM injection site and is slowly and erratically absorbed. Wide distribution to all tissues with highest concentrations in liver and fat; 70 to 95% **bound to plasma proteins** (mainly albumin). **Half-life:** 8 to 60 (average: 20 to 30) hours after initiation of therapy with oral daily dose of 300 mg (may be longer in black patients). Biotransformation in liver primarily, with excretion in bile as inactive metabolites which are reabsorbed from GI tract (enterohepatic circulation). Renal excretion (enhanced by alkaline urine) as glucuronides. Less than 5% excreted unchanged. Crosses placenta; enters breast milk.

CONTRAINDICATIONS AND PRECAUTIONS   Hypersensitivity to hydantoin products, skin rash, seizures due to hypoglycaemia, during lactation, sinus bradycardia, complete or incomplete heart block, Adams-Stokes syndrome. **Cautious Use:** impaired hepatic or renal function, alcoholism, blood dyscrasias, hypotension, heart block, bradycardia, myocardial insufficiency, impending or frank heart failure, elderly, debilitated, gravely ill patients; pancreatic adenoma, pregnancy, diabetes mellitus, hyperglycaemia, respiratory depression.

ADVERSE/SIDE EFFECTS   These include: nystagmus, diplopia, blurred or dimmed vision, lethargy, drowsiness, ataxia, dizziness, slurred speech, mental confusion, tre-

PHENYTOIN (continued)

mors, insomnia, headache; peripheral neuropathy, encephalopathy. With rapid IV injection: ventricular fibrillation, bradycardia, hypotension, cardiovascular collapse, cardiac (and respiratory) arrest. Also: phlebitis, injection site pain, nausea, vomiting, constipation, epigastric pain, dysphagia, loss of taste, weight loss, hepatitis, liver necrosis, thrombocytopenia, leucopenia, leucocytosis, agranulocytosis, pancytopenia, eosinophilia, macrocytosis, megaloblastic anaemia, hyperglycaemia, glycosuria, transient increase in serum thyrotropic level, photophobia, conjunctivitis, visual disturbances, gingival hyperplasia, hirsutism (especially young females), keratosis, oedema, osteomalacia or rickets associated with hypocalcaemia and elevated alkaline phosphatase activity; pulmonary fibrosis, periarteritis nodosum; acute systemic lupus erythematosus; tissue necrosis; lymphadenopathy, craniofacial abnormalities (especially in young people) after long-term use, neonatal haemorrhage.

NURSING IMPLICATIONS

- **Therapeutic serum concentration**: 10 to 20 mcg/ml; *toxic levels*: 30 to 50 mcg/ml; *lethal level*: 100 mcg/ml. Steady state therapeutic levels are not achieved for at least 7 to 10 days.
- If patient cannot take a whole tablet or capsule, the table may be crushed or the capsule may be emptied prior to administration. Drug should be mixed with food or fluid; have patient swallow a fluid first, then follow with the diluted or mixed drug along with a full glass of water, milk, or with food. This drug is strongly alkaline, and should not be swallowed without prior preparation prevent oesophageal and gastric direct contact.
- Shake suspension vigorously before pouring to ensure uniform distribution of drug.
- Inform patient that drug may impart a harmless pink or red to red-brown colouration to urine.
- Do not interchange preparations of phenytoin; capsules, Infatabs and Syrup are not equivalent.
- Chewable tablets are not intended for once-a-day dosage since drug is too quickly bioavailable and can therefore lead to toxic serum levels.
- Intramuscular injection is not recommended because of high alkalinity of solution (pH 12). If used however, when patient is returned to oral regimen, dosage is reduced by 50% of original oral dosage for 1 week to compensate for sustained release of medication.
- Solubility of phenytoin is pH dependent; therefore, avoid mixing with other drugs or adding to any infusion solution, to prevent precipitation.
- A slightly yellowed injectable solution may be used safely. Precipitation may be caused by refrigeration, but slow warming to room temperature restores clarity. Do not administer unclear solution.
- During IV phenytoin administration, observe injection site frequently to prevent increase in rate of infusion and infiltration.
- To minimize local venous irritation, 0.9% saline solution is introduced after the drug injection through the same in-place catheter or needle.
- To reduce side effects, lower doses than the usual adult range are given to geriatric, severely ill, debilitated patients or those with liver damage and the flow rate is reduced to 50 mg over a 2- to 3-minute period.

P

PHENYTOIN (continued)

- Margin between toxic and therapeutic IV dose is relatively small. Closely monitor vital signs and symptoms during IV infusion and for an hour afterward. If patient is elderly or has cardiac disease constant observation and a cardiac monitor are necessary.
- Observe patient closely for CNS side effects. Have on hand oxygen, atropine, vasopressor, assisted ventilation, seizure precaution equipment (padded side rails, suction apparatus).
- Phenytoin can unmask a low thyroid reserve. Advise patient on long-term therapy to report symptoms of fatigue, dry skin, deepening voice.
- Caution patient to report promptly onset of liver dysfunction as evidenced by jaundice. Since the drug is largely metabolized in the liver, impairment of function leads to increased serum levels of phenytoin, and toxicity. Early recognition of a toxic reaction may save the patient's life.
- Liver and thyroid function tests, blood counts, and urinalyses are recommended prior to therapy, at monthly intervals during early therapy, and at regular periods during prolonged therapy.
- Caution patient not to alter prescribed drug regimen. Abrupt drug discontinuation may precipitate seizures and status epilepticus.
- Withdrawal and discontinuation of phenytoin must be done gradually, over a period of 1 to 3 or more months and in relation to serum drug levels and EEGs.
- Gingival hyperplasia appears most commonly in children and adolescents; never occurs in edentulous patients. Condition can be minimized by daily brushing with soft toothbrush, careful flossing to remove dental plaque, and gum massage. Parents must brush and floss teeth (waxed floss) for children once daily up to at least 6 to 8 years of age when children should be able to do it alone. Advise patient/parent to inform dentist that patient is taking phenytoin, gingivectomy is sometimes necessary.
- Use of electric toothbrush may assure better compliance in young children.
- Caution patient to avoid hazardous activities particularly during early therapy, and not to drive a car until approval is given by physician.
- Warn patient about the effects of alcohol: alcohol intake may increase phenytoin serum levels leading to phenytoin toxicity. The chronic alcoholic may decrease serum levels of the drug with alcohol ingestion leading to loss of or erratic seizure control. Doses will need to be higher than for the nonalcoholic patient.
- Phenytoin should be discontinued immediately if a measles-like skin rash appears. Therapy may be resumed when rash disappears. If exfoliative, purpuric, or bullous, drug treatment is not usually resumed.
- Anticonvulsant therapy during pregnancy lactation or in the woman of childbearing age must be weighed carefully as to benefit—risk to both mother and unborn child. Multiple congenital anomalies in the newborn of a mother on phenytoin during pregnancy have been reported.
- Notify physician if pregnancy is suspected or planned. Seizure frequency during pregnancy increases in a large number of women because of changes in absorption or metabolism of phenytoin.
- If patient is receiving phenytoin to prevent major seizures it probably will not be

PHENYTOIN (continued)

stopped during pregnancy because of the risk of precipitated status epilepticus with attendant hypoxia, a danger to both mother and foetus.

■ Be certain patient realizes she needs the drug and counsel her about risk to foetus if she interrupts drug therapy without physician's advice. Urge her to keep appointments for frequent serum concentration evaluations during pregnancy.

■ An attempt may be made to discontinue anticonvulsant treatment before and during pregnancy if the nature, frequency, and severity of seizures do not pose a threat to the woman. Whether or not slight seizures affect the foetus is not clearly established.

■ Anticonvulsants taken during pregnancy appear to pose a threat of coagulation defect that may cause neonatal bleeding (usually within 24 hours). Vitamin K_1 may be given to the mother one month before and during delivery amd to the infant (IV) immediately after birth.

■ Marked hypoglycaemic states may cause severe convulsive seizures. If hypoglycaemia is present or suspected as with pancreatic adenoma, blood sugar studies should be followed.

■ Patients with diabetes should be monitored regularly for symptoms of hyperglycaemia (polydipsia, polyuria, lethargy, drowsiness, psychotic manifestations, glycosuria). Adjustment of phenytoin dosage (for patients on insulin) or adjustment of oral hypoglycaemic dosage may be necessary.

■ Hydration may be a sufficient factor in seizure control. Mild dehydration has been associated with decline in number of seizures. Discuss with physician.

■ A well balanced diet is an important adjunct to effective anticonvulsant therapy. Collaborate with dietitian, patient/family in diet planning. Urge patient to eat regularly and to avoid overeating.

Food/nutrient–drug interactions

■ Patients on prolonged therapy should have adequate intake of vitamin D containing foods (e.g., fortified milk, margarine, butter, liver, egg yolk, fish such as salmon, sardines, herring), and sufficient exposure to sunlight.

■ Periodic checks are indicated for decrease in serum Ca levels (sign of bone demineralization and potential rickets or osteomalacia). Particularly susceptible: black children, patients receiving other anticonvulsants concurrently, patients who are inactive, have limited exposure to sunlight, or whose dietary intake is inadequate.

■ Hydantoin derivatives interfere with metabolism of folic acid, a nutrient with doubled requirements during pregnancy (could lead to megaloblastic anaemia). Observe patient for symptoms of folic acid deficiency: neuropathy, mental dysfunction, psychiatric disorders. Serum folate levels should be determined at onset of symptoms.

■ Daily supplements (if required) with phenytoin therapy: vitamin K, vitamin D, folic acid may be prescribed.

■ Influenza vaccine during phenytoin treatment may cause an increase in seizure activity. The patient should be alerted in case a change in dose is necessary.

■ After patient has been well stabilized on maintenance regimen of divided doses, physician may prescribe single daily phenytoin dose of same amount.

P

PHENYTOIN (continued)

■ Duration of phenytoin treatment is extremely variable. In some patients, a lifetime of drug therapy is necessary; in others, physician may attempt to withdraw drug after a seizure-free period (including auras) of 2 to 5 years.

■ Instruct responsible family member how to take care of patient during a seizure, what to observe and record. Advise to call for emergency help if patient has one seizure after another, has trouble breathing, or has sustained an injury. *General instructions*: Do not attempt to restrain patient, but protect from injury, e.g., pillow, blanket, or clothing under head, loosen constricting clothing. If teeth are clenched, do not force them open because they could be broken and aspirated. After convulsion is over, turn patient on side to facilitate drainage of oropharyngeal secretions. Record sequence of various phenomena during seziure (describe location and type movements; position of head, eyes, extremities; pupil size; duration of seizure, behaviour following seizure to help physician to localize area of brain involved) Notify physician that patient had a seizure.

■ Patient/family may require help with emotional reaction to epilepsy, problems of stigmatized discrimination that may occur, and require life style adjustments.

Patient–family teaching plan Construct plan in collaboration with physician, dietitian, and other relevant health team members emphasizing the following points:

☐ Reason for taking medication.
☐ Take drug precisely as prescribed.
☐ Adverse reactions.
☐ What to do in the event of a seizure.
☐ Avoid colds, infections: if they occur, notify physician.
☐ Importance of regularity and moderation in life style.
☐ Well-balanced diet; avoid overeating and overhydration.
☐ Avoid OTC drugs.
☐ Alcohol restriction (consult physician regarding allowable amount).
☐ Moderation in physical activity; avoid high risk sports.
☐ Avoid emotional stress; talk problems out with physician, nurse, or significant other.
☐ Keep follow-up appointments.
☐ Carry identification card or jewellery with pertinent medical data.

Diagnostic test interferences Phenytoin (hydantoins) may produce lower than normal values for dexamethasone or methyrapone tests; may increase serum levels of glucose, BSP and alkaline phosphatase; and may decrease PBI levels and urinary steroid levels.

DRUG INTERACTIONS   *Phenytoin*_____

Decreased serum levels: decreased phenytoin effects

Alcohol, chronic abuse
Antacids (aluminium, calcium magnesium compounds)
Antihistamines (H_1-receptor antagonists)
Anti neoplastics (cisplatin, vinblastine, bleomycin)
Barbiturates

Calcium gluconate
Carbamazepine
CNS depressants
Folic acid
Reserpine
Rifampicin

PHENYTOIN (continued)

Increased serum levels: increased risk of toxicity; loss of seizure control; increased phenytoin effects

Alcohol (acute intake)
Aminosalicylic acid (PAS)
Amiodarone
Anticoagulants, coumarins
Anticonvulsants, other e.g., trimethoidione, ethotoin
Benzodiazepines (e.g., diazepam, flurazepam)
Chloramphenicol
Cimetidine
Dexamethasone
Disulphiram
Lignocaine ⎱
Propranolol ⎰
Sympathomimetics
Valproic acid

Oestrogens (including oral contraceptives)
Ethosuximide
Halothane
Isoniazid
Methylphenidate
Phenothiazines (e.g., chlorpromazine, thioridazine)
Pyrazolones (e.g., phenylbutazone)
Salicylates
Sulphonamides
Tolbutamide

Additive cardiac depressant effects

Sudden hypotension and bradycardia
May cause increased or decreased phenytoin serum concentration

Physostigmine sulphate ▬▬▬▬▬▬▬▬▬▬▬▬▬▬▬▬

Cholinergic, ophthalmic; miotic

ACTIONS AND USES   Reversible anticholinesterase and tertiary amine. Used topically to eye to reduce intraocular tension in glaucoma.

ROUTE AND DOSAGE   **Topical:** *Ophthalmic solution* (0.25% or 0.5%): 1 or 2 drops, three times daily.

ABSORPTION AND FATE   Readily absorbed from mucous membranes, muscle, and subcutaneous tissue. Onset of action following instillation into conjunctival sac, action begins within 2 minutes, peaks in 1 to 2 hours, and persists 12 to 36 hours. Renal impairment does not require dose adjustment.

NURSING IMPLICATIONS
- The patient with brown or hazel irides may require a stronger ophthalmic solution, or more frequent instillation for desired effects than the patient with blue irides.
- When used as topical agent, be alert to symptoms of systemic absorption. Dosage should be reduced or drug discontinued.
- Inform patient that physostigmine ophthalmic preparations may produce annoying lid twitching, temporary blurring of vision, and difficulty in seeing in dimmed light; therefore, necessary safety precautions should be taken. Hospitalized patients will require supervised ambulation.
- Emphasize the need for following prescribed drug regimen for glaucoma, and

PHYSOSTIGMINE SULPHATE (continued)

urge patient to remain under medical supervision. Untreated glaucoma can cause blindness.

■ Tolerance may develop with long-term use. Effectiveness can be regained by substituting another miotic for a short time and then resuming treatment with physostigmine.

■ Teaching plan for patients with glaucoma should include the following:
   □ Proper administration of eyedrops;
   □ Adverse symptoms to be reported;
   □ Caution about not wearing constricting clothing, such as tight collar, belt, or girdle;
   □ Activities to avoid that could provoke increase in intraocular pressure, such as heavy exertion, forceful nose blowing or coughing, straining at stool, crying, and emotionally upsetting situations.

■ Patient should be advised to wear identification tag indicating the presence of glaucoma and the medication being taken.

■ Store at temperature between 15° and 30°C (59° and 86°F).

■ *See also neostigmine.*

DRUG INTERACTIONS   *Physostigmine*

PLUS	INTERACTIONS
Ecothiophate, isoflurophate	Actions inhibited by prior instillation

Phytomenadione

(Konakion)

ACTIONS AND USES   Vitamine K, used to treat deficiency in neonates and excessive reduction in clotting ability due to oral anticoagulants such as warfarin.

ROUTE AND DOSAGE   *Deficiency in neonate*: 1 mg by iminjection. *Reduced clotting abilities* Oral: 5–10 mg.

Pilocarpine hydrochloride

(Ispoto Carpine, Ocusert, Opulets pilocarpine, Sno pilo)   *Cholinergic (parasympathomimetic); miotic*

ACTIONS AND USES   Tertiary amine derived from chief alkaloid of *Pilocarpus jaborandi*. Acts directly on cholinergic receptor sites, thus, mimicking acetylcholine.

Used for medical management of open-angle and angle-closure glaucomas:

PILOCARPINE HYDROCHLORIDE *(continued)*

ROUTE AND DOSAGE   Ophthalmic solution: (many strengths ranging from 0.5 to 4%), apply 3–6 times a day.

ABSORPTION AND FATE   Penetrates cornea rapidly. Miosis begins in 10 to 30 minutes, peaks in about 30 minutes and lasts 4 to 8 hours and is continuously maintained for 7 days. Tolerance may develop with prolonged use.

CONTRAINDICATIONS AND PRECAUTIONS   Hypersensitivity to drug components, secondary glaucoma, acute iritis, acute inflammatory disease of anterior segment of eye. Safe use during pregnancy and lactation has not been established. **Cautious Use**: bronchial asthma, hypertension. Ocular therapeutic system: not used in acute infectious conjunctivitis, keratitis, retinal detachment, or when intense miosis is required.

ADVERSE/SIDE EFFECTS   Generally well tolerated, Ciliary spasm with brow ache, twitching of eyelids, eye pain with change in eye focus, miosis, diminished vision in poorly illuminated areas, blurred vision, reduced visual acuity, sensitivity. **Infrequent**: contact allergy, lacrimation, follicular conjunctivitis, conjunctival irritation, cataract, retinal detachment. **Systemic**: nausea, vomiting, abdominal cramps, diarrhoea, epigastric distress, salivation, bronchospasm, tachycardia, tremors, increased sweating.

NURSING IMPLICATIONS

- Wash hands thoroughly with soap and water before and after instilling eyedrops or placing the ocular therapeutic system in the cul-de-sac.
- When instilling eye drops, care should be taken to prevent contamination of dropper tip and solution, and to avoid touching eyelids or surrounding area with the dropper tip.
- Immediately after instillation of drops, apply gentle digital pressure to periphery of nasolacrimal drainage system for 1 to 2 minutes to prevent delivery of drug to nasal mucosa and general circulation. Excess solution around eye or on hands should be removed immediately with a tissue. (*See Index: Drug administration for additional notes about ophthalmic instillation.*)
- The patient should understand that therapy for glaucoma is prolonged and that adherence to established regimen is crucial to prevent blindness.
- Since drug causes blurred vision and difficulty in focusing, caution patient to avoid hazardous activities such as driving a car or operating machinery until vision clears.
- Brow pain and myopia tend to be more prominent in younger patients and generally disappear with continued use of drug.
- Inform patient to withhold medication if symptoms of irritation or sensitization persist and to report to physician/ophthalmologist.
- Advise patient to keep follow-up appointments.
- Store ocular system form at 2° to 8°C (35° to 46°F); avoid freezing. Store solutions in tight, light-resistant containers.

Drug interactions   The actions of pilocarpine and carbarchol are additive when used concomitantly.

Pimozide

(Orap)

Psychotropic; antipsychotic
agent (neuroleptic);
butyrophenone

ACTIONS AND USES   Neuroleptic agent; analogue of the butyrophenones and derivative of pethidine-like analgesics. A potent central dopamine antagonist that causes altered release and turnover of central dopamine stores; has no effect on turnover of noradrenaline.

Used to treat schizophrenia and related psychoses.

ROUTE AND DOSAGE   (Slow, gradual introduction.) **Oral:** 2–20 mg/day according to response. Maximum dose 60 mg/day.

ABSORPTION AND FATE   More than 50% of dose absorbed after ingestion; significant first-pass metabolism. Peak serum levels attained in 6 to 8 hours after dose is administered. Metabolized chiefly in liver with production of two major metabolites. **Half-life:** about 55 hours. Excreted in urine.

CONTRAINDICATIONS AND PRECAUTIONS   Hypersensitivity to pimozide, history of cardiac dysrrhythmias and conditions marked by prolonged QT syndrome, patient taking drugs that may prolong QT interval (e.g., quinidine), severe toxic CNS depression. Safe use in children under 12 years of age, during pregnancy, and by nursing mothers not established. **Cautious Use:** renal and hepatic dysfunction; patients receiving anticonvulsant therapy.

ADVERSE/SIDE EFFECTS   These include: headache, sedation, drowsiness, insomnia, akathisia, speech disorder, handwriting changes, akinesia, grand mal seizures, fainting, hyperpyrexia, persistent tardive dyskinesia, oculogyric crisis, hyperreflexia; neuroleptic malignant syndrome: extrapyramidal dysfunction, hyperthermia, autonomic dysfunction; tachycardia, labile blood pressure, diaphoresis, dyspnoea, urinary incontinence; elevated CPK, WBC, liver function enzymes; respiratory failure, acute renal failure, stupor, prolongation of QT interval, inverted or flattened T-wave, appearance of U-wave, sweating, skin irritation, visual disturbances, photosensitivity, decreased accommodation, blurred vision cataracts, loss of libido, impotence, nocturia, urinary frequency, weight changes, asthenia, chest pain, periorbital oedema.

NURSING IMPLICATIONS
- Advise patient to adhere to established drug regimen, i.e., dose or intervals should not be changed and dose should be discontinued only with physician's guidance.
- Risk to tardive dyskinesia appears to be greatest in women, in the elderly, and those on high dosage. Both patient and family should be alerted to the earliest symptom ('flycatching'—an involuntary movement of the tongue) which should be reported promptly to the physician.
- When drug is to be discontinued, the regimen should be adjusted by prescription: slow, gradual changes over a period of days or weeks (drug has a long half-life). Sudden withdrawal may cause reemergence of original symptoms (motor and phonic tics) and of neuromuscular side effects of the drug.

P

PIMOZIDE (continued)

- If neuromuscular reactions are too distressing, an antiparkinsonian agent may be prescribed.
- The syndrome of tardive dyskinesia can be unmasked by reinstitution of drug therapy after a drug holiday, by increasing dosage, or by switching to another antipsychotic drug. Be alert to symptoms at these particular times.
- Pseudoparkinsonian symptoms (drooling, mask facies, rigidity and tremors especially of hands) are usually mild and reversible with dose adjustment.
- ECG baseline data should be obtained at beginning of therapy and checked periodically, especially during period of dosage adjustment.
- Urge patient to return for periodic assessments of therapy benefit and cardiac status.
- Anticholinergic effects (dry mouth, constipation) may increase as dose is increased. Check with patient about their occurrence. Discuss measures to help patient tolerate dry mouth (frequent rinsing with water, saliva substitute, increased fluid intake) and constipation (increased dietary fibre, drink 6 to 8 glasses of water daily). Other anticholinergic symptoms (urinary retention, ataxia, dizziness) are indicators for dose adjustment or drug therapy. Discuss with physician.
- The physician will periodically attempt to reduce pimozide dosage to see if tics persist. An increase in frequency and intensity may be due to a withdrawal-like phenomenon rather than reemergence of disease symptoms. Usually 1 to 2 weeks are allowed to elapse before clinical differentiation between drug withdrawal or disease aetiology can be made.
- Moderation or abstinence from alcohol is advised, to prevent augmenting CNS depressant effects of pimozide.
- *See also haloperidol for nursing implications of drug therapy with an antipsychotic agent.*

DRUG INTERACTIONS   *Pimozide*

PLUS	INTERACTIONS
Alcohol, sedatives, hypnotics	Increased CNS depressant action of pimozide
Anticholinergics	Increased anticholinergic effects of pimozide
Phenothiazines, tricyclic antidepressants, antiarrhythmics	Increased risk of QT prolongation
Anticonvulsants	Loss of seizure control; increased CNS depressant effects

Pindolol

(Visken)

Antihypertensive; beta-adrenergic blocking agent (nonselective)

ACTIONS AND USES   Nonselective beta-adrenergic blocking agent. Possesses slight intrinsic sympathomimetic activity (ISA) or partial beta-agonist effect in therapeutic dose ranges. Thus pindolol exerts vasodilator as well as hypotensive effects. Hypotensive

PINDOLOL (continued)

action mechanism similar to that of propranolol (q.v.) competitively blocks beta-adrenergic receptors primarily in myocardium, and beta receptors within bronchial and smooth muscle. Membrane-stabilizing or anaesthetic-like action has been demonstrated but only at plasma levels above therapeutic safety. Has negative chronotropic and inotropic properties and slows conduction in AV node (but to lesser extent than other beta-blockers). Does not consistently affect cardiac output, resting heart rate, or renin release; it does, however, decrease peripheral vascular resistance, perhaps and major factor in pindolol's hypotensive effect. The ISA effect can be completely reversed by other beta-antagonists.

Used in the management of hypertension concurrently with a thiazide diuretic or as single agent. Used in patient who has failed to respond to diet, exercise, and/or weight reduction. Stress/exercise-induced chronic stable angina pectoris.

ROUTE AND DOSAGE   Oral: Adult: *Hypertension*: 5 mg two or three times a day. Maximum dosage of 45 mg/day. *Angina pectoris*: 2.5 to 5 mg up to three times a day.

ABSORPTION AND FATE   Rapid absorption from GI tract. Bioavailability 50 to 95% (less in uraemic patient). Peak plasma concentrations achieved 1 to 2 hours after administration of a single 20 mg dose. **Action duration**: begins within 3 hours after administration and lasts for 24 hours. 40 to 60% protein bound. **Half-life**: 3 to 4 hours; increased to 3 to 11 hours in renal failure, 7 to 15 hours in geriatric patient, and varies from 2½ to 30 hours in hepatic cirrhosis. 60 to 65% of dose metabolized in liver to glucuronide and sulphate metabolites. 35 to 50% excreted unchanged. Secreted into breast milk.

CONTRAINDICATIONS AND PRECAUTIONS   Bronchospastic diseases, severe brady-cardia, cardiogenic shock, cardiac failure. Safe use in pregnancy, nursing mothers, and children not established. **Cautious Use**: nonallergic bronchospasm, CHF, diabetes mellitus, hyperthyroidism, impaired hepatic and renal function. *See also propranolol.*

ADVERSE/SIDE EFFECTS   *See propranolol.*

NURSING IMPLICATIONS
- Food does not decrease bioavailability but may increase rate of absorption. Advise patient to take drug at same time of day each day with respect to time of food intake.
- Pindolol masks the dizziness and sweating premonitory symptoms of hypoglycaemia less than other beta-blockers; however, this drug action should be understood by the patient/primary care provider as a potential problem during regulation period of antidiabetic therapy.
- Hypotensive effect may begin within 7 days but is not therapeutically maximum until about 2 weeks after beginning of treatment with pindolol.
- Abrupt withdrawal of drug might precipitate a thyroid crisis in a patient with hyperthyroidism, and angina in the patient with ischaemic heart disease and lead to an MI. Warn any patient on pindolol to adhere to the prescribed drug regimen. If a change is desired, consult physician first.
- Withdrawal or discontinuation of treatment is gradual over a period of 1 to 2 weeks.

PINDOLOL (continued)

- Because of the vasodilating action of this drug, the cold extremities side effect observed with other beta-blockers is rarely a problem.
- *See propranolol*.

Piperacillin sodium

(Pipril)

Antibiotic (beta-lactam); penicillin

ACTIONS AND USES   Extended-spectrum parenteral penicillin with antibiotic activity against most gram-negative and many gram-positive anaerobic and aerobic organisms including members of *Clostridium*, *Bacteroides*, *Klebsiella*, *Enterobacter*, *Pseudomonas*, *Proteus*, *Serratia* species, and the anaerobic and aerobic cocci. Action mechanism is similar to that of other penicillins: used to treat susceptible organisms. Also used prophylactically prior and during surgery, and as empiric antiinfective therapy in granulocytopenic patients.

ROUTE AND DOSAGE   **Intramuscular; intravenous: Adult**: 100–150 mg/kg day in divided doses. Increased to a maximum of 16 gm/day in severe life-threatening infections.

ABSORPTION AND FATE   Approximately 70 to 80% IM dose absorbed from injection site. Peak serum concentrations attained within 30 to 50 minutes (30 to 36 mcg/ml after a 2 g dose). Distribution (after both IV and IM dose) into pleural, peritoneal, wound and synovial fluids, sputum, and bone (low concentrations). Minimal distribution to CSF unless meninges are inflamed. (Concurrent administration with oral probenecid increases CSF concentration.) **Protein binding**: 16 to 22%; hepatic metabolism is slight. **Half-life** is biphasic: initial, 0.7 to 0.33 hours; terminal, 0.6 to 1.35 hours; prolonged in severe renal and hepatic impairment. Rapidly excreted in urine and partly in faeces via bile. Readily crosses placenta; distributed into milk. Removed by haemodialysis, but not appreciably by peritoneal dialysis.

CONTRAINDICATIONS AND PRECAUTIONS   Hypersensitivity to penicillins, cephalosporins, or other drugs. Safe use in children younger than 12 years, lactating mother, and during pregnancy not established. **Cautious Use**: hepatic and renal dysfunction. *See also penicillin G*.

ADVERSE/SIDE EFFECTS   *Rare*: abnormal platelet aggregation and prolonged prothrombin time (with high doses). *See also penicillin G*.

NURSING IMPLICATIONS

- Duration of therapy depends on type and severity of infection but usually continues for at least 48 to 72 hours after patient is asymptomatic and evidence that infection is eradicated has been obtained.

P

PIPERACILLIN SODIUM (continued)

- Doses and frequency are usually modified if creatinine clearance is less than 40 ml/minute.
- Patients undergoing haemodialysis usually receive a maximum dosage of 2 g piperacillin every 8 hours and an additional 1 g dose after each dialysis period.
- IM injections should be limited to 2 g/site. Use the gluteal muscle, preferably. The deltoid muscle should be used only if well developed.
- Do not mix piperacillin with an aminoglycoside in a syringe or infusion bottle; aminoglycoside will be inactivated.
- Store reconstituted solution at room temperature for 24 hours; up to 48 hrs refrigerated.
- *See penicillin G.*

Piperazine

(Antepar, Ascalix, Pripsen)   *Anthelmintic*

ACTIONS AND USES   Appears to act by producing muscle paralysis in parasite, thus promoting elimination through intestinal peristalsis.

Used in treatment of thread worm disease (*Enterobius vermicularis*) and roundworm or ascariasis (*Ascaris lumbricoides*) infestations.

ROUTE AND DOSAGE   Piperazine hydrate 100 mg = piperazine citrate 125 mg = 104 mg piperazine phosphate. **Adult and child (over 12 yrs):** 2 g; **Child (up to 2 yrs):** 50–75 mg; **(2–4 yrs):** 750 mg; **(5–12 yrs):** 1.5 g daily for 7 days.

ABSORPTION AND FATE   Variable GI absorption. Excreted essentially unchanged in urine within 24 hours.

CONTRAINDICATIONS AND PRECAUTIONS   Hypersensitivity to piperazine or its salts, impaired renal or hepatic function, convulsive disorders. Safe use during pregnancy not established. **Cautious Use:** malnutrition, anaemia.

ADVERSE/SIDE EFFECTS   Low toxicity. Usually with excessive dosage. Side effects include: headache, vertigo, ataxia, tremors, choreiform movements, muscular weakness, hyporeflexia, paraesthesia, sense of detachment, memory defect, EEG abnormalities, convulsions, blurred vision, paralytic strabismus, nystagmus, cataracts, lacrimation, rhinorrhoea, accomodative defects, nausea, vomiting, abdominal cramps, diarrhoea. **Hypersensitivity:** urticaria, erythema multiforme, photosensitivity, purpura, fever, productive cough, bronchospasm, arthralgia.

NURSING IMPLICATIONS
- Drug may be given with food to reduce gastric distress.
- Use of laxatives or enema and dietary restrictions are usually not necessary.
- Caution patient or parent not to exceed recommended schedule because of danger of neurotoxicity with high dosages.

PIPERAZINE (continued)

■ Instruct patient to withhold medication if CNS, GI, or hypersensitivity reactions occur and report to physician.

■ In severe infections, course of therapy may be repeated after 1-week rest period.

■ It is not unusual for an entire family to be infested with pinworms. Positive diagnosis in one family member warrants stool examination of other members to prevent reinfestation.

■ Specimens for thread worms are best obtained immediately on arising in the morning (female worm lays eggs at night around anal region). Obtain specimen by applying cellulose tape swab to perianal region; eggs can then be transferred to glass slide and examined microscopically.

■ Roundworm ova are examined in routine stool specimens.

■ Threadworms and roundworms are transmitted by direct and indirect transfer or ova, e.g., by hands, food, and contaminated articles. *Instruct patient and family in personal hygiene*: washing hands after defaecation and before touching food; sanitary disposal of faeces; daily change of underwear and bedding (for pinworms). Ova are destroyed by household washing machine.

■ Store at controlled room temperature protected from heat and light.

Drug interactions   There is a possibility that piperazine may exaggerate extrapyramidal effects of **phenothiazines**.

Piperazine oestrone sulphate

(Harmogen)   *Hormone; oestrogen*

ACTIONS AND USES   Water-soluble preparation of pure crystalline oestrone (responsible for therapeutic actions conjugated as the sulphate and stabilized with piperazine). Has same actions, absorption, fate, contraindications, precautions, and adverse reactions as oestradiol (q.v.)

Used in oestrogen substitution therapy.

ROUTE AND DOSAGE   Oral: 1.5–4.5 mg/day for 21–28 days, repeated if necessary after 5–7 days.

NURSING IMPLICATIONS

■ See oestradiol.

Pipothiazine palmitate

(Piportil depot)

PIPOTHIAZINE PALMITATE (continued)

ACTIONS AND USES   Antipsychotic drug used in the long-term treatment of schizophrenia.

ROUTE AND DOSAGE   IM: deep IM injection 50–100 mg at 4 weekly intervals.
For further informations: *see chlorpromazine*.

Pirbuterol

(Exirel)

ACTIONS AND USES   Adrenoceptor stimulant used for bronchial dilatation.

ROUTE AND DOSAGE   Oral: **Adult**: 10–15 mg three to four times a day. **Child** (6–12 years): 7.5 mg up to four times a day.
For further information: *see salbutamol*.

Pirenzepine

(Gastrozepin)

ACTIONS AND USES   Anticholinergic used to treat gastric ulceration. May be used in conjunction with H_2 blocking drugs.

ROUTE AND DOSAGE   Oral: **Adult**: 50 mg twice a day increased to a maximum of 150 mg/day in three doses if necessary for 4–6 weeks. Dose should be taken 30 minutes before meals.
For further information: *see atropine*.

Piretanide

(Arelix)

ACTIONS AND USES   Loop diuretic used to treat hypertension.

ROUTE AND DOSAGE   Oral: **Adult**: 6–12 mg in the morning.
For further information: *see frusemide*.

Piroxicam

(Feldene, Larapam)

NSAID; analgesic; antipyretic;
antirheumatic

ACTIONS AND USES   Oxicam nonsteroidal antiinflammatory drug with analgesic, antipyretic, as well as antiinflammatory properties. Exact mechanism of action not clear. Drug-induced reduction in prostaglandin levels is associated with decreased inflammatory processes in bone–joint disease (including crystal disorders), and with possible interference with platelet aggregation. Habituation, tolerance, and addiction data not reported.

Used for acute and long-term relief of mild to moderate pain and for symptomatic treatment of osteoarthritis and rheumatoid arthritis.

ROUTE AND DOSAGE   Oral: Adult: 10–30 mg/day. If desired, may be given in divided doses.

ABSORPTION AND FATE   Well-absorbed after oral administration. Analgesic action begins in about 1 hour, peaks in 3 to 5 hours, and last 48 to 72 hours. **Antirheumatic action: onset**, up to 7 days; **peak action**, 2 to 4 weeks. Hepatic metabolism; highly protein bound. **Half-life**: 30 to 86 hours (average 50 hours); is unaffected by age but effects of impaired renal or hepatic disease have not been established. Piroxicam and its metabolites are excreted primarily in urine; small amounts in faeces. Less than 5% of dose excreted unchanged.

CONTRAINDICATIONS AND PRECAUTIONS   Hypersensitivity to piroxicam, haemophilia; syndrome (bronchospasm, nasal polyps, angioedema) precipitated by aspirin, active peptic ulcer, GI bleeding. Safe use in children, during pregnancy, and during lactation not established. **Cautious Use**: history of upper GI disease including ulcerative colitis, renal dysfunction, compromised cardiac function, hypertension or other conditions predisposing to fluid retention; coagulation disorders.

ADVERSE/SIDE EFFECTS   These include: somnolence, dizziness, vertigo, depression, insomnia, nervousness. Causal relationships not established: akathisia, depression, hallucinations, dream abnormalities, mental confusion paraesthesias, peripheral oedema, hypertension, worsening of congestive heart failure, exacerbation of angina, urticaria, erythema multiforme, maculopapular, vesiculobullous rash; photosensitivity, sweating, Stevens-Johnson syndrome, bruising, dermatitis, tinnitus, hearing loss, nausea, vomiting, dyspepsia, GI bleeding, diarrhoea, constipation, flatulence, dry mouth, peptic ulceration, anorexia, jaundice, hepatitis, anaemia, decreases in Hgb, Hct; leucopenia, eosinophilia, aplastic anaemia; thrombocytopenia, blurred vision, reduced visual acuity, changes in colour vision, scotomata, corneal deposits, retinal disturbances, bronchospasm, allergic rhinitis, angioedema, fever, hypoglycaemia, hyperglycaemia, hyperkalaemia, weight gain; causal relationships not established: dysuria, dyspnoea, palpitations, syncope, muscle cramps, fever, hypersensitivity reactions.

NURSING IMPLICATIONS
■ Patient should take drug at the same time every day.

P

PIROXICAM (continued)

- Administration of capsule with food or fluid may help to reduce GI irritation.
- Concomitant administration of an antacid to reduce gastric distress; does not interfere with piroxicam absorption or action.
- Clinical evidence of benefits from drug therapy: pain relief in motion and in rest, reduction in night pain, stiffness, and swelling; increased range of motion in all joints.
- Check to be sure patient is not self-dosing with aspirin or any other OTC drug without physician's advice. For example: there is no evidence that aspirin in combination with piroxicam increases relief from pain; but the possibility of intensified side effects has not been completely ruled out.
- If patient misses a dose, advise taking the drug when omission is discovered if it is 6 to 8 hours before the next scheduled dose. Otherwise, omit the dose and reestablish regimen at next scheduled hour.
- Warn patient not to increase dosage beyond prescribed regimen. Patient should understand the reasons for delayed therapeutic effect and need to adhere to the established regimen. Higher than recommended doses are associated with increased incidence of GI irritation and peptic ulcer. If dose appears to be ineffective, physician should be consulted.
- Incidence of GI bleeding with this drug is relatively high. Instruct patient to promptly report symptoms of melaena, haematemesis, or severe gastric pain.
- Be alert to symptoms of drug-induced anaemia: profound fatigue, skin and mucous membrane pallor, lethargy. Drug will be discontinued if diagnosis is confirmed (Hgb, Hct studies).
- Because most of the drug is excreted by the kidneys, impaired renal function could increase danger of toxicity and overdose. Encourage patient to maintain adequate fluid intake, i.e., at least 6 to 8 full glasses of water daily (if allowed) and to report signs of compromised renal function: peripheral oedema, changed intake and output ratio and pattern, dysuria, unusual weight gain.
- Advise patient to report immediately to the physician the onset of eye problems; ophthalmological studies may be indicated.
- If piroxicam is used concomitantly with an anticoagulant be alert to signs of hypoprothrombinaemia during and for several days after therapy has been discontinued: ecchymoses, petechiae, unexplained bleeding, epistaxis, haematuria.
- Since side effects, i.e., blurred vision, vertigo dizziness, may impair ability to perform activities requiring mental alertness, caution patient to avoid driving a car or engaging in hazardous activities until response to drug is known.
- Since alcohol may intensify the risk of gastric mucosal erosion (GI bleeding), it is advisable to avoid or at least to moderate its use.
- Overdosage reports are few. If it occurs, treatment would follow standard procedures: evacuate stomach promptly by emesis or gastric lavage and administer symptomatic and supportive treatment as indicated. If absorption has already occurred, patient should be observed for 4 to 6 days after overdosage because of the long plasma half-life.
- Store in tightly closed container at 15° to 30°C (59° to 86°F), unless otherwise directed by manufacturer.

PIROXICAM (continued)
DRUG INTERACTIONS   *Piroxicam*_____

PLUS	INTERACTIONS
Alcohol	May augment risk of GI bleeding
Anticoagulants (coumarins)	Slight increase in hypoprothrombinaemic response
Aspirin	Slight reduction in piroxicam plasma level
Diazepam Propranolol Phenylbutazone Other highly protein-bound drugs	May be displaced by piroxicam leading to their increase therapeutic and toxic serum levels
Lithium	Possible increase in therapeutic and toxic levels of lithium

Similar drug azapropazone (Rheumox).

Pivampicillin————————————————————

(Pondocillin)

For further information: *see ampicillin.*

Pivmecillinam————————————————————

(Selexid)

For further information: *see mecillinam.*

Pizotifen————————————————————

(Sanomigran)

ACTIONS AND USES   Antihistamine, antispasmodic used in migraine.

ROUTE AND DOSAGE   Adult: 1.5 mg at night according to response. Child: up to 1.5 mg/day or 1 mg at night.

Plicamycin _____

(Mithracin, Mithramycin)   *Antineoplastic hypocalcaemic*
                                                      agent

ACTIONS AND USES   Cytotoxic antibiotic produced by *Streptomyces plicatus*, with minimal immunosuppressive activity. High toxicity with low therapeutic index limits clinical use.

Used to treat hospitalized patients with hypercalcaemia or hypercalciuria associated with advanced neoplasms.

ROUTE AND DOSAGE   **Intravenous**: dosage and duration of therapy highly individualized on basis of haematologic and clinical responses.

ABSORPTION AND FATE   Information on absorption, fate, and excretion is limited. Crosses blood–brain barrier, and appears to localize in areas of active bone resorption; excreted in urine. Has cumulative and irreversible toxicity.

CONTRAINDICATIONS AND PRECAUTIONS   Bleeding and coagulation disorders, myelosuppression, electrolyte imbalance (especially hypocalacemia, hypokalaemia, hypophosphataemia), pregnancy, women of childbearing age. **Cautious Use**: patients with prior abdominal or mediastinal radiology; liver or renal impairment.

ADVERSE/SIDE EFFECTS   These include: stomatitis, anorexia, nausea, vomiting, diarrhoea, widespread intestinal haemorrhage, thrombocytopenia, bleeding and coagulation disorders (dose related) leucopenia (mild), fever, drowsiness, irritability, dizziness, weakness, headache, mental depression, marked facial flushing, haemoptysis, nonspecific or acneiform skin rash, phlebitis, hypophosphataemia, hypokalaemia, hypocalciuria, abnormal liver and renal function (reflected in laboratory values).

NURSING IMPLICATIONS

- Terminate infusion if extravasation occurs. Apply moderate heat to disperse the drug and to minimize tissue irritation. Infusion should be restarted in another vein.
- Inspect skin daily for signs of purpura. Haemoptysis may occur because of bleeding into metastasis; report this immediately.
- Rebound hypercalcaemia may follow induced hypocalcaemia. *Hypercalcaemia symptoms*: nausea, vomiting, GI atony, polyuria, nocturia, thirst, skeletal muscle weakness, confusion, drowsiness, shortened Q-T interval, bradycardia.
- The hypercalcaemia patient may be dehydrated. Monitor fluid intake–output ratio to assure adequate fluid intake. Encourage increased oral intake.
- A single intravenous dose may be sufficient to reduce elevated serum calcium to normal level within 24 to 48 hours for 3 to 15 days.
- Signs of antiblastic action on GI mucosal cells (haematemesis, melaena) necessitate stopping drug use.
- Check patient's bowel function daily to prevent high faecal impaction due to diminished action of intestinal musculature.
- Consult physician about dietary calcium intake, and coordinate dietary planning with dietitian patient, and family.

PLICAMYCIN (continued)
Drug interactions   Concomitant administration of **vitamin D** may enhance hyper-calcaemia.

Poldine methylsulphate ▬▬▬▬▬▬▬▬▬▬▬▬

(Nacton)

ACTIONS AND USES   Anticholinergic used to treat gastrointestinal disorders. For further information: *see atropine*.

ROUTE AND DOSAGE   Oral: **adult**: 2–4 mg, 3 times a day and at bed time. Increased to a maximum tolerated.

Polyestradiol phosphate ▬▬▬▬▬▬▬▬▬▬▬

(Estradurin)   *Antineoplastic; hormone;*
                                                     oestrogen

ACTIONS AND USES   Oestrogen derivative. Provides a continuous active level of ex-ogenous oestradiol that functions to alter the hormonal milieu of a tumour originating from hormone-responsive tissue. Polyestradiol suppresses pituitary secretion of luteiniz-ing or interstitial cell stimulating hormone, an action that in turn depresses ('turns off') androgen secretion by the testes (antitumour effect). Tumour growth is interrupted, but existing neoplastic cells are not killed.

Used as palliative treatment of an inoperable, progressing prostatic carcinoma.

ROUTE AND DOSAGE   Intramuscular: individualized.

ABSORPTION AND FATE   Injected solution leaves bloodstream within 24 hours; pas-sively stored in reticuloendothelial system. As circulating oestradiol level drops, more enters bloodstream from storage sites to provide continuous therapeutic effects. *See oestradiol for contraindications, adverse/side effects.*

NURSING IMPLICATIONS
- Reconstitute solution with sterile diluent; swirl gently to produce clear solution; do not shake vigorously. Discard cloudy solution.
- Administer drug deeply into large muscle mass (gluteus). A transitory burning sensation may occur, but this usually dose not continue with subsequent doses. If it continues, thereafter the dose may be given with local anaesthetic.
- Increasing the dosage prolongs action but does not increase blood level.

P

POLYESTRADIOL PHOSPHATE (continued)

- Clinical response should be apparent within 3 months. Hormone should be continued until, disease is again progressive, then stopped. 30% of patients may have another period of improvement (rebound regression).
- Store reconstituted solution at room temperature, away from direct light. Stability remains about 10 days, as long as solution is clear.
- *See oestradiol.*

Polymyxin B sulphate

(Aerosporin)

Antibiotic (polypeptide); polymyxin

ACTIONS AND USES   Basic polypeptide antibiotic of the polymyxin group derived from strains of *Bacillus polymyxa*. Bactericidal against susceptible gram-negative organisms, particularly most strains of *Pseudomonas aeruginosa*, *Escherichia coli*, *Haemophilus influenzae*, *Enterobacter aerogenes*, and *Klebsiella pneumoniae*.

Used topically for bladder irrigation, in eye, ear and skin infections. Few indications for use.

ABSORPTION AND FATE   Does not appear to be significantly absorbed from normal GI tract, mucous membranes or skin.

ADVERSE/SIDE EFFECTS   **Hypersensitivity**: drug fever, dermatoses, pruritus, urticaria, local irritation and burning (topical use), eosinophilia, anaphylactoid reaction (rarely). **Neurotoxicity**: rising blood drug levels without increase in dosage; albuminuria, cylinduria, azotaemia, heamaturia. **Other**: irritability, facial flushing, drowsiness, dizziness, vertigo, ataxia, circumoral, lingual, and peripheral paraesthesias (stocking-glove distribution); blurred vision, nystagmus, slurred speech, dysphagia, ototoxicity (vestibular and auditory) with high doses; convulsions, coma; neuromuscular blockade (generalized muscle weakness, respiratory depression or arrest); meningeal irritation, increased protein and cell count in cerebrospinal fluid, fever, headache, stiff neck (intrathecal use).

P

Polythiazide

(Nephril)

Diuretic; antihypertensive; thiazide

POLYTHIAZIDE (continued)

ACTIONS AND USES Benzothiadiazine (thiazide) derivative. Similar to chlorothiazide (q.v.) in actions, uses, contraindications, adverse reactions, and interactions.

Used as primary agent in stepped care approach to antihypertensive treatment, and adjunctively in the management of oedema associated by congestive heart failure, renal pathology, and hepatic cirrhosis. *See also chlorothiazide.*

ROUTE AND DOSAGE Oral: **Adult**: *diuretic*: 1 to 4 mg daily, *Antihypertensive*: 500 mcg/day.

ABSORPTION AND FATE Diuretic effect begins in 2 hours, peaks in 6 hours, and lasts 24 to 48 hours. Highly bound to plasma proteins. Excreted unchanged in urine. *See chlorothiazide.*

CONTRAINDICATIONS AND PRECAUTIONS Hypersensitivity to other thiazides or sulphonamides; anuria, pregnancy, lactation. **Cautious Use**: renal and hepatic dysfunction, gout, diabetes mellitus. *See chlorothiazide.*

ADVERSE/SIDE EFFECTS Agranulocytosis, vascular thrombosis, hyperuricaemia, hypokalaemia, hyperglycaemia, orthostatic hypotension, hepatic encephalopathy, photosensitivity. *See also chlorothiazide.*

NURSING IMPLICATIONS
- Elderly patients may be more sensitive to the average adult therapeutic dose. Excessive diuresis may induce sudden hypotension and serious electrolyte imbalance.
- Counsel patient to avoid OTC drugs unless approved by the physician. Many preparations contain both potassium and sodium and if misused, or if patient overdoses, electrolyte side effects could be induced.
- Store drug in tightly closed container at temperature between 15° and 30°C (59° and 86°F) unless otherwise instructed by manufacturer.
- *See chlorothiazide.*

Potassium salts

(Kay-Cee-L, K-Contin Continus, Kloref, Leo K, Nu-K, Slow-K)

Electrolyte replenisher

ACTIONS AND USES Potassium (K), the principle intracellular cation, is essential for maintenance of intracellular isotonicity, transmission of nerve impulses, contraction of cardiac, skeletal and smooth muscles, maintenance of normal renal function, and for enzyme activity.

Used to prevent and treat K deficit secondary to diuretic or corticosteroid therapy. Also indicated when K is depleted by severe vomiting, diarrhoea; intestinal drainage, fistulas, or malabsorption; prolonged diuresis, diabetic acidosis. Effective in the treatment of hypokalaemic alkalosis (chloride, not the gluconate).

POTASSIUM SALTS (continued)
ROUTE AND DOSAGE *Highly individualized.* Oral: *prophylactic* 2–4 g/day.

ABSORPTION AND FATE Nearly all dietary K absorbed from upper GI tract; enters cells from extracellular fluid by active transport. Excreted by kidneys (90%) and in faeces (10%). Amount of K excreted in urine essentially equals dietary K intake. During excessive K intake, amount secreted into colon and excreted in faeces increases.

CONTRAINDICATIONS AND PRECAUTIONS Severe renal impairment, severe haemolytic reactions, untreated Addison's disease, crush syndrome, early postoperative oliguria (except during GI drainage); adynamic ileus, acute dehydration, heat cramps, hyperkalaemia, patients receiving K-sparing diuretics, digitalis intoxication with AV conduction disturbance. **Cautious Use:** cardiac or renal disease, systemic acidosis, slow-release K preparations in presence of delayed GI transit or Meckel's diverticulum; extensive tissue breakdown (such as severe burns).

ADVERSE/SIDE EFFECTS Nausea, vomiting, diarrhoea, abdominal distention and pain, skin rash (rare), oliguria. *Hyperkalaemia*: mental confusion, irritability, listlessness, paraesthesias of extremities, muscle weakness and heaviness of limbs, difficulty in swallowing, flaccid paralysis, anuria, respiratory distress, hypotension, bradycardia; cardiac depression, arrhythmias, or arrest; altered sensitivity to digitalis glycosides. *ECG changes* (in hyperkalaemia): tenting (peaking) of T-wave (especially in right precordial leads), lowering of R- with deepening of S-waves and depression of RST; prolonged P-R interval, widened QRS complex, decreased amplitude and disappearance of P-waves, prolonged Q-T interval, signs of right and left bundle block, deterioration of QRS contour and finally ventricular fibrillation and death.

NURSING IMPLICATIONS
- Some patients find it difficult to swallow the large sized KCl tablet. Be sure it is taken while patient is sitting up or standing (never in recumbent position) to prevent drug-induced oesophagitis.
- No potassium salt tablets should be crushed and then taken dry, or chewed. Be certain patient does not suck tablet (oral ulcerations have been reported if tablet is allowed to dissolve in mouth). Whole tablet should be swallowed with large glass of water or fruit juice (if allowed, since it is another source of K) to wash drug down and to start oesophageal peristalsis. Liquids, powders, and effervescent tablets must be completely dissolved in a large glass of water or fruit juice before administration. Allow 'fizzing' to stop, then sip slowly with meal or immediately after eating, over a 5 to 10 minute period. Dilution minimizes saline cathartic effect, gastric distress and unpleasant taste.
- The extended-release tablet (e.g., Slow-K) utilizes a wax matrix as carrier for KCl crystals. After absorption of drug, the tablet carcass appears in the stool. Inform the patient that this is no cause for alarm.
- Use of extended-release tablets reduces the danger of bowel ulcerations and potential compliance problems. However, oesophageal and gastric ulceration in cardiac patients with oesophageal compression from left atrial enlargement have been reported

POTASSIUM SALTS *(continued)*

with use of this formulation. Report signs of oesophageal or epigastric pain or haematemesis). A liquid preparation in such a patient could be more tolerable.

- An antacid may improve the tolerance of KCl by decreasing its irritating effect on GI mucosa. 10 ml KCl flavoured syrup mixed with 15 ml antacid has given relief. Consult physician.

- Before discharge from medical supervision, help patient to design an acceptible, feasible dosing schedule for KCl and other drugs being taken concomitantly (e.g., digitalis, diuretics).

- Patient should be well informed about sources of K with special reference to foods and OTC drugs, because their selection and intake are controlled by the patient.

- The physician may want to augment therapeutic K intake by diet. Arrange an opportunity for patient/family to discuss diet with dietitian before patient is discharged.

- Suggested daily requirement for K is 0.8 to 1.3 g. The normal diet provides 2 to 4 g daily. K-rich foods include avocado, lima-beans, broccoli, carrots, potato, peanut butter, nuts, fruits (especially banana, orange, grapefruit, apricot, melons, prunes); whole grain cereals; instant coffee, cocoa, molasses.

- Advise patient to include a banana (about 370 mg K) and at least 6 ounces orange juice (about 330 mg K) in diet each day. Patient should avoid liquorice, since large amounts can cause both hypokalaemia and sodium retention.

- Salt substitutes contain a substantial amount of K and electrolytes other than Na. Excessive use can be dangerous for the patient who borders on the hyperkalaemic state. Instruct patient not to use any substitute unless it is specifically ordered by the physician.

- Discuss self-medication habits with patient. Point out that many OTC drugs contain K: multiple vitamin preparations, antacids (Alka-Seltzer), analgesics. Advise consulting physician before continuing or starting to use any OTC preparation.

- Caution patient not to self-prescribe laxatives. Chronic laxative use has been associated with diarrhoea-induced K loss.

- Large losses of K can also occur because of persistent vomiting. If this occurs, notify physician.

- Urge patient on long-term replacement therapy to report continuing signs of K deficit: weakness, fatigue, disturbances in cardiac rhythm, polyuria, polydipsia.

- If K supplement is given in conjunction with a diuretic it may be preferable to give the K on days other than when diuretic is given.

- The risk of hyperkalaemia with K supplement increases: (1) in the elderly because of decremental changes in kidney function associated with ageing, (2) when dietary intake of K suddenly increases, and (3) when renal function is significantly compromised.

- Potassium intoxication (hyperkalaemia) may result from any therapeutic dosage and the patient may be asymptomatic. Monitoring of K level is of extreme importance. Urge patient to keep appointments for periodic evaluation of electrolyte status.

- When detected, hyperkalaemia demands immediate attention since lethal levels can be reached in a few hours.

- ***Treatment of K intoxication*** Eliminate all K-containing foods and medications. Have available parenteral calcium to overcome cardiotoxicity (not used in patient

POTASSIUM SALTS (continued)

receiving digitalis); parenteral sodium bicarbonate, glucose infusion with regular insulin (facilitates shift of K into cell), cation exchange resins (hasten K elimination). Haemodialysis and peritoneal dialysis may be required.

- Counsel patient to assume responsibility for informing dentist or new physician that a potassium drug has been prescribed as maintenance therapy.
- Foil-wrapped powders and tablets should not be opened before use.
- Unless manufacturer advises otherwise, store all preparations of KCl at temperatures between 15° and 30°C (59° and 86°F). Protect from light, and do not freeze.
- Colour in some commercial oral solutions fades with exposure to light, but drug effectiveness is reportedly not altered.

DRUG INTERACTIONS   *Potassium Chloride*

PLUS	INTERACTIONS
K-sparing diuretics (triamterene, spironolactone)	Severe hyperkalaemia
Penicillin G potassium	

Practolol

(Eraldin)

ACTIONS AND USES   Beta-adrenergic blocking drug used in emergency treatment of supraventricular tachycardia and ventricular tachycardia after myocardial infarction.

ROUTE AND DOSAGE   IV by slow injection: 5 mg repeated as required.

Pralidoxime chloride

ACTIONS AND USES   Used in the treatment of organophosphorus poisoning.

Prazepam

(Centrax)

Antianxiety agent (minor tranquillizer); benzodiazepine

PRAZEPAM (continued)

ACTIONS AND USES   Benzodiazepine derivative structurally and pharmacologically related to chlordiazepoxide (q.v.). Has hypnotic and sedative effects.

Used for management of anxiety disorders or for short-term relief of symptoms of anxiety.

ROUTE AND DOSAGE   Oral: 30 mg, **Elderly debilitated**: *initial* dose: 10 to 15 mg daily in divided doses.

NURSING IMPLICATIONS

- Continued effectiveness of response to prazepam should be reassessed at end of 4 months. Urge patient to keep appointments with physician.
- Store in tightly closed container at temperature between 15° and 30°C (59° and 86°F) unless otherwise specified by manufacturer.
- See *also chlordiazepoxide.*

Praziquantel

(Biltricide)

ACTIONS AND USES   Used in schistomosiasis.

ROUTE AND DOSAGE   Oral: 40 mg/kg as a single dose.

Prazosin hydrochloride

(Hypovase)   *Antihypertensive; alpha-*
                                              adrenergic blocking agent

ACTIONS AND USES   Quinazoline derivative and alpha-adrenergic blocking agent structurally unrelated to other antihypertensive drugs. Does not significantly change cardiac output, heart rate, renal blood flow, or glomerular filtration, and does not increase plasma renin activity.

Used in treatment of hypertension as initial agent or in conjunction with a diuretic and/or another antihypertensive drug, and conjunctively in treatment of congestive heart failure.

ROUTE AND DOSAGE   Oral: 500 mcg 2–3 times a day, maintenance 4–20 mg/day.

ABSORPTION AND FATE   **Peak plasma levels** in 2 to 3 hours in fasting patients (plasma levels usually to not correlate with therapeutic effect). **Plasma half-life**: 2 to 3 hours. Approximately 97% **bound to plasma proteins**. Blood pressure begins to

P

PRAZOSIN HYDROCHLORIDE (continued)

decrease within 2 hours, with maximum reduction in 2 to 4 hours; antihypertensive effect lasts less than 24 hours. Widely distributed to body tissues. Probably metabolized in liver and excreted mainly in bile and faeces; about 6 to 10% excreted in urine.

CONTRAINDICATIONS AND PRECAUTIONS Hypersensitivity to prazosin. **Cautious Use:** chronic renal failure. Safe use in women of childbearing potential, during pregnancy and lactation, and in children not established.

ADVERSE/SIDE EFFECTS These include: oedema, dyspnoea, syncope, orthostatic hypotension, tachycardia, angina, rash, pruritis, alopecia, lichen planus, blurred vision, epistaxis, tinnitus, reddened sclerae, dry mouth, nasal congestion, vomiting, diarrhoea, constipation, abdominal discomfort, and/or pain, urinary frequency, incontinence, priapism (especially patients with sickle cell trait), impotence, dizziness, lightheadedness, headache, drowsiness, fatigue, weakness, palpitation, nausea, diaphoresis, arthralgia, transient leucopenia, increased serum uric acid and BUN.

NURSING IMPLICATIONS
- Reportedly, food may delay absorption, but does not affect degree of absorption. It has been suggested that the frequency of faintness and dizziness may be reduced by taking drug with food.
- 'First-dose phenomenon' is a transient, dose-related syndrome manifested by dizziness, weakness, lightheadedness, and syncope. It may be especially severe in patients with low serum sodium. It commonly occurs within 30 minutes to 2 hours after initial dose is given, and may usually be prevented by administering initial dose at bedtime.
- Caution patient to avoid situations that would result in injury should syncope occur. In most cases, effect does not recur after initial period of therapy; however, it has occurred during acute febrile episodes.
- Syncope is also associated with rapid dosage increases or addition of another antihypertensive drug to regimen.
- Instruct patient to make position changes slowly, particularly from recumbent to upright posture, and to dangle legs and move ankles a few minutes before standing.
- Caution patient to lie down immediately if feeling weak or faint and to avoid potentially hazardous activities such as driving a car or operating machinery until reaction to drug is known. Side effects usually disappear with continuation of therapy, but they may require dosage reduction.

Patient-teaching points
- ☐ Take drug at same times each day.
- ☐ Maintain optimum weight.
- ☐ Control sodium intake.
- ☐ Comply with established medical regimen.
- ☐ Keep follow-up appointments.

- Advise patient not to take OTC medications, especially those that may contain a

PRAZOSIN HYDROCHLORIDE (continued)

sympathomimetic agent (e.g., remedies for coughs, colds, allergy) without first consulting physician.

- Full therapeutic effect of prazosin may not be achieved until after 4 to 6 weeks of therapy.

Drug interactions   Hypotensive effect of prazosin is increased when given concomitantly with other **antihypertensive agents**, particularly **propranolol** (may be used therapeutically; permits reduction in dosage of each drug).

Prednisolone

(Codelsol, Delta-Phoricol, Deltacortil Enteric,   *Corticosteroid; glucocorticoid*
    Deltastab, Precortisyl, Prednesol, Sintisone)

ACTIONS AND USES   Intermediate-acting synthetic dehydrogenated analogue of hydrocortisone (q.v.) with three to five times greater potency. Mineralocorticoid properties are minimal and potential for sodium and water retention and potassium loss is reduced. **HPA suppression**: 24 to 36 hours; **half-life**: about 130 minutes. Side effects minimal, but insomnia sometimes occurs during first few days of treatment. Compared with hydrocortisone, prednisolone and its esters have greater tendency to produce gastric irritation, gastroduodenal ulceration, ecchymotic skin lesions, vasomotor symptoms. Safe use during pregnacy, by lactating women, or children not established.

Used principally as an antiinflammatory and immunosuppressant agent.

ROUTE AND DOSAGE   Oral: Adult: *Initial*: Up to 30 mg/day in divided doses. **IM**: *(acetate)*: 25–100 mg one or two times a week. *(Sodium phosphate)*: 4–60 mg/day in divided doses.

ADVERSE/SIDE EFFECTS   Hirsutism (occasional), perforation of cornea (with topical drug), sensitivity to heat, fat embolism, adverse effects on growth and development of the individual and on spermatozoa; hypotension and shocklike reactions. *See also hydrocortisone.*

NURSING IMPLICATIONS

- Administer with meals to reduce gastric irritation. If distress continues, consult physician about possible adjunctive antacid therapy.
- Advise patient to adhere to established dosage regimen, i.e, should not increase, decrease, or omit doses; or change dose intervals.
- Since topical corticosteroid treatment may increase intraocular pressure in susceptible individuals, it is usual to have frequent tonometric exams during prolonged therapy.
- In diseases caused by microorganisms, infection may be masked, activated, or enhanced by corticosteroids. Be alert to subclinical signs of lack of improvement such as continued drainage, low-grade fever, and interrupted healing. Observe and report exacerbation of symptoms after short period of therapeutic response.

P

PREDNISOLONE (continued)

- Temporary local discomfort may follow injection of prednisolone into bursa or joint.
- Reconstituted solution should not be autoclaved.
- Preserve in airtight containers; protect from light. Store at temperature 15° to 30°C (59° to 86°F); do not freeze.
- *See hydrocortisone for contraindications, additional nursing implications, and drug interactions.*

Prednisone

(Decortisil)   *Corticosteroid; glucocorticoid*

ACTIONS AND USES   Immediate acting synthetic analogue of hydrocortisone (q.v.). Effect depends on biotransformation to prednisolone, a conversion that may be impaired in patient with liver dysfunction. Safe use by pregnant women, children, or during lactation, not established.

Used as single agent or conjunctively with antineoplastics in cancer therapy; also used in treatment of myasthenia gravis. *See hydrocortisone.*

ROUTE AND DOSAGE   Oral: **Adult:** Initial up to 30 mg/day.

ABSORPTION AND FATE   **Peak effect:** 1 to 2 hours; duration, 1 to 1½ days. **Plasma half-life:** 3.4 to 3.8 hours; **HPA (hypothalamic–pituitary–adrenal)** axis suppression: 24 to 36 hours.

NURSING IMPLICATIONS
- Tablet may be crushed before administration and taken with fluid of patient's choice.
- Administer prednisone after meals and at bedtime.
- Alternate day drug administration may be advised to keep daily dose at minimal levels and to reduce degree of 'steroid rebound' with withdrawal.
- Periodic blood K levels are recommended. Urge patient to keep scheduled appointments for medical supervison.
- Monitor weight to detect onset of fluid accumulation, especially if patient is on unrestricted salt intake and does not receive K supplement. Report if weight gain is more than 2 kg/week.
- When patient is on an extended therapy regimen, incidence of oral candida infection is high. Inspect mouth daily for symptoms: white patches, black furry tongue, painful membranes and tongue.
- Advise patient to report symptoms of K deficit (anorexia, paresthesias, drowsiness, muscle weakness, nausea, polyuria, postural hypotension, mental depression).
- Protect drug from light and air in tightly closed dark container.
- Store at temperature between 15° and 30°C (59° and 86°F).
- *See hydrocortisone for contraindications, additional nursing implications and drug interactions.*

P

Prenylamine

ACTIONS AND USES   Calcium channel blocker.

ROUTE AND DOSAGE   Oral: Adult: 60 mg three times a day.
For further information: *see verapamil*.

Prilocane

(Citanest)

ACTIONS AND USES   Local anaesthetic.
See lignocaine.

Primaquine

Antimalarial

ACTIONS AND USES   Synthetic 8-aminoquinoline that acts on primary exoerythrocytic forms of *Plasmodium vivax* and *P. falciparum* by an incompletely known mechanism. Destroys late tissue forms of *P. vivax* and thus effects radical cure (prevents relapse). Also has gametocidal activity against all species of plasmodia that infect man, and thus can interrupt transmission of malaria. For treatment of acute attacks, always used in conjunction with a 4-aminoquinolone schizontocide such as chloroquin, which destroys erythrocytic parasites.
    Used to prevent relapse ('radical' or 'clinical' cure) of *P. vivax* and *P. ovale* malarias and to prevent attacks after departure from areas where *P. vivax* and *P. ovale* malarias are endemic.

ROUTE AND DOSAGE   Oral: *Relapse prevention*: Adult: 15 mg (base). Child: 7.5 mg (base). Doses given daily for 14 days concomitantly or consecutively with chloroquine, hydroxychloroquine, or amodiaquine which are given on first 3 days of an acute attack. Each 13.2 mg tablet = 7 mg base.

ABSORPTION AND FATE   Absorbed well from intestine. Peak plasma levels in about 6 hours; only trace amounts detectable after 24 hours. Biodegradation products of primaquine are the active antimalarial and haemolytic agents. Concentrates in liver, lungs, heart, brain, and skeletal muscle. About 1% excreted unchanged in urine.

CONTRAINDICATIONS AND PRECAUTIONS   Rheumatoid arthritis, lupus erythematosus, haemolytic drugs, concomitant or recent use of agents capable of bone marrow

P

PRIMAQUINE (continued)

depression, e.g., quinacrine; patients with G6PD deficiency. NADH methaemoglobin reductase deficiency, pregnancy.

ADVERSE/SIDE EFFECTS   Haematological reactions including granulocytopenia and acute haemolytic anaemia in patients with G6PD deficiency. *Overdosage*: nausea, vomiting, epigastric distress, abdominal cramps, pruritus, methaemoglobinaemia (cyanosis): headache, confusion, mental depression, hypertension, arrhythmias (rare), moderate leucocytosis or leucopenia, anaemia, granulocytopenia, agranulocytosis, disturbances of visual accommodation.

NURSING IMPLICATIONS

- Administration of drug at mealtime or with an antacid (prescribed) may prevent or relieve gastric irritation. Notify physician if GI symptoms persist.
- Primaquine may precipitate acute haemolytic anaemia in persons with G6PD deficiency, an inherited error of metabolism carried on the X chromosome, present in about 10% American black males and certain Caucasian ethnic groups: Sardinians, Sephardic Jews, Greeks, and Iranians and those with personal or family history of favism. Caucasians manifest more intense expression of haemolytic reaction than do blacks.
- Patients whose ethnic origin indicate the possibility of G6PD deficiency should be screened prior to initiation of therapy.
- Advise all patients to examine urine after each voiding and to report darkening of urine, red-tinged urine and decrease in urine volume. Also report chills, fever, precordial pain, cyanosis (all are suggestive signs of haemolytic reaction). Sudden reductions in haemoglobin or erythrocyte count suggest impending haemolytic reaction.
- Repeated haematological studies (particularly blood cell counts and haemoglobin) and urinalyses should be performed during therapy.
- Preserve in well-closed, light-resistant containers.

Drug interactions   Quinacrine potentiates toxicity of primaquine and other 8-aminoquinolone antimalarial agents.

Primidone ————————————————

(Mysoline)   *Anticonvulsant*

ACTIONS AND USES   Not a true barbiturate, but closely related chemically and with similar mechanism of action. Converted in body to phenobarbitone (q.v.) metabolite. Appears to increase metabolism of vitamin D so that more is needed to fulfill normal requirements. May also impair calcium, folic acid and vitamin B_{12} metabolism and utilization.

Used alone or concomitantly with other anticonvulsant agents in the prophylactic

PRIMIDONE (continued)

management of complex partial (psychomotor) and generalized tonic–clonic (grand mal) seizures.

ROUTE AND DOSAGE Oral: **Adult and Children (over 8 years):** *Initial:* 125 mg daily; increased by 125 mg every 3 days to tolerance or therapeutic effect, or to maximum of 500 mg daily divided into 2 to 4 doses. **Children (under 8 years):** 20–30 mg/kg/ day in 2 divided doses.

ABSORPTION AND FATE Approximately 60 to 80% of dose absorbed from GI tract. Peak serum levels reached in 4 hours. Slowly metabolized in liver to two active metabolites: phenobarbitone and phenylethylmalonamide. Protein binding varies from 0 to 19%, but phenobarbitone metabolite is 50% bound. Primidone plasma half-life varies from 3 to 24 hours. Excreted in urine, approximately 15 to 25% as unchanged drug (40% in children). Appears in breast milk.

CONTRAINDICATIONS AND PRECAUTIONS Safe use in women of childbearing potential, during pregnancy, and in nursing mothers not established. Hypersensitivity to barbiturates, porphyria. **Cautious Use:** chronic lung disease, hepatic or renal disease, hyperactive children.

ADVERSE/SIDE EFFECTS These include: drowsiness, sedation, vertigo, ataxia, headache, excitement (children), confusion, unusual fatigue, hyperirritability, emotional disturbances, acute psychoses (usually patients with psychomotor epilepsy), nausea, vomiting, anorexia, leucopenia, thrombocytopenia, eosinophilia, decreased serum folate levels, megaloblastic anaemia (rare), diplopia, nystagmus, swelling of eyelids, alopecia, impotence, maculopapular or morbilliform rash oedema, lupus erythematosus-like syndrome, lymphadenopathy, osteomalacia.

NURSING IMPLICATIONS

- Tablet may be crushed before administration and taken with fluid of patient's choice.
- If drug causes GI distress, take it with meals.
- Because drowsiness, dizziness, and ataxia may be severe at beginning of treatment, advise patient to avoid driving and other potentially hazardous activities. Symptoms tend to disappear with continued therapy; if they persist, dosage reduction or drug withdrawal may be necessary.
- Transition from another anticonvulsant to primidone should not be completed in less than 2 months.
- Dosage may be adjusted with reference to primidone or phenobarbitone metabolite plasma levels (concentrations of primidone greater than 10 mg/ml are usually associated with significant ataxia and lethargy).
- Therapeutic response may not be evident for several weeks.
- Neonatal haemorrhage has been reported in newborns whose mothers were taking primidone. Monitor closely for bleeding.
- Presence of unusual drowsiness in nursing newborns of primidone-treated mothers is an indication to discontinue nursing.
- Pregnant women should receive prophylactic vitamin K therapy for 1 month prior to and during delivery to prevent neonatal haemorrhage.

P

PRIMIDONE (continued)

- Observe for signs and symptoms of folic acid deficiency: mental dysfunction, psychiatric disorders, neuropathy, megaloblastic anaemia. When indicated, serum folate levels should be determined.
- Megaloblastic anaemia responds to folic acid 15 mg daily, without necessity of interrupting primidone therapy.
- Caution patient not to take OTC medications unless approved by physician.
- Primidone withdrawal should be done gradually to avoid precipitating status epilepticus.
- Advise patient to avoid alcohol and other CNS depressants unless otherwise directed by physician.
- Advise patient to carry medical information card or jewellery with name of drug, physician's name, and telephone number.

Drug interactions   Concomitant use of **barbiturates** may result in excessive phenobarbitone blood levels (*see Absorption and Fate*). **Isoniazid** may inhibit primidone metabolism with resulting high blood levels. **Phenytoin** may cause increase in phenobarbitone blood levels probably by stimulating conversion of primidone to phenobarbitone. *See also phenobarbitone.*

Probenecid ━━━━━━━━━━━━━━

(Benemid)

Antigout agent; uricosuric;
sulphonamide derivative

ACTIONS AND USES   Sulphonamide-derivative renal tubular blocking agent. In sufficiently high doses, competitively inhibits renal tubular reabsorption of uric acid, thereby promoting its excretion and reducing serum urate levels (subtherapeutic doses may depress uric acid excretion). Prevents formation of new tophaceous deposits, and causes gradual shrinking of old tophi. Since it has no analgesic or antiinflammatory activity, it is of no value in acute gout, and may exacerbate and prolong acute phase. Increases plasma levels of weak organic acids, including beta-lactam antibiotics, by competitively inhibiting their renal tubular secretion.

Used for treatment of hyperuricaemia in chronic gouty arthritis and tophaceous gout, and as adjuvant to therapy with penicillin G and penicillin analogues to elevate and prolong plasma concentrations of these antibiotics.

ROUTE AND DOSAGE   Oral: *Gout therapy*: first week 0.25 g twice daily for 1 week, followed by 0.5 g twice daily. For patients with renal impairment: 1 g; daily dosage may be increased by 0.5 g increments every 4 weeks (usually not above 2 gm/day) if symptoms are not controlled or 24-hour urate excretion is not above 700 mg. *Penicillin or cephalosporin therapy*: **Adults**: 2 g in divided doses daily. **Children (2 to 14 years)**: *Initial*: 25 mg/kg; maintenance 40 mg/kg/day divided into 4 doses; children weighing over 50 kg may receive adult dosage.

PROBENECID (continued)

ABSORPTION AND FATE   Rapidly and completely absorbed from GI tract. Maximal renal clearance of uric acid in 30 minutes; effect on penicillin levels after about 2 hours. Plasma levels peak in 2 to 4 hours and persist for 8 hours. *Plasma half-life* 8 to 10 hours. About 75 to 95% bound to plasma proteins. Metabolized by liver. Excreted in urine after 2 days as metabolites and unchanged drug. Urine alkalinization decreases reabsorption of probenecid and increases uric acid solubility. Crosses placenta.

CONTRAINDICATIONS AND PRECAUTIONS   Hypersensitivity to probenecid, blood dyscrasias, uric acid kidney stones, during or within 2 to 3 weeks of acute gouty attack, overexcretion of uric acid (over 1,000 mg/day), patients with creatinine clearance less than 50 mg/minute, use with penicillin in presence of known renal impairment, use for hyperuricaemia secondary to cancer chemotherapy. Safe use during pregnancy, in nursing mothers, and in children under 2 years of age not established. **Cautious Use**: history of peptic ulcer.

ADVERSE/SIDE EFFECTS   Headache, nausea, vomiting, anorexia, sore gums, urinary frequency, flushing, dizziness, anaemia, haemolytic anaemia (possibly related to G6PD deficiency). Nephrotic syndrome, hepatic necrosis, and aplastic anaemia (rare). Exacerbations of gout, uric acid kidney stones. **Hypersensitivity**: dermatitis, pruritus, fever, anaphylaxis. **Overdosage**: CNS stimulation, convulsions, respiratory depression.

NURSING IMPLICATIONS

- GI side effects minimized by taking drug after meals, with food, milk, or with antacid (prescribed). If symptoms persist, dosage reduction may be required.
- Increased uric acid excretion promoted by probenecid predisposes to renal calculi. Therefore, during early therapy, high fluid intake (approximately 3,000 ml/day) is recommended to maintain daily urinary output of at least 2,000 ml or more.
- Oral sodium bicarbonate (3 to 7.5 g/day) or potassium citrate (7.5 g/day) may be prescribed to alkalinize urine until serum uric acid levels return to normal range (178.5 to 416.4 mmol/L).
- When urinary alkalinizers are used, periodic determinations of acid–base balance are advised. Some physicians prescribe acetazolamide at bedtime to keep urine alkaline and dilute throughout night.
- Physician may advise restriction of high-purine foods during early therapy until uric acid level stabilizes. Foods high in purine: organ-meats (sweetbreads, liver, kidney), meat extracts, meat soups, gravy, anchovies, sardines. Moderate amounts in other meats, fish, seafood, asparagus, spinach, peas, dried legumes, wild game.
- Alcohol may increase serum urate levels and therefore should be avoided.
- Caution patient not to stop taking drug without consulting physician. Irregular dosage schedule may cause sharp elevation of serum urate level and precipitation of acute gout.
- Urate tophaceous deposits should decrease in size with probenecid therapy. Classic locations are in cartilage of ear pinna and big toe, but they can occur in bursae, tendons, skin, kidneys, and other tissues.
- Because frequency of acute gouty attacks may increase during first 6 to 12 months of therapy, physician may prescribe concurrent prophylactic doses of colchicine for first

P

PROBENECID (continued)

3 to 6 months of probenecid therapy (probenecid alone aggravates acute gout). Probenecid is available in combination with colchicine.

- When gouty attacks have been absent for 6 months or more and serum urate levels are controlled, daily dosage may be cautiously decreased by 0.5 g every 6 months to lowest effective dosage that maintains stable serum urate levels.
- Lifelong therapy is usually required in patients with symptomatic hyperuricaemia. Advise patient to keep scheduled appointments with physician and appointments for studies of renal function and haematology.
- Instruct patient to report symptoms of hypersensitivity to physician. Discontinuation of drug is indicated.
- Patients taking oral hypoglycaemics may require dosage adjustment. Probenecid enhances hypoglycaemic actions of these drugs. *See also Diagnostic Test Interferences*.
- Advise patient not to take aspirin or other OTC medications without consulting physician. If a mild analgesic is required, paracetamol is usually allowed.
- Tablets should be stored in well-closed containers at 15° to 30°C (59° to 86°F). Expiration date is 3 to 5 years after date of manufacture.

Diagnostic test interferences   Probenecid may decrease excretion of **urinary 17-ketosteroids** and may increase **BSP** retention and inhibit **urinary PSP** excretion. False-positive results **urine glucose** tests are possible with Clinitest (glucose oxidase methods not affected, e.g., Clinistix).

DRUG INTERACTIONS   *Probenecid*

PLUS	INTERACTIONS
Aminosalicylic acid (PAS), dapsone, clofibrate, pantothenic acid, indomethacin, rifampicin methotrexate, naproxen Sulphonylureas Sulphonamides	Probenicid inhibits renal excretion and raises the plasma concentration of these drugs thus increasing their potential for toxicity
Nitrofurantoin Alcohol Diazoxides Diuretics Salicylates	Decreased antiinfective activity of nitrofurantoin Increased serum urate levels, therefore increased dosage of probenecid may be necessary

P

Probucol

(Lurselle)   *Antilipaemic*

ACTIONS AND USES   Lowers serum cholesterol levels by reducing low density lipoprotein concentrations.

ROUTE AND DOSAGE   Oral: Adult: 500 mg twice daily.

PROBUCOL (continued)
NURSING IMPLICATIONS

- Administer drug with morning and evening meals to enhance its action.
- The patient should fully understand that this drug does not reduce necessity to adhere to special diet.
- Store in light- and moisture-proof container at temperature between 15° and 30°C (59° and 86°F) unless otherwise specified by the manufacturer.

Diagnostic test interferences   Probucol therapy is accompanied by transient elevations in serum transaminases (AST, ALT), bilirubin, alkaline phosphatase, creatine, phosphokinase, uric acid, BUN and blood glucose. Haematocrit, haemoglobin and eosinophil values may be decreased.

Procainamide hydrochloride ━━━━━━━━━━━━

(Pronestyl)   *Antiarrhythmic; vasodilator*

ACTIONS AND USES   Amide analogue of procaine hydrochloride with cardiac actions very similar to those of quinine. Depresses excitability of myocardium to electrical stimulation, reduces conduction velocity in atria, ventricles and His–Purkinje system. Increases duration of refractory period especially in the atria. Unless myocardial damage is present, contractility of cardiac muscle and cardiac output are changed only slightly by procainamide; however, automaticity of His–Purkinje-ventricular muscle is suppressed. In the absence of dysrhythmia, therapeutic doses may accelerate heart rate, suggesting that procainamide may have anticholinergic properties. Produces peripheral vasodilation and hypotension, especially with IV use. Larger doses can induce AV block and ventricular extrasystoles that may proceed to ventricular fibrillation.

Used prophylactically to maintain normal sinus rhythm following conversion of atrial flutter or fibrillation by other methods. Also used to prevent recurrence of paroxysmal atrial fibrillation and tachycardia.

ROUTE AND DOSAGE   Oral: 250 mg 4–6 hrly. **Slow IV injection** 25–50 mg/min until arrhythmia is controlled. Maximum 1 g. **Maintenance IM**: 100–250 mg 4–6 hrly.

ABSORPTION AND FATE   Rapidly absorbed, except for extended-release form. **Plasma levels peak** within 15 to 60 minutes after IM; within 30 to 60 minutes after PO administration; **duration of effects** about 3 hours (about 8 hours for extended release form). **Protein binding** 20%; **plasma half-life**: about 3 hours (5 to 8 hours in patients with cardiac disease, 11 to 20 hours in presence of renal dysfunction). Approximately 25% of dose acetylated in liver to produce active metabolite N-acetylprocainamide with half-life of 6 hours. About 60% of drug excreted in urine unchanged.

CONTRAINDICATIONS AND PRECAUTIONS   Myasthenia gravis, hypersensitivity to procainamide or procaine; blood dyscrasias, complete AV block, second and third degree

P

PROCAINAMIDE HYDROCHLORIDE (continued)

AV block unassisted by pacemaker. **Cautious Use**: patient who has undergone electrical reversion to sinus rhythm, hypotension, cardiac enlargement, congestive heart failure, myocardial infarction, coronary occlusion, ventricular dysrhythmia from digitalis intoxication, hepatic or renal insufficiency, electrolyte imbalance, bronchial asthma, history of systemic lupus erythematosis. Safe use in pregnancy or lactation not established.

ADVERSE/SIDE EFFECTS These include: dizziness, mental depression, psychosis with hallucinations, severe hypotension, pericarditis, ventricular fibrillation (parenteral use); tachycardia, flushing, (mostly oral); bitter taste, nausea, vomiting, diarrhoea, anorexia, agranulocytosis with repeated use; thrombocytopenia, polyarthralgias, pleuritic pain, pleural effusion, erythema, skin rash, myalgia, fever.

NURSING IMPLICATIONS

- Patients at particular risk to adverse effects are those with severe heart, hepatic or renal disease, and hypotension. Dosage adjustment is based on individual requirements, response, general condition and cardiovascular status.
- Administer oral preparation on empty stomach 1 hour before or 2 hours after meals with a full glass of water to enhance absorption. If drug causes gastric distress, administer with food.
- Instruct patient to swallow sustained-release tablet whole. It uses a wax matrix which is not absorbed but appears in the stool.
- Fever sometimes occurs during the first few days of therapy and may necessitate discontinuation of drug. Monitor temperature and report elevation.
- Procainamide administration by IV infusion pump requires constant monitoring by qualified personnel to maintain desired flow rate and to detect special problems. Keep patient in supine position. Be alert to signs of 'speed shock' (because of too rapid administration of drug): irregular pulse, tight feeling in chest, flushed face, headache, loss of consciousness, shock, cardiac arrest.
- A complication of procainamide infusion given to treat atrial dysrhythmia is the onset of ventricular tachycardia (a lethal arrhythmia) evidence by increased rate to as high as 200 beats per minute.
- If symptoms of ventricular dysrhythmia develop during IV therapy, talk with patient to gauge responsiveness. Be prepared to defibrillate immediately if beginning to lose consciousness.
- Ventricular dysrhythmias are usually abolished within a few minutes after IV dose and within an hour after oral or IM administration.
- IV dosage over a period of several hours in controlled by assessment of procainamide plasma levels: effective nontoxic therapeutic level: 3 to 10 mcg/ml. (Eight to 16 mcg/ml is potentially toxic and toxicity is common at plasma levels about 16 mcg/ml).
- Drug is temporarily discontinued when the following occur: (1) arrhythmia is interrupted, (2) severe toxic effects present, (3) QRS complex is excessively widened, (greater than 50%) (4) PR interval is prolonged, or (5) blood pressure drops 15 mm Hg or more. Obtain rhythm strip and notify physician.
- Hypotensive effects of IV infusion are treated with dopamine phenylephredine or

P

PROCAINAMIDE HYDROCHLORIDE (continued)

noradrenaline overdosage is managed by fluid volume replacement, vasopressors, · haemodialysis or resin haemoperfusion.

■ When patient with acute myocardial infarction is changed from parenteral to oral dosage form, the first oral dose may coincide with one elimination half-life. Consult physician about precise time.

■ Apical-radial pulses should be checked before each dose of procainamide during period of adjustment to the oral route.

■ Digitalization may precede procainamide in patients with atrial arrhythmias. Cardiotonic glycosides may induce sufficient increase in atrial contraction to cause dislodgement of atrial mural emboli with subsequent pulmonary embolism. Report promptly patient complaints of chest pain, dyspnoea and anxiety.

■ Procainamide blood levels and that of its active metabolite are reached in approximately 24 hours if kidney function is normal, but are delayed several days in presence of renal impairment.

■ In renal pathology or congestive heart failure dosage may be reduce to prevent procainamide build-up (and potential toxicity).

■ Urge the patient on long-term therapy to keep appointments for periodic evaluations of blood counts, hepatic and renal function, and ECG studies.

■ Instruct patient on maintenance doses to record and report date, time and duration of fibrillation episodes (lightheadedness, giddiness, weakness, or syncope): such symptoms suggest changed ventricular rhythm. Evaluation of ECG rhythm strips and procainamide plasma levels will be necessary.

■ Consult with physician regarding patient monitoring own pulse and how often it should be done.

Patient-teaching points for pulse-taking

☐ Establish a base-line pulse range for comparison purposes.
☐ Show patient how to 'feel' and count radial pulse rate.
☐ Take a resting pulse rate, i.e., just before getting out of bed each AM.
☐ Count pulse for 1 full minute.
☐ Avoid taking carotid pulse: may cause arrhythmias or asytole.
☐ Keep a record of pulse rates.
☐ Report changes in rate or quality (i.e., if pulse is too rapid or too slow, faint or irregular).

■ Instruct patient or family to report to the physician if signs of reduced procainamide control occur: weakness, irregular pulse, unexplained fatigue, anxiety.

■ Adequacy of oral dosage may be evaluated by 24-hour ECG recordings.

■ The characteristic symptoms of agranulocytosis (soreness of mouth, gums and throat; upper respiratory tract infection, fatigue and unexplained fever) should be reported promptly to permit appropriate differential diagnosis (leucocyte counts) and treatment. Discontinuation of procainamide therapy may be required because of the danger of severe or even fatal infection.

■ Although bleeding disorders are uncommon, the patient should be aware of the possibility. Any unexplainable bleeding (melaena, petechiae, purpura, ecchymosis, bruising, epistaxis) should be investigated.

P

PROCAINAMIDE HYDROCHLORIDE (continued)

- Consult physician about whether patient should discontinue drinking caffeine beverages (tea, coffee, cola, hot chocolate).
- Caution the patient to adhere to dosage schedule as planned by the physician. At no time should a dose be doubled nor should an interval be changed because a previous dose was missed. Procainamide should be taken at evenly spaced intervals around the clock unless otherwise prescribed.
- Before discharge, work with patient to design a 24-hour dosing schedule for procainamide and all other prescribed drugs that will best fit into activities of daily living at home.
- Check patient's self-medication habits. If patient has been in the habit of taking OTC medications for nasal congestion, allergy, pain, or obesity, instruct patient to discuss with physician about continued need and safe substitutes, if necessary.
- If surgery is anticipated, and in an emergency situation, the patient should inform doctor or dentist that procainamide is being taken.
- Caution patient to avoid driving car until risk of lightheadedness and fainting has been eliminated.
- Advise patient to carry medical identification card or bracelet stating that procainamide is being taken.
- Store tablets in dark airtight containers. Procainamide is hygroscopic: therefore do not store in bathroom medicine cabinet or in refrigerator where moisture levels are high.

Diagnostic test interferences   Procainamide increases the plasma levels of **alkaline phosphatase, bilirubin, lactic dehydrogenase** and **SGOT** (serum glutamic oxaloacetic transaminase). It may also alter results of the **edrophonium test**.

DRUG INTERACTIONS *Procainamide hydrochloride*_____

PLUS	INTERACTIONS
Acetazolamide	Increases effect of procainamide
Antiarrhythmics	Additive effect of both procainamide and the other antiarrhythmics
Anticholinergic agents	Additive anticholinergic effects
Antihypertensives	Additive hypotensive effect
Cholinergics	Antagonizes effects of cholinergic drugs
Kanamycin, magnesium salts, Neomycin	
Neuromuscular blockers (nondepolarizing and depolarizing)	Enhances muscle relaxation produced by these agents
Sodium bicarbonate	

Procarbazine ▬▬▬▬▬▬▬▬▬▬▬▬▬▬▬▬▬▬▬▬▬▬▬▬▬▬▬▬▬▬▬▬

(Natulan)   *Antineoplastic; hydrazine*

PROCARBAZINE (continued)

ACTIONS AND USES   Hydrazine derivative with antimetabolite properties; cell-cycle-specific for the S phase of cell division. Precise mechanism of action unknown. Suppresses mitosis at interphase, and causes chromatin derangement. Highly toxic to rapidly proliferating tissue. Has immunosuppressive properties, and exhibits MAO inhibitory activity. May cause delayed myelosuppression. No cross-resistance with radiotherapy, steroids, or other antineoplastics has been demonstrated. Reportedly does not affect survival time, but may produce remissions of at least 1 month's duration.

Used as adjunct in palliative treatment of Hodgkin's disease.

ROUTE AND DOSAGE   Oral: individualized.

ABSORPTION AND FATE   Readily absorbed from GI tract. Wide distribution through body fluids, with concentrations in liver, kidneys, intestinal wall, and skin. Half-life in plasma and cerebrospinal fluid about 1 hour. Metabolized in liver; excreted in urine (25 to 42% appearing during first 24 hours after administration) as unchanged drug and metabolites, and from respiratory tract as methane and CO_2.

CONTRAINDICATIONS AND PRECAUTIONS   Hypersensitivity to procarbazine; myelosuppression; alcohol ingestion; foods high in tyramine content; sympathomimetic drugs. MAO inhibitors should be discontinued 14 days prior to therapy; tricyclic antidepressants, 7 days before therapy. Safe use during pregnancy and lactation and in women of childbearing potential not established. **Cautious Use**: concomitant administration with CNS depressants; hepatic or kidney impairment; following radiation or chemotherapy before at least 1 month has elapsed, hepatic and renal impairment, infection, diabetes mellitus.

ADVERSE/SIDE EFFECTS   These include: myalgia, arthralgia, paraesthesias, weakness, fatigue, lethargy, drowsiness, dermatitis, pruritus, herpes, hyperpigmentation, flushing, alopecia, severe nausea and vomiting (common), anorexia, stomatitis, dry mouth, dysphagia, diarrhoea, constipation, jaundice, bone marrow suppression (leucopenia, anaemia, thrombocytopenia), haemolysis, bleeding tendencies, ascites, pleural effusion, cough, hoarseness, hypotension, tachycardia, chills, fever, sweating, gynaecomastia, depressed spermatogenesis, atrophy of testes; (rare): oedema, nystagmus, photophobia, retinal haemorrhage, diplopia, papilloedema; altered hearing; photosensitivity; intercurrent infections.

NURSING IMPLICATIONS

- Toxicity is a serious problem and demands that patient be hospitalized and under close medical and nursing supervision during treatment induction period.
- Haematological status (haemoglobin, haematocrit, WBC, differential, reticulocyte, and platelet counts) should be determined initially and at least every 3 to 4 days. Hepatic and renal studies (transaminase, alkaline phosphatase, BUN, urinalysis) are also indicated initially and at least weekly during therapy.
- Start flow sheet, and record baseline blood pressure, weight, temperature, pulse, and intake–fluid, output ratio and pattern.
- Since procarbazine has MAO inhibitory activity, OTC nose drops, cough medicines, and antiobesity preparations containing sympathomimetic drugs (e.g., ephedrine, amphetamine, adrenaline) and tricyclic antidepressants should be avoided because

PROCARBAZINE (continued)

they may cause hypertensive crises. Warn patient not to use OTC preparations without physician's approval.

- Intake of foods high in tyramine content should also be avoided (*see Index: Food sources*). Warn patient that ingestion of any form of alcohol may precipitate a disulphiram-like reaction.
- Be alert to signs of hepatic dysfunction: jaundice (yellow skin, sclerae, and soft palate), frothy or dark urine, clay-coloured stools.
- Patient's haematological status should be monitored carefully for indicators that suggest special nursing interventions and need for dosage adjustment or drug withdrawal.
- As patient approaches nadir of leucopenia, protect patient from exposure to infection and trauma. Visitors and personnel with common colds should be visit. Alert patient to report any sign of impending infection. Note and report changes in voiding pattern, haematuria, and dysuria (possible signs of urinary tract infection) fluid. Intake–output ratio and temperature should be closely monitored.
- Tolerance to nausea and vomiting (most common side effects) usually develops by end of first week of treatment. Doses are kept at a minimum during this time. If vomiting persists, therapy will be interrupted.
- Symptoms of pleural effusion, an allergic reaction to procarbazine (chills, fever, weakness, shortness of breath, productive cough) should be reported promptly. Drug will be discontinued.
- Instruct patient to report immediately signs of haemorrhagic tendencies: bleeding into skin and mucosa, epistaxis, haemoptysis, haematemesis, haematuria, melaena, ecchymoses, petechiae. Bone marrow depression often occurs 2 to 8 weeks after start of therapy.
- Prompt cessation of therapy is usual with appearance of CNS signs and symptoms (paraesthesias, neuropathies, confusion), leucopenia, thrombocytopenia, hypersensitivity reaction, the first small ulceration or persistent spot soreness of oral cavity, diarrhoea, and bleeding. Patient should be warned to report promptly any signs and symptoms of toxicity.
- *See mustine for nursing implications of stomatitis and xerostomia.*
- Advise patient to avoid excessive exposure to the sun because of potential photosensitivity reaction: cover as much skin area as possible with clothing, and use sunscreen lotion (SPF above 12) on all exposed skin surfaces.
- Since drowsiness, dizziness, and blurred vision are possible side effects, warn patient to use caution while driving or performing hazardous tasks until response to drug is known.
- Advise use of contraceptive measures during procarbazine therapy.

Diagnostic test interference   Procarbazine may enhance the effects of **CNS depressants**. A disulphiram-like reaction may occur following ingestion of alcohol.

DRUG INTERACTIONS   *Procarbazine hydrochloride*

PLUS	INTERACTIONS
Alcohol	Additive CNS depressant effects; disulphiramlike reaction

PROCARBAZINE (continued)

Antidepressants, tricyclics, MAO inhibitors, tyramine foods	Hypertensive crisis, hyperpyrexia, convulsions and death
Antihistamines, belladonna alkaloids, antiparkinsonism agents	Potentiate atropinelike effects of procarbazine
Antihypertensives	Enhance hypotensive effects of procarbazine
Guanethidine, levodopa, methyldopa, reserpine	Excitement and hypertension
Insulin, oral hypoglycaemics	Augmented hypoglycaemic effects
Phenothiazines	Increased CNS depression
Sympathomimetics (indirect-acting) e.g., amphetamines, ephedrine, phenylpropanoline	Severe hypertension and hyperpyrexia
Thiazide diuretics	Enhance hypotensive effects of procortrozine

Prochlorperazine

(Stemetil, Vertigon)

*Psychotropic; antipsychotic
(neuroleptic); antiemetic;
phenothiazine*

ACTIONS AND USES   Piperazine phenothiazine derivative with similar actions, contraindications, and interactions as chlorpromazine (q.v.). Has greater extrapyramidal effects and antiemetic potency but less sedative, hypotensive and anticholinergic effects than chlorpromazine.

Used in management of vertigo and to control severe nausea and vomiting.

ROUTE AND DOSAGE   Adult: *Severe nausea*: **Oral**: *acute attack*: *initial*: 20 mg, then 10 mg after 2 hrs. *Prevention* 5–10 mg, 2–3 times a day. **Child**: 250 mcg/kg 2–3 times a day. **Adult: IM**: deep injection 12.5 mg as required. Suppositories: 25 mg as required.

ABSORPTION AND FATE   Onset of action: oral tablet: 30 to 40 minutes (duration 3 to 4 hours); extended-release form: 30 to 40 minutes (duration 10 to 12 hours); rectal suppository: 60 minutes (duration 3 to 4 hours); IM: 10 to 20 minutes (duration up to 12 hours). Crosses placenta; appears in breast milk.

CONTRAINDICATIONS AND PRECAUTIONS   Hypersensitivity to phenothiazines, bone marrow depression, comatose or severely depressed states, children under 10 kg or 2 years of age, paediatric surgery, short-term vomiting in children or vomiting of unknown etiology, Reye's syndrome or other encephalopathies, history of dyskinetic reactions or epilepsy. *See also chlorpromazine.*

ADVERSE/SIDE EFFECTS   Drowsiness, dizziness, hypotension, contact dermatitis, galactorrhoea, amenorrhoea, blurred vision, cholestatic jaundice, leucopenia, agranulocytosis, extrapyramidal reactions (akathesia, dystonia or parkinsonism), persistent tardive dyskinesia, acute catatonia. *See also chlorpromazine.*

P

PROCHLORPERAZINE (continued)
NURSING IMPLICATIONS

- Minimum effective dosage is advised. Keep physician informed of patient's response to drug therapy.
- Most elderly and emaciated patients and children, especially those with dehydration or acute illness, appear to be particularly susceptible to extrapyramidal effects. Be alert to onset of symptoms: in early therapy watch for pseudoparkinsonism and acute dyskinesia. After 1 to 2 months, be alert to akathisia. *See Chlorpromazine.*
- Dosage for elderly, emaciated patients, and for children should be advanced very slowly.
- Counsel patient to take drug as prescribed and not to alter dose or schedule. Consult physician before stopping the medication.
- Keep in mind that the antiemetic effect may mask toxicity of other drugs or make it difficult to diagnose conditions with a primary symptom of nausea, such as intestinal obstruction, brain disease.
- IM injection in adults should be made deep into the upper outer quadrant of the buttock. Do not mix IM solution in the same syringe with other agents.
- Postoperative patients who have received prochlorperazine should be carefully positioned to prevent aspiration of vomitus. Keep in mind that the cough reflex is depressed.
- ***Treatment of overdosage***   Early gastric lavage, airway maintenance, general supportive measures. Have available antiparkinsonian drugs, barbiturates, and diphenhydramine. Emesis should not be induced because it may precipitate dystonic reactions of head and neck with possible aspiration of vomitus.
- Instruct patient to withhold dose and report to the physician if the following symptoms persist more than a few hours: tremor, involuntary twitching, exaggerated restlessness. Other reportable symptoms include: light-coloured stools, changes in vision, sore throat, fever, rash.
- Slight yellowing does not appear to alter potency; however, markedly discoloured solutions should be discarded. Protect drug from light; do not freeze. Store at temperature between 15° and 30°C (59° and 86°F) unless otherwise instructed by manufacturer.
- *See chlorpromazine.*

Procyclidine hydrochloride ———————————————

(Arpicolin, Kemadrin)

Anticholinergic (parasympatholytic); antimuscarinic; antiparkinsonian agent

ACTIONS AND USES   Centrally acting synthetic anticholinergic agent with actions similar to those of atropine (q.v.); closely related to benzhexal.

PROCYCLIDINE HYDROCHLORIDE (continued)

Used to relieve parkinsonism, including postencephalitic, arteriosclerotic, and idiopathic types, and drug-induced extrapyramidal symptoms.

ROUTE AND DOSAGE   Oral: *initial*: 2.5 mg three times daily after meals: Maximum 30 mg/day. **IM/IV**: 5–10 mg repeated after 20 min if required. Maximum 20 mg/day.

ABSORPTION AND FATE   Onset of action in 30 to 45 minutes; duration 4 to 6 hours.

CONTRAINDICATIONS AND PRECAUTIONS   Angle-closure glaucoma. Safe use during pregnancy and use in women of childbearing potential, in nursing mothers, and in children not established. **Cautious Use**: hypotension, mental disorders, tachycardia, prostatic hypertrophy.

ADVERSE/SIDE EFFECTS   Dry mouth, blurred vision, mydriasis, palpitation, tachycardia, flushing of skin, headache, lightheadedness, nausea, vomiting, epigastric distress, dizziness, urinary retention, feeling of muscle weakness, constipation, acute suppurative parotitis, skin eruptions; (occasionally): mental confusion, psychotic-like symptoms.

NURSING IMPLICATIONS
- Side effects may be minimized by administration of drug during or after meals.
- Drug occasionally causes mental confusion, disorientation, agitation, and psychotic-like symptoms, particularly in elderly patients who have low blood pressure. Report these symptoms to physician.
- Report palpitation, tachycardia, or decreasing blood pressure. Dosage adjustment or discontinuation of drug may be indicated.
- Since dosage is guided by clinical response, observe and record improvement (or lack of it) that accompanies therapy.
- Advise patient to avoid alcohol and not to take other CNS depressants unless otherwise advised by physician.
- Procyclidine is usually more effective in controlled rigidity than tremors. Tremors may temporarily appear to be exaggerated as rigidity is relieved, especially in patients with severe spasticity.
- Store in tightly closed containers at controlled room temperature, preferably between 15° and 30°C (59° and 86°F) unless otherwise directed by manufacturer.

Drug interactions   Procyclidine may partially inhibit the therapeutic effects of **haloperiodol** (possibly by delaying gastric emptying time and increasing its metabolism in GI tract) and **phenothiazines** (possible by interfering with their absorption). *See also atropine sulphate.*

Progesterone ━━━━━━━━━━━━━━━━━━━━━━━━━━

(Cyclogest, Gestone)   *Progestogen; hormone*

PROGESTERONE (continued)

ACTIONS AND USES   Steroid hormone synthesized and released by testes, ovary, adrenal cortex, and placenta. Has antioestrogenic, anabolic, and androgenic activity. Physiological precursor to oestrogens, androgens, and adrenocortical steroids. Transforms endometrium from proliferative to secretory state; suppresses pituitary gonadotropin secretion thereby blocking follicular maturation and ovulation. Sudden drop in blood levels of progestogen (and oestradiol) causes 'withdrawal bleeding' from endometrium. Intrauterine placement of progesterone (intrauterine progesterone contraceptive system) hypothetically inhibits sperm capacity or survival, alters uterine milieu so as to prevent nidation and suppresses endometrial proliferation (antioestrogenic effect).

Used to treat secondary amenorrhoea, functional uterine bleeding, endometriosis, and investigationally to treat premenstrual syndrome.

ROUTE AND DOSAGE   Intramuscular: *Habitual abortion*: 10–20 mg twice a week for the first 4 months of pregnancy. *Dysfunctional bleeding*: 5–10 mg/day for 5–10 days prior to anticipated menstruation. **Rectal or vaginal**: for premenstrual syndrome: 200 mg/day to 400 mg twice a day from day 12–14 of the cycle continued until menstruation starts.

ABSORPTION AND FATE   Rapid absorption follows injection. **Plasma half-life** approximately 5 minutes; **duration of action** about 24 hours. Biotransformation takes place during one pass through liver; after enterohepatic circulation, portion of metabolites excreted in faeces. Urinary excretion of remainder as pregnanediol provides indirect index of natural progesterone secretion. Small amounts excreted in breast milk.

CONTRAINDICATIONS AND PRECAUTIONS   Hypersensitivity to progestogens known or suspected breast or genital malignancy; thrombophlebitis, thromboembolic disorders; cerebral apoplexy (or its history), impaired liver function or disease, undiagnosed vaginal bleeding, missed abortion, first 4 months of pregnancy, nursing mother. Progestasert: pregnancy or suspicion of pregnancy. **Cautious Use**: anaemia, diagnostic test for pregnancy; diabetes mellitus, cardiac and renal dysfunction, epilepsy, asthma, migraine, history of psychological depression; persons susceptible to acute intermittent porphyria, previous ectopic pregnancy, presence or history of salpingitis, venereal disease, unresolved abnormal Pap smear, genital bleeding of unknown etiology, previous pelvic surgery.

ADVERSE/SIDE EFFECTS   These include: partial or complete loss of vision, proptosis, diplopia, migraine, mental depression, thromboembolic disorders, pulmonary embolus, mammary nodules, benign and malignant; gynaecomastia, galactorrhoea, masculinization of female foetus, changes in cervical erosion and secretions, and in menstrual pattern; amenorrhoea, breakthrough bleeding, spotting, pruritus vulvae, changes in libido, fatigue, headache, acne, alopecia, hirsutism, urticaria, photosensitivity, allergic rash, pruritus cholestatic jaundice, oedema, changes in weight, candidiasis, pain at injection site, melasma or chloasma.

NURSING IMPLICATIONS
■ Protect medication vial from light.

PROGESTERONE (continued)

- Immerse vial in warm water momentarily to redissolve crystals and to facilitate aspiration of drug into syringe.
- Inject deeply IM. Injection site may be irritated by drug in oil. Inspect used sites carefully and rotate areas systematically.
- A physical examination with special reference to pelvic organs, breasts, as well as Pap smear should precede therapy with a progestogen. Urge patient to keep appointments for physical check-ups at established intervals.
- Baseline data for comparative value about patient's weight fluid intake–output ratio, blood pressure, and pulse should be recorded at onset of progestogen therapy. Deviations should be reported promptly.
- Progestogens may cause some degree of fluid retention. Monitor conditions that may be worsened by oedema: epilepsy, migraine, asthma, cardiac or renal dysfunction.
- Treatment with a progestogen may mask onset of the climacteric.
- Progestogens reportedly may precipitate attack of acute intermittent porphyria in susceptible patients. (Common manifestations include acute colicky, severe abdominal pain; vomiting, distention, diarrhoea, constipation.)
- Instruct patient to notify physician if she suspects pregnancy while receiving progestational therapy. She should be apprised of the potential risk to the foetus from progestogen exposure.
- Serious mental depression may signal a recurrence of previous psychiatric disorder. Alert family or significant other to this potential side effect and give instructions for prompt reporting. The drug will be discontinued if mental changes are severe.
- Instruct a diabetic user of progestogen or progestogen combination drug to monitor clinical signs of loss of diabetes control. If urine tests become positive, or hypoglycaemic symptoms occur, the physician should be consulted.
- Caution patient to avoid exposure to ultraviolet light and prolonged periods of time in the sun. Photosensitivity severity is related to both time of exposure and dose. A phototoxic drug reaction usually looks like an exaggerated sunburn but may also produce acute eczematous or urticarial reactions. The reaction can occur within 5 to 18 hours after exposure to sun and is maximal by 36 to 72 hours.
- Advise use of sunscreen lotion (SPF above 12) which contains para-amino-benzoic acid (PABA) on exposed skin surfaces whenever patient goes outdoors, even on dark days.
- Side effects that warrant medical attention should be clearly identified for the patient. Inform physician promptly if any of the following occur: sudden severe headache or vomiting, dizziness or fainting, numbness in an arm or leg, pain in calves accompanied by swelling, warmth and redness; visual disturbance, acute chest pain or dyspnoea.
- Progestogens can affect endocrine and hepatic function tests. An interval of up to 60 days following cessation of therapy with the drug may be necessary before laboratory results can be considered definitive.
- Progestogens are no longer recommended for use in pregnancy tests because of potential teratogenic effects.
- Inform pathologist of progestogen therapy when relevant specimens are submitted.

P

PROGESTERONE (continued)

Instruct patient to tell the dentist if extraction is anticipated and the surgeon in an emergency situation.

■ Store drug at temperature between 15° and 30°C (59° and 86°F) unless otherwise specified by manufacturer. Protect from freezing and light.

Diagnostic test interferences Progestogens may increase levels of **urinary pregnanediol, serum alkaline phosphatase, plasma amino acids, urinary nitrogen.** They also decrease **glucose tolerance** (may cause false-positive urine glucose tests) and lower **HDL** (high density lipoprotein) levels.

Proguanil

(Paludrine)

ACTIONS AND USES   Used in chemoprophylaxis of malaria.

ROUTE AND DOSAGE   Usual adult dose, 200 mg/day alone or in combination with chloroquine. Drug choice depends on risk and local factors.

For further information: *see chloroquine.*

Promazine hydrochloride

(Sparine)   *Antipsychotic; (neuroleptic);*
phenothiazine

ACTIONS AND USES   Aliphatic (ethylamino) derivative of phenothiazine. Compared with chlorpromazine (q.v.) has weak antipsychotic activity and extrapyramidal effects occur less frequently. Although drug-induced agranulocytosis is rare, it occurs more often than with other phenothiazines.

Used in management of manifestations of psychotic disorders and for reducing agitation and paranoia association with alcohol withdrawal.

ROUTE AND DOSAGE   Oral: Adult: 25–200 mg 4 times a day according to response. Reduce dose in the elderly.

CONTRAINDICATIONS AND PRECAUTIONS   Hypersensitivity to phenothiazines, myelosuppression, CNS depression, children under 12 years of age, Reye's syndrome. Safe use during pregnancy and by nursing mothers not established. **Cautious Use**: prostatic hypertrophy, cardiovascular or hepatic disease, paralytic ileus, xerostomia, angle closure glaucoma, persons exposed to extremes in temperature or to organophosphorous insecticides, convulsive disorders. *See also chlorpromazine.*

PROMAZINE HYDROCHLORIDE (continued)

ADVERSE/SIDE EFFECTS   *Common*: Drowsiness, orthostatic hypotension. Also, blurred vision, constipation, epileptic seizures in susceptible individuals, leucopenia, agranulocytosis (rare). *See also chlorpromazine*.

NURSING IMPLICATIONS

- Oral route should be used whenever possible. Parenteral administration is reserved for acutely disturbed or uncooperative patients or those who cannot tolerate an oral preparation.
- Store medication in light-resistant container at temperature between 15° and 30°C (59° and 86°F) unless otherwise directed by manufacturer.
- *See chlorpromazine*.

Promethazine hydrochloride ━━━━━━━━━━━━━━━━

(Phenergan)   *Antihistamine; phenothiazine*

ACTIONS AND USES   Long-acting ethylamino derivative of phenothiazine with marked antihistaminic activity and prominent sedative, amnesic, antiemetic, and anti-motion-sickness actions. Unlike other phenothiazine derivatives, it is relatively free of extrapyramidal side effects; however, in high doses it carries same potential for toxicity. In common with other antihistamines, exerts antiserotonin, anticholinergic, and local anaesthetic action. Prevents most actions of histamine by competing with it for H_1-receptor sites on effector cells. Antiemetic action thought to be due to depression of CTZ in medulla. Reported to have slight antitussive activity, but this may be due to anticholinergic and CNS depressant effects.

Used for symptomatic relief of various allergic conditions, to ameliorate and prevent reactions to blood and plasma, in prophylaxis and treatment of motion sickness, and for preoperative sedation.

ROUTE AND DOSAGE   Adults: Oral: 20–75 mg/day in divided doses or as a single dose at night. **Child (6–12 mth)**: 5–10 mg; **(1–5 yrs)**: 5–15 mg; **(6–10 yrs)**: 10–25 mg/ml solution in water for injection. *Premedication*: **Oral: Child (6–12 mths)**: 10 12.5 mg. **Slow IV injection in emergency**: 25–50 mg, maximum 100 mg as 2.5 mg/ml solution in water for injection. *Premedication*: **Oral: Child (6–12 mths)**: 10 mg; **(1–5 yrs)**: 15–20 mg; **(6–10 yrs)**: 20–25 mg; **deep IM injection** (one hour preoperatatively) **Child (5–10 yrs)**: 6.25–12.5 mg.

ABSORPTION AND FATE   Well absorbed from GI tract and parenteral routes. Antihistaminic effects occur within 20 minutes following oral, rectal, and IM and within 3 to 5 minutes after IV administration. Duration of action generally 4 to 6 hours; antihistaminic activity sometimes persists for 12 hours. Widely distributed in body tissues. Metabolized by liver; excreted slowly in urine and faeces, primarily as inactive metabolites.

P

PROMETHAZINE HYDROCHLORIDE (continued)

CONTRAINDICATIONS AND PRECAUTIONS Hypersensitivity to phenothiazines, narrow-angle glaucoma, stenosing peptic ulcer, pyloroduodenal obstruction, prostatic hypertrophy, bladder neck obstruction, epilepsy, bone marrow depression, comatose or severely depressed states, pregnancy (except labour), nursing mothers, newborn or premature infants, acutely ill or dehydrated children. **Cautious Use:** impaired hepatic function, cardiovascular disease, asthma, acute or chronic respiratory impairment (particularly in children), hypertension, elderly or debilitated patients.

ADVERSE/SIDE EFFECTS These include: sedation drowsiness, confusion, dizziness, disturbed coordination, restlessness, tremors, transient mild hypotension or hypertension, anorexia, nausea, vomiting, constipation, leucopenia, agranulocytosis, photosensitivity, irregular respiration, blurred vision, urinary retention; dry mouth, nose, or throat.

NURSING IMPLICATIONS

- Administration of oral medication with food, milk or a full glass of water may minimize GI distress.
- Oral doses for allergy are generally prescribed before meals and on retiring or as single dose at bedtime.
- When administered as prophylaxis against motion sickness, initial dose should be taken 30 minutes to 1 hour before anticipated travel and repeated at 8 to 12 hour intervals if necessary. For duration of journey, repeat dose on arising and again at evening meal.
- Inspect parenteral drug before preparation. Discard if it is darkened or contains precipitate.
- IM injection is made deep into large muscle mass. Aspirate carefully before injecting drug. Intraarterial injection can cause arterial or arteriolar spasm, with resultant gangrene. Subcutaneous injection (also contraindicated) can cause chemical irritation and necrosis. Rotate injection sites and observe daily.
- Promethazine injection is reportedly incompatible with several drugs, especially those with alkaline pH. Consult pharmacist for specific information.
- Promethazine sometimes produces marked sedation and dizziness. Cot sides and supervision of ambulation may be advisable.
- Advise ambulatory patient to avoid driving a car or engaging in other activities requiring mental alertness and normal reaction time until reponse to drug is known.
- Bear in mind that antiemetic action may mask symptoms of unrecognized disease and signs of drug overdosage as well as dizziness, vertigo, or tinnitus associated with toxic doses of aspirin or other ototoxic drugs.
- Patients in pain may develop involuntary (athetoid) movement of upper extremities following parenteral administration. These symptoms usually disappear after pain is controlled.
- Respiratory function should be monitored in patients with respiratory problems, particularly children. Promethazine may suppress cough reflex and cause thickening of bronchial secretions.
- Dry mouth may be relieved by frequent rinses with warm water or by increasing

P

PROMETHAZINE HYDROCHLORIDE (continued)

noncaloric fluid intake (if allowed), or by sugarless gum or lemon drops. If these measures fail a saliva substitute may help.

■ Promethazine may cause photosensitivity. Advise patient to avoid sunlamps or prolonged exposure to sunlight. A sunscreen lotion may be advisable during initial drug therapy.

■ Advise patient not to take OTC medications without physician's approval, and caution against alcohol and other CNS depressants.

■ *Treatment of overdosage* Early gastric lavage (endotracheal tube with cuff in place to prevent aspiration of vomitus). Emesis should not be induced because dystonic reactions of head and neck may result in aspiration. Have on hand: antiparkinson drugs, barbiturates, diazepam, diphenhydramine, phenylephrine, nor adrenaline.

■ Store in tight, light-resistant container at controlled room temperature, preferably between 15° and 30°C (59° and 86°F) unless otherwise directed by manufacturer.

Diagnostic test interferences Promethazine may interfere with **blood grouping** in ABO system and may produce false results with **urinary pregnancy tests.** Promethazine can cause significant alterations of flare response in **intradermal allergen tests** if performed within 4 days of receiving promethazine, and can cause elevations in **blood glucose.**

Drug interactions Additive sedative action may result when promethazine is given concurrently with drugs that have CNS depressant effect, e.g., **alcohol,** other **antihistamines, barbiturates, narcotic analgesics,** and antipsychotics. Promethazine reverses vasopressor effect of adrenaline and may cause further lowering of blood pressure in patients with hypotension. **MAO inhibitors** intensify and prolong the anticholinergic effects of promethazine.

Propantheline bromide

(Pro-Banthine)　　　　　　　　　　　　　　　　*Anticholinergic; antimuscarinic*

ACTIONS AND USES　Synthetic quaternary ammonium compound. Similar to atropine (q.v.) in peripheral effects, contraindications, precautions, and adverse reactions. Potent in antimuscarinic activity and in nondepolarizing ganglionic blocking action. Very high doses block neurotransmission at myoneural junction.

Used as adjunct in treatment of peptic ulcer, irritable bowel syndrome, pancreatitis, ureteral and urinary bladder spasm. Also used prior to radiological diagnostic procedures to reduce duodenal motility.

ROUTE AND DOSAGE　Adult: **Oral:** 15 mg with meals and 30 mg at bedtime. Usual adult prescribing limit: 120 mg daily.

ABSORPTION AND FATE　Incompletely absorbed from GI tract. Onset of effects fol-

PROPANTHELINE BROMIDE (continued)

lowing oral administration in 30 to 45 minutes, persisting 4 to 6 hours. Metabolism: 50% in GI tract before absorption; 50% hepatic. Excreted through all body fluids, but chiefly in urine and bile.

ADVERSE/SIDE EFFECTS   Constipation, difficult urination, dry mouth, blurred vision, mydriasis, increased intraocular pressure, drowsiness, decreased sexual activity. *See atropine.*

NURSING IMPLICATIONS

- Oral preparation is generally administered 30 to 60 minutes before meals and at bedtime. Advise the patient not to chew tablet; drug is very bitter.
- If patient is also receiving an antacid (or antidiarrhoeal agent), propantheline should be taken at least 1 hour before or 1 hour after the other drug.
- Alcoholic beverages should be avoided while patient is receiving propantheline.
- Store dry powder and tablets at temperature between 15° and 30°C (59° and 86°F), protected from freezing and moisture.
- *See atropine.*

Propranolol hydrochloride

(Angilol, Apsolol, Berkolol, Inderal, Sloprolol)

Antihypertensive; beta-adrenergic blocking agent (non-selective); antiarrhythmic

ACTIONS AND USES   Nonselective beta-blocker of both cardiac (beta$_1$) and bronchial (beta$_2$) adrenoreceptors which competes with adrenaline and noradrenaline for available beta-receptor sites. Blocks cardiac effects of beta-adrenergic stimulation; as a result, reduces heart rate, myocardial irritability and force of contraction, depresses automaticity of sinus node and ectopic pacemaker, and decreases AV and intraventricular conduction velocity. In higher doses, exerts direct quinidine-like effects which depress cardiac function. Propranolol also blocks bronchodilator effect of catecholamines and reduces plasma levels of free fatty acids, and tends to promote retention of sodium; therefore, a diuretic is frequently given concurrently. Inhibition of adrenaline, the result of beta-adrenergic blockade, prevents premonitory signs of hypoglycaemia in the diabetic and may also augment hypoglycaemia by interfering with catecholamine-induced glycogenolysis. Propranolol may also block insulin release from pancreas with resulting hyperglycaemia. Lowers both supine and standing blood pressures in hypertensive patients. Hypotensive effect (i.e., lowered systolic and diastolic blood pressure) is associated with decreased cardiac output, suppressed renin activity, as well as beta-blockade. Increases exercise tolerance by blocking sympathetic effects of exertion and decreases myocardial oxygen requirements in patients with frequent anginal attacks. Also decreases platelet aggregability. Mechanism of antimigraine action unknown but thought to be related to inhibition of cerebral vasodilation and arteriolar spasms.

PROPRANOLOL HYDROCHLORIDE (continued)

Used in management of cardiac arrhythmias, myocardial infarction, tachyarrhythmias associated with digitalis intoxication, anaesthesia, and thyrotoxicosis, hypertrophic subaortic stenosis, angina pectoris due to coronary atherosclerosis, phaeochromocytoma; also treatment of hypertension alone, but generally with a thiazide or other antihypertensive agent.

ROUTE AND DOSAGE   Oral: *Hypertension*: 80 mg twice daily, increased until optimum response obtained. *Maintenance*: 160 to 320 mg/day in divided doses; up to 640 mg/day be required. *Angina pectoris*: *initial*: 40 mg two or three times daily; dosage gradually increased at 3 to 7 day intervals until optimum response obtained (average optimum dosage: 160 mg/day). *Arrhythmias and thyrotoxicosis*: 10 to 40 mg three to four times daily. *Migraine prevention*: *initial*: 120 mg daily in divided doses. *Maintenance*: 80 to 160 mg daily in divided doses. *Intravenous (for life-threatening arrhythmias)*: 1 mg/minute; may be repeated after 2 minutes, if necessary. Maximum 10 mg.

ABSORPTION AND FATE   Almost completely absorbed from GI tract following oral administration. Much of drug is metabolized during first pass through liver; about 30 to 60% may reach systemic circulation. With chronic administration less drug is removed during first pass; accordingly half-life gradually increases. Onset of action within 30 minutes, peak plasma levels in 1 to 1½ hours (marked interindividual variations in plasma levels); duration about 6 hours. following IV administration, action begins within 2 minutes, peaks in about 15 minutes, with duration of 3 to 6 hours; plasma levels more consistent. Half-life: 3 to 5 hours. Widely distributed in body tissues; more than 90% bound to plasma proteins. Excreted in urine as free and conjugated propranolol, and active metabolites; 1 to 4% excreted in faeces. Crosses placenta and blood–brain barrier; small amounts may appear in breast milk.

CONTRAINDICATIONS AND PRECAUTIONS   Greater than first degree heart block, congestive heart failure, right ventricular failure secondary to pulmonary hypertension; sinus bradycardia, cardiogenic shock, significant aortic or mitral valvular disease, bronchial asthma or bronchospasm, severe chronic obstructive airways disease, allergic rhinitis during pollen season; concurrent use with adrenergic-augmenting psychotropic drugs or within 2 weeks of MAO inhibition therapy. Safe use in women of childbearing potential, during pregnancy, in nursing mothers and in children not established. **Cautious Use**: peripheral arterial insufficiency, history of allergy, history of systemic insect sting reaction, patients prone to nonallergenic bronchospasm (e.g., chronic bronchitis, emphysema); major surgery; renal or hepatic impairment, diabetes mellitus, patients prone to hypoglycaemia, myasthenia gravis, Wolff–Parkinson–White syndrome.

ADVERSE/SIDE EFFECTS   These include: drug-induced psychosis, sleep disturbances, depression, confusion, agitation, giddiness, light-headedness, fatigue, vertigo, syncope, weakness, drowsiness, insomnia, vivid dreams, visual hallucinations, delusions, reversible organic brain syndrome, palpitation, profound bradycardia, AV heart block, cardiac standstill, hypotension, angina pectoris, tachyarrhythmia, acute congestive

PROPRANOLOL HYDROCHLORIDE (continued)

heart failure, peripheral arterial insufficiency resembling Raynaud's disease, myotonia, paraesthesia of hands, reversible alopecia; hyperkeratoses of scalp, palms, feet; nail changes, dry skin, dry eyes (gritty sensation), visual disturbances, conjunctivitis, tinnitus, hearing loss, nasal stuffiness, dry mouth, cheilostomatitis, nausea, vomiting, heartburn, diarrhoea, constipation, flatulence, abdominal cramps, mesenteric arterial thrombosis, ischaemic colitis, transient eosinophilia, thrombocytopenic or nonthrombocytopenic purpura, agranulocytosis, hypoglycaemia, hyperglycaemia (rare); hypocalcaemia (patients with hyperthyroidism), dyspnoea, laryngospasm, bronchospasm, brown discolouration of tongue (rare), pancreatitis, weight gain, impotence or decreased libido, Peyronie's disease (rare), LE-like reaction, acid extremities, leg fatigue.

NURSING IMPLICATIONS

- Manufacturer recommends giving oral propranolol before meals and at bedtime. Reports to date are conflicting relative to whether food enhances or delays bioavailability of propranolol. Advise patient to be consistent with regard to taking propranolol with food or on an empty stomach, to minimize variations in absorption.
- Careful medical history and physical examination are essential to rule out allergies, asthma, and other obstructive pulmonary disease. Propranolol can cause bronchiolar constriction even in normal subjects.
- Take apical pulse before administering drug; if blood pressure is not stabilized, also take this reading before giving drug.
- Apical pulse, respiration, blood pressure, and circulation of extremities should be closely monitored throughout period of dosage adjustment. Consult physician regarding acceptable parameters.
- Patient receiving propranolol at home should be informed about usual pulse rate and should be instructed to take radial pulse before each dose. Advise patient to report to physician if it is slower than base level or becomes irregular.
- Response to propranolol is reported to be associated with a high degree of individual variability. Therefore, sensitive observations are critically essential for establishing the patient's optimal dosage level.
- For patients being treated for hypertension, checking blood pressure near end of dosage interval or before administration of next dose is a way of evaluating if control is adequate or whether more frequent dosage intervals are indicated.
- Bradycardia is the most common adverse cardiac effect especially in patients with digitalis intoxication and Wolff–Parkinson–White syndrome.
- When administered by IV route careful monitoring must be made of ECG, blood pressure, and pulmonary wedge pressure. Reduction in sympathetic stimulation caused by beta blocking action can result in cardiac standstill.
- Adverse reactions generally occur most frequently following IV administration; however, incidence is also high following oral use in the elderly and in patients with impaired renal function. Reactions may or may not be dose-related and commonly occur soon after therapy is initiated.
- Treatment of toxicity or exaggerated response may include use of the following drugs: atropine, adrenaline, isoprenaline, aminophylline, dobutamine, and glucagon. Cardiac failure is treated by digitalization and diuresis.

P

PROPRANOLOL HYDROCHLORIDE (continued)

- Fluid intake and output ratio and weight are significant indices for detecting fluid retention and developing heart failure: dyspnoea on exertion, orthopnoea, night cough, pulmonary rales, distended neck veins, oedema (tight shoes or rings, puffiness).
- Plasma volume may increase with consequent risk of congestive failure if dietary sodium is not restricted in patients receiving propranolol without concomitant diuretic therapy. Consult physician regarding allowable salt intake.
- Patients with diabetes should be closely monitored. Propranolol suppresses clinical signs of hypoglycaemia (e.g., blood pressure changes, increased pulse rate) and may prolong hypoglycaemia. Patient should be alert to other possible signs of hypoglycaemia not affected by propranolol such as excessive sweating, hunger, fatigue, inability to concentrate. Instruct patient to report these easily overlooked and tolerated symptoms. Adjustment in dosage of insulin or other hypoglycaemic agents may be necessary.
- Fasting for more than 12 hours may induce hypoglycaemic effects fostered by propranolol.
- Because of beta-blocking action, usual rise in pulse rate may not occur response to stress situations, such as fever or following vigorous exercise. Activity programmes must be highly individualized. Consult physician for guidelines.
- In patients taking propranolol for angina pectoris, exercise performance studies and ECGs are recommended before therapy to establish baseline data, and during therapy to determine dosage requirements and need to continue treatment. Therapy is not continued unless there is reduced pain and increased work capacity.
- When propranolol is to be discontinued, dosage is reduced gradually over a period of 1 to 2 weeks and patient closely monitored.
- Abrupt discontinuation of propranolol can precipitate withdrawal syndrome: tremulousness, sweating, severe headache, malaise, palpitation, rebound hypertension, myocardial infarction, and life-threatening arrhythmias (in patients with angina pectoris), and hyperthyroidism in patients with thyrotoxicosis.
- Anaesthetist should be informed about propranolol use prior to general anaesthesia.
- Caution patient to avoid prolonged exposure of extremities to cold. If patient complains of cold, painful, or tender feet or hands examine them carefully for evidence of impaired circulation. Peripheral pulses may still be present even though circulation is impaired.
- Stress importance of compliance and warn patient not to alter established regimen, i.e., not to omit, increase or decrease dosage, or change dosage intervals.
- Normotensive patients on prolonged therapy should be cautioned that propranolol may cause mild hypotension (experienced as dizziness or light-headedness). Advise patient to make position changes slowly and to avoid prolonged standing and to notify physician if these symptoms persist.
- Since propranolol may cause dizziness and light-headedness, caution patient to avoid driving and other potentially hazardous activities until reaction to drug is known.
- When given for prolonged periods, periodic determinations should be made of haematological, renal, hepatic, and cardiac function.
- Counsel patient to avoid excesses of alcohol. Heavy alcohol consumption (i.e., more than 60 mls/day) may elevate arterial pressure; therefore to maintain treatment

P

PROPRANOLOL HYDROCHLORIDE (continued)

effectiveness, patient should either avoid alcohol or drink moderately (less than 60 mls/day). Consult physician.

- Moderation in sodium (salt) intake is advisable for the hypertensive patient. Give information about food sources to be avoided (*see Index: Food sources*). A consultation with the dietician regarding a diet for weight control (if necessary) should be arranged before patient is discharged.
- ***Smoking–drug interaction***   Smoking has a direct and adverse effect on the myocardium: (increased heart rate and myocardial oxygen requirements). Additionally it increases hepatic metabolism of propranolol leading to unpredictable or lack of drug effects. Advise patient to stop smoking; but if it continues, more frequent monitoring for clinical effects of the drug is indicated.
- Advise patient to consult physician before self-medicating with OTC drugs.
- It is advisable for patient on prolonged propranolol therapy to wear or carry medical identification such as Medic Alert. Instruct patient to inform dentist, surgeon, or ophthalmologist (propranolol lowers normal and elevated intraocular pressure) that he or she is taking propranolol.

Patient-teaching points   (**Pharmacological therapy of hypertension**, *see Index: Nursing Intervention: hypertension*.) **Nonpharmacological therapy of hypertension**: Discuss the following with the patient:
- □ Weight reduction.
- □ Modification of dietary sodium intake.
- □ Moderation of alcohol consumption.
- □ Avoidance of tobacco.
- □ Controlled exercise programme.
- □ Behaviour modification (biofeedback, relaxation therapy).

- Preserve in tightly closed, light-resistant containers at temperature 15° to 30°C (59° to 86°F).

Diagnostic test interferences   Beta-adrenergic blockers may produce false-negative test results in exercise tolerance ECG tests, and elevations in: **serum potassium, peripheral platelet** count, **serum uric acid, serum transaminase, alkaline phosphatase, lactate dehydrogenase, serum creatinine, BUN**, and an increase or decrease in **blood glucose** levels in diabetic patients.

DRUG INTERACTIONS   *Propranolol hydrochloride*

PLUS	INTERACTIONS
Antacids	Delay absorption if administration concomitantly; space several hours apart
Antiarrhythmics, other: e.g., lignocaine, phenytoin, procainamide, quinidine	Additive cardiac depressant effects; additive toxic effects
Antidiabetic drugs (insulins and oral hypoglycaemics)	Prolonged hypoglycaemic effects of insulin and coumarins

PROPRANOLOL HYDROCHLORIDE (continued)

PLUS	INTERACTIONS
(continued)	
Barbiturates ⎫ Rifampicin ⎬	Enhance metabolism of propranolol (by inducing hepatic microsomal enzymes), thereby reducing pharmacological effects of propranolol
Clonidine	Severity of rebound hypertension caused by abrupt discontinuation of clonidine may be increased
Digitalis glycosides	Potentiation of bradycardic effect (additive depression of AV conduction)
Adrenaline (intravenous)	Possibility of hypertension and excessive bradycardia
Cimetidine ⎫ Chlorpromazine ⎪ Contraceptives, oral ⎬ Frusemide ⎪ Hydralazine ⎭	Increased hypotensive effects (inhibition of hepatic metabolism therefore increased bioavailability of propranolol).
Ergot alkaloids	Possible additive peripheral vasoconstrictors
Glucagon	Propranolol may partially inhibit glucagon-induced hyperglycaemia
Indomethacin ⎫ Salicylates ⎬	May inhibit antihypertensive response (inhibition of prostaglandin synthesis)
Isoprenaline ⎫ Dobutamine ⎪ Adrenaline ⎬ Dopamine ⎭	May reverse beta blockade; severe hypotension is possible
Phenothiazines	Additive hypotensive effects
Reserpine (and other catecholamine-depleting drugs)	Additive hypotensive and bradycardic effects
Skeletal muscle relaxants, e.g, gallamine, pancuronium, tubocurarine	Intensified neuromuscular blockade
Tricyclic antidepressants ⎫ Antimuscarinics (e.g., atropine) ⎬	May antagonize cardiac depressive activity of propranolol

Propylthiouracil ━━━━━━━━━━━━━━━━━━━━━━━━━━━

Antithyroid agent

ACTIONS AND USES   Relatively nontoxic thioamide. Interferes with organification of iodine and blocks synthesis of thyroxine (T_4) and triiodothyronine (T_3). Does not interfere with release and utilization of stored thyroid; thus antithyroid action is delayed days and weeks until preformed T_3 and T_4 are degraded. Drug-induced hormone reduction results in compensatory release of thyrotropin, which causes marked hyperplasia and vascularization of thyroid gland. With good adherence to drug regimen, chemical euthyroidism can be achieved 6 to 12 weeks after start of thioamide therapy.

Used in medical treatment of hyperthyroidism, to established euthyroid. State prior

PROPYLTHIOURACIL (continued)

to surgery or radioative iodine treatment, and for palliative control of toxic nodular goitre. Also used to treat iodine-induced thyrotoxicosis and hyperthyroidism associated with thyroiditis.

ROUTE AND DOSAGE   Oral: Adults: *initial*: 300 to 450 mg/day. **Maintenance**: 100 to 150 mg.

ABSORPTION AND FATE   Absorption of effective amounts within 30 minutes after oral dose. **Duration of action** 2 or 3 hours; **plasma half-life**: 3 to 5 hours; **protein binding**: 80%. 30 to 35% of drug is excreted in urine within 24 hours; some excretion through bile. Crosses placenta, inhibits foetal thyroid function, and is excreted in breast milk.

CONTRAINDICATIONS AND PRECAUTIONS   Hypersensitivity or idiosyncrasy to propylthiouracil, last trimester of pregnancy, lactation, concurrent administration of sulphonamides or coal tar derivatives such as aminopyrine or antipyrine. **Cautious Use**: infection, concomitant administration of anticoagulants or other drugs known to cause agranulocytosis; bone marrow depression, impaired hepatic function.

ADVERSE/SIDE EFFECTS   These include: paraesthesias, headache, vertigo, drowsiness, neuritis, skin rash, urticaria, pruritus, hyperpigmentation, lightening of hair colour, abnormal hair loss, nausea, vomiting, diarrhoea, dyspepsia, loss of taste, sialoadenitis, hepatitis, myelosuppression, lymphadenopathy, periarteritis, hypoprothrombinaemia, thrombocytopenia, leucopenia, agranulocytosis, enlarged thyroid, reduced GI motility, periorbital oedema, puffy hands and feet, bradycardia, cool and pale skin, worsening of ophthalmopathy, sleepiness, fatigue, mental depression, dizziness, vertigo, sensitivity to cold, paraesthesias, nocturnal muscle cramps, changes in menstrual periods, unusual weight gain, drug fever, lupus like syndrome, arthralgia, myalgia.

NURSING IMPLICATIONS

- Administer at the same time each day with relation to meals. Food may alter drug response by changing absorption rate.
- Objective signs of clinical response (usually within 2 or 3 weeks): significant weight gain, reduced pulse rate, reduced serum T_4.
- When thyroid gland is greatly enlarged, satisfactory euthyroid state may be delayed for several months.
- Generally duration of therapy covers a period of 6 months to several years, followed by remission in 25% of patients. Medication is then stopped in the hope that natural remission will occur.
- Long-term therapy is usually monitored by follow-up examinations and haematological studies every 2 to 3 months. As soon as patient is euthyroid, thyroid hormone (especially T_3) may be added to regimen to prevent goitrogenic-induced hypothyroidism and to suppress thyrotrophin production.
- If surgery fails to render patient euthyroid, treatment may be reinstituted.
- If given during pregnancy may be withdrawn 2 or 3 weeks before delivery to prevent

P

PROPYLTHIOURACIL (continued)

excess drug passage across the placenta and the accompanying danger of cretinism and goiter in foetus.

- To prevent hypothyroidism in mother, thyroid may be given concomitantly with propylthiouracil throughout pregnancy and after delivery with little effect on foetus.
- Postpartum patients should not nurse their babies. Exacerbation of hyperthyroidism 3 to 4 months postpartum in the mother is common.
- The goitrogenic hypothyroid state (excess dosage) develops insidiously, and in some cases it may be noted only after an infrequent observer calls attention to changes such as periorbital oedema.
- Important diagnostic signs of excess dosage: contraction of a muscle bundles when pricked, mental depression, hard and nonpitting oedema, and need for high thermostat setting and extra blankets in winter (cold intolerance).
- Urticaria may occur (3 to 7% of patients) during period from second to eighth week of treatment. If mild, symptomatic treatment with an antihistamine may be started; switching to another thioamide is usual if rash is severe.
- Advise patient to report severe skin rash or swelling of cervical lymph nodes. Therapy may be discontinued.
- Warn patient to report sore throat, fever, and rash immediately (most apt to occur in first few months of treatment). Drug will be discontinued and haematological studies initiated. If agranulocytosis is diagnosed, patient may be given broad-spectrum antibiotics and placed on reverse isolation.
- Be alert to signs of hypoprothrombinaemia: ecchymoses, purpura, petechiae, unexplained bleeding. Warn ambulatory patients to report these signs promptly.
- Advise patients to avoid use of OTC drugs for asthma, coryza, or cough treatment without checking with the physician. Iodides sometimes included in such preparations are contraindicated.
- Teach patient how to take pulse accurately. Advise daily check.
- Clinical response is monitored through changes in weight and pulse. Advise patient to chart weight two or three times weekly. Continued tachycardia, diarrhoea, fever, irritability, listlessness, vomiting, weakness, should be reported as signs of inadequate therapy or thyrotoxicosis.
- Instruct patient in remission to continue monitoring and recording weight and pulse rate. Patient should report onset of tremor, anxiety state, gradual ascending pulse rate, and loss of weight to the physician (signs of hormone deficiency).
- Some young females may have been 'outeating' their hyperthyroidism and gaining weight prior to seeking treatment. Restoration of euthyroid state may be accompanied by further obesity; reduced caloric intake may be prescribed for these patients. Consult dietician.
- Urge patient not to alter drug regimen: not to increase, decrease or omit doses nor change administration intervals.
- If compliance is a problem, the physician may prescribe a once-a-day regimen.
- Check with physician about use of iodized salt and inclusion of seafood in the diet.
- Store drug in light-resistant container at temperature between 15° and 30°C (59° and 86°F).

PROPYLTHIOURACIL *(continued)*
Diagnostic test interferences   Propylthiouracil may elevate prothrombin time and serum alkaline phosphatase, SGOT (AST), SGPT (ALT) levels.

DRUG INTERACTIONS   *Propylthiouracil*

PLUS	INTERACTIONS
Anticoagulants, oral ⎱ Heparin ⎰	May enhance anticoagulant effect

Protamine sulphate

Antidote

ACTIONS AND USES   Used to counteract heparin overdose.

ROUTE AND DOSAGE   IV: determined by coagulation tests.

Protriptyline hydrochloride

(Concordin)
*Psychotropic, antidepressant
tricyclic*

ACTIONS AND USES   Dibenzocycloheptene derivative tricyclic antidepressant with more rapid onset of action than imipramine (q.v.).

Used for symptomatic treatment of endogenous depression.

ROUTE AND DOSAGE   Oral: *Initial*: 5–10 mg, 3–4 times a day. **Elderly patients**: maximum 5 mg three times a day.

NURSING IMPLICATIONS
- Tablet may be crushed before administration and taken with fluid or mixed with food.
- Has fairly rapid onset of initial effect characterized by increased activity and energy, usually within 1 week after therapy is initiated.
- Increase in dosage should be made in the morning dose to prevent sleep interference, and because this TCA has psychological energizing action.
- Last dose of day should be taken no later than midafternoon; insomnia rather than drowsiness is a frequent side effect.
- *See imipramine.*

Pseudoephedrine hydrochloride

*Adrenergic agonist
(sympathomimetic);
decongestant*

ACTIONS AND USES   Sympathomimetic amine that, like ephedrine, produces decongestion of respiratory tract mucosa by action on sympathetic nerve endings. Unlike ephedrine, also acts directly on smooth muscle and constricts renal and vertebral arteries. Has fewer side effects, less pressor action and longer duration of effects than ephedrine. Produces little, if any, congestive rebound or irritation that occur with nasal sprays and solutions.

Used for symptomatic relief of nasal congestion associated with rhinitis, coryza, and sinusitis and for eustachian tube congestion in proprietory preparations.

ROUTE AND DOSAGE   Oral: depends on the preparation.

ABSORPTION AND FATE   Onset of action within 15 to 30 minutes, and persists for 4 to 6 hours; 8 to 12 hours after extended-release form. Partially metabolized in liver. Enters breast milk.

CONTRAINDICATIONS AND PRECAUTIONS   Hypersensitivity to sympathomimetic amines, severe hypertension, coronary artery disease, use within 14 days of MAO inhibitors, nursing mother, glaucoma, hyperthyroidism, prostatic hypertrophy. Safe use during pregnancy, lactation, and in children under 6 not established. **Cautious Use**: hypertension, heart disease.

ADVERSE/SIDE EFFECTS   Transient stimulation, tremulousness, difficulty in voiding, arrhythmias, palpitation, tachycardia, nervousness, dizziness, headache, sleeplessness, numbness of extremities, anorexia, dry mouth, nausea, vomiting.

NURSING IMPLICATIONS
- Since drug may act as a stimulant, advise patient to avoid taking it within 2 hours of bedtime.
- *See ephedrine sulphate.*

P

Pyrantel pamoate

(Combantrin)   *Antiinfective; anthelmintic*

ACTIONS AND USES   Exerts selective depolarizing neuromuscular blocking action, which results in spastic paralysis of worm; also inhibits cholinesterases.

Used to treat roundworm and threadworm infestations.

ROUTE AND DOSAGE   Oral: **Adults and Children**: 10 mg/kg body weight administered in a single dose. Maximum total dose 1 g.

PYRANTEL PAMOATE (continued)

ABSORPTION AND FATE   Partially absorbed from GI tract. Plasma levels of unchanged drug, which are low, peak in 1 to 3 hours. Metabolized in liver. Over 50% excreted in faeces unchanged within 24 hours; about 7% eliminated in urine as free drug and metabolites.

CONTRAINDICATIONS AND PRECAUTIONS   Safe use during pregnancy and in children under 6 months of age not established. **Cautious Use**: liver dysfunction, malnutrition, dehydration, anaemia.

ADVERSE/SIDE EFFECTS   CNS: dizziness, headache, drowsiness, insomnia. **GI**: anorexia, nausea, vomiting, abdominal distention, diarrhoea, tenesmus, transient elevation of SGOT (AST). **Other**: skin rashes.

NURSING IMPLICATIONS

- May be taken with milk or fruit juices and without regard to prior ingestion of food or time of day.
- Purging is not necessary before, during, or after therapy.
- Store at temperature below 30°C (86°F). Protect from light.
- *See mebendazole for patient-teaching points.*

Drug interactions   There is a possibility that pyrantel and **piperazine** are mutually antagonistic.

Pyrazinamide ─────────────────────────

(Zinamide)   *Antituberculosis agent*

ACTIONS AND USES   Pyrazinoic acid amide, analog of nicotinamide and bacteriostatic against *Mycobaterium tuberculosis*. When employed alone, resistance may develop in 6 to 7 weeks; therefore, administration with other effective agents is recommended. Appears to interfere with renal capacity to concentrate and excrete uric acid; thus may cause hyperuricaemia.

Used for short-term therapy of advanced tuberculosis before surgery and to treat patients unresponsive to primary agents (e.g., isoniazid, streptomycin).

ROUTE AND DOSAGE   Oral: 20 to 30 mg/kg/day in 3 or 4 divided doses; maximal dose 3 g/day.

ABSORPTION AND FATE   Readily absorbed from GI tract. Peak serum concentrations in about 2 hours, declining thereafter; **half-life**: 9 to 10 hours, prolonged in patient with impaired hepatic and renal function. Metabolized in liver. Slowly excreted in urine; 30% eliminated as metabolites and 4% as unchanged drug within 24 hours.

CONTRAINDICATIONS AND PRECAUTIONS   Severe hepatic damage. Safe use in children not established. **Cautious Use**: presence or family history of gout or diabetes mellitus, impaired renal function, history of peptic ulcer, acute intermittent porphyria.

PYRAZINAMIDE (continued)

ADVERSE/SIDE EFFECTS   Arthralgia, active gout, difficulty in urination, headache, photosensitivity, urticaria, skin rash (rare), sideroblastic or haemolytic anaemia, splenomegaly, lymphadenopathy, fatal haemoptysis, aggravation of peptic ulcer, rise in serum uric acid, hepatotoxicity, abnormal liver function tests, acute yellow atrophy of liver, decreased plasma prothrombin.

NURSING IMPLICATIONS

- The patient receiving pyrazinamide requires close observation and medical supervision. He or she should receive at least one other effective antituberculosis agent concurrently.
- Drug should be discontinued if hepatic reactions (jaundice, pruritis, icteric, sclerae, yellow skin), or hyperuricaemia with acute gout (severe pain in great toe and other joints) occur. (Normal serum uric acid: 178.5−416.4 mmol/L.)
- Patients should be examined at regular intervals and questioned about possible signs of toxicity: liver enlargement or tenderness, jaundice, fever, anorexia, malaise, impaired vascular integrity (ecchymoses, petechiae, abnormal bleeding).
- Hepatic reactions appear to occur more frequently in patients receiving high doses.
- Liver function tests (especially AST, ALT, serum bilirubin) should be done prior to and at 2- to 4-week intervals during therapy. Blood uric acid determinations are advised before, during, and following therapy.
- Report to physician the onset of difficulty in voiding. Patient should be urged to keep fluid intake at a 2,000 ml/day level, if possible.
- Aspirin in large doses (e.g., 3 to 5 g/day) or other uricosuric agents may prescribed to control hyperuricaemia.
- Patients with diabetes should be closely monitored for possible loss of control.
- Store tablets in well-closed container at temperature 15° to 39°C (59° to 56°F).

Diagnostic test interferences   Pyrazinamide may produce a temporary decrease in 17-ketosteroids and an increase in **protein-bound iodine**.

Pyridostigmine bromide

(Mestinon)

*Cholinergic
(parasympathomimetic);
cholinesterone inhibitor*

ACTIONS AND USES   Indirect-acting cholinergic with anticholinesterase activity. Synthetic quaternary ammonium compound similar to neostigmine (q.v.) in actions, contraindications, precautions, and adverse reactions. Has longer duration of action than does neostigmine, and reportedly produces less GI and other muscarinic side effects.

Used to improve muscle strength in symptomatic treatment of myasthenia gravis. Used parenterally to reverse the effects of neuromuscular blocking agents.

ROUTE AND DOSAGE   Oral (myasthenia gravis): Adults: dosage range 30 mg to

PYRIDOSTIGMINE BROMIDE (continued)

120 mg spaced according to requirements and response of patient. Total daily dose should not exceed 720 mg. **Neonate:** 5–10 mg/4 hrly. **Child (up to 6 yrs):** *initial:* 30 mg; **6–12 yrs:** 60 mg. Usual daily dose: 30–360 mg. **SC/IM: Adult:** 1–4 mg at intervals spread throughout the day (usual 10–40 mg). **Neonate:** 200–400 mcg 4 hrly by IM injection. **Child:** 1–12 mg/day.

ABSORPTION AND FATE   Poorly absorbed from GI tract; **onset of action** (improved muscle strength) in 20 to 30 minutes, with **duration** of 3 to 6 hours. Action begins within 15 minutes following IM and 2 to 5 minutes after IV injection. Metabolized in liver. Excreted in urine as metabolites and free drug up to 72 hours after a single IV dose. Reportedly metabolized and excreted more rapidly in patients with severe myasthenia. Crosses placenta.

CONTRAINDICATIONS AND PRECAUTIONS   Hypersensitivity to anticholinesterase agents or to bromides. Safe use in women of childbearing potential and use during pregnancy or lactation not established. **Cautious Use:** bronchial asthma, cardiac dysrhythmias. *See neostigmine.*

ADVERSE/SIDE EFFECTS   Acneiform (bromide) rash, thrombophlebitis (following IV administration). **With large doses:** *Muscarinic effects:* nausea, vomiting, diarrhoea, miosis, excessive salivation and sweating, increased bronchial secretion, bronchoconstriction, bradycardia, weakness, fasciculation and hypotension. *See also neostigmine.*

NURSING IMPLICATIONS

- Failure of patient to show improvement may reflect either underdosage or overdosage. Report increasing muscular weakness, cramps, or fasciculations. *See neostigmine for differentiation between myasthenic and cholinergic crises.*
- Neonates of myasthenic mothers who have received pyridostigmine should be closely observed for difficulty in breathing, swallowing, or sucking.
- When used as muscle relaxant antagonist, patient should be continuously observed. Airway and respiratory assistance must be maintained until full recovery of voluntary respiration and neuromuscular transmission is assured. Complete recovery usually occurs within 30 minutes.
- Report onset of rash. Drug discontinuation may be indicated.
- *See neostigmine.*

Drug interactions   Pyridostigmine antagonizes the effect of nondepolarizing muscle relaxants (e.g., tubocurarine, gallamine, pancuronium). Atropine antagonizes the muscarinic effects of pyridostigmine. *See also neostigmine.*

Pyridoxine hydrochloride ——————————————————

(Benadon, Comploment continus, Paxadon)   *Vitamin B6*

PYRIDOXINE HYDROCHLORIDE (continued)

ACTIONS AND USES   Water-soluble complex of three closely related compounds (pyridoxine and its active derivatives pyridoxamine and pyridoxal) with B_6 activity. Considered essential to human nutrition, although a deficiency syndrome is not well defined. Converted in body to pyridoxal, a coenzyme that functions in protein, fat, and carbohydrate metabolism and in facilitating release of glycogen from liver and muscle. In protein metabolism, participates in many enzymatic transformations of amino acids and conversion of tryptophan to niacin and serotonin. Aids in energy transformation in brain and nerve cells, and is thought to stimulate haeme production.

Used in prophylaxis and treatment of pyridoxine deficiency. Also used to treat peripheral neuritis caused by isoniazid and sideroblastic anaemia associated with high serum iron concentration.

ROUTE AND DOSAGE   Oral: *Neuritis and deficiency*: 20–50 mg three times a day. *Isoniazid neuropathy*: 50 mg three times a day, and *prophylaxis*: 10 mg/day. *Sideroblastic anaemia*: 100–400 mg/day in divided doses.

ABSORPTION AND FATE   Readily absorbed following oral and parenteral administration. **Half-life**: 15 to 20 days. Degraded in liver and excreted in urine primarily as 4-pyridoxic acid.

CONTRAINDICATIONS AND PRECAUTIONS   History of hypersensitivity to pyridoxine. Safe use of large doses in pregnancy, during lactation, and in children not established.

ADVERSE/SIDE EFFECTS   Rarely: paraesthesias, somnolence (particularly following large parenteral doses), slight flushing or feeling of warmth, low folic acid levels, temporary burning or stinging pain in injection site.

NURSING IMPLICATIONS

- Normal serum concentrations of vitamin B_6 are 30 to 80 ng/ml. Total body store is estimated to be 16 to 27 ng.
- Therapeutic effectiveness of vitamin B_6 therapy is evaluated by improvement of deficiency manifestations: nausea, vomiting, skin lesions resembling those of riboflavin and niacin deficiency (seborrhoea-like lesions about eyes, nose, and mouth, glossitis, stomatitis), oedema, CNS symptoms (depression, irritability, peripheral neuritis, convulsions), hypochromic microcytic anaemia.
- Collaborate with physician, dietitian, patient, and a responsible family member in planning for diet teaching. A complete dietary history should be recorded so that poor eating habits can be identified and corrected (a single vitamin deficiency is rare; patient can be expected to have multiple vitamin deficiencies).
- Rich dietary sources of vitamin B_6 include yeast, wheat germ, whole grain cereals, offal and meat (especially liver), legumes, green vegetables, bananas.
- Advise patient not to self-medicate with vitamin combinations (OTC) without first consulting physician.
- Preserved in tight, light-resistant containers at temperature 15° to 30°C (59° to 86°F). Avoid freezing.

P

PYRIDOXINE HYDROCHLORIDE (continued)

Drug interactions   Pyridoxine (in doses of 5 mg or more daily) appears to enhance the peripheral metabolism of **levodopa** and thus may greatly reduce or abolish its therapeutic effects; may decrease serum concentrations of phenobarbital and phenytoin. Pyridoxine requirements may be increased by INH, cycloserine, penicillamine, hydralazine, and oral contraceptives.

Pyrimethamine ——————————————

(Daraprim, Fansidar, Maloprim)   *Antimalarial; folic acid*
                                                       antagonist

ACTIONS AND USES   Long-acting folic acid antagonist chemically related to metabolite of chloroguanide. Selectively inhibits action of dehydrofolic reductate in parasite with resulting blockade of folic acid metabolism. Available in fixed combination with sulphadoxine (Fansidar), and dapsone (Maloprim).

Used for prophylaxis of malaria due to susceptible strains of plasmodia. May be used conjointly with fast-acting schizonticide (e.g., chloroquine, quinacrine, quinine) to initiate transmission control and suppressive cure.

ROUTE AND DOSAGE   Oral: depends on the preparation.

ABSORPTION AND FATE   Well-absorbed from GI tract; peak plasma concentrations in about 2 hours. Concentrates mainly in kidneys, lungs, liver, spleen. Slowly excreted in urine; excretion may extend over 30 days or longer. Appears in breast milk.

CONTRAINDICATIONS AND PRECAUTIONS   Chloroguanide-resistant malaria. Safe use during pregnancy not established. **Cautious Use**: patients with convulsive disorders receiving high doses of an anticonvulsant (e.g., phenytoin).

ADVERSE/SIDE EFFECTS   With large doses or prolonged therapy: anorexia, vomiting, atrophic glossitis, skin rashes, folic acid deficiency (megaloblastic anaemia, leucopenia, thrombocytopenia, pancytopenia, diarrhoea). Acute toxicity: CNS stimulation including convulsions, respiratory failure.

NURSING IMPLICATIONS
- GI distress may be minimized by taking drug with meals. If symptoms persist, dosage reduction may be necessary.
- For malaria prophylaxis, drug should be taken on same day each week. Administration should begin when individual enters malarious area and should continue for 10 weeks after leaving the area.
- Some physicians prescribe leucovorin concurrently for patients on high-dosage therapy to prevent the haematological complications of folic acid deficiency.

Drug interactions   Antitoxoplasmic effects of pyrimethamine may be decreased by **folic acid** and **para-aminobenzoic acid**. Pyrimethamine may increase quinine blood levels (displaces quinine from plasma blinding sites).

Quinidine

(Kiditard)   *Antiarrhythmic*

ACTIONS AND USES   Dextro isomer of quinine and alkaloid of *Cinchona*. Like quinine, exhibits some antimalarial, antipyretic, and oxytocic properties. Contains 83% anhydrous quinidine alkaloid. Cardiac actions similar to those of procainamide. At the cellular level, decreases sodium influx during depolarization and potassium efflux in repolarization; also reduces calcium transport across cell membrane. Depresses myocardial excitability, contractility, automaticity, and conduction velocity, and prolongs effective refractory period. Anticholinergic action blocks vagal stimulation of AV node, thus tending to increase ventricular rate, particularly in large doses. Also exerts muscle relaxant action by decreasing effective transmission across neuromuscular junction. Hypotensive effect is produced primarily by peripheral vasodilation and in part by alpha-adrenergic blockade.

Used in treatment of supraventricular tachycardia and ventricular arrhythmias.

ROUTE AND DOSAGE   Dosages individualized according to patient's requirements and responses. **Oral: Adults:** *Quinidine sulphate*: 200–400 mg three to four times a day. *Quinidine sulphate* 200 mg is equipotent to 250 mg quinidine bisulphate.

ABSORPTION AND FATE   Almost completely absorbed following oral administration. **Peak plasma level** within ½ to 1 hour; persisting 6 to 8 hours or more; (about 12 hours for extended-release form). Widely distributed in body tissues, except brain. At therapeutic serum levels (3 to 6 mcg/ml) about 60 to 80% strongly bound to plasma albumin. Unbound fraction is increased in hepatic insufficiency. Accumulation occurs in most tissues except brain. **Plasma half-life**: 4 to 10 hours (prolonged in congestive heart failure and in the elderly). Metabolized in liver. Approximately 10 to 30% excreted in urine within 24 hours as unchanged drug, and remainder as metabolites. Urinary pH influences excretion rate (alkalinization decreases and acidification increases excretion).

CONTRAINDICATIONS AND PRECAUTIONS   Hypersensitivity or idiosyncrasy to quinidine or *Cinchona* derivatives; safe use during pregnancy, during lactation, or in children not established. Thrombocytopenic purpura resulting from prior use of quinidine, intraventricular conduction defects, complete AV block, ectopic impulses and rhythms due to escape mechanisms, thyrotoxicosis, acute rheumatic fever, subacute bacterial endocarditis, extensive myocardial damage, frank congestive heart failure, hypotensive states, myasthenia gravis, digitalis intoxication. **Cautious Use**: incomplete heart block, impaired renal or hepatic function, bronchial asthma or other respiratory disorders, myasthenia gravis, potassium imbalance.

ADVERSE/SIDE EFFECTS   These include: headache, fever, tremors, apprehension, delirium, syncope with sudden loss of consciousness, and ventricular arrhythmias, disturbed hearing (tinnitus, auditory acuity), hypotension, congestive heart failure, widened QPS complex, bradycardia, heart block, atrial flutter, ventricular flutter, fibrillation or tachycardia; quinidine syncope, rash, urticaria, cutaneous flushing with

QUINIDINE (continued)

intense pruritus, photosensitivity, nausea, vomiting, diarrhoea, abdominal pain, hepatic dysfunction, acute haemolytic anaemia, hypoprothrombinaemia, leucopenia, blurred vision, disturbed colour perception, reduced visual field, photophobia, diplopia, night blindness, scotomata, optic neuritis. Cinchonism: nausea, vomiting, headache, dizziness, fever, tremors, vertigo, tinnitus, visual disturbances. **Overdosage**: hypokalaemia, cinchonism, tachyarrhythmias, seizures.

NURSING IMPLICATIONS

- Test dose (200 mg) is used to determine idiosyncrasy before establishing full dosage schedule.
- For optimum absorption, quinidine is taken preferably with a full glass of water on an empty stomach (i.e., 1 hour before or 2 hours after meals). If GI symptoms occur (nausea, vomiting, diarrhoea are most common), administer drug with food.
- Sustained-release tablet is usually reserved for maintenance and prophylactic therapy.
- Dosage is adjusted to maintain plasma concentration between 3 and 6 mcg/ml. Levels of 8 mcg/L or more are associated with myocardial toxicity.
- During acute treatment, monitor vital signs every 1 to 2 hours (frequency depends on individual patient requirements and dosage used). Count apical pulse for a full minute. Report any change in pulse rate, rhythm, or quality or any fall in blood pressure.
- Severe hypotension is most likely to occur in patients receiving high oral doses or parenteral quinidine.
- Reversion to sinus rhythm in long-standing fibrillation, or when complicated by congestive failure, involves some risk of embolization from dislodgement of atrial mural emboli.
- Quinidine can cause unpredictable rhythm abnormalities in the digitalized heart. Patients with atrial flutter or fibrillation may be pretreated with digitalis (until ventricular rate is 100 bpm) to increase AV nodal block and thus reduce possibility of paradoxic tachycardia.
- Monitor fluid intake and output. Diarrhoea occurs commonly during early therapy; most patients become tolerant to this side effect. If symptoms become severe, serum electrolytes and acid–base, and fluid balance should be evaluated. Dosage adjustment may be required.
- During long-term therapy, periodic blood counts, serum electrolyte determinations, and kidney and liver function tests are advised.
- **Food–drug interaction**   A diet high in alkaline ash foods (vegetables, citrus fruit, milk) renders urine alkaline may prolong half-life of quinidine by decreasing its excretion and increasing danger of toxicity. Advise patient to eat a balanced diet: i.e., no excesses in fruit or fruit juices, milk, or a vegetarian diet.
- Hypersensitivity reactions usually appear 3 to 20 days after drug is started. Fever occurs commonly and may or may not be accompanied by other symptoms.
- Instruct patient to report feeling of faintness ('quinidine syncope') caused by quinidine-induced changes in ventricular rhythm resulting in decreased cardiac output and syncope.
- Advise patient not to self-medicate with OTC drugs without advice from physician.

QUINIDINE (continued)

- Discuss medication schedule with patient. Advise patient not to increase, decrease, skip, or discontinue doses without consulting physician.
- Also advise patient to notify physician immediately of disturbances in vision, ringing in ears, sense of breathlessness, onset of palpitation, and unpleasant sensation in chest and to note time of occurrence and duration of chest symptoms.
- **Overdosage treatment**   Induce vomiting or give lavage; charcoal (even many hours after ingestion because of quinidine long half-life). Monitor CV status. Prepare for seizures (IV diazepam); sodium bicarbonate IV, adrenergic stimulants; haemodialysis or resin haemoperfusion.

Patient-teaching points should be included in the discharge plan (consult physician)
- ☐ Reason for taking drug.
- ☐ Specific dosage schedule.
- ☐ Use of calendar check-off sheet when dose is taken.
- ☐ Symptoms to report.
- ☐ Allowable planned physical activities.
- ☐ Importance of spaced rest periods.
- ☐ Diet and weight control.
- ☐ Things to avoid, e.g., fatigue, excessive caffeine (coffee, tea, cola), alcohol, smoking, heavy meals, (avoid excessive citrus juices) stressful situations, OTC medications (unless approved by physician).
- ☐ Advisability of wearing medical identification

- Preserve in tight, light-resistant containers away from excessive heat.

Diagnostic test interferences   Possibility of false increases in **urinary catechol-amines**. Quinidine may also interfere with **urinary steroid (17-OHCS)** determinations.

DRUG INTERACTIONS   *Quinidine sulphate*

PLUS	INTERACTIONS
Antiarrhythmics (other) Phenothiazines, reserpine	Additive cardiac depressant effects
Anticholinergic blocking agents	Additive vagolytic effect
Anticoagulants: coumarins	Decreased prothrombin levels and clotting factor concentrations possibly resulting in haemorrhage
Anticonvulsant (hydantoins): Phenobarbitone Rifampicin	Quinidine half-life shortened by up to 50%; dose adjustment of quinidine may be necessary when adding any one of these agents to quinidine regimen
Carbonic anhydrase inhibitors: Sodium bicarbonate Thiazide diuretics Antacids	Prolonged half-life of quinidine leading to decreased excretion and increased potential for toxicity
Cholinergics	Antagonized by quinidine
Digoxin	Increased digoxin levels leading to necessity to decrease dose of digoxin or use another antiarrhythmic

Q

QUINIDINE (continued)

PLUS (continued)	INTERACTIONS
Nifedipine	Decreased quinidine serum concentrations with breakthrough ventricular tachycardia
Skeletal muscle relaxants (e.g., tubocurarine, decamethonium, succinylcholine)	Potentiates neuromuscular blocking effects in ventilatory depression of patient receiving relaxants
Verapamil	Significant hypotensive effects

Quinine

Antimalarial

ACTIONS AND USES   Chief alkaloid from bark of cinchoma tree. Exact mechanism of antimalarial action uncertain. Inhibits protein synthesis, and depresses many enzyme systems in malaria parasite. Has schizonticidal action and is gametocidal with *Plasmodium vivax* and *P. malariae*, but not *P. falciparum*. Generally replaced by less toxic and more effective agents in treatment of malaria.

Used for treatment of chloroquine-resistant falciparum malaria and in combination with other antimalarials for radical cure of relapsing vivax malaria; also used for relief of nocturnal recumbency leg cramps.

ROUTE AND DOSAGE   Oral: **Adults:** 600 mg every 8 hours for 5 days. **Children:** up to one tenth of the adult dose, older children calculated: $\dfrac{age\ (yrs)}{20} \times$ adult dose for 5 days. **IV:** *severe chloroquine resistant infection:* 10 mg/kg by infusion over 4 hours. **Nocturnal cramps:** 200–300 mg at bedtime.

ABSORPTION AND FATE   Rapidly and completely absorbed from GI tract. **Peak plasma concentrations** in 1 to 3 hours. Oral dose of 1 g/day produces therapeutic plasma concentration of 7 mcg/ml. Approximately 70% bound to plasma proteins. **Plasma half-life:** 4 to 5 hours. Metabolized primarily in liver. Excreted in urine in about 24 hours, mostly as inactive metabolites; small amount eliminated in saliva, gastric juice, bile, and faeces. Renal excretion is decreased when urine is alkaline. Crosses placenta. Dialyzable by haemodialysis and by haemoperfusion.

CONTRAINDICATIONS AND PRECAUTIONS   Hypersensitivity or idiosyncrasy to quinine, patients with tinnitus, optic neuritis, myasthenia gravis, G6PD deficiency and pregnancy. **Cautious Use:** cardiac arrhythmias. Same precautions as for quinidine when used in patients with cardiovascular conditions.

ADVERSE/SIDE EFFECTS   **Cinchonism:** tinnitus, decreased auditory acuity, dizziness, vertigo, headache, visual impairment, nausea, vomiting, diarrhoea, fever. **Hypersensitivity:** visual impairment, pruritus, skin rash, fever, gastric distress, dyspnoea, tinnitus. **Toxicity:** decrease in blood pressure and respiration, tachycardia, hypo-

Q

QUININE (continued)

thermia, convulsions, cardiovascular collapse, coma, blackwater fever (extensive intravascular haemolysis with renal failure), death. **Other**: urticaria, acute asthma, confusion, excitement, apprehension, syncope, delirium, angina, leucopenia, thrombocytopenia, agranulocytosis, hypoprothrombinaemia, haemolytic anaemia.

NURSING IMPLICATIONS

- Administer drug with or after meals or a snack to minimize gastric irritation. Quinine has potent local irritant effect on gastric mucosa. Advise patients not to crush capsule; drug is not only irritating but also extremely bitter.
- Patients should be informed about possible adverse reactions and advised to report promptly the onset of any unusual symptom.
- Be alert to rising plasma concentration of quinine: tinnitus and hearing impairment usually do not occur until concentration is 10 mcg/ml or more.
- **Treatment of overdosage** Prompt emesis or gastric lavage is imperative because drug is rapidly absorbed; oxygen, support of respiration, and blood pressure.
- Preserved in tight, light-resistant containers.

Diagnostic test interferences Quinine may interfere with determinations of **urinary catecholamines**

Drug interactions Quinine absorption from GI tract may be delayed by **aluminium containing antacids**. Quinine enhances hypoprothrombinaemic action of **oral anticoagulants** and may decrease anticoagulant action of heparin. Excessive quinine blood levels may result from concomitant use of **pyrimethamine**, or **quinidine** or urinary alkalizers (decrease urinary excretion of quinine). Use of quinine with *skeletal muscle relaxants* may prolong respiratory depression and apnoea.

Ranitidine hydrochloride ─────────────────────

(Zantac)

Antihistamine;
H₂-receptor antagonist

ACTIONS AND USES A potent antiulcer drug that competitively and reversibly inhibits histamine action at H_2-receptor sites on parietal cells. Blocks daytime and nocturnal basal gastric acid secretion stimulated by histamine and reduces gastric acid release in response to food, pentogastrin, and insulin. Indirectly reduces pepsin secretion but appears to have minimal effect on fasting and postprandial serum gastrin concentrations, or secretion of gastric intrinsic factor or mucus. It is not known whether ranitidine alters ulcer recurrence rates; however, it appears that the clinical response it produces outlasts that of cimetidine (H_2-receptor inhibitor), permitting a twice daily regimen.

Used for short-term treatment of active duodenal ulcer; to treat pathological GI hypersecretory conditions (e.g., Zollinger–Ellison syndrome, systemic mastocytosis, and postoperative hypersecretion), and reflux oesophagitis.

R

RANITIDINE HYDROCHLORIDE (continued)

ROUTE AND DOSAGE   Oral: Adult: 150 mg twice a day or 300 mg at night. *Zollinger –Ellison syndrome*: 150 mg 3 times a day, increased to 6 g/day in divided doses if necessary. *Maintenance* 150 mg at night. **Child (8–18 yrs)**: up to 150 mg twice a day. **Intramuscular or slow IV injection**: 50 mg 6–8 hourly. **IV infusion**: 25 mg/hour for 2 hours repeated if necessary after 6–8 hours.

ABSORPTION AND FATE   Absorption rate following 150 mg oral dose is slow but constant, promoting maintenance of blood levels for up to 8 hours. Bioavailability is low (50%); peak levels of 440 to 545 ng/ml reached in 2 to 3 hours; **duration of action**: 8 to 12 hours. **Half-life**: 2 to 3 hours. Minimal penetration of CSF. Excreted in the urine with 30% dose collected in the urine as unchanged drug in 24 hours. Metabolites make up 6% of dose; remainder is found in the stool. Secreted in human milk; removed by haemodialysis.

CONTRAINDICATIONS AND PRECAUTIONS   Known hypersensitivity to ranitidine. Safe use during pregnancy, lactation, and in children under age 12 not established. **Cautious Use**: hepatic and renal dysfunction.

ADVERSE/SIDE EFFECTS   These include: tachycardia, bradycardia, PVCs, constipation, nausea, abdominal pain, diarrhoea; headache, malaise, dizziness, somnolence, insomnia, vertigo. Rare: mental confusion, agitation, depression, hallucinations in elderly patients; increased intraocular pressure (ocular pain, blurred vision). Others: gynaecomastia, impotence, rash, reversible decreases in WBC and platelet counts (clinically unimportant); hypersensitivity reactions, anaphylaxis (rare).

NURSING IMPLICATIONS
- It has been shown that to inhibit 50% of the stimulated gastric acid secretion, serum concentrations of ranitidine need to be 36 to 94 ng/ml. Concentrations in this range are maintained after a 150 mg dose for up to 12 hours.
- If patient is having haemodialysis treatments, the scheduled ranitidine dose should coincide with the end of haemodialysis.
- Long duration of action provides ulcer pain relief that is maintained through the night as well as the day.
- Adjunctive antacid treatment of pain may be necessary and can be given without affecting action of ranitidine. Administer the antacid 2 hours before or after ranitidine.
- Endoscopic examination is usually performed at end of 2 weeks of therapy because about 37% of patients have been completely healed in that time.
- Most patients have healed ulcers by 4 weeks; however, if healing cannot be confirmed endoscopically, treatment may be continued for up to 8 weeks.
- Even if symptomatic relief is provided by ranitidine, this should not be interpreted as absence of gastric malignancy. Follow-up examinations will be scheduled after therapy is discontinued.
- The potential for toxicity resulting from decreased clearance (elimination) and therefore prolonged action, is greatest in the elderly patient or the patient with hepatic or renal dysfunction.
- Creatinine clearance is monitored if renal dysfunction is present or suspected. When clearance is less than 50 ml/min, manufacturer recommends reduction of the dose

RANITIDINE HYDROCHLORIDE (continued)

to 150 mg once every 24 hours with cautious and gradual reduction of the interval to every 12 hours or less, if necessary.

- **Smoking–drug interaction** Smoking has been shown to decrease ranitidine efficacy and adversely affect ulcer healing, i.e., it has been associated with increased frequency of duodenal ulcers and decreased rate of ulcer healing. Smoking itself, rather than the number of cigarettes smoked per day, is the key factor. Urge patient to stop smoking, informing him or her that giving it up may be more important in preventing ulcer recurrence than the medication.
- **Food–drug interaction** Long-term ranitidine therapy may lead to vitamin B_{12} deficiency.
- Overdosage is treated by removing unabsorbed drug from GI tract (emesis, lavage), clinical monitoring, supportive treatment and haemodialysis if necessary.
- Store tablets in light-resistant, tightly capped container at controlled room temperature in a dry place.

Drug test interferences Ranitidine may produce slight elevations in **serum creatinine** (without concurrent increase in BUN); increases in **AST**, **ALT**, **phosphatase**, **LDH** and total **bilirubin**.

Drug interactions Propantheline delays absorption and increases peak concentration of ranitidine, thus increasing its bioavailability.

Razoxane

(Razoxin)

ACTIONS AND USES Antineoplastic with limited action in leukaemia. Little used.

Reproterol

(Bronchodil)

ACTIONS AND USES Bronchial dilator used in reversible airways obstruction. *See salbutamol.*

ROUTE AND DOSAGE **Oral: Adult:** 10–20 mg three times a day. **Child (6–12 yrs):** 10 mg three times a day. **Aerosol:** 0.5–1 mg (1–2 puffs) three times a day. **Child (6–12 yrs):** 500 mg (1 puff) three times a day. **Nebulizer:** 10–20 mg in 3 ml sterile saline over 10 minutes.

R

Reserpine/Rauwolfia alkaloids

(Decaserpyl, Hypercal, Serpasil)

Antihypertensive; rauwolfia alkaloid

ACTIONS AND USES   Derived from *Rauwolfia serpentina*. Used orally in treatment of mild essential hypertension and as adjunctive therapy with other antihypertensive agents in the more severe forms of hypertension.

ROUTE AND DOSAGE   Adults: Oral: depends on the preparation.

NURSING IMPLICATIONS
- Reserpine is administered with meals or with milk or other food to minimize possibility of gastric irritation (drug increases gastric secretions).
- Take blood pressure and pulse at intervals prescribed by physician. Both should be taken before each parenteral dose. Compared readings with baseline determinations and keep physician informed. (Note: drop in blood pressure may be accompanied by bradycardia.)
- Advise patient to take drug at the same time each day, not to skip or double doses, and not to stop therapy without advice of physician.
- Since drowsiness, sedation, and dizziness are possible side effects, caution patient to avoid driving and other potentially hazardous activities until reaction to drug has been determined.
- Counsel patient regarding possible side effects and importance of prompt reporting. Untoward effects are usually minimal with proper dosage and adequate supervision.
- Because rauwolfia alkaloids are cumulative and have a long duration of action, dosage adjustments when necessary are usually made at 7- to 14-day intervals.
- Full therapeutic effect of oral drug for hypertension may not occur until 2 to 3 weeks of therapy, and effects may persist for as long as 4 to 6 weeks after drug is discontinued. Special precautions should be observed when reserpine is prescribed for the elderly and the obese patient (half-life is reportedly prolonged in obese patients).
- Mental depression is a serious side effect and may be sufficiently severe to lead to suicide.
- Now rarely used.

Riboflavine

(Vitamin B$_2$)

Vitamin B$_2$

ACTIONS AND USES   Water-soluble vitamin and component of the flavoprotein enzymes that work together with a wide variety of proteins to catalyze many cellular respiratory reactions by which the body derives its energy.

RIBOFLAVINE (continued)

Used as supplement to other B vitamins in treatment of pellagra and beriberi.

ROUTE AND DOSAGE   Depends on the preparation.

Rifampicin ────────────────────────

(Rifadin, Rifater, Rifinah, Rimactazid)   *Antibiotic; antituberculosis agent*

ACTIONS AND USES   Semisynthetic derivative of rifamycin B, an antibiotic derived from *Streptococcus mediterranei*, with bacteriostatic and bactericidal actions. Inhibits DNA-dependent RNA polymerase activity in susceptible bacterial cells, thereby suppressing RNA synthesis. Active against *Mycobacterium tuberculosis, Neisseria meningitidis*, and a wide range of gram-negative and gram-positive organisms. Since resistant strains emerge rapidly when it is employed alone, it is used in conjunction with other antitubercular agents in treatment of tuberculosis.

Used primarily as adjuvant with other antituberculosis agents in initial treatment and retreatment of clinical tuberculosis, also alone or in combination with dapsone in treatment of leprosy.

ROUTE AND DOSAGE   **Oral: Adult:** 10 mg/kg/day before breakfast. Reduce dose to 8 mg/kg/day in hepatic impairment. **Child:** up to 20 mg/kg/day. Maxmium 600 mg/day.

ABSORPTION AND FATE   Well absorbed from GI tract. Peak plasma concentrations in 2 to 4 hours following 600-mg dose; still detectable for 24 hours. Widely distributed in body tissues and fluids, including CSF and saliva, with highest concentrations in liver, gall-bladder wall, and kidneys. About 80 to 90% protein bound. **Half-life:** about 3 hours (higher and more prolonged in hepatic dysfunction, and may be decreased in patients receiving isoniazid concomitantly). Rapidly deacetylated in liver to active and inactive metabolites; enters bile via enterohepatic circulation; 60 to 65% excreted in faeces. Up to 30% of dose is excreted in urine, about half as free drug. Rifampicin induces microsomal enzymes and thus may inactivate certain drugs. Crosses placenta; appears in breast milk.

CONTRAINDICATIONS AND PRECAUTIONS   Hypersensitivity to rifamycin derivatives; obstructive biliary disease, intermittent rifampin therapy. Safe use during pregnancy and in children under 5 years of age not established. **Cautious Use:** hepatic disease, history of alcoholism, concomitant use of other hepatotoxic agents.

ADVERSE/SIDE EFFECTS   These include: fatigue, drowsiness, headache, ataxia, confusion, dizziness, inability to concentrate, generalized numbness, pain in extremities, muscular weakness, visual disturbances, transient low-frequency hearing loss

RIFAMPICIN (continued)

(infrequent), conjunctivitis, heartburn, epigastric distress, nausea, vomiting, anorexia, flatulence, cramps, diarrhoea, pseudomembranous colitis, thrombocytopenia, transient leucopenia, anaemia, including haemolytic anaemia, haemoglobinuria, haematuria, acute renal failure, haemoptysis, light-chain proteinuria, flu-like syndrome, menstrual disorders, hepatorenal syndrome (with intermittent therapy), transient elevations in liver function tests (bilirubin, BSP, alkaline phosphatase, SGOT (AST), SGPT (ALT), pancreatitis (infrequent). **Overdosage**: GI symptoms, increasing lethargy, liver enlargement and tenderness, jaundice, brownish-red or orange discolouration of skin, sweat, saliva, tears, and faeces; unconsciousness.

NURSING IMPLICATIONS

- Capsule may be emptied and contents swallowed with fluid or mixed with food, if desired.
- Administered 1 hour before or 2 hours after a meal. Peak serum levels are delayed and may be slightly lower when given with food.
- A desiccant should be kept in bottle containing capsules; they become unstable with moisture.
- Caution patient not to interrupt prescribed dosage regimen. Hepatorenal reaction with flu-like syndrome has occurred when therapy has been resumed following interruption.
- Serology and sensitivity testing should be performed prior to and in the event of positive cultures.
- Inform patients that drug may impart a harmless red-orange colour to urine, faeces, sputum, sweat, and tears. Soft contact lenses may be permanently stained.
- Periodic hepatic function tests are advised. Patients with hepatic disease must be closely monitored.
- Instruct patients to report onset of jaundice (yellow skin, sclerae, and posterior portion of hard palate; pruritus), hypersensitivity reactions, and persistence of GI adverse effects.
- Patients taking oral contraceptives should consider alternative methods of contraception (see Drug Interactions). Concomitant use of rifampicin leads to decreased effectiveness of the contraceptive and to menstrual disturbances (spotting, breakthrough bleeding).
- If patient is also receiving an anticoagulant, prothrombin times should be performed daily or as necessary to establish and maintain required anticoagulant activity.
- Caution patient to keep drug out of reach of children.
- **Treatment of overdosage** Gastric lavage in absence of vomiting, followed by activated charcoal slurry; antiemetic to control severe nausea and vomiting. Forced diuresis, with measurement of fluid intake and output ratio, to promote drug excretion. Haemodialysis may be required.

Diagnostic test interferences Rifampicin interferes with contrast media used for **gall bladder study**, therefore test should precede daily dose of rifampicin. May also cause retention of **BSP**. Inhibits standard assays for **serum folate** and **vitamin B$_{12}$**. Possible interference with **contrast media** used for gall bladder study; may also caused retention of **BSP**.

RIFAMPICIN (continued)
DRUG INTERACTIONS   *Rifampicin*

PLUS	INTERACTIONS
Alcohol	Increased risk of hepatotoxicity
Aminosalicylic acid	Decreased serum concentration of rifampicin
Barbiturates, benzodiazepines, clofibrate, corticosteroids, dapsone, digitoxin, methadone, metoprolol; oral anticoagulants, antidiabetic agents and contraceptives; progestogens, propranolol, quinidine	Decreased plasma concentrations of these drugs leading to potential of treatment failure and necessity to adjust dosage
Isoniazid	May result in hepatotoxicity

Rimiterol

(Pulmadil)

ACTIONS AND USES   Bronchial dilator used in reversible airways obstruction.

ROUTE AND DOSAGE   Adult and child: Aerosol: 200–600 mcg (1–3 puffs) repeated after 30 min (Maximum 8 doses per day). *See salbutamol.*

Ritodrine hydrochloride

(Yutopar)   *Adrenergic agonist (sympathominetic), uterine relaxant*

ACTIONS AND USES   Beta$_2$-adrenergic agonist clinically effective in preventing or delaying of preterm labour. Preferentially stimulates beta$_2$-receptors in uterine smooth muscle resulting in reduced intensity and frequency of uterine contractions and lengthening gestation period.

Used to manage premature labour in selected patients.

ROUTE AND DOSAGE   Intravenous: 50 to 100 mcg/minute administered by means of a calibrated constant-rate infusion pump. Dose gradually increased by 50 mcg/minute every 10 minutes until adequate uterine relaxation is achieved. Effective dose range: 150 to 350 mcg/minute. May be continued for 12 hours after uterine contractions cease. **Oral (started 30 minutes prior to termination of infusion):** 10 mg every 2 hours for first 24 hours; thereafter, 10 to 20 mg every 4 to 6 hours up to but not exceeding 120 mg daily. **IM:** 10 mg/3–8 hourly continued for 12–48 hours after contractions have ceased.

R

RITODRINE HYDROCHLORIDE (continued)

ABSORPTION AND FATE   Following oral administration, 30% of drug absorbed; maximum serum levels of 5 to 15 ng/ml reached within 30 to 60 minutes. Serum levels of 32 to 52 ng/ml reached after IV infusion at rate of 0.15 mg/minute for 1 hour. 32% protein-bound. **Half-life** (triphasic): initial: 6.9 minutes, second phase: 1.7 to 2.6 hours, third phase: more than 10 hours. Metabolized in liver. 90% excretion completed in 24 hours. Crosses placenta.

CONTRAINDICATIONS AND PRECAUTIONS   Mild to moderate preeclampsia or eclampsia, intrauterine infection, cervix dilated 4 or more centimeters (in a singleton pregnancy); hypertension, diabetes mellitus; use prior to twentieth week or after 36 weeks of pregnancy or if continuation of pregnancy would be hazardous to mother and foetus (e.g., antepartum haemorrhage, eclampsia, intrauterine foetal death, maternal cardiac disease, pulmonary hypertension, maternal hyperthyroidism, severe diabetes mellitus). Also hypovolaemia, cardiac arrhythmias associated with tachycardia or digitalis intoxication, uncontrolled hypertension, thyrotoxicosis, bronchial asthma being treated with betamimetics and/or steroids. **Cautious Use:** concomitant use of potassium depleting diuretics, cardiac disease.

ADVERSE/SIDE EFFECTS   More pronounced and frequent following IV infusion: altered maternal and foetal heart rates and maternal blood pressure (dose-related); temporary hyperglycaemia, palpitations, arrhythmias, tremor, nausea, vomiting, headache, erythema; nervousness, restlessness, anxiety, malaise, chest pain, pulmonary oedema. Infrequent: anaphylactic shock, rash, epigastric distress, ileus, bloating, constipation, diarrhoea, dyspnoea, hyperventilation, glycosuria, haemolytic icterus, sweating, chills, drowsiness, weakness, myotomic muscular dystrophy.

NURSING IMPLICATIONS
- Hospitalization is advised during treatment with ritodrine.
- Preparation of IV solution: 150 mg ritodrine is added to 500 ml 5% dextrose or normal saline solution giving a final concentration of 0.3 mg/ml.
- IV solution should be clear and should not be administered if cloudy or if a precipitate is present.
- Place patient in left lateral recumbent position throughout the infusion period to reduce risk of hypotension.
- Monitor IV infusion flow rate to prevent circulation overload.
- Pronounced dose-related side effects in cardiovascular system require continuous monitoring of maternal and foetal heart rates and maternal blood pressure while infusion is running.
- Occult cardiac disease has been unmasked by use of ritodrine.
- Uterine contractions will decrease in frequency and intensity during treatment.
- If patient is also on steroid therapy, hospitalization for treatment with ritodrine is advised.
- Be alert to signs and symptoms of pulmonary oedema *(see Index)*.
- Store drug at controlled room temperature preferably below 30°C (80°F). Do not freeze.

RITODRINE HYDROCHLORIDE (continued)

Diagnostic test interferences   Ritodrine (intravenous route) may produce an increase in serum levels of **glucose, insulin** and **free fatty acids**, and a decrease in **serum potassium.** It temporarily elevates results of **glucose tolerance test.**

DRUG INTERACTIONS   *Ritodrine hydrochloride*

PLUS	INTERACTIONS
Anaesthetics, general	Potentiated hypotensive effects of general anaesthetic
Corticosteroids	Pulmonary oedemia in mother; action is antagonized by beta-adrenergic blocking agents, e.g., propranolol, and is potentiated by other sympathomimetics

Salbutamol

(Salbolin, Ventolin)

Beta-adrenergic agonist;
bronchodilator

ACTIONS AND USES   Moderately selective beta-2-adrenergic agonist with comparatively long action. Has more prominent effect on beta-2-receptors (particularly bronchial, uterine, and vascular smooth muscle, and mast cells) than on beta-1-(heart) and alpha-adrenergic receptors. Produces bronchodilation, regardless of administration route, by relaxing smooth muscles of bronchial tree. This decreases airway resistance, facilitates mucus drainage, and increases vital capacity. As effective as isoprenaline and orciprenaline, but produces more prolonged bronchodilation and causes little direct cardiac stimulation. Reportedly improved cardiac output due to lowered left ventricular afterload.

Used to relieve bronchospasm in patients with reversible obstructive airway disease (e.g., asthma).

ROUTE AND DOSAGE   **Adults: Inhalation:** two metered inhalations or 200−400 mcg rotacaps 3−4 times a day. **Child:** 100 mcg. **Inhalation of nebulized solution:** 2.5 mg (2.5 ml of a solution containing 1 mg/ml) repeated up to 4 times a day. Administer with air *only* (unless physician has prescribed oxygen) at 8 litres and no lower than 6 litres, per minute. **Oral: Adults:** 2−8 mg, 3−4 times a day. **Child (2−6 yrs):** 1−2 mg, 3−4 times a day; **(6−12 yrs):** 2 mg, 3−4 times a day; **(over 12 yrs):** 2−4 mg, 3−4 times a day. **Subcutaneous or intramuscular:** 0.5 mg every 4 hrs as required. **Intravenous injections:** 250 mcg. **Intravenous infusion:** 3−20 mcg/min.

ABSORPTION AND FATE   *Inhalation:* Gradually absorbed from bronchi; (small swallowed portions absorbed from GI tract). **Onset of bronchodilation** in 5 to 15 minutes with physiological effects related to topical action rather than to blood levels. **Peak**

SALBUTAMOL (continued)

effect in ½ to 2 hours; duration: 3 to 6 hours; half-life: 3.8 hours. About 65 to 90% of dose excreted in urine within 24 hours, as unchanged drug (28%) and metabolite (44%). *Oral tablet*: Onset of bronchodilation within 30 minutes. Peak plasma levels in 2½ hours. Peak effect in 2 to 3 hours; duration: 4 to 6 or more hours; half-life: 2.7 to 5 hours; metabolized in liver. Approximately 76% of dose excreted in urine over 3 days (most is eliminated in first 24 hours). Apparently does not cross blood–brain barrier, but may cross placenta. Distribution to breast milk not known.

CONTRAINDICATIONS AND PRECAUTIONS   Safe use during pregnancy and in breast feeding not established. **Cautious Use**: cardiovascular disease, hypertension, hyperthyroidism, diabetes mellitus, hypersensitivity to sympathomimetic amines or to fluorocarbon propellant used in inhalation aerosols.

ADVERSE/SIDE EFFECTS   These include: tremor (most commonly with oral drug), dizziness, vertigo, stimulation, nervousness, restlessness, irritability, insomina, weakness, headache, hallucinations, paranoia, palpitation, increased or decreased blood pressure; reflex tachycardia, angina (with high doses), nausea, vomiting, heartburn, paradoxical bronchospasm, difficulty in voiding, unusual taste; hyperaemia, drying and irritation of oropharynx; muscle cramps, aggravation of preexisting diabetes mellitus and ketoacidosis; inhibition of uterine contractions; hypokalaemia (theoretically possible).

NURSING IMPLICATIONS

- Patient should receive explicit directions on use of medication and inhaler and follow them precisely. Review patient instruction sheet dispensed with medication. Caution patient to avoid contact of drug with eyes.
- Summary of instructions for using metered dose inhalers:
    - Shake container well before using.
    - Place mouthpiece well into mouth and close lips firmly around it.
    - Exhale.
    - Take slow deep breath through mouth while actuating the inhaler.
    - After holding breath as long as possible, remove mouthpiece and exhale slowly.
    - Remove drug canister from inhaler assembly following treatment.
    - Wash inhaler assembly with warm running water at least daily. Dry thoroughly.
- If patient is also receiving beclomethasone, inhalation treatments with salbutamol should be administered 20 to 30 minutes before, to allow deeper penetration of beclomethasone into lungs, unless otherwise directed by physician.
- Significant subjective improvement in pulmonary function should occur within 60 to 90 minutes after drug administration.
- All patients with asthma should have a thorough initial history and physical examination to help identify factors that provoke attacks.
- Baseline and periodic evaluation of pulmonary function should be done to monitor patient's progress.
- The most common adverse effect associated with the oral drug is fine tremor in fingers, which may interfere with precision handwork (believed to be caused by direct

SALBUTAMOL (continued)

stimulation of skeletal muscles). Keep physician informed of any unusual symptoms.
- Drug-induced dry mouth and throat may be relieved by rinsing mouth well with water immediately after each inhalation treatment.
- If paradoxical bronchospasm (wheezing) occurs discontinue drug immediately, and notify physician.
- Emphasize dangers of using self-prescribed OTC drugs without physician's approval. Many remedies (e.g., cold medicines) contain sympathomimetics that may intensify salbutamol action.
- The ideal approach in asthma management is to prevent relapses, to maintain good pulmonary function, and to provide prompt therapy when an emergency situation arises.
- Advise patient to maintain optimal health in order to prevent an overlay of stress on respiratory tract: e.g., avoid crowds and individuals with known respiratory infections; adhere to immunization schedules for influenza and pneumonia.

Patient-teaching plan for chronic obstructive airways disease Constructed in collaboration with physician, respiratory therapist, patient and responsible family member(s) should include the following guidelines and advice:
- ☐ Review of drug action and expected effects.
- ☐ Importance of precise compliance with drug regimen.
- ☐ Avoid environmental irritants (e.g., dust, smoke, animal dander, sprays, feathers).
- ☐ Maintain optimum environmental humidification, especially in winter.
- ☐ Avoid temperature extremes.
- ☐ Planned rest and physical reconditioning programme: balanced diet.
- ☐ Prevent respiratory tract infections.
- ☐ No smoking.
- ☐ Keep follow-up appointments.
- ☐ Carry medical identification.

- Salbutamol tablets should be stored between 2° and 30°C (36° and 86°F) in tight, light-resistant container, unless otherwise directed by manufacturer.
- Store canisters between 15° and 30°C (59° and 86°F) away from heat and direct sunlight. Since contents of inhalers are under pressure, do not puncture and never throw container into incinerator or fire for disposal.

Diagnostic test interferences Transient small increases in **plasma glucose** may occur.

DRUG INTERACTIONS *Salbutamol*

PLUS	INTERACTIONS
Adrenaline and other adrenergic aerosol bronchodilators	Possibility of additive effects. Concurrent use not recommended
MAO inhibitors, tricyclic antidepressants	Potentiate salbutamol action on vascular system
Propranolol and other beta-adrenergic blocking agents	Mutual inhibitory effect

Salcatonin

For further informaton: *see calctonin*.

Salsalate

(Disalcid)   NSAID; salicylate

ACTIONS AND USES   Action similar to those of other salicylates. *See aspirin.* Clinical studies suggest that salsalate does not produce significant gastric irritation, and it has not been associated with reactions causing asthmatic attacks in susceptible individuals. The incidence of side effects in general appears to be lower than that of other salicylates. Unlike aspirin it does not appear to inhibit platelet aggregation.

Used for symptomatic treatment rheumatoid arthritis, osteoarthritis, and related rheumatic disorders.

ROUTE AND DOSAGE   Oral: 1.5–4 g daily in divided doses adjusted to the individual.

ABSORPTION AND FATE   Insoluble in gastric acid. Completely absorbed from small intestine and partially hydrolyzed in liver; almost totally excreted in urine. **Half-life:** about 1 hour.

CONTRAINDICATIONS AND PRECAUTIONS   Hypersensitivity to salicylates, chronic renal insufficiency, peptic ulcer, pregnancy, children under 12 years. *See also aspirin.*

ADVERSE/SIDE EFFECTS   Occasionally, nausea, dyspepsia, heartburn. **Overdosage:** (salicylism) tinnitus, hearing loss (reversible), vertigo, flushing, headache, confusion, drowsiness, hyperventilation, sweating, vomiting, diarrhoea. *See also aspirin.*

NURSING IMPLICATIONS
- Administer with a full glass of water or with food or milk to reduce GI side effects.
- Symptom relief is gradual (may require 3 to 4 days to establish steady-state salicylate level).
- Warn patient not to take another salicylate (e.g., aspirin) while on salicylate therapy.
- *See aspirin.*

Scopolamine

For further information: *see hyocine*.

Selegiline

(Eldepryl)

ACTIONS AND USES Selective MAOI used with levodopa to treat Parkinson's disease.

ROUTE AND DOSAGE 5 mg in the morning increased to 10 mg as required.

NURSING IMPLICATIONS
- The dietary restrictions applied to MAOI's do not apply to selegiline.

Senna

(Agiolax, Senokot, X-Prep)   *Laxative (stimulant);*
                                                           anthraquinone

ACTIONS AND USES Anthraquinone derivative prepared from dried leaflet of *Cassia acutifolia* or *Cassia angustifolia*. Similar to cascara sagrada, but with more potent action. Senna glycosides are converted in colon to active aglycones, which stimulate Auerbach's plexus to induce peristalsis.

Used for relief of acute constipation and for preoperative and preradiographic bowel evacuation.

ROUTE AND DOSAGE Oral: Depends on the preparation.

ABSORPTION AND FATE Cathartic action usually occurs in 6 to 10 hours; may not act before 24 hours in some patients; metabolized in liver; excreted in faeces (some may be eliminated in urine).

CONTRAINDICATIONS AND PRECAUTIONS Irritable colon, nausea, vomiting, abdominal pain, intestinal obstruction, nursing mothers.

ADVERSE/SIDE EFFECTS Abdominal cramps, flatulence, nausea. *Prolonged use*: watery diarrhoea, excessive loss of water and electrolytes, weight loss, melanotic segmentation of colonic mucosa (reversible).

NURSING IMPLICATIONS
- Generally administered at bedtime for relief of constipation.
- When given for preoperative or prediagnostic bowel preparation, usually prescribed to be taken between 1400 hrs and 1600 hrs on day prior to procedure. Diet is then confined to clear liquids.
- Some patients may experience considerable griping; if medication is to be repeated, dose reduction may be indicated.
- Inform patient that drug may impart yellowish brown colour (in acid urine) or reddish brown colour (in alkaline urine). Faeces may be similarly coloured.

S

SENNA (continued)

- Caution patient that continued use may lead to dependence. If constipation persists, consult physician.
- Avoid exposure of drug to excessive heat; fluid extracts should be protected from light.
- *See bisacodyl for patient-teaching points.*

Sodium aurothiomalate

(Myocrisin)

Gold compound;
antiinflammatory

ACTIONS AND USES   Slow-acting preparation of approximately 50% gold. Available commercially as a suspension in anhydrous vegetable oils to delay absorption and prolong action. Major effect is suppression of joint inflammation in early arthritic disease; has no effect on separative process, but may significantly slow or arrest progression of the disease. Mechanism of antiinflammatory action not clearly understood. Gold uptake by macrophages with subsequent inhibition of phagocytosis and lysosomal enzyme activity may be a principle mechanism. Other proposed mechanisms include altered immune response and inhibition of prostaglandin synthesis.

Used in treatment of adult and juvenile rheumatoid arthritis.

ROUTE AND DOSAGE   Intramuscular (only): **Adults**: Usual dose 50 mg weekly to a total of 1 g. Dose reduced if a reaction occurs. **Child**: *Stills disease*: weekly doses according to body weight: under 20 kg–10 mg; 20–50 kg 20 mg; 50 kg or more 30 mg.

ABSORPTION AND FATE   Slowly and irregularly absorbed from IM injection site. Widely distributed in body, especially to synovial fluid, eyes, skin, bone marrow, reticuloendothelial system (liver, spleen), kidneys. Does not cross blood–brain barrier. **Peak blood levels** in 2 to 6 hours. About 95% bound to plasma proteins. **Half-life:** 3 to 27 days for 50 mg dose (varies with dose and duration of therapy). Metabolism unknown. Eliminated slowly; 85% of each dose is retained for at least 1 week. Almost 60 to 90% of dose ultimately excreted in urine and 10 to 40% in faeces. (May be found in urine for more than 1 year following a course of therapy.) Crosses placenta; appears in breast milk.

CONTRAINDICATIONS AND PRECAUTIONS   Gold allergy or severe toxicity from previous therapy with gold or other heavy metals; severely debilitated patients, uncontrolled diabetes mellitus; renal or hepatic insufficiency, history of infectious hepatitis; congestive heart failure, tuberculosis, abnormalities of haematopoietic system, severe anaemia, haemorrhagic conditions; disseminated lupus erythematosus, recent radiation therapy, colitis, urticaria, eczema, history of exfoliative dermatitis. Safe use during pregnancy, in nursing women, and in children under 6 years not established. **Cautious Use**: elderly patients, history of drug allergies, history of blood dyscrasias,

S

SODIUM AUROTHIOMALATE (continued)

history of renal or hepatic disease, marked hypertension, compromised cerebral or cardiovascular circulation.

ADVERSE/SIDE EFFECTS   These include: pruritus, erythema, 'gold dermatitis,' fixed-drug eruptions, exfoliative dermatitis with alopecia and shedding of nails; Stevens-Johnson syndrome, grey to blue pigmentation (chrysiasis), photosensitivity, nausea, vomiting, abdominal cramps, anorexia, diarrhoea, ulcerative enterocolitis, agranulocytosis, thrombocytopenia with or without purpura, leucopenia, eosinophilia, panmyelopathy, haemorrhagic diathesis, aplastic and hypoplastic anaemia, nephrotic syndrome with proteinuria, haematuria, dyspnoea, gold bronchitis, interstitial pneumonitis, pulmonary fibrosis, peripheral neuritis, headache, hepatitis, cholestatic jaundice, acute yellow atrophy of liver, EEG abnormalities, encephalitis, immunological destruction of synovial fluid; arthralgia, myalgia (rare), fever. **Mucous membranes**: ulcerative stomatitis, glossitis or gingivitis (may be preceded by metallic taste), pharyngitis, tracheitis, gastritis, colitis, vaginitis.

NURSING IMPLICATIONS

- Before initiation of treatment, patient should be well-informed regarding dangers associated with gold therapy and requirements for compliance in receiving scheduled doses, for keeping laboratory appointments, and for prompt reporting of adverse effects. Minor or moderate transient toxicity occurs in 25 to 50% of patients, and serious toxicity in about 10% of patients.
- Hold vial horizontally and shake thoroughly to assure uniform suspension. Heating vial to body temperature (by placing in a warm water bath) facilitates withdrawal. Aurothioglucose must not be injected intravenously. Needle and syringe must be dry.
- Administer drug deep into upper outer quadrant of gluteal muscle. An 18- or 20-gauge, 1½-inch needle is recommended (for obese patients a 2-inch needle may be preferable). During early therapy some patients complain of arthralgia for 1 or 2 days postinjection.
- Patient should remain recumbent for 10 minutes after injection to overcome possible nitritoid reaction (manufacturer's recommendation although reaction occurs infrequently). Observe patient for about 30 minutes after injection for anaphylactic shock, bradycardia oedema of tongue, face, eyelids, difficulty in breathing or swallowing.
- Clinical observation and interview remain the most effective means for regulating dosage, and for predicting therapeutic effectiveness and gold toxicity. Provide patient with a list of possible adverse reactions that should be reported. If therapy is interrupted at the onset of gold toxicity, serious reactions can be avoided. Note that elderly patients are particularly sensitive to the effects of gold therapy.
- Reactions are most likely to occur during second and third months of therapy, but they may appear at any time during therapy and for several weeks after treatment has been discontinued.
- Instruct patient to report any unusual colour or odour to urine, or change in fluid intake and output ratio and pattern.
- Advise patient to report early signs of infection that may indicate onset of agranulocytosis (unusual fatigue or weakness, malaise, chills, fever, sore throat), and

SODIUM AUROTHIOMALATE (continued)

unusual bleeding (possible signs of thrombocytopenia): bleeding gums, nosebleeds, dark urine (haematuria), petechiae, easy bruising. Thrombocytopenia can occur abruptly or gradually and it can appear several months after gold therapy has been terminated.

- Be alert to vulnerability of patient to secondary infection because of the possible immunosuppressive effect of gold. Caution patient to avoid contact with persons who have colds or other communicable diseases.
- Therapeutic effectiveness may not be apparent before 6 to 8 weeks of gold therapy. There is little agreement regarding how long to continue therapy following a remission. Some rheumatologists prefer to continue patient indefinitely on gold treatment; others discontinue drug after a year of therapy.
- Inform patient that the necessity to increase the amount of aspirin for analgesia is a significant indication of diminishing response to gold therapy, and therefore should be reported to physician.
- **Treatment of toxicity**   Antihistamines and systemic corticosteroids, e.g., prednisone, may be prescribed for rash and mucous membrane ulcerations. Grey-blue pigmentation (chrysiasis) of mucous membranes and light-exposed skin areas may be treated with Lugol's solution (strong iodine solution); advise patient to avoid sunlight. Severe toxic reactions are treated with dimercaprol, a chelating agent.
- Gold therapy is contraindicated following a severe reaction, but may be attempted at reduced initial dosage schedule and careful monitoring after a mild reaction.
- **Symptomatic treatment of stomatitis**   Use a soft tooth brush (may be softened with hot water) or finger covered with moistened cotton or moistened gauze (rub gently), to clean teeth after meals; floss gently with waxed dental floss once daily. Rinse mouth frequently with warm water, tea, or saline (if allowed). Some clinicians prefer occasional use of hydrogen peroxide (H_2O_2) diluted with normal saline or water 1:1 to 1:4; prepare solution immediately before use. Have patient rinse mouth with clear water or normal saline after using H_2O_2 and avoid overuse (can cause gum sponginess and decalcification of tooth surfaces). Other agents that might provide relief of discomfort include solutions of Mylanta or milk of magnesia. Avoid overuse of commercial mouth washes especially those that are bactericidal. Many contain alcohol which enhances drying and irritation and can change mouth flora. Advise patient to avoid concentrated fruit juices, hard or dry foods, smoking, and alcohol.
- Stored in light-resistant containers at room temperature, preferably between 15° and 30°C (59° and 86°F) unless otherwise directed by manufacturer. Protect from freezing and light.

Diagnostic test interferences   Low **PBI** (by chloric acid method); test interference may persist for several weeks after gold therapy is discontinued.

DRUG INTERACTIONS   *Aurothiomalate*

PLUS	INTERACTIONS
Antimalarials Cytotoxic agents Immunosuppressants Oxyphenbutazone Phenylbutazone	Possibility of increased risk of blood dyscrasias. Concurrent use generally avoided

Sodium bicarbonate

Antacid used alone or in combination for dyspepsia and in electrolyte replacement therapy.

Metabolic acidosis: By slow IV injection (up to 8.4% solution) or by infusion (1.26% solution) dose depends on requirements.

S

Sodium cromoglycate

(Intal)   *Antiasthmatic; mast cell stabilizer*

ACTIONS AND USES   Synthetic asthma-prophylactic agent with unique action. Inhibits release of bronchoconstrictors—histamine and slow-reacting substance of anaphylaxis—from sensitized pulmonary mast cells, thereby suppressing an allergic response. Has no direct bronchodilator, antihistaminic, or antiinflammatory properties. Particularly effective for IgE-mediated or 'extrinsic asthma' (precipitated by exposure to specific allergen, e.g., pollen, dust, animal dander). Has also benefited many patients with nonatopic or 'intrinsic asthma' which is triggered by nonallergic factors such as infections, irritants, emotions. Patient response is reportedly unpredictable. Believed to act by interfering with calcium transport across mast cell membrane and by promoting phosphorylation of mast cell protein.

Used prophylactically as adjunct in management of severe perennial bronchial asthma, and allergic ocular disorders. Of no value in acute asthmatic attack, especially status asthmaticus. Does not obviate the need for usual therapy with bronchodilators, expectorants, antibiotics or corticosteroids, but the amount and frequency of use of these agents may be appreciably reduced.

ROUTE AND DOSAGE   Oral Inhalation: depends on the preparation.

ABSORPTION AND FATE   Peak plasma concentrations within 15 minutes, following inhalation. Duration of action: 4 to 6 hours but carryover effect (unexplainable) may be as long as 2 to 3 weeks. About 8% of dose reaches lungs and is readily absorbed into systemic circulation. The rest is deposited in mouth and back of throat and is then swallowed, and excreted unchanged in bile (faeces) and urine in approximately equal amounts. **Elimination half-life:** 80 minutes. Small amounts exhaled.

CONTRAINDICATIONS AND PRECAUTIONS   Hypersensitivity to sodium cromoglycate or lactose; acute asthma, status asthmaticus, dyspnoea; patients unable to coordinate actions or follow instructions. Safe use during pregnancy and in nursing women not established. **Cautious Use:** renal or hepatic dysfunction, long-term use.

ADVERSE/SIDE EFFECTS   Generally well tolerated. Side effects include: headache, dizziness, vertigo, peripheral neuritis, irritation of throat, trachea; cough, hoarseness; nasal congestion, bronchospasm, wheezing, laryngeal oedema (rare), swelling of parotid glands, dry mouth, slightly bitter after taste, nausea, vomiting oesophagitis, dysuria,

S

SODIUM CROMOGLYCATE (continued)

urinary frequency, nephrosis, itchy, puffy eyes, lacrimation, transient burning, stinging, tamponade, fever, haemoptysis, anaemia. Related to the delivery system: inhalation of gelatin particles, mouthpiece, or propellant.

NURSING IMPLICATIONS

- Pulmonary function test recommended prior to initiation of therapy. (Candidate for therapy must have a significant bronchodilator-reversible component to the airway obstruction.)
- Patient should receive detailed instructions for loading the turbo-inhaler and administering preparation (see manufacturer's instructions) and must demonstrate correct use of apparatus. Therapeutic effect is largely dependent on proper scheduling of treatments and use of inhaler.
- Advise patient to clear as much mucus as possible before inhalation treatments.
- Instruct patient to exhale as completely as possible before placing inhaler mouthpiece between lips, tilt head backwards and inhale rapidly and deeply with steady, even breaths. Remove inhaler from mouth, hold breath for a few seconds then exhale into the air. Repeat until entire dose is taken.
- Caution patient not to exhale into inhaler, because moisture from breath will interfere with its proper operation. Also inform patient that capsule is intended for inhalation only and is ineffective if swallowed because it is not absorbed from GI tract.
- Throat irritation, cough, and hoarseness, possible adverse effects from inhaling sodium cromoglycate can be minimized by gargling with water, drinking a few swallows of water or by sucking on a lozenge after each treatment oesophageal irritation manifested as substernal burning sensation may be prevented by prophylactic administration of an antacid (consult physician) or a glass of milk before each treatment.
- Patient should be provided with specific instructions regarding what to do in the event of an acute asthmatic attack.
- Advise patient to report any unusual signs or symptoms. Hypersensitivity reactions can be severe and life-threatening. Eosinophil count is a reliable indicator of developing allergy and therefore should be monitored. Drug should be discontinued if an allergic reaction occurs.
- Instruct patient to pay careful attention to general health and to protect against colds and flu.
- Prior treatment 15 minutes before doing protracted exercise (e.g. jogging) reportedly blunts the effects of vigorous exercise as well as cold air.
- Therapeutic effects may be noted within a few days but generally not until after 2 to 4 weeks of therapy: reduced number of asthmatic attacks; decreased cough, sputum, wheezing, and breathlessness; increased exercise tolerance; decreased requirement for concomitant drug (e.g., bronchodilators, corticosteroids) therapy. Keep physician informed.
- Patient should be advised not to wear soft contact lenses during ocular therapy. They may be worn within a few hours after therapy is terminated.
- Protect from moisture and heat. Store at temperature in well-closed, light-resistant

SODIUM CROMOGLYCATE (continued)

container preferably between 15° and 30°C (59° and 86°F) unless otherwise directed by manufacturer.

Sodium fusidate

(Fucidin) *Antimicrobial*

ACTIONS AND USES   Sodium fusidate is the sodium salt of fusidic acid, a substance produced by *Fusidium coccineum* with antimicrobial properties. It has a steroid structure and is chemically related to cephalosporin P. It is highly effective against gram-positive bacteria and gram-negative cocci including *Staphylococcus aureus* strains resistant to penicillin and other similar antimicrobials. These actions are due to interference with bacterial protein synthesis. *In vitro* sodium fusidate enhances the action of benzyl penicillin against resistant strains of penicillinase producing staphylococci. This may be due to the delay in inactivation of penicillin rather than a true synergistic action. True synergism with novobiocin and erythromycin causes bacteriostasis.

Used to treat infections caused by penicillin resistant staphylococci including osteomyelitis, wound infections, septicaemia, endocarditis and soft tissue infections.

ROUTE AND DOSAGE   Oral: **Adult**: 500 mg/8 hourly; **Child (under one year)**: 50 mg/kg/day in divided doses, (1–5 yrs): 250 mg three times a day. **Intravenous**: **Adult**: 500 mg over 6 hours/3 times a day; **Child**: 20 mg/kg/day in divided doses. Ointment or medicated gauze is applied to infected wounds up to four times a day.

ABSORPTION AND FATE   Well absorbed by the gastrointestinal tract, 500 mg producing plasma concentrations of 30 mcg/ml after 2 to 4 hours. In plasma, sodium fusidate is 95% protein bound, it is widely distributed in the tissues but does not penetrate into the cerebrospinal fluid. Excretion is mainly in the bile, 2% is excreted unchanged in the faeces, little is excreted in breast milk or urine.

CONTRAINDICATIONS AND PRECAUTIONS   Cautious use: abnormal liver function. Tests should also be performed when high doses are given.

ADVERSE/SIDE EFFECTS   Mild gastrointestinal upsets, rashes, jaundice and changes in liver function which resolve when treatment is terminated.

NURSING IMPLICATIONS
- Sodium fusidate should never be given by intramuscular or subcutaneous routes. Caution should be taken to prevent extravasation when the drug is given intravenously: severe tissue reaction may occur.
- Reconstitute powder for intravenous use with diluent provided.
- Protect suspension from direct light.
- Discard any unused prepared drug after 24 hours.
- Check infecting organism for sensitivity.

S

SODIUM FUSIDATE (continued)
- Sodium fusidate has few side effects other than those on the liver, patients on high doses or with known liver impairment should have regular function checks.
- Store at room temperature.

Sodium nitroprusside

(Nipride)

*Antihypertensive; vasodilator
(peripheral)*

ACTIONS AND USES   Potent, rapid-acting hypotensive agent with effects similar to those of nitrates. Acts directly on vascular smooth muscle to produce peripheral vasodilation, with consequent marked lowering of arterial blood pressure, associated with slight increase in heart rate, mild decrease in cardiac output, and moderate lowering of peripheral vascular resistance. Thiocyanate metabolite may inhibit uptake and binding of iodine, with prolonged therapy.

Used for short-term, rapid reduction of blood pressure in hypertensive crises and for producing controlled hypotension during anaesthesia to reduce bleeding.

ROUTE AND DOSAGE   **Intravenous infusion (only)**: Initial dose 0.1–1 mcg/kg/min average dose 3 mcg/kg/minute.

ABSORPTION AND FATE   Onset of hypotensive effect usually occurs within 2 minutes; effect lasts 1 to 10 minutes after infusion is terminated. Rapidly converted to cyanogen (cyanides) in erythrocytes and tissue, which is metabolized to thiocyanate in liver. Excreted in urine, primarily as thiocyanate metabolite.

CONTRAINDICATIONS AND PRECAUTIONS   Use in treatment of compensatory hypertension, as in atriovenous shunt or coarctation of aorta, or for producing controlled hypotension in patients with inadequate cerebral circulation. Safe use during pregnancy and in women of childbearing potential and children not established. **Cautious Use**: hepatic insufficiency, hypothyroidism, severe renal impairment, hyponatraemia, elderly patients with low vitamin B_{12} plasma levels or with Leber's optic atrophy.

ADVERSE/SIDE EFFECTS   Usually associated with too rapid reduction in blood pressure: nausea, retching, abdominal pain, nasal stuffiness, diaphoresis, headache, dizziness, apprehension, restlessness, muscle twitching, retrosternal discomfort, palpitation, increase or transient lowering of pulse rate, irritation at infusion site, hypothyroidism with prolonged therapy (rare), increase in serum creatinine, fall or rise in total plasma cobalamins. **Overdosage (thiocyanate toxicity)**: profound hypotension, tinnitus, blurred vision, fatigue, metabolic acidosis, pink skin colour, absence of reflexes, faint heart sounds, loss of consciousness.

NURSING IMPLICATIONS
- Solutions must be freshly prepared and used no later than 4 hours after reconstitution.

SODIUM NITROPRUSSIDE (continued)

- Following reconsitution, solutions usually have faint brownish tint; if highly coloured do not use. Promptly wrap container with aluminum foil or other opaque material to protect drug from light.
- Administered by infusion pump, micro-drip regulator, or similar device that will allow precise measurement of flow rate.
- Constant monitoring is required to titrate IV infusion rate to blood pressure response. If concomitant oral hypertensive therapy is given, IV infusion rate will require further adjustment.
- Adverse effects (*see Adverse/Side Effects*) are usually relieved by slowing IV rate or by stopping drug; they may be minimized by keeping patient supine.
- Monitor fluid intake and output.
- Monitoring blood thiocyanate level is recommended in patients receiving prolonged treatment or in patients with severe renal dysfunction (levels usually are not allowed to exceed 10 mg/dl). Determination of plasma cyanogen level following 1 or 2 days of therapy is advised in patients with impaired hepatic function (*see Absorption and Fate*).
- No other drug should be added to sodium nitroprusside infusion.
- Protect drug from light, heat, and moisture; store preferably at 15° to 30°C (59° to 86°F) unless otherwise directed by manufacturer.

S

Sodium salicylate ━━━━━━━━━━━━━━━━━━━━━━━

NSAID; salicylate

ACTIONS AND USES   Properties similar to those of aspirin (q.v.), but less effective. *See aspirin.*

ROUTE AND DOSAGE   Oral: Adult: 0.5–2 g.

Sodium valproate ━━━━━━━━━━━━━━━━━━━━━━━

(Epilim)   *Anticonvulsant*

ACTIONS AND USES   Antiepileptic agent unrelated chemically to other drugs used to treat seizure disorders. Mechanism of action unknown; may be related to increased bioavailability of the inhibitory neurotransmitter gamma-aminobutyric acid (GABA) to brain neurones. Inhibits secondary phase of platelet aggregation.

Used alone or with other anticonvulsants in management of epilepsy.

ROUTE AND DOSAGE   Oral: Adults: *initial*: 600 mg/day. Increase at 3 day intervals by 200 mg/day until seizures are controlled or side effects preclude more increases.

SODIUM VALPROATE (continued)

Maximum recommended dose: 2.5 g/day. Divide doses (2 or more times daily). **Child (up to 20 kg):** *initial* 20 mg/kg/day maximum 40 mg/kg/day; **(over 20 kg):** *initial* 400 mg/day in divided doses increased to 30 mg/kg/day according to need.

ABSORPTION AND FATE   Absorbed rapidly and almost completely from GI tract. **Peak plasma levels** (wide interindividual variation) are usually reached in 1 to 4 hours following single oral dose. **Half-life:** 8 to 16 hours; may be increased in patient with cirrhosis or acute hepatitis. Protein binding: 85 to 95%. Widely distributed; may enter enterohepatic circulation. Metabolized in liver; excreted primarily as glucuronic conjugates in urine. Small amount excreted in faeces and expired air. Crosses placenta, enters breast milk.

CONTRAINDICATIONS AND PRECAUTIONS   Hypersensitivity to valproic acid; patient with bleeding disorders, hepatic dysfunction or disease. **Cautious Use:** women who are or may become pregnant, nursing mothers, history of renal disease, adjunctive treatment with other anticonvulsants, angina pectoris, active recovery period following myocardial infarction.

ADVERSE/SIDE EFFECTS   These include: breakthrough seizures, sedation, drowsiness, dizziness, decreased alertness, ataxia, headache, nystagmus, diplopia, 'spots before eyes,' tremors, asterixis, dysarthria, muscle weakness, incoordination, paraesthesias, nausea, vomiting, indigestion (transient), hypersalivation, anorexia with weight loss, increased appetite with weight gain, abdominal cramps, diarrhoea, constipation, acute pancreatitis, hepatic failure, prolonged bleeding time, leucopenia, lymphocytosis, thrombocytopenia, hypofibrinogenaemia, bone marrow depression, anaemia, depression, hallucinations, hyperactivity, behavioural deterioration in children, aggression, emotional upset, enuresis, skin rash, transient hair loss, curliness or waviness of hair, irregular menses, secondary amenorrhoea; hyperammonaemia (usually asymptomatic); tremor. **Overdosage:** deep coma, pulmonary oedema, death.

NURSING IMPLICATIONS

- Patient should avoid using a carbonated drink as diluent for the syrup because it will release drug from delivery vehicle. Free drug painfully irritates oral and pharyngeal membranes.
- Serious GI side effects can lead to discontinuation of therapy with valproic acid. To reduce gastric irritation administer drug with food. Enteric-coated tablet or syrup formulation are usually well tolerated.
- Effective therapeutic serum levels of valproic acid: 50 to 100 mcg/ml.
- Inform the diabetic patient that this drug may cause a false-positive test for urine ketones.
- Warn patient to avoid alcohol and self-medicating with other depressants during therapy. The use of all OTC drugs should be approved by the physician during anticonvulsant therapy. Particularly unsafe are combination drugs containing aspirin, sedatives, medications for hay fever or other allergies.
- If spontaneous bleeding and/or bruising (petechiae, ecchymotic areas, otorrhagia, epistaxis, melaena), occur, notify physician promptly.

SODIUM VALPROATE (continued)

- Monitor alertness in patient on multiple drug therapy for seizure control. Plasma levels of the adjunctive anticonvulsants should be evaluated periodically as indicators for possible neurological toxicity.
- Patients on multiple drug therapy are at risk from hyperammonaemia (lethargy, anorexia, asterixis, increased seizure frequency, vomiting. These symptoms should be reported promptly.
- Advise patient not to drive a car or engage in other activities requiring mental alertness and physical coordination until reaction to drug is known.
- The syrup is red and tasty. Keep out of the reach of children.
- Advise patient to carry medical identification card or jewellery bearing information about medication in use and the epilepsy diagnosis.
- Instruct patient to withhold dose and report to the physician if the following symptoms appear: visual disturbances, rash, jaundice, light-coloured stools, protracted vomiting, diarrhoea. Fatal hepatic failure has occurred in patients receiving this drug.
- Increased dosage increases frequency of adverse effects. Monitor patient carefully when dose adjustments are being made and report promptly if side effects persist.
- Before any kind of surgery (including dental surgery), the patient should inform the doctor or dentist of taking this drug.
- Inform patient that abrupt discontinuation of therapy can lead to loss of seizure control. Warn patient not to stop or alter dosage regimen without consulting physician. He or she should also refrain from giving any of the drug to another person.

Diagnostic test interferences Sodium valproate produces false-positive results for urine ketones, elevated SGOT (AST), SGPT (ALT), LDH, and serum alkaline phosphatase, prolonged bleeding time, altered thyroid function tests.

DRUG INTERACTIONS *Sodium valporate*

PLUS	INTERACTIONS
Alcohol	Potentiated depressant effects of alcohol
Anticonvulsants	Increased anticonvulsant action
Antidepressants, tricyclic	Potentiated CNS depressant effects
Aspirin	Potentiated platelet aggregation (increases possibility of spontaneous bleeding)
Barbiturates	Increased serum levels of barbiturates; severe CNS depression
Clonazepam	Absence seizures may occur
CNS depressants	Increased depressant action
Dipyridamole	*See aspirin*
MAO inhibitor	Potentiated CNS depressant effects
Phenytoin	May increase or decrease phenytoin plasma levels; breakthrough seizures may occur. Adjust phenytoin dosage accordingly

SODIUM VALPROATE (continued)

PLUS	INTERACTIONS
(continued)	
Primidone	*See barbiturates*
Salicylates	Increased valproic acid serum level; increased toxicity
Sulphinpyrazone	*See aspirin*
Warfarin	*See aspirin*

Sotalol ━━━━━━━━━━━━━━━━━━━━━━━━━━━━━━━━━━━━━━━

(Beta Cardone, Sotacor)   *Antihypertensive; beta-adrenergic blocking drug*

ACTIONS AND USES   Beta-adrenergic blocking drug with similar action and uses to propranolol (q.v.).

ROUTE AND DOSAGE   Oral: Adult; *hypertension and angina*: 160 mg as a single or divided dose. Maximum 600 mg/day. *Arrhythmias and thyrotoxicosis*: 120–240 mg/day as a single or divided dose. *Prophylaxis after myocardial infarction*: 320 mg/day commencing 5–14 days post infarction. **IV**: slow injection 20–60 mg over 2–3 min repeated as required at 10 min intervals up to 100 mg in total.

NURSING IMPLICATIONS
- Monitor ECG during IV injection.
- *See propranolol.*

Spectinomycin ━━━━━━━━━━━━━━━━━━━━━━━━━━━━━━━━━

(Trobicin)   *Antibiotic; aminoglycoside*

ACTIONS AND USES   Aminocyclitol antibiotic produced by *Streptomyces spectabilis*. Antibacterial action results from selective binding of 30S subunits of bacterial ribosomes, thereby inhibiting protein synthesis. Variable activity against a wide variety of gram-negative and gram-positive organisms. Inhibits majority of *Neisseria gonorrhoeae* strains. Not effective against syphilis.

   Used only for treatment of uncomplicated gonorrhoea, particularly in patients sensitized or resistant to penicillin or other effective drugs.

ROUTE AND DOSAGE   **Intramuscular**: (2 g for men and 4 g for women). Reconstitute with accompanying diluent.

SPECTINOMYCIN (continued)

ABSORPTION AND FATE   Rapidly absorbed after IM injection. Plasma concentration peaks in 1 to 2 hours; appreciable levels persist 8 hours or more. **Half-life:** 1 to 3 hours; minimal binding to plasma proteins. Active form excreted in urine within 48 hours after injection.

CONTRAINDICATIONS AND PRECAUTIONS   Hypersensitivity to spectinomycin. Safe use during pregnancy and in infants and children not established. **Cautious Use:** history of allergies.

ADVERSE/SIDE EFFECTS   Soreness at injection site, urticaria, dizziness, nausea, chills, fever, insomnia. Following multiple doses: decrease in haemoglobin, haematocrit, or creatinine clearance; elevated alkaline phosphatase, SGPT (ALT), BUN; decrease in urine output.

NURSING IMPLICATIONS

- Shake vial vigorously immediately after adding diluent and before withdrawing drug. Following reconsitution, solution should be used within 24 hours.
- Administer IM injection deep to upper outer quadrant of buttock. No more than 5 ml should be injected into single site (20-gauge needle is recommended). Injection may be painful.
- Observe patient for 45 to 60 minutes after injection. Systemic anaphylaxis has been reported (apprehension, pruritus, hypertension, abdominal pain, collapse).
- All patients with gonorrhoea should have serological tests for syphilis at time of diagnosis and again after 3 months.
- Clinical effectiveness of drug should be monitored to detect antibiotic resistance.

Spironolactone ▬▬▬▬▬▬▬▬▬▬▬▬▬▬▬▬▬▬▬▬▬▬

(Aldactone, Diatensec, Laractone, Spiretic, Spiroctan, Spirolone)

Diuretic (potassium-sparing); aldosterone antagonist

ACTIONS AND USES   Steroidal compound and specific pharmacological antagonist of aldosterone. Presumably acts by competing with aldosterone for cellular receptor sites in distal renal tubule. Promotes sodium and chloride (and water) excretion without concomitant loss of potassium. Diuretic effect reportedly not associated with hyperuricaemia or hyperglycaemia. Activity depends on presence of endogenous or exogenous aldosterone. Lowers systolic and diastolic pressures in hypertensive patients by unknown mechanism. Potentially mutagenic and tumourigenic.

Used in clinical conditions associated with augmented aldosterone production, as in essential hypertension, refractory oedema due to congestive heart failure, hepatic cirrhosis, nephrotic syndrome, and idiopathic oedema. May be used to potentiate actions of other diuretics and antihypertensive agents or for its potassium-sparing effect.

SPIRONOLACTONE (continued)
ROUTE AND DOSAGE   Oral: 100–200 mg/day increased to 400 mg as required. Child: 3 mg/kg/day in divided doses.

ABSORPTION AND FATE   Rapidly and extensively metabolized. Peak plasma levels of active metabolite (canrenone) within 2 to 4 hours. **Half-life** following multiple doses: between 13 and 24 hours. (90% protein bound.) Maximal diuretic effect attained in about 3 days; activity persists 2 or 3 days after discontinuation of drug. Metabolites excreted slowly, primarily in urine, and also in bile. Crosses placental barrier.

CONTRAINDICATIONS AND PRECAUTIONS   Anuria, acute renal insufficiency, progressing impairment of renal function, hyperkalaemia. Safe use in women of childbearing potential, during pregnancy and lactation not established. **Cautious Use:** BUN of 14 mmol/L or greater, hepatic disease.

ADVERSE/SIDE EFFECTS   These include: lethargy, mental confusion, fatigue (with rapid weight loss), headache, drowsiness, ataxia, maculopapular or erythematous rash, urticaria, gynaecomastia (both sexes), inability to achieve or maintain erection, androgenic effects (hirsutism, irregular menses, deepening of voice); parathyroid changes, decreased glucose tolerance, abdominal cramps, nausea, vomiting, anorexia, diarrhoea, fluid and electrolyte imbalance (particularly hyperkalaemia and hyponatraemia); evelated BUN, mild acidosis, drug fever, agranulocytosis, SLE, hypertension (postsympathectomy patient), hyperuricaemia, gout.

NURSING IMPLICATIONS
- Administer with food to enhance absorption.
- Tablet may be crushed before administration and taken with fluid of patient's choice.
- Serum electrolytes should be monitored, especially during early therapy.
- *Food–drug interaction*   Potassium supplementation is not indicated in spironolactone therapy (unless patient is also receiving another diuretic and a corticosteroid). Patient is generally instructed to avoid excessive intake of high-potassium foods and salt substitutes (*see Index: Food sources*). If hyperkalaemia develops, patient is usually placed on restricted dietary intake of potassium. Consult physician regarding allowable potassium and sodium intake.
- Inform patient that maximal diuretic effect may not occur until third day of therapy and that diuresis may continue for 2 or 3 days after drug is withdrawn.
- Monitor daily fluid intake and output and check for oedema. Report lack of diuretic response or development of oedema; both may indicate tolerance to drug action.
- Weigh patient under standard conditions before therapy begins and throughout therapy. Weight is a useful index of need for dosage adjustment. For patients with ascites, physician may want measurements of abdominal girth.
- Check blood pressure before initiation of therapy and at regular intervals throughout therapy.
- Be alert for signs of fluid and electrolyte imbalance, and instruct patient to report dry mouth, thirst, abdominal cramps, lethargy, and drowsiness (symptoms of hyponatraemia, most likely to occur in patients with severe cirrhosis), as well as paraesthesias, confusion, weakness, or heaviness of legs (symptoms of hyperkalaemia).

SPIRONOLACTONE (continued)

- Observe for and report immediately the onset of mental changes, lethargy, or stupor in patients with hepatic disease.
- Adverse reactions are generally reversible with discontinuation of drug. Gynaecomastia appears to be related to dosage level and duration of therapy; it may persist in some patients even after drug is stopped.
- Presumptive diagnosis of primary aldosteronism is made if short test produces serum potassium increase during spironolactone administration followed by decrease when it is discontinued or if long test results in correction of hypertension and hypokalaemia with spironolactone.
- Preserved in tight, light-resistant containers. Suspension formulation is stable for 1 month under refrigeration.

Diagnostic test interferences   Spironolactone may produce marked increases in **plasma cortisol determinations** by Mattingly fluorometric method; these may persist for several days after termination of drug (spironolactone metabolite produces fluorescence). There is the possibility of false elevations in measurements of **digoxin serum levels** by radioimmunoassay procedures.

Drug interactions   Combinations of spironolactone and acidifying doses of **ammonium chloride** may produce systemic acidosis; use these combinations with caution. Diuretic effect of spironolactone may be antagonized by **aspirin** and other **salicylates** (possibly by competing for same receptor sites). Spironolactone potentiates the actions of other **antihypertensives**, particularly **ganglionic blocking agents** (dosage of these drugs should be reduced by at least 50% when spironolactone is added), and other **diuretics**. Patients receiving spironolactone and **digitoxin** or similar **cardiac glycosides** concurrently should be monitored for decreased effect of cardiac glycoside (spironolactone shortens its half-life, possibly by acting as enzyme inducing agent). Hyperkalaemia may result with **potassium supplements** (spironolactone conserves potassium).

Stanozolol

(Stromba)   *Anabolic*

ACTIONS AND USES   Synthetic steroid with relatively strong anabolic and weak androgenic activity.

Used primarily to increase protein synthesis for example after surgery or in hereditary angioedema.

ROUTE AND DOSAGE   Oral: Adults: *Anabolic effect*: 5 mg/day. *Hereditary angioedema*: 2.5–10 mg/day. **IM**: 50 mg every 2–3 weeks.

NURSING IMPLICATIONS
- Give IM dose deep in the gluteal muscle.
- Administer just before or with meals to reduce incidence of gastric distress.

STANOZOLOL (continued)

- Smaller dose for young women is given to prevent virilizing effects of the drug. If such effects appear (early sign: change of voice), physician should be notified.
- Patient may need to have a restricted salt intake. Check with the physician.
- Used with high caloric, high protein diet unless contraindicated.
- Be alert to symptoms of hypercalcaemia. (*See Index: Clinical sign, symptoms.*)
- Stanozolol does not enhance athletic ability.
- *See oethylestrenol.*

Stilboestrol

Oestrogen; antineoplastic

ACTIONS AND USES Reportedly the most potent nonsteroidal syntheticoestrogen compound. Has strong teratogenic potential; may cause vaginal or cervical cancer in offspring if mother is treated with stilboestrol during pregnancy. Interferes with implantation of fertilized ovum in uterus by unclear mechanism; does not terminate pregnancy. Suppresses lactation. Excessive or prolonged use may inhibit anterior pituitary secretions. Long-term therapy with 5 mg/daily for prostatic carcinoma reportedly associated with increased risk of cardiovascular deaths.

Used in treatment of advanced metastatic carcinoma of the breast in men and post-menopausal women, and inoperable carcinoma of prostate.

ROUTE AND DOSAGE Oral: *cancer palliation* (breast) 10–20 mg daily; (prostate): 1 to 3 mg daiily.

ABSORPTION AND FATE *See oestradiol.*

CONTRAINDICATIONS AND PRECAUTIONS Birth control, except emergency post-coital contraception; malignancies or precarcinomatous lesions (vagina, vulva, or breasts), pregnancy, blood clotting disorders, hepatic dysfunction, undiagnosed vaginal bleeding, long-term use during menopause. **Cautious Use:** hypertension, migraine, diabetes mellitus, asthma. *See also oestradiol.*

NURSING IMPLICATIONS
- Reassure the male patient that drug-induced loss of libido and development of feminine characteristics will disappear with termination of therapy.
- Urge patient to maintain established regimen, i.e., the dose should not be increased, decreased, or omitted, without physician's advice.
- Review package insert with patient to assure complete understanding about stilboestrol therapy.
- Store tablets at temperature between 15° and 30°C (59° and 86°F) in a well-closed container, and suppositories between 8° and 30°C (46° and 86°F) in a tight container, unless otherwise directed by manufacturer.
- *See oestradiol.*

Streptokinase

(Kabikinase, Streptase)   *Thrombolytic; enzyme*

ACTIONS AND USES   Derivative of the purified filtrates of beta-haemolytic strepto-cocci. Promotes thrombolysis by activating the conversion of plasminogen to plasmin, the enzyme that degrades fibrin, fibrinogen, and other procoagulant proteins into soluble fragments. This fibrinolytic activity is effective both outside and within the formed thrombus/embolus. Decreases blood and plasma viscosity and erythrocyte aggre-gation tendency thus increasing perfusion of collateral blood vessels. Bacterial source bestows strong antigenic properties: support of antibody formation and high potential for allergic reactions. Use has been associated with altered platelet function. Strep-tokinase activity is expressed in international units (IU): one IU equals amount of drug required to activate enough blood plasminogen to lyse a standard fibrin clot within 10 minutes under standard conditions.

Used for treatment of acute extensive deep venous thrombosis, acute arterial throm-bosis or embolism, acute pulmonary embolus, coronary artery thrombosis, and arterio-venous cannula occlusion.

ROUTE AND DOSAGE   **Intravenous: infusion:** 250,000–600,000 units over 30–60 min, then 100,000 units hourly for up to 48–72 hours. **Intracoronary:** *initial:* 10,000 to 20,000 IU followed by 2,000 to 4,000 IU/minute until lysis occurs, then 2,000 IU/minute for 1 hour.

ABSORPTION AND FATE   Plasminogen activation begins promptly with infusion or instillation; streptokinase is rapidly removed from circulation by antibodies and reticu-loendothelial system. Biphasic half-life: initial, 18 minutes (due to antibody action); then 83 minutes. Does not cross placenta but its antibodies do. Anticoagulation effect may persist 12 to 24 hours after infusion is discontinued.

CONTRAINDICATIONS AND PRECAUTIONS   Active internal bleeding, very recent cardiopulmonary resuscitation; recent (within 2 months) intraspinal, intracranial, intra-arterial procedures; intracranial neoplasm; CVA, severe uncontrolled hypertension; history of allergic response, recent streptococcal infection, obstetrical delivery; diabetic haemorrhagic retinopathy, ulcerative colitis, diverticulitis; any condition in which bleeding presents a hazard or would be difficult to manage because of location; pregnancy, safe use during lactation or in children, not established. **Cautious Use:** patient with preexisting haemostatic deficits, conditions accompanied by risk of cerebral embolism, septic thrombophlebitis, uraemia, hepatic failure.

ADVERSE/SIDE EFFECTS   **Allergic:** major (12%) (bronchospasm, periorbital swel-ling, angioneurotic oedema, anaphylaxis); mild (urticaria, itching, headache, musculo-skeletal pain, flushing, nausea, pyrexia). **Haematological:** phlebitis, bleeding or oozing at sites of percutaneous trauma; prolonged systemic hypocoagulability; spontaneous bleeding, unstable blood pressure; reperfusion atrial or ventricular dysrhythmias, acute CVA or MI (causal relationship not established).

STREPTOKINASE (continued)
NURSING IMPLICATIONS

- Prolonged infusion time may seriously deplete plasminogen pool leading to reduced fibrinolytic capacity of the blood (reduced drug response).
- Effectiveness of intracoronary instillation to prevent extension of myocardial infarct decreases rapidly after 5 to 6 hours.
- Before treatment is started, heparin is discontinued and baseline control levels are established for thrombin time, activated partial thromboplastin time, prothrombin time Hct, and platelet count.
- The patient is frequently premedicated with a corticosteroid that can be repeated during the treatment to minimize pyrogenic or allergic reaction.
- Heparin is contraindicated during IV infusion of streptokinase, but may be continued during intracoronary administration. After intracoronary use, heparin therapy is continued (or instituted). Eventually an oral anticoagulant is substituted for heparin.
- Streptokinase is reconstituted with 5 ml water for injection. Roll or tilt vial; avoid shaking to prevent foaming or increase in flocculation. Reconstituted solution may be carefully diluted again, avoiding shaking or agitation of the solution. Slight flocculation does not interfere with drug action; discard solution with large amount of flocculant.
- Spontaneous bleeding occurs about twice as often with streptokinase as with heparin. Protect patient from invasive procedures: IM injections are contraindicated. Also prevent undue manipulation during thrombolytic therapy to prevent bruising.
- Support thrombosed extremity for proper alignment and reduce unnecessary movement to prevent infusion site bleeding.
- Report signs of potential serious bleeding; gum bleeding, epistaxis, haematoma, spontaneous ecchymoses, oozing at catheter site, increased pulse, pain from internal bleeding, infusion should be interrupted, then resumed when bleeding stops.
- Observe infusion site frequently. If phlebitis occurs, it can usually be controlled by diluting the infusion solution.
- Monitor for excessive bleeding every 15 minutes for the first hour of therapy, every 30 minutes for second to eighth hour, then every 8 hours.
- Complete bed rest is usual during entire treatment.
- Check patient's temperature during treatment. A slight elevation, $0.8°C$ ($1.5°F$), perhaps with chills, occurs in about one-third of the patients. An elevation to $40°C$ ($104°F$) or more requires symptomatic treatment.
- If an analgesic/antipyretic is indicated, avoid giving aspirin because of its antiplatelet action; instead acetaminophen or corticosteroids may be prescribed.
- Monitor blood pressure. Mild changes can be expected, but report substantial changes (greater than $\pm$ 25 mm Hg). Therapy may be discontinued.
- Report promptly symptoms of a major allergic reaction; therapy will be discontinued and emergency treatment instituted. Minor symptoms (e.g., itching, nausea) respond to concurrent antihistamine and/or corticosteroid treatment without interruption of streptokinase administration.
- Check pulse frequently. Be alert to changes in cardiac rhythm, especially during intracoronary instillation. Dysrhythmias signal need to stop therapy at once.
- Have readily available for treatment of serious bleeding: typed and cross-matched

STREPTOKINASE (continued)

fresh whole blood, packed RBCs, cryoprecipitate or fresh frozen plasma (dextran should not be used); tranexamic acid (antidote).

- Patient is at risk for postthrombolytic bleeding for 2 to 4 days after intracoronary streptokinase treatment. Continue monitoring vital signs until laboratory tests confirm anticoagulant control.
- Reconstituted solution should be stored at 2° to 4°C (36° to 39°F). Discard after 24 hours.
- Store unopened vials at 15° to 30°C (59° to 86°F).

Diagnostic test interferences   Streptokinase promotes increases in TT, APTT, and PT.

DRUG INTERACTIONS   *Streptokinase*

PLUS	INTERACTIONS
Tranexamic acid	Inhibition of streptokinase-induced activation of plasminogen
Anticoagulants (including oral anticoagulants) Antiplatelet agents (e.g., indomethacin, phenylbutazone, salicylates)	Increased risk of haemorrhage

Streptomycin sulphate

Antituberculostatic; aminoglycoside

ACTIONS AND USES   Aminoglycoside antibiotic derived from *Streptomyces griseus*, with bactericidal and bacteriostatic actions. Appears to act by interfering with normal protein synthesis in susceptible bacteria by binding to 30S subunits of ribosomes. Active against a variety of gram-positive, gram-negative, and acid-fast organisms. Because of rapid emergence of resistant strains when used alone, most commonly used concurrently with other antimicrobial agents. Reportedly, the least nephrotoxic of aminoglycosides. In common with other aminoglycosides, has weak neuromuscular blocking effect.

Used in treatment of all forms of active tuberculosis.

ROUTE AND DOSAGE   Intramuscular: **Adults:** 1 g/day, patients over 40 yrs 750 mg/day; small patients 500 mg/day.

ABSORPTION AND FATE   Following IM administration, peak serum levels in 1 to 2 hours; levels slowly diminish by about 50% after 5 to 6 hours, but are still measurable up to 8 to 12 hours. About one-third of dose is bound to plasma proteins. **Half-life:** about 2 to 3 hours for young adults; longer in newborns, and up to 27 hours in impaired renal function. Diffuses rapidly into most body tissues and extracellular fluids and penetrates tuberculous cavities and caseous tissue. Does not diffuse into CSF unless

STREPTOMYCIN SULPHATE (continued)

meninges are inflamed. Excreted rapidly, primarily by glomerular filtration; 30 to 90% of dose is excreted within 24 hours. Small amounts excreted in saliva, sweat, tears, bile, and milk. Crosses placenta.

CONTRAINDICATIONS AND PRECAUTIONS History of toxic reaction or hypersensitivity to aminoglycosides, labyrinthine disease, during pregnancy or lactation, myasthenia gravis, concurrent or sequential use of other neurotoxic and/or nephrotoxic agents. **Cautious Use**: impaired renal function (given in reduced dosages), use in the elderly and in prematures, neonates, and children.

ADVERSE/SIDE EFFECTS These include: labyrinthine damage (most frequent), auditory damage paraesthesias (peripheral, facial, myocarditis (rare), nephrotoxicity (uncommon), hepatotoxicity, transient bleeding (due to inhibition of factor and especially circumoral), headache, inability to concentrate, lassitude, muscular weakness, optic nerve toxicity (scotomata, V), systemic lupus erythematosus, pain and irritation at IM site, superinfections, neuromuscular blockade (respiratory dimmed or blurred vision), arachnoiditis, encephalopathy, CNS depression syndrome (infants): stupor, flaccidity, coma, paralysis, cardiac arrest). respiratory depression.

NURSING IMPLICATIONS

- Administer IM deep into large muscle mass to minimize possibility of irritation. Injections are painful.
- Avoid direct contact with drug; sensitization can occur. Rubber or plastic gloves are advised when preparing drug.
- Culture and sensitivity tests are done prior to and periodically during course of therapy.
- Patient should be instructed to report any unusual symptom. Adverse reactions should be reviewed periodically, especially in patients on prolonged therapy.
- In patients with impaired renal function, drug accumulation reportedly occurs if administered more frequently than every 8 to 12 hours (intervals of 1 to 2 days are recommended if creatinine clearance is 10 ml/minute or greater, and 3 to 4 days if less than 10 ml/minute.
- Be alert for and report immediately symptoms suggestive of ototoxicity. Symptoms are most likely to occur in patients with impaired renal function, patients receiving high doses (1.8 to 2 g daily) or other ototoxic or neurotoxic drugs, and the elderly. If drug is not discontinued promptly, irreversible damage may occur.
- Damage of vestibular portion of eighth cranial nerve (higher incidence than auditory toxicity) appears to occur in three stages: *Acute stage*: may be preceded for 1 or 2 days by moderately severe headache, then followed by nausea, vomiting, vertigo in upright position, difficulty in reading, unsteadiness, and positive Romberg; lasts 1 to 2 weeks and ends abruptly. *Chronic stage*: characterized by difficulty in walking or in making sudden movements and ataxia; lasts approximately 2 months. *Compensatory stage*: symptoms are latent and appear only when eyes are closed. Full recovery may take 12 to 18 months; residual damage is permanent in some patients.
- Auditory nerve damage is usually preceded by vestibular symptoms and high-pitched tinnitus, roaring noises, impaired hearing (especially to high-pitched sounds), sense

STREPTOMYCIN SULPHATE (continued)

of fullness in ears. Audiometric test should be done if these symptoms appear, and drug should be discontinued if indicated. Hearing loss can be permanent if damage is extensive. Tinnitus may persist several days to weeks after drug is stopped.

- Solutions made from streptomycin sulphate powder are preferably used immediately after reconstitution. Check package insert.
- Exposure to light may cause slight darkening of solution, with no apparent loss of potency.

Diagnostic test interferences   Streptomycin reportedly produces false-positive **urinary glucose** tests using copper sulphate methods (Clinitest), but not with glucose oxidase methods (e.g., Clinistix). **Culture and sensitivity** tests may be affected if patient is taking salts such as sodium and potassium chloride, sodium sulphate and tartrate, ammonium acetate, calcium and magnesium ions.

Drug interactions   Streptomycin may produce additive anticoagulant effect in patients receiving **oral anticoagulants** (it is thought that streptomycin interferes with synthesis of intestinal vitamin K and stimulates production of factor V inhibitor). *See gentamicin.*

Sucralfate ————————————————————————

(Antepsin)   *Enzyme inhibitor*

ACTIONS AND USES   A complex of aluminium hydroxide and sulphated sucrose structurally related to heparin but lacks its anticoagulant activity. Its action is chemically unlike any other drug used for antiulcer therapy. Following oral administration, sucralfate and gastric acid react to form a viscous, adhesive, paste-like substance that is resistant to further reaction with acid. This 'paste' adheres to the GI mucosa with a major portion binding electrostatically to the positively charged protein molecules in the damaged mucosa of an ulcer crater or an acute gastric erosion caused by alcohol or other drugs. Sucralfate absorbs bile, inhibits (inactivates) the enzyme pepsin, and blocks back diffusion of H^+ ions (acid). These actions plus adherence of the pastelike complex protect damaged mucosa against further destruction from ulcerogenic secretions and drugs. The aluminium ions released as sucralfate reacts with HCl are partly responsible for sucralfate-poor absorption from GI tract. May decrease rate of gastric emptying; has no effect on activity of trypsin or pancreatic amylase.

Used for treatment of duodenal gastric ulcer.

ROUTE AND DOSAGE   Oral: **Adult:** 1 g four times daily on empty stomach (1 hour before meals and at bedtime). Maximum 8 g for 4–12 weeks.

ABSORPTION AND FATE   Minimally absorbed from GI tract (less than 5% of dose). Duration of action (depends on contact time with damaged tissue) up to 6 hours. 30% of dose retained in GI tract for at least 3 hours; the small amount that is systemically

SURCRALFATE (continued)

absorbed is excreted unchanged within 48 hours. It is not known if sucrose sulphate crosses placenta or is distributed into milk.

CONTRAINDICATIONS AND PRECAUTIONS   Safe use during pregnancy, by nursing mothers, or by children has not been established.

ADVERSE/SIDE EFFECTS   These include: nausea, gastric discomfort, constipation, diarrhoea, dry mouth, dizziness, sleepiness, vertigo, rash, pruritus, back pain, hypophosphataemia (rare).

NURSING IMPLICATIONS

- Antacids may be prescribed for pain relief if needed. Administer ½ hour before or after sucralfate.
- Successful short-term course of sucralfate therapy dose not seem to alter the tendency of the duodenal ulcer to heal and then to recur.
- Sucralfate apparently binds to certain compounds (*see Drug Interactions*) in the intestinal tract, thereby reducing their bioavailability. To prevent this action separate administration of these agents from that of sucralfate by 2 hours.
- Although healing has occurred within the first 2 weeks of therapy, treatment is usually continued 4 to 8 weeks (in absence of healing as demonstrated by radiographic or endoscopic examination).
- If constipation is a drug-related problem, investigate patient's food–fluid–exercise habits. Relief and prevention of constipation may result from the following measures (unless contraindicated): increase water intake to 8 to 10 glasses/day; increase physical exercise, increase dietary bulk, avoid laxative abuse. Consult physician: a suppository or bulk-producing laxative may be prescribed.
- Emphasize need to adhere to sucralfate regimen: patient should not omit, increase, or decrease dosage or change administration times.
- Advise patient to stop smoking. Research findings indicate that smoking is a major factor in recurrence of duodenal ulcer. Further, it is suggested that giving up smoking may be more important in prevention of recurrence of the ulcer than medication.
- Store in tight container at room temperature. Stable for 2 years after manufacture.

DRUG INTERACTIONS   *Sucralfate*

PLUS	INTERACTIONS
Cimetidine Phenytoin Tetracyclines }	Decreased bioavailability of these drugs

Sulconazole nitrate

(Exelderm)

SULCONAZOLE NITRATE (continued)

ACTIONS AND USES   Used for fungal infections of the skin.

ROUTE AND DOSAGE   Topical, apply 1−2 times a day continuing for 2−3 weeks after lesions have healed.

For further information: *see clotrimazole.*

Sulfametopyrazine

(Kelfizine W)

ACTIONS AND USES   Sulphonamide used to treat urinary tract infection and chronic bronchitis.

ROUTE AND DOSAGE   Oral: **Adult**: 2 g once a week.

For further information: *see sulphadiazine.*

Sulindac

(Clinoril)   *Analgesic; antipyretic; NSAID*

ACTIONS AND USES   Indene acetic acid derivative structurally and pharmacologically related to indomethacin. Pharmacological properties are similar to those of aspirin (q.v.) but chemically unrelated. In common with these drugs, exhibits antiinflammatory, analgesic, and antipyretic, properties. Exact mechanism of antiinflammatory action not known but thought to result from inhibition of prostaglandin synthesis. Sulindac is an inactive prodrug converted to an active sulphide metabolite in the liver. Comparable to aspirin in antiinflammatory activity, but has longer half-life, lower incidence of GI intolerance and tinnitus, and less effect on bleeding time and platelet function. May prolong bleeding time, but prothrombin time, whole blood clotting time, and platelet count are not affected. Serum uric acid lowering effect is less than that of aspirin. Cross-sensitivity to other nonsteroidal antiinflammatory drugs (NSAID) has been reported.

Used for acute and long-term symptomatic treatment of osteoarthritis, rheumatoid arthritis, ankylosing spondylitis; for acute painful shoulder (acute subacromial bursitis or supraspinatus tendinitis), and acute gouty arthritis.

ROUTE AND DOSAGE   Oral: **Adult**: 200 mg twice daily for 7 to 14 days then reduced according to patient's response. Maximum 400 mg/day.

ABSORPTION AND FATE   Approximately 90% absorbed following oral administration. Plasma concentration peaks within 2 hours in fasting state and within 3 to 4 hours

SULINDAC (continued)

if drug is taken with food. About 99% protein bound. Metabolized in liver to active (sulphide) and to inactive (sulphone) metabolites. Half-life of unchanged drug and active sulphide metabolite: 7.8 and 16.4 hours, respectively. Sulindac and its metabolites undergo extensive enteroheptic recirculation. Approximately 50% excreted in urine as unchanged drug and inactive metabolites, and about 25% excreted in faeces primarily as active and inactive metabolites. Minimal, if any, passage of drug across placenta; enters breast milk.

CONTRAINDICATIONS AND PRECAUTIONS   Hypersensitivity to sulindac; hypersensitivity to aspirin (patients with 'aspirin triad': acute asthma, rhinitis, nasal polyps) or to other NSAIDs; significant renal or hepatic dysfunction. Safe use during pregnancy, in nursing mothers, and in children not established. **Cautious Use**: history of upper GI tract disorders, compromised cardiac function, hypertension, haemophilia or other bleeding tendencies.

ADVERSE/SIDE EFFECTS   These include: drowsiness, dizziness, headache, anxiety, nervousness, palpitation, peripheral oedema, congestive heart failure (patients with marginal cardiac function), blurred vision, amblyopia, vertigo, tinnitus, decreased hearing, abdominal pain, dyspepsia, nausea, vomiting, constipation, diarrhoea, ulceration, flatulence, anorexia; stomatitis, sore or dry mucous membranes, dry mouth; rarely: gastritis, gastroenteritis, peptic ulcer, GI bleeding, prolonged bleeding time, aplastic anaemia, thrombocytopenia, Stevens-Johnson toxic epidermal necrolysis syndrome. Causal relationship unknown: hypertension, epistaxis, paraesthesias, vaginal bleeding, haematuria.

NURSING IMPLICATIONS

- If patient cannot swallow tablet, it may be crushed prior to administration.
- May be administered with food, milk, or antacid (if prescribed) to reduce possibility of GI upset. However, food retards absorption and results in delayed and lower peak concentrations.
- A detailed drug history should be elicited before initiation of therapy. *See Contraindications and Precautions*.

Sulphacetamide sodium ━━━━━━━━━━━━━━━━━━━━━━━━

(Albucid, Isopto Cetamide, Ocusol)   *Sulphonamide*

ACTIONS AND USES   Highly soluble sulphonamide effective against a wide range of gram-positive and gram-negative microorganisms. Exerts bacteriostatic effect by interfering with bacterial utilization of para-aminobenzoic acid, thereby inhibiting folic acid biosynthesis required for bacterial growth.

   Used for treatment of conjunctivitis, corneal ulcers, and other superficial ocular infections.

SULPHACETAMIDE SODIUM (continued)

ROUTE AND DOSAGE   Ophthalmic solution (10, 20, 30%): *Initial*: 1 or 2 drops into lower conjunctival sac every 1 to 4 hours during the day and less frequently during the night. Interval increased as condition responds. **Ophthalmic ointment** 2.5%, 6%, 10%: ½ to 1 inch into lower conjunctival sac every 6 hours and at bedtime.

NURSING IMPLICATIONS

Instruct patient or responsible family member how to instill eye drops

- Wash hands thoroughly with soap and running water (before and after instillation).
- Patient should be sitting or lying down if another person is to administer medication. If patient is to instill own medication, the patient should sit in front of a mirror.
- Examine eye medication; discard if cloudy or dark in colour. Avoid contaminating any part of eye dropper that is inserted in bottle.
- With head tilted back, pull down lower lid. At the same time, have patient look up while drop is being instilled into conjunctival sac.
- Immediately apply gentle pressure to punctum (inner canthus next to nose) for 1 minute.
- As soon as pressure is applied to punctum, patient should close eyes gently, so as not to squeeze out medication.
- Blot excess medication with clean facial tissue.
- Drug should be discontinued if symptoms of hypersensitivity appear (erythema, skin rash, pruritus, urticaria).

Sulphadiazine ▄▄▄▄▄▄▄▄▄▄▄▄▄▄▄▄▄▄▄▄▄▄▄▄▄▄

Sulphonamide

ACTIONS AND USES   Short-acting sulphonamide. In common with other sulphonamides, has broad antimicrobial spectrum against both gram-positive and gram-negative organisms. Bacteriostatic action believed to be by competitive inhibition of *p*-aminobenzoic acid, thereby interfering with folic acid biosynthesis required for bacterial growth. Increase in resistant organisms is a limitation to usefulness of sulphonamides; cross-resistance to other sulphonamides is possible. Since sulphafurazole and its derivatives are highly soluble in alkaline urine and slightly acidic urine and are excreted rapidly, the risk of crystalluria is small.

Used in treatment of meningococcal meningitis.

ROUTE AND DOSAGE   Adult: *initial*: **IV or IM**: 1–1.5 g every 4 hours for 2 days then oral treatment.

ABSORPTION AND FATE   Sulphafurazole and diolamine forms readily absorbed. Peak blood levels within 2 to 4 hours after oral and IM administration and within 30 minutes after IV injection; wide variations in blood levels. About 85% protein-bound (65 to 72% in nonacetylated form). Distributed only into extracellular fluids. Half-life: 4 to 7

SULPHADIAZINE (continued)

hours. Metabolized chiefly in liver. Up to 95% of single dose is excreted in urine within 24 hours (70% as free drug). Small amounts eliminated in faeces, sweat, saliva, tears, breast milk, and intestinal and other secretions. Crosses placenta.

CONTRAINDICATIONS AND PRECAUTIONS   History of hypersensitivity to sulphonamides, salicylates, or chemically related drugs; use in treatment of group A beta-haemolytic streptococcal infections; infants less than 2 months of age, pregnant women at term, nursing mothers; porphyria; advanced renal or hepatic disease; intestinal and urinary obstruction. **Cautious Use:** impaired renal or liver function, severe allergy, bronchial asthma, blood dyscrasias, patients with G6PD deficiency.

ADVERSE/SIDE EFFECTS   Low toxicity level, but may include the following: acute haemolytic anaemia (especially in patients with G6PD deficiency), aplastic anaemia, methaemoglobinaemia, agranulocytosis, thrombocytopenia, leucopenia, eosinophilia, hypoprothrombinaemia, headache, peripheral neuritis, peripheral neuropathy, tinnitus, hearing loss, vertigo, insomnia, drowsiness, mental depression, acute psychosis, ataxia, convulsions, kernicterus (newborns), nausea, vomiting, diarrhoea, abdominal pains, hepatitis, jaundice pancreatitis, stomatitis, impaired folic acid absorption crystalluria, haematuria, proteinuria, anuria, toxic nephrosis, conjunctivitis, goitre hypoglycaemia, diuresis, overgrowth of nonsusceptible organisms, lupus erythematosus phenomenon, retardation of corneal healing (ophthalmic ointment), alopecia, reduction in sperm count, lymphadenopathy, local reaction following IM injection, fixed drug eruptions.

NURSING IMPLICATIONS
- Tablet may be crushed before administration and taken with full glass of water (or other fluid) of patient's choice.
- Administration with food appears to delay, but reportedly does not reduce amount of drug absorbed.
- Monitor fluid intake and output. Report oliguria and changes in intake and output ratio. Fluid intake should be adequate to support urinary output of at least 1,500 ml/day to prevent crystalluria and stone formation.
- Since a fall in urinary pH (more acidic) increases risk of crystalluria, daily check of urine pH with Labstix is advisable.
- Report increasing acidity. If urine is highly acidic, physician may prescribe a urinary alkalinizer, e.g., acetazolamide (routine alkalinization of urine not necessary).
- Monitor temperature. Sudden appearance of fever may signify sensitization (serum sickness) or haemolytic anaemia (frequent in patients with G6PD deficiency, which is most common among black males and Mediterranean ethnic groups). These reactions generally develop within 10 days after start of drug. Agranulocytosis may develop after 10 days to 6 weeks of therapy.
- Fever with sore throat, malaise, unusual fatigue, joint pains, pallor, bleeding tendencies, rash, and jaundice are early manifestations of blood dyscrasias or hypersensitivity reactions.
- Frequent kidney function tests and urinalyses (including microscopic examination) are recommended; complete blood tests and hepatic function tests are advised, especially in patients receiving sulphonamides for longer than 2 weeks.

S

SULPHADIAZINE (continued)

■ Determinations of drug blood levels are advised, particularly in patients receiving high doses. Therapeutically effective blood level ranges from 5 to 15 mg/dl; levels above 20 mg/dl are usually associated with adverse reactions.

■ Bacterial sensitivity tests are not always reliable and therefore must be closely correlated with bacteriological studies and accurate assessments of clinical response.

■ Diabetic patients receiving oral hypoglycaemic agents should be closely observed for hypoglycaemic reactions (*see Drug Interactions*). Monitor urine and blood sugar frequently, as necessary, during and after concurrent treatment. Determinations of blood glucose levels are advised before and shortly after initiation of sulphonamide therapy.

■ Advise patients to avoid exposure to ultraviolet light and excessive sunlight to prevent photosensitivity reaction, during therapy and for several months after treatment is discontinued.

■ The patient should understand clearly that the established dosage regimen must be followed: patient should not omit, increase, interrupt, or decrease dose. The full course of treatment should be completed.

■ Caution patients not to take OTC medications without consulting physician. Many proprietary analgesic mixtures contain aspirin in combination with *p*-aminobenzoic acid (*see Drug Interactions*). Inform patients that excessive doses of vitamin C acidify urine and therefore should be avoided (to prevent crystalluria).

■ Recent studies suggest that recurrent dysuria may be due to overuse of soap when washing female genitalia, rather than to bacteriuria. Cleansing with water only may prevent this 'urethral syndrome.'

■ Oral contraceptives may be unreliable while patient is receiving a sulphonamide. Advise abstinence from intercourse or use of an alternate method of contraception. Breakthrough bleeding should be considered evidence of an interaction.

■ Preserved in tight, light-resistant containers. Store at 15° to 30°C (59° to 86°F).

Diagnostic test interferences   Sulphonamides may interfere with **BSP** retention and **PSP** excretion tests and may affect results of **thyroid function tests** (I-131 may be decreased for about 7 days). Large doses of sulphonamides reportedly may produce false-positive **urine glucose** determinations with copper reduction methods (e.g., Clinitest). Sulphonamides may produce false-positive results for **urinary protein** (with sulphosalicylic acid test) and may interfere with **urine urobilinogen** determinations using Ehrlich's reagent. Follow-up cultures are unreliable unless *p*-aminobenzoic acid is added to culture medium.

DRUG INTERACTIONS   *Sulphonamides*

PLUS	INTERACTIONS
Alkalinizing agents, urinary	Increased excretion of sulphonamide
Anaesthetics, local (derived from *p*-aminobenzoic acid)	Antagonize antibacterial activity of sulphonamide
Antacids	May decrease absorption of sulphonamide
Anticoagulants, oral	Increased or prolonged anticoagulant effects

SULPHADIAZINE (continued)

PLUS (continued)	INTERACTIONS
Anticonvulsants (hydantoins)	Increased anticonvulsant effects and potential increase in toxicity of anticonvulsant
Digoxin, folic acid	Decreased absorption when used concurrently with a sulphonamide; dose adjustment may be necessary
Hypoglycaemics, oral; methotrexate, phenotoin, thiopental	Increased or prolonged clinical effects leading to increase in potential for toxicity
Acidifying agents	Increased danger of sulphonamide crystallization in urine
Oral contraceptives ⎫ Oestrogens ⎭	May increase risk of pregnancy because of increased hepatic metabolism and reduced absorption of oestrogen
Oxyphenbutazone, phenylbutazone	Potentiated effects of the agents
PABA and local anaesthetics	May antagonize sulphonamide action
Phenothiazines	May increase toxic effects of sulphonamide
Probenecid, sulphinpyrazone	Decreased excretion of sulphonamide resulting in prolonged antibacterial level and increased potential for toxicity

Sulphadimidine

ACTIONS AND USES   Sulphonamide used to treat urinary tract infection; meningococcal meningitis and for prophylaxis.

ROUTE AND DOSAGE   Oral/IV/IM: **Adult:** *initial* 2 g then 0.5–1 g 6–8 hrly.
For further information: *see sulphadiazine.*

Sulphamethoxazole

Sulphonamide

ACTIONS AND USES   Used with trimethoprim (q.v.) in Cotrimoxazole.
For further information: *see cotrimoxazole.*

Sulphasalazine

Sulphonamide

SULPHASALAZINE (continued)

ACTIONS AND USES   Locally acting sulphonamide. Believed to be converted by intestinal microflora to sulphapyridine (which has antibacterial action) and 5-aminosalicylic acid (with may exert antiinflammatory effect). Other proposed mechanisms of action include: inhibition of prostaglandins known to cause diarrhoea and affect mucosal transport, interference with absorption of fluids and electrolytes from colon, and reduction in *Clostridium* and *Escherichia coli* in the stools. Contraindications, precautions, and adverse/side effects are as for other sulphonamides.

Used in treatment of ulcerative colitis, Crohn's disease, and rheumatoid arthritis.

ROUTE AND DOSAGE   **Oral: Adults:** Acute attack 1–2 g 4 times a day. **Child:** 40 mg/kg/day in divided doses. *Maintenance:* 20–30 mg/kg/day. ***Rheumatoid arthritis***: *initial* 500 mg/day increased by 500 mg at weekly intervals to a maximum of 2–3 g/day. **Suppositories:** 0.5–1 g morning and evening. **Enema:** 3 g at night retained for 1 hr.

ABSORPTION AND FATE   About one-third of dose absorbed from small intestine as unchanged drug; remaining two-thirds absorbed from colon, where it is converted to sulphapyridine (SP) most of which is absorbed, and 5-aminosalicylic acid (5-ASA), 30% of which is absorbed, with remainder being excreted in urine. Peak serum levels in 1.5 to 6 hours for parent drug and 6 to 24 hours for SP (serum levels tend to be higher in slow acetylator phenotypes). **Half-life:** 5 to 10 hours. Excreted in urine as unchanged drug, SP, 5-ASA, and acetyl derivatives.

CONTRAINDICATIONS AND PRECAUTIONS   Sensitivity to sulphonamides, agranulocytosis, children under 2 years of age, intestinal and urinary tract obstruction.

ADVERSE/SIDE EFFECTS   Frequent: nausea, vomiting, bloody diarrhoea; anorexia, arthralgia, rash, anaemia, infertility (reversible), blood dyscrasias, hepatic injury, infectious mononucleosis-like reaction, SLE (rare), allergic reactions (common).

NURSING IMPLICATIONS
- If possible, drug should be administered after eating food to provide longer intestine transit time for the drug.
- Should be given in evenly divided doses over each 24-hour period. Intervals between night time doses should not exceed 8 hours.
- If GI intolerance occurs after first few doses, symptoms are probably due to irritation of stomach mucosa. Symptoms may be relieved by spacing total daily dose more evenly over the day or by administration of enteric-coated tablets.
- High doses (more than 2 g/day) reduce tissue folate stores. In addition the disease condition itself compromises an adequate dietary intake of folates. Therefore, food sources cannot be depended upon to restore normal levels. A daily supplement may be prescribed.
- Desensitization of patient who has an allergic reaction to sulphasalazine can be accomplished safely to permit continued use of the drug. Usually the process is started with one-eighth tablet daily; dose is doubled every 3 to 7 days.
- Preserved in tight, light-resistant containers; store at 15° to 30°C (59° to 86°F).
- *See sulphadiazine.*

SULPHASALAZINE (continued)

Drug interactions Antibiotics may alter metabolism of sulphasalazine by altering intestinal flora. By chelating iron, sulphasalazine absorption may be inhibited, with resulting lower blood levels. *Sulphasalazine inhibits* **folic acid** absorption. **Phenobarbital** administered concomitantly may decrease urinary excretion of sulphasalazine. *See also drug interactions for sulphadiazine.*

Sulphaurea

(Uromide)   *Sulphonamide*

ACTIONS AND USES   Used to treat urinary tract infection. *See sulphadiazine.*

Sulphinpyrazone

(Anturan)   *Uricosuric; pyrazolone*

ACTIONS AND USES   Potent pyrazolone-derivative renal tubular blocking agent structurally related to phenylbutazone. At therapeutic doses, promotes urinary excretion of uric acid and reduces serum urate levels by competitively inhibiting tubular reabsorption of uric acid. Like all uricosurics, low doses may inhibit tubular secretion of uric acid and cause urate retention. Inhibits release of adenosine diphosphate and 5-hydroxytryptophan, and thus decreases platelet adhesiveness and increases platelet survival time; has no effect on prothrombin or blood clotting time. May cause slight but significant decrease in serum cholesterol. Since it has no apparent analgesic or anti-inflammatory activity, it is not used for relief of acute gout. Reportedly not associated with cumulative effects, development of tolerance, or electrolyte imbalance.

Used for maintenance therapy in chronic gouty arthritis and tophaceous gout, to treat drug-induced hyperuricaemia, to decrease platelet aggregation and increase survival after myocardial infarction.

ROUTE AND DOSAGE   Oral: Adult (first week of therapy): 100 to 200 mg initially daily, gradually increased as needed to full maintenance range of 200 to 400 mg twice daily; after serum urate levels are controlled, dosage may be reduced to 200 mg daily in divided doses.

ABSORPTION AND FATE   Readily and completely absorbed from GI tract. **Peak plasma levels** in 1 to 2 hours. **Duration of action** 4 to 6 hours, but may persist to 10 hours. About 98% bound to plasma proteins. **Half-life**: 3 hours (range 1 to 9 hours). Rapidly metabolized by liver to active and inactive metabolites. After 2 days, 45% of single dose is excreted as unchanged drug and metabolites.

SULPHINPYRAZONE (Continued)

CONTRAINDICATIONS AND PRECAUTIONS Known hypersensitivity to pyrazoline derivatives, active peptic ulcer, concurrent administration of salicylates, patients with creatinine clearance less than 50 mg/minute, treatment of hyperuricaemia secondary to neoplastic disease or cancer chemotherapy. **Cautious Use:** impaired renal function, pregnancy, history of healed peptic ulcer, use in conjunction with sulphonamides and sulphonylurea, hypoglycaemic agents.

ADVERSE/SIDE EFFECTS GI disturbances (common): nausea, vomiting, diarrhoea, epigastric pain, blood loss, reactivation or aggravation of peptic ulcer, ataxia, dizziness, vertigo, tinnitus; oedema, laboured respirations, convulsions, coma, hypersensitivity, reactions (skin rashes, fever), blood dyscrasias (rare: anaemia, leucopenia, agranulocytosis, thrombocytopenia), jaundice, precipitation of acute gout, urolithiasis, renal colic.

NURSING IMPLICATIONS

- Administered with meals, milk, or antacid (prescribed) to prevent local drug irritant effect. Severity and frequency of symptoms increase with dosage. Persistence of GI symptoms may require discontinuation of drug.
- During early therapy, fluid intake should be sufficient to support urinary output of at least 2,000 to 3,000 ml/day (consult physician), and urine should be alkalinized (e.g., with large doses vitamin C) to increase solubility of uric acid and minimize risk of uric acid stones.
- Serum urate levels are used to monitor therapy. Aim of therapy is to lower serum urate levels to about 2 mmol/L and thus to reduce joint changes, tophi formation, and frequency of acute attacks and to improve renal function.
- Patient must remain under close medical supervision while taking sulphinpyrazone. Therapy is continued indefinitely.
- Caution patient to avoid experimentation with dosage, since subtherapeutic doses may enhance urate retention, and large doses may increase risk of toxicity.
- Periodic blood cell counts are advised during prolonged therapy. Patients with impaired renal function should have period aassessments of renal function.
- May increase the frequency of acute gouty attacks during first 6 to 12 months of therapy, even when serum urate levels appear to be controlled. Physician may prescribe prophylactic doses of colchicine concurrently during first 3 to 6 months of treatment to prevent or at least lessen severity of attacks.
- Sulphinpyrazone therapy should be continued without interruption even when patient has an acute gouty attack, which may be treated with full therapeutic doses of colchicine or other antiinflammatory agent.
- Caution patient to avoid aspirin-containing medications (*see Drug Interactions*). If an analgesic is required (in patients with normal renal function), generally paracetamol is recommended.
- Patients receiving oral hypoglycaemic agents should be supervised closely (*see Drug Interactions*).

Drug interactions Possibility of additive uricosuric effects with **allopurinol** (may be used therapeutically). The uricosuric action of sulphinpyrazone is antagonized by **aspirin** and other **salicylates**. May affect urinary excretion of weak organic acids with

SULPHINPYRAZONE (continued)

resulting higher serum levels, e.g., **aminosalicylic acid, cephalosporins, dapsone, indomethacin, nitrofurantoin, penicillins. Probenecid** may increase toxicity of sulphinpyrazone by inhibiting its renal excretion. May potentiate hypoglycaemia by interfering with renal excretion of **sulphonylurea** hypoglycaemic agents. There is the possibility that sulphinpyrazone may enhance hypoprothrombinaemic effect of **warfarin** and **other coumarin-type anticoagulants.** Concomitant administration of drugs that tend to increase serum urate levels may necessitate higher sulphinpyrazone dosage, e.g., **alcohol, aluminium nicotinate, diazoxide,** most **diuretics, mecamylamine, pyrazinamide.** Cholestyramine may delay absorption of sulphinpyrazone (administer sulphinpyrazone at least 1 hour before or 4 to 6 hours after cholestyramine). There is the possibility of increased risk of blood dyscrasias with concomitant use of sulphinpyrazone and colchicine.

Sulpiride▬▬▬▬▬▬▬▬▬▬▬▬▬▬▬▬▬▬▬▬

(Domatil)

ACTIONS AND USES   Antipsychotic drug used to treat schizophrenia.

ROUTE AND DOSAGE   Oral: Adult: 200–400 mg twice a day–maximum 800 mg/day in patients with mainly negative symptoms. Patients with predominantly positive symptoms up to 2.4 g/day.
   For further information: *see chlorpromazine.*

Suxamethonium▬▬▬▬▬▬▬▬▬▬▬▬▬▬▬▬

(Anectine, Scoline)   *Skeletal muscle relaxant*
                                                                      (depolarizing);
                                                                      neuromuscular
                                                                      blocking agent

ACTIONS AND USES   Synthetic, ultrashort-acting depolarizing neuromuscular blocking agent with high affinity for acetylcholine receptor sites. Initial transient contractions and fasciculations are followed by sustained flaccid skeletal muscle paralysis produced by state of accomodation that develops in adjacent excitable muscle membranes. Rapidly hydrolyzed by plasma pseudocholinesterase.
   Used to produce skeletal muscle relaxation as adjunct to anaesthesia, to facilitate intubation and endoscopy, to increase pulmonary compliance in assisted or controlled respiration, and to reduce intensity of muscle contractions in pharmacologically-induced or electroshock convulsions.

SUXAMETHONIUM (continued)

ROUTE AND DOSAGE   Intravenous: 20–100 mg according to need. **Child:** *initial* 1–1.5 mg/kg then one third of the initial dose.

ABSORPTION AND FATE   Following IV administration, complete muscle relaxation occurs within 1 minute, persists 2 or 3 minutes, returns to normal in 6 to 10 minutes. Following IM injection, action begins in 2 to 3 minutes and lasts 10 to 30 minutes. Plasma level falls rapidly by redistribution. Rapidly hydrolyzed by plasma pseudocholinesterases to succinylmonocholine (a mildly active nondepolarizing muscle relaxant), and then more slowly to succinic acid and choline. Excreted in urine primarily as active and inactive metabolites; 10% excreted as unchanged drug. Does not readily cross placenta.

CONTRAINDICATIONS AND PRECAUTIONS   Hypersensitivity to succinylcholine; family history of malignant hyperthermia. Safe use in pregnancy and in women of childbearing potential not established.

ADVERSE/SIDE EFFECTS   These include: bradycardia, tachycardia, hypotension, hypertension, arrhythmias, sinus arrest, muscle fasciculations, profound and prolonged muscle relaxation, muscle pain, respiratory depression, bronchospasm, hypoxia, apnoea, malignant hyperthermia, increased intraocular pressure, excessive salivation, enlarged salivary glands, myoglobinaemia, hyperkalaemia; hypersensitivity reactions (rare); decreased tone and motility of GI tract (large doses).

NURSING IMPLICATIONS

- Transient apnoea usually occurs at time of maximal drug effect (1 to 2 minutes); spontaneous respiration should return in a few seconds, or at most, 3 or 4 minutes.
- Facilities for emergency endotracheal intubation, artificial respiration, and assisted or controlled respiration with oxygen should be immediately available. A nerve stimulator may be used to assess nature and degree of neuromuscular blockage.
- Selective muscle paralysis following drug administration develops in the following sequence: levator eyelid muscles, mastication, limbs, abdomen, glottis, intercostals, diaphragm. Recovery generally occurs in reverse order.
- Adverse effects are primarily extensions of pharmacological actions.
- Patient may experience postprocedural muscle stiffness and pain (caused by initial fasciculations following injection) for as long as 24 to 30 hours. Inform patient that hoarseness and sore throat are common even when pharyngeal airway has not been used.
- Monitor vital signs and keep airway clear of secretions. Observe for and report residual muscle weakness.
- Tachyphylaxis (reduced response) may occur after repeated doses. Expiration date and storage before and after reconstitution varies with the manufacturer.

Drug interactions   Agents that may potentiate or prolong neuromuscular blockage of skeletal muscle relaxants: **acetylcholine, certain antibiotics** (gentamicin, kanamycin, neomycin, streptomycins); **benzodiazepines, cholinesterase inhibitors, colistin, cyclophosphamide, cyclopropane, echothiophate iodide, halothane, magnesium salts, methotrimeprazine, narcotic analgesics, organophosphamide insecticides,**

SUXAMETHONIUM (continued)
pantothenyl alcohol, phenelzine, phenothiazines, lignocaine polymixins, procainamide (possibly); procaine, propranolol quinidine, quinine. Succinylcholine may increase risk of cardiac arrhythmias in patients receiving digitalis glycosides. Diazepam may decrease neuromuscular blockade of succinylcholine.

Talampicillin

(Talpen)

ACTIONS AND USES   Antibiotic closely related to ampicillin.

ROUTE AND DOSAGE   Oral: Adult: 250–500 mg/8 hourly.
For further information: *see ampicillin*.

Tamoxifen citrate

(Noltam, Nolvadex, Tamofen)   *Antineoplastic; antioestrogen*

ACTIONS AND USES   Nonsteroid gonad-stimulating principle with potent antioestrogenic activity. Competes with oestradiol at oestrogen receptor sites in target tissues such as breast, uterus, vagina, anterior pituitary, tumour with high concentration of oestrogen receptors. Tamoxifen-receptor complexes move into nucleus resulting in decreased DNA synthesis and oestrogen responses. Ovulation may be induced by stimulation of the release of hypothalamic gonadotropic-releasing factor. May have oncogenic activity.

Used in palliative treatment of advanced breast cancer in postmenopausal women, and increasingly used as a first line treatment in premenopausal women.

ROUTE AND DOSAGE   Oral: individualized.

ABSORPTION AND FATE   Blood level following single oral dose reaches peak values approximately 4 to 7 hours after dose administration with only 20 to 30% of drug remaining as tamoxifen. **Biphasic half-life**: initial: 7 to 14 hours; terminal: 7 days. Hepatic metabolism; enters enterohepatic circulation and is excreted primarily in faeces.

CONTRAINDICATIONS AND PRECAUTIONS   Pregnancy especially during first trimester. **Cautious Use**: lactation, vision disturbances, cataracts, leucopenia, thrombocytopenia.

TAMOXIFEN CITRATE (continued)

ADVERSE/SIDE EFFECTS These include: depression, lightheadedness, dizziness, headache, mental confusion, sleepiness, thrombosis, nausea and vomiting (about 25% of patients), distaste for food, anorexia, leucopenia, thrombocytopenia, retinopathy, corneal changes (infrequent), decreased visual acuity, blurred vision, changes in menstrual period, milk production and leaking from breasts, vaginal discharge and bleeding, pruritus vulvae, swelling and pain in legs, hands or feet; skin rash or dryness, excessive growth of hair, increased bone pain, and transient local disease flair; loss of hair, weight gain, shortness of breath, photosensitivity, hot flashes, hypercalcaemia.

NURSING IMPLICATIONS

- An objective response may require 4 to 10 weeks of therapy, longer if there is bone metastasis.
- Bone and tumour pain and local disease flair often necessitate administration of analgesics for pain relief. Reassure patient that this discomfort frequently signals a good tumour response.
- Soft tissue disease response to tamoxifen may be local swelling and marked erythema over preexisting lesions and/or the development of new lesions. These symptoms rapidly subside after tamoxifen treatment is initiated.
- Complete blood counts including platelet counts are periodically assessed. Transient leucopenia and thrombocytopenia (50,000 to 100,000/mm^3) without haemorrhagic tendency have been reported, but it is uncertain if these effects are caused by tamoxifen.
- If side effects are severe, sometimes a simple reduction in dosage gives sufficient relief without losing control of disease.
- Report to physician if marked weakness, sleepiness, mental confusion, oedema, dyspnoea, and blurred vision occur.
- Discuss the possibility of drug-induced menstrual irregularities with patient before starting treatment. She should be advised not to conceive while taking tamoxifen and to notify physician if she suspects pregnancy.
- Avoid prolonged sun exposure especially if skin is unprotected. Sun-screen lotions (SFP 12 and above) are available and should be applied to all exposed skin surfaces before going outdoors.
- Caution patient not to change established dose schedule, i.e., not to omit, double, interrupt, or divide doses, or change length of dose intervals.
- OTC drugs should be avoided unless specifically prescribed by the physician. Discuss with patient, particularly with respect to OTC analgesics.
- Report onset of tenderness or redness in an extremity.
- Urge patient to adhere to scheduled appointments for clinical evaluation. Medical supervision is necessary during tamoxifen therapy.
- Store drug at temperature between 15° and 30°C (59° and 86°F) in container that protects drug from light.

Diagnostic test interferences Tamoxifen may produce transient increase in **serum** calcium.

Temazepam

(Normison)

Sedative/hypnotic;
benzodiazepine

ACTIONS AND USES   Benzodiazepine derivative with hypnotic, anxiolytic, sedative effects. Principal effect is significant improvement in sleep parameters as evidenced by: reduced night awakenings and early morning awakening, increased total sleep times and absence of rebound effects. Sleep latency is not reduced, and there is minimal change in REM sleep.

Used to relieve insomnia associated with frequent nocturnal awakenings and/or early AM awakenings.

ROUTE AND DOSAGE   Oral: **Adult:** 10 to 30 mg at bedtime increased if necessary to 60 mg. **Elderly:** 5–15 mg.

ABSORPTION AND FATE   Absorption nearly complete with detectable blood levels in 20 to 40 minutes and peak concentration reached in 2 to 3 hours; minimal first-pass metabolism. Hepatic metabolism nearly complete with formation of metabolites. **Half-life:** 10 hours; protein binding: 96%. 80 to 90% dose excreted in urine as inactive metabolites.

CONTRAINDICATIONS AND PRECAUTIONS   Pregnancy, safe use in children below age of 18 not established; narrow angle glaucoma; psychoses. **Cautious Use:** nursing mother, severely depressed patient or one with suicidal ideation, history of drug abuse or dependence, acute intoxication, hepatic or renal dyfunction, elderly patients.

ADVERSE/SIDE EFFECTS   (Usually mild and transient.) These include: anorexia, diarrhoea, drowsiness, dizziness, lethargy, confusion, euphoria, relaxed feeling, weakness; (rare): tremor, ataxia, lack of concentration, loss of equilibrium, hallucination, horizontal nystagmus, paradoxical reaction, palpitations.

NURSING IMPLICATIONS
- If dreams or nightmares (usually occurring during REM sleep) interfere with rest, notify physician. An alternate drug or reduced dose may be prescribed.
- Since temazepam affects little change in sleep latency, patient may still have difficulty getting to sleep. Drug effect is evidenced by the increased amount of rest once asleep.
- If insomnia continues in spite of medication, physician should be consulted. It is possible the complaint is related to a condition for which a more specific treatment is indicated.
- Discuss patient's presleep routine and mental activity during attempts to fall asleep. Propose some measures that might help shorten sleep latency:
  - □ Allow time to 'unwind' from physical/mental activity of day.
  - □ Avoid engaging in mentally stimulating activity just before bedtime.
  - □ Go to bed only when sleepy and arise at regular time in the AM.

TEMAZEPAM *(continued)*
- ☐ Gradually increase physical exercise during day (if allowed) but avoid it just before bedtime.
- ☐ Avoid use of alcohol as a sedative.
- ☐ Take a warm beverage (e.g., milk) or light snack before bedtime.
- ☐ Sit upright in bed for 20 to 30 minutes after taking drug; (this may help patient to experience the onset of natural sleepiness).
- ■ If patient is elderly, suggest to avoid daytime 'catnaps'; but if patient does nap, the time should be added to night-time sleep (i.e., patient should not believe that 7 to 8 hours of sleep at night are needed in addition to an afternoon nap).
- ■ Psychoactive drugs are the most frequent cause of acute confusion in the elderly. Be alert to signs of paradoxical reaction (excitement, hyperactivity, and disorientation) in this age group.
- ■ As with any hypnotic drug (and even without medication), onset of sleep is associated with temporally unpredictable process of relaxation. The danger of a lighted cigarette is obvious; therefore no smoking should be allowed after patient begins to prepare for sleep nor after medication is taken.
- ■ CNS side effects are more apt to occur in the patient with hypoalbuminaemia, liver disease, and the elderly patient. Report promptly incidence of bradycardia, drowsiness, dizziness, clumsiness, lack of coordination. Supervise ambulation, especially at night.
- ■ If patient becomes pregnant, she should be advised to stop taking temazepam. If she intends to become pregnant while taking the drug she should discuss the potential risks to the foetus with the physician.
- ■ Use by nursing mothers may cause sedation and possibly feeding problems and weight loss in the infant. Neonates metabolize benzodiazepines more slowly than adults, leading to accumulation of both unchanged drug and metabolites.
- ■ With long-term use of this drug, hepatic and renal function tests are advised.
- ■ Gradual reduction of dose may be necessary to avoid withdrawal symptoms.
- ■ Use of alcohol and other CNS depressants should be avoided.
- ■ Advise patient about using extreme caution when operating machinery or driving a car, because this drug may depress psychomotor skills, and causes sedation.
- ■ Signs of overdose include weakness, bradycardia, somnolence, confusion, slurred speech, ataxia, coma with reduced or absent reflexes, hypertension, respiratory depression. Treatment includes use of an emetic (if patient is conscious), gastric lavage, and measures to support adequate respiratory function, fluids to encourage diuresis.
- ■ Store between 15° and 30°C (59° and 86°F) in tight container, unless otherwise specified by manufacturer.

DRUG INTERACTIONS   *Temazepam*

PLUS	INTERACTIONS
Alcohol and other CNS depressants	Increased sedation; increased effects of both drugs
Hydantoin anticonvulsants (e.g., phenytoin)	Increased serum concentration of hydantoin, leading to toxicity.

TEMAZEPAM (continued)

PLUS	INTERACTIONS
(continued)	
Levodopa	Decreased antiparkinsonian effect of levodopa
	Interferon
Contraceptives, oral	Pharmacological effect of temazepam may be increased

Terazosin

(Hytrin)

ACTIONS AND USES   New selective alpha-blocker used to treat mild to moderate hypertension.

ROUTE AND DOSAGE   Oral: **Adult**: 1 mg at bedtime increased according to response. Usual maintenance 2–10 mg/day. Report adverse reactions to the Committee on Safety of Medicines.

For further information: *see prazosin.*

Terbutaline sulphate

(Bricanyl)

Adrenergic agonist (sympathomimetic); bronchodilator

ACTIONS AND USES   Synthetic adrenergic stimulant with selective beta$_2$- and negligible beta$_1$-agonist (cardiac) activity. Exerts preferential effect on beta$_2$-receptors in bronchial smooth muscles, inhibits histamine release from mast cells, and increases ciliary motility. These effects lead to relief of bronchospasm in chronic obstructive airways disease and significant increase in vital capacity. Other adrenergic effects include relaxation of vascular smooth muscle, contraction of GI, and urinary sphincters, increase in renin, pancreatic beta-cell secretion, and increase in serum HDL–cholesterol concentration. Increases uterine relaxation (thereby preventing or abolishing high intrauterine pressure).

Used orally or subcutaneously as a bronchodilator in bronchial asthma and for reversible airway obstruction associated with bronchitis and emphysema.

ROUTE AND DOSAGE   Oral: **Adult**: 2.5 to 5 mg two to three times daily at 6 hour intervals; not to exceed 15 mg daily. **Children (7 to 15 years)**: 2.5 mg three times

TERBUTALINE SULPHATE (continued)

daily at 6 hour intervals not to exceed 7.5 mg in 24 hours. **Subcutaneous, IM or slow IV injection: Adult:** 250–500 mcg up to 4 times a day. **Child:** 2–15 yrs 10 mcg/kg maximum 300 mcg. **IV infusion: Adult:** 3–5 mcg/ml solution at a rate of 1.5–5 mcg/min for 8–10 hours. Reduce the dose in children. **Inhalation: Adult and child (over 12 yrs):** 250–500 mcg (1–2 puffs) 4 hrly. **Nebulizer: Adult:** 5–10 mg, 2–4 times a day. **Child (up to 3 yrs):** 2 mg; **(3–6 yrs);** 3 mg; **(6–8 yrs):** 4 mg; **(over 8 yrs):** 5 mg; all 2–4 times a day.

ABSORPTION AND FATE   Bioavailability is less with oral than SC dose. **Onset of action:** 30 minutes after oral administration, 6 to 15 minutes after SC, and 5 to 30 minutes after inhalation. **Duration of action** (bronchodilation): 4 to 8 hours after oral, 1½ to 4 hours after SC, 3 to 6 hours after inhalation. **Elimination half-life:** 3 to 4 hours; **protein binding:** 25%. Metabolized in liver and excreted in urine (small amount in faeces). Distributed into breast milk.

CONTRAINDICATIONS AND PRECAUTIONS   Known hypersensitivity to sympatho-mimetic amines, severe hypertension and coronary artery disease, tachycardia with digitalis intoxication, use within 14 days of MAO inhibitor therapy, children under 12 years of age, angle closure glaucoma. Used only after evaluation of risk–benefit ratio in pregnancy, lactation, and in women of childbearing years. **Cautious Use:** angina, stroke, hypertension, diabetes mellitus, thyrotoxicosis, history of seizure disorders, cardiac arrhythmias, the elderly patient, renal and hepatic dysfunction.

ADVERSE/SIDE EFFECTS   (Dose-related.)   These include: tachycardia, hypotension or hypertension, palpitation, maternal and foetal tachycardia, nausea, vomiting, nervousness, tremor, headache, light-headedness, drowsiness, fatigue, seizures, sweating, muscle cramps, tinnitus (rare).

NURSING IMPLICATIONS

- Tablet may be crushed before administration and taken with fluid of patient's choice.
- *Be certain about recommended doses*: oral preparation: 2.5 mg; SC: 0.25 mg. A decimal point error can be fatal.
- If GI symptoms occur, advise patient to take the tablets with food.
- Onset and degree of effect, incidence and severity of side effects of the SC formulation resemble those of adrenaline. Oral terbutaline appears to be equally as effective as ephedrine; however, onset of action is more rapid and it has longer duration of effects.
- Teach the ambulatory patient on oral terbutaline how to take own pulse and the limits of change that indicate need to notify the physician.
- SC injection is usually administered into lateral deltoid area.
- Most side effects are transient and disappear without treatment. However, rapid heart rate may persist for a relatively long time.
- Cardiovascular side effects are more apt to occur when drug is given by SC route and

TERBUTALINE SULPHATE (continued)

when it is used by a patient with cardiac arrhythmia. Check pulse and BP before each dose. If perceptively altered from baseline level, consult physician.

- Terbutaline appears to have a short clinical period for sustained effectiveness. Advise patient to keep appointments with physician for evaluation of continued drug effectiveness and clinical condition.

- Tolerance can develop with chronic use of terbutaline. Consult physician if symptomatic relief wanes. Usually a substitute agent will be prescribed.

- Instruct patient to consult the physician if breathing difficulty is not relieved or if it becomes worse within 15 minutes after an oral dose of terbutaline.

- Muscle tremor is a fairly common side effect that appears to subside with continued use.

- Be alert to the pattern of self-dosing established by the patient on long-term therapy. Caution patient that in the face of waning response increasing the dose may cause overdosage and will not improve the clinical condition. The patient should understand that decreasing relief with continued treatment indicates need for another bronchodilator, not an increase in dose.

- Warn the patient not to use OTC drugs unless the physician approves. Many cold and allergy remedies, for example, contain a sympathomimetic agent that when combined with terbutaline may be deleterious to the patient.

- Overdosage resulting in enhanced adverse reactions (*see Adverse/Side Effects*) in the alert patient is treated by emptying the stomach (induced emesis and gastric lavage). In the unconscious patient, a cuffed endotracheal tube secures the airway before beginning the lavage. Activated charcoal slurry may be instilled to reduce terbutaline absorption; respiratory and cardiac supportive measures should be readily available.

- Contents of the aerosol are under pressure. Warn patient not to puncture container, not to use or store it near heat or open flame, and not to expose it to temperature above 49°C (120°F) may cause bursting. Can should not be discarded into a fire or incinerator. Keep it out of reach of children.

- Store medication at temperature between 15° and 30°C (59° and 86°F). Protect from light and freezing.

Diagnostic test interferences   Terbutaline may increase **blood glucose** and free **fatty acids.**

DRUG INTERACTIONS   *Terbutaline sulphate*_____

PLUS	INTERACTIONS
MAO inhibitors	Concurrent use may cause severe hypertensive crisis
Propranolol	Antagonizes bronchodilating effect of terbutaline
Sympathomimetics, other	May increase effects and potential side effects of sympathomimetics and/or terbutaline; does not preclude, however, use of a stimulant adrenergic bronchodilator for acute bronchospasm (*see Nursing Implications*)

Terodiline hydrochloride

(Terolin)

ACTIONS AND USES   Anticholinergic drug used to reduce frequency in patients with urge incontinence and detrusor instability.

ROUTE AND DOSAGE   Oral: Adult: 12.5–25 mg twice a day.

Terfenadine

(Triludan)

ACTIONS AND USES   Antihistamine used to treat hay fever and urticaria. Reported to be non-sedating.

ROUTE AND DOSAGE   Oral: Adult: 60 mg twice a day. **Child (6–12 yr):** 30 mg twice a day.

Terlipressin

(Glypressin)

ACTIONS AND USES   Derivative of vasopressin used to control bleeding from oesophageal varices.

ROUTE AND DOSAGE   IV injection: 2 mg initially followed by 1–2 mg every 4–6 hours until bleeding is under control. Treatment continued for up to 72 hours.
    For further information: *see vasopressin.*

Testosterone and testosterone esters

(Primoteston depot, Restanol, Sustanon, Virormone)

Androgen; anabolic steroid; hormone

ACTIONS AND USES   Synthetic steroid compound with both androgenic and anabolic activity (1:1). Controls development and maintenance of secondary sexual characteristics. Androgenic activity: responsible for the growth spurt of the adolescent and for

TESTOSTERONE AND TESTOSTERONE ESTERS (continued)

growth termination by epiphyseal closure. Anabolic activity: increases protein metabolism and decreases its catabolism. Large doses suppress spermatogenesis, thereby causing testicular atrophy. Unlike other androgens, testosterone and its esters do not produce cholestatic hepatitis or creatinuria.

Used primarily as androgen replacement in male sex hormone deficiency states, e.g., male climacteric, postpubertal cryptorchidism, oligospermia, impotence.

ROUTE AND DOSAGE   Intramuscular: depends on the preparation. **Implant:** 200–600 mg effective for 7–8 months.

ABSORPTION AND FATE   Rapid absorption following oral administration; more prolonged absorption from IM site. In plasma, 98% bound to sex hormone-binding globulin (transcortin) and albumin. Remainder is free and represents magnitude of androgen effects. **Serum half-life:** 10 to 100 minutes. Metabolites (including andosterone and etiocholanolone) conjugated and excreted through enterohepatic route (about 10%) and urinary route (90%). Crosses placenta; appears in breast milk.

CONTRAINDICATIONS AND PRECAUTIONS   Hypersensitivity or toxic reactions to androgens; pregnancy, lactation, women of childbearing potential (possibility of virilization of female infant); hypercalcaemia; known or suspected prostatic or breast cancer in male; benign prostatic hypertrophy with obstruction; patients easily stimulated sexually; elderly, asthenic males who may react adversely to androgenic overstimulation; conditions aggravated by fluid retention; hypertension. **Cautious Use:** cardiac, hepatic and renal disease; prepubertal males, geriatric patients, acute intermittent porphyria.

ADVERSE/SIDE EFFECTS   **Both sexes:** hypersensitivity, anaphylactoid reaction (rare), increased libido, skin flushing and vascularization, acne, excitation and sleeplessness, chills, leucopenia, sodium and water retention (especially in the elderly) with oedema; nausea, vomiting, anorexia, diarrhoea, gastric pain, jaundice, bladder irritability, hypercalcaemia, renal calculi in bedfast or partially immobilized patient, hypercholesterolaemia, precipitation of acute intermittent porphyria, aggravation of disease being treated, site irritation and sloughing (pellet implantation), hepatocellular carcinoma (rare). **Female:** suppression of ovulation, lactation, or menstruation; virilism: hoarseness or deepening of voice (often irreversible); hirsutism; oily skin; acne; clitoral enlargement; regression of breasts; male-pattern baldness (in disseminated breast cancer). **Male (post-pubertal):** testicular atrophy, decreased ejaculatory volume, azoospermia, oligospermia (after prolonged administration or excessive dosage), impotence, epididymitis, priapism, gynaecomastia; (prepubertal): phallic enlargement, priapism, premature epiphyseal closure.

NURSING IMPLICATIONS

- IM injections should be made deep into gluteal muscle.
- Check fluid intake and output and weigh patient regularly during dose adjustment period.
- Sodium and water retention respond to diuretic therapy; therefore, use of a diuretic differentiates skeletal growth from oedema weight gain.

TESTOSTERONE AND TESTOSTERONE ESTERS (continued)

- Restoration of positive nitrogen balance, as in patients with metastatic carcinoma, is supported by a diet high in protein and carlories. Sodium restriction may be prescribed to control oedema. Collaborate with physician and dietitian in developing a dietary teaching plan that includes patient and responsible family members.
- Periodic serum cholesterol and calcium determinations as well as cardiac and liver function tests should be performed throughout testosterone therapy.
- Testosterone-induced anabolic action enhances hypoglycaemia (hyperinsulinism). Instruct diabetic patient to report sweating, tremor, anxiety, diplopia, vertigo. Dosage adjustment of antidiabetic agent may be required.
- Be sensitive to the fact that the patient may find it embarrassing to initiate questions or report symptoms related to sexual organs and functions. Attention to such symptoms should not be delayed by hesitant reporting, since many signify overdosage.
- Instruct male patient to report priapism (sustained and often painful erections occurring especially in early replacement therapy), reduced ejaculatory volume, and gynaecomastia. The symptoms indicate necessity for temporary withdrawal or discontinuation of testosterone therapy.
- Instruct patient to notify physician promptly if pregnancy is suspected or planned. Masculinization of the foetus is most likely to occur if testosterone (androgen) therapy is provided during first semester of pregnancy.
- Observe the patient who is on concomitant anticoagulant treatment for signs of overdosage (e.g., ecchymoses, petechiae). Report promptly to physician; anticoagulant dose may need to be reduced.
- Prepubertal or adolescent males should be monitored by radiology throughout therapy to avoid precocious sexual development and premature epiphyseal closure. Skeletal stimulation may continue 6 months beyond termination of therapy.
- Alterations in clinical laboratory test values persist 2 to 3 weeks after drug discontinuation. Notify laboratory and pathologist that patient is on testosterone.

Diagnostic test interferences   Testosterone alters **glucose** tolerance tests; decreases **PBI, thyroxine-binding globulin concentration, creatinine** and **creatinine** excretion (lasting up to 2 weeks after therapy is discontinued), and alters response to **metyrapone test.** It suppresses **clotting factors II, V, VII, X; haematocrit,** increases uptake of **triiodothyronine** by RBC and excretion of **17-ketosteroids.** May increase or decrease **serum cholesterol.**

DRUG INTERACTIONS   *Testosterone*

PLUS	INTERACTIONS
Adrenal steroids, ACTH	Increased testosterone-induced oedema
Anticoagulants	Enhanced effect may necessitate reduced dose of anticoagulant
Antidiabetic agents	Additive hypoglycaemic effect; decreased doses of hypoglycaemic may be necessary
Oxyphenbutazone	Antiflammatory effects may be enhanced by testosterone (conflicting evidence)

Tetracosactrin

(Synacthen)

ACTIONS AND USES   Synthetic corticotrophin mainly used as a diagnostic agent.

Tetracycline

(Anchromycin, Deteclo, Economycin, Sustamycin,   *Antibiotic; tetracycline*
  Telrabid-Organon, Tetrachel, Tetrex)

ACTIONS AND USES   Broad-spectrum antimicrobial effective against a variety of gram-positive and gram-negative bacteria, certain *Mycoplasma*, *Rickettsiae*, protozoa. Believed to act by inhibiting phosphorylation and protein synthesis by susceptible microorganisms. Oral administration results in suppression of intestinal flora, therefore has been used in treatment of vitamin B malabsorption and steatorrhea.
    Used in treatment of acne, bronchitis, syphilis and other injections.

ROUTE AND DOSAGE   Oral: **Adults:** 1 to 2 g/day in divided doses. **Intramuscular:** Adults: 100 mg every 8–12 hours (4–6 hours in severe infections). **Intravenous:** Adult: 500 mg every 12 hours, maximum 2 g/day.

ABSORPTION AND FATE   Irregularly absorbed from GI tract. Peak levels reached in 2 to 4 hours; effective blood levels maintained for at least 6 hours. IM administration produces lower blood levels than oral administration, 20 to 66% protein bound. **Half-life:** 6 to 10 hours. Well distributed in tissues and body fluids; lower levels in spinal and joint fluids, and higher than plasma concentrations in bile. Excreted mainly in faeces and urine. Crosses placenta; enters breast milk.

CONTRAINDICATIONS AND PRECAUTIONS   Liver and renal impairment, hypersensitivity to tetracyclines, use during pregnancy, lactation, infancy and during period of tooth development (from the fourth foetal month to the child of 12 years; concomitant administration of potentially hepatotoxic drugs, and penicillins. **Cautious Use:** undernourished patients.

ADVERSE/SIDE EFFECTS   Nausea, anorexia, vomiting, diarrhoea, dizziness, thrombophlebitis at site of injection, fever, hypersensitivity reactions, photosensitivity, superimposed candidal growth (skin eruptions, gingivitis, stomatitis, pharyngitis, dysphagia, lingua nigra, anal pruritus, proctitis, vaginal discharge); hepatotoxicity, nephrotoxicity, blood dyscrasias; intracranial hypertension (pseudotumour cerebri): bulging fontanels, impaired vision, papilloedema, severe headache; permanent discoloration and inadequate calcification of deciduous teeth, enamel hypoplasia, onycholysis and discolouration of nails; fixed drug eruptions.

TETRACYCLINE (continued)
NURSING IMPLICATIONS

- Therapy should be designed on basis of culture studies.
- Check expiry date before administering drug. Renal injury has been attributed to administration of outdated tetracyclines.
- Tetracycline absorption is inhibited by iron, aluminium, calcium and magnesium. Therefore administer oral doses on an empty stomach (at least 1 hour before or 2 hours after eating).
- Avoid concurrent use of antacids; if necessary, however, administer 2 hours before or after tetracycline.
- If nausea, anorexia, and diarrhoea occur, they are controlled by administering drug with some food (exception: foods high in calcium, such as milk, interfere with absorption of tetracycline preparations) or by reducing drug dosage. Consult physician. If symptoms persist, drug should be discontinued.
- Deep IM injection into body of a large muscle is recommended. Inadvertent injection into subcutaneous or fat layer may result in painful local irritation; may be relieved by an ice pack.
- IV tetracycline is an irritant. Inspect IV site frequently to prevent extravasation. At particular risk are the very young (cannot communicate pain at site), the debilitated and the elderly (ageing causes loss of skin elasticity), thereby promoting leakage around the needle.
- Be alert for evidence of overgrowth of *nonsensitive organisms (superinfection)*. Inspect tongue regularly to note development of black, furry appearance. The incidence of infection by candida may be reduced by meticulous hygienic care of skin and mouth, and by allowing patient to wash perineal area several times a day, particularly after each bowel movement. If superinfection develops, drug is discontinued.
- It is important to distinguish between frequent stools resulting from local irritant effect of drug (usually occur early during therapy) and those due to superinfection, which require immediate discontinuation of therapy.
- Monitor fluid intake and output. Report oliguria or changes in intake−output ratio (patient can be taught to make rough estimates).
- Advise patient to avoid exposure to direct or artificial sunlight during use of tetracyclines. Certain hypersensitive persons develop a phototoxic reaction (exaggerated sunburn) precipitated by exposure to sun or ultraviolet light. Advise use of sun screen lotion (SPF above 12). At the first sign of skin discomfort, drug should be discontinued.
- Tetracycline may combine with calcium of developing teeth to cause yellow-grey-brownish discolouration. Its use during bone formation and tooth development periods (prenatally, neonatally, and in childhood) is generally avoided.
- The drug is generally administered for 24 to 72 hours after fever and other symptoms have subsided. Warn patient to discard unused tetracycline after therapy is completed.
- Solutions prepared for IM injection should be used within 24 hours. Initial reconstituted IV solutions are stable at room temperature for 12 hours, but when final dilution is made, they should be administered immediately.
- Tetracyclines decompose with age, with exposure to light, and when improperly

TETRACYCLINE (continued)

stored under conditions of extreme humidity and heat. The resulting product may be toxic.

Diagnostic test interferences   Possibility of false increases in **urinary catecholamines** (Hungert method) and false decreases in **urinary urobilinogen**. Parenteral tetracycline containing ascorbic acid may produce false-positive **urinary glucose** determinations by copper reduction methods (e.g., Benedict's and Clinitest) and false-negative values with glucose oxidase methods (e.g., Clinistix)

DRUG INTERACTIONS   *Tetracycline*

PLUS	INTERACTIONS
Antacids (aluminium, magnesium, calcium) ⎫ Iron preparations ⎬	Chelation and interference with tetracycline absorption
Anticoagulants (oral, and heparin)	Augmented anticoagulant effects
Penicillins	Possible decrease in bacterial action of penicillin
Sodium bicarbonate	Interference with tetracycline absorption

Theophylline

(Biophylline, Nuelin, Lasma, Pro-Vent, Slo-Phyllin, Theo-Dur, Theograd, Uniphyllin Continus)

Smooth muscle relaxant; bronchodilator; xanthine

ACTIONS AND USES   Methyl xanthine derivative with pharmacological actions qualitatively similar to those of other xanthines e.g., caffeine, theobromine; occurs naturally in tea. Relaxes, smooth muscle by direct action, particularly of bronchi and pulmonary vessels, and stimulates medullary respiratory centre with resulting increase in vital capacity. Also relaxes smooth muscles of biliary and GI tracts. Stimulates myocardium, thereby increasing force of contractions and cardiac output, and stimulates all levels of CNS, but to a lesser degree than caffeine. Produces mild diuresis by increasing renal blood flow and by inhibiting sodium and chloride reabsorption at proximal tubule.

Used for prophylaxis and symptomatic relief of bronchial asthma, as well as bronchospasm associated with chronic bronchitis and emphysema.

ROUTE AND DOSAGE   Theophylline: **Adults: Oral:** 125 to 250 mg, 3–4 times a day. Sustained-release forms: depends on the preparation. **Children: Oral:** 4 to 6 mg/kg every 6 hours.

ABSORPTION AND FATE   Rate of absorption depends on drug solubility. Oral solution and uncoated tablet are well absorbed from GI tract; peak blood levels in 1 to 2 hours. Absorption following sustained-release forms is variable and incomplete. Peak plasma levels occur in about 5 hours for sustained-release form but this varies with manufacturer. Rapidly distributed throughout extracellular fluid and tissues. About

THEOPHYLLINE (continued)

60% bound to plasma proteins. **Plasma elimination half-life**: approximately 7 to 9 hours in nonsmokers, 4 to 5 hours in smokers, and 2 to 9 hours in children and 15 to 58 in premature infants. Partially demethylated and oxidized in liver (individual variability in rate of metabolism). About 10% excreted unchanged in urine. Small amount excreted in faeces. Readily crosses placenta; appears in breast milk in high concentrations.

CONTRAINDICATIONS AND PRECAUTIONS Hypersensitivity to xanthines; coronary artery disease or angina pectoris when myocardial stimulation might be harmful; severe renal or liver impairment. Safe use during pregnancy and lactation and in women of childbearing potential not established. **Cautious Use**: children, compromised cardiac or circulatory function, hypertension, hyperthyroidism, peptic ulcer, prostatic hypertrophy, glaucoma, diabetes mellitus, in the elderly (particularly males) and neonates.

ADVERSE/SIDE EFFECTS These include: irritability, restlessness, insomnia, dizziness, headache, hyperexcitability, muscle twitching, drug-induced seizures, palpitation, tachycardia, extrasystoles, flushing, marked hypotension, circulatory failure, nausea, vomiting, anorexia, epigastric or abdominal pain, diarrhoea, activation of peptic ulcer, transient urinary frequency, albuminuria, kidney irritation, tachypnoea, respiratory arrest, fever, dehydration, possibility of increased urinary catecholamine excretion.

NURSING IMPLICATIONS

- Therapeutic theophylline plasma level ranges from 10 to 20 mcg/ml (a narrow therapeutic range). Levels exceeding 20 mcg/ml are associated with toxicity.
- Oral preparations should preferably be administered with a full glass of water and may be given after meals to minimize gastric irritation. Food, and antacids delay but do not reduce extent of absorption. Physician may prescribe an antacid if GI symptoms continue. Dosage reduction may also be indicated.
- Timing of dose is critically important. Be certain patient understands the food and drug relationships and the necessity to adhere to the proper intervals between doses.
- Once a-day administration provides patient convenience and increased compliance. However, such a schedule may not adequately control asthmatic patients, smokers, or children.
- In the neonate of a mother using this drug, slight tachycardia, jitteriness, and apnoea have been observed.
- If theophylline is given to a patient with severe cardiac disease, monitor for tachycardia. Conversely, keep in mind that theophylline toxicity may be masked in patients with tachycardia.
- Plasma clearance of xanthines may be reduced in patients with heart failure, renal or hepatic dysfunction, alcoholism, high fever. Dosage regulation must be closely monitored particularly in these patients.
- Monitor vital signs and fluid intake and output. Improvement in quality of pulse and respiration and diuresis are expected clinical effects.
- *Observe and report early signs of possible toxicity*: anorexia, nausea, vomiting, dizziness, shakiness, restlessness, abdominal discomfort, irritability, palpitation, tachycardia, marked hypotension, cardiac arrhythmias, seizures.

THEOPHYLLINE (continued)

- During early therapy, dizziness is a relatively common side effect in the elderly. Take necessary safety precautions and forewarn patient of this possibility.
- Urge patient to drink adequate fluids (at least 2,000 ml/day) to decrease viscosity of airway secretions.
- Warn patient to avoid self-dosing with OTC medications, especially cough suppressants. The physician may prescribe one for short periods, but unsupervised use may cause retention of secretions and CNS depression.
- Since theophylline is distributed into breast milk it may be advisable for the infant to be nursed just before mother takes the drug.
- Theophylline metabolism in the infant under 6 months and in prematures is prolonged as is the half-life, therefore close monitoring for side effects is especially crucial in this age-group.

Food–drug interactions

- Methylxanthines derivatives (coffee, tea, chocolate) can change theophylline metabolism.
- A low carbohydrate, high protein diet is said to increase theophylline elimination (shortens half-life) therefore interfering with dosing. Conversely, a high carbohydrate, low protein diet increases the half-life.

Smoking–drug interactions

- Cigarettes and marijuana-smoking induce hepatic microsomal enzyme activity, decreasing serum half-life and increasing body clearance of theophylline. This effect plus the narrow therapeutic range requires close monitoring of drug level in the heavy smoker who will need a larger dose for therapeutic effects. An increase of dosage from 50 to 100% is usual in heavy smokers.
- The heavy smoker may suffer less from drug side effects than nonsmokers because of increased theophylline metabolism.
- Chest physiotherapy (postural drainage with rapid percussion of thorax, instruction in coughing, training to prevent airway collapse during expiration, and improved diaphragmatic movement) is a necessary concomitant to adequate response to this drug. Consult physiotherapist or respiratory therapist.
- If patient has exacerbations of bronchial symptoms, exposure to unknown or unsuspected environmental allergens should be ruled out.
- Overdose with prolonged release preparation necessitates observing patient for a longer period of time than if conventional formulation had been ingested. Continued slow absorption leads to sustained high plasma concentrations for a prolonged period. Avoid discharge of the patient from medical supervision too soon.
- **Treatment of overdosage**   Induce vomiting with ipecacuanha syrup (gastric lavage if patient has had seizures); activated charcoal; cathartic. IV diazepam for convulsions. Maintain airway, oxygenation, and hydration, tepid sponging for hyperpyrexia. Monitor vital signs.

Patient-teaching points   Clarify or emphasize:

- ☐ Drug action and expected responses to drug.
- ☐ Dosage schedule: stress adherence to established regimen.

THEOPHYLLINE (continued)

- ☐ Food–drug and smoking–drug interactions.
- ☐ Adequate fluid intake.
- ☐ Humidified environment especially in winter months.
- ☐ Postural drainage (4 to 6 times daily).
- ☐ Planned physical conditioning programme.
- ☐ Avoidance of exposure to infection, chilling, environmental pollutants including smoke and sprays.
- ☐ Avoidance of smoking.
- ☐ Do not accept brand changes as tablet content differs.
- ☐ Maintenance of follow-up appointments.

Diagnostic test interferences   False-positive elevations of **serum uric acid** (Bittner or colourimetric methods). **Probenecid** may cause false high serum theophylline readings, and spectrophometric methods of determining **serum theophylline** are effected by a frusemide, phenylbutazone, probenecid, theobromine.

DRUG INTERACTIONS *Theophylline*_____

PLUS	INTERACTIONS
Adrenergics Allopurinol Cimetidine Frusemide Influenza virus vaccine	Excessive CNS stimulation especially in children
Macrolide antibiotics (e.g., erythromycin) Thiabendazole Troleandomycin	Increased serum concentrations of theophylline (increased pharmacological effects and risk of toxicity)
Antacids (aluminium and magnesium products) Anticoagulants, oral	Slowed absorption rate of theophylline (with high doses of theophylline): increased anticoagulant effect
Barbiturates (e.g., phenobarbitone)	Decreased therapeutic effects of theophylline
Beta-adrenergic blocking agents (e.g., propranolol)	Antagonistic effects: theophylline produces beta-adrenergic stimulation
Halothane	Cardiac arrhythmias, reduced therapeutic effects of lithium
Phenytoin	Increased theophylline clearance requiring larger than usual doses
Reserpine	Produces tachycardia
Skeletal muscle relaxants, nondepolarizing (e.g., pancuronium)	Reversal of neuromuscular blockade of skeletal muscle relaxants

Thiabendazole_____

(Mintezol)   *Anthelmintic; enzyme inhibitor*

THIABENDAZOLE (continued)

ACTIONS AND USES   Benzimadazole with vermicidal properties, structurally related to mebendazole.

Used in treatment of ascariasis (roundworm), strongyloidiasis (threadworm), cutaneous larva migrans (creeping eruption), and hookworm infestations. Used during invasive stage of trichinosis to relieve symptoms and for mixed helminthic infestations.

ROUTE AND DOSAGE   Oral: 25 mg/kg every 12 hrs for 3 days.

ABSORPTION AND FATE   Oral dose rapidly absorbed from GI tract (can also be absorbed from skin). Peak plasma concentration reached in 1 to 2 hours after dose. Metabolized almost completely with most of drug out of plasma within 8 hours; major excretion in first 24 hours. 48 hours after dose about 5% administered dose is recovered from faeces and about 90% from urine as glucuronide or sulphate conjugates.

CONTRAINDICATIONS AND PRECAUTIONS   Safe use during pregnancy and lactation not established. **Cautious Use:** hepatic or renal dysfunction, when vomiting can be dangerous, severe dehydration or malnutrition, anaemia, children weighing less than 15 kg.

ADVERSE/SIDE EFFECTS   These include: hypotension, bradycardia, anorexia, nausea, vomiting, epigastric distress, jaundice, cholestasis, parenchymal liver damage, diarrhoea, perianal rash, weariness, drowsiness, headache; rarely: tinnitus, abnormal sensation in eyes, blurred vision, zanthopsia, malodour of urine, crystalluria, haematuria, nephrotoxicity, enuresis, transient rise in cephalin flocculation and AST, transient leucopenia, hypersensitivity, hyperglycaemia, pruritus.

NURSING IMPLICATIONS

- If patient is anaemic, dehydrated, or malnourished, supportive treatment is indicated prior to start of thiabendazole therapy.
- Administer drug after meals. Tablets should be chewed before swallowing. Shake suspension well before pouring.
- Adverse/side effects generally occur 3 to 4 hours after administration, are mild and last for 2 to 8 hours. Incidence tends to be related to dose and duration of treatment.
- If hypersensitivity occurs, drug should be discontinued immediately. Symptoms: fever, facial flush, chills, conjunctival injection, skin rashes, erythema, multiforme (including Stevens-Johnson syndrome), which can be fatal.
- CNS side effects occur frequently and may prevent the patient from driving a car or engaging in activities requiring mental alertness. Warn patient of the possibility.
- *See mebendazole for additional Nursing Implications related to drug therapy of helminthic infestation.*

Thiamine hydrochloride ————————————————

Vitamin

THIAMINE HYDROCHLORIDE (continued)

ACTIONS AND USES   Water-soluble vitamin and member of B-complex group. Functions as an essential coenzyme in carbohydrate metabolism. Also has role in conversion of tryptophan to nicotinamide.

Used in treatment and prophylaxis of beriberi, to correct anorexia due to thiamine deficiency states. Therapy generally includes other members of vitamin B complex, since thiamine deficiency rarely occurs alone.

ROUTE AND DOSAGE   *Oral or IM*: 10–300 mg/day.

ABSORPTION AND FATE   Limited absorption following oral administration, as compared with IM injection, which is rapid and complete. Wide distribution to most body tissues, with highest concentrations in liver, brain, kidney, and heart. Minimal body storage. Excreted in urine as pyrimidine and, with excessive intake, as unchanged drug.

ADVERSE/SIDE EFFECTS   Feeling of warmth, weakness, urticaria, pruritus, sweating, nausea, restlessness, tightness of throat, angioneurotic oedema, cyanosis, pulmonary oedema, GI haemorrhage, cardiovascular collapse, anaphylaxis. Following rapid IV administration: slight fall in blood pressure.

NURSING IMPLICATIONS

- IM injections may be painful. Rotate sites and apply cold compresses to area if necessary for relief of discomfort.
- Careful recording of patient's dietary history is an essential part of vitamin replacement therapy. Collaborate with physician, dietitian, patient, and responsible family member in developing a diet teaching plan that can be sustained by patient.
- Therapeutic effectiveness is evaluated by improvement of clinical manifestations of thiamine deficiency: anorexia, gastric distress, depression, irritability, insomnia, palpitation, tachycardia, loss of memory, paraesthesias, muscle weakness and pain, elevated blood pyruvic acid level (diagnostic test for thiamine deficiency), elevated lactic acid level. Severe deficiency: ophthalmoplegia, polyneuropathy, muscle wasting ('dry' beriberi) oedema, serous effusions, congestive heart failure ('wet' beriberi).
- Body requirement of thiamine is directly proportional to carbohydrate intake and metabolic rate; thus, requirement increases when diet consists predominantly of carbohydrates. Total absence of dietary thiamine can produce a deficiency state in about 3 weeks.
- Rich thiamine food sources: yeast, pork, beef, liver, wheat and other whole grains, fresh vegetables, especially peas and dried beans.
- Preserved in tight, light-resistant, nonmetallic containers. Thiamine is unstable in alkaline solutions (e.g., solutions of acetates, barbiturates, bicarbonates, carbonates, citrates) and neutral solutions.

Thiethylperazine maleate

(Torecan)   *Antiemetic; phenothiazine*

THIETHYLPERAZINE MALEATE (continued)

ACTIONS AND USES   Piperazine phenothiazine derivative with contraindications, precautions, and toxic effects similar to those of chlorpromazine (q.v.). Reported to have higher ratio of antiemetic action to tranquillizing action than other phenothiazines. Acts directly on chemoreceptor trigger zone as well as the vomiting centre.

Used to control nausea and vomiting, and for the treatment of vertigo.

ROUTE AND DOSAGE   **Oral:** 10 mg two to three times a day. **Rectal suppository:** 6.5 mg twice a day. **Intramuscular:** 6.5 mg as required.

ABSORPTION AND FATE   Onset of effects in less than 1 hour following oral or rectal administration and within 30 minutes following IM injection. *See chlorpromazine.*

CONTRAINDICATIONS AND PRECAUTIONS   Hypersensitivity to phenothiazines, CNS depression or comatose states, pregnancy, IV administration. Safe use in children under age 1.5 in nursing mothers, or following intracardiac or intracranial surgery not established. **Cautious Use:** renal or hepatic disease. *See also chlorpromazine.*

ADVERSE/SIDE EFFECTS   Drowsiness, dizziness, headache, dry mouth and nose, blurred vision, tinnitus, restlessness, fever, orthostatic hypotension. Occasionally: extrapyramidal symptoms including convulsions; sialorrhoea with altered taste sensations, cholestatic jaundice. *See chlorpromazine.*

NURSING IMPLICATIONS
- Examine parenteral solution and administer only if it is clear and colourless.
- Stored at room temperature, away from heat, in light-resistant containers. Suppositories should be stored below 77°F.
- *See chlorpromazine.*

Thioguanine ———————————————————

(Lanvis)   *Antineoplastic; antimetabolite*

ACTIONS AND USES   Antimetabolite and purine antagonist with immunosuppressive activity. Qualitatively and quantitatively similar to mercaptopurine (q.v.). A highly toxic drug with a low therapeutic index; therapeutic response is normally accompanied by evidence of toxicity. Delays myelosuppression; has potential mutagenic and carcinogenic properties. Cross-resistance exists between mercaptopurine and thioguanine. *For Contraindications and Adverse/Side Effects, see mercaptopurine.*

Used in combination witha other antineoplastics for remission induction in acute myelogenous leukaemia and as treatment of chronic myelogenous leukaemia. Has little advantage over mercaptopurine.

ROUTE AND DOSAGE   Oral dosage depends on clinical and haematological responses and is highly individualized.

THIOGUANINE (continued)

ABSORPTION AND FATE   Partially (30%) absorbed from GI tract, with maximum blood levels achieved in 10 to 12 hours. Rapidly detoxified in liver. **Biphasic half-life**: initial, 15 minutes; terminal, 11 hours; excreted in faeces and urine as metabolites. Toxicity is not reduced by hemodialysis.

NURSING IMPLICATIONS

- Unlike mercaptopurine, thioguanine dose schedule may be maintained during concomitant administration of allopurinol.
- Blood counts are determined weekly; monitor reports as indicators for adaptations in nursing and drug regimens.
- Patient receiving this drug experiences an increased incidence of infections, and possibly haemorrhage complications. Therapy should be discontinued at first sign of altered blood cell counts.
- Maintenance doses are continued throughout remissions.
- Monitor fluid intake and output ratio and report oliguria.
- Observe patient's skin and sclera for jaundice. It is thought to be a reversible clinical sign, but it should be reported promptly as a symptom of toxicity; drug will be discontinued promptly.
- Expect that the leucocyte count descent may be slow over a period of 2 to 4 weeks. Treatment is interrupted if there is a rapid fall within a few days.
- Contraceptive measures should be used during therapy with this drug.
- Because there is no known antagonist to thioguanine, prompt discontinuation of the drug is essential in avoiding irreversible myelosuppression when toxicity develops.
- Store drug in airtight containers at temperature 15° to 30°C (59° to 86°F).
- *See mercaptopurine.*

Thiopentone sodium

(Intraval sodium)
*Anaesthetic; sedative/hypnotic;
barbiturate*

ACTIONS AND USES   Ultra-short-acting barbiturate. CNS depressant action produces anaesthesia, without analgesia, and with insignificant effects at myoneural junctions.

Used to induce hypnosis and anaesthesia prior to or as supplement to other anaesthetic agents, or as sole agent for brief (15-minute) operative procedures.

ROUTE AND DOSAGE   Intravenous: Highly individualized by titration against patient's requirements as governed by age, sex, and body weight, preexisting disease, premedication, concurrent nitrous oxide administration.

ABSORPTION AND FATE   Hypnotic action within 30 to 40 seconds following IV administration. Absorption from rectum is unpredictable, with onset of action in 8 to 10 minutes and duration of about 1 hour. With repeated doses, fatty tissue acts as

THIOPENTONE SODIUM (continued)

reservoir (concentrations 6 to 12 times that of plasma), from which slow release of drug prolongs anaesthesia. Metabolized in liver. **Half-life:** 11.5 hours (increases with age, and during pregnancy). Crosses placenta.

CONTRAINDICATIONS AND PRECAUTIONS Absolute contraindications; hypersensitivity to barbiturates, absence of suitable veins for IV administration, status asthmaticus, acute intermittent or other hepatic porphyrias. **Cautious Use:** severe cardiovascular disease, hypotension or shock, conditions that may potentiate or prolong hypnotic effect (excessive premedication, Addison's disease, hepatic or renal dysfunction, myxoedema, increased BUN, severe anaemia, increased intracranial pressure, asthma, myasthenia gravis).

ADVERSE/SIDE EFFECTS Respiratory and myocardial depression, cardiac arrhythmias, retrograde amnesia, prolonged somnolence and recovery, sneezing, coughing, bronchospasm, laryngospasm, shivering, muscle irritability, hypersensitivity reactions, pain, neurosis, neuritis, thrombosis, and sloughing at site of IV extravasation, anaphylaxis (rare). *See also phenobarbitone.*

NURSING IMPLICATIONS

- Solution should be freshly prepared and used promptly. If a precipitate is present, discard solution. Unused portions should be discarded within 24 hours.
- Resuscitation equipment, endotracheal tube, suction, and oxygen should be readily available for treatment of respiratory depression.
- Shivering or twitching muscles sometimes progressing to localized or generalized tremors may result from increased sensitivity to cold or from pain. Control environment and provide additional external heat, if necessary.
- Monitor for signs of pain (e.g., increased pulse, restlessness). Administer prescribed analgesic before pain is intense.
- *See phenobarbitone.*

Thioridazine

(Melleril)

Antipsychotic; neuroleptic; phenothiazine

ACTIONS AND USES Piperidine phenothiazine with actions, uses, limitations and interactions similar to those of chlorpromazine (q.v.).

ROUTE AND DOSAGE Oral: Adults: *Psychotic manifestations*: 150–600 mg/day in divided doses maximum 800 mg daily for up to 4 weeks. *Moderate to severe nonpsychotic emotional disturbance*: 75 to 200 mg/day. **Elderly:** *initial*: 10 mg three times daily; increments up to 200 mg/day if needed and tolerated. Recommended maximum single dose: 100 mg. **Children** (2–5 yr): 1 mg/kg/day; **(5–12 yrs):** 75–150 mg/day (severe cases 300 mg/daily).

THIORIDAZINE (continued)
NURSING IMPLICATIONS
- Periodic blood and hepatic function tests are advised during therapy.
- May turn urine pink-red to reddish brown colour.
- Preserved in tightly covered, light-resistant containers at temperature between 15° and 30°C (59° and 86°F), unless otherwise indicated by the manufacturer.
- *See chlorpromazine.*

Thiotepa

Antineoplastic; alkylating agent

ACTIONS AND USES   Ethylenimine cell cycle nonspecific alkylating agent that selectively reacts with DNA phosphate groups to produce chromosome cross-linkage and consequent blocking of nucleoprotein synthesis. Nonvesicant, highly toxic haematopoietic agent with a low therapeutic index. Myelosuppression is cumulative and unpredictable, and may be delayed. Has some immunosuppressive activity. Like all alkylating agents thiotepa is carcinogenic, and potentially mutagenic.

Used occasionally in the treatment of breast cancer and intracavity for the treatment of bladder cancer and neoplastic effusions.

ROUTE AND DOSAGE   **Intracavitary**: 10–30 mg in 20–60 mg water for injection. (usually through same tubing used for parencentesis) given at intervals of at least 1 week. **Intravesicular**: 60 mg in 60 ml distilled water instilled into bladder by catheter; to be retained 2 hours. Maintenance: once a week for 4 weeks, then once monthly.

ABSORPTION AND FATE   Rapidly cleared from plasma following intravenous administration. Slow onset of action, with therapeutic response becoming increasingly evident over period of several weeks. Slowly bound to tissues; significant amounts remain in blood 72 hours after IV administration. Extensively metabolized. About 60% of IV dose eliminated in urine within 24 to 72 hours.

CONTRAINDICATIONS AND PRECAUTIONS   Hypersensitivity to drug; acute leukaemia, pregnancy. **Cautious Use** (if at all): chronic lymphocytic leukaemia, myelosuppression produced by radiation, with other antineoplastics; bone marrow invasion by tumour cells, impaired renal or hepatic function.

ADVERSE/SIDE EFFECTS   These include: anorexia, nausea, vomiting, stomatitis, ulceration of intestinal mucosa, leucopenia, thrombocytopenia, anaemia, pancytopenia, amenorrhoea, interference with spermatogenesis, headache, febrile reactions, pain and weeping of injection site, hyperuricaemia, alopecia (rare), slowed or lessened response in heavily irradiated area, sensation of throat tightness. Reported with intravesical administration: lower abdominal pain, haematuria, haemorrhagic chemical cystitis, vesical irritability.

THIOTEPA (continued)
NURSING IMPLICATIONS

- Used only under constant supervision by physicians experienced in therapy with cytotoxic agents.
- Reconstitute with sterile water for injection.
- Avoid exposure of skin and respiratory tract to particles of thiotepa during solution preparation.
- Following reconstitution, solution may be clear to slightly opaque. If markedly opaque or contains a precipitate do not use.
- Powder for injection and reconstituted solutions should be stored in refrigerator at 2° to 8°C (35° to 46°F) and protected from light. Reconstituted solutions are stable for 5 days under refrigeration.
- Most patients will manifest some evidence of toxicity; therefore close monitoring is essential.
- Because of cumulative effects, maximum myelosuppression may be delayed 3 or 4 weeks after termination of therapy. Warn patient to report onset of fever, bleeding, a cold or illness, no matter how mild; medical supervision may be necessary.
- **Treatment of bladder tumour**   Patient is dehydrated 8 to 12 hours prior to treatment; 60 mg in 60 ml distilled water are instilled into bladder by catheter to be retained for 2 hours (if patient cannot retain 60 ml solution, 30 ml dilution is used); if desired, patient is repositioned every 15 minutes for maximal area contact. Usual course of treatment is once a week for 4 weeks; repeated beyond this with caution, because bone marrow depression may increase.
- *See mustine.*

Drug interactions   Thiotepa increases pharmacological and toxic effects of **succinylcholine** by decreasing pseudocholinesterase levels.

Thymoxamine

(Opilon)

ACTIONS AND USES   Peripheral vasodilator used in the treatment of Raynaud's syndrome.

ROUTE AND DOSAGE   Oral: Adult: 40 mg four times a day. IV: 100 mcg/kg/four times a day, continued by oral therapy. **Intraarterial injection**: 5 mg.
   For further information: *see nicotinic acid.*

Thyroxine sodium

(Eltroxin)   *Hormone, thyroid*

THYROXINE SODIUM *(continued)*

ACTIONS AND USES Synthetically prepared monosodium salt and levo isomer of thyroxine, with similar actions and uses: 0.1 mg is equivalent to 65 mg desiccated thyroid and is about 600 times more potent.

Used as specific replacement therapy for diminished or absent thyroid function resulting from primary or secondary atrophy of gland, surgery, excessive radiation or antithyroid drugs, congenital defect.

ROUTE AND DOSAGE All doses individualized and initiated cautiously according to age, physical condition, severity, and duration of hypothyroidism. **Oral** (thyroid replacement): **Adults:** *Initial:* not more than 100 mcg/day (**elderly patient** 25–50 mcg) increased by 25–50 mcg at 2–4 weekly intervals. *Usual maintenance dose:* 100–200 mcg/day. **Infants:** 10 mcg/kg, maximum 50 mcg/day, increased to 100 mcg/day at 5 yrs and to the adult dose by 12 yrs.

ABSORPTION AND FATE Following absorption, binds to plasma protein. **Circulation half-life:** 6 or 7 days. Distributed widely; gradually released into tissue cells, where it causes increased metabolic rate, usually after 12 to 48 hours. One mg of levothyroxine increases heat production about 1,000 calories.

CONTRAINDICATIONS AND PRECAUTIONS Thyrotoxicosis, acute myocardial infarction uncomplicated by hypothyroidism, cardiovascular disease, morphologic hypogonadism, nephrosis, uncorrected hypoadrenalism. **Cautious Use:** angina pectoris, hypertension, elderly patients who may have occult cardiac disease, renal insufficiency, pregnancy, concomitant administration of catecholamines, diabetes mellitus, hyperthyroidism (history of), malabsorption states.

ADVERSE/SIDE EFFECTS Chronic overdosage: hyperthyroidism. **Massive overdosage:** thyroid storm: high temperature (as high as 106°F: 41°C) tachycardia, vomiting, shock, coma. **Overdosage (thyrotoxicosis):** staring expression in eyes, congestive heart failure, angina, cardiac arrhythmias, palpitation, tachycardia; weight loss, tremors, headache, nervousness, fever, diarrhoea or abdominal cramps, insomnia, warm and moist skin, heat intolerance, leg cramps, menstrual irregularities, shock, changes in appetite, hyperglycaemia (usually offset by increased tissue oxidation of sugar).

NURSING IMPLICATIONS

- Administered as single dose, preferably before breakfast.
- During institution of treatment, observe patient carefully for untoward reactions such as angina, palpitation, cardiac pain.
- Generally dosage is initiated at low level and systematically increased in small increment to desired maintenance dose.
- Be alert for symptoms of overdosage (*see Adverse/Side Effects*) that may occur 1 to 3 weeks after therapy is started. If they develop, treatment should be interruptd for several days and restarted with reduced dosage.
- Hypothyroidism is common in the elderly. Women generally require less thyroxine replacement than men; however, if replacement dosage is required the regimen is: initial: 25 mcg/daily with gradual increments, as indicated. Monitor response until regimen is stabilized (e.g., thyroid function tests, weight changes) to prevent

THYROXINE SODIUM (continued)

iatrogenic hyperthyroidism. In drug-induced hyperthyroidism, there may also be increased bone loss. Such a patient is vulnerable to pathological fractures. If back or chest (rib) pain is experienced, the physician should be consulted.

- Toxic effects of thyroid develop slowly and disappear gradually. T_4 effects require up to 3 to 6 weeks to dissipate; T_3 effects last 6 to 14 days after drug withdrawal.
- If patient has taken hormone during pregnancy, dose is frequently discontinued in the postpartum period, with evaluation of thyroid function 6 weeks later.
- Serial height measurement of the juvenile being treated with thyroid is an important means of monitoring influence of thyroid on growth. Too rapid growth rate results in premature epiphyseal closure. Urge parent to keep accurate record of height measurements for reporting to physician.
- Useful guides of thyroid therapy in children include sleeping pulse and basal morning temperature.
- Prepare parent and juvenile hypothyroid for a dramatic response to therapy: excessive shedding of hair, increased assertiveness of previously passive child, initial rapid weight loss and rapid catch-up growth. Symptoms usually disappear with continued therapy.
- Earliest clinical response to thyroid (adult) is diuresis, accompanied by loss of weight and puffiness, followed by sense of well-being, increased pulse rate, increased pulse pressure, increased appetite, increased psychomotor activity, loss of constipation, normalization of skin texture and hair, and increased T_3 and T_4 serum levels.
- Instruct patient to adhere to established dosage regimen: patient should not double, decrease or omit doses and the dose intervals should not be changed without approval of the physician.
- In patient-teaching, emphasize that replacement therapy for hypothyroidism is life-long; therefore, continued follow-up surveillance is important. Regular yearly appointments for evaluation are recommended.
- Keep in mind that these patients tend to discontinue their medication when they begin to feel well.
- Thyroid hormone is no longer used as a therapeutic agent for treatment of obesity, reproductive disorders (e.g., habitual abortion), breast cancer, and depression. The patient should not be taking thyroid at home without medical supervision.
- Pulse rate is an important clue to drug effectiveness. Count pulse before each dose during period of dosage adjustment. Consult physician if rate is 100 or more, or if there has been a marked change in rate or rhythm.
- When patient is euthyroid, teach to take own pulse and to record it periodically. If rate begins to increase or if rhythm changes, patient should notify physician.
- Thyroxine may aggravate severity of previously obscured symptoms of diabetes mellitus, Addison's disease, or diabetes insipidus. Therapeutic measures directed at these disorders may require adjustment.
- There is great urgency in achieving full thyroid replacement in infants or children because of the critical importance of the hormone in sustaining growth and development; therefore doses are generally higher than adult doses.
- Therapy with thyroxine results in euthyroidism, and a return to normal of laboratory values.

THYROXINE SODIUM (continued)

■ Store in dark bottle to minimize spontaneous deiodination. Keep desiccated thyroid dry. Potency in this form reportedly persists for as long as 17 years.

Diagnostic test interferences Thyroid increases basal metabolic rate; may increase blood glucose levels, creatine phosphokinase, AST, LDH, PBI. It may decrease serum uric acid, cholesterol, thyroid stimulating hormone (TSH), I-131 uptake. Many medications may produce false results in thyroid function tests.

DRUG INTERACTIONS *Thyroxine*

PLUS	INTERACTIONS
Antidiabetics (coumarins, warfarin)	Anticoagulant effect may be potentiated (reduction of anticoagulant may be necessary)
Cholestyramine	May decrease thyroid action by interfering with absorption
Digitalis glycosides adrenaline and other catecholamines	Thyroxine may increase toxic effects of the glycosides Increased risk of coronary insufficiency
Oestrogens	Increases serum thyroxine binding globulin (TBg). Increased dose of thyroid may be necessary
Insulin and oral hypoglyaemics	Increases need for antidiabetic agent
Sympathomimetic agents ⎱ Tricyclic antidepressants ⎰	May increase effects of these medications and of thyroxine

Tiaprofenic acid

(Surgam)

ACTIONS AND USES NSAID used to treat rheumatic disease.

ROUTE AND DOSAGE Oral: Adult: up to 600mg 2–3 times a day in divided doses. For further information: *see aspirin.*

Ticarcillin disodium

(Ticar) *Penicillin*

ACTIONS AND USES Antibiotic used to treat infections due to *pseudomonas* and *proteus* spp.

ROUTE AND DOSAGE IV infusion: Adult: 15–20 g/day in divided doses over

TICARCILLIN DISODIUM (continued)

30–40 min. **Child**: 200–300 mg/kg/day in divided doses. *Urinary tract infection*: **IM**: 3–4 g/day in divided doses. **Child**: 50–100 mg/kg/day in divided doses.
For further information: *see penicillin G.*

Timolol maleate————————————————

(Blocadren, Betim, Timoptol)

Antihypertensive; beta-adrenergic blocking agent (nonselective); antiglaucoma agent

ACTIONS AND USES   Nonselective beta-adrenergic blocking agent similar to propranolol (q.v.) in actions, but approximately 5 to 10 times as potent. Like propranolol, demonstrates antihypertensive, antiarrhythmic, and antianginal properties, and suppresses plasma renin activity. Unlike propranolol, appears to lack quinidine-like (local anaesthetic or membrane-stabilizing) effects. When applied topically lowers elevated and normal intraocular pressure by unknown mechanism, but presumed to act by decreasing formation of aqueous humour and possibly by increasing outflow. In contrast to pilocarpine and other miotics, timolol does not constrict pupil and therefore does not cause night blindness, nor does it affect accommodation or visual acuity. Reportedly as effective as pilocarpine or epinephrine in reducing intraocular pressure and produces fewer and less severe adverse effects.

Used topically (ophthalmic solution) to reduce elevated intraocular pressure in chronic, open-angle glaucoma, aphakic glaucoma, secondary glaucoma, and ocular hypertension. May be used alone or in conjunction with pilocarpine or a carbonic anhydrase inhibitor such as acetazolamide. Oral preparation is used alone or in combination with a thiazide diuretic to prevent reinfarction after MI, and to treat mild hypertension, with a thiazide diuretic to prevent reinfarction after MI, and to treat mild hypertension, prophylactic management of stable, uncomplicated angina pectoris and migraine headaches.

ROUTE AND DOSAGE   Topical (ophthalmic solution): *Glaucoma*: **Adult**: 1 drop of 0.25% solution twice a day, if no response 0.5% solution 1 drop twice a day. **Oral**: **Adult**: *hypertension*: *initial* 5 mg twice a day to maximum of 60 mg/day. *Angina*: *initial* 5 mg, 2–3 times a day. *Maintenance* 15–45 mg/day. *Migraine prophylaxis*: 10–20 mg/day. *Prophylaxis after infarction*: *initial* 5 mg twice a day increased to 10 mg after 2 days, starting 7–28 days postinfarction.

ABSORPTION AND FATE   Reduction in intraocular pressure usually occurs in 15 to 30 minutes following instillation into eye. Effects peak in 1 to 2 hours; duration of effects about 24 hours. Over 98% absorbed following oral administration. Hepatic metabolism. **Peak action** in ½ to 3 hours; **duration**: approximately 4 hours. **Half-life**: 4

TIMOLOL MALEATE (continued)

hours (prolonged with renal failure); 10% protein bound. About 15% excreted in urine as unchanged drug. Not dialyzable.

CONTRAINDICATIONS AND PRECAUTIONS Hypersensitivity to timolol or to any components in product; chronic obstructive airways disease, bronchial asthma, heart failure. Safe use during pregnancy, lactation and in children not established. **Cautious Use**: bronchitis, patients subject to bronchospasms; sinus bradycardia, greater than first degree heart block, cardiogenic shock, right ventricular failure secondary to pulmonary hypertension, myasthenia gravis; concomitant use with adrenergic augmenting psychotropic drugs, e.g., MAO inhibitors.

ADVERSE/SIDE EFFECTS **Topical**: fatigue, lethargy, weakness, somnolence, anxiety, headache, dizziness, confusion, psychic dissociation, depression, anorexia, dyspepsia, nausea. **Hypersensitivity**: rash, urticaria. **Ophthalmic**: eye irritation including conjunctivitis, blepharitis, keratitis, blurred vision (rare), superficial punctate keratopathy. **Systemic**: palpitation, bradycardia, hypotension, syncope, AV conduction disturbances, congestive heart failure, difficulty in breathing, bronchospasm, hypoglycaemia, hypokalaemia, aggravation of peripheral vascular insufficiency, brown discolouration of finger and toe nails.

NURSING IMPLICATIONS
- Tablet may be crushed before administration and taken with fluid of patient's choice.
- Check pulse before administering timolol, topical or oral.
- Inform patient that drug may cause slight reduction in resting heart rate. Patient should be informed about usual pulse rate and should be instructed to report significant changes in pulse rate and rhythm.
- Monitor pulse rate and blood pressure at regular intervals in patients with severe heart disease.
- Apply gentle pressure to lacrimal sac during and immediately following drug instillation, for about 1 minute, to lessen possibility of systemic absorption. *See Index: Drug administration: eye drops.*
- Intraocular pressure must be monitored throughout ophthalmic therapy. Normal IOP is in the range of 12 to 20 mm Hg. Readings may vary during the day; pressure tends to be higher at time or waking and lowest in the evening.
- Because of diurnal variations in intraocular pressure, patients on once a day drug dosage should have measurements taken at various times during the day.
- When drug is instilled in one eye only, intraocular pressure in opposite eye may be reduced slightly also.
- Emphasize importance of adhering to prescribed regimen and of keeping follow-up appointments.
- Advise patient to report difficulty in breathing promptly. Drug withdrawal may be indicated.
- Some patients develop tolerance during long-term therapy.
- *Systemic use: see propranolol, nursing implications.*

TIMOLOL MALEATE (continued)
- Store between 15° and 30°C (59° and 86°F) in tight, light-resistant container unless otherwise directed by manufacturer.
- *See propranolol.*

Tinidazole ──────────────────

(Fasigyn)

ACTIONS AND USES   Antimicrobial used to treat anaerobic and protozoal infections.

ROUTE AND DOSAGE   Oral: **Adult:** *initial* 2 g followed by 1 g/day as a single or divided dose, for 5–6 days. **IV:** 800 mg/day.
  For further information: *see metronidazole.*

Tobramycin sulphate ──────────────────

(Nebcin, Tobralex)   *Antibiotic; aminoglycoside*

ACTIONS AND USES   Aminoglycoside antibiotic derived from *Streptomyces tenebrarius*. Closely related to gentamicin (q.v.) in spectrum of antibacterial activity and pharmacological properties. Reportedly causes less nephrotoxicity.
  Used in treatment of severe infections caused by susceptible organisms.

ROUTE AND DOSAGE   **Intramuscular, intravenous: Adults, children, and older infants with normal renal function:** 3–5 mg/kg/day in 3 equal doses every 8 hours. **Infant (up to 1 week):** 2 mg/kg twice a day; **(over one week):** 2–2.5 mg/kg every 8 hrs. **Topical** (ophthalmic): 1 or 2 drops in affected eye every 4 hours. If infection is severe: 2 drops in the infected eye two hourly.

ABSORPTION AND FATE   Following IM injection, peak serum concentrations in 30 to 90 minutes in adults and 1 to 2 hours in children. Measurable levels persist up to 8 hours. Serum concentrations higher and more prolonged in patients with reduced kidney function and infants. Widely distributed to body tissues and fluids; significant levels in CSF usually not achieved. Minimal protein binding. **Half-life:** 2 hours. Not appreciably metabolized in body. Eliminated by glomerular filtration; up to 93% of dose is excreted in urine in 24 hours. Crosses placenta.

CONTRAINDICATIONS AND PRECAUTIONS   History of hypersensitivity to tobramycin and other aminoglycoside antibiotics, concurrent use with other neurotoxic and/ or nephrotoxic agents or potent diuretics. Safe use during pregnancy and in nursing

TOBRAMYCIN SULPHATE (continued)

mothers not established. **Cautious Use**: impaired renal function, premature and neonatal infants. *See also gentamicin.*

ADVERSE/SIDE EFFECTS   Neurotoxicity (including ototoxicity), nephrotoxicity, increased SGOT (AST), and SGPT (ALT), LDH, increased serum bilirubin; anaemia, granulocytopenia, thrombocytopenia, fever, rash, pruritis, urticaria, nausea, vomiting, headache, lethargy, superinfections. **Ophthalmic**: burning, stinging of eye after drug instillation; lid itching and oedema. Hypersensitivity. *See also gentamicin.*

NURSING IMPLICATIONS

- Weigh patient before treatment for calculation of dosage (by physician).
- Bacterial culture and sensitivity tests are advised prior to and during tobramycin therapy.
- As with other aminoglycosides, patient receiving tobramycin must remain under close clinical observation because of the high potential for toxicity, even in conventional doses.
- Monitoring of serum drug concentrations is advised to minimize rise of toxicity. Prolonged serum concentrations above 12 mcg/ml are not recommended.
- Renal, auditory, and vestibular functions should also be closely monitored, particularly in patients with known or suspected renal impairment and patients receiving high doses.
- Drug induced auditory changes are irreversible (may be partial or total); usually bilateral. In cochlear damage, the patient may be asymptomatic and partial or bilateral deafness may continue to develop even after therapy has been discontinued.

Ophthalmic

- Prolonged use may encourage development of superinfection with nonsusceptible organisms including fungi.
- Wash hands before and after instillation of medication. (*See Index: Drug administration: eye drops.*)
- Apply gentle finger pressure to lacrimal sac for 1 minute after drug has been instilled.
- Overdosage: increased lacrimation, keratitis, oedema and itching of eye lids. Report symptoms to physician.

- Advise patient to report symptoms of superinfections (black furry tongue or white patches on oral membranes, stomatitis, malodourous vaginal discharge, anorectal itching and irritation). Prompt treatment with an antibiotic or antifungal medication may be necessary.
- Monitor patient with neuromuscular disorder (e.g., myasthenia gravis) for muscular weakness. Observe ambulation and assist, if necessary.
- Evidence of impaired renal function (increasing BUN or NPN, increasing creatinine, cylinduria, proteinuria, cells, oliguria), auditory toxicity (hearing impairment, tinnitus), or vestibular damage (dizziness, vertigo, nystagmus, ataxia) indicates need for discontinuation of drug or dosage adjustment.
- Monitor fluid intake and output. Report oliguria, changes in intake−output ratio, and cloudy or frothy urine (may indicate proteinuria). The elderly patient is especially

TOBRAMYCIN SULPHATE (continued)

susceptible to renal toxicity. Patient is usually kept well hydrated to prevent chemical irritation in renal tubules. Consult physician.

- Therapy is generally continued for 7 to 10 days. Complicated infection may require longer course of therapy, in which case close monitoring of renal, auditory, and vestibular function and serum drug concentrations is essential.
- Tobramycin should not be mixed with other drugs.
- *See gentamicin.*

Tocainide hydrochloride ─────────────────────

(Tonocard)

Antiarrhythmic; anaesthetic (local)

ACTIONS AND USES   Antiarrhythmic agent and analogue of lignocaine (q.v.), with similar electrophysiological characteristics and haemodynamic properties. Effective orally. Suppresses PVCs and may have particular use in arrhythmias associated with a prolonged QT interval that do not respond to quinidine-like antiarrhythmics.

Used in treatment of ventricular arrhythmia.

ROUTE AND DOSAGE   **Oral**: 1.2 g/day in 2–3 divided doses. Maximum 2.4 g/day. **Intravenous**: 500–750 mg over 15–30-minute period; directly followed by 600–800-mg oral dose.

ABSORPTION AND FATE   Absorption nearly complete from GI tract followed by 95 to 100% bioavailability. Peak plasma levels in approximately 1 hour (range ½ to 3 hours) oral, in 10 to 15 minutes IV. Metabolized in liver; about 10 to 20% protein bound. **Elimination half-life**: 10 to 17 hours (increases in renal failure to 22 hours and in hepatic dysfunction to 27 hours). About 35 to 40% excreted unchanged by kidneys; remainder excreted as metabolites. Renal elimination of unchanged drug increased by alkalynization of urine.

CONTRAINDICATIONS AND PRECAUTIONS   Hypersensitivity to tocainide and to local anaesthetics of the amide type, second- or third-degree AV block (in absence of artificial ventricular pacemaker), hypokalaemia, myasthemia gravis, pregnancy, and nursing mothers. Safe use in children not established. **Cautious Use**: during multiple drug therapy, known heart failure patient with minimum cardiac reserve, renal or hepatic disease.

ADVERSE/SIDE EFFECTS   These include: exacerbation of arrhythmias, complete heart block, sinus node slowing (in patient with preexisting conduction system disease); hypotension, palpitation, bradycardia, chest pain, left ventricular failure, PVCs, hot flashes, nausea, vomiting, anorexia, abdominal pain, diarrhoea, tremors, dizziness, lightheadedness, visual disturbances, vertigo, tinnitus hearing loss, ataxia, paraesthesia; (rare): agitation, memory loss, confusion, convulsions, pulmonary fibrosis, oedema, embolism and alveolitis; pneumonia, dyspnoea, alopecia, sweating, night

TOCAINIDE HYDROCHLORIDE (continued)

sweats, tiredness/drowsiness, sleepiness, hot/cold feelings, haematological disorders (leucopenia, agranulocytosis, thrombocytopenia, hypoplastic anaemia), lupus, claudication, cold extremities, leg cramps, urinary retention, polyuria, metallic or menthol taste, hiccoughs.

NURSING IMPLICATIONS

- Prior to beginning treatment, patient should be evaluated by ECG and clinically. Periodic reevaluations during treatment produces essential data to support decision to continue therapy.
- Administer with food to decrease GI distress. This also protects against high peak concentration and toxicity because absorption rate is slowed. Bioavailability is not affected by food.
- When steady-state drug level is attained (usually in about 70 hours), plasma level monitoring is recommended, especially if patient has renal or hepatic dysfunction.
- Onset of tremors is a good clinical indicator that maximum dose is being approached.
- Blood pressure should be checked before administration of drug. It may be slightly increased within 5 minutes of IV tocainide but usually returns to normal in about 15 minutes. If patient is hypotensive, question continuing drug administration.
- The patient and/or primary care-giver should fully understand what an irregular pulse signifies and how often it should be checked.
- Since drug may cause dizziness and drowsiness, warn patient to use caution while driving a car until drug response is known.
- Symptomatic bradycardia (pulse below 60, lightheadedness, syncope) should be reported. Dose adjustment or discontinuation will follow.
- In patient with kidney or hepatic dysfunction, drug elimination is significantly decreased.
- Monitor fluid intake–output ratio and pattern. Instruct patient on self-care to report to physician if symptoms of renal dysfunction occur.
- Advise patient to report promptly: chest pain, exertional dyspnoea, wheezing, and cough even if no fever is present. Pulmonary fibrosis is a serious side effect and should be ruled out by chest radiograph or pulmonary function tests. Drug is discontinued if pulmonary symptoms persist or if pulmonary disorder is diagnosed.
- Drug-induced lupus-like syndrome (rare) may first be evidenced as an inflammatory facial photosensitivity dermatitis with butterfly configuration on malar surfaces.
- Anticipate and report evidence of blood dyscrasia: unexplained bruising or bleeding, flu-like symptoms (fever, sore throat, chills).
- Blood counts may be monitored during first 6 months of treatment; abnormal counts usually stabilize within 1 month after discontinuing treatment.

DRUG INTERACTIONS *Tocainide hydrochloride*

PLUS	INTERACTIONS
Allopurinol	Extends half-life (increases blood level of tocainide)
Metoprolol	Additive effects on wedge pressure and cardiac index
Propranolol	May lead to paranoia

Tolazamide ———————————————————————

(Tolanase) *Antidiabetic; sulphonylurea*

ACTIONS AND USES   Orally effective sulphonylurea hypoglycaemic structurally and pharmacologically related to tolbutamide (q.v.), but about 5 times more potent in action (potency is about equal to that of chlorpropamide).

Used in management of mild to moderately severe non-insulin-dependent diabetes mellitus which cannot be controlled by diet and weight reduction, and which is uncomplicated by acidosis, ketosis, coma. Effective in primary or secondary failures to other sulphonylurea.

ROUTE AND DOSAGE   Oral: (individualized): 100 mg to 1 g once daily with breakfast; doses exceeding 500 mg should be divided and given twice daily.

NURSING IMPLICATIONS
- Unlike tolbutamide, tolazamide is effective in some patients with a history of ketoacidosis or coma; close observation of these patients is especially important during the early adjustment period.
- Store below 40°C (104°F) preferably between 15° and 30°C (59° and 86°F) in a well-closed container, unless otherwise directed by manufacturer. Keep drug out of the reach of children.
- *See tolbutamide.*

Tolbutamide ———————————————————————

(Glyconon, Pramidex, Rastinon) *Antidiabetic; sulphonylurea*

ACTIONS AND USES   Short-acting and sulphonylurea compound chemically related to sulphonamides, but without antiinfective activity. Lowers blood glucose concentration by stimulating pancreatic beta cells to synthesize and release insulin. No action demonstrated if functional beta cells are absent. During long-term use it is proposed that extrapancreatic effects (increased number of insulin receptors on cell membranes, decreased hepatic uptake of insulin, and increased peripheral utilization of insulin) also contribute to hypoglycacmic effect of the sulphonylurea drugs. Responsiveness to blood glucose lowering effects with long-term therapy may decline in some patients. Alternatively, patient who has become poorly responsive to other sulphonylureas may be responsive to tolbutamine. May be mildly goitrogenic without producing clinical hypothyroidism or thyroid enlargement. It has not been established that long-term cardiovascular or neural complications of diabetes can be prevented by the sulphonylureas.

Used in management of mild to moderately severe, stable non-insulin-dependent diabetes which is not controlled by diet and/or weight reduction alone.

TOLBUTAMIDE *(continued)*

ROUTE AND DOSAGE   Oral (highly individualized): 0.5 to 1.5 g daily. *Maintenance dose*: no more than 2 g.

ABSORPTION AND FATE   Rapidly absorbed from GI tract; detected in blood in 20 to 60 minutes with peak concentrations in 3 to 5 hours; only small amount detectable in 24 hours. Onset of hypoglycaemic action is gradual with peak antidiabetic activity occurring within 5 to 8 hours and lasting 6 to 12 hours. Blood glucose level then gradually returns to pretreatment level within 24 hours. About 95% protein bound. **Half-life** (considerable interindividual difference): 4 to 25 hours (average: 7 hours). Oxidized in liver to inactive metabolites. Eliminated in urine (85%); about 9% excreted in faeces via bile.

CONTRAINDICATIONS AND PRECAUTIONS   Hypersensitivity to sulphonylureas or to sulphonamides, history of repeated episodes of diabetic ketoacidosis (with or without coma), diabetes; as sole therapy; diabetic coma; severe stress, infection, trauma, or major surgery; severe renal insufficiency, hepatic or endocrine disease. Safe use during pregnancy or use in children not established. **Cautious Use:** cardiac, thyroid, pituitary, or adrenal dysfunction, history of peptic ulcer, women of childbearing age who may become pregnant, alcoholism; the elderly, debilitated, malnourished or uncooperative patient.

ADVERSE/SIDE EFFECTS   These include: allergic skin reactions: pruritus, erythema, urticaria, morbilliform or maculopapular eruptions; porphyria cutanea tarda, photosensitivity, cholestatic jaundice (rare); (dose related): nausea, epigastric fullness, heartburn, anorexia constipation, diarrhoea, agranulocytosis, thrombocytopenia, leucopenia, haemolytic anaemia, aplastic anaemia, pancytopenia, hepatic porphyria, disulphiram-like reactions, taste alterations, headache. **Overdosage:** *Hypoglycaemia (mild)* without loss of consciousness or neurological symptoms: unusual fatigue, tremulousness, hunger, drowsiness, GI distress, sweating, anxiety, headache; *(severe)*: visual disturbances, ataxia, paraesthesias, confusion, tachycardia, seizures, coma.

NURSING IMPLICATIONS

- Treatment with an oral antidiabetic agent is generally preceded by an appropriate trial of dietary management, including weight control.
- Tolbutamide is neither oral insulin nor a substitute for insulin; however, the same diagnostic and therapeutic measures required to insure optimum insulin control of diabetes are required for control by tolbutamide.
- Impress on the patient and family that oral antidiabetic drug therapy controls diabetes, but will never cure it.
- Total dose may be taken before breakfast but preferably in divided doses after meals.
- Tablet may be crushed and taken with full glass of water if patient desires.
- Because of danger of noctural hypoglycaemia, tolbutamide should not be taken at bedtime unless specifically prescribed.
- Elderly patients may be hyperresponsive to oral antidiabetic therapy; thus the initial dose should be low and given before breakfast. If blood and urine glucose tests are negative during first 24 hours of therapy, initial dose may be continued on a daily

TOLBUTAMIDE (continued)

basis; if hypoglycaemia occurs, dose is reduced to minimum level or discontinued.

- During initial period of therapy, patient should be under close medical supervision until dosage is established (using negative tests for glucosuria, ketonuria, and blood glucose level as criteria). One or 2 weeks of therapy may be required before full therapeutic effect is achieved.

- If a patient stabilized on tolbutamide is exposed to stress (e.g., infection, surgery), loss of blood glucose control may occur. Tolbutamide may be discontinued and replaced by insulin.

- The patient/family member should fully understand that symptoms of hypergly-caemia and ketoacidosis (representing loss of diabetes control) must be reported to the physician promptly. Symptoms include flushed, dry skin, weight loss, fatigue, Kussmaul respiration, double or blurred vision, soft eyeballs, irritability, fruity smelling breath, abdominal cramps, nausea, vomiting, diarrhoea, dyspnoea, polydipsia, polyphagia, polyuria, headache, hypotension, weak and rapid pulse, positive ketonuria and glycosuria). Report symptoms promptly so that emergency antidiabetic therapy can be instituted.

- *Hypoglycaemia* is frequently caused by overdosage of hypoglycaemic drug, inadequate or irregular food intake, nausea, vomiting, diarrhoea, and added exercise without caloric supplement or dose adjustment. *See Adverse/Side Effects.* Its occurrence indicates need for immediate reevaluation of patient's diet, medication regimen, and compliance. It is most likely to appear in patients over 50 years of age. Report to physician.

- A beta-adrenergic agent (e.g., propranolol) blocks hypoglycaemia-induced tachycardia, but does not inhibit hypoglycaemia sweating. Detection of a hypoglycaemic reaction in a diabetic patient also receiving a beta-blocker, especially if elderly, is difficult. Monitor closely during adjustment period watching for other symptoms (e.g., unexplained fatigue, hunger, nausea) of impending hypoglycaemia.

- Early hypoglycaemic reactions can be stemmed quickly by ingestion of soluble glucose (such as orange juice, or other fruit juices, sugar cubes, or table sugar dissolved in water, soft drinks). If symptoms do not subside in 10 to 15 minutes, repeat glucose; if after another 10 to 15 minutes patient still has symptoms and urine test for sugar is negative, notify physician. If feeling faint, advise patient to go to the doctor or hospital.

- When hypoglycaemic reaction has progressed to grogginess, the patient can be given a teaspoon of honey or corn syrup; the sugar will be rapidly absorbed by oral membranes, and patient should revive enough to drink a glass of fruit juice. Unconsciousness should be treated in the hospital, where IV dextrose in water and clinical supervision will be given until maintenance dose is reestablished. Patient should be observed closely for at least 3 to 5 days.

- Hypoglycaemic symptoms may be especially vague in the elderly; therefore, check out nondefinitive expressions such as 'I don't feel well today' to discover real meaning. Observe patient carefully, especially 2 to 3 hours after eating, check urine for sugar and ketone bodies and capillary blood glucose.

- Repetitive complaints of headache and weakness a few hours after eating may signal incipient hypoglycaemia. Dosage adjustment may be indicated.

TOLBUTAMIDE (continued)

- Teach patient that undereating is as hazardous as overeating. Warn that a self-directed, weight-loss regimen, redistribution of dietary carbohydrate, or skipped meals interfere with drug control of diabetes.
- Patients using oral contraceptives should be advised to use another form of birth control (*see Drug Interactions*).
- Pruritus and rash, frequently reported side effects, may clear spontaneously; however, if they persist, drug will be discontinued.
- Instruct patient to avoid self-medication with OTC drugs unless approved or prescribed by physician.
- Alcohol, even in moderate amounts, can precipitate a disulphiram reaction (flushing, sweating, slurred speech, palpitations, headache abdominal cramps, nausea, vomiting). The patient should be aware of becoming hypoglycaemic after ingesting alcohol; an observer may mistakenly think he or she is inebriated and therefore patient may be deprived of necessary emergency treatment.
- Because of potential photosensitivity (especially in the alcoholic), it may be wise for the patient to protect exposed skin areas from the sun with a sunscreen lotion (SPF 12 to 15) when outdoors for several hours.
- Transient alterations in certain liver function tests during initial period of sulphonylurea therapy reportedly have little clinical significance; fluctuating abnormalities of liver function frequently occur in patients with diabetes.
- Advise patient to report promptly signs of hepatic dysfunction (pruritus, jaundice, dark urine, abdominal discomfort), renal sufficiency (dysuria, anuria, haematuria), or blood dyscrasia (easy bruising, unexplained bleeding). All indicate probable reasons for terminating treatment with tolbutamide (perhaps only temporarily).
- Advise patient to weigh self at least weekly and to report a progressive gain, especially if oedema is present. These signs indicate the necessity to discontinue tolbutamide.
- *Urine testing*: In stabilized patients urine blood is tested for glucose usually once a day about 2 hours after largest meal. Instruct patient to keep record and to show physician at next visit.
- When a drug that effects the hypoglycaemic action of sulphonyureas (*see Drug Interaction*) is withdrawn or added to the tolbutamide regimen the patient should be alerted to the added danger of loss of control (hyperglycaemia). Urine tests and blood glucose tests and test for ketone bodies should be carefully monitored and possibly increased in frequency for several days to determine if antidiabetic drug dose adjustment is indicated.
- A careless, casual attitude toward oral antidiabetic regimen leads to noncompliance and lack of diabetic control. Encourage and support the patient in accepting responsibility for keeping his or her condition under control and for maintaining scheduled visits to the physician for periodic clinical evaluation.
- Instruct the patient to carry medical identification card or jewellery with self at all times. Card information should include patient and physician's names and addresses, diagnosis, medication, and dose being taken.
- Store below 40°C (104°F), preferably between 15° and 30°C (59° and 86°F) in well-closed container; avoid freezing.
- *For summary of patient/family teaching plan, see insulin.*

TOLBUTAMIDE (continued)

Diagnostic test interferences The sulphonylureas may produce abnormal **thyroid function test** results, and reduced **RAI uptake** (after long-term administration). A tolbutamide metabolite may cause false-positive **urinary protein** values when turbidity procedures are used (such as heat and acetic acid or sulphosalicylic and); Ames reagent strips reportedly not affected.

DRUG INTERACTIONS   *Tolbutamide*

PLUS	INTERACTIONS
Alcohol	Disulphiram-like reactions with concomitant use
Anticoagulants, oral Chloramphenicol MAO inhibitors Probenecid Salicylates and other NSAIDs Sulphonamides	May displace tolbutamide from binding site potentiating its hypoglycaemic effects
Beta adrenergic blockers: (e.g., propranolol)	Suppresses rebound increase in blood sugar following tolbutamide-induced hypoglycaemia. Concomitant use with caution
Digitalis glycosides (e.g., digoxin)	May decrease metabolism of digitalis agents
Calcium channel blockers (e.g., verapamil) Corticosteroids Contraceptives, oral Oestrogens Hydantoins (e.g., phenytoin) Isoniazid Nicotinic acid Phenothiazines Thiazide diuretics Thyroid products	May cause hyperglycaemia leading to loss of control (secondary failure)
Pyrazolones (e.g., phenylbutazone)	Inhibit tolbutamide metabolism leading to enhanced hypoglycaemic effects

Tranylcypromine

(Parnate)   *Psychotropic; antidepressant; MAO inhibitor*

ACTIONS AND USES Potent nonhydrazine MAO inhibitor structurally similar to amphetamine. Actions and toxicity similar to those of hydrazine MAO inhibitors, but also has rapid and direct amphetamine-like CNS stimulatory action, is less likely to cause hepatotoxicity, and does not produce prolonged MAO inhibition.

Owing to its toxic potential, use is reserved for treatment of severe mental depression in hospitalized patients who have not responded to other antidepressant therapy. *See phenelzine.*

TRANYLCYPROMINE (continued)
ROUTE AND DOSAGE   Oral: *initial*: 10 mg in morning and 10 mg in afternoon. This dosage may be continued for 2 weeks. If no response, dosage may be adjusted to 10 mg in morning and 20 mg in afternoon for another week. *Maintenance* 10 mg/day.

NURSING IMPLICATIONS
- Tablet may be crushed before administration and taken with fluid or mixed with food, if patient has difficulty swallowing a pill.
- Because of possibility of insomnia, usually not given in the evening.
- Incidence of severe hypertensive reactions appears to be greater with tranylcypromine than with other MAO inhibitors.
- **Food–drug interactions**   Emphasize importance of avoiding tyramine-containing foods (e.g., aged cheeses, Chianti wine, raisins). (*See Index*: *Food sources*.)
- Inform patient that excessive use of caffeine-containing beverages (chocolate, coffee, tea, cola) can contribute to development of rapid heart beat, arrhythmias, and hypertension.
- Instruct patient to make position changes slowly, particularly from recumbent to upright posture.
- Usually produces therapeutic response within 3 days, but full antidepressant effects may not be obtained until 2 or 3 weeks of drug therapy.
- *See phenelzine sulphate*

Trazodone hydrochloride ─────────────

(Molipaxin)

Psychotropic (antidepressant); alpha-adrenergic blocking agent

ACTIONS AND USES   Centrally acting triazolepyridine derivative, chemically and structurally unrelated to tricyclic, tetracyclic, or other antidepressants but has its own profile of actions. Does not stimulate CNS; causes fewer anticholinergic genitourinary and neurological effects when compared with incidence with other antidepressants. Produces varying degrees of sedation in normal and mentally depressed patient, increases total sleep time, decreases number and duration of awakenings in depressed patient, and decreases REM sleep. Has anxiolytic effect in severely depressed patient and exhibits mild analgesic, antihistaminic and skeletal muscular relaxant action. Has no anticonvulsant action.

Used to treat major depression with or without prominent anxiety.

ROUTE AND DOSAGE   (Individualized.) **Oral: Adult:** *Initial*: 150 mg/day in divided doses. Drug may be increased by 50 mg every 3 to 4 days (depending on clinical response and tolerance). Maximum dosage: not to exceed 600 mg/day (400 mg/day for

TRAZODONE HYDROCHLORID (continued)

outpatient). *Maintenance*: lowest dose to preserve attained antidepressive effect. Reduce dose in the elderly.

ABSORPTION AND FATE   Well-absorbed from GI tract. Peak blood concentrations reached in 1 hour if taken on empty stomach, 2 hours if taken with food. Multidose regimen steady state plasma level reached in about 4 days. Extensive hepatic metabolism (oxidation and hydroxylation); 89 to 95% protein-bound. **Biphasic half-life**: 4.4 hours for first 3 to 10 hours after drug ingestion; 7.5 hours for next 10 to 34 hours. Approximately 75% drug and metabolites are excreted in urine within 72 hours; remainder in faeces via bile.

CONTRAINDICATIONS AND PRECAUTIONS   Hypersensitivity to trazodone, initial recovery phase of MI, ventricular ectopy, electroshock therapy. Safe use in children below 18 years of age not established; pregnancy. **Cautious Use**: patient with suicidal ideation, cardiac arrhythmias or disease; nursing mother.

ADVERSE/SIDE EFFECTS   (Appear to be dose-related.) These include: hypotension (including orthostatic hypotension), hypertension, syncope, shortness of breath, chest pain, tachycardia, palpitations, bradycardia, PVCs, ventricular tachycardia (short episodes of 3 to 4 beats), skin eruptions, rash, pruritus, acne, photosensitivity, nasal and sinus congestion, blurred vision, eye irritation, sweating or clamminess, tinnitus, dry mouth, anorexia, constipation, abdominal distress, nausea, vomiting, dysgeusia, flatulence, diarrhoea, haematuria, increased frequency, delayed urine flow, early or absent menses, male priapism, ejaculation inhibition, anaemia, decreased and neutrophil counts (infrequent), skeletal aches and pains, muscle twitches, drowsiness, lightheadedness, tiredness, dizziness, insomnia, headache, agitation, impaired memory and speech, disorientation; rarely: hypomania, nightmares, seizures, hallucinations, paraesthesias, akathisia, increased alkaline phosphatase, AST and ALT; weight gain or loss.

NURSING IMPLICATIONS

Food–drug interferences   Drug taken with food rather than on an empty stomach increases amount of absorption by 20% and appears to decrease incidence of dizziness or lightheadedness. Urge patient to maintain the same schedule for food–drug intake throughout treatment period to prevent variations in serum concentration (i.e., always with food or snack, or always before or after food intake).

- Therapeutic effects usually begin in 1 week but may require 2 to 4 weeks to reach maximum levels. This period, i.e., waiting for desired symptom relief, is the most vulnerable for noncompliant drug-taking behaviour. Teach patient importance of adhering to regimen and have family member reenforce this teaching with patient in the home.
- Therapy is usually continued on minimum dosage several months beyond optimum clinical response to prevent recurrence of depression.
- Urge patient not to alter dose or intervals between doses.

TRAZODONE HYDROCHLORID (continued)

- Adherence to follow-up appointment is important to permit dose adjustment or discontinuation, as indicated.
- If patient has preexisting cardiac disease, monitor pulse rate and regularity before administration of drug.
- When trazodone is given at the same time as an MAO inhibitor, therapy is initiated cautiously and dose is adjusted according to clinical response. No interaction has been documented but the potential for hypertensive crisis is recognized until ruled out.
- Adverse/side effects generally are mild and tend to decrease and disappear after the first few weeks of treatment.
- Observe patient's level of activity and compare with base or admission level. If it appears to be increasing toward sleeplessness and agitation, with changes in reality orientation report to physician. Manic episodes have been reported.
- Ask male patient if he is having inappropriate or prolonged penile erections. If he is, the drug should be discontinued and physician consulted.
- Check patient for symptoms of hypotension. If orthostatic, hypotension is troublesome (and it may be, especially in the elderly), suggest measures to reduce danger of falling and to help patient to tolerate the effects. *See Index: Nursing Interventions: hypotension.* Discuss with physician; a reduction of dose or discontinuation of the drug may be prescribed.
- Advise patient to limit or abstain from alcohol use. The depressant effects of CNS depressants and alcohol may be potentiated by this drug.
- Warn patient not to self-medicate with OTC drugs for colds, allergy, or insomnia treatment without advice of physician. Many of these drugs contain CNS depressants.
- Overdosage causes extension of common adverse/side effects: vomiting, lethargy, drowsiness and exaggerated anticholinergic effects. Seizures or arrhythmias are unusual. Death rarely occurs except when other drugs are being given concomitantly (such as alcohol, meprobamate).
- Treatment of overdosage (no antidote) is symptomatic and supportive. It is not known whether drug is dialyzable but high protein binding suggests that haemodialysis would not be effective.
- Alert dentist, surgeon, or emergency personnel that drug is being used. Trazodone is discontinued as long as possible prior to elective surgery.
- Store drug in tightly closed, light-resistant container at temperature of 15° to 30°C (59° to 86°F).

DRUG INTERACTIONS   *Trazodone hydrochloride*

PLUS	INTERACTIONS
Antihypertensives	May inhibit hypotensive effects requiring reduction of antihypertensive dose
CNS depressants (e.g., alcohol, opiates, barbiturates, anaesthetics)	Potentiated or additive depressant effects
Digoxin	Increased digoxin level
MAO inhibitors (e.g., isocarboxazid, phenelzine)	Intensified hypertensive effect of trazodone
Phenytoin	Increased serum phenytoin level

Triamcinolone

(Adcortyl, Kenalog, Ledercort)   *Corticosteroid; glucocorticoid*

ACTIONS AND USES   Immediate acting synthetic fluorinated adrenal corticosteroid with glucocorticoid and antirheumatic activity 7 to 13 times more potent than that of hydrocortisone (q.v.). Possesses minimal sodium and water retention properties in therapeutic doses. Differs from other corticosteriods in that it does not increase appetite.
    Used as an inflammatory or immunosuppressant agent.

ROUTE AND DOSAGE   **Oral:** up to 24 mg/day in divided doses. IM: 40 mg (acetonide) repeated according to response. Maximum single dose 100 mg. **Topical:** apply sparingly 2–4 times a day.

ABSORPTION AND FATE   Oral preparation rapidly absorbed. IM slowly absorbed. **Onset of action** (oral, IM), 24 to 48 hours; **peak effect:** 1 to 2 hours. **Duration of action:** oral; 2.25 days; IM, 1 to 6 weeks; intralesional, intraarticular (hexacetonide) 3 to 4 weeks. Plasma half-life: 2 to 5 hours; **HPA axis suppression:** 18 to 36 hours.

CONTRAINDICATIONS AND PRECAUTIONS   Safe use during pregnancy, by lactating women, and by children under 6 not established. Renal dysfunction. *See also hydrocortisone.*

ADVERSE/SIDE EFFECTS   Muscle weakness and loss of tissue mass. Local: burning, itching, folliculitis, hypertrichosis, hypopigmentation. *See also hydrocortisone.*

NURSING IMPLICATIONS
- Tablet may be crushed before administration and taken with fluid of patient's choice.
- This preparation may cause natriuresis, negative nitrogen balance, with weight loss in most patients (along with headache, fatigue, and dizziness) and sodium retention with weight gain and moon facies in others. Adequate diet to counter these effects should be designed. Plan with dietician, patient, and physician. High protein, high K diet is often needed.
- Caution patient to adhere to drug regimen: i.e., not to increase or decrease established regimen and not to abruptly discontinue taking or using the drug.
- Postural hypotension may accompany sodium and weight loss. It may be necessary to keep patient in supine position for 30 minutes after triamcinolone is given. Warn patient to keep this possibility in mind as ambulating.
- Give IM dose deep into the gluteal muscle for depot effect.
- Protect drug from light. Store at temperature 15° to 30°C (59° to 86°F).
- *See hydrocortisone for nursing implications and nursing interactions.*

Triamterene

(Dytac)   *Diuretic (potassium-sparing)*

TRIAMTERENE (continued)

ACTIONS AND USES Pteridine derivative structurally related to folic acid. Like spironolactone, has weak diuretic action and a potassium-sparing effect. Promotes excretion of sodium, chloride (to lesser extent), and carbonate, with no excretion or slight excretion of potassium ion. Unlike spironolactone, blocks potassium secretion by direct action on distal renal tubule rather than by inhibiting aldosterone; activity is independent of aldosterone levels. May cause decrease in alkali reserve and slight increase in urinary pH. Does not appear to inhibit excretion of uric acid, but serum uric acid levels may increase in predisposed individuals. Decreased glomerular filtration rate and elevated BUN are associated with daily administration, but seldom with intermittent (every other day) therapy. Has mild hypotensive effect and is a weak competitive inhibitor of dihydrofolate reductase.

Used as adjunct in the management of oedema. Also used alone or in conjunction with a thiazide or loop diuretic in patients with hypertension because of its potassium-sparing activity.

ROUTE AND DOSAGE Oral: Adult: *initial*: 150–200 mg daily; titrated to needs of patient. Total daily dosage (adult and paediatric) not to exceed 300 mg. *Maintenance*: 100 mg/day or every other day.

ABSORPTION AND FATE Rapidly and irregularly absorbed from GI tract (individual variability). Onset of diuretic action in 2 to 4 hours; usually tapers off 7 to 9 hours later. Approximately 40 to 70% bound to plasma proteins. **Plasma half-life**: 90 to 100 minutes. Metabolized by liver to active and inactive metabolites. Excreted by renal filtration and tubular secretion; 10 to 18% of dose is eliminated within 24 hours.

CONTRAINDICATIONS AND PRECAUTIONS Hypersensitivity to drug; anuria, severe or progressive kidney disease or dysfunction, severe hepatic disease, elevated serum potassium. Safe use during pregnancy, in women of childbearing potential, and in nursing mothers not established. **Cautious Use**: impaired renal or hepatic function, history of gouty arthritis, diabetes mellitus.

ADVERSE/SIDE EFFECTS Diarrhoea, nausea, vomiting, and other GI disturbances; dizziness, headache, dry mouth, pruritus, rash, anaphylaxis, photosensitivity, weakness and hypotension (large doses), muscle cramps, hyperkalaemia and other electrolyte imbalances, elevated BUN, elevated uric acid (patients predisposed to gouty arthritis), hyperchloraemic acidosis, blood dyscrasias: granulocytopenia, eosinophilia, megaloblastic anaemia, patients with reduced folic acid stores (e.g., hepatic cirrhosis).

NURSING IMPLICATIONS
- If patient cannot swallow capsule, it may be emptied and contents swallowed with fluid or mixed with food.
- Give drug with or after meals to prevent or minimize nausea. Note that nausea and vomiting are also symptoms of electrolyte imbalance and renal failure and therefore, require careful evaluation. Dosage reduction or discontinuation of drug may be indicated.
- Schedule doses to prevent interruption of sleep from diuresis, e.g., with or after

TRIAMTERENE (continued)

breakfast if a single dose is taken, or no later than 18.00 hours if more than one dose is prescribed. Consult physician.

- Monitor blood pressure during period of dosage adjustment. Hypotensive reactions, although rare, have been reported. Implications for ambulation should be noted, particularly for elderly patients.
- Weigh patient under standard conditions (preferably before breakfast, after voiding, same scale, same clothing), prior to drug initiation and during therapy.
- Diuretic response usually occurs on first day of therapy, but maximum effect may not occur for several days.
- Monitor and report oliguria and unusual changes in fluid intake–output ratio. Hyperkalaemia is reportedly not as likely to occur in patients with adequate urinary output. Consult physician regarding allowable fluid intake.
- Unlike most diuretics, triamterene promotes potassium retention. Therefore, potassium supplements, potassium-rich diet, and salt substitutes are usually not prescribed.
- Generally salt restriction is not stressed because of the possibility of low-salt syndrome (hyponatraemia). Consult physician.
- Observe for signs and symptoms of hyperkalaemia (*see Index*), particularly in patients with renal insufficiency, in patients on high-dose or prolonged therapy, in the elderly, and in patients with diabetes. Baseline and periodic determinations of serum potassium and other electrolytes should be done.
- Periodic blood studies are advised in patients on prolonged therapy and in patients with cirrhosis since they are prone to develop megaloblastic anaemia, symptoms of which may include: burning, inflamed mouth with bright red tongue, cracked corners of lips, weakness.
- Instruct patient to report overpowering fatigue or weakness, malaise, fever, sore throat, or mouth (possible symptoms of granulocytopenia) and unusual bleeding or bruising (thrombocytopenia).
- Drug should be withdrawn gradually in patients on prolonged therapy, or patients who have received high doses, in order to prevent rebound kaliuresis (increased urinary excretion of potassium).
- Triamterene may increase blood glucose, therefore, it should not be given to a diabetic patient unless blood glucose is controlled, primarily in patients with diabetes. Patients should be closely monitored.
- Warn patient that triamterene may cause photosensitivity and therefore to avoid exposure to sun and sunlamps.
- Inform patient that triamterene may impact a harmless pale blue fluorescence to urine.
- Preserved in tight, light-resistant containers, preferably between 15° and 30°C (59° and 86°F), unless otherwise directed by manufacturer.

Diagnostic test interferences   Pale blue fluorescence in urine interferes with fluoro-metric assay of **quinidine** and **lactic dehydrogenase activity**. Triamterene may cause increases in **blood glucose** levels (diabetic patients), **BUN, serum potassium, magnesium,** and **uric acid** and **urinary calcium excretion**.

TRIAMTERENE (continued)
DRUG INTERACTIONS *Triamterene*

PLUS	INTERACTIONS
Antihypertensives	Additive hypotensive effect
Digitalis glycosides	Effects may be decreased by triamterene
Lithium	Possibility of lithium toxicity due to decreased renal clearance
Indomethacin and other NSAIDs	Combined therapy can cause marked decrease in creatinine clearance
Whole blood and plasma	May contain a significant amount of potassium when stored for more than 10 days. Possibility of hyperkalaemia

Triazolam

(Halcion)   *Hypnotic; benzodiazepine*

ACTIONS AND USES   Benzodiazepine derivative with hypnotic effects similar to those of flurazepam but with fewer residual daytime effects. Drug-induced effects on sleep include decreased sleep latency and number of nocturnal awakenings, decreased total nocturnal wake time, and increased duration of sleep. Reduction of daytime anxiety and carry-over CNS depression is minimal.

Used for short-term management of insomnia characterized by difficulty in falling asleep, frequent wakeful periods and/or early morning wakefulness. Following long-term use, tolerance or adaptation may develop.

ROUTE AND DOSAGE   Carefully individualized. **Oral: Adults:** 250 mcg. **Elderly, debilitated patient:** 125 mcg, 15–20 min before retiring.

ABSORPTION AND FATE   Readily absorbed from GI tract. **Onset of action** in 15 to 30 minutes with peak effect, 1.3 hours after single dose. **Duration of action:** 6 to 8 hours. **Half-life:** 1.7 to 3 hours; **protein-binding (high):** 89%. Metabolized in liver; excreted with its metabolites in urine.

CONTRAINDICATIONS AND PRECAUTIONS   Hypersensitivity to triazolam and benzodiazepines; pregnancy. **Cautious Use:** depression, elderly and debilitated patients, patient with suicidal tendency, impaired renal or hepatic function, chronic pulmonary insufficiency. *See also chlordiazepoxide.*

ADVERSE/SIDE EFFECTS   These include: drowsiness, lightheadedness, headache, dizziness, ataxia, visual disturbances, confusional states, memory impairment, 'rebound insomnia,' euphoria, anterograde amnesia, nausea, vomiting, constipation, and taste alterations (rare), paradoxical reactions, minor changes in EEG patterns, tinnitus (rare). *See also chlordiazepoxide.*

TRIAZOLAM (continued)
NURSING IMPLICATIONS

- Because of short half-life, under normal circumstances dose is usually cleared before next bedtime dose; therefore 'morning after' grogginess rarely occurs.
- Warn patient not to stop taking drug suddenly, especially if patient is subject to seizures. Withdrawal symptoms may occur. These range from mild dysphoria to more serious symptoms such as tremors, abdominal and muscle cramps, convulsions. Consult physician about schedule for discontinuing therapy.
- Signs of developing tolerance or adaptation (with long-term use) include increased daytime anxiety, increased wakefulness during last one third of the night.
- Habituation and dependence can occur.
- **Symptoms of overdosage** Slurred speech, somnolence, confusion, impaired co-ordination, coma. Treatment: immediate gastric lavage; support of respiratory and cardiovascular systems by maintenance of patent airway, and IV fluids if necessary.
- **Smoking–drug interaction** As with other benzodiazepines, smoking may decrease hypnotic effects of triazolam. When preparing patient for sleep, remove cigarettes, not only to assure maximum drug effect but to prevent accidental fire by smoking while drowsy.
- Caution patient not to increase dose without physician's advice.
- Store at controlled room temperature 15° to 30°C (59° to 86°F).
- See also *chlordiazepoxide*.

Drug interactions Triazolam CNS depressant effects are augmented if coadministered with any of the following: **anticonvulsants, antihistamines, ethanol, other psychotropics, other CNS depressants.**

Tricloflos sodium

ACTIONS AND USES Sedative with similar action and uses to chloral hydrate. Now rarely used.

ROUTE AND DOSAGE Oral: Adult: 1–2 g. Child (up to 1 yr): 100–200 mg; (1–5 yrs): 250–500 mg; (6–12 yrs): 0.5–1 g: all 30 minutes before retiring. For further information: *see chloral hydrate*.

Trifluoperazine

(Stelazine)

Antipsychotic (neuroleptic); phenothiazine

TRIFLUOPERAZINE (continued)

ACTIONS AND USES   Piperazine phenothiazine similar to chlorpromazine (q.v.) in most actions, uses, limitations, and interactions. Produces less sedative, cardiovascular and anticholinergic effects and more prominent antiemetic and extrapyramidal effects than other phenothiazines. Total pharmacological effects are more prolonged than those of chlorpromazine. Lowers convulsive threshold.

Used in management of schizophrenia and excessive anxiety and tension associated with neuroses or somatic conditions.

ROUTE AND DOSAGE   Oral: Adult: *Psychoses*: *initial*: 5 mg twice daily: increased by 5 mg after one week, then increased by 5 mg every 3 days according to response. *Severe anxiety*: Adult: 2–4 mg/day in divided doses, increased to 6 mg/day if required. Child (3–5 yrs): up to 1 mg; (6–12 yrs): up to 4 mg a day in divided doses. IM: Adult: 1–3 mg/day in divided doses maximum 6 mg/day. Child: 50 mcg/kg/day in divided doses.

ABSORPTION AND FATE   Rapid onset of action; effects persist for more than 12 hours. Optimum therapeutic dose level reached in 2 to 3 hours. *See also chlorpromazine.*

CONTRAINDICATIONS AND PRECAUTIONS   Hypersensitivity to phenothiazines, comatose states, CNS depression, blood dyscrasias, children under 6, bone marrow depression, preexisting hepatic disease, pregnancy. **Cautious Use**: previously detected breast cancer; patient with compromised respiratory function; seizure disorders. *See also chlorpromazine.*

ADVERSE/SIDE EFFECTS   Nasal congestion, dry mouth, sweating, blurred vision, drowsiness, insomnia, dizziness, agitation, extrapyramidal effects, agranulocytosis, photosensitivity, skin rash, constipation, tachycardia, hypotension, pigmentary retinopathy, depressed cough reflex, gynaecomastia, galactorrhoea. See also *chlorpromazine.*

NURSING IMPLICATIONS

- Separate antacid and phenothiazine doses by at least 2 hours.
- Administer IM injection deep into upper outer quadrant of buttock. Unlike other phenothiazines this drug apparently causes little if any pain and irritation at injection site. Rotate sites.
- Intervals between injections should be no less than 4 hours because of possible cumulative effects. Oral therapy is substituted for IM treatment as soon as feasible.
- Hypotension and extrapyramidal effects (especially akathisia and dystonia) are most likely to occur in patients receiving high doses or parenteral administration and in the elderly patient. Stop drug if patient has dysphagia, neck muscle spasm, or if tongue protrusion occurs.
- Reduction in dosage or temporary discontinuation of drug usually reverses extrapyramidal symptoms.
- Counsel patient to take drug as prescribed and not to alter dosing regimen or stop medication without consulting physician. Additionally, patient should not give any of the drug to another person.
- Advise patient to consult physician about use of any OTC drugs during therapy.
- Alcohol and other depressants should not be taken during phenothiazine therapy.

TRIFULOPERAZINE (continued)

■ Drug-induced antiemetic effect may mask toxicity of other drugs or block diagnosis of conditions with nausea as the primary symptom (e.g., brain tumour, intestinal obstruction, or Reye's syndrome).

■ Monitor fluid intake—output ratio and bowel elimination pattern. Check for abdominal distention and pain. Encourage adequate fluid intake as prophylaxis for constipation and xerostomia. The depressed patient may not seek help for either symptom or for urinary retention.

■ Patient may be unable to adjust to temperature extremes because of drug effect on thermoregulatory centre. If patient complains of being cold even at average room temperature, heed complaints, and furnish additional clothing or blankets, if necessary. Do not apply heating pad or hot water bottles; because of depressed conditioned avoidance behaviours, a severe burn may result.

■ Caution patient to avoid potentially hazardous activities such as driving a car or operating machinery, especially during first days of therapy. (Drowsiness and dizziness may be prominent during this time.)

■ Since trifluoperazine potentiates analgesics, its use may reduce amount of narcotic required in painful long-term illness such as cancer.

■ Agitation, jitteriness, and sometimes insomnia may simulate original neurotic or psychotic symptoms. (They may disappear spontaneously.) Dosage should not be increased until side effects have subsided.

■ Increase in mental and physical activity is an expected result of therapy. Caution patients with angina to avoid overexertion and to report increase in frequency of original pain.

■ Advise patient to cover as much skin surface as possible with clothing when he or she must be in direct sunlight. A sun screen lotion (SPF above 12) should be applied to exposed skin.

■ Inform patient that urine may be discoloured or reddish brown, and that this is harmless.

■ Maximum therapeutic response generally occurs within 2 to 3 weeks after initiation of therapy.

■ Slight yellow discolouration of injectable drug reportedly does not alter potency. If colour markedly changed, discard solution.

■ Store drug in light-resistant container at temperature between 15° and 30°C (59° and 86°F), unless otherwise directed by manufacturer.

■ *See chlorpromazine for drug interactions.*

Trifluperidol ————————————————————

(Triperidol)

ACTIONS AND USES Antipsychotic drug with similar action and uses to trifluoperazine.

TRIFLUPERIDOL (continued)
ROUTE AND DOSAGE   Oral: **Adult:** *initial*: 500 mcg/day increased by 500 mcg every 3–4 days according to response. Maximum 6–8 mg/day. **Child** (6–12 yrs): *initial* 250 mcg increased according to response. Maximum 2 mg/day.

Trimeprazine tartrate

(Vallergan)

ACTIONS AND USES   Antihistamine used for symptomatic relief in allergy. Also used as a premedication for anaesthesia.

ROUTE AND DOSAGE   Oral: **Adult:** 10 mg 3–4 times a day maximum 100 mg/day. **Child:** 2.5–5 mg. 3–4 times a day. *Premedication*: **Oral: Adult:** 3–4.5 mg/kg, **child (2–7 yrs):** 2–4 mg/kg given 1–2 hours preoperatively.

Trimetaphan camsylate

(Arfonad)   *Antihypertensive;*
                                                     ganglionic blocking agent

ACTIONS AND USES   Potent, short-acting nondepolarizing ganglionic blocking agent. Blocks transmission in both adrenergic and cholinergic ganglia by competing with acetylcholine for receptor sites on postganglionic membranes.

Used to produce controlled hypotension for certain surgical procedures (e.g., neurological, ophthalmic, and plastic surgery)

ROUTE AND DOSAGE   Intravenous infusion: *Initial*: 3–4 mg/min adjusted according to response.

ABSORPTION AND FATE   Effects appear almost immediately following IV administration and may persist 10 to 30 minutes. Thought to be metabolized by pseudocholinesterases. About 20 to 40% excreted in urine. Crosses placenta.

CONTRAINDICATIONS AND PRECAUTIONS   Anaemia, hypovolaemia, shock, asphyxia, respiratory insufficiency, glaucoma; during pregnancy. **Cautious Use:** history of allergy; elderly and debilitated patients, children, cardiac disease, arteriosclerosis, hepatic or renal disease, degenerative CNS disease, Addison's disease, diabetes mellitus, patients receiving steroids, antihypertensives, anaesthetics (especially spinal), and diuretics.

ADVERSE/SIDE EFFECTS   These include: tachycardia or decrease in heart rate,

TRIMETAPHAN CAMSYLATE (continued)

orthostatic hypotension, angina, nausea, vomiting, anorexia, restlessness, extreme weakness; respiratory depression, respiratory arrest (following large doses).

NURSING IMPLICATIONS

- Continue to monitor vital signs at regular intervals after completion of treatment. Since blood pressure returns to pretreatment level within 10 minutes after the infusion is terminated an oral antihypertensive is usually initiated in patients with hypertension as soon as desired blood pressure level is achieved with trimethaphan.
- *Note*: Pupillary dilatation may not necessarily indicate anoxia or depth of anaesthesia, but may represent a specific effect of the drug.
- Facilities for resuscitation and maintenance of oxygenation and ventilation should be immediately available.
- Some patients become refractory to trimethaphan (tachyphylaxis) within 48 hours after initiation of therapy. Notify physician promptly if blood pressure fails to respond.
- Monitor fluid intake and output. Ganglionic blockade may reduce renal blood flow initially as well as voiding contractions and urge to void. Check lower abdomen for bladder distention.
- Trimethaphan is stable under refrigeration, but freezing should be avoided. Infusion solution should be freshly prepared and any unused portion discarded. Storage: controlled room temperature: 15° to 30°C (59° to 86°F).

Diagnostic test interferences   Trimethaphan may decrease **serum potassium** and may prevent elevation of **blood glucose** that usually occur during postoperative period.

DRUG INTERACTIONS   *Trimethaphan*

PLUS	INTERACTIONS
Antihypertensives, other diuretics ⎫ Anaesthetics ⎬	Additive hypotensive effects

Trimethoprim

(Monotrim, Syraprim, Tiempe, Trimogal, Trimopan)   *Antiinfective, urinary;*
folate antagonist

ACTIONS AND USES   Antiinfective and folate antagonist with slow bactericidal action. Binds to and reversibly blocks enzyme reduction of folic acid to its active metabolite tetrahydrofolic acid, thus preventing bacterial synthesis of thymidine, an essential nucleoside in DNA. This binding and interference with cell growth is 1,000 times stronger in bacterial than in mammalian cells. Emergence of trimethoprim-resistant organisms occurs more frequently when it is used alone than when used in

TRIMETHOPRIM *(continued)*

combination therapy. Efficacy as treatment of UTI appears to match that of amoxicillin, ampicillin, nitrofurantoin, or sulphafurazole. Available in fixed combination with sulphamethoxazole (1 part trimethoprim to 5 parts sulphamethoxazole) as co-trimoxazole.

Used to treat initial episodes of acute uncomplicated UTIs and in the treatment and prophylaxis of chronic and recurrent UTI in both men and women, also for acute and chronic bronchitis.

ROUTE AND DOSAGE   Oral: Adult: 200 mg every 12 hours. *Urinary tract infection*: 300 mg/day as a single or divided dose. Child (2–5 months): 25 mg; (6 months–5 yrs): 50 mg; (6–12 yrs): 100 mg all twice a day. IV: Adult: 150–250 mg 12 hrly. Child (under 12 yrs): 6–9 mg/kg/day in 2–3 divided doses.

ABSORPTION AND FATE   Readily and almost completely absorbed from GI tract. Peak serum concentration of approximately 1 mcg/ml reached in 1 to 4 hours after single 100-mg dose. Widely distributed into most body tissues and fluids including CSF. (If meninges are inflamed, concentration in CSF increases.) **Elimination half-life**: 8 to 11 hours in adult with normal renal function; metabolized in liver; 50 to 60% oral dose rapidly excreted in urine unchanged within 24 hours. Drug concentration in urine decreased in patient with impaired renal function. Crosses placenta and enters amniotic fluid and breast milk. Partial removal by haemodialysis.

CONTRAINDICATIONS AND PRECAUTIONS   Hypersensitivity to trimethoprim, megaloblastic anaemia secondary to folate deficiency, creatinine clearance less than 15 ml/min, impaired renal or hepatic function, possible folate deficiency, pregnancy, nursing mothers, children with fragile X chromosome associated with mental retardation. Safe use in infants less than 2 months old and efficacy in children under 12 years old has not been established.

ADVERSE/SIDE EFFECTS   Most serious: hypersensitivity and haematological reaction (0.5%). **Others**: rash, pruritus, exfoliative dermatitis, epigastric discomfort, nausea, vomiting, glossitis, abnormal taste sensation, thrombocytopenia, neutropenia, megaloblastic anaemia, methemoglobinaema, fever, increased serum transaminases (ALT, AST), bilirubin, creatinine, BUN.

NURSING IMPLICATIONS
- Culture of the causative organism and sensitivity tests are conducted before trimethoprim therapy is initiated; however, therapy may be started before test results have been received.
- Antiinfective treatment of acute uncomplicated UTIs is usually continued 10 to 14 days.
- Recurrent UTI may reflect noncompliance with drug therapy. Reinforce initial teaching about importance of adhering to drug regimen at time of checkup visits.
- Trimethoprim may worsen the psychomotor regression associated with mental retardation because of potential drug-induced folate deficiency.

TRIMETHOPRIM (continued)

- Monitor *creatinine clearance tests*. Usually dose reduction is prescribed when clearance values are 15 to 30 ml/minute. (*Normal*: 90 to 120 ml/minute.)
- Periodic urine cultures are recommended during therapy for recurrent or chronic UTIs.
- Leucovorin (folinic acid) will be administered if bone marrow suppression occurs ('leucovorin rescue'). Usually 3 to 6 mg only for 3 days restores normal haematopoiesis.
- Discuss fluid intake pattern with the patient. Ordinarily, the elderly tend to restrict fluids; therefore teaching needs to emphasize that amount and frequency of drinking water and other fluids is an important adjunct to drug therapy.
- Usually the adult patient should attempt to maintain fluid intake of 2,000 to 3,000 ml/day (if not contraindicated) to help flush out urinary bacteria.
- Assess urinary pattern during treatment. Altered pattern (frequency, urgency, nocturia, retention, polyuria) may reflect emerging drug resistance, necessitating change of drug regimen. Periodically inspect bladder area for distension.
- Pain and haematuria should be reported immediately.
- Before full drug effects are experienced, patient may have pain and discomfort with voiding which can be relieved by a urinary analgesic.
- Tell the male patient not to postpone voiding even though increases in fluid intake may cause more frequent urination.
- If patient (especially the elderly) has oedema, urge elevation of legs when sitting and physical exercise as tolerated. When patient goes to bed at night, fluid accumulated in the legs during the day reenters the circulatory system and is excreted during the night, resulting in nocturia.
- Elderly, malnourished, alcoholic, pregnant, or debilitated patients are especially susceptible to the haematologic toxic effects.
- Drug-induced rash, a common side effect, is usually maculopapular, pruritic, or morbilliform and appears 7 to 14 days after start of therapy with daily doses of 200 mg or less.
- To prevent nosocomial infections, aseptic technique during catheter insertion and care is essential. Thoroughly wash hands before and after any procedural interventions.
- Inspect perineal areas for evidence of inflammation (sore, red excoriated mucosa). Warm baths may give relief. Warn patient not to use douching, sprays, or bubble baths during treatment period, and stress careful perineal hygiene to prevent reinfection. Cleansing areas with water (no soap) is advised. Vaginal discharge, dysuria, and pruritus should be reported.
- The female patient with recurrent UTIs should be advised to cleanse genital area before sex and to urinate afterwards. If this is not possible, advise her to drink a glass of water before sex.
- Overdosage of 1 g or more produces symptoms of nausea, vomiting, diarrhoea, mental depression, confusion, facial swelling, bone marrow depression, elevated serum transaminases. *Treatment*: induce emesis, lavage stomach, administer supportive and symptomatic treatment, and acidify urine. Haemodialysis is moderately effective.

TRIMETHOPRIM (continued)

Drug interaction When trimethoprim and phenytoin are given concomitantly, incidence of folate deficiency increases.

Trimipramine maleate

(Surmontil)

Psychotropic, antidepressant; tricyclic

ACTIONS AND USES Tricyclic antidepressant pharmacologically similar to imipramine (q.v.) in actions, uses, absorption and fate, limitations, and interactions.

ROUTE AND DOSAGE Highly individualized. **Oral: Adults:** *Initial*: 50–75 mg/day in divided doses. Maximum 300 mg/day if required. *Maintenance*: 75–150 mg at bedtime. **Elderly patients and adolescents:** 10–25 mg three times a day.

NURSING IMPLICATIONS

- Administer drug with food to decrease gastric distress.
- The severely depressed patient may need assistance with personal hygiene, particularly because of excessive sweating caused by the drug.
- Inspect oral membranes daily if patient is on high doses. Urge outpatient to report symptoms of stomatitis, sialoadenitis, xerostomia.
- Report signs of hepatic dysfunction: yellow skin and sclerae, light-coloured stools, pruritus, abdominal discomfort.
- Alert patient to the fact that because TCAs have a 'lag period' of 2 to 4 weeks, therapeutic response will be delayed. (Increased dosage does not shorten period but rather increases incidence of adverse reactions). This period is one that fosters noncompliance. Monitor drug intake to see that therapy is not interrupted.
- Store drug in tightly closed container at temperature between 15° and 30°C (59° and 86°F), unless otherwise specified by the manufacturer.
- *See imipramine for additional Nursing Implications and Drug Interactions.*

Triprolidine hydrochloride

(Actidil)

ACTIONS AND USES Antihistamine used to treat allergies such as hay fever and urticaria.

ROUTE AND DOSAGE **Oral: Adult:** 2.5–5 mg three times a day. **Child (up to 1 yr):** 1 mg; **(1–5 yrs):** 2 mg; **(6–12 yrs):** 3 mg all three times a day. For further information: *see diphenhydramine.*

Tropicamide

(Mydriacyl)

*Anticholinergic
(parasympatholytic);
mydriatic*

ACTIONS AND USES Derivative of tropic acid, with pharmacological properties similar to those of atropine (q.v.), but mydriatic and cycloplegic effects occur more rapidly and are less prolonged. Duration of action about 3 hours.

Used to induce mydriasis and cycloplegia for ophthalmological diagnostic procedures.

ROUTE AND DOSAGE Ophthalmic: solution 0.5 and 1%. *See also atropine.*

Tubocurarine chloride

(Jexin)

*Skeletal muscle relaxant
(nondepolarizing);
neuromuscular blocking
agent*

ACTIONS AND USES Curare alkaloid, nondepolarizing neuromuscular blocking agent extracted from the plant *Chondodendron tomentosum*. Produces skeletal muscle relaxation or paralysis by competing with acetylcholine at cholinergic receptor sites on skeletal muscle endplate, and thus blocks nerve impulse transmission.

Used to induce skeletal muscle relaxation as adjunct to general anaesthesia, to facilitate management of mechanical ventilation, to reduce intensity of muscle contractions in tetanus and in pharmacologically or electrically induced convulsions.

ROUTE AND DOSAGE Intravenous: Adult: 20−45 mg according to requirements. Child: average dose 300−500 mcg/kg.

ABSORPTION AND FATE Following IV injection, muscle relaxation begins within seconds. Maximal effects in 2 to 3 minutes; effects usually last 25 to 90 minutes. IM injection is slowly and irregularly absorbed; action time unpredictable. Approximately 40% protein-bound. Half-life: 1 to 3 hours. Minimally degraded in liver and kidney. Approximately 35 to 75% excreted unchanged in urine within 24 hours; about 10% excreted in bile. Crosses placenta.

CONTRAINDICATIONS AND PRECAUTIONS Hypersensitivity to curare preparations; when histamine release is a hazard; hyperthermia; electrolyte imbalance; acidosis; neuromuscular disease; renal disease. Safe use in women of childbearing potential or during pregnancy not established. Cautious Use: impaired cardiovascular, renal, hepatic, pulmonary, or endocrine function; hypotension; carcinomatosis; thyroid disorders; collagen diseases; porphyria; familial periodic paralysis; history of allergies; myasthenia gravis; elderly or debilitated patients.

TUBOCURARINE CHLORIDE (continued)

ADVERSE/SIDE EFFECTS Slight dizziness, feeling of warmth, profound and prolonged muscle weakness and flaccidity, respiratory depression, hypoxia, apnoea, increased bronchial and salivary secretions, bronchospasm, decreased GI motility, hypotension, circulatory collapse, malignant hyperthermia, hypersensitivity reactions.

NURSING IMPLICATIONS

- Preparations should be made in advance for endotracheal intubation, suction, or assisted or controlled respiration with oxygen administration. Have on hand atropine and antagonists neostigmine or edrophonium (cholinesterase inhibitors). A nerve stimulator may be used to assess nature and degree of neuromuscular blockade.
- Selective muscle paralysis following drug administration occurs in the following sequence: jaw muscles, levator eyelid muscles and other muscles of head and neck, limbs, intercostals and diaphragm, abdomen, trunk. Facial and diaphragm muscles are first to recover, followed in order by legs, arms, shoulder girdle, trunk, larynx, hands, feet, pharynx. Muscle function is usually restored within 90 minutes.
- Monitor blood pressure, vital signs, and airway until assured of patient's recovery from drug effects. Ganglionic blockade (hypotension) and histamine liberation (increased salivation, bronchospasm) and neuromuscular blockade (respiratory depression) are known effects of tubocurarine.
- Tubocurarine is retained in the body long after effects of neuromuscular blockade appear to have dissipated. Observe for and report residual muscule weakness.
- Patient may find oral communication difficult until muscles of head and neck recover.
- Measure and record fluid intake–output ratio during day of drug administration. Renal dysfunction will prolong drug action. Peristaltic action may be suppressed. Check for bowel sounds.
- Test for myasthenia gravis is considered positive if muscle weakness is exaggerated.
- Solutions of drug should not be used if more than faintly discoloured.
- Tubocurarine is incompatible with solutions that have a high pH such as barbiturates; therefore, do not mix in same syringe.

Drug interactions Drugs that may potentiate or prolong neuromuscular blocking action of (curariform) skeletal muscle relaxants: **certain inhalation anaesthetics** (cyclopropane, ether, halothane, methoxyflurane); **certain antibiotics**, e.g., amikacin, aminoglycosides, amphotericin B, bacitracin, clindamycin, lincomycin, tetracyclines; also **diazepam**; **potassium-depleting diuretics**, **magnesium salts**, narcotic analgesics, **phenothiazines, procainamide, propranolol, quinidine**.

Urea ▬▬▬▬▬▬▬▬▬▬▬▬▬▬▬▬▬▬▬▬▬▬▬▬▬▬▬▬▬▬▬▬▬▬▬▬▬▬

(Ureaphil)   *Diuretic; keratolytic*

UREA (continued)

ACTIONS AND USES   Diamide salt of carbonic acid. When present in high concentrations in blood, induces diuresis by elevating osmotic pressure of glomerular filtrate, with subsequent decrease in sodium and water reabsorption and promotion of chloride and (to a lesser extent) potassium excretion. Increased blood toxicity results in transudation of fluid from tissue including brain, cerebrospinal, and intraocular fluid, into the blood. Topical applications increase water binding capacity of stratum corneum and thus may soften dry scaly skin conditions.

Used to reduce or prevent intracranial pressure (cerebral oedema) and intraocular pressure and to prevent acute renal failure during prolonged surgery or trauma. Also used to induce abortion in the mid trimester of pregnancy. Topical preparation used to promote hydration and removal of excess keratin in dry skin and hyperkeratotic conditions.

ROUTE AND DOSAGE   Intravenous infusion: Adults (30% solution): *Cerebral oedema*: 40–80 g as a 30% solution by slow infusion at a rate of 3–4 ml/min. **Topical**: in proprietory creams (Calmurid, Aquadrate, Nutraplus) apply to the affected part 1–3 times a day.

ABSORPTION AND FATE   Following IV administration, maximum reduction of intraocular and intracranial pressures and diuretic effect occur in 1 or 2 hours. Diuresis and intracranial pressure reduction may persist 3 to 10 hours; intraocular pressure lasts 5 to 6 hours then returns to pretreatment levels. Distributed widely; good ocular penetration. **Half-life**: about 1 hour. Excreted in urine essentially unchanged; 50% may be reabsorbed. Crosses placenta; excreted in breast milk.

CONTRAINDICATIONS AND PRECAUTIONS   Severely impaired renal or hepatic function; congestive heart failure; active intracranial bleeding; marked dehydration; IV injection into lower extremeties, especially in elderly patients, topical use for viral skin diseases, or impaired circulation. Safe use in pregnancy, lactation or in children not established. (Contraindications for intraamniotic urea: impaired renal function, frank liver failure, active intracranial bleeding; marked dehydration, diabetes mellitus, sickle cell anemia.) **Cautious Use**: women of childbearing potential; use on face or broken skin.

ADVERSE/SIDE EFFECTS   These include: somnolence (prolonged use in patients with renal dysfunction), headache, acute psychosis, confusion, disorientation, nervousness, tachycardia, hypotension, syncope, nausea, vomiting, increased thirst, fluid and electrolyte imbalance, dehydration, intraocular haemorrhage (rapid IV), pain, irritation, sloughing, venous thrombosis, chemical phlebitis at injection site (infrequent); hyperthermia, skin rash.

NURSING IMPLICATIONS
- Solution should be freshly prepared for each patient; discard unused portion. May be reconstituted with 5 or 10% dextrose injection.
- Reconstituted solution should be used within a few hours if stored at room temperature.

UREA (continued)

- Urea should not be administered by same IV set through which blood is being infused.
- Urea has the potential for causing tissue damage because of its osmotic properties. Extreme care must be taken to avoid extravasation; thrombosis and tissue necrosis can occur. Inspect injection site frequently. If extravasation is suspected, discontinue the IV line stat. Consult physician about removal of needle or cannula. Institute local treatment (according to hospital policy). Elevate part even if extravasation is minor. Use of heat or cold is debatable. Heat induces vasodilation and increases drug distribution and absorption. Cold may decrease circulation and reentry of drug into circulation.
- Dosage is individualized on basis of water and electrolyte balance, urinary volume, clinical signs.
- Determinations of serum and urinary sodium should be performed every 12 hours. Frequent kidney function studies are advised, particularly in patients suspected of having renal dysfunction.
- Be alert for signs of hyponatraemia, hypokalaemia, dehydration, or transient over-hydration (due to hyperosmotic activity).
- Monitor vital signs and mental status; promptly report any changes.
- Observe postoperative patients closely for signs of haemorrhage. Urea reportedly may increase prothrombin time and promote internal oozing at suture sites.
- Patient should be encouraged to drink fluids so as to hasten excretion or urea. However, if patient complains of a headache do not allow him or her to drink as this will counteract the osmotic effects of the drug. Consult physician about fluid volume parameters.
- Comatose patients receiving urea should have an indwelling catheter to insure satisfactory bladder emptying.
- Action of topical preparation is enhanced by applying it to skin while still moist following washing or bathing.
- *See also mannitol.*

Drug interactions   Urea may increase excretion rate of lithium, thereby decreasing its effectiveness.

Urokinase ────────────────────────────

(Ukidan)   *Enzyme;*
                                          plasminogen activator

ACTIONS AND USES   Enzyme produced by kidneys and isolated from human kidney tissue cultures. Promotes thrombolysis by direct action on the endogenous fibrinolytic system which results in conversion of plasminogen to the enzyme plasmin, an action that occurs within as well as on the surface of thrombus/embolus. (Plasmin degrades

UROKINASE (continued)

fibrin, fibrinogen, and other procoagulant plasma proteins.) Urokinase also has an anticoagulant effect because its action leads to high plasma levels of fibrin and fibrinogen degradation products. Activity expressed in international units (IU): i.e., ability to cause lysis of a fibrin clot via the *in vivo* plasmin system. Most effective action is on fresh, recently formed thrombi.

Used for lysis of emboli, in arteriovenous shunts and occular thrombosis.

ROUTE AND DOSAGE   *Arteriovenous shunt*: instillation of 5,000–37,500 IU in 2–3 ml 0.9% saline for infusion. *Occular*: 5,000–37,500 IU in 2 ml 0.9% saline for injection.

ABSORPTION AND FATE   Following IV infusion, rapidly cleared from circulation. Adequate activation of fibrinolytic system usually established within 3 to 4 hours after start of therapy. **Half-life**: 10 to 20 minutes (longer in presence of hepatic dysfunction). Small amount excreted in urine and bile. It is not known if drug crosses placenta. Fibrinolytic effects usually disappear in a few hours after treatment is discontinued, but increased thrombin time (TT), decreased fibrinogen and plasminogen levels, and increased degradation products may persist for 12 to 24 hours.

CONTRAINDICATIONS AND PRECAUTIONS   Pregnancy, during lactation, children. *See also streptokinase*.

ADVERSE/SIDE EFFECTS   *See streptokinase*.

NURSING IMPLICATIONS

- Measurable signs of clinical response may not occur for 6 to 8 hours after therapy is started.
- Urokinase should be reconstituted immediately before use. Since the product contains no preservatives discard unused portion.
- Avoid adding other medication to urokinase solution.
- Anticoagulant therapy with heparin is reinstituted at end of urokinase therapy and when thrombin time has decreased to less than twice normal control value (usually within 3 to 4 hours).
- Severe spontaneous bleeding, including fatality from cerebral haemorrhage, has occurred during urokinase treatment. Risk is estimated to be twice that associated with heparin therapy.
- Store vials at 2° to 8°C (35° to 47°F).
- *See also Streptokinase for additional Nursing Implications, Diagnostic Test Interferences, and Drug Interactions.*

Ursodeoxycholic acid _____

(Destolit, Ursofalk)

URSODEOXYCHOLIC ACID (continued)

ACTIONS AND USES   Antilithic drug with similar action and use to chenodeoxycholic acid.

ROUTE AND DOSAGE   Oral: Adult: 8–12 mg/kg/day as a single dose at bedtime.

Vancomycin

(Vancocin)   *Antibiotic*

ACTIONS AND USES   Glucopeptide antibiotic prepared from *Streptomyces orientalis*, with bactericidal and bacteriostatic actions. Action interferes with cell membrane synthesis in multiplying organisms. Active against many gram-positive organisms, including group A beta-haemolytic streptococci, staphylococci, pneumococci, enterococci, clostridia, and corynebacteria. Gram-negative organisms, mycobacteria, and fungi are highly resistant. Cross-resistance with other antibiotics, or resistance to vancomycin has not been reported.

Used parenterally for potentially life-threatening infections in patient allergic, nonsensitive, or resistant to other less toxic antimicrobial drugs. Used in treatment of antibiotic associated pseudomembranous colitis and for prophylaxis and treatment of endocarditis.

ROUTE AND DOSAGE   Oral: 125 mg/6 hourly for 7–10 days. **IV infusion**: 500 mg over 60 minutes/6 hourly; or 1 g/12 hourly. *Endocarditis prophylaxis*: 1 g IV over 60 min.

ABSORPTION AND FATE   Poorly absorbed from GI tract. Peak serum levels of 49 mcg/ml achieved in 5 minutes following IV injection of 1 g; trough level of 2 mcg/ml after 12 hours. Oral doses of 2 g/day produce serum concentrations less than 1 mcg/ml. Diffuses into pleural, ascitic, pericardial and synovial fluids; penetrates noninflamed meninges, but does not enter CSF if meninges are inflamed. About 10% protein bound. **Half-life**: 4 to 8 hours in adults; 2 to 3 hours in children; increased to 7 to 8 days in the anuric patient. Accumulation occurs with renal dysfunction. About 80 to 90% of dose excreted in active form in urine within 24 hours. Readily crosses placenta. Not significantly removed by haemodialysis or continuous ambulatory peritoneal dialysis.

CONTRAINDICATIONS AND PRECAUTIONS   Known hypersensitivity to vancomycin, previous hearing loss, concurrent or sequential use of other ototoxic or nephrotoxic agents, IM administration. Safe use during pregnancy not established. **Cautious Use**: neonates, impaired renal function.

ADVERSE/SIDE EFFECTS   Ototoxicity (auditory portion of eighth cranial nerve), nephrotoxicity leading to uraemia, hypersensitivity reactions (chills, fever, skin rash,

VANCOMYCIN (continued)

urticaria, shocklike state); transient leucopenia, eosinophilia, anaphylactic reaction with vascular collapse; superinfections, severe pain, thrombophlebitis at injection site; nausea, warmth, and generalized tingling following rapid IV infusion.

NURSING IMPLICATIONS

- Rapid infusion may cause sudden hypotension. Monitor BP and heart rate continuously through period of drug administration.
- Extravasation of IV infusion must be avoided; severe irritation and necrosis can result.
- Periodic urinalyses, renal and hepatic function tests, and haematologic studies are advised in all patients.
- Serial tests of vancomycin blood levels are recommended in patients with borderline renal function and in patients over age 60 (generally maintained at 10 to 20 mg/ml).
- Vancomycin may cause damage to auditory branch (not vestibular branch) of eighth cranial nerve, with consequent deafness, which may be permanent.
- Serum levels of 60 to 80 mcg/ml are associated with ototoxicity. Tinnitus and high tone hearing loss may precede deafness which may progress even after drug is withdrawn. The elderly and those on high doses are especially susceptible. Warn patient to report ringing in ears promptly.
- Instruct patient to adhere to drug regimen: i.e., not to increase, decrease, or interrupt dosage. The full course of prescribed drug therapy should be completed.
- Monitor fluid intake and output; report changes in intake and output ratio and pattern. Oliguria or cloudy or pink urine may be a sign of nephrotoxicity (also manifested by transient elevations in BUN, albumin, and hyaline and granular casts in urine).

Drug interactions   Possibility of additive toxicity with other ototoxic and/or nephrotoxic drugs (e.g., **aminoglycoside antibiotics, cephaloridine, colistin, polymyxin B, viomycin**).

Vasopressin injection ─────────────────────────────

(Pitressin)   *Hormone; antidiuretic*

ACTIONS AND USES   Polypeptide hormone extracted from animal posterior pituitaries. Possesses pressor and antidiuretic principles, but is relatively free of oxytocic properties. Produces concentrated urine by increasing tubular reabsorption of water, thus preserving up to 90% water. May increase Na and decrease K reabsorption, but plays no causative role in oedema formation.

Used as an antidiuretic to treat diabetes insipidus, and for emergency control of massive GI haemorrhage.

ROUTE AND DOSAGE   Adults: *Vasopressin Injection*: **Intramuscular, subcuta-**

VASOPRESSIN INJECTION (continued)

neous: *Diabetes insipidus*: 5 to 20 units 4 hrly. **IV infusion**: *oesophageal varices*: 20 units over 15 min.

ABSORPTION AND FATE   Following IM or SC injection of aqueous preparation, antidiuretic activity maintained 2 to 8 hours. IV infusion: pressor response for 30 to 60 minutes. Distributed throughout extracellular fluid, with little evidence of plasma protein binding; **Half-life**: 10 to 20 minutes. Most of drug is destroyed in liver and kidneys. Approximately 5% of subcutaneous dose of aqueous vasopressin is excreted unchanged after 4 hours; following IV administration, 5 to 15% of dose appears in urine.

CONTRAINDICATIONS AND PRECAUTIONS   Intravenous injection, chronic nephritis accompanied by nitrogen retention, ischaemic heart disease, PVCs, advanced arteriosclerosis, during first stage of labour. **Cautious Use**: epilepsy, migraine, asthma, heart failure, angina pectoris; any state in which rapid addition to extracellular fluid may be hazardous; vascular disease, preoperative and postoperative polyuric patients, renal disease, goitre with cardiac complications, elderly patients, children, pregnancy.

ADVERSE/SIDE EFFECTS   Infrequent with low doses. **Hypersensitivity reactions**: rash, urticaria, anaphylaxis, tremor, sweating, bronchoconstriction, circumoral and facial pallor, angioneurotic oedema, eructations, passage of gas, nausea, vomiting, pounding in head, anginal (in patient with coronary vascular disease), cardiac arrest, uterine cramps, water intoxication (especially with tannate). **Intraarterial infusion**: cardiac arrhythmia, pulmonary oedema, bradycardia, gangrene at injection site. **Intranasal**: congestion, rhinorrhoea, irritation, mucosal ulceration and pruritus, headache, conjunctivitis, heartburn, postnasal drip, abdominal cramps, increased bowel movements secondary to excessive use. **Large doses**: blanching of skin, abdominal cramps, nausca (almost spontaneously reversible), hypertension, bradycardia, minor arrhythmias, premature atrial contraction, heart block, peripheral vascular collapse, coronary insufficiency, myocardial infarction.

NURSING IMPLICATIONS

- Polyuria and thirst of diabetes insipidus are usually controlled for 36 to 48 hours with a single dose.
- At beginning of therapy, establish baseline data of blood pressure, weight fluid intake and output pattern and ratio. Monitor both blood pressure and weight throughout therapy. Report sudden changes in pattern to physician.
- Patient with vascular disease and diabetes insipidus may receive small doses of vasopressin. Patient should be prepared for possibility of anginal attack and should have available a coronary vasodilator. Such pain should be reported to the physician.
- Be alert to the fact that even small doses of vasopressin may precipitate myocardial infarction or coronary insufficiency, especially in elderly patients. Emergency equipment and drugs (antiarrhythmics) should be readily available.
- Use of intraarterial vasopressin for emergency treatment of GI haemorrhage should not preclude other measures usually employed: e.g., blood transfusion, oesophageal tamponade, ice water gavage, emergency surgery.

V

VASOPRESSIN INJECTION (continued)

- Intraarterial infusion constricts the splanchnic and peripheral vasculature and may cause gangrene in the peripheral entry vessel. Inspect infusion site and catheter at hourly intervals for blanching of skin. If noted, stop infusion immediately and notify the physician.
- Dose used to stimulate diuresis has little effect on blood pressure.
- Check patient's alertness and orientation frequently during therapy. Lethargy and confusion associated with headache may signal onset of water intoxication. Although insidious in rate of development, symptoms can lead to convulsions and terminal coma.
- If water intoxication occurs (drowsiness, listlessness, headache, confusion, anuria, weight gain), vasopressin is withdrawn and fluid intake is restricted until specific gavity is at least 1.015 and polyuria occurs. With severe overhydration, osmotic diuresis is effected by drug therapy (e.g., mannitol, alone or in conjunction with frusemide).
- Urine output, specific gravity and serum osmolality are monitored while patient is hospitalized.

Diagnostic test interferences   Vasopressin increases **plasma cortisol** levels.

DRUG INTERACTIONS   *Vasopressin*

PLUS	INTERACTIONS
Alcohol, cyclophosphamide, demeclocycline, adrenaline, heparin, lithium	Decrease antidiuretic activity of vasopressin
Antidiabetic agents, paracetomol fluodrocortisone, ganglionic blocking agents (e.g., guanethidine), neostigmine	Increase action of vasopressin
Chlorpropamide, clofibrate, carbamazepine	Increase antidiuretic activity of vasopressin

Vecuronium bromite

(Norcuron)

Skeletal muscle relaxant (nondepolarizing); neuromuscular blocking agent

ACTIONS AND USES   Intermediate-acting nondepolarizing skeletal muscle relaxant.

Used as adjunct for general anaesthesia to produce skeletal muscle relaxation during surgery. Also used to facilitate endotracheal intubation.

ROUTE AND DOSAGE   **IV injection:** *initial* 80–100 mcg/kg then 30–50 mcg/kg as required. For further information: *see tubocurarine.*

Verapamil hydrochloride

(Berkatens, Cordilox, Securon)

Vasodilator; antiarrhythmic; calcium channel blocking agent

ACTIONS AND USES   Calcium channel blocking agent with short duration of action. Inhibits calcium ion (Ca) influx through slow channels into contractile and conductile myocardial cells and vascular smooth muscle cells. Inhibits exercise-induced broncho-constriction and may slow and convert multifocal atrial tachycardia to normal sinus rhythm. Vasodilation effect is reflected by transient, usually asymptomatic reduction in normal systemic arterial pressure, vascular resistance, and contractility and slight increase in left ventricular filling pressure. Coronary vasodilation improves blood flow and oxygen supply to myocardium leading to reduced anginal pain. Does not alter total serum Ca levels. Has local anaesthetic action 1.6 times that of procaine but significance to man is unclear.

Used for treatment of supraventricular tachyarrhythmias and temporary control of rapid ventricular rate in atrial flutter or atrial fibrillation and to relieve hypertension and effort angina.

ROUTE AND DOSAGE   Oral: *Hypertension*: 240–480 mg/day in 2–3 divided doses; *Angina*: 80–120 mg three times a day. *Arrhythmia*: 40–120 mg three times a day. **IV**: *initial* 5–10 mg as a bolus over 2 min followed as required by 5 mg after 5–10 min. Administer the drug more slowly in elderly patients. **Infant and neonate: IV**: 0.75–1 mg. **Child (1–5 yrs)**: 2–3 mg; **(6–15 yrs)**: 2.5–5 mg.

ABSORPTION AND FATE   Bolus IV dose produces therapeutic effects in 3 to 5 minutes with duration of action, 10 to 20 minutes. Use in atrial arrhythmias: onset of action on AV node, 1 to 5 minutes; peak action in 10 to 15 minutes with duration of 6 hours. Oral dose almost completely absorbed from GI tract; only 10 to 20% is bioavailable after first-pass hepatic metabolism. **Elimination half-life** is biphasic: initial: 4 minutes; terminal: 2 to 5 hours. Therapeutic plasma level ranges from 80 to 300 ng/ml. 90% **protein binding**. Approximately 70% excreted in urine and 16% or more in faeces within 5 days. About 3 to 4% excreted as unchanged drug.

CONTRAINDICATIONS AND PRECAUTIONS   Severe hypotension, cardiogenic shock, cardiomegaly, digitalis toxicity, second- or third-degree AV block, severe congestive heart failure, concomitant IV beta-blockers (unless hours apart), sick sinus syndrome (except in patient with functioning artificial ventricular pacemaker). Safe use during pregnancy or lactation not established. **Cautious Use**: concomitant digitalis, pro-cainamide and quinidine therapy; disopyramide unless administered at least 48 hours before or 24 hours after verapamil, hepatic and renal impairment.

ADVERSE/SIDE EFFECTS   These include: dizziness, headache; (rarely): vertigo, sleepi-ness, rotary nystagmus, depression, hypotension (symptomatic), congestive heart failure, bradycardia, severe tachycardia, nausea, abdominal discomfort, constipation, ankle oedema, pruritus, flushing, pulmonary oedema, muscle fatigue, diaphoresis.

VERAPAMIL HYDROCHLORIDE (continued)
NURSING IMPLICATIONS

■ The initial use of verapamil should be in a treatment setting with facilities for monitoring and resuscitation.

■ Establish baseline data before treatment is started: blood pressure, pulse, and laboratory evaluations of hepatic and renal function.

■ Transient asymptomatic hypotension may accompany IV bolus. Instruct patient to remain in recumbent position for at least 1 hour after the dose is given to diminish subjective effects of hypotension.

■ Adverse reactions occur most frequently after IV administration, in the elderly or in patients with impaired renal function.

■ During early treatment for hypertension, check blood pressure near end of dosage interval or before administration of next dose to evaluate degree of control or whether dose intervals need to be changed.

■ Patient receiving verapamil at home should be informed about his or her usual pulse rate and instructed to take radial pulse before each dose. An irregular pulse or one slower than base level should be reported.

■ Warn patient to adhere to established guidelines for exercise programme. Reduced anginal pain because of verapamil action can give a false interpretation of tolerance.

■ Caution against driving or operating dangerous equipment until patient's response to verapamil is established. Dizziness (experienced as lightheadedness) during early treatment period is common.

■ Advise patient to decrease caffeine-containing beverage intake (i.e., coffee, tea, chocolate). (*See Drug Interactions*.)

■ Until tolerance to reduced blood pressure is established, advise patient to change positions slowly from recumbent to standing to prevent falls because of vertigo.

■ Verapamil should decrease angina frequency and requirement for glyceryl trinitrate.

■ If anginal pain (rest or effort) is not reduced by this drug therapy, the patient should notify the physician.

■ Stress importance of compliance. Caution patient not to alter established drug regimen, i.e., not to increase, omit or decrease dosage, or change dose intervals without consulting the physician.

■ Advise patient not to use OTC drugs unless they are specifically prescribed.

■ Emphasize importance of keeping appointments made for periodic evaluation of efficacy of verapamil and cardiovascular status.

■ *Treatment of overdosage* is supportive and may include: beta-adrenergic stimulation or IV Ca solutions to increase transmembrane influx of Ca ion through slow channels; vasopressor agents, cardiac pacing or cardiopulmonary rescusitation.

■ Inspect parenteral drug preparation before administration. Solution should be clear and colourless.

■ Store at 15° to 30°C (59° to 86°F) and protect from light.

Diagnostic test interferences   Verapamil may cause elevations of serum AST, AST, alkaline phosphase.

VERAPAMIL HYDROCHLORIDE (continued)
DRUG INTERACTIONS   *Verapamil*

PLUS	INTERACTIONS
Beta-adrenergic agonists (e.g., adrenaline, isoprenaline)	May oppose calcium blocking action of verapamil
Beta-adrenergic blocking agents (e.g., propranolol, metoprolol)	May augment cardiodepressant activity of verapamil
Highly protein-bound drugs: e.g., oral anticoagulants, hydantoins salicylates, sulphonamides, sulphonylureas	Verapamil could be displaced by or could displace these agents from protein binding sites thus increasing risk of toxicity. Concurrent use with caution
Methylxanthines (caffeine, theophylline)	May oppose Ca blocking effects of verapamil
Digoxin, possibly digitoxin	May elevate digoxin and digitoxin blood levels and increase risk of digitalis toxicity
Quinidine	Increased incidence of symptomatic hypotension

Vidarabine

(Vira-A)   *Antiviral*

ACTIONS AND USES   Pyrimidine nucleoside obtained from fermentation cultures of *Streptomyces antibioticus*. Has antiviral activity against herpes simplex virus types 1 and 2, varicella zoster, vaccinia, cytomegalovirus, hepatitis B virus, and Epstein–Barr virus. A degree of immunocompetence must be present if drug is to be effective. Potentially mutagenic and oncogenic.

Used systemically for treatment of herpes simplex encephalitis and herpes zoster infections in patients with suppressed immunological responses. Used topically (ophthalmic) for treatment of acute keratoconjunctivitis and recurrent epithelial keratitis caused by herpes simplex virus types 1 and 2.

ROUTE AND DOSAGE   **Ophthalmic:** approximately ½ inch ribbon into lower conjunctival sac five times daily at 3-hour intervals. **Intravenous:** 10 mg/kg daily for at least 5 days.

ABSORPTION AND FATE   Following topical application to eye, a trace amount of the major metabolite Ara-Hx (ara-hypoxanthine) is found in aqueous humour, no appreciable systemic absorption. Following IV administration, rapidly deaminated to Ara-Hx, which is less active than parent drug; it has mean **half-life** of 3.3 hours and is 0 to 3% protein-bound. Accumulates in plasma in patient with impaired renal function. Vidarabine half-life: 1.5 hours; 20 to 30% protein bound. Parent drug and metabolite widely distributed in body tissues and fluid and both cross blood–brain barrier. Excreted primarily by kidneys, mostly as the metabolite. Probably crosses placenta. Secretion into breast milk not determined.

VIDARABINE (continued)

CONTRAINDICATIONS AND PRECAUTIONS   Hypersensitivity to vidarabine. Safe use during pregnancy, and breast feeding not established. **Cautious Use**: impaired renal or hepatic function, patients susceptible to fluid overload or cerebral oedema.

ADVERSE/SIDE EFFECTS   Intravenous: (with high doses): hallucinations, confusion, psychosis, dizziness, ataxia, weakness, tremor, fatal metabolic encephalopathy. **Others**: nausea, vomiting, anorexia, diarrhoea, weight loss, anaemia, thrombocytopenia, neutropenia, decrease in WBC, Hgb, Hct, elevated bilirubin and SGOT (AST) malaise, pruritus, painful injection site. *Ophthalmic use*: burning, itching, mild irritation, lacrimation, foreign body sensation, pain, photophobia, punctal occlusion, superficial punctate keratitis. Association with ophthalmic vidarabine not determined: uveitis, stromal oedema, secondary glaucoma, trophic defects, corneal vascularization, and hyphaema.

NURSING IMPLICATIONS

Intravenous administration

- Dilute the vidarabine just before administration and use within 48 hours.
- Shake vial well before withdrawing dose, and transfer it to appropriate IV fluid. Most IV infusion fluids are suitable. Blood products, protein, or other colloidal fluids should not be used. Follow manufacturer's directions.
- A large volume of fluid is required to dissolve vidarabine since it is only slightly soluble (1 L of IV infusion fluid will solubilize a maximum of 450 mg of vidarabine, or 1 mg of drug to 2.22 ml of IV fluid). Agitate thoroughly until drug is completely dissolved. Prewarming the IV infusion fluid to 35° to 40°C (95° to 100°F) will facilitate dissolution. Once dissolved, subsequent shaking is unnecessary. *Do not refrigerate the dilution*.
- Final dilution is administered through an in-line membrane filter (pore size of 0.45 μ or smaller).
- Infusion should be administered at a constant rate over 12 to 24 hours.

Ophthalmic use

- Instruct patient to wash hands before and after treatment.
- Caution patient that vision may be temporarily hazy following instillation, and to avoid potentially hazardous activities until vision clears.
- Advise patient that drug may cause sensitivity to bright lights, and to use sunglasses, if necessary.
- Generally, epithelial healing begins in 2 to 4 days with complete healing in 1 to 3 weeks. If patient deviates from this expected course, other forms of therapy may be prescribed. Keep physician informed.
- Caution patient not to exceed recommended dose, frequency and duration of treatment.
- *See Index: Drug administration: eye ointment*.

Drug interaction   Concurrent therapy with **allopurinol** increases potential for CNS side effects.

Viloxazine

(Vivalan)

ACTIONS AND USES Tricyclic antidepressant with similar action and uses to amitriptyline.

ROUTE AND DOSAGE Oral: **Adult**: *initial*: 50–100 mg three times a day increased to a maximum of 400 mg/day as required. For further information: *see amitriptyline*.

Vinblastine sulphate

(Velbe)   *Antineoplastic; mitotic inhibitor*

ACTIONS AND USES Cell cycle specific alkaloid, extracted from periwinkle plant *Vinca rosea*. Arrests mitosis in metaphase by combination with microtubule proteins; may also interfere with other microtubular functions such as phagocytosis and cell mobility. It contrast to vincristine, has potent myelosuppressive and immunosuppressive properties, but produces less neurotoxicity. Spectrum of activity not completely established.

Used for palliative treatment of Hodgkin's disease and non-Hodgkin's lymphomas, choriocarcinoma, lymphosarcoma, neuroblastoma, mycosis fungoides, advanced testicular germinol cell cancer, histiocytosis and other malignancies resistant to other chemotherapy. Used singly or in combination with other chemotherapeutic drugs.

ROUTE AND DOSAGE **IV**: highly individualized.

ABSORPTION AND FATE Following IV administration, rapidly clears bloodstream and concentrates primarily in liver where it is partially metabolized. About 75% protein-bound with additional localization on platelets and leucocytes. **Half-life**: initial phase: 53 to 98 minutes; terminal phase: 24 hours. Toxicity increases if liver disease is present. Poor penetration of blood-brain barrier. Excreted in bile to faeces; less than 5% of dose excreted in urine.

CONTRAINDICATIONS AND PRECAUTIONS Leucopenia, bacterial infection, pregnancy, men and women of childbearing potential, elderly patients with cachexia or skin ulcers. **Cautious Use**: malignant cell infiltration of bone marrow, obstructive jaundice, hepatic impairment, history of gout; use of small amount of drug for long periods; use in eyes.

ADVERSE/SIDE EFFECTS Generally dose-related and short-lived. Side effects include: mental depression, peripheral neuritis, numbness and paraesthesias of tongue and extremities, loss of deep tendon reflexes, headache, convulsions, alopecia (reversible), vesiculation, vesiculation of mouth, stomatitis, pharyngitis, anorexia, nausea, vomiting, diarrhoea, ileus, abdominal pain, constipation, rectal bleeding, haemorrhagic

V

VINBLASTINE SULPHATE (continued)

enterocolitis, bleeding of old peptic ulcer, leucopenia (most common), agranulocytosis, thrombocytopenia and anaemia (infrequent), phlebitis, cellulitis, and sloughing following extravasation (at injection site); fever, weight loss, muscular pains, weakness, urinary retention, hyperuricaemia, parotid gland pain and tenderness, tumour site pain, aspermia, Raynaud's phenomenon, photosensitivity.

NURSING IMPLICATIONS

- Drug is usually injected into tubing of running IV infusion over period of 1 minute. If given directly into vein, fresh, dry needle is used (discard needle used to withdraw drug).
- If extravasation occurs, stop infusion promptly; applications of moderate heat and local injection of hyaluronidase are advised to help disperse extravasated drug. Infusion should be restarted in another vein. Observe injection site; sloughing may occur.
- Avoid contact with eyes. Severe irritation and persisting corneal changes may occur. Copious amounts of water should be applied immediately and thoroughly. Wash both eyes; don't assume one eye escaped contamination.
- Recovery from leucopenic nadir follows rapidly, usually within 7 to 14 days. With high doses, total leucocyte count may not return to normal for 3 weeks.
- Even if 7 days have passed, drug is not administered unless WBC count has not returned to at least 4,000/mm^3.
- Thrombocyte reduction seldom occurs unless patient has had prior treatment with other antineoplastics. However, be alert to unexplained bruising or bleeding which should be promptly reported.
- An antiemetic given before the injection may help to control nausea and vomiting.
- Course of therapy may be continued 12 weeks or more for adequate clinical trial. Encourage community-based patient to keep all appointments so that course of treatment is not interrupted.
- With exception of epilation, leucopenia and neurological side effects, adverse reactions seldom persist beyond 24 hours.
- Temporary mental depression sometimes occurs on second or third day after treatment begins.
- Monitor bowel elimination pattern and bowel sounds to recognize severe constipation or paralytic ileus. A stool softener may be necessary.
- Instruct patient to avoid exposure to infection, injury to skin or mucous membranes, and excessive physical stress, especially during leucocyte nadir period.
- Alopecia is frequently not total; in some patients, regrowth begins during maintenance therapy period. Arrange for wigs to be ordered if desired.
- Instruct patient to report promptly onset of symptoms of agranulocytosis: profound weakness, high fever, chills, rapid and weak pulse, sore throat, dysphagia, pharyngeal and buccal ulcerations. Appropriate treatment should not be delayed.
- Skin surfaces over pressure areas should be inspected daily if patient is not ambulating. Note condition of skin of the elderly especially, since normal ageing changes of integument (thinning, decrease in subcutaneous fatty tissue and microcirculation, diminished hydration) promote breakdown under stressed conditions.

VINBLASTINE SULPHATE (continued)

- Avoid exposure to sunlight unless protected with sunscreen lotion (SPF above 12), and clothing.
- *See mustine for nursing care of stomatitis.* Drug should be stopped if oral tissues breakdown.
- Preserved in tight, light-resistant containers in refrigerator. Reconstituted solution may be refrigerated up to 30 days without loss of potency.

Vincristine sulphate ━━━━━━━━━━━━━━━━━━━━━━━━━━━━

(Oncovin)   *Antineoplastic; mitotic inhibitor*

ACTIONS AND USES   Cell cycle specific vinca alkaloid (obtained from periwinkle plant *Vinca rosea*); analogue of vinblastine. Antineoplastic mechanism unclear; arrests mitosis at metaphase, thereby inhibiting cell division. In contrast to vinblastine, has relatively low toxic effect on normal cells and thus produces minimal myelosuppression; however, neurological and neuromuscular effects are more severe.

Used in treatment of acute lymphoblastic and other leukaemias, Hodgkin's disease, lymphosarcoma, neuroblastoma, Wilm's tumour and rhabdomyosarcoma.

ROUTE AND DOSAGE   Various schedules have been used; all are highly individualized. **Intravenous: Adult:** Highly individualized.

ABSORPTION AND FATE   Following IV administration, rapidly distributed with extensive tissue binding; about 75% plasma protein bound with additional binding to formed blood elements. **Half-life:** initial: 50 to 155 minutes; terminal: 23 to 85 hours. Hepatic dysfunction increases toxicity. Hepatic metabolism; poor penetration into CSF. Excreted primarily in faeces via bile.

CONTRAINDICATIONS AND PRECAUTIONS   Obstructive jaundice, pregnancy, men and women of childbearing age. **Cautious Use:** leucopenia, preexisting neuromuscular disease, hypertension, infection, patients receiving drugs with neurotoxic potential.

ADVERSE/SIDE EFFECTS   Usually dose-related and reversible. Side effects include: peripheral neuropathy, neuritic pain, paraesthesias, especially of hands and feet; foot and hand drop, sensory loss, athetosis, ataxia, loss of deep tendon reflexes, muscle atrophy, dysphagia, weakness in larynx and extrinsic eye muscles, ptosis, diplopia, mental depression, vrticaria, rash, alopecia, cellulitis and phlebitis following extravasation (at injection site), stomatitis, pharyngitis, anorexia, nausea, vomiting, diarrhoea, abdominal cramps, severe constipation (upper-colon impaction), paralytic ileus, (especially in children), rectal bleeding; hepatotoxicity, urinary retention, polyuria, dysuria, high urinary Na excretion, hyponatraemia, dehydration, hypotension, uric acid nephropathy, thrombocytopenia, anaemia, leucopenia, optic atrophy with blindness; transient cortical

VINCRISTINE SULPHATE (continued)

blindness, ptosis, diplopia, photophobia, convulsions with hypertension, malaise, fever, headache, pain in parotid gland area, hyperuricaemia, hyperkalaemia, weight loss.

NURSING IMPLICATIONS

- Administration directly into vein or into running infusion should be over a 1 minute period. Syringe and needle should be rinsed with venous blood before needle is withdrawn.
- If extravasation occurs, drug administration is discontinued immediately and restarted in another vein. Check hospital policy or consult physician.
- Reconstitute with provided solution or with sterile water or physiological saline to concentrations of 0.01 to 1.0 mg/ml.
- Classical MOPP treatment of advanced Hodgkin's disease combines administration of mechlorethamine and vincristine by rapid IV injection on days 1 and 8 of each cycle, and oral procarbazine and oral prednisone each day for 14 days only during each cycle.
- Monitor fluid intake—output ratio and pattern, blood pressure, and temperature daily. Record on flow chart as indicators for adaptations in nursing and drug regimen.
- Regularly scheduled serum uric acid determinations, adequate hydration, and administration of a uricosuric agent may be prescribed to prevent uric acid nephropathy. Advise patient to report promptly stomach, bone or joint pain, and swelling of lower legs and ankles.
- Weigh patient under standard conditions weekly or more often if ordered. In the presence of oedema or ascites, patient's ideal weight is used to determine dosage. Report a steady gain or sudden weight change to physician.
- A prophylactic regimen against constipation and paralytic ileus (adequate fluids, high fibre diet, laxatives) is usually started at beginning of treatment with vincristine. Encourage patient to report changes in bowel habit as soon as manifested. Paralytic ileus is most likely to occur in young children.
- Note that while fluid intake should be encouraged to prevent constipation, if hyponatraemia is a problem, fluid deprivation may be necessary. Consult physician for guidelines.
- An empty rectum with colicky pain may be misdiagnosed.
- Care should be taken to distinguish between the depression associated with realization of neoplastic disease and that which is drug-induced.
- Toxicity with vincristine occasionally follows an irreversible sequence: sensory impairment and paraesthesias, neuritic pain, more difficulties.
- Neuromuscular side effects, most apt to appear in the patient with preexisting neuromuscular disease, usually disappear after 6 weeks of treatment. Occasionally, however, side effects persist for prolonged periods of time after therapy is terminated.
- Children are especially susceptible to neuromuscular side effects.
- Grasp hands of patient each day to detect onset of hand muscular weakness, and check deep tendon reflexes (depression of Achilles reflex is the earliest sign of neuropathy). Also observe for and report promptly: mental depression, ptosis, double vision, hoarseness, paraesthesias, neuritic pain, and motor difficulties.
- If patient is bedridden, provide prophylactic measures to prevent footdrop; inspect skin over pressure areas frequently to prevent tissue breakdown.

VINCRISTINE SULPHATE (continued)

- Walking may be impaired; check patient's ability to ambulate, and supply support if necessary.
- Dental caries or periodontal disease should be treated since patient is highly susceptible to superinfections.
- *See mustine for nursing care of stomatitis.*
- Alopecia (reversible) (up to 70% of patients) is reportedly the most common adverse reaction any may persist for the duration of therapy. However, regrowth of hair may start before end of treatment. Before therapy begins, discuss this side effect with patient so that plans for providing a wig or hair piece can be made if desired. Inform patient that scalp hair will drop out in large clumps on pillow at night. This is a very distressing side effect. Many patients avoid all social contacts because of the loss of hair (self-image problems).
- Wigs should be ordered before hair is lost.
- Leucopenia occurs in a significant number of patients; leucocyte count in children usually reaches nadir on fourth day and begins to rise on fifth day after drug administration. Provide special protection against infection or injury during leucopenic days.
- Reconstituted solution may be refrigerated for 14 days without loss of potency. Both dry form and solutions should be protected from light. Refrigerate dry powder.

Vindesine

(Eldisine)

ACTIONS AND USES   Vinca alkaloid with similar action and use to vincristine.

ROUTE AND DOSAGE   IV: Highly individualized.

Vitamin A

(Halycitrol, Retinol)   *Vitamin*

ACTIONS AND USES   Synthetic fat-soluble vitamin available for clinical use. Vitamin A is essential for normal growth and development of bones and teeth, for integrity of epithelial and mucosal surfaces and for synthesis of rhodopsin (visual purple) necessary for visual dark adaptation.

Used in treatment of vitamin A deficiency.

ROUTE AND DOSAGE   Oral: Adults and children (over 8 years): 50,000 units/day to treat deficiency, 4,000 units for prevention. Children (4 to 8 years): 15,000 IU

VITAMIN A (continued)

daily; **Children (under 4 years):** 10,000 IU daily. **Intramuscular: Adults:** 150,000 to 300,000 IU monthly.

ABSORPTION AND FATE   Readily absorbed from GI tract (in presence of bile salts, pancreatic lipase, and dietary fat). Aqueous formulations produce more rapid and higher blood concentrations than oil form; absorption of emulsion is moderate. Stored mainly in liver; small amounts also found in kidney and body fat. Metabolites excreted in faeces and urine. Does not readily cross placenta, but passes into breast milk.

CONTRAINDICATIONS AND PRECAUTIONS   History of sensitivity to vitamin A or to any ingredient in formulation, hypervitaminosis A, oral administration to patients with malabsorption syndrome. Safe use in amounts exceeding 6,000 IU during pregnancy not established. **Cautious Use:** women on oral contraceptives, high doses in nursing mothers.

ADVERSE/SIDE EFFECTS   These include: irritability, headache, intracranial hypertension (pseudotumour cerebri), increased intracranial pressure, bulging fontanelles, papilloedema, exophthalmos, miosis, nystagmus, gingivitis, lip fissures, excessive sweating, drying or cracking of skin, pruritus, increase in skin pigmentation, massive desquamation, brittle nails, alopecia. **Hypervitaminosis A syndrome** (general manifestations): malaise, lethargy, abdominal discomfort, anorexia, vomiting. **Skeletal:** slow growth; deep tender hard lumps (subperiosteal thickening) over radius, tibia, occiput; migratory arthralgia; retarded growth; premature closure of epiphyses. **Other:** hypomenorrhoea, hepatosplenomegaly, hypercalcaemia, polydipsia, polyurea, jaundice, leucopenia, hypoplastic anaemias.

NURSING IMPLICATIONS

- Evaluation of dosage is made with consideration of patient's average daily intake of vitamin A. Dietary and drug history is advisable, e.g., intake of fortified foods, dietary supplements, self-administration or prescription drug sources. Women taking oral contraceptives tend to have significantly high plasma vitamin A levels.
- Vitamin A deficiency is often associated with protein malnutrition as well as other vitamin deficiencies. May be manifested by night blindness, retardation of growth and development, epithelial alterations, susceptibility to infection, abnormal dryness of skin, mouth, and eyes (xerophthalmia) progressing to keratomalacia (ulceration and necrosis of cornea and conjunctiva), urinary tract calculi.
- Cause of deficiency should be clearly identified for patient, and he or she and responsible family members should be included in dietary planning.
- About half of vitamin A activity in the average diet comes from carotene (provitamin A), found in yellow and green (leafy) vegetables and yellow fruits. Sources of preformed vitamin A are supplied primarily from livers of cod, halibut, tuna, fat of dairy products, fortified margarine and milk, and egg yolk.
- Avoid use of mineral oil while on vitamin A therapy.
- Instruct patient to report symptoms of overdosage: nausea, vomiting, anorexia, drying and cracking of skin or lips, headache, loss of hair.

VITAMIN A (continued)

- Patients receiving therapeutic doses should be closely supervised. Inform patient and family that self-medication with vitamin A is potentially harmful.
- **Treatment of overdosage**   Drug should be discontinued immediately. Most signs and symptoms (*see Adverse/Side Effects*) subside within a week, but tender, hard swellings in extremities and occiput may remain for several months.
- Caution patient to keep drug out of reach of children. Toxicity from a large dose of vitamin A is more common in a child than an adult.
- Preserved in tight, light-resistant containers.

Diagnostic test interferences   Vitamin A may falsely increase **serum cholesterol** determinations (Zlatkis-Zak reaction); may falsely elevate bilirubin determination (with Ehrlich's reagent).

Drug interactions   Concomitant administration of **mineral oil** may decrease absorption of vitamin A. **Corticosteroids** may increase plasma vitamin A levels.

Vitamin E/alpha tocopheryl acetate —————————————————

(Ephynal)   *Vitamin*

ACTIONS AND USES   Vitamin E refers to a group of naturally occurring fat-soluble substances known as tocopherols (alpha, beta, gamma, and delta). Alpha tocopheryl, comprising 90% of the tocopherols, is the most biologically potent and has been synthesized. Vitamin E deficiency causes no specific disease in humans. Low serum tocopherol in adults and children appears to be associated with creatinuria, muscle weakness, and decreased RBC survival—conditions that are completely reversed by the administration of vitamin E. Although vitamin E has not been shown to have any therapeutic value, it is prescribed for a number of clinical problems: anaemia associated with protein-calorie malnutrition (kwashiorkor), infertility, impotence, habitual abortion, menopausal syndrome, chronic cystic mastitis, peptic ulcer, burns, cancer prevention, skin disorders, heart diseases.

ROUTE AND DOSAGE   Oral: Adult: 3–15 mg/day.

W

Warfarin sodium ————————————————————————

(Marevan)   *Anticoagulant, oral; coumarin*

ACTIONS AND USES   Indirectly interferes with blood clotting by depressing hepatic synthesis of vitamin K-dependent coagulation factors: II (prothrombin), VII (procon-

WARFARIN SODIUM (continued)

vertin), IX (Christmas factor or plasma thromboplastin component), and X (Stuart–Prower factor). Deters further extension of existing thrombi and prevents new clots from forming. Has no effect on already synthesized circulating coagulation factors, or on circulating thrombi but may prevent extension of existing thrombi. Does not reverse ischaemic tissue damage and has no effect on platelets. Unlike heparin, action is cumulative and more prolonged. Warfarin is not cross allergenic with other coumarin derivatives. Some patients have an inherited resistance to warfarin and other oral anticoagulants and thus require larger than usual doses to achieve therapeutic effects.

Used for prophylaxis and treatment of deep venous thrombosis, and its extension, pulmonary embolism, transient cerebral ischaemic attacks, and as a prophylactic in patients with prosthetic cardiac valves.

ROUTE AND DOSAGE   Oral: **Adult or child**: dose adjusted according to clotting time. Usual adult maintenance dose 3–9 mg/day.

ABSORPTION AND FATE   Onset of action in 2 to 12 hours; peak prothrombin activity (i.e., after circulating functional coagulation factors are depleted) in 0.5 to 3 days. **Duration of action**: 2 to 5 days following single dose. **Half-life**: ½ to 3 days, is independent of dose. Approximately 99% weakly bound to plasma albumin. Accumulates mainly in liver where it is metabolized; also distributed to lungs, spleen, kidney. Excreted in urine and faeces via bile as inactive metabolites and traces of unchanged drug. Marked individual differences in metabolism and excretion rates. Crosses placenta. Amount in breast milk is negligible.

CONTRAINDICATIONS AND PRECAUTIONS   Haemorrhagic tendencies: vitamin C or K deficiency, haemophilia, coagulation factor deficiencies, dyscrasias; active bleeding, open wounds, active peptic ulcer, visceral carcinoma, oesophageal varices, malabsorption syndromes, hypertension (diastolic BP > 110 mm Hg), cerebral vascular disease, pregnancy, pericarditis with acute MI, severe hepatic or renal disease, continuous tube drainage of any orifice, subacute bacterial endocarditis, recent surgery of brain, spinal cord, eye, regional or lumbar block anaesthesia, threatened abortion, unreliable patients; **Cautious Use**: alcoholism, allergic disorders, during menstruation, nursing mother, elderly, debilitated patients; in *endogenous factors that may increase prothrombin time response* (enhance anticoagulant effect): carcinoma, congestive heart failure, collagen diseases, hepatic and renal insufficiency, diarrhoea, fever, pancreatic disorders, malnutrition, vitamin K deficiency, alcoholism, *endogenous factors that may decrease prothrombin time response* (decrease anticoagulant response): oedema, hypothyroidism, hyperlipidaemia, hypercholesterolaemia, chronic alcoholism, hereditary resistance to coumarin therapy.

ADVERSE/SIDE EFFECTS   Major or minor haemorrhage from any tissue or organ anorexia, nausea, vomiting, abdominal cramps, diarrhoea, steatorrhoea, stomatitis, increased serum transaminase levels, hepatitis, jaundice, priapism (rare), burning sensation of feet, transient hair loss. With prolonged use of high doses: myalgia, bone pain, osteoporosis. **Overdosage**: internal or external bleeding, paralytic ileus; skin necrosis

WARFARIN SODIUM (continued)

of toes (purple toes syndrome), tip of nose, buttocks, thighs, calves, female breast, abdomen, and other fat-rich areas.

NURSING IMPLICATIONS

- Tablet may be crushed before administration and taken with fluid of patient's choice.
- Prothrombin time (PT) should be determined before initiation of therapy and then daily until maintenance dosage is established. Daily checks should be made by physician to verify or change dose order.
- When patient is receiving maintenance dosage, PT determinations may be ordered at 1- to 4-week intervals depending upon patient's response. Periodic urinalyses, and liver function tests are also usually performed. Optimum time to draw blood sample: 12 to 18 hours after last dose.
- Since so many drugs interfere with the activity of anticoagulant drugs, a careful medication history should be obtained before start of therapy and whenever interpreting altered responses to therapy.
- Continued anticoagulant therapy is not advised in the absence of laboratory facilities or patient compliance.
- Elderly, psychotic, or alcoholic patient require close monitoring because they present serious noncompliance problems.
- Patients with greatest risk of haemorrhage include those who are difficult to regulate, who have an aortic valve prostheses, who are receiving long-term anticoagulant therapy and the elderly and debilitated.
- Inform patient, without frightening, that bleeding can occur even though PT is within therapeutic range. Advise patient to withhold dose and to notify physician immediately if bleeding or signs of bleeding appear: haematuria, bright red or black tarry stools, haematemesis, gingival bleeding with toothbrushing, petechiae (often occurs in ankle areas), epistaxis, bloody sputum, chest pain, abdominal or lumbar pain or swelling (retroperitoneal bleeding), menorrhagia, pelvic pain, severe or continuous headache, faintness or dizziness (intracranial bleeding); prolonged oozing from any minor injury (e.g., nicks from shaving).
- Instruct patient to use a soft toothbrush and to floss teeth gently with waxed floss. Also advise use of electric razor for shaving.
- Menstrual flow is generally normal, but may be slightly increased or prolonged. Advise patient to notify physician if there is an unusual increase in bleeding.
- If patient becomes pregnant while on anticoagulant therapy, she should be informed of the potential risk of congenital malformations.
- **Antidote**   In the event of bleeding, anticoagulant effect usually is reversed by omitting one or more doses of warfarin and by administration of specific antidote phytomenadione (vitamin K_1) 2.5 to 10 mg orally. If bleeding persists or progresses to a severe level, vitamin K_1 5 to 25 mg IV is given or a fresh whole blood transfusion may be necessary.
- Resumption of anticoagulant therapy reverses the effect of vitamin K_1 and a therapeutic hypothrombinaemic level can be obtained.
- Instruct patient/family to withhold dose and to report immediately: symptoms of hepatitis (dark urine, itchy skin, jaundice, abdominal pain, light stools), or hypersensitivity reaction.

W

WARFARIN SODIUM (continued)

- Suspect skin necrosis (local gangrene) and report immediately if area is painful and skin appears purple-black surrounded by redness. Lesions usually occur within 3 days after initiation of therapy. Incidence is high in elderly, obese patients.
- **Smoking–drug interaction** Smoking increases metabolism and therefore may increase dose requirement. Patient should stop smoking or at least greatly modify amount of smoking during anticoagulant therapy.
- Influenza vaccine decreases hepatic metabolism of warfarin, leading to augmented anticoagulant effect as evidenced by haemorrhage. Monitor patient. It is believed that the patient is at risk of bleeding for up to 1 month after receiving the vaccine.

Patient-teaching points Alert patient to factors that may affect anticoagulant response:
- □ Prothrombin time may be *lengthened* (enhanced anticoagulant affect) by fever, prolonged hot weather, malnutrition, diarrhoea, exposure to radiography.
- □ Prothrombin time may be *shortened* (decreased anticoagulant effect) by: oedema (reduces drug absorption and distribution), exposure to DDT or chlordane. (*See also contraindications and precautions.*)

- **Food–drug interactions** PT may be shortened by a high-fat diet, sudden increase in vitamin K-rich foods: cabbage, cauliflower, broccoli, asparagus, lettuce, onions, spinach, kale, fish, liver, and coffee or green tea (caffeine), or by tube feedings with high vitamin K content.
- Resistance to effects of warfarin may result from a vegetable-rich reducing diet because of high vitamin K content (see above). Some commercial dietary supplements have sufficient vitamin K content to produce resistance.
- If a coumarin is administered before, during, or immediately following minor dental or surgical procedures, the dose is adjusted to maintain PT at about 1½ to 2½ times control level.
- When emergency surgery is necessary for a patient receiving a coumarin, blood coagulation can be brought to normal by administration of fresh, whole blood or plasma.
- Advise patient to inform dentist or any new physician about anticoagulant therapy and duration of treatment.
- Warn patient against taking any other drug unless specifically approved by physician or pharmacist. Anticoagulant action is affected by many prescription drugs as well as commonly used OTC preparations: e.g., antacids, antihistamines, aspirin, liquid paraffin, oral contraceptives or vitamin C (in large doses).
- Urge patient to maintain a well-balanced diet and to avoid excess intake of alcohol. Consult physician regarding allowable amount. Generally an occasional drink is allowed.
- Misuse of sodium bicarbonate (self-dosed to decrease dyspepsia) causes the urine to be alkaline, which may result in red-orange colouration of urine.
- Patient should carry on his or her person medical identification card or jewellery.
- Recent studies suggest that anticoagulant therapy can be stopped abruptly rather than tapered over a few weeks.
- The risk of recurrence of venous thrombosis or thrombophlebitis can be lessened by measures that prevent venous stasis. Discuss the following points with physician before developing a teaching plan for the patient:

WARFARIN SODIUM (continued)

- ☐ Avoid standing still.
- ☐ Elevate legs when sitting (avoid jackknife position); interrupt sitting periods with walk breaks about every ½ hour.
- ☐ Do not cross legs; avoid garters, tight girdles, tight trousers, and narrow band Pop socks.
- ☐ Wear support hose or antiembolic stockings (must be prescribed by physician and patient must be measured for them). To be put on before getting out of bed in the morning and removed just before going to bed at night. (Review proper foot hygiene.)
- ☐ Planned exercise: have physician specify type (walking, bicycling, etc.), frequency, length of time, and rate of increase of exercise.
- ☐ Maintain optimum weight.
- ☐ Avoid injuring legs.

- ■ The patient and a significant family member of friend should be provided with explicit information and guidelines, verbally and in writing, concerning oral anti-coagulant therapy.
  - ☐ Why drug was prescribed and its expected action. Proper drug storage.
  - ☐ Dosage and time of administration. Emphasize importance of taking drug at same time each day (usually late afternoon) and not skipping or changing a dose.
  - ☐ Use of OTC drugs only with physician's approval.
  - ☐ Assist patient in setting up a system for keeping track of drug administration and drug-related events, such as a check-off drug calendar or diary.
  - ☐ Importance of adhering to schedule of PT determinations, other laboratory procedures, and doctor's appointments: give patient next laboratory date and date patient is to call doctor following laboratory visit, for directions concerning dosage.
  - ☐ Adverse drug effects and reportable symptoms.
  - ☐ Drug interactions.
  - ☐ Factors that may affect anticoagulant response. Importance of maintaining consistency in diet and life-style. Allowable intake of fat, vitamin K-rich foods, alcohol.
  - ☐ Necessity of carrying medical information card or jewellery.
  - ☐ Keep drug out of the reach of children.

- ■ Protect all tablets from light and moisture.

Diagnostic test interferences   Warfarin (coumarins) may cause alkaline urine to be red-orange in colour, may enhance **uric acid** excretion, cause elevation of **serum transaminases** and may increase **lactic dehydrogenase** activity.

DRUG INTERACTIONS

In addition to the listed drugs, many other drugs have been reported to alter the expected response to warfarin (prototype coumarin); however, clinical importance of these reports has not been substantiated. The addition or withdrawal of any drug to an established drug regimen should be made cautiously, with more frequent PT determinations than usual, with careful observation of the patient and dose adjustment as indicated.

WARFARIN SODIUM (continued)

Drugs that may increase response (i.e., enhance anticoagulant effect):

Acetohexamide
Alcohol-acute intoxication*
Alkylating agents
Allopurinol
Aminoglycosides
Aminosalicylic acid
Amiodarone
Anabolic steroids[†]
Antibiotics (oral)
Antimetabolites
Antiplatelet drugs
Aspirin
Asparaginase

Bezafibrate

Chloral hydrate*,[†]
Chloramphenicol[†]
Chlorpropamide
Chymotrypsin
Cimetidine
Cephamandole
Clofibrate
Co-trimoxazole

Danazol
Dextran
Dextropropoxyphene
Diazoxide
Dietary deficiencies
Disulphiram[†]
Diuretics*
Drugs affecting blood elements

Erythromycin
Ethacrynic acid

Glucagon
Guanethidine
Gemfibrozil

Hepatotoxic drugs

Influenza vaccine
Isoniazid

Ketoconazole

Latamoxef
Liquid paraffin

MAO inhibitors
Mefenamic acid
Methyldopa
Metronidazole[†]
Miconazole

Nalidixic acid
Neomycin (oral)
NSAIDs (except ibuprofen, naproxen, tolmetin)

Paracetomol
Phenylbutazone
Plicamycin
Potassium products
Prolonged narcotics
Propylthiouracil
Pyrazolones[†]

Quinidine
Quinine

Salicylates[†]
Streptokinase[†]
Sulindac
Sulphonamides
Sulphonylureas

Tetracyclines
Thiazides
Tolbutamide
Tricyclic antidepressants
Thyroxine

Urokinase

Vitamine E

Drugs that may decrease response (i.e., reduce anticoagulant effect):

Alcohol (chronic alcoholism)*,[†]

Barbiturates[†]

Carbamazepine
Chloral hydrate*,[†]
Cholestyramine[†]
Corticosteroids
Corticotropin

Diuretics
Dichloralphenazone

Glutethimide[†]
Griseofulvin

Laxatives

Mercaptopurine

Oral contraceptives (containing oestrogens)[†]

Primidone

Rifampicin

Spironolactone

Vitamin C
Vitamin K (dietary)

[†] Avoid concurrent use if possible.
* Increased or decreased response.

Xipamide

(Diurexan)

ACTIONS AND USES Thiazide diuretic used to treat oedema and hypertension.

ROUTE AND DOSAGE Oral: Adult: *Oedema*: *initial* 40 mg in the morning increased to 80 mg as required. *Maintenance* 20 mg in the morning. *Hypertension*: 20–40 mg in the morning.

For further information: *see chlorothiazide.*

Zidovudine

(Retrovir)   *Antiviral*

ACTIONS AND USES Interferes with retroviral replication by inhibiting reverse transcriptase. Prevents replication of the human immunodeficiency virus (HIV) but cannot eliminate the infection. Used to treat serious manifestations of HIV and for patients with acquired immune deficiency syndrome (AIDS).

ROUTE AND DOSAGE Oral: Adult: 200–300 mg/4 hourly (6 doses in 24 hours).

CONTRAINDICATIONS AND PRECAUTIONS Patients with low haemoglobin and neutrophil counts, myelosuppression, hepatic or renal insufficiency, elderly patients. Safe use in pregnancy and for children not established.

ADVERSE/SIDE EFFECTS Anaemia, neutropenia, leucopenia, nausea, vomiting, anorexia, abdominal pain, headache, rashes, fever, insomnia, paraesthesia, myalgia.

NURSING IMPLICATIONS
- Doses should be regularly spaced 4 hrly day and night. Blood tests should be undertaken every 2 weeks during the first 3 months of treatment, then monthly.
- Warn patient not to self medicate with OTC drugs. Counsel patient that zidovudine cannot be regarded as a cure for AIDS.
- Report adverse reactions to the Committee on Safety of Medicines.

Drug interactions Paracetomol, probenecid and drugs causing hepatic or renal toxicity, myelosuppressants.

XYZ

Zuclopenthixol

(Clopixol)

ZUCLOPENTHIXOL (continued)

ACTIONS AND USES   Antipsychotic drug used to treat schizophrenia and related psychoses where the patient presents with aggressive behaviour.

ROUTE AND DOSAGE   Oral: Adult: 20–30 mg/day in divided doses. Maximum 150 mg/day. *Maintenance*: 20–50 mg/day. **IM (depot injection)**: 200–400 mg at weekly intervals. A test dose of 100 mg should be given followed by 100–200 mg after 7–28 days to establish effective dose. Maximum 600 mg/week.

For further information: *see chlorpromazine*.

XYZ

BIBLIOGRAPHY

BOOKS

ABPI, (1986–7): *Data Sheet Compendium*, Datapharm Publications: London.

Avery GS (ed.) (1980): *Drug treatment: The Principles and Practice of Clinical Pharmacology and Therapeuticals*, 2nd ed., Churchill Livingstone: Edinburgh.

Bayliss PFC (1980): *Law on Poisons, Medicines and Related Substances*, 3rd ed., Ravenswood Publications: Beckenham.

Booth J (1983): *Handbook of Investigations*, Harper and Row: London.

Boore JRP, Champion R and Ferguson MC (1987): *Nursing the Physically Ill Adult*, Churchill Livingstone: Edinburgh.

British National Formulary (Biannual publication): British Medical Association and the Pharmaceutical Press: London.

Central Health Services Council (1958): *Report of Joint Sub-Committee on the Control of Dangerous Drugs and Poisons in Hospitals*, Chairman JK Aitken, HMSO: London.

Currey SH (1980): *Drug Disposition and Pharmco-kinetics*, Blackwell Scientific Publications: Oxford.

Dale JR and Applebe GE (1983): *Pharmacy, Law and Ethics*, 3rd ed., The Pharmaceutical Press: London.

David JA and Pritchard AP (eds) (1988): *Royal Marsden Handbook of Clinical Procedures*, 2nd ed., Harper and Row: London.

Dorr R and Fritz W (1980): *Cancer Chemotherapy Handbook*, Kimpton: London.

Downie G, Machenqie J and Williams A (1987): *Drug Management for Nurses*, Churchill Livingstone: Edinburgh.

Garrod LP, Lambert HP and O'Grady F (1981): *Antibiotic and Chemotherapy*, 5th ed., Churchill Livingstone: Edinburgh.

Gilman AG, Goodman LS and Gilman A (eds) (1980): *Goodman and Gilman's Pharmacological Basis of Therapeutics*, 6th edition, Macmillan: London.

King EM *et al.* (1981): *Illustrated Manual of Nursing Techniques*, 2nd ed., Lippincott: Philadelphia.

Laurence DR (1973): *Clinical Pharmacology*, 4th edition, Churchill Livingstone: Edinburgh.

Li Wan Po A (1982): *Non-Prescription Drugs*, Blackwell Scientific Publications: Oxford.

Lydiate PWH (1977): *The Law Relating to the Misuse of Drugs*, Butterworth: London.

Plant MA (1987): *Drugs in Perspective*, Hodder and Stoughton: London.

Sears WG and Winwood RS (1980): *Materia Medica for Nurses*, 9th ed., Edward Arnold: London.

Stockley I (1981): *Drug Interactions*, Blackwell Scientific Publications: Oxford.

Trounce JR (1985): *Clinical Pharmacology for Nurses*, 11th edition, Churchill Livingstone: Edinburgh.

Twycross RG and Lack SA (1984): *Therapeutics in Terminal Cancer*, Pitman: London.

BIBLIOGRAPHY (continued)

Wade A (ed.) (1982): *Martindale — The Extra Pharmacopea*, 28th edition, The Pharmaceutical Press: London.

Wade A (1980): *Pharmaceutical Handbook* 19th ed., Pharmaceutical Press: London.

Wellington FM, Hoare DV, Hyde J, Knight BM, Montague-Johnson D and Roberts D (eds) (1987): *Baillière's Pharmacology and Drug Information for Nurses*, 2nd ed., Bailliere Tindall: Eastbourne.

Whincup MH (1982): *Legal Rights and Duties in Medical and Nursing Service* 3rd ed., Ravenswood Publications: Beckenham.

JOURNALS

Adverse Drug Reaction Bulletin
Prescribes Journal
Drugs and Therapeutics Bulletin
Monthly Index of Medical Specialities (MIMS)

INDEX